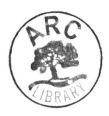

The GALE ENCYCLOPEDIA of NEUROLOGICAL DISORDERS

SECOND EDITION

The GALE
ENCYCLOPEDIA *of*
NEUROLOGICAL
DISORDERS

SECOND EDITION

VOLUME

2

M–Z
GLOSSARY
INDEX

BRIGHAM NARINS, EDITOR

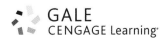

GALE
CENGAGE Learning·

Detroit • New York • San Francisco • New Haven, Conn • Waterville, Maine • London

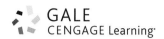

Gale Encyclopedia of Neurological Disorders, Second Edition

Project Editor: Brigham Narins

Image Editors: Kristin Key and Alejandro Valtierra

Editorial: Donna Batten, Kristin Key, Jacqueline Longe, Kristin Mallegg, Jeffrey Wilson, Alejandro Valtierra

Product Manager: Anne Marie Sumner

Editorial Support Services: Andrea Lopeman

Indexing Services: Cathy Goddard and Laura Dorricott, Dorricott Information Services

Rights Acquisition and Management: Margaret Chamberlain

Composition: Evi Abou-El-Seoud

Manufacturing: Wendy Blurton

Imaging: John Watkins

For product information and technology assistance, contact us at **Gale Customer Support, 1-800-877-4253.**
For permission to use material from this text or product, submit all requests online at **www.cengage.com/permissions.**
Further permissions questions can be emailed to **permissionrequest@cengage.com**

While every effort has been made to ensure the reliability of the information presented in this publication, Gale, a part of Cengage Learning, does not guarantee the accuracy of the data contained herein. Gale accepts no payment for listing; and inclusion in the publication of any organization, agency, institution, publication, service, or individual does not imply endorsement of the editors or publisher. Errors brought to the attention of the publisher and verified to the satisfaction of the publisher will be corrected in future editions.

Library of Congress Cataloging-in-Publication Data

The Gale encyclopedia of neurological disorders / Brigham Narins, editor. --2nd ed.
p. cm.
Summary: "A two-volume set designed for allied health students, patients, and the general public. The collection of alphabetically arranged entries covers rare and well-known neurological disorders, related medications and drug classes, patient and caregiver support, as well as background articles on the brain and nervous system anatomy"-- Provided by publisher.
Includes bibliographical references and index.
ISBN 978-1-4144-9008-3 (hardback) -- ISBN 978-1-4144-9009-0 (v. 1) -- ISBN 978-1-4144-9010-6 (v. 2)
1. Neurology–Encyclopedias. I. Narins, Brigham, 1962- II. Title: Encyclopedia of neurological disorders.
RC334.G34 2012
616.8003–dc23   2011035435

Gale
27500 Drake Rd.
Farmington Hills, MI, 48331-3535

ISBN-13: 978-1-4144-9008-3 (set)   ISBN-10: 1-4144-9008-9 (set)
ISBN-13: 978-1-4144-9009-0 (vol. 1)   ISBN-10: 1-4144-9009-7 (vol. 1)
ISBN-13: 978-1-4144-9010-6 (vol. 2)   ISBN-10: 1-4144-9010-0 (vol. 2)

This title is also available as an e-book.
978-1-4144-9011-3
Contact your Gale, Cengage Learning sales representative for ordering information.

Printed in China
1 2 3 4 5 6 7 16 15 14 13 12

CONTENTS

LIST OF ENTRIES

A

Abulia
Acetazolamide
Acupuncture
Acute disseminated
  encephalomyelitis
Adrenoleukodystrophy
Affective disorders
Agenesis of the corpus callosum
Agnosia
Agraphia
AIDS
Alcohol-related neurologic
  disease
Alexander disease
Alpers' disease
Alternating hemiplegia
Alzheimer's disease
Amantadine
Amnestic disorders
Amyotrophic lateral sclerosis
Anatomical nomenclature
Anencephaly
Aneurysms
Angelman syndrome
Angiography
Anosmia
Anticholinergics
Anticoagulant antiplatelet drugs
Antiepileptic drugs
Antimigraine drugs
Antiparkinson drugs
Antiviral drugs
Anxiolytics

Aphasia
Apraxia
Arachnoid cysts
Arachnoiditis
Arnold-Chiari malformation
Arteriovenous malformations
Asperger syndrome
Assistive communicative
  technologies
Assistive mobile devices
Ataxia
Ataxia-telangiectasia
Atomoxetine
Attention-deficit hyperactivity
  disorder (ADHD)
Autism
Autoimmune diseases
Autonomic dysfunction

B

Back pain
Balance and gait disorders
Bassen-Kornzwieg syndrome
Batten disease
Behcet's syndrome
Bell's palsy
Benign positional vertigo
Benzodiazepines
Beriberi
Binswanger disease
Biopsy
Blepharospasm
Botulinum toxin
Botulism

Brachial plexus injury
Brain anatomy
Brain and spinal tumors
Brain death
Brain edema, cerebral edema
Brown-Sequard syndrome

C

Canavan disease
Carbamazepine
Carotid endarterectomy
Carotid stenosis
Carpal tunnel syndrome
Catechol-o-methyltransferase
Central cord syndrome
Central nervous system
Central nervous system
  stimulants
Central pain syndrome
Cerebellum
Cerebral angiitis
Cerebral cavernous
  malformation
Cerebral circulation
Cerebral dominance
Cerebral hematoma
Cerebral palsy
Channelopathies
Charcot Marie Tooth disease
Cholinergic stimulants
Cholinesterase inhibitors
Chorea
Chronic inflammatory
  demyelinating polyneuropathy

Lee Silverman voice treatment
Leigh disease
Lennox-Gastaut syndrome
Lesch-Nyhan syndrome
Leukodystrophy
Levetiracetam
Lewy body dementia
Lidocaine patch
Lissencephaly
Locked-in syndrome
Lumbar puncture
Lupus
Lyme disease

M

Machado-Joseph disease
Magnetic resonance imaging
Megalencephaly
Melodic intonation therapy
Ménière's disease
Meninges
Mental retardation
Meralgia paresthetica
Metachromatic leukodystrophy
Microcephaly
Mitochondrial myopathies
Modafinil
Moebius syndrome
Monomelic amyotrophy
Motor neuron diseases
Movement disorders
Moyamoya disease
Mucopolysaccharidoses
Multi-infarct dementia
Multifocal motor neuropathy
Multiple sclerosis
Multiple system atrophy
Muscular dystrophy
Myasthenia gravis
Myoclonus
Myofibrillar myopathy
Myopathy
Myotonic dystrophy

N

Narcolepsy
Nerve compression
Nerve conduction study
Neurocysticercosis
Neurofibromatosis
Neuroleptic malignant syndrome
Neurological emergencies
Neurologist
Neuromuscular blockers
Neuronal migration disorders
Neuropathologist
Neuropsychological testing
Neuroradiology
Neurosarcoidosis
Neurosurgery
Neurotransmitters
Niemann-Pick disease

O

Occipital neuralgia
Olivopontocerebellar atrophy
Opsoclonus myoclonus
Organic voice tremor
Orthostatic hypotension
Overactive bladder
Oxazolindinediones

P

Pain
Pallidotomy
PANDAS
Pantothenate kinase-associated
    neurodegeneration
Paramyotonia congenita
Paraneoplastic syndromes
Parkinson's disease
Paroxysmal hemicrania
Parsonage-Turner syndrome
Perineural cysts
Periodic paralysis
Peripheral nervous system

Peripheral neuropathy
Periventricular leukomalacia
Phantom limb
Pharmacotherapy
Phenobarbital
Pick's disease
Piriformis syndrome
Plexopathies
Poliomyelitis
Polymyositis
Pompe disease
Porencephaly
Positron emission tomography
    (PET)
Postpolio syndrome
Primary lateral sclerosis
Primidone
Prion diseases
Progressive multifocal
    leukoencephalopathy
Progressive supranuclear palsy
Pseudobulbar palsy
Pseudotumor cerebri
Psychogenic neurological
    disorders

R

Radiation
Radiculopathy
Ramsay-Hunt syndrome
    type II
Rasmussen encephalitis
Reflex sympathetic dystrophy
Refsum disease
Repetitive motion disorders
Respite
Restless legs syndrome
Rett syndrome
Reyes syndrome

S

Sandhoff disease
Schilders disease
Schizencephaly

PLEASE READ—IMPORTANT INFORMATION

The *Gale Encyclopedia of Neurological Disorders, Second Edition* is a health reference product designed to inform and educate readers about a wide variety of diseases, disorders, syndromes, and conditions, as well as treatments, diagnostic tests, therapies, and medications. Gale, Cengage Learning believes the product to be comprehensive, but not necessarily definitive. It is intended to supplement, not replace, consultation with a physician or other healthcare practitioners. While Gale, Cengage Learning has made substantial efforts to provide information that is accurate, comprehensive, and up-to-date, Gale, Cengage Learning makes no representations or warranties of any kind, including without limitation, warranties of merchantability or fitness for a particular purpose, nor does it guarantee the accuracy, comprehensiveness, or timeliness of the information contained in this product. Readers should be aware that the universe of medical knowledge is constantly growing and changing, and that differences of opinion exist among authorities. Readers are also advised to seek professional diagnosis and treatment for any medical condition, and to discuss information obtained from this book with their healthcare provider.

INTRODUCTION

The Gale Encyclopedia of Neurological Disorders, Second Edition (GEND2) is a one-stop source for medical information that covers diseases, syndromes, drugs, treatments, therapies, and diagnostic equipment. It keeps medical jargon to a minimum, making it easier for the layperson to use. *The Gale Encyclopedia of Neurological Disorders* presents authoritative and balanced information and is more comprehensive than single-volume family medical guides.

SCOPE

Almost 400 full-length articles are included in *The Gale Encyclopedia of Neurological Disorders*. Articles follow a standardized format that provides information at a glance. Rubrics include:

Diseases

• Definition

• Description

• Demographics

• Causes and symptoms

• Diagnosis

• Treatment team

• Treatment

• Recovery and rehabilitation

• Clinical trials

• Prognosis

• Special concerns

• Resources

• Key terms

Drugs

• Definition

• Purpose

• Description

• Recommended dosage

• Precautions

• Side effects

• Interactions

• Resources

• Key terms

Treatments

• Definition

• Purpose

• Precautions

• Description

• Preparation

• Aftercare

• Risks

• Normal results

• Resources

• Key terms

INCLUSION CRITERIA

A preliminary topic list was compiled from a wide variety of sources, including professional medical guides, consumer guides, and textbooks and encyclopedias. The advisory board, made up of several medical and healthcare experts, evaluated the topics and made suggestions for inclusion. Final selection of topics to include was made by the medical advisors in conjunction with Gale editors.

ABOUT THE CONTRIBUTORS

The essays were compiled by experienced medical writers, physicians, nurses, and pharmacists. GEND2 medical advisors reviewed most of the completed essays to insure that they are appropriate, up-to-date, and medically accurate.

HOW TO USE THIS BOOK

The Gale Encyclopedia of Neurological Disorders has been designed with ready reference in mind:

• Straight alphabetical arrangement allows users to locate information quickly.

• Bold-faced terms function as print hyperlinks that point the reader to full-length entries in the encyclopedia.

• A list of key terms is provided where appropriate to define unfamiliar words or concepts used within the context of the essay.

• Cross-references placed throughout the encyclopedia direct readers to where information on subjects without their own entries can be found. Cross-references are also used to assist readers looking for information on diseases that are now known by other names; for example, there is a cross-reference for the rare childhood disease commonly known as Hallervorden-Spatz disease that points to the entry entitled Pantothenate kinase-associated neurodegeneration.

• A Resources section directs users to sources of further information, which include books, periodicals, websites, and organizations.

• A glossary is included to help readers understand unfamiliar terms.

• A comprehensive general index allows users to easily target detailed aspects of any topic.

GRAPHICS

The Gale Encyclopedia of Neurological Disorders is enhanced with over 100 images, including photographs, tables, and customized line drawings.

ADVISORY BOARD

An advisory board made up of prominent individuals from the medical and healthcare communities provided invaluable assistance in the formulation of this encyclopedia. They defined the scope of coverage and reviewed individual entries for accuracy and accessibility; in some cases they contributed entries themselves. We would therefore like to express our great appreciation to them:

CONTRIBUTORS

Margaret Alic, PhD
Science Writer
Eastsound, WA

Lisa Maria Andres, MS, CGC
Certified Genetic Counselor and Medical Writer
San Jose, CA

Paul Arthur
Science writer
London, England

Bruno Verbeno Azevedo
Espirito Santo University
Vitória, Brazil

Deepti Babu, MS, CGC
Genetic Counselor
Marshfield Clinic
Marshfield, WI

Laurie Barclay, MD
Neurologist and writer
Tampa, FL

Julia Barrett
Science Writer
Madison, WI

Danielle Barry, MS
Graduate Assistant
Center of Alcohol Studies
Rutgers University
Piscataway, NJ

Maria Basile, PhD
Neuropharmacologist and Medical Writer
Roselle, NJ

Tanja Bekhuis, PhD
Science Writer and Psychologist
TCB Research
Boalsburg, PA

Juli M. Berwald, PhD
Geologist (Ocean Sciences)
Chicago, IL

Robert G. Best, PhD
Director
Division of Genetics
University of South Carolina
School of Medicine
Columbia, SC

Michelle Lee Brandt
Medical Writer
San Francisco, CA

Dawn J. Cardeiro, MS, CGC
Genetic Counselor
Fairfield, PA

Francisco de Paula Careta
Espirito Santo University
Vitória, Brazil

Rosalyn Carson-DeWitt, MD
Physician and Medical Writer
Durham, NC

Laura Jean Cataldo, RN, EdD
Medical Writer
Myersville, MD

Stacey L. Chamberlin
Science Writer and Editor
Fairfax, VA

Bryan Richard Cobb, PhD
Institute for Molecular and
Human Genetics
Georgetown University
Washington, D.C.

Adam J. Cohen, MD
Craniofacial Surgery, Eyelid and Facial Plastic Surgery, Neuro-Ophthalmology
Downers Grove, IL

Tish Davidson, AM
Medical Writer
Fremont, CA

James Paul Dworkin, PhD
Professor
Department of Otolaryngology,
Voice/Speech Pathology
Program and Laboratory
Wayne State University
Detroit, MI

L. Fleming Fallon, Jr., MD, PhD, DrPH
Professor and Director of Public Health
College of Health and Human Services
Bowling Green State University
Bowling Green, OH

Antonio Farina, MD, PhD
Department of Embryology,
Obstetrics, and Gynecology
University of Bologna
Bologna, Italy

Karl Finley
Medical Writer
West Bloomfield, MI

Kevin Fitzgerald
Science Writer and Journalist
South Windsor, CT

Paula Anne Ford-Martin
Medical Writer
Warwick, RI

Lisa A. Fratt
Medical Writer
Ashland, WI

Rebecca J. Frey, PhD
Medical Writer
New Haven, CT

Sandra L. Friedrich, MA
Science Writer, Clinical Psychologist
Chicago, IL

Sandra Galeotti, MS
Science Writer
Sao Paulo, Brazil

Larry Gilman, PhD
Electrical Engineer and Science Writer
Sharon, VT

Laith Farid Gulli, MD
Consulting Psychotherapist
Lathrup Village, MI

Stephen John Hage, AAAS, RT(R), FAHRA
Medical Writer
Chatsworth, CA

Brook Ellen Hall, PhD
Science Writer
Loomis, CA

Dan Harvey
Medical Writer
Wilmington, DE

Hannah M. Hoag, MSc
Science and Medical Writer
Montreal, Canada

Fran Hodgkins
Medical Writer
Sparks, MD

Brian Douglas Hoyle, PhD
Microbiologist
Nova Scotia, Canada

Cindy L. Hunter, CGC
Genetic Counselor
Medical Genetics Department
Indiana University School of Medicine
Indianapolis, IN

Alexander I. Ioffe, PhD
Senior Scientist
Geological Institute of the Russian Academy of Sciences
Moscow, Russia

Holly Ann Ishmael, MS, CGC
Genetic Counselor
The Children's Mercy Hospital
Kansas City, MO

Joel C. Kahane, PhD
Professor, Director of the Anatomical Sciences Laboratory
The School of Audiology and Speech-Language Pathology
The University of Memphis
Memphis, TN

Kelly Karpa, PhD, RPh
Assistant Professor
Department of Pharmacology
Pennsylvania State University College of Medicine
Hershey, PA

Karen M. Krajewski, MS, CGC
Genetic Counselor, Assistant Professor of Neurology
Wayne State University
Detroit, MI

Judy Leaver, MA
Behavioral Health Writer and Consultant
Washington, D.C.

Adrienne Wilmoth Lerner
Science Writer
University of Tennessee College of Law
Knoxville, TN

Brenda Wilmoth Lerner, RN
Nurse, Writer, and Editor
London, UK

K. Lee Lerner
Fellow (rt)
Science Policy Institute
London, UK

Agnieszka Maria Lichanska, PhD
Department of Microbiology and Parasitology
University of Queensland
Brisbane, Australia

Peter T. Lin, MD
Research Assistant; Member: American Academy of Neurology, American Association of Electrodiagnostic Medicine
Department of Biomagnetic Imaging
University of California, San Francisco
Foster City, CA

Iuri Drumond Louro, MD, PhD
Adjunct Professor, Human and Molecular Genetics
Espirito Santo University
Vitória, Brazil

Nicole Mallory, MS, PA-C
Medical Student
Wayne State University
Detroit, MI

Igor Medica, MD, PhD
Assistant Professor
School of Medicine
University of Rijeka
Pula, Croatia

Michael Mooney, MA, CAC
Consultant Psychotherapist
Warren, MI

Alfredo Mori, MD, FACEM, FFAEM
Emergency Physician
The Alfred Hospital
Victoria, Australia
Oxford's Program in Evidence-Based Health Care
University of Oxford
Oxford, England

Marcos do Carmo Oyama
Espirito Santo University
Vitória, Brazil

Greiciane Gaburro Paneto
Espirito Santo University
Vitória, Brazil

Borut Peterlin, MD, PhD
Neurologist; Consultant Clinical Geneticist; Director
Division of Medical Genetics
University Medical Center
Lubiana, Slovenia

Toni I. Pollin, MS, CGC
Research Analyst
Division of Endocrinology, Diabetes, and Nutrition
University of Maryland School of Medicine
Baltimore, MD

J. Ricker Polsdorfer, MD
Medical Writer
Phoenix, AZ

Scott J. Polzin, MS, CGC
Medical Writer
Buffalo Grove, IL

Jack Raber, PharmD
Principal
Clinipharm Services
Seal Beach, CA

Robert Ramirez, DO
Medical Student
University of Medicine and
    Dentistry of New Jersey
Stratford, NJ

Richard Robinson
Medical Writer
Tucson, AZ

Jennifer Ann Roggenbuck, MS, CGC
Genetic Counselor
Hennepin County Medical Center
Minneapolis, MN

Nancy Ross-Flanigan
Science Writer
Belleville, MI

Stephanie Dionne Sherk
Medical Writer
University of Michigan
Ann Arbor, MI

Lee Alan Shratter, MD
Consulting Radiologist
Kentfield, CA

Genevieve T. Slomski, PhD
Medical Writer
New Britain, CT

Amie Stanley, MS
Genetic Counselor
Medical Genetics
The Cleveland Clinic
Cleveland, OH

Constance K. Stein, PhD
Director of Cytogenetics,
Assistant Director of Molecular
Diagnostics
SUNY Upstate Medical
    University
Syracuse, NY

Roger E. Stevenson, MD
Senior Clinical Geneticist, Senior
Clinical Laboratory Geneticist
Greenwood Genetic Center
Greenwood, SC

Roy Sucholeiki, MD
Physician
Neurosciences Institute
Central DuPage Hospital
Winfield, IL

Kevin M. Sweet, MS, CGC
Cancer Genetic Counselor
James Cancer Hospital, Ohio
    State University
Columbus, OH

David Tulloch
Science Writer
Wellington, New Zealand

Carol A. Turkington
Medical Writer
Lancaster, PA

Samuel D. Uretsky, PharmD
Medical Writer
Wantagh, NY

Chitra Venkatasubramanian, MBBS, MD
Clinical Assistant Professor,
Neurology & Neurological
Sciences
Stanford Neurocritical Care Program
Stanford School of Medicine
Palo Alto, CA

Bruno Marcos Verbeno
Espirito Santo University
Vitória, Brazil

Beatriz Alves Vianna
Espirito Santo University
Vitória, Brazil

SYMBOL GUIDE FOR PEDIGREE CHARTS

Pedigree charts are visual tools for documenting biological relationships in families and the presence of disorders. Using these charts, medical professionals such as geneticists and genetic counselors can analyze the genetic risk in a family for a particular trait or condition by tracking which individuals have the disorder and determining how it is inherited.

A standard set of symbols has been established for use in creating pedigree charts. Those found within the body of several entries in the encyclopedia follow the symbol guide explained on the next page. The exact style and amount of information presented on the chart varies for each family and depends on the trait or condition under investigation. Typically, only data that is directly related to the disorder being analyzed will be included.

Symbol Guide for Pedigree Charts

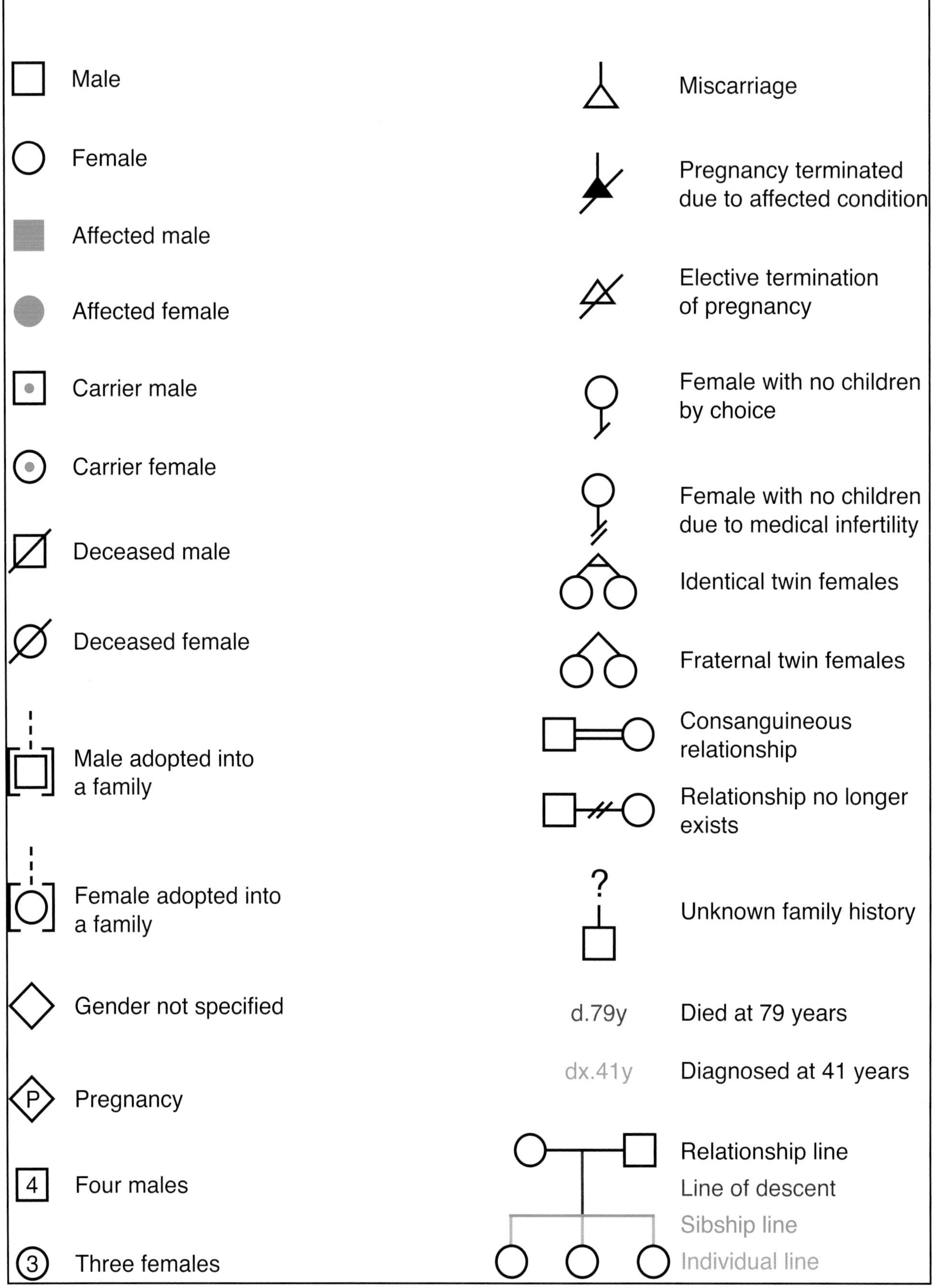

☐ Male

○ Female

▪ Affected male

● Affected female

⊡ Carrier male

⊙ Carrier female

⧄ Deceased male

⦸ Deceased female

⌷ Male adopted into a family

⟦○⟧ Female adopted into a family

◇ Gender not specified

◇P Pregnancy

4 Four males

③ Three females

△ Miscarriage

◣ Pregnancy terminated due to affected condition

⧄ Elective termination of pregnancy

○ Female with no children by choice

○ Female with no children due to medical infertility

○○ Identical twin females

○○ Fraternal twin females

☐══○ Consanguineous relationship

☐─⫰○ Relationship no longer exists

? ☐ Unknown family history

d.79y Died at 79 years

dx.41y Diagnosed at 41 years

○───☐ Relationship line

Line of descent

Sibship line

Individual line

○ ○ ○

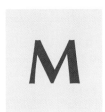

Machado-Joseph disease

Definition

Machado-Joseph Disease (MJD), also known as **spinocerebellar ataxia** Type 3 (SCA 3), is a rare hereditary disorder affecting the **central nervous system**, especially the areas responsible for movement coordination of limbs, facial muscles, and eyes. The disease involves the slow and progressive degeneration of brain areas involved in motor coordination, such as the cerebellar, extrapyramidal, pyramidal, and motor areas. Ultimately, MJD leads to paralysis or a crippling condition, although intellectual functions usually remain normal. Other names of MJD are Portuguese-Azorean disease, Joseph disease, and Azorean disease.

Description

Machado-Joseph disease was first described in 1972 among the descendants of Portuguese-Azorean immigrants to the United States, including the family of William Machado. In spite of differences in symptoms and degrees of neurological degeneration and movement impairment among the affected individuals, it was suggested by investigators that in at least four studied families the same gene mutation was present. In early 1976, investigators went to the Azores Archipelago to study an existing neurodegenerative disease in the islands of Flores and São Miguel. In a group of 15 families, they found 40 people with neurological disorders with a variety of different symptoms among the affected individuals.

Another research team in 1976 reported an inherited neurological disorder of the motor system in Portuguese families, which they named Joseph disease. During the same year, the two groups of scientists published independent evidence suggesting that the same disease was the primary cause for the variety of symptoms observed. When additional reports from other countries and ethnic groups were associated

with the same inherited disorder, it was initially thought that Portuguese-Azorean sailors had been the probable disseminators of MJD to other populations around the world during the sixteenth-century period of Portuguese colonial explorations and commerce. At present, MJD is found in Brazil, United States, Portugal, Macau, Finland, Canada, Mexico, Israel, Syria, Turkey, Angola, India, United Kingdom, Australia, Japan, and China. Because MJD continues to be diagnosed in a variety of countries and ethnic groups, there are current doubts about its exclusive Portuguese-Azorean origin.

Causes and symptoms

The gene responsible for the MJD appears at chromosome 14, and the first symptoms usually appear in early adolescence. Dystonia (**spasticity** or involuntary and repetitive movements) or gait **ataxia** is usually the initial symptom in children. Gait ataxia is characterized by unstable walk and standing, which slowly progresses with the appearance of some of the other symptoms, such as hand dysmetria, involuntary eye movements, loss of hand and superior limbs coordination, and facial dystonia (abnormal muscle tone). Another characteristic of MJD is clinical anticipation, which means that in most families the onset of the disease occurs progressively earlier from one generation to the next. Among members of one same family, some patients may show a predominance of muscle tone disorders, others may have loss of coordination, some may have bulging eyes, and yet another sibling may be free of symptoms during that person's entire life. In the late stages of MJD, some people may experience **delirium** or **dementia**.

According to the affected brain area, MJD is classified as Type I, with extrapyramidal insufficiency; Type II, with cerebellar, pyramidal, end extrapyramidal insufficiency; and Type III, with cerebellar insufficiency. Extrapyramidal tracts are networks of uncrossed motor nerve fibers that function as relays between the motor areas and corresponding areas of the brain. The pyramidal tract consists of groups of crossed nerves located in the white matter of the spinal cord that conduct motor impulses originated in the opposite area of the brain to the arms and legs. Pyramidal tract nerves regulate both voluntary and reflex muscle movements. However, as the disease progresses, both motor systems tracks will eventually suffer degeneration.

Diagnosis

Diagnosis depends mainly on the clinical history of the family. Genetic screening for the specific mutation that causes MJD can be useful in cases of persons at risk or when the family history is not known or a person has symptoms that raise suspicion of MJD. Initial diagnosis may be difficult, as people have symptoms easily mistaken for other neurological disorders such as Parkinson's and Huntington's diseases or even **Multiple Sclerosis**.

Treatment

Although there is no cure for Machado-Joseph disease, some symptoms can be relieved. The medication Levodopa or L-dopa often succeeds in lessening muscle rigidity and tremors and is often given in conjunction with the drug Carbidopa. However, as the disease progresses and the number of neurons decreases, this palliative (given for comfort) treatment becomes less effective. Antispasmodic drugs such as baclofen are also prescribed to reduce spasticity. **Dysarthria**, or difficulty to speak, and dysphagia, difficulty to swallow, can be treated with proper medication and speech therapy. Physical therapy can help patients with unsteady gait, and walkers and wheelchairs may be needed as the disease progresses. Other symptoms also require palliative treatment, such as muscle cramps, urinary disorders, and sleep problems.

Clinical Trials

Further basic research is needed before clinical trials become a possibility for MDJ. Ongoing genetic and molecular research on the mechanisms involved in the genetic mutations responsible for the disease will eventually yield enough data to provide for future development and design of experimental gene therapies and drugs specific to treat those with MJD.

Prognosis

The frequency with which such genetic mutations trigger the clinical onset of disease is known as penetrance. Machado-Joseph disease has a 94.5%

> ## KEY TERMS
>
> **Autosomal**—Relating to any chromosome besides the X and Y sex chromosomes. Human cells contain 22 pairs of autosomes and one pair of sex chromosomes.
>
> **Cerebellar**—Involving the part of the brain (cerebellum) that controls walking, balance, and coordination.
>
> **Dysarthria**—Slurred speech.
>
> **Dystonia**—Painful involuntary muscle cramps or spasms.
>
> **Extrapyramidal**—Refers to brain structures located outside the pyramidal tracts of the central nervous system.
>
> **Genotype**—The genetic makeup of an organism or a set of organisms.
>
> **Mutation**—A permanent change in the genetic material that may alter a trait or characteristic of an individual or manifest as disease. This change can be transmitted to offspring.
>
> **Penetrance**—The degree to which individuals possessing a particular genetic mutation express the trait that this mutation causes. One hundred percent penetrance is expected to be observed in truly dominant traits.
>
> **Phenotype**—The physical expression of an individual's genes.
>
> **Spasticity**—Increased mucle tone, or stiffness, which leads to uncontrolled, awkward movements.
>
> **Trinucleotide**—A sequence of three nucleotides.

penetrance, which means that 94.5% of the mutation carriers develop the symptoms during their lives, and less than 5% remain free of symptoms. Because the intensity and range of symptoms are highly variable among the affected individuals, it is difficult to determine the prognosis for a given individual. As MJD progresses slowly, most patients survive until middle age or older.

Resources

BOOKS

Subramony, Sankara H., and Alexandra Dürr, eds. *Ataxic Disorders Vol. 103: Handbook of Clinical Neurology.* Elsevier: 2011.

OTHER

"Machado-Joseph Disease Information Page." National Institute of Neurological Disorders and Stroke

(NINDS) (August 16, 2011). http://www.ninds.nih.gov/ disorders/machado_joseph/machado_joseph.htm (accessed October 21, 2011).

ORGANIZATIONS

Dystonia Medical Research Foundation. 1 East Wacker Drive, Suite 2430, Chicago, IL 60601-1905. Phone: (312) 755-0198. Fax: (312) 803-0138. Email: dystonia@ dystoniafoundation.org. http://www.dystonia-foundation.org.

International Machado-Joseph Disease Foundation, Inc. PO Box 994268, Redding, CA 96099-4268. Phone: (530) 246-4722. Email: MJD@ijdf.net. http://www.ijdf.net.

National Ataxia Foundation (NAF). 2600 Fernbrook Lane, Suite 119, Minneapolis, MN 55447-4752. Phone: (763) 553-0020. Fax: (763) 553-0167. Email: naf@ataxia.org. http://www.ataxia.org.

National Organization for Rare Disorders (NORD). PO Box 1968 (55 Kenosia Avenue), Danbury, CT 06813-1968. Phone: (203) 744-0100. Fax: (203) 798-2291. Tollfree phone: (800) 999-NORD (6673). Email: orphan@ rarediseases.org. http://www.rarediseases.org.

Worldwide Education & Awareness for Movement Disorders (WE MOVE). 204 West 84th Street, New York, NY 10024. Phone: (212) 875-8312. Fax: (212) 875-8389. Tollfree phone: (800) 437-MOV2 (6682). Email: wemove@ wemove.org. http://www.wemove.org.

Sandra Author Galeotti

Macrencephaly *see* **Megalencephaly**
Mad cow disease *see* **Creutzfeldt-Jakob disease**

Magnetic resonance imaging

Definition

Magnetic resonance imaging (MRI) is the newest and perhaps most versatile medical imaging technology available. Doctors can get highly refined images of the body's interior without surgery using MRI. By using strong magnets and pulses of radio waves to manipulate the natural magnetic properties in the body, this technique makes better images of organs and soft tissues than those of other scanning technologies. MRI is particularly useful for imaging the brain and spine, as well as the soft tissues of joints and the interior structure of bones. The entire body is visible to the technique, which poses few known health risks.

Purpose

MRI was developed in the 1980s. Recent additions to MRI technology are angiography (MRA) and spectroscopy (MRS). MRA was developed to study blood flow, whereas MRS can identify the chemical composition of diseased tissue and produce color images of brain function. The many advantages of MRI include:

- Detail. MRI creates precise images of the body based on the varying proportions of magnetic elements in different tissues. Very minor fluctuations in chemical composition can be determined. MRI images have greater natural contrast than standard x rays, computed tomography (CT) scan, or ultrasound, all of which depend on the differing physical properties of tissues. This sensitivity lets MRI distinguish fine variations in tissues deep within the body. It also is particularly useful for spotting and distinguishing diseased tissues (tumors and other lesions) early in their development. Often, doctors prescribe an MRI scan to more fully investigate earlier findings of the other imaging techniques.

- Scope. The entire body can be scanned, from head to toe and from the skin to the deepest recesses of the brain. Moreover, MRI scans are not obstructed by bone, gas, or body waste, which can hinder other imaging techniques; the scans can be degraded by motion such as breathing, heartbeat, and normal bowel activity. The MRI process produces cross-sectional images of the body that are as sharp in the middle as on the edges, even of the brain through the skull. A close series of these two-dimensional images can provide a three-dimensional view of a targeted area.

- Safety. MRI does not depend on potentially harmful ionizing radiation, as do standard x ray and CT scan. There are no known risks specific to the procedure, other than for people who might have metal objects in their bodies.

MRI is being used increasingly during surgical operations, particularly those involving very small structures in the head and neck, as well as for preoperative assessment and planning. Intraoperative MRIs have shown themselves to be safe as well as feasible and to improve the surgeon's ability to remove an entire tumor or other abnormality.

Given all the advantages, doctors would undoubtedly prescribe MRI as frequently as ultrasound scanning, but the MRI process is complex and costly. The process requires large, expensive, and complicated equipment; a highly trained operator; and a doctor specializing in radiology. Generally, MRI is prescribed only when serious symptoms and/or negative results from other tests indicate a need. Many times another test is appropriate for the type of diagnosis needed.

Doctors may prescribe an MRI scan of different areas of the body.

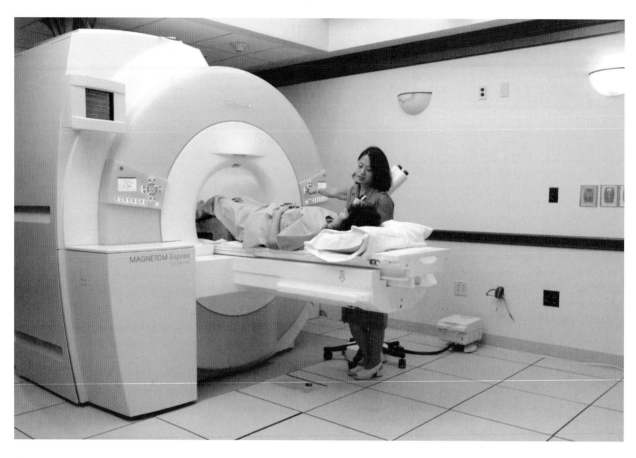

Technician conducting an MRI. (© *Michael Ventura/Alamy*)

- Brain and head. MRI technology was developed because of the need for brain imaging. It is one of the few imaging tools that can see through bone (the skull) and deliver high quality pictures of the brain's delicate soft tissue structures. MRI may be needed for patients with symptoms of a brain tumor, stroke, or infection (such as meningitis). MRI also may be needed when cognitive and/or psychological symptoms suggest brain disease (such as Alzheimer's or Huntington's diseases, or multiple sclerosis), or when developmental retardation suggests a birth defect. MRI can also provide pictures of the sinuses and other areas of the head beneath the face. Recent refinements in MRI technology may make this form of diagnostic imaging even more useful in evaluating patients with brain cancer, stroke, schizophrenia, or epilepsy. In particular, a new 3-D approach to MRI imaging known as diffusion tensor imaging (DTI) measures the flow of water within brain tissue, allowing the radiologist to tell where the normal flow of fluid is disrupted and to distinguish more clearly between cancerous and normal brain tissue. The introduction of DTI has led to a technique known as fiber tracking, which allows the neurosurgeon to tell whether a space-occupying brain

tumor has damaged or displaced the nerve pathways in the white matter of the brain. This information in turn improves the surgeon's accuracy during an operation. MRI is also being used to treat intractable seizure disorders targeting causative lesions with destructive lasers, utilizing real-time MRI-guided thermal imaging.

- Spine. Spinal problems can create a host of seemingly unrelated symptoms. MRI is particularly useful for identifying and evaluating degenerated or herniated spinal discs. It can also be used to determine the condition of nerve tissue within the spinal cord.

- Joint. MRI scanning is most commonly used to diagnose and assess joint problems. MRI can provide clear images of the bone, cartilage, ligament, and tendon that comprise a joint. MRI can be used to diagnose joint injuries due to sports, advancing age, or arthritis. MRI can also be used to diagnose shoulder problems, such as a torn rotator cuff. MRI can detect the presence of an otherwise hidden tumor or infection in a joint and can be used to diagnose the nature of developmental joint abnormalities in children.

- Heart. MRI scans are increasingly being used to image the heart and its blood vessels. "Black blood" MRI scans reveal the presence of atherosclerotic plaques within blood vessels, helping to distinguish between stable and unstable plaques.

- Skeleton. The properties of MRI that allow it to see through the skull also allow doctors to view the inside of bones. It can be used to detect bone cancer, inspect the marrow for leukemia and other diseases, assess bone loss (osteoporosis), and examine complex fractures.

- Prostate. MRI is used to map the prostate, allowing for more exact and accurate biopsy.

- The rest of the body. While CT and ultrasound satisfy most chest, abdominal, and general body imaging needs, MRI may be needed in certain circumstances to provide better pictures or when repeated scanning is required. The progress of some therapies, such as liver cancer therapy, needs to be monitored, and the effect of repeated radiation exposure from x ray and CT scan is a concern.

Description

In essence, MRI produces a map of hydrogen distribution in the body. Hydrogen is the simplest element known, the most abundant in biological tissue, and one that can be magnetized. It will align itself within a strong magnetic field, like the needle of a compass. The earth's magnetic field is not strong enough to keep a person's hydrogen atoms pointing in the same direction, but the superconducting magnet of an MRI machine can. This comprises the "magnetic" part of MRI.

Once a patient's hydrogen atoms have been aligned in the magnet, pulses of very specific radio wave frequencies are used to knock them back out of alignment. The hydrogen atoms alternately absorb and emit radio wave energy, vibrating back and forth between their resting (magnetized) state and their agitated (radio pulse) state. This comprises the "resonance" part of MRI.

The MRI equipment records the duration, strength, and source location of the signals emitted by the atoms as they relax and translate the data into an image on a television monitor. The state of hydrogen in diseased tissue differs from healthy tissue of the same type, making MRI particularly good at identifying tumors and other lesions. In some cases, chemical agents such as gadolinium can be injected to improve the contrast between healthy and diseased tissue.

A single MRI exposure produces a two-dimensional image of a slice through the entire target area. A series of these image slices closely spaced (usually less than half an inch) makes a virtual three-dimensional view of the area.

Magnetic resonance spectroscopy (MRS) is different from MRI because MRS uses a continuous band of radio wave frequencies to excite hydrogen atoms in a variety of chemical compounds other than water. These compounds absorb and emit radio energy at characteristic frequencies, or spectra, which can be used to identify them. Generally, a color image is created by assigning a color to each distinctive spectral emission. This comprises the "spectroscopy" part of MRS. As of 2011 MRS was still experimental and available in only a few research centers.

Doctors primarily use MRS to study the brain and disorders, such as epilepsy, Alzheimer's disease, brain tumors, and the effects of drugs on brain growth and metabolism. The technique is also useful in evaluating metabolic disorders of the muscles and nervous system.

Magnetic resonance angiography (MRA) is another variation of standard MRI. MRA, like other types of angiography, looks specifically at fluid flow within the blood (vascular) system but does so without the injection of dyes or radioactive tracers. Standard MRI cannot make a good picture of flowing blood, but MRA uses specific radio pulse sequences to capture usable signals. The technique is generally used in combination with MRI to obtain images that show both vascular structure and flow within the brain and head in cases of stroke or when a blood clot or aneurysm is suspected.

Regardless of the exact type of MRI planned or area of the body targeted, the procedure involved is basically the same and occurs in a special MRI suite. The patient usually lies on a narrow table and is made as comfortable as possible. Transmitters are positioned on the body and the cushioned table that the patient is laying on moves into a long tube that houses the magnet. The tube is as long as an average adult lying down, and the tube is narrow and open at both ends. Once the area to be examined has been properly positioned, a radio pulse is applied. Then a two-dimensional image corresponding to one slice through the area is made. The table then moves a fraction of an inch and the next image is made. Each image exposure takes several seconds, and the entire exam lasts 30–90 minutes. During this time, the patient is not allowed to move. If the patient moves during the scan, the picture will not be clear.

An open MRI scanner is less restrictive and is usually open on two or three sides. Although this type of machine accommodates larger or claustrophobic persons with greater ease, high-field or closed MRI machines usually generate more accurate and detailed images. The stand-up type of open MRI generates images of the spine, allowing the physician to evaluate images made in the weight-bearing state.

Depending on the area to be imaged, the radio-wave transmitters will be positioned in different locations.

• For the head and neck, a helmet-like hat is worn.
• For the spine, chest, and abdomen, the patient will be lying on the transmitters.
• For the knee, shoulder, or other joint, the transmitters will be applied directly to the joint.

Additional probes will monitor vital signs, including pulse and respiration.

The process is very noisy and confining. The patient hears a thumping sound for the duration of the procedure. Since the procedure is noisy, music supplied via earphones is often provided. Some patients become anxious or panic because they are in the small, enclosed tube. This is why vital signs are monitored and the patient and medical team can communicate between each other. If the chest or abdomen are to be imaged, patients are asked to hold their breath as each exposure is made. Other instructions may be given to the patient, as needed. In many cases, the entire examination will be performed by an MRI operator who is not a doctor, but the supervising radiologist should be available to consult as necessary during the exam and will view and interpret the results sometime later.

Preparation

In some cases (such as for MRI brain scanning or an MRA), a chemical designed to increase image contrast may be given by the radiologist immediately before the exam. If a patient suffers from anxiety or claustrophobia, drugs may be given to help the patient relax.

The patient must remove all metal objects (watches, jewelry, eye glasses, hair clips, etc.). Any magnetized objects (like credit and bank machine cards) should be kept far away from the MRI equipment because they can be erased. Patients cannot bring their wallet or keys into the MRI machine. The patient may be asked to wear clothing without metal snaps, buckles, or zippers, unless a medical gown is worn during the procedure. The patient may be asked to remove any hair spray, hair gel, or cosmetics that could interfere with the scan.

Aftercare

No aftercare is necessary, unless the patient received medication or had a reaction to a contrast agent. Normally, patients can immediately return to

---

KEY TERMS

Angiography—Any of the different methods for investigating the condition of blood vessels, usually via a combination of radiological imaging and injections of chemical tracing and contrasting agents.

Diffusion tensor imaging (DTI)—A refinement of magnetic resonance imaging that allows the doctor to measure the flow of water and track the pathways of white matter in the brain. DTI is able to detect abnormalities in the brain that do not show up on standard MRI scans.

Gadolinium—A very rare metallic element useful for its sensitivity to electromagnetic resonance, among other things. Traces of it can be injected into the body to enhance the MRI pictures.

Hydrogen—The simplest, most common element known in the universe. It is composed of a single electron (negatively charged particle) circling a nucleus consisting of a single proton (positively charged particle). It is the nuclear proton of hydrogen that makes MRI possible by reacting resonantly to radio waves while aligned in a magnetic field.

Ionizing radiation—Electromagnetic radiation that can damage living tissue by disrupting and destroying individual cells. All types of nuclear decay radiation (including x rays) are potentially ionizing. Radio waves do not damage organic tissues they pass through.

Magnetic field—The three-dimensional area surrounding a magnet, in which its force is active. During MRI, the patient's body is permeated by the force field of a superconducting magnet.

Radio waves—Electromagnetic energy of the frequency range corresponding to that used in radio communications, usually 10,000 cycles per second to 300 billion cycles per second. Radio waves are the same as visible light, x rays, and all other types of electromagnetic radiation, but are of a higher frequency.

---

their daily activities. If the exam reveals a serious condition that requires more testing and/or treatment, appropriate information and counseling will be needed.

Risks

MRI poses no known health risks to the patient and produces no physical side effects. Again, the potential effects of MRI on an unborn baby are not well known. Any woman who is, or may be, pregnant, should carefully discuss this issue with her doctor and radiologist before undergoing a scan. The most common problems are minor bleeding and bruising at the site of contrast injection. Since these are not reportable events, morbidity can only be estimated. Occasionally, an unknown allergy to seafood is discovered after injecting contrast. No deaths have been reported from MRI tests.

MRI scanning should not be used when there is the potential for an interaction between the strong MRI magnet and metal objects that might be imbedded in a patient's body. The force of magnetic attraction on certain types of metal objects (including surgical steel) could move them within the body and cause serious injury. Metal may be imbedded in a person's body for several reasons.

- Medical. People with implanted cardiac pacemakers, metal aneurysm clips, or who have had broken bones repaired with metal pins, screws, rods, or plates must tell their radiologist prior to having an MRI scan. In some cases (like a metal rod in a reconstructed leg) the difficulty may be overcome.

- Injury. Patients must tell their doctors if they have bullet fragments or other metal pieces in their body from old wounds. The suspected presence of metal, whether from an old or recent wound, should be confirmed before scanning.

- Occupational. People with significant work exposure to metal particles (working with a metal grinder, for example) should discuss this with their doctor and radiologist. The patient may need pre-scan testing—usually a single x ray of the eyes to see if any metal is present.

Chemical agents designed to improve the picture and/or allow for the imaging of blood or other fluid flow during MRA may be injected. In rare cases, patients may be allergic to or intolerant of these agents, and these patients should not receive them. If these chemical agents are to be used, patients should discuss any concerns they have with their doctor and radiologist.

The potential side effects of magnetic and electric fields on human health remain a source of debate. In particular, the possible effects on an unborn baby are not well known. Any woman who is, or may be, pregnant should carefully discuss this issue with her doctor and radiologist before undergoing a scan.

As with all medical imaging techniques, obesity greatly interferes with the quality of MRI.

Results

Normal results

A normal MRI, MRA, or MRS result is one that shows the patient's physical condition to fall within normal ranges for the target area scanned.

Abnormal results

Generally, MRI is prescribed only when serious symptoms and/or negative results from other tests indicate a need. There often exists strong evidence of a condition that the scan is designed to detect and assess. Thus, the results will often be abnormal, confirming the earlier diagnosis. At that point, further testing and appropriate medical treatment is needed. For example, if the MRI indicates the presence of a brain tumor, an MRS may be prescribed to determine the type of tumor so that aggressive treatment can begin immediately without the need for a surgical biopsy.

Resources

BOOKS

Bradley, W, et al. *Neurology in Clinical Practice*. 5th ed. Philadelphia: Butterworth-Heinemann, 2008.

Culbreth, L.J., and C. Watson. *Magnetic Resonance Imaging Technology*. New York: Cambridge University Press, 2007.

Goetz, C.G. *Goetz's Textbook of Clinical Neurology*. 3rd ed. Philadelphia: Saunders, 2007.

Kastler, B. *Understanding MRI*. 2nd ed. Berlin: Springer-Verlag, 2008.

McRobbie, D.W., E.A. Moore, M. J. Graves, and M.R. Prince. *MRI from Picture to Proton*. 2nd ed. New York: Cambridge University Press, 2007.

Weishaupt, D., V.D. Koechli, and B. Marincek. *How Does MRI Work? An Introduction to the Physics and Function of Magnetic Resonance Imaging*. 2nd ed. Berlin: Springer-Verlag, 2008.

PERIODICALS

Hara, H., et al. "Magnetic Resonance Imaging of Medullary Bone Infarction in the Early Stage." *Clinical Imaging* 32, no. 2 (2008): 147–51.

Wada, R., and W. Kucharczyk. "Prion Infections of the Brain." *Neuroimaging Clinics of North America* 18, no. 1 (2008): 183–91.

Zhao, W., J.H. Choi, G.R. Hon, and M.A. Vannan. "Left Ventricular Relaxation." *Heart Failure Clinics* 4, no. 1 (2008): 37–46.

WEBSITES

"Magnetic Resonance Imaging (MRI)." WebMD. http://www.webmd.com/a-to-z-guides/magnetic-resonance imaging-mri (accessed August 26, 2011).

"MRI." Medline Plus. http://www.nlm.nih.gov/medlineplus/ency/article/003335.htm (accessed August 26, 2011).

ORGANIZATIONS

American College of Radiology (ACR), 1891 Preston White Drive, Reston, VA 20191, (703) 648-8900, (800) 227-5463, info@acr.org, http://www.acr.org.

Kurt Richard Sternlof
L. Fleming Fallon, Jr, MD, DrPH
Rosalyn Carson-DeWitt, MD
Brenda W. Lerner

Megalencephaly

Definition

Megalencephaly (also called macrencephaly) describes an enlarged brain whose weight exceeds the mean (the average weight for that age and sex) by at least 2.5 standard deviations (a statistical measure of variation). Megalencephaly may also be defined in terms of volume rather than weight. Hemimegalencephaly (or unilateral megalencephaly) is a related condition in which brain enlargement occurs in one hemisphere (half) of the brain.

Description

A person with megalencephaly has a large, heavy brain. In general, a brain that weighs more than 1600 grams (about 3.5 pounds) is considered megalencephalic. The heaviest brain on record weighed 2850 grams (about 6.3 pounds). Macrocephaly, a related condition, refers to an abnormally large head. Macrocephaly may be due to megalencephaly or other causes such as hydrocephalus (an excess accumulation of fluid in the brain), and **brain edema**. Megalencephaly may be an isolated finding in an otherwise normal individual, or it can occur in association with neurological problems (such as seizures or **mental retardation**) and/or somatic abnormalities (physical problems or birth defects of the body). Dysmorphic facial features (abnormal shape, position or size of facial features) may also be observed in an affected individual.

According to the National Institute of Neurological Disorders and Stroke (NINDS), megalencephaly is one of the cephalic disorders, congenital conditions due to damage to or abnormal development of the nervous system. There have been various attempts to classify megalencephaly into subcategories based on etiology (cause) and/or pathology (the condition of the brain tissue and cells). Dekaban and Sakurgawa (1977) proposed three main categories: primary megalencephaly, secondary megalencephaly, and hemimegalencephaly. DeMyer (1986) proposed two main categories: anatomic and metabolic. Gooskens and others (1988) modified these classifications and added a third category: dynamic megalencephaly. The existence of different classification systems highlights the inherent difficulty in categorizing a condition that has a wide range of causes and associated pathology.

Demographics

The incidence of megalencephaly is estimated at between 2% and 6%. There is a preponderance of affected males; megalencephaly affects males three to four times more often than it does females. Among individuals with macrocephaly, estimates of megalencephaly are between 10% and 30%. Hemimegalencephaly is a rare condition and occurs less frequently than megalencephaly.

Causes and symptoms

Causes

Both genetic and non-genetic factors may produce megalencephaly. Most often, megalencephaly is a familial trait that occurs without extraneural (outside the brain) findings. Familial megalencephaly may occur as an autosomal dominant (more common) or autosomal recessive condition. The autosomal recessive form is more likely than the autosomal dominant form to result in mental retardation. Other genetic causes for megalencephaly include single gene disorders such as **Sotos syndrome** (an overgrowth syndrome), **neurofibromatosis** (a neurocutaneous syndrome), and **Alexander disease** (a leukodystrophy); or a chromosome abnormality such as Klinefelter syndrome. Non-genetic factors such as a transient disorder of cerebral spinal fluid may also contribute to the development of megalencephaly. Finally, megalencephaly can be idiopathic (due to unknown causes).

The cells that make up the brain (neurons and other supporting cells) form during the second to fourth months of pregnancy. Though the precise mechanisms behind megalencephaly at the cellular level are not fully understood, it is thought that the condition results from an increased number of cells, an increased size of cells, or an accumulation of a metabolic byproduct or abnormal substance due to an inborn error of metabolism. It is possible that more than one of these processes may explain megalencephaly in a given individual.

Symptoms

There is variability in age of onset, symptoms present, rate of progression, and severity of megalencephaly. The disorder typically presents as a large head circumference (distance around the head) either prenatally (before birth), at birth, or within the first few years of life. The head circumference may increase rapidly in the span of a few months or may progress slowly over a longer period of time. Head shape may be abnormal and skull abnormalities such as widened or split sutures (fibrous joints between the bones of the head) may occur. There may also be increased cranial pressure and bulging fontanels (the membrane covered spaces at the juncture of an infant's cranial bones which later harden).

From a neurological standpoint, the clinical picture of megalencephaly varies widely. Manifestations may range from normal intellect, as in the case of benign familial megalencephaly, to severe mental retardation and seizures, as with Alexander disease, an inherited leukodystrophy (disease of the brain's white matter). Neurological symptoms that may be present or develop in a person with megalencephaly include:

• delay of motor milestones such as holding up head, rolling over, or sitting
• mental retardation
• speech delay
• poor muscle tone
• body asymmetry
• paralysis of one or both sides of the body
• poor coordination
• involuntary movements
• visual disturbances

Brain abnormalities that may be seen in individuals with megalencephaly include:

• gyral abnormalities
• neuronal heterotopias
• corpus callosum dysgenesis
• myelum dysplasia
• abnormal or an excess amount of neurons
• abnormal or an excess amount of glia cells

Diagnosis

A diagnosis of megalencephaly is based on clinical findings and results of brain imaging studies. Since megalencephaly can be a benign condition, there may well be many individuals who never come to medical attention. Though no longer used as a primary means of diagnosing megalencephaly, an autopsy may provide additional evidence to support this diagnosis. The evaluation of a patient with suspected megalencephaly will usually consist of questions about medical history and family history, a physical exam that includes head measurements, and a developmental and/or neurological exam. It may be necessary to obtain head circumference measurements for first-degree relatives (parents, siblings, children). Depending upon the history and clinical findings, a physician may recommend imaging studies such as CT (computed tomography) scan or MRI (magnetic resonance imaging). Findings on CT scan or MRI consistent with a diagnosis of megalencephaly are an enlarged brain with normal-sized ventricles and subarachnoid spaces. The volume (size) of the brain may be calculated or estimated using measurements from the CT or MRI. A patient with megalencephaly may be referred to specialists in neurology or genetics for further evaluation. Laboratory testing for a genetic condition or chromosome abnormality may also be performed.

Treatment

There is no cure for megalencephaly. Management of this condition largely depends upon the presence and severity of associated neurological and physical problems. In cases of benign familial megalencephaly, additional management beyond routine health care maintenance may consist of periodic head measurements and patient education about the inheritance and benign nature of the condition. For patients with neurological and/or physical problems, management may include anti-epileptic drugs for seizures, treatment of medical complications related to the underlying syndrome, and rehabilitation for neurological problems such as speech delay, poor muscle tone, and poor coordination. Placement in a residential care facility may be necessary for those cases in which megalencephaly is accompanied by severe mental retardation or uncontrollable seizures.

Treatment team

The types of professionals involved in the care of patients is highly individualized because the severity of symptoms varies widely from patient to patient. For patients with associated neurological and/or physical

KEY TERMS

Autosomal dominant—A pattern of inheritance in which only one of the two copies of an autosomal gene must be abnormal for a genetic condition or disease to occur. An autosomal gene is a gene that is located on one of the autosomes or non-sex chromosomes. A person with an autosomal dominant disorder has a 50% chance of passing it to each of their offspring.

Autosomal recessive—A pattern of inheritance in which both copies of an autosomal gene must be abnormal for a genetic condition or disease to occur. An autosomal gene is a gene that is located on one of the autosomes or non-sex chromosomes. When both parents have one abnormal copy of the same gene, they have a 25% chance with each pregnancy that their offspring will have the disorder.

Chromosome—A microscopic thread-like structure found within each cell of the human body and consisting of a complex of proteins and DNA. Humans have 46 chromosomes arranged into 23 pairs. Chromosomes contain the genetic information necessary to direct the development and functioning of all cells and systems in the body. They pass on hereditary traits from parents to child (like eye color) and determine whether the child will be male or female.

Gene—A building block of inheritance, which contains the instructions for the production of a particular protein, and is made up of a molecular sequence found on a section of DNA. Each gene is found on a precise location on a chromosome.

Inborn error of metabolism—One of a group of rare conditions characterized by an inherited defect in an enzyme or other protein. Inborn errors of metabolism can cause brain damage and mental retardation if left untreated. Phenylketonuria, Tay-Sachs disease, and galactosemia are inborn errors of metabolism.

problems, the treatment team may include specialists in neonatology, neurology, radiology, orthopedics, rehabilitation, and genetics. Genetic counseling may be helpful to the patient and family, especially at the time of diagnosis. Participation in a support group may also be beneficial to those families adversely affected by megalencephaly.

Recovery and rehabilitation

The optimal remedial strategies for individuals with megalencephaly depend upon the presence and severity of associated neurological and physical problems. Interventions such as speech, physical, and occupational therapy may be indicated for individuals with megalencephaly. Early intervention services for young children and special education or other means of educational support for school-aged children may be recommended if developmental delays, learning disabilities, or other barriers to learning are present. The goal of these therapies is to maximize the patient's success in school, work, and life in general. A child with megalencephaly may be eligible to have an Individual Education Plan (IEP). An IEP provides a framework within which administrators, teachers, and parents can meet the educational needs of a child with learning disabilities. Depending upon severity of symptoms and the degree of learning difficulties, some children with megalencephaly may be best served by special education classes or a private educational setting.

Clinical trials

There are no active clinical trials specifically designed to study megalencephaly. Patients with underlying syndromes that produce megalencephaly may be candidates for clinical trials that relate to that particular syndrome. Current information about clinical trials can be found at ClinicalTrials.gov.

Prognosis

The prognosis for megalencephaly varies according to the presence and severity of associated problems such as intractable seizures, paralysis and mental retardation. Hemimegalencephaly is often associated with severe seizures, hemiparesis (paralysis of one side of the body), and mental retardation, and as such, it carries a poor prognosis. In the case of a fetus diagnosed with megalencephaly, prediction of outcome remains imprecise.

Resources

BOOKS

Garel, C., et al. *MRI of the Fetal Brain: Normal Development and Cerebral Pathologies.* Springer: 2004.

Holmes, Gregory. *Pediatric Neurology (What Do I Do Now?).* Oxford University Press: 2010.

Raymond, Gerald V., and Florian S. Eichler, Ali Fatemi, Sakkubai Naidu, eds. *Leukodystrophies* (International Child Neurology Association). Mac Keith Press: 2011.

PERIODICALS

Batla, Amit, Ravi Nehru, and Sanjay Pandey. "Megalencephalic leukoencephalopathy with subcortical cysts: A report of four cases." *Journal of Pediatric Neurosciences* 6.1 (2011): 74.

Baybis, Marianna, et al. "STRAD alpha deficiency results in aberrant mTORC1 signaling during corticogenesis in humans and mice." *Journal of Clinical Investigation* 120.5 (2010): 1591.

Osborne, Lucy R. "Caveat mTOR: aberrant signaling disrupts corticogenesis." *Journal of Clinical Investigation* 120.5 (2010): 1392.

WEBSITES

National Institute of Neurological Disorders and Stroke (NINDS). Cephalic Disorders Fact Sheet. http://www.ninds.nih.gov/health_and_medical/pubs/cephalic_disorders.htm.

National Institute of Neurological Disorders and Stroke (NINDS). *Megalencephaly Information Page.* http://www.ninds.nih.gov/health_and_medical/disorders/megalencephaly.htm.

Online Mendelian Inheritance In Man (OMIM). *Megalencephaly.* http://www.ncbi.nlm.nih.gov/entrez/dispomim.cgi?id = 155350.

ORGANIZATIONS

National Institute of Child Health and Human Development (NICHD) Information Resource Center. P. O. Box 3006, Rockville, MD 20847. Fax: (301) 496-7101. Tollfree phone: (800) 370-2943. Email: NICHDInformationResourceCenter@mail.nih.gov. http://www.nichd.nih.gov.

National Institute of Neurological Disorders and Stroke (NINDS). P.O. Box 5801, Bethesda, MD 20824. Phone: (301) 496-5751. Tollfree phone: (800) 352-9424. http://www.ninds.nih.gov.

National Organization for Rare Disorders (NORD). PO Box 1968, 55 Kensonia Avenue, Danbury, CT 06813. Phone: (203) 744-0100. Fax: (203) 798-2291. Tollfree phone: 800-999-NORD (6673) voice mail. http://www.rarediseases.org.

Dawn J. Cardeiro, MS, CGC

Meige syndrome *see* **Hemifacial spasm**

Melodic intonation therapy

Definition

Melodic intonation therapy (MIT) uses melodic and rhythmic components to assist in speech recovery for patients with **aphasia**.

Purpose

Although MIT was first described in the 1970s, it is considered a relatively new and experimental therapy. Few research studies have been performed to analyze the effectiveness of treatment with large numbers of patients. Despite this, some speech therapists use the method for children and adults with aphasia as well as for children with developmental **apraxia** of speech.

The effectiveness of MIT derives from its use of the musical components melody and rhythm in the production of speech. A group of researchers from the University of Texas have discovered that music stimulates several different areas in the brain, rather than just one isolated area. They also found a strong correlation between the right side of the brain that comprehends music components and the left side of the brain that comprehends language components. Because music and language structures are similar, it is suspected that by stimulating the right side of the brain, the left side will begin to make connections as well. For this reason, patients are encouraged to sing words rather than speak them in conversational tones in the early phases of MIT. Studies using **PET (positron emission tomography)** scans have shown Broca's area (a region in the left frontal brain controlling speech and language comprehension) to be reactivated through repetition of sung words.

Precautions

Patients and caregivers should be aware that there is little research to support consistent success with MIT. Theoretically, this form of therapy has the potential to improve speech communication to a limited extent.

Description

Melodic intonation therapy was originally developed as a treatment method for speech improvements in adults with aphasia. The initial method has had several modifications, mostly adaptations for use by children with apraxia. The primary structure of this therapy remains relatively consistent however.

There are four steps, or levels, generally outlining the path of therapy.

- Level I: The speech therapist hums short phrases in a rhythmic, singsong tone. The patient attempts to follow the rhythm and stress patterns of phrases by tapping it out. With children, the therapist uses signing while humming and the child is not initially expected to participate. After a series of steps, the child gradually increases participation until they sign and hum with the therapist.
- Level II: The patient begins to repeat the hummed phrases with the assistance of the speech therapist.

KEY TERMS

Aphasia—Loss of the ability to use or understand language, usually as a result of brain injury or disease.

Apraxia—Loss of the ability to carry out a voluntary movement despite being able to demonstrate normal muscle function.

Pitch—The property of sound that is determined by the frequency of sound wave vibrations reaching the ear.

Children at this level are gradually weaned from therapist participation.

- Level III: For adults, this is the point where therapist participation is minimized and the patient begins to respond to questions still using rhythmic speech patterns. In children, this is the final level and the transition to normal speech begins. *Sprechgesang* is the technique used to transition the constant melodic pitch used up to this point with the variable pitch in normal conversational speech.

- Level IV: The adult method incorporates *sprechgesang* at this level. More complex phrases and longer sentences are attempted.

Preparation

Preparation for MIT involves some additional research into the therapy and discussions with a neurologist and a speech pathologist. It is important to have an understanding of the affected brain areas. MIT is most likely to be successful for patients who meet certain criteria such as non-bilateral brain damage, good auditory aptitude, non-fluent verbal communication, and poor word repetition. The speech pathologist should be familiar with the different MIT methodologies as they relate to either adults or children.

Aftercare

There is no required aftercare for MIT.

Risks

There are no physical risks associated with the use of melodic intonation therapy.

Normal results

The expected outcome after completion of the MIT sequence is increased communication through production of intelligible word groups. Patients are typically able to form short sentences of 3–5 words, but more complex communication may also be possible depending on the initial cause of speech impairment.

Resources

BOOKS

Aldridge, David. *Music Therapy in Dementia Care*. Philadelphia: Jessica Kingsley, 2008.

PERIODICALS

Goldfarb, Robert. "Operant conditioning and programmed instruction in aphasia rehabilitation." *The Journal of Speech-Language Pathology and Applied Behavior Analysis* 1.1 (2006): 56.

Marchina, Sarah, et al. "From singing to speaking: facilitating recovery from nonfluent aphasia." *Future Neurology* 5.5 (2010): 657.

Orest, Marianne R. "Alternate Therapies in the Treatment of Brain Injury and Neurobehavioral Disorders: A Practical Guide." *Physical Therapy* Dec. 2006: 1714.

Rapposelli, Dee. "INTENSIVE MIT CURES APHASIA, 'REWIRES' BRAIN." *Applied Neurology* 1 June 2007: 16.

ORGANIZATIONS

Center for Music Therapy. 404-A Baylor Street, Austin, TX 78703. Phone: (512) 472-5016. Fax: (512) 472-5017. Tollfree Email: info@centerformusictherapy.com. http://www.centerformusictherapy.com.

American Speech-Language-Hearing Association. 10801 Rockville Pike, Rockville, MD 20852. Phone: (301) 897-5700. Fax: (301) 571-0457. Tollfree phone: (800) 638-8255. Email: actioncenter@asha.org. http://www.nsastutter.org.

Music Therapy Association of British Columbia. 2055 Purcell Way, North Vancouver, British Columbia, Canada V7J 3H5. Phone: (604) 924-0046. Fax: (604) 983-7559. Email: info@mtabc.com. http://www.mtabc.com.

Stacey L. Chamberlin

Ménière's disease

Definition

Ménière's disease is a condition characterized by recurrent **vertigo (dizziness)**, **hearing loss**, and **tinnitus** (a roaring, buzzing or ringing sound in the ears).

Description

Ménière's disease was named for the French physician Prosper Ménière, who first described the illness in 1861. It is an abnormality within the inner ear. A fluid called endolymph moves in the membranous labyrinth or semicircular canals within the bony labyrinth inside the inner ear. When the head or body moves, the endolymph moves, causing nerve receptors in the membranous labyrinth to send signals to the brain about the body's motion. A change in the volume of the endolymph fluid or swelling or rupture of the membranous labyrinth is thought to result in Ménière's disease symptoms.

Causes and symptoms

Causes

The cause of Ménière's disease is unknown however, scientists are studying several possible causes, including noise pollution, viral infections, or alterations in the patterns of blood flow in the structures of the inner ear. Since Ménière's disease sometimes runs in families, researchers are also looking into genetic factors as possible causes of the disorder.

One area of research that shows promise is the possible relationship between Ménière's disease and **migraine headache**. Dr. Ménière himself suggested the possibility of a link, but early studies yielded conflicting results. A rigorous German study reported that the lifetime prevalence of migraine was 56% in patients diagnosed with Ménière's disease as compared to 25% for controls. The researchers noted that further work is necessary to determine the exact nature of the relationship between the two disorders.

A study published in late 2002 reported that there is a significant increase in the number of CD4 cells in the blood of patients having an acute attack of Ménière's disease. CD4 cells are a subtype of T cells, which are produced in the thymus gland and regulate the immune system's response to infected or malignant cells. Further research is needed to clarify the role of these cells in Ménière's disease.

Another possible factor in the development of Ménière's disease is the loss of myelin from the cells surrounding the vestibular nerve fibers. Myelin is a whitish fatty material in the cell membrane of the Schwann cells that form a sheath around certain nerve cells. It acts like an electrical insulator. A team of researchers at the University of Virginia reported in 2002 that the vestibular nerve cells in patients with unilateral Ménière's disease are demyelinated; that is, they have lost their protective "insulation." The researchers are investigating the possibility that a viral disease or disorder of the immune system is responsible for the demyelination of the vestibular nerve cells.

Symptoms

The symptoms of Ménière's disease are associated with a change in fluid volume within the labyrinth of the inner ear. Symptoms include severe dizziness or vertigo, tinnitus, hearing loss, and the sensation of pain or pressure in the affected ear. Symptoms appear suddenly, last up to several hours, and can occur as often as daily to as infrequently as once a year. A typical attack includes vertigo, tinnitus, and hearing loss; however, some individuals with Ménière's disease may experience a single symptom, like an occasional bout of slight dizziness or periodic, intense ringing in the ear. Attacks of severe vertigo can force the sufferer to have to sit or lie down and may be accompanied by headache, nausea, vomiting, or diarrhea. Hearing tends to recover between attacks but becomes progressively worse over time.

Ménière's disease usually starts between the ages of 20 and 50 years; however, it is not uncommon for elderly people to develop the disease without a previous history of symptoms. Ménière's disease affects men and women in equal numbers. In most patients only one ear is affected but in about 15% both ears are involved.

Diagnosis

An estimated 3–5 million people in the United States have Ménière's disease, and almost 100,000 new cases are diagnosed each year. Diagnosis is based on medical history, physical examination, hearing and balance tests, and medical imaging with magnetic resonance imaging (MRI).

Several types of tests may be used to diagnose the disease and to evaluation the extent of hearing loss. In patients with Ménière's disease, audiometric tests (hearing tests) usually indicate a sensory type of hearing loss in the affected ear. Speech discrimination or the ability to distinguish between words that sound alike is often diminished. In about 50% of patients, the balance function is reduced in the affected ear. An electronystagnograph (ENG) may be used to evaluate balance. Since the eyes and ears work together through the nervous system to coordinate balance, measurement of eye movements can be used to test the balance system. For this test, the patient is seated in a darkened room and recording electrodes, similar to those used with a heart monitor, are placed near the eyes. Warm and cool water or air are gently introduced into the each ear canal and eye movements are recorded.

Another test that may be used is an electrocochleograph (EcoG), which can measure increased inner ear fluid pressure.

Treatment

There is no cure for Ménière's disease, but medication, surgery, and dietary and behavioral changes, can help control or improve the symptoms.

Medications

Symptoms of Ménière's disease may be treated with a variety of oral medicine or through injections. Antihistamines, like diphenhydramine, meclizine, and cyclizine, can be prescribed to sedate the vestibular system. A barbiturate medication such as pentobarbital may be used to completely sedate the patient and relieve the vertigo. Anticholinergic drugs, like atropine or scopolamine, can help minimize nausea and vomiting. **Diazepam** has been found to be particularly effective for relief of vertigo and nausea in Ménière's disease. There have been some reports of successful control of vertigo after antibiotics (gentamicin or streptomycin) or a steroid medication (dexamethasone) are injected directly into the inner ear. Some researchers have found that gentamicin is effective in relieving tinnitus as well as vertigo.

A newer medication that appears to be effective in treating the vertigo associated with Ménière's disease is flunarizine, which is sold under the trade name Sibelium. Flunarizine is a calcium channel blocker and anticonvulsant used to treat **Parkinson's disease**, migraine headache, and other circulatory disorders that affect the brain.

Surgical procedures

Surgical procedures may be recommended if the vertigo attacks are frequent, severe, or disabling and cannot be controlled by other treatments. The most common surgical treatment is insertion of a small tube or shunt to drain some of the fluid from the canal. This treatment usually preserves hearing and controls vertigo in about one-half to two-thirds of cases, but it is not a permanent cure in all patients.

The vestibular nerve leads from the inner ear to the brain and is responsible for conducting nerve impulses related to balance. A vestibular neurectomy is a procedure where this nerve is cut so the distorted impulses causing dizziness no longer reach the brain. This procedure permanently cures the majority of patients and hearing is preserved in most cases. There is a slight risk that hearing or facial muscle control will be affected.

A labyrinthectomy is a surgical procedure in which the balance and hearing mechanism in the inner ear are destroyed on one side. This procedure is considered when the patient has poor hearing in the affected ear. Labyrinthectomy results in the highest rates of control of vertigo attacks, however, it also causes complete deafness in the affected ear.

Alternative treatment

Changes in diet and behavior are sometimes recommended. Eliminating caffeine, alcohol, and salt may relieve the frequency and intensity of attacks in some people with Ménière's disease. Reducing stress levels and eliminating tobacco use may also help.

Acupuncture is an alternative treatment that has been shown to help patients with Ménière's disease. The World Health Organization (WHO) lists Ménière's disease as one of 104 conditions that can be treated effectively with acupuncture.

Prognosis

Ménière's disease is a complex and unpredictable condition for which there is no cure. The vertigo associated with the disease can generally be managed or eliminated with medications and surgery. Hearing tends to become worse over time, and some of the surgical procedures recommended, in fact, cause deafness.

Prevention

Since the cause of Ménière's disease is unknown, there are no current strategies for its prevention. Research continues on the environmental and biological factors that may cause Ménière's disease or induce an attack, as well as on the physiological components of the fluid and labyrinth system involved in hearing and balance. Preventive strategies and more effective treatment should become evident once these mechanisms are better understood.

Resources

BOOKS

Harris, Jeffrey, and Quyen T. Nguyen. *Meniere's Disease, An Issue of Otolaryngologic Clinics.* Saunders: 2010.

Ruckenstein, Michael. *Meniere's Disease: Evidence and Outcomes,* Plural Publishing: 2010.

PERIODICALS

Aita, Maria, Gino Marioni, and Marina Savastano. "Psychological characteristics of patients with Meniere's disease compared with patients with vertigo, tinnitus, or hearing loss." *Ear, Nose and Throat Journal* Mar. 2007: 148

Aran, Ismael, et al. "Polymorphisms of CD16A and CD32 Fcγ receptors and circulating immune complexes in Meniere's disease: a case-control study." *BMC Medical Genetics* 12 (2011): 2.

Bellini, C., et al. "Efficacy of low-level laser therapy in Meniere's disease: a pilot study of 10 patients." *Photomedicine and Laser Surgery* 26.4 (2008): 349.

Bhuta, Sunita, et al. "Histopathological and ultrastructural analysis of vestibular endorgans in Meniere's disease reveals basement membrane pathology." *BMC Ear, Nose and Throat Disorders* 9.4 (2009): 4.

Candiloros, D., et al. "Meniere's disease: Still a mystery disease with difficult differential diagnosis." *Annals of Indian Academy of Neurology* 14.1 (2011): 12.

Cronin, Gaye W., Robin B. Hardin, and Ronald Leif Steenerson. "Gentamicin injections for Meniere disease: comparison of subjective and objective end points." *Ear, Nose and Throat Journal* Aug. 2008: 452.

Djalilian, Hamid R., et al. "HLA-B27-associated bilateral Meniere disease." *Ear, Nose and Throat Journal* Mar. 2010: 122.

Goto, Fumiyuki, et al. "Case report: a case of intractable Meniere's disease treated with autogenic training." *BioPsychoSocial Medicine* 2.3 (2008): 3.

Warren, Ed. "ENT in primary care: part 4 vertigo: vertigo implies a problem with the inner-ear balance organs. Common causes are vestibular neuronitis, benign positional vertigo and Meniere's disease." *Practice Nurse* 23 May 2008: 36.

ORGANIZATIONS

American Academy of Otolaryngology-Head and Neck Surgery, Inc. One Prince St., Alexandria VA 22314-3357. (703) 836-4444. http://www.entnet.org.

Ménière's Network. 2000 Church St., P.O. Box 111, Nashville, TN 37236. (800) 545-4327. http://www.healthy.net/pan/cso/cioi/mn.htm.

On-Balance, A Support Group for People with Ménière's Disease. http://www.midwestear.com/onbal.htm.

Vestibular Disorders Association. P.O. Box 4467, Portland, OR 97208-4467. (800) 837-8428.

Altha Roberts Edgren
Rebecca J. Frey, PhD

Meninges

Definition

Meninges (singular is meninx) is the collective term for the three membranes covering the brain and spinal cord. The meninges are composed of the dura mater (outer), the arachnoid (middle), and the pia mater (inner). In common usage, the membranes are often referred to as simply the dura, pia, and arachnoid.

Description

"Dura" is the Latin word for "hard," while "pia" in Latin means "soft." The dura mater was so-named because of its tough, fibrous consistency. The pia mater is thinner and more delicate than the dura mater and is in direct contact with the neural tissue of the brain and spinal cord. Along with the arachnoid layer and the cerebrospinal fluid (CSF), the dura and pia membranes help cushion, protect, and nourish the brain and spinal cord.

"Mater" is Latin for "mother" and thus refers to the membranes' protective and nourishing functions. Each of the meninges can also be classified as to the portion that covers the brain (e.g., dura mater cerebri or dura mater encephali) or that portion lining the spinal cord (e.g., pia mater spinalis). "Arachnoid" means "spidery," referring to the membrane's webbed appearance and consistency. The space between the arachnoid membrane and pia mater contains many fibrous filaments and blood vessels that attach the two layers.

Anatomy

The outer surface of the dura adheres to the skull, while the inner surface is loosely connected to the arachnoid layer. The exception is the spinal canal, where there is normally a thin layer of fat and a network of blood vessels between the dura and the bony portion of the vertebrae. There is normally no space between the dura and skull on one side, and the dura and arachnoid on the other. However, these are sometimes called "potential" spaces because abnormal conditions may create "actual" spaces there. Anything in the space between the dura and skull is called epidural (above the dura), while the space between the dura and arachnoid is considered subdural (below the dura).

There *is* normally an actual space between the arachnoid layer and the pia mater known as the subarachnoid space. As noted, it contains many fibrous filaments, known as trabeculae (little beams), joining and stabilizing the two layers. The importance of the subarachnoid space is that it contains the circulating CSF. It is this layer of fluid that helps to cushion the brain and protect it from sudden movements and impacts to the skull.

The pia mater has the appearance of a thin mesh, with a network of tiny blood vessels interlacing it. It is always in contact with the neural tissue of the brain and spinal cord, much like a skin. It follows all of the grooves, folds, and fissures of the brain's various lobes and prominences.

All of the meninges are composed of connective tissue, which is made up of relatively few cells, with an abundance of structural and supportive proteins.

Function

Given the singular importance of the **central nervous system** (CNS) to both basic and higher-level functions of the body, it is not surprising that a system evolved to help protect it. Thicker skull bones would certainly afford more protection against skull fracture and open head injury but would come at the cost of greater weight for the spine to bear. If the head is struck or strikes some other object, even unbreakable skull bones would not protect the brain from the injury that results as brain tissue impacts the inside of the skull (concussion). The layer of CSF that circulates in the subarachnoid space helps to lower this risk, although it cannot eliminate it. Wearing a sports helmet composed of a hard, plastic outer shell with firm padding inside simply mimics and augments the safety mechanism already present in the skull and outer lining of the brain.

The dura mater is the tough, but flexible, second line of defense for the brain after the skull. The flexibility of the dura is important in that most skull fractures, other than those involving severe penetrating injuries, will not result in loss of CSF

through the injury site which, before the days of antibiotics and emergency medicine, would pose a serious risk for infection and death.

The arachnoid membrane provides a stable substrate and space through which the CSF can circulate, and also provides specialized tissue necessary for absorption of the CSF back into the bloodstream. The arachnoid trabeculae help to anchor the surrounding membranes and keep the subarachnoid space at a constant depth.

While the CSF is normally sterile and mostly inert—containing glucose, proteins, electrolytes (necessary minerals), and very few cells—the brain and spinal neurons nonetheless need some protection from direct contact with the fluid, which is provided by the pia mater. As blood vessels pass through the dura mater and then the subarachnoid space, they pierce the pia mater as they enter the CNS. The membrane follows the blood vessel down and becomes the external portion of the blood vessel wall.

CSF Production and Circulation

In a sense, the CSF can be thought of as a fourth layer of the meninges. The fluid is produced in, circulates through, and is reabsorbed by the meningeal layers, thus creating a self–contained system. The volume of fluid in adults is normally 100–150 ml. About 500 ml of new fluid is produced and reabsorbed each day, which means the CSF is "turned over" three times in 24 hours. It is important for the body to maintain CSF volume within the normal range, since there is limited space within the skull and spinal column. It is also important for the fluid to remain at a constant pressure. Increased fluid pressure typically leads to compression of the surrounding neural tissue, which then leads to increased fluid volume. Since the bones of the skull are not fused in a developing fetus or newborn infant, increased fluid pressure in the brain may cause the head to grow to an abnormally large size (see Hydrocephalus), called macrocephaly. The skull bones are fused after about 2 years of age, so increased fluid pressure and volume after that point will most likely result in compression of, and damage to, neural tissue.

The CSF is produced by a layer of densely packed capillaries and supporting cells known as the choroid plexus. It lines the upper portion of the lateral (cerebral), third, and fourth ventricles. Once produced, the CSF flows down through the fourth ventricle and then through openings at the base of the brain and around the brain stem. Some of the fluid

KEY TERMS

Arachnoid membrane—One of the three membranes that sheath the spinal cord and brain; the arachnoid is the middle membrane. Also called the arachnoid mater.

Cerebrospinal fluid—The clear, normally colorless fluid that fills the brain cavities (ventricles), the subarachnoid space around the brain, and the spinal cord and acts as a shock absorber.

Choroid plexus—Specialized cells located in the ventricles of the brain that produce cerebrospinal fluid.

Dura mater—The strongest and outermost of three membranes that protect the brain, spinal cord, and nerves of the cauda equina.

Hydrocephalus—An abnormal accumulation of cerebrospinal fluid within the brain. This accumulation can be harmful by pressing on brain structures and damaging them.

Meningitis—An infection or inflammation of the membranes that cover the brain and spinal cord. It is usually caused by bacteria or a virus.

Pia mater—The innermost of the three meninges covering the brain.

Ventricles—The four fluid-filled chambers, or cavities, found in the two cerebral hemispheres of the brain, at the center of the brain, and between the brain stem and cerebellum. They are linked by channels, or ducts, allowing cerebral fluid to circulate through them.

circulates down through the subarachnoid space encircling the length of the spinal cord, while the remainder flows up to the subarachnoid space around the brain.

Most of the fluid is absorbed back into the bloodstream through vessels lining branched projections from the arachnoid membrane called arachnoid villi, or granulations. These arachnoid granulations extend into the dura, primarily at points where large blood veins lie within the dural membrane itself. These veins traveling through the dura that drain blood and absorbed CSF from the brain are collectively known as the venous sinuses of the dura mater. The remainder of the CSF is absorbed through small lymph sacs scattered around the CNS known as perineural lymphatics.

Causes and symptoms

Infection/inflammation of the meninges is covered elsewhere (see **Meningitis**). Other abnormalities of the meninges typically involve situations in which a fluid occupies and expands the epidural, subdural, or subarachnoid spaces. For instance, blood accumulation that separates the dura from the inner side of the skull is known as an **epidural hematoma** (blood swelling). The same occurrence between the dura and arachnoid layers is a **subdural hematoma**. Both of these conditions are most frequently caused by head trauma but may also result from a bleeding disorder or defect in a cranial blood vessel (aneurysm).

A hemorrhage between the arachnoid membrane and the pia mater is called a subarachnoid bleed and is usually caused by the rupture of a congenital aneurysm, hypertension, or trauma. Unlike conditions affecting the epidural and subdural spaces, a bleed into the subarachnoid space is less likely to affect its volume and increase pressure. A subarachnoid (CSF) infection (abscess), however, may cause increased pressure.

Meningitis may also cause bleeding into the subdural or epidural spaces but more often results in the accumulation of fluid and pus, which are consequences of the body's response to the infection.

Resources

BOOKS

Blumenfeld, Hal. *Neuroanatomy Through Clinical Cases, Second Edition.* Sinauer Associates, Inc.: 2010.
Goldberg, Stephen. *Clinical Neuroanatomy Made Ridiculously Simple.* MedMaster Inc.: 2010.
Waxman, Stephen. *Clinical Neuroanatomy,* 26th Edition. McGraw-Hill Medical: 2009.

Scott J Polzin, MS, CGC

Meningitis *see* **Encephalitis and meningitis**

Mental retardation

Definition

Mental retardation is a developmental disability that first appears in children under the age of 18. It is defined as an intellectual functioning level (as measured by standard tests for intelligence quotient) that is well below average and significant limitations in daily living skills (adaptive functioning).

Description

Mental retardation occurs in 2.5–3% of the general population. About 6–7.5 million mentally retarded individuals live in the United States alone. Mental retardation begins in childhood or adolescence before the age of 18. In most cases, it persists throughout adulthood. A diagnosis of mental retardation is made if an individual has an intellectual functioning level well below average and significant limitations in two or more adaptive skill areas. Intellectual functioning level is defined by standardized tests that measure the ability to reason in terms of mental age (intelligence quotient or IQ). Mental retardation is defined as IQ score below 70–75. Adaptive skills are the skills needed for daily life. Such skills include the ability to produce and understand language (communication); home-living skills; use of community resources; health, safety, leisure, self-care, and social skills; self-direction; functional academic skills (reading, writing, and arithmetic); and work skills.

In general, mentally retarded children reach developmental milestones such as walking and talking much later than the general population. Symptoms of mental retardation may appear at birth or later in childhood. Time of onset depends on the suspected cause of the disability. Some cases of mild mental retardation are not diagnosed before the child enters preschool. These children typically have difficulties with social, communication and functional academic skills. Children who have a neurological disorder or illness such as **encephalitis** or **meningitis** may suddenly show signs of cognitive impairment and adaptive difficulties.

Mental retardation varies in severity. *The Diagnostic and Statistical Manual of Mental Disorders, Fourth Edition (DSM-IV)* is the diagnostic standard for mental healthcare professionals in the United States. The *DSM-IV* classifies four different degrees of mental retardation: *mild, moderate, severe,* and *profound*. These categories are based on the functioning level of the individual.

Mild mental retardation

Approximately 85% of the mentally retarded population is in the mildly retarded category. These individuals have IQ score ranges from 50–75, and they can often acquire academic skills up to the 6th grade level. They can become fairly self-sufficient and in some cases live independently, with community and social support.

Moderate mental retardation

About 10% of the mentally retarded population is considered moderately retarded. Moderately retarded individuals have IQ scores ranging from 35–55. They can carry out work and self-care tasks with moderate supervision. They typically acquire communication skills in childhood and are able to live and function successfully within the community in a supervised environment such as a group home.

Severe mental retardation

About 3–4% of the mentally retarded population is severely retarded. Severely retarded individuals have IQ scores of 20–40. They may master very basic self-care skills and some communication skills. Many severely retarded individuals are able to live in a group home.

Profound mental retardation

Only 1–2% of the mentally retarded population is classified as profoundly retarded. Profoundly retarded individuals have IQ scores under 20–25. They may be able to develop basic self-care and communication skills with appropriate support and training. Their retardation is often caused by an accompanying neurological disorder. The profoundly retarded need a high level of structure and supervision.

The American Association on Mental Retardation (AAMR) has developed another widely accepted diagnostic classification system for mental retardation. The AAMR classification system focuses on the capabilities of the retarded individual rather than on the limitations. The categories describe the level of support required. They are: *intermittent support, limited support, extensive support,* and *pervasive support*. To some extent, the AAMR classification mirrors the *DSM-IV* classification. Intermittent support, for example, is support needed only occasionally, perhaps during times of stress or crisis. It is the type of support typically required for most mildly retarded individuals. At the other end of the spectrum, pervasive support, or life-long, daily support for most adaptive areas, would be required for profoundly retarded individuals.

Causes and symptoms

Low IQ scores and limitations in adaptive skills are the hallmarks of mental retardation. Aggression, self-injury, and mood disorders are sometimes associated with the disability. The severity of the symptoms and the age at which they first appear depend on the cause. Children who are mentally retarded reach developmental milestones significantly later than expected, if at all. If retardation is caused by chromosomal or other genetic disorders, it is often apparent from infancy. If retardation is caused by childhood illnesses or injuries, learning and adaptive skills that were once easy may suddenly become difficult or impossible to master.

In about 35% of cases, the cause of mental retardation cannot be found. Biological and environmental factors that can cause mental retardation include the following.

Genetics

About 5% of mental retardation is caused by hereditary factors. Mental retardation may be caused by an inherited abnormality of the genes, such as fragile X syndrome. Fragile X, a defect in the chromosome that determines sex, is the most common inherited cause of mental retardation. Single gene defects such as phenylketonuria (PKU) and other inborn errors of metabolism may also cause mental retardation if they are not found and treated early. An accident or mutation in genetic development may also cause retardation. Examples of such accidents are development of an extra chromosome 18 (trisomy 18) and Down syndrome. Down syndrome, also called mongolism or trisomy 21, is caused by an abnormality in the development of chromosome 21. It is the most common genetic cause of mental retardation.

Prenatal illnesses and issues

Fetal alcohol syndrome affects one in 600 children in the United States. It is caused by excessive alcohol intake in the first twelve weeks (trimester) of pregnancy. Some studies have shown that even moderate alcohol use during pregnancy may cause learning disabilities in children. Drug abuse and cigarette smoking during pregnancy have also been linked to mental retardation.

Maternal infections and illnesses such as glandular disorders, rubella, toxoplasmosis, and cytomegalovirus infection may cause mental retardation. When the mother has high blood pressure (hypertension) or blood poisoning (toxemia), the flow of oxygen to the fetus may be reduced, causing brain damage and mental retardation.

Birth defects that cause physical deformities of the head, brain, and **central nervous system** frequently cause mental retardation. Neural tube defect, for example, is a birth defect in which the neural tube that forms the spinal cord does not close completely. This defect may cause children to develop an accumulation of cerebrospinal fluid on the brain (hydrocephalus). Hydrocephalus can cause learning impairment by putting pressure on the brain.

Childhood illnesses and injuries

Hyperthyroidism, whooping cough, chickenpox, measles, and Hib disease (a bacterial infection) may cause mental retardation if they are not treated adequately. An infection of the membrane covering the brain (meningitis) or an inflammation of the brain itself (encephalitis) causes swelling that in turn may cause brain damage and mental retardation. **Traumatic brain injury** caused by a blow or a violent shake to the head may also cause brain damage and mental retardation in children.

Environmental factors

Ignored or neglected infants who are not provided the mental and physical stimulation required for normal development may suffer irreversible learning impairments. Children who live in poverty and suffer from malnutrition, unhealthy living conditions, and improper or inadequate medical care are at a higher risk. Exposure to lead can also cause mental retardation. Many children have developed lead poisoning by eating the flaking lead-based paint often found in older buildings.

Diagnosis

If mental retardation is suspected, a comprehensive physical examination and medical history should be done immediately to discover any organic cause of symptoms. Conditions such as hyperthyroidism and PKU are treatable. If these conditions are discovered early, the progression of retardation can be stopped and, in some cases, partially reversed. If a neurological cause such as brain injury is suspected, the child may be referred to a neurologist or neuropsychologist for testing.

A complete medical, family, social, and educational history is compiled from existing medical and school records (if applicable) and from interviews with parents. Children are given intelligence tests to measure their learning abilities and intellectual functioning. Such tests include the Stanford-Binet Intelligence Scale, the Wechsler Intelligence Scales, the Wechsler Preschool and Primary Scale of Intelligence, and the Kaufmann Assessment Battery for Children. For infants, the Bayley Scales of Infant Development may be used to assess motor, language, and problem-solving skills. Interviews with parents or other

KEY TERMS

Amniocentesis—A test usually done between 16 and 20 weeks of pregnancy to detect any abnormalities in the development of the fetus. A small amount of the fluid surrounding the fetus (amniotic fluid) is drawn out through a needle inserted into the mother's womb. Laboratory analysis of this fluid can detect various genetic defects, such as Down syndrome, or neural tube defects.

Developmental delay—The failure to meet certain developmental milestones, such as sitting, walking, and talking, at the average age. Developmental delay may indicate a problem in development of the central nervous system.

Down syndrome—A disorder caused by an abnormality at chromosome 21. One symptom of Down syndrome is mental retardation.

Extensive support—Ongoing daily support required to assist an individual in a specific adaptive area, such as daily help with preparing meals.

Hib disease—An infection caused by *Haemophilus influenza* type b (Hib). This disease mainly affects children under the age of five. In that age group, it is the leading cause of bacterial meningitis, pneumonia, joint and bone infections, and throat inflammations.

Inborn error of metabolism—A rare enzyme deficiency; children with inborn errors of metabolism do not have certain enzymes that the body requires to maintain organ functions. Inborn errors of metabolism can cause brain damage and mental retardation if left untreated.

Limited support—A predetermined period of assistance required to deal with a specific event, such as training for a new job.

Phenylketonuria (PKU)—An inborn error in metabolism that prevents the body from using phenylalanine, an amino acid necessary for normal growth and development.

Trisomy—An abnormality in chromosomal development. Chromosomes are the structures within a cell that carry its genetic information. They are organized in pairs. Humans have 23 pairs of chromosomes. In a trisomy syndrome, an extra chromosome is present so that the individual has three of a particular chromosome instead of the normal pair. An extra chromosome 18 (trisomy 18) causes mental retardation.

Ultrasonography—A process that uses the reflection of high-frequency sound waves to make an image of structures deep within the body. Ultrasonography is routinely used to detect fetal abnormalities.

caregivers are used to assess the child's daily living, muscle control, communication, and social skills. The Woodcock-Johnson Scales of Independent Behavior and the Vineland Adaptive Behavior Scale (VABS) are frequently used to test these skills.

Treatment

Federal legislation entitles mentally retarded children to free testing and appropriate, individualized education and skills training within the school system from ages 3–21. For children under the age of three, many states have established early intervention programs that assess, recommend, and begin treatment programs. Many day schools are available to help train retarded children in basic skills such as bathing and feeding themselves. Extracurricular activities and social programs are also important in helping retarded children and adolescents gain self-esteem.

Training in independent living and job skills is often begun in early adulthood. The level of training depends on the degree of retardation. Mildly retarded individuals can often acquire the skills needed to live independently and hold an outside job. Moderate to profoundly retarded individuals usually require supervised community living.

Family therapy can help relatives of the mentally retarded develop coping skills. It can also help parents deal with feelings of guilt or anger. A supportive, warm home environment is essential to help the mentally retarded reach their full potential.

Prognosis

Individuals with mild to moderate mental retardation are frequently able to achieve some self-sufficiency and to lead happy and fulfilling lives. To reach these goals, they need appropriate and consistent educational, community, social, family, and vocational supports. The outlook is less promising for those with severe to profound retardation. Studies have shown that these individuals have a shortened life expectancy. The diseases that are usually associated with severe retardation may cause the shorter life span. People with Down syndrome will develop the brain changes that characterize **Alzheimer's disease** in later life and may develop the clinical symptoms of this disease as well.

Prevention

Immunization against diseases such as measles and Hib prevents many of the illnesses that can cause mental retardation. In addition, all children should undergo routine developmental screening as part of their pediatric care. Screening is particularly critical for those children who may be neglected or undernourished or may live in disease-producing conditions. Newborn screening and immediate treatment for PKU and hyperthyroidism can usually catch these disorders early enough to prevent retardation.

Good prenatal care can also help prevent retardation. Pregnant women should be educated about the risks of drinking and the need to maintain good nutrition during pregnancy. Tests such as amniocentesis and ultrasonography can determine whether a fetus is developing normally in the womb.

Resources

OTHER

"Developmental Disabilities." National Institutes of Health (NIH) (April 7, 2011). http://health.nih.gov/topic/DevelopmentalDisabilities (accessed October 21, 2011).

ORGANIZATIONS

American Association on Mental Retardation (AAMR). 444 North Capitol St., NW, Suite 846, Washington, D 20001-1512. (800) 424-3688. http://www.aamr.org.

The Arc. 900 Varnum Street NE, Washington, D 20017. (202) 636-2950. http://thearc.org.

Paula Anne Ford-Martin

Meralgia paresthetica

Definition

Meralgia paresthetica is a condition characterized by numbness, tingling, or pain along the outer thigh.

Description

Meralgia paresthetica occurs when the lateral femoral cutaneous nerve, which supplies sensation to the outer part of the thigh, is compressed or entrapped at the point where it exits the pelvis. Usually, only one thigh is affected. Obese, diabetic, or pregnant people are more susceptible to this disorder. Tight clothing may exacerbate or cause the condition.

Demographics

Overweight individuals are more likely to develop meralgia paresthetica; men are more commonly affected than women. The disorder tends to occur in middle-aged individuals.

Causes and symptoms

Meralgia paresthetica is the result of pressure on the lateral femoral cutaneous nerve, and subsequent inflammation of the nerve. The point of pressure or entrapment is usually where the nerve exits the pelvis, running through the inguinal ligament. Being overweight, having diabetes or other risk factors for nerve disorders, wearing tight clothing or belts, previous surgery in the area of the lateral femoral cutaneous nerve, or injury (such as pelvic fracture) predispose individuals to meralgia paresthetica.

Symptoms of meralgia paresthetica include numbness, tingling, stinging, or burning pain along the outer thigh. The skin of the outer thigh may be particularly sensitive to touch, resulting in increased pain. Many people note that their symptoms are initiated or worsened by walking or standing.

Diagnosis

The diagnosis is usually evident based on the patient's description of symptoms and the physical examination. Neurological testing will usually reveal normal thigh-muscle strength and normal reflexes, but there will be numbness or extreme sensitivity of the skin along the outer aspect of the thigh.

Treatment team

Depending on its severity, meralgia paresthetica may be treated by a family medicine doctor, internal medicine specialist, neurologist, or orthopedic surgeon.

Treatment

Patients with meralgia paresthetica are usually advised to lose weight and to wear loose, light clothing. Sometimes medications can ameliorate some of the symptoms (amitriptyline, **carbamazepine**, or **gabapentin**, for example). In patients with severe pain, temporary relief can be obtained by injecting lidocaine (a local anesthetic) and steroids (an anti-inflammatory agent) into the lateral femoral cutaneous nerve. In very refractory cases, surgery to free the entrapped lateral femoral cutaneous nerve may be required in order to improve symptoms.

Prognosis

Many cases of meralgia paresthetica resolve spontaneously, usually within two years of onset.

Resources

BOOKS

Lotke, Paul A., and Joseph A. Abboud, Jack Ende, eds. *Lippincott's Primary Care Orthopaedics.* Lippincott Williams & Wilkins: 2008.

Waldman, Stephen D. *Pain Review.* Saunders: 2009.

PERIODICALS

Shetty, Gautam M., and Vijay D. Shetty. "Persistent bilateral anterior hip pain in a young adult due to meralgia paresthetica: a case report." *Cases Journal* 1.396 (2008): 396.

WEBSITES

National Institute of Neurological Disorders and Stroke (NINDS). *NINDS Meralgia Paresthetica Disease Information Page.* January 28, 2003. http://www.ninds.nih.gov/health_and_medical/disorders/meralgia_paresthetica.htm (June 3, 2004).

Rosalyn Carson-DeWitt, MD

Metachromatic leukodystrophy

Definition

Metachromatic leukodystrophy (MLD) is a rare degenerative neurological disease and is the most common form of the leukodystrophies, a group of disorders affecting the fatty covering that acts as an insulator around nerve fibers known as the myelin sheath. With destruction of the myelin sheath, progressive deterioration of muscle control and intellectual ability occur. Metachromatic leukodystrophy is inherited as an autosomal recessive trait, meaning that that the disease is inherited from parents that are both carriers but do not have the disorder. There are three forms of MLD, distinguished by the age of onset and by the molecular defect in the gene underlying the disease.

Description

The late infantile form of metachromatic leukodystrophy, which is the most common form, usually begins in the second year of life (ranges 1–3 years). After normal early development, the infant displays irritability and an unstable walk. As the disease progresses, physical and mental deterioration occur. Developmental milestones, such as language development, are not met, and muscle wasting eventually gives way to spastic movements then profound **weakness**. Seizures usually occur, followed by paralysis.

The juvenile form of MLD usually begins between the ages of 4 and 10 (ranges 3–20 years) and presents with disturbances in the ability to walk (gait disturbances), urinary incontinence, mental deterioration, and emotional difficulties. Some scientists distinguish between early and late juvenile MLD. Late juvenile MLD is similar to the adult form of the disease. Adult MLD begins after the age of 20 (ranges 16–30 years) and presents mainly with emotional disturbances and psychiatric symptoms, leading to a diagnosis of psychosis. Disorders of movement and posture appear later. **Dementia** (loss of mental capacity), seizures, and decreased visual function also occur.

Demographics

The frequency of MLD is estimated to be 1 in 40,000 persons in the United States. No differences have been identified on the basis of race, sex, or ethnic origin.

Causes and symptoms

MLD is caused by a deficiency of the enzyme arylsulfatase A (ARSA). Without properly functioning ARSA, a fatty substance known as sulfatide accumulates in the brain and other areas of the body such as the liver, gall bladder, kidneys, and/or spleen. The buildup of sulfatide in the **central nervous system** causes demyelination, the destruction of the myelin protective covering on nerve fibers. With progressive demyelination, motor skills and mental function diminish.

MLD is an autosomal recessive inherited disease and can be caused by mutations in two different genes, the ARSA and the prosaposin gene. Mutations in the ARSA gene are far more frequent. So far, about 50 mutations have been identified in ARSA gene.

Diagnosis

Diagnosis of MLD is suspected in a person displaying its symptoms. Magnetic resonance imaging may be used to identify lesions and atrophy (wasting) in the white matter of the brain that are characteristic of MLD. Urine tests usually show elevated sulfatide levels. Some psychiatric disorders coupled with difficulty walking or muscle wasting suggest the possibility of MLD. Blood testing can show a reduced activity of the ARSA enzyme.

Deficiency of the ARSA enzyme alone is not proof of MLD, because a substantial ARSA deficiency without any symptoms or clinical consequences is frequent in the general population. During diagnosis and genetic counseling, these harmless ARSA enzyme deficiencies must be distinguished from those causing MLD. The only diagnostic test that solves this problem and is definitive for MLD diagnosis is analysis of the genetic mutation.

Treatment team

The treatment team usually involves a neurologist, a pediatrician, an ophthalmologist, an orthopedist, a genetic counselor, a neurodevelopmental psychologist, a bone marrow transplant physician, a genetic and/or metabolic disease specialist, and also a physical and an occupational therapist.

Treatment

No effective treatment is available to reverse the course of MLD. Drug therapy is part of supportive care for symptoms such as behavioral disturbances, feeding difficulties, seizures, and constipation. Bone marrow transplantation has been tried, and there is evidence that this treatment might slow the progression of the disease. In infants, during a symptom-free phase of the late infantile form, neurocognitive function may be stabilized, but the symptoms of motor function loss progress. Persons with the juvenile and adult forms of MLD and with mild or no symptoms are more likely to be stabilized with bone marrow transplantation. Gene therapy experimentation on animal models as a possible therapy is still under consideration, and there are not yet any gene therapy-related clinical trials for MLD.

Recovery and rehabilitation

MLD patients require follow-up evaluation and treatment. Physical therapists, occupational therapists, orthopedists, ophthalmologists, and neuropsychologists are often involved in helping maintain optimal function for as long as possible.

Clinical trials

Current information about clinical trials can be found at ClinicalTrials.gov.

Prognosis

In young children with the late infantile form of MLD, progressive loss of motor and cognitive functions is rapid. Death usually results within five years

---

KEY TERMS

Autosomal recessive disorder—A genetic disorder that is inherited from parents that are both carriers, but do not have the disorder. Parents with an affected recessive gene have a 25% chance of passing on the disorder to their offspring with each pregnancy

Demyelination—Loss of the myelin covering of some nerve fibers resulting in their impaired function.

Enzyme—A protein produced by living cells that regulates the speed of the chemical reactions that are involved in the metabolism of living organisms, without itself being altered in the process.

---

after the onset of clinical symptoms. In the early juvenile form of MLD, although progression is less rapid, death usually occurs within 10–15 years of diagnosis, and most young people with the disease die before the age of 20. Persons with the late juvenile form often survive into early adulthood, and patients with the adult form may have an even slower progression.

Special concerns

Genetic counseling is important to inform the family about the risk of occurrence of MLD in future offspring. Prenatal testing may be available on an experimental basis in some centers.

Resources

BOOKS

The Official Parent's Sourcebook on Metachromatic Leukodystrophy: A Revised and Updated Directory for the Internet Age. San Diego: Icon International, 2002.

Von Figura, K., V. Gieselman, and J. Jaeken. "Metachromatic leukodystrophy." In *The Metabolic and Molecular Bases of Inherited Disease.* 8th ed. Edited by C. Scriver et al. New York: McGraw-Hill Professional, 2001.

PERIODICALS

Giesselmann, V. "Metachromatic leukodystrophy: recent research developments." *Journal of Child Neurology* 18, no. 9 (September 2003): 591–594.

OTHER

"NINDS Metachromatic Leukodystrophy Information Page." *National Institute of Neurological Disorders and Stroke.*http://www.ninds.nih.gov/health_and_medical/disorders/meta_leu_doc.htm (March 4, 2004).

ORGANIZATIONS

National Tay-Sachs and Allied Diseases Association . 2001 Beacon Street , Suite 204, Brighton, MA 02135. Phone: (617) 277-4463. Tollfree phone: (800) 90-NTSAD (906-8723). Email: info@ntsad.org. http://www.ntsad.org.

United Leukodystrophy Foundation. 2304 Highland Drive, Sycamore, IL 60178. Phone: (815) 895-3211. Fax: (815) 895-2432. Tollfree phone: (800) 728-5483. Email: ulf@tbcnet.com. http://www.ulf.org.

Igor Medica, M, Ph

Methylphenidate *see* **Central nervous system stimulants**

Methylprednisolone *see* **Glucocorticoids**

Microcephaly

Definition

Microcephaly is a neurological disorder where the distance around the largest portion of the head (the circumference) is less than should normally be the case in an infant or a child. The condition can be evident at birth or can develop within the first few years following birth. The smaller than normal head restricts the normal growth and development of the brain.

Description

The word microcephaly comes from the Greek *micros* meaning small, and *kephale* meaning head. The small head circumference that is a hallmark of microcephaly has been defined as that which is either two or three standard deviations (a statistical measure of variability) below the normal average head circumference for the age, gender, and race of the child. Put another way, the head size is markedly smaller than the expected size for about 97–99% of other children.

The condition can be present at birth or may develop during the first few years of life. In the latter situation, the growth of the head fails to keep to a normal pace. This produces a small head, relatively large face (since the face keeps growing at a normal rate), and a forehead that slopes backward. The smallness of the head becomes even more pronounced with age. An older child with microcephaly also has a body that is smaller and lighter than normal. This may be a consequence of the restricted brain development.

Demographics

Microcephaly is a rare neurological condition and occurs worldwide. Little detailed information on the prevalence of the disorder is available. Microcephaly does not appear to be more prevalent in any race or one gender.

Causes and symptoms

Microcephaly may have a genetic basis. If the gene defect(s) are expressed during fetal development, the condition is present at birth. This is the congenital form of the disorder. The microcephaly that develops after birth may still reflect genetically based developmental defects. As well, the delayed microcephaly can be caused if the normal openings in the skull close too soon after birth, preventing normal head growth. This condition is also referred to as **craniosynostosis**.

Other possible causes of microcephaly include infections during pregnancy (rubella, cytomegalovirus, toxoplasmosis), adverse effects of medication, and the excessive use of alcohol by the mother during pregnancy (fetal alcohol syndrome).

The damage from microcephaly comes because of the cramped interior of the skull. This lack of space exerts pressure on the growing brain. This causes impairment and delayed development of functions such as speech and control of muscles. The impaired muscle control can produce effects ranging from a relatively minor clumsiness in body movement to the more serious and complete loss of control of the arms and legs. A child can also be hyperactive and mentally retarded, although the latter is not always present. As a child grows older, seizures may occur.

It should be noted that at times it is diminished growth of the brain that results in microcephaly. Without proper brain growth, the surrounding skull does not expand and microcephaly results.

Diagnosis

Diagnosis of craniosynostosis and microcephaly is made by a physician, typically during examination after birth. A physician may also be alerted to the presence of microcephaly based on the appearance of the head at birth. Other clues in the few years after birth can be the failure to achieve certain developmental milestones and the appearance of the distinctive facial appearance.

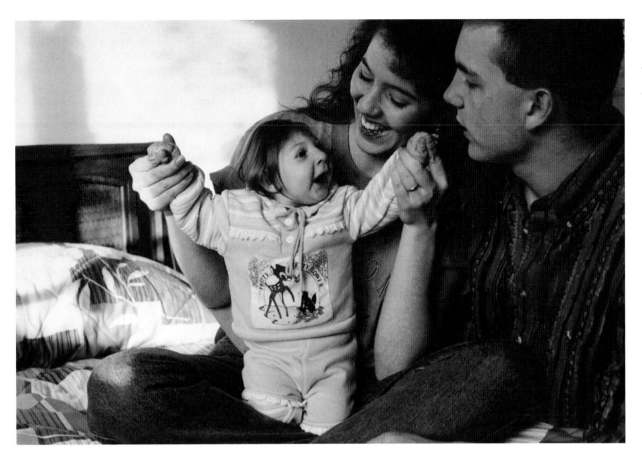

A Gulf War veteran sits with his wife and daughter who has microcephaly due to Seckel syndrome. The veteran suspects his service in the Gulf War had an influence in his daughter's condition. *(© Taro Yamasaki/Time & Life Pictures/Getty Images)*

Treatment team

The medical treatment team can consist of family and more specialized physicians and nurses. Parents and caregivers play an important role in supportive care. As various developmental challenges present themselves, physical therapists and special education providers may become part of the treatment team.

Treatment

In the case of craniosynostosis, surgery can be accomplished to reopen the prematurely closed regions of the skull. This allows the brain to grow normally. There is no such treatment for the congenital form of microcephaly. Treatment then consists of providing for the person's comfort and strategies to compensate for physical and mental delays.

Recovery and rehabilitation

Recovery from craniosynostosis can be complete if surgery is done at an early enough age. For a child with other forms of microcephaly, few treatment options are available. Emphasis, therefore, is placed upon maximizing mobility and mental development, rather than recovery. Speech therapists and audiologists can help with hearing and language development. Physical and occupational therapists provide aid in walking and adaptive equipment such as wheelchairs. Special education teachers coordinate educational goals and strategies based upon the child's abilities.

Clinical trials

There are no ongoing clinical trials for the study or treatment of microcephaly; however, research is being done to explore and understand the mechanisms, particularly genetic, of brain and skull development. By understanding the nature of the developmental malfunctions, it is hoped that corrective or preventative strategies might be developed. Current information about relevant clinical trials can be found at ClinicalTrials.gov.

KEY TERMS

Craniosynostosis—A birth defect of the brain characterized by the premature closure of one or more of the cranial sutures, the fibrous joints between the bones of the skull

Microcephaly—A rare neurological disorder in which the circumference of the head is smaller than the average for the age and gender of the infant or child.

Prognosis

With surgery, the prognosis for children with craniosynostosis can be good. However the outlook for children with other forms of microcephaly is poor, and the likelihood of having normal brain function is likewise poor.

Special concerns

As microcephaly is often associated with chromosomal abnormalities, the specific genetic cause for a person's microcephaly should be determined, if possible. Genetic counseling is available to help parents with information about their child with microcephaly and to plan for future pregnancies.

Resources

BOOKS

Abdel-Salam, Ghada, and Andrew Czeizel. *Microcephaly: Clinical and Epidemiological Studies: Microcephaly: An overview.* LAP LAMBERT Academic Publishing: 2011.

PERIODICALS

Ahmad, Wasim, Muhammad J. Hassan, and Saqib Mahmood. "Autosomal recessive primary microcephaly (MCPH): clinical manifestations, genetic heterogeneity and mutation continuum." *Orphanet Journal of Rare Diseases* 6 (2011): 39.

OTHER

National Institute of Neurological Disorders and Stroke. *NINDS Microcephaly Information Page.*http://www.ninds.nih.gov/health_and_medical/disorders/microcephaly.htm (April 9, 2004).

ORGANIZATIONS

National Institute for Child Health and Human Development (NICHD). 31 Center Drive, Rm. 2A32 MSC 2425, Bethesda, MD 20892-2425. Phone: (301) 496-5133. Fax: (301) 496-7101. Tollfree http://www.nichd.nih.gov.

National Institute for Neurological Diseases and Stroke (NINDS). 6001 Executive Blvd., Bethesda, MD 20892. Phone: (301) 496-5751. Tollfree phone: (800) 352-9424. http://www.ninds.nih.gov.

National Organization for Rare Disorders. 55 Kenosia Avenue, Danbury, CT 06813-1968. Phone: (203) 744-0100. Fax: (203) 798-2291. Tollfree phone: (800) 999-6673. Email: orphan@rarediseases.org. http://www.rarediseases.org.

March of Dimes Birth Defects Foundation. 1275 Mamaroneck Avenue, White Plains, NY 10605. Phone: (914) 428-7100. Fax: (914) 428-8203. Tollfree phone: (888) 663-4637. Email: askus@marchofdimes.com. http://www.marchofdimes.com.

Brian Douglas Hoyle, Ph

Migraine headache *see* **Headache, migraine**
Miller-Fisher syndrome *see* **Fisher syndrome**
Mini-strokes *see* **Transient ischemic attack**

Mitochondrial myopathies

Definition

Mitochondrial myopathies are a group of neuromuscular disorders that result from defects in the function of the mitochondrion, a small organelle located inside many cells that are responsible for fulfilling energy requirements of the tissue. These structures serve as "power plants" and are particularly important for providing energy for both muscle and brain function due to the large requirement for energy in these tissues.

People affected with one of these disorders usually have muscle symptoms such as **weakness**, breathlessness, exercise intolerance, heart failure, **dementia**, stroke-like symptoms, deafness, blindness, seizures, heavy eyelids or eye problems, and/or vomiting. Originally, mitochondrial myopathies were recognized based solely on clinical findings. Later genetic explanations provided additional information that was usually consistent with the clinical diagnosis and could, in some cases, help determine the long-term prognosis. Mitochondrial myopathies can also result as secondary effects from other diseases.

Description

Myopathy means a disorder of the muscle tissue or muscle. Mitochondrial myopathies are, therefore, disorders of the muscle tissue caused by abnormalities of the mitochondria.

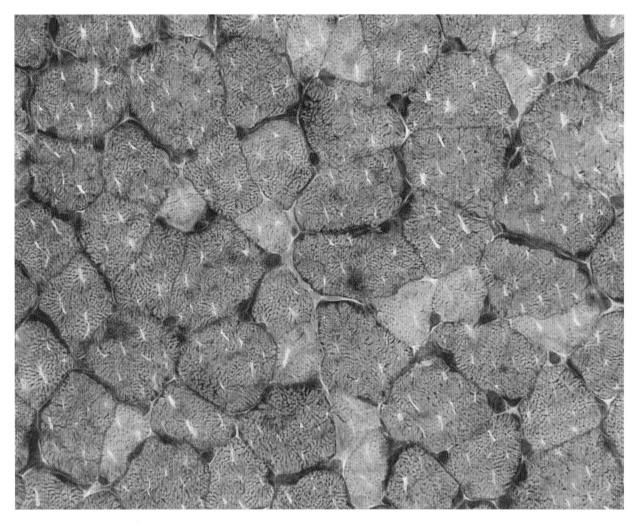

Fat accumulation in muscle. The focal ragged red fibers are consistent with mitochondrial myopathy. *(© Custom Medical Stock Photo, Inc. Reproduced by permission.)*

The following disorders are the most common mitochondrial myopathies:

- NARP: neuropathy, ataxia and retinitis pigmentosa

- KS: Kearns-Sayre syndrome

- Leigh's syndrome

- PEO: progressive external ophthalmoplegia

- MILS: maternally inherited Leigh's syndrome

- MELAS: mitochondrial encephalomyopathy, lactic acidosis, and strokelike episodes

- MERFF: myoclonus epilepsy with ragged-red fibers

- Pearson syndrome

- MNGIE: mitochondrial neurogastrointestinal encephalopathy

- LHON: Leber hereditary optic neuropathy

Demographics

The initial disease-causing or disease-related (pathogenic) alterations in mitochondrial DNA (mtDNA) were first identified in the early 1990s. Currently, more than 50 different single-base pathogenic mutations in the mtDNA sequence and more than 100 different pathogenic rearrangements within the genome have been identified. These include large deletions or duplications in the mtDNA sequence of bases. With the high mutation rate, it would seem that the prevalence of mitochondrial myopathies would be high; however, mitochondrial myopathies are relatively rare, having an incidence of approximately six out of every 100,000 individuals to as high as 16 out of 100,000 individuals. But there is evidence that, as part of the normal aging process, the accumulation of mtDNA mutations leads to neurological changes and abnormalities such as **hearing loss** or diabetes, which are normally considered to be associated with aging.

Causes and symptoms

In most cases, the primary defect in mitochondrial myopathies results from mutations in important genes that determine (encode) the structure of proteins that function in the mitochondria. Mutations can be found in DNA from the nucleus of the cell. This DNA is known as nuclear DNA, which is the DNA that most people consider with respect to human genetic diseases, but DNA is also found in the mitochondrial genome. Mitochondrial myopathies can be caused by defects in nuclear and mitochondrial DNA.

Mitochondrial DNA (mtDNA) is much smaller than nuclear DNA (nDNA). Nuclear DNA has approximately 3.9 billion base pairs in its entire sequence; mtDNA has only 16.5 thousand pairs. Although mtDNA is much smaller in size, each cell contains anywhere from 2–100 mitochondria, and each mitochondria has 5–10 copies of its genome.

Unlike nDNA that is twisted into a double helix, mtDNA has a circular structure. Mitochondrial DNA also has a high mutation rate, almost 20 times that of the nDNA. All of these factors are important in understanding the role of mtDNA mutations in the development of inherited or other mitochondrial myopathies.

A unique feature of mtDNA is that out of the more than 1,000 mtDNA genomes within the cell, a new mutation in one of the mtDNA genomes can be replicated each time the cell divides, thus increasing the number of defective mtDNA genomes. Because the distribution of the newly replicated mtDNA into the two daughter cells is random, one of the daughter cells may contain mtDNA that is not mutated (a condition referred to as homoplasmy), while the other daughter cell inherits both mutation genomes (known as heteroplasmy, or a mixture of mutated and normal genomes). Knowing the percentage of heteroplasmy for different mutations is often helpful in determining whether the disorder will manifest symptoms, as well as how severe they might be. As a result of the heteroplasmic nature of mitochondrial myopathies, the range of symptoms and severity of symptoms is often highly variable.

Mitochondrial myopathies are caused by mutations in either the nDNA or the mtDNA. These mutations generally affect tissues that have a high demand for metabolic energy production. Some disorders only affect a single organ, but many involve multiple organ systems. Generally, nDNA mutations result in clinical symptoms that develop during early childhood, while mtDNA mutations (either directly or as secondary effects from a nDNA mutation) lead to clinical manifestations that develop in late childhood or early adulthood. The genes that comprise the mtDNA genome encode proteins that function inside the mitochondria. For example, sugar broken down from food is used for fuel to manufacture a specific molecule, adenosine triphosphate (ATP), which is used by the cell to accomplish a variety of essential functions. ATP is produced by charged particles called electrons that come from digested food products to harness the energy. This is accomplished through five, highly organized protein complexes. The first four complexes (complex I, II, III, and IV) are part of the electron transport chain and function to move the electrons towards the fifth complex (complex V), which produces the ATP molecule. A defect in any one of these complexes can lead to mitochondrial myopathies. Both DNA from the nucleus and the mitochondria are required to assemble the many subunits that make up these complexes.

The process of producing ATP requires oxygen. This is essentially why humans cannot live without it. In the absence of a properly functioning electron transport chain, precursor molecules as well as unused oxygen begin to accumulate. One molecule in particular, called lactic acid, accumulates normally during strenuous exercise when tissue demands for energy cannot be met, resulting in muscle fatigue. This occurs essentially by accumulation of lactic acid, or lactic acidosis. Persons with a deficiency in the electron transport chain, therefore, have symptoms similar to an athlete's muscle fatigue, but without the factor of strenuous exercise. Both muscle contraction and nerve cell stimulation requires ATP; thus, these cells are particularly sensitive to defects in mitochondrial function. Furthermore, oxygen that is not metabolized can be converted into toxic compounds called reactive oxygen species (ROS). ROS can lead to many symptoms that an individual with a mitochondrial myopathy will experience.

Inheritance and medical significance

Mitochondrial DNA is inherited almost entirely from the maternal sex cell (the egg). Therefore, mutations or alterations in the mtDNA can be transmitted from a maternal sex cell to all the mother's children, regardless of gender.

Heteroplasmy, or the condition of having both normal and mutated mtDNA genomes, has several clinically important implications. If mtDNA molecules are deleted, they are generally not transmitted from the mother to her offspring for reasons that are currently unclear. If the mtDNA is duplicated (or various sequences are repeated with the same sequences such that the total size of the genome increases by exactly the number of repeated bases) or there is a mutation that only affects one base in the sequence, there usually is some of the mutant mtDNA molecules that gets transmitted. Additionally, a phenomenon called the mitochondrial genetic bottleneck occurs during the production of the mother's sex cells (eggs). This term refers to a reduction in the number of mtDNA molecules followed by an amplification of this reduced mtDNA that occurs during maturation of the mother's eggs. The result is considerable variability in the amount of mutated mtDNA molecules that each of the offspring inherits. However, in general, mothers that have a higher amount of mutated molecules are more likely to have offspring that are more severely affected compared to mothers that have a lower mutant load.

Inheritance and the nuclear genome

Not all mitochondrial proteins are produced by the mitochondrial genome. In fact, the majority is produced by the nuclear genome. Therefore, mitochondrial myopathies can be caused by mutations in both the nDNA and the mtDNA. This has important implications for genetic counselors that assess the recurrence risks in families with affected offspring. If the defect is of nuclear origin, it is typically recessive. In this case, there is a 25% chance of having an affected baby if both parents are carriers. There are also dominant disorders leading to mitochondrial myopathies that are characterized by a carrier parent passing on the mutant nuclear gene to 50% of the offspring. There are many mitochondrial myopathies that do not have a mtDNA mutation, and there are no nDNA mutations known.

Scientists are increasing their understanding of the intercommunication between the nucleus and the mitochondria. The identification of nDNA mutations that cause mitochondrial myopathies was first made when a nuclear gene involved in mtDNA replication was found to be defective in a disorder involving a patient with a mitochondrial myopathy.

Symptoms

Symptoms of mitochondrial myopathies are largely variable from person to person, even within the same family, and are dependent on the amount and type of genetic mutations present. These disorders can occur in infancy, childhood, or adulthood. In general, individuals with mitochondria dysfunction have abnormalities in the **central nervous system**. Defects can involve seizures, movement disorders, headaches, and cognitive (thought) disorders such as developmental delay or dementia (forgetfulness, senility). People with mitochondrial myopathies can also have hearing loss.

It is common that symptoms become apparent in a specific cluster of abnormalities and are thus considered a syndrome. For example, Kearns-Sayre syndrome can be recognized clinically due to similar symptoms that patients have. These symptoms include ocular abnormalities (degeneration of the retina and external opthamaloplegia, or droopy eyelids), dysphagia (swallowing problems), progressive myopathy, and various central nervous system abnormalities such as hearing loss. Confirmation of this disorder can be performed by genetic analysis that looks for large deletions in mtDNA.

Due to the nature of the genetic and biophysical defects, mitochondrial myopathies have symptoms related to muscle weakness and atrophy. Droopy eyelids and loss of the ability to control eye movements indicate muscle wasting, which leads to paralysis and compensatory attempts at correcting eye movements by tilting the head. Visual loss often occurs.

Muscle wasting, or myopathy, is not restricted to the eyes. The face and neck can also be affected, leading to incomprehensible speech and swallowing difficulties. Overall musculature wasting pervades many affected individuals, requiring wheelchairs and, in severe cases, assisted living requirements. Exercise-induced pain can also result.

Diagnosis

The diagnosis of mitochondrial myopathies is initially clinical, which means that it is based on the observable clinical manifestations that the patient shows versus results obtained from genetic analysis or laboratory tests. The physician will make careful observations of the affected child and interview the parents, in particular the mother, as it is common that she has the same mtDNA mutation, though usually at a lower percent load. Persons with mitochondrial myopathies are referred to a clinical geneticist for management and further evaluation, particularly in the absence of a confident clinical diagnosis. If there is a positive test after a genetic evaluation, genetic counseling is critical for understanding the nature of the disease and the implications for future offspring.

Diagnostic criteria

Any multi-system progressive disorder should lead a physician to suspect a mitochondrial disorder. A diagnosis can be particularly difficult if there is only one symptom. The diagnostic criteria for mitochondrial myopathies involve phenotypic evaluation (or evaluation of observable traits), followed by laboratory evaluation. A clinical diagnosis can be confirmed by laboratory studies, muscle **biopsy**, and molecular genetic evaluation, in which a geneticist analyzes the mtDNA. If a mtDNA mutation is detected, diagnosis is much more straightforward. In the absence of a mtDNA mutation, diagnosis becomes difficult.

There are several classical clinical manifestations that warrant DNA studies, such as in the case of MELAS, MERRF or LHON. Other disorders such as MNGIE require nDNA studies. In the absence of specific clinical criteria characteristic of a mitochondrial myopathy, blood plasma or cerebral spinal fluid is measured for lactic acid concentration, ketone bodies, plasma acylcarnitines, and organic acids in the urine. These are metabolites that are typically abnormal in an individual with a mitochondrial myopathy. If they are abnormal, a muscle biopsy is performed. Molecular genetic testing can often confirm a clinical diagnosis with or without positive laboratory results.

Treatment team

Treatment for patients with mitochondrial myopathies is best performed by a neurologist and a clinical geneticist or specialist that has experience diagnosing, treating, and managing patients with mitochondrial myopathies.

Treatment

There is no cure for mitochondrial myopathies. Therefore, treatment is solely for the purposes of minimizing pain and symptoms, and increasing mobility. Due to the wide variability in the disorders, treatment is usually individualized. Although the diseases are rare, many of their clinical symptoms are common and treatable. There are medications and lifestyle modifications that can help treat conditions such as headaches, diabetes, stroke-like symptoms, and seizures that are often associated with mitochondrial myopathies.

Medications are tailored to reduce the specific symptoms that the patient is experiencing (anticonvulsant medication may be required, for example, for an individual suffering from seizures). Dietary supplements are often used, although they have not been investigated in long-term studies. Creatine, coenzyme Q10, and carnitine are naturally occurring supplements that are thought to enhance ATP production.

Recovery and rehabilitation

Because there is no cure for mitochondrial myopathies, the focus is on maintaining optimum function for as long as possible, rather than recovery. Physical therapy helps extend the range of muscle movement. Occupational therapy helps with positioning and mobility devices and trains the affected individual in strategies designed to accomplish self-care and activities of daily living. Speech therapy can help children and adults who have difficulty in speaking, as well as help them to safely eat and swallow food. Hearing and visual aids (glasses) are often necessary and helpful.

Clinical trials

There are a few clinical trials to develop therapies to treat mitochondrial myopathies. One study investigated the role of dichloroacetate to lower lactate levels in patients diagnosed with MELAS at the National Institutes of Health (NIH). Lactic acidosis has been shown to be associated with nerve cell and muscle cell impairment in patients who have MELAS. Decreasing the levels of lactate might help prevent severe lactic acidosis. Current information about relevant clinical trials can be found at ClinicalTrials.gov.

Prognosis

Mitochondrial myopathies are extremely variable in the symptoms produced, and so the prognosis for those affected with mitochondrial myopathies also varies. The adverse affects on muscle function are often progressive, and persons often show physical deterioration over time. Occasionally, affected persons are mentally delayed. It is difficult to determine the exact course that each individual will endure, and in many cases the symptoms are relatively mild. Life expectancy for a person with a mitochondrial myopathy depends on many different circumstances, including the percentage of mtDNA that is mutated, the type of mutation, and the tissue in which it is mutated. If it is a nDNA defect, the physical and developmental effects depend on the gene that is mutated, the location of the mutation in the gene, the importance this gene has on the function of the mitochondria, and whether there are compensatory mechanisms. Overall, the prognosis is dependent on the involvement of vital organs.

Special concerns

Perhaps one of the most problematic issues that patients with mitochondrial myopathies experience is

KEY TERMS

Mitochondria—A part of the cell that is responsible for energy production.

Mitochondrial DNA (mtDNA)—The genetic material found in mitochondria, the organelles that generate energy for the cell. Because reproduction is by cloning, mtDNA is usually passed along female lines, as part of the egg's cytoplasm.

Myopathy—A disorder of the muscle or muscle tissue.

Nucleic DNA (nDNA)—The genetic material found in the nucleus of the cell.

the absence of an explanation for why the symptoms developed. This is especially challenging for determining recurrence risks for parents considering future pregnancies. Mitochondrial myopathic disorders can pose challenges for the entire family, especially since many affected children and adults are not born with the disorder, but the condition worsens with time. Support groups are available through various national disease foundations and local community organizations.

Resources

PERIODICALS

El-Sayed, Y.Y., et al. "Successful pregnancy and cesarean delivery via noninvasive ventilation in mitochondrial myopathy." *Journal of Perinatology* 29.2 (2009): 166.

Iizuka, Takahiro, and Fumihiko Sakai. "Pathophysiology of stroke-like episodes in MELAS: neuron-astrocyte uncoupling in neuronal hyperexcitability." *Future Neurology* 5.1 (2010): 61.

Northrop, Jennifer L., and Fernando Scaglia. "The mitochondrial myopathy encephalopathy, lactic acidosis with stroke-like episodes (MELAS) syndrome: a review of treatment options." *CNS Drugs* 20.6 (2006): 443.

OTHER

"MELAS." Genetics Home Reference (November 2006). http://ghr.nlm.nih.gov/condition/mitochondrial-encephalomyopathy-lactic-acidosis-and-stroke-like-episodes (accessed October 24, 2011).

"Mitochondrial Myopathies Information Page." National Institute of Neurological Disorders and Stroke (NINDS) (May 4, 2007). http://www.ninds.nih.gov/disorders/mitochondrial_myopathy/mitochondrial_myopathy.htm (accessed October 24, 2011).

ORGANIZATIONS

National Organization for Rare Disorders (NORD). P.O. Box 1968 (55 Kenosia Avenue), Danbury, CT 06813-1968. Phone: (203) 744-0100. Fax: (203) 798-2291. Tollfree phone: (800) 999-NORD (6673). Email: orphan@ rarediseases.org. http://www.rarediseases.org. United Mitochondrial Disease Foundation. 8085 Saltsburg Road Suite 201, Pittsburgh, PA 15239. Phone: (412) 793-8077. Fax: (412) 793-6477. Email: info@umdf.org. http://www.umdf.org.

Bryan R. Cobb, PhD

▌ Modafinil

Definition

Modafinil is a **central nervous system** (CNS) stimulant. It is primarily used to promote wakefulness and alertness in persons with **narcolepsy**, a condition that causes excessive sleepiness and cataplexy (episodes of sudden loss of muscle control.)

Purpose

Modafinil is an improvement over amphetamines in the treatment of narcolepsy. It promotes wakefulness but has fewer pronounced side effects than amphetamines. Modafinil acts to combat excessive daytime sleepiness (EDS) and cataplexy, the leading symptoms of narcolepsy, by stimulating sleep-suppressing peptides (orexins) in the brain.

Description

Although primarily indicated for the treatment of narcolepsy, modafinil is also used to treat some forms of sleep apnea. Experimentally, modafinil is being evaluated in the treatment of **Alzheimer's disease**, **depression**, attention-deficit disorder (ADD), and **fatigue** associated with **multiple sclerosis**.

Recommended dosage

Modafinil is taken by mouth in tablet form. It is prescribed by physicians in varying dosages and is usually taken once a day, in the morning.

Precautions

In some patients, modafinil may be habit forming. When taking the medication, it is important to follow physician instructions precisely. Modafinil may cause clumsiness and impair clarity of thinking. Persons taking this medication should not drive a car or operate machinery until they know how the stimulant affects them. Patients should avoid alcohol while

KEY TERMS

Cataplexy—A symptom of narcolepsy in which there is a sudden episode of muscle weakness triggered by emotions. The muscle weakness may cause the person's knees to buckle or the head to drop. In severe cases, the patient may become paralyzed for a few seconds to minutes.

Narcolepsy—A life-long sleep disorder marked by four symptoms: sudden brief sleep attacks, cataplexy (a sudden loss of muscle tone usually lasting up to 30 minutes), temporary paralysis, and hallucinations. The hallucinations are associated with falling asleep or the transition from sleeping to waking.

Orexin—Another name for hypocretin, a chemical secreted in the hypothalmus that regulates the sleep/wake cycle. Narcolepsy is sometimes described as an orexin deficiency syndrome.

taking modafinil. It can exacerbate the side effects of alcohol and other medications.

Modafinil may not be suitable for persons with a history of liver or kidney disease, mental illness, high blood pressure, angina (chest pain), irregular heartbeats, or other heart problems. Before beginning treatment with modafinil, patients should notify their physicians if they consume a large amount of alcohol, have a history of drug use, are pregnant, or plan to become pregnant. Patients who become pregnant while taking modafinil should inform their physicians immediately.

Side effects

Research indicates that modafinil is generally well tolerated. However, modafinil may case a variety of usually mild side effects. Headache, nausea, and upset stomach are the most frequently reported side effects of modafinil. Other possible side effects include excessive difficulty sleeping, nervousness, depression, diarrhea, dry mouth, runny nose, neck pain or stiffness, **back pain**, loss of appetite, and confusion.

Other, uncommon side effects of modafinil can be potentially serious. Persons taking modafinil who experiences any of the following symptoms should immediately contact their physician: irregular heartbeat, unusually rapid heartbeat, shortness of breath, hives or rashes, chest pain, persistent or severe headache, and persistent fever, pain, or other sign of infection.

Interactions

Modafinil may have negative interactions with some anticoagulants (blood thinners), antidepressants, antifungals, antibiotics, and monoamine oxidase inhibitors (MAOIs). Seizure prevention medication, **diazepam** (Valium), **phenobarbital** (Luminal, Solfoton), phenytoin (Dilantin), propranolol (Inderal), and rifampin (Rifadin, Rimactane) may also adversely react with Modafinil.

Furthermore, modafinil may decrease the effectiveness of oral contraceptives (birth control pills). Patients should consult their physicians about using alternative methods of birth control while taking modafinil, and for at least one month after ending treatment.

Resources

BOOKS

Berry, Richard B. *Fundamentals of Sleep Medicine.* Saunders: 2011.

OTHER

"Modafinil." MedlinePlus Drug Information (September 9, 2008). http://www.nlm.nih.gov/ medlineplus/druginfo/meds/a602016.html (accessed October 24, 2011).

ORGANIZATIONS

Center for Narcolepsy. 701B Welch Road, Room 146, Palo Alto, CA 94304-5742. Phone: (650) 725-6517. Fax: (650) 725-4913. http://www-med.stanford.edu/school/Psychiatry/narcolepsy/.

Adrienne Wilmoth Lerner

Moebius syndrome

Definition

Moebius syndrome is a condition in which the facial nerve is underdeveloped, causing paralysis or **weakness** of the muscles of the face. Other nerves to the facial structures may also be underdeveloped.

Description

Moebius syndrome has been called "life without a smile" because the paralysis of the facial muscles, the most constant feature, leads to the physical inability to form a smile even when happy feelings are experienced. The facial nerve is one of a group of 12 nerves known as the cranial nerves because they originate in the brain. The facial nerve is also known as the seventh cranial nerve. The sixth cranial nerve, also called the abducens, controls blinking and back-and-forth eye movement and is the second most commonly affected cranial nerve in Moebius syndrome. Additional cranial nerves affected in some patients control other eye movements and other functions such as hearing, balance, speech, and feeding.

Individuals with Moebius syndrome may also have abnormalities of their limbs, chest muscles, and tongue. The chance of **mental retardation** appears to be increased in people with Moebius syndrome, but most people with the disorder have normal intelligence.

Genetic profile

Most cases of Moebius syndrome are isolated and do not appear to be genetic, but occurrence in multiple individuals within some families indicates that there are multiple genetic forms. One study in 1991 suggested that forms of Moebius syndrome that included abnormalities of the limbs and skeleton were less likely than other types to be genetic. During pregnancy, certain exposures, such as to the drug misoprostol, appear to increase the risk of Moebius syndrome.

Chromosomes 13, 3, and 10 appear to contain genes causing forms of Moebius syndrome, now named, respectively, types 1, 2, and 3. The presence of a gene on chromosome 13 was first suggested based on a family in which several members had facial weakness and finger abnormalities along with a chromosome rearrangement called a balanced translocation involving chromosomes 1 and 13. In a balanced translocation, two chromosomes have broken and exchanged pieces. Balanced translocations are usually not associated with physical abnormalities unless (1) material has been lost or gained during the breaks, or (2) a gene is disrupted by one of the breaks. When a child with Moebius syndrome in an unrelated family was found to have a deletion (missing piece) of chromosome 13 in the same area as the break in the first family, this suggested that there might be a gene causing Moebius syndrome on chromosome 13 rather than on 1.

The genes on chromosomes 3 and 10 were localized using a technique called linkage mapping, which involves using molecular genetics and statistical methods to look throughout all of the chromosomes in families with several affected members for areas associated with the disease. The actual genes on chromosomes 3, 10, and 13 have not been identified. These three forms of the disease are inherited in an autosomal dominant manner, which means that only one altered copy of the gene is required to have the disease, and people with the disease have a 50% chance of having an affected child with each pregnancy.

However, in the chromosome 3 and 10 families, some individuals who appear to carry a gene do not show signs of Moebius syndrome, suggesting that factors other than genetics, such as uterine environment, are involved even in these highly familial cases.

One family was reported in which two brothers and their male cousin who were the sons of sisters all had Moebius syndrome along with other physical abnormalities and mental retardation. Boys only have one X chromosome and can inherit an X-linked disease from their unaffected mothers, who have two X chromosomes. The pattern of affected children in this family is therefore typical of X-linked inheritance, so it is suggested that there may be a gene involved in Moebius syndrome on the X chromosome as well. If this is the case, the son of a woman with an altered Moebius gene on one X-chromosome would have a 50% chance of inheriting the gene and having the condition. A man with this type of Moebius syndrome would be unlikely to have affected children since his daughters would likely have one normal X chromosome from their mother and his sons would not receive his X chromosome but his Y chromosome. In another family, a brother and sister with unaffected parents had Moebius syndrome, suggesting autosomal recessive inheritance, in which two altered copies of a gene are required to have the disorder. In an autosomal recessive disorder, a couple in which each parent carries one altered copy of the disease gene has a 25% chance of having a child with the condition with each pregnancy.

Demographics

Moebius syndrome is extremely rare and does not seem to affect any particular ethnic group more than others. The families in which genes on chromosomes 3 and 10 were mapped were Dutch.

Signs and symptoms

The first sign of Moebius syndrome in newborns is an inability to suck, sometimes accompanied by excessive drooling and crossed eyes. Also seen at birth in some patients are abnormalities of the limbs, tongue, and jaw. Children also often have low muscle tone, particularly in the upper body. The lack of facial expression and inability to smile become apparent as children get older.

When cranial nerve palsy is associated with limb reduction abnormalities and the absence of the pectoralis muscles, the condition is known as Poland-Moebius or Moebius-Poland syndrome. Common limb abnormalities are missing or webbed fingers and clubfoot.

The prevalence of mental retardation in Moebius syndrome is uncertain. It has been estimated to be between 10% and 50%, but these numbers are thought to be overestimates resulting from the lack of facial expression and drooling seen in people with Moebius syndrome. In one study of familial cases of Moebius syndrome, 3% were reported to be mentally retarded.

Diagnosis

Diagnosis of Moebius syndrome is made on the basis of clinical symptoms, especially the lack of facial expression. Since exact genes involved in Moebius syndrome have not yet been identified molecular genetic testing is not available at this time.

Treatment and management

The ability to smile has been restored in some cases of Moebius syndrome by surgery that transfers nerve and muscle from the thigh to the face. Other surgeries can be used to treat eye, limb, and jaw problems. In children with feeding problems, special bottles or feeding tubes are used. Physical and speech therapy are used when necessary to improve control over coordination, speech, and eating.

Prognosis

Moebius syndrome does not appear to affect life span, and individuals who are treated for their symptoms can lead normal lives.

Resources

WEBSITES

"Moebius Syndrome Information Page." National Institute of Neurological Disorders and Stroke (NINDS) (June 23, 2011). http://www.ninds.nih.gov/disorders/mobius/moebius.htm (accessed October 24, 2011).

ORGANIZATIONS

Moebius Syndrome Foundation (MSF). PO Box 993, Larchmont, NY 10538. (914) 834-6008. http://www.ciaccess.com/moebius.

Toni I. Pollin, MS, CGC

Monomelic amyotrophy

Definition

Monomelic amyotrophy (MMA) is a rare disease of the nerves that control voluntary movements of the limbs.

Description

One of the motor neuron diseases (MND), degenerative conditions that involve the nerves of the upper or lower parts of the body, MMA is generally a benign disease associated with minimal disability. Onset of MMA primarily occurs between the ages of 15 and 25. The main features of the disease are wasting and **weakness** of a single upper or lower limb. Generally, MMA progresses slowly over a period of 2–4 years and then reaches a stationary phase during which the disease remains stable for years.

Monomelic amyotrophy may also be known as benign focal amyotrophy, single limb atrophy, Hirayama syndrome or Sobue disease. Descriptive terms such as brachial monomelic amyotrophy (MMA confined to an arm), monomelic amyotrophy of the lower limb (MMMA of a leg) may be used to specify the type of limb affected. O'Sullivan-McLeod syndrome, a variant of MMA, is a slowly progressive form of the disease that causes weakness and wasting of the small muscles of the hand and forearm.

Demographics

Monomelic amyotrophy occurs worldwide and is most prevalent in Asia, and especially in Japan and India. According to a report in 1984, MMA of the lower limb occurs in about four in a million people in India. There is a preponderance of males with MMA; estimates of the male to female ratio range from 5:1 to 13:1.

Causes and symptoms

Causes

The underlying cause or causes for MMA remain unresolved. Most cases are sporadic and occur in an individual without a family history of MMA. Numerous factors such as viral infection, vascular insufficiency (inadequate blood supply) of the spinal cord, heavy physical activity, radiation injury, traumatic injury, and atrophy of the spinal cord have been suggested as possible causes of MMA. There are a few reports of familial cases of MMA.

Symptoms

Symptoms of MMA appear slowly and steadily over a period of time. The main features of MMA are muscle weakness and atrophy (wasting) in a portion of one limb. The weakness and wasting progresses slowly and may spread to the corresponding limb on the opposite side of the body. Symptoms can develop elsewhere in the affected limb or another limb at the same time or later in the course of the disease. Patients may notice worsening of symptoms on exposure to the cold. Other symptoms of MMA include: **tremor**, fasciculations, cramps, mild loss of sensation, excessive sweating, and an abnormal sympathetic skin response. It is rare that individuals with MMA experience significant functional impairment.

Diagnosis

Diagnosis of MMA is based on physical exam and medical history. Physical findings include reduced muscle girth (width around the arm or leg) and decreased strength in the affected limb. Tendon reflexes tend to be normal or sluggish. Cranial nerves, pyramidal tracts, sensory, cerebellar or extrapyramidal systems are not affected. Patients may report or display symptoms described above. They may also indicate difficulty carrying out activities of daily living such as writing, lifting, getting dressed, or walking.

Tests that may aid in diagnosis of MMA include **electromyography** (EMG), imaging studies such as magnetic resonance imaging (MRI) and computed tomography (CT) scans, and muscle **biopsy**. EMG shows chronic loss of nerve cells confined to specific areas of the affected limb. MRI has been reported to be a useful means of determining which muscles are affected in a given patient. Muscle biopsy shows evidence of atrophy of the neurons. EMG, muscle biopsy, or isometric strength testing may also reveal significant findings in seemingly normal muscles of the affected and the contralateral limb.

Treatment

There is no known cure for MMA. The goal of treatment, which is largely supportive, is to help patients optimize function and manage any disability associated with the disorder. Treatment primarily consists of rehabilitation measures such as physical therapy and occupational therapy. Severe muscle weakness (present in a minority of cases) may require orthopedic intervention such as splinting.

Treatment team

In addition to routine health care through their primary care practitioners, individuals with MMA generally see specialists in neurology and rehabilitation. Some patients with MMA may receive comprehensive services through a muscular dystrophy association (MDA) clinic or another type of neuromuscular clinic. Given the rarity of MMA, the potential for rehabilitation in this disorder is unknown.

Recovery and rehabilitation

Rehabilitation for MMA consists of physical and occupational therapy. The goal of these therapies is to make full use of the patient's existing functions. Physical therapy can help a patient with MMA to strengthen muscles in a weak arm or leg. Occupational therapy can teach patients to use adaptive techniques and devices that may help compensate for difficulty with everyday tasks such as writing, buttoning, or tying shoes. Depending upon the degree of weakness in the affected limb, a person with MMA may need to use the unaffected limb for activities previously performed by the now atrophied limb.

Clinical trials

There are no clinical trials for patients with MMA. As more is learned about how MMA or related motor neuron diseases develop, it is hoped that novel therapies will be developed. Information about relevant clinical trials can be found at ClinicalTrials.gov.

Prognosis

MMA is generally a benign condition. Disability associated with MMA is typically mild. In the majority of cases, the disorder usually ceases to progress within five years of onset. People with MMA can expect to have a normal life span.

Special concerns

Initially, symptoms of MMA can be similar to early signs of other, more serious neurological disorders such as **amyotrophic lateral sclerosis** (ALS or Lou Gherig's disease) and **spinal muscular atrophy**. For this reason, periodic neurological evaluation may be recommended to be sure that no symptoms of these or other motor neuron diseases develop.

Resources

BOOKS

Amato, Anthony, and James Russell. *Neuromuscular Disorders*. McGraw-Hill Professional: 2008.

PERIODICALS

Aktas, Liknur, et al. "Monomelic amyotrophy: case report/ Monomelik amyotrofi: olgu sunumu." *Turkish Journal of Physical Medicine and Rehabilitation* (2008): 116.

Atchayaram, Nalini, Gaurav Goel, and M. Vasudev. "Familial monomelic amyotrophy (Hirayama disease): Two brothers with classical flexion induced dynamic changes of the cervical dural sac." *Neurology India* 57.6 (2009): 810.

Ebenezer, Beulah, et al. "Multichannel somato sensory evoked potential study demonstrated abnormalities in cervical cord function in brachial monomelic amyotrophy." *Neurology India* 56.3 (2008): 368.

Moglia, C., et al. "Monomelic amyotrophy is not always benign: a case report." *Amyotroph Lateral Scler.* 12, 4 (July 2011): 307-8.

WEBSITES

"Monomelic Amyotrophy Information Page." National Institute of Neurological Disorders and Stroke (NINDS) (February 13, 2007). http://www.ninds.nih. gov/disorders/monomelic_amyotrophy/monomelic_ amyotrophy.htm (accessed October 24, 2011).

ORGANIZATIONS

Muscular Dystrophy Association. 3300 East Sunrise Drive, Tucson, AZ 85718. Phone: (520) 529-2000. Fax: (520) 529-5300. Tollfree phone: (800) 572-1717. Email: mda@mdausa.org. http://www.mdausa.org.

National Organization for Rare Disorders. P.O. Box 1968, 55 Kensonia Avenue, Danbury, CT 06813. Phone: (203) 744-0100. Fax: (203) 798-2291. Tollfree phone: (800) 999-NORD. Email: orphan@rarediseases.org. http://www.rarediseases.org.

Dawn J. Cardeiro, MS, CGC

Motor Neuron Diseases

Definition

Motor neuron diseases are progressive disorders involving the nerve cells responsible for carrying impulses that instruct the muscles in the upper and lower body to move. Motor neuron diseases are varied and destructive in their effect. They commonly have distinctive differences in their origin and causation, but a similar result in their outcome for the patient: severe muscle weakness. Amyotrophic lateral sclerosis (ALS), spinal muscular atrophy, poliomyelitis, and primary lateral sclerosis are all examples of motor neuron diseases.

Description

A motor neuron is one of the largest cells in the body. It has a large cell body with many extensions reaching out 360° from the cell body (soma). These extensions are called dendrites and are chemically able to receive instructions from adjacent neurons. These instructions are received in the form of an impulse stimulation of a particular protein channel on the dendrite by a neurotransmitter termed acetycholine (ACh). Extending from the soma of the motor neuron is a long portion of the cell called the axon. When conditions are favorable, an electrical signal passes down the axon to a region of the cell identified as the axon terminals. These terminals also branch in many directions and have, at their tips, a region called the synaptic end bulb. This region releases ACh that crosses a small gap until it reaches a protein on another dendrite.

When motor neurons line up in a tract, they allow an electrical signal to spread from the brain to the intended muscle. There are a huge number of nerve tracts that extend to all the muscles of the body that are responsible for contraction and relaxation of all types of muscles, including smooth and cardiac, as well as skeletal muscle. When the motor neuron is affected or damaged and it cannot perform at peak performance, the muscles of the body are affected. Often, a disorder of the motor neurons results in progressive muscle atrophy (shrinking and wasting) of some, if not all, the muscles of the body. Muscle twitching (fasciculation) is common among these disorders. Motor neuron diseases are difficult to treat, debilitating to movement, and, in some cases, fatal.

Amyotrophic lateral sclerosis (ALS) is a disorder that generally involves either the lower or upper motor systems of the body. In advanced stages, both regions of the body are affected. This disease is commonly known as Lou Gehrig's disease after the famous baseball player who died from the condition. It is caused by sclerosis (a hardening of the surrounding fibrous tissues) in the corticospinal tracts. Associated with the sclerosis is a loss of the tissue of the anterior horns (gray matter) in the spinal cord, including the brainstem. ALS is characterized by a wasting of the muscles that, in turn, produce weakness. The bulbar, or facial/mouth muscles can initially become involved, which may lead to slurring of speech and drooling. The significance of this involvement is that, with rapid progression, the patient may not be able to swallow properly. This may lead to the risk of choking and other difficulties with obtaining nutrition and proper respiration. Death from complications of ALS is common within five years.

Spinal muscular atrophies (SMAs) are genetic disorders characterized by primary degeneration of the anterior horn cells of the spinal cord, resulting in progressive muscle weakness. Spinal muscular atrophies affect only lower motor neurons. In babies and children, many SMAs are rapidly progressive with paralysis of the legs, trunk, and eventually, the respiratory muscles. In teenagers and adults, SMAs are usually slowly progressive. Kennedy's disease, an X-linked (carried by women and passed on to male offspring) SMA, features similar wasting of facial muscles as seen in ALS, with characteristic difficulty speaking and swallowing.

Primary lateral sclerosis (PLS) is a rare motor neuron disease that resembles ALS. Primary lateral sclerosis often begins after age 50 and results in slowly progressive weakness and stiffness in the leg muscles, clumsiness, and difficulty maintaining balance. Symptoms worsen over a period of years. Muscle spasms in the legs may also occur, but in PLS, there is no evidence of the degeneration of spinal motor neurons or muscle wasting (amyotrophy) that occurs in ALS.

Unlike most motor neuron diseases, poliomyelitis results from infection with a virus. Contamination occurs through fecal or oral exposure. Once inside the body, the virus uses the cells of the gastrointestinal tract to enter the bloodstream and move throughout the body. Eventually, the poliovirus invades the nerve cells of the spinal cord and kills the motor neurons. When the motor neurons are destroyed, the muscles they connect to become damaged and weaken. The result is varying degrees of paralysis, including difficulty swallowing, walking, breathing, and control of speech.

Demographics

Motor neuron diseases are uncommon, as about one person in 50,000 is diagnosed with a motor neuron disease in the United States each year. In total, about 5,500 people in the United States each year receive a diagnosis of a motor neuron disease.

About 20,000 Americans are living with ALS and nearly 4,500 new cases are reported annually. The peak time for onset is around 55 years of age, but younger patients have been observed. Spinal muscular atrophies and primary lateral sclerosis are rare diseases.

The occurrence of poliomyelitis is seen in records of epidemics that were intricately documented in the last 100 years. A description of an epidemic in recent times in the United States discussed a low of 4,197 cases in the early 1940s to a high of 42,033 in 1949. By 1952, the number of case had reached over 58,000. In 1955, a vaccine was developed that used weakened forms of the virus. This vaccine and the subsequent Sabin vaccine nearly wiped out polio in the world. The Americas were declared free of polio in the 1990s. In 2002, there were fewer than 500 cases worldwide, and in 2003, that number decreased to fewer than 100 cases. According the World Health Organization (WHO), "Poliomyelitis" (http://www.who.int/mediacentre/factsheets/fs114/en/index.html), "in 2010, only four countries in the world remain polio-endemic, down from more than 125 in 1988. The remaining countries are Afghanistan, India, Nigeria and Pakistan." WHO also notes that "in 2009–2010, 23 previously polio-free countries were re-infected due to imports of the virus."

Causes and symptoms

Causes of many motor neuron diseases are unknown, and others have varying causes according to the specific motor neuron disease. Most cases of ALS occur sporadically for an unknown reason, but up to 10% of ALS cases are inherited. Most spinal muscular atrophies are inherited. A virus causes poliomyelitis. Additionally, environmental factors and toxin are under study as causes or triggers for motor neuron diseases.

Muscle weakness is the symptom common to all motor neuron diseases. Muscles of the legs are most often affected, leading to clumsiness, unstable gait, or lower limb paralysis. Muscle cramps and fasciculations (twitching) occur with most motor neuron diseases. Facial muscles may also be affected, leading to difficulty with speech (dysarthria). Later in the course of some motor neuron diseases, the muscles involved with swallowing and breathing may be impaired (dysphagia).

Diagnosis

Diagnosis of motor neuron disease is often based upon symptoms and exclusion of other neurological diseases. Nerve conduction studies can help distinguish some forms of peripheral neuropathy from motor neuron disease. Electromyelogram (EMG), a test measuring the electrical activity in muscles, can support the diagnosis of ALS and some other motor neuron diseases. Although computed tomography (CT) scans and magnetic resonance imaging (MRI) are often normal in persons with motor neuron disease, they may help exclude spinal malformations or tumors that could be responsible for similar symptoms. A muscle biopsy can exclude myopathies. Diagnosis of primary lateral sclerosis is especially difficult and often delayed, as it is frequently misdiagnosed as ALS. Polio may be diagnosed by recovering the virus from a stool or throat culture, examining antibodies in the blood or, rarely, by spinal fluid analysis. Finally, molecular genetic studies can aid in the diagnosis of spinal muscular trophies and the small percentage of inherited ALS cases.

Treatment team

Caring for a person with a motor neuron disease requires a network of health professionals, community resources, and friends or family members. A neurologist usually makes the diagnosis, and the neurologist and primary physician coordinate ongoing treatment and symptom relief. Physical, occupational, and respiratory therapists provide specialized care, as do nurses. Social service and mental health consultants organize support services.

Treatment

There are few specific treatments for motor neuron diseases, and efforts focus on reducing the symptoms of muscle spasm and pain, while maintaining the highest practical level of overall health. Riluzole, the first drug approved by the U.S. Food and Drug Administration for the treatment of ALS, has extended the life of ALS patients by several months and also extended the time a person with ALS can effectively use his or her own muscles to breathe, although it provides no symptom relief. Symptom relief can be obtained from muscle relaxants such as baclofen, tiznidine, and benzodiazepine. Salivation can be improved with glycopyrrolate and atropine. Pain can be improved with anticonvulsants and non-steroidal anti-inflammatory medications, and in later stages with morphine and other opiates. Panic attacks often respond to benzodiazepines.

Other medications used to treat persons with motor neuron disease are designed to relieve symptoms and improve the quality of life for patients. These include medicines to help with depression, sleep disturbances, and constipation.

Recovery and rehabilitation

Recovery from motor neuron diseases depends on the type of disease and the amount of muscle degeneration present. In diseases such as ALS, the emphasis is placed upon maintaining mobility and function for as long as possible, rather than recovery. With all motor neuron diseases, physical therapy can teach exercises to help with range of motion and prevent contractures (stiff muscles at the joints). Occupational therapy provides assistive devices for mobility such as wheelchairs, positioning devices, braces, and other orthotics for performing daily activities such as reaching and dressing. Respiratory therapists and speech therapists help prevent pneumonia by maintaining lung function and promoting safe eating strategies. Speech therapists also help with alternate forms of communication if facial muscles are involved.

Recovery from polio may be complete or only partial, depending on the degree of lower motor neuron damage. Years or decades after recovering from polio, persons may again experience muscle weakness and pain. This is known as postpolio syndrome. Vigorous exercise has been shown to cause additional weakness in postpolio syndrome, and physicians recommend energy conservation and lifestyle changes for these patients.

Clinical trials

As of August 2011, there were 89 active clinical trials examining various motor neuron diseases. Details and up-to-date information about patient recruiting can be found at ClinicalTrials.gov.

Prognosis

The prognosis of persons with motor neuron diseases depends on the type of the disease and the mount and progression of muscle degeneration. Most persons with ALS die from complications of respiratory failure within five years of developing symptoms. About one out of ten persons with ALS live a decade or longer with the disease. The prognosis for a person with spinal muscular atrophy varies greatly, according to the severity of the disease. Some forms result in immobility and death within a few years, while others impede movement, but do not affect a normal lifespan.

KEY TERMS

Amyotrophy—A type of neuropathy resulting in pain, weakness, and/or wasting in the muscles.

Atrophy—Shrinking or wasting of muscles or tissues.

Contractures—Abnormal, usually permanent contraction of a muscle due to atrophy of muscle fibers, extensive scar tissue over a joint, or other factors.

Dysarthria—Imperfect articulation of speech due to muscular weakness resulting from damage to the central or peripheral nervous system.

Dysphagia—Difficulty swallowing.

Fasciculations—Fine muscle tremors or twitches.

Gait—Posture and manner of walking.

Motor neuron—A neuron conducting impulses outwards from the brain or spinal cord with the specific job of controlling a muscle movement.

Special concerns

It is important to remember that even in the most severe motor neuron diseases, a person's personality, intelligence, reasoning ability, or memory are not impaired. The person with motor neuron disease also retains the senses of sight, smell, hearing taste, and in the unaffected areas, touch.

Resources

BOOKS

Bradley, W, et al. *Neurology in Clinical Practice.* 5th ed. Philadelphia: Butterworth-Heinemann, 2008.

Goetz, C.G. *Goetz's Textbook of Clinical Neurology.* 3rd ed. Philadelphia: Saunders, 2007.

PERIODICALS

Chang, P.A. "Motor neuron diseases and neurotoxic substances: a possible link?" *Chemico-Biological Interactions* 180 (2009): 127–30.

Tripodoro, V.A. "Management of dyspnea in advanced motor neuron diseases." *Current Opinions in Supportive and Palliative Care* 2 (2008): 173–79.

WEBSITES

"NINDS Motor Neuron Diseases Information Page." National Institute of Neurological Disorders and Stroke. http://www.ninds.nih.gov/health_and_medical/disorders/motor_neuron_diseases.htm (accessed August 26, 2011).

ORGANIZATIONS

ALS Association, 1275 K Street NW, Suite 1050, Washington, DC, United States, 20005, (202) 407-8580, (800) 782-4747, Fax: (202) 289-6801, alsinfo@alsa-national.org, http://www.alsa.org.

Families of SMA, 925 Busse Road, Elk Grove Village, IL, United States, 60007, (847) 367-7620, (800) 886-1762, Fax: (847) 367-7623, info@fsma.org, http://www.fsma.org.

Brook Ellen Hall, PhD
Rosalyn Carson-DeWitt, MD

▌Movement disorders

Definition

Movement disorders are neurological diseases and syndromes that involve the motor and movement systems' ability to produce and control movement.

Description

Though it seems simple and effortless, normal movement actually requires an astonishingly complex system of control. Disruption of any portion of this system can cause a person to produce movements that are too weak, too forceful, too uncoordinated, or too poorly controlled for the task at hand. Unwanted movements may occur at rest. Intentional movement may become impossible. These conditions are examples of movement disorders.

Abnormal movements themselves are symptoms of underlying disorders. In some cases, the abnormal movements are the only symptoms. The more common diseases causing motor disorders are:

- spinal cord injury (SCI)
- stroke
- multiple sclerosis (MS)
- muscular dystrophy (MD)
- Huntington's chorea (HC)
- cerebral palsy (CP)
- dystonias
- tremor
- myasthenia gravis (MG)
- parkinsonism (PD)
- Tourette syndrome

Other causes of motor disorders are Wilson's disease (WD), inherited ataxias (Friedreich's ataxia), Machado-Joseph disease, and spinocerebellar ataxias, and encephalopathies.

Causes and symptoms

Causes

Movement is produced and coordinated by several interacting brain centers, including the motor cortex, the cerebellum, and a group of structures in the inner potions of the brain called the basal ganglia. Sensory information provides critical input on the current position and velocity of body parts, and spinal nerve cells (neurons) help prevent opposing muscle groups from contracting simultaneously.

To understand how movement disorders occur, it is helpful to consider a normal voluntary movement, such as reaching to touch a nearby object with the right index finger. To accomplish the desired movement, the arm must be lifted and extended. The hand must be held out to align with the forearm, and the forefinger must be extended while the other fingers remain flexed.

THE MOTOR CORTEX. Voluntary motor commands begin in the motor cortex located on the outer, wrinkled surface of the brain. Movement of the right arm is begun by the left motor cortex, which generates a large volley of signals to the involved muscles. These electrical signals pass along upper motor neurons, through the midbrain, to the spinal cord (SC). Within the SC, these signals connect to lower motor neurons, which convey the signals from the SC to the surface of the muscles involved. Neural activation of the muscles causes contraction, and the force of contraction pulling on the skeleton causes movement of the arm, hand, and fingers.

Damage to, or death of any of the neurons along this path, can cause weakness or paralysis of the affected muscles.

THE CEREBELLUM. Once the movement of the arm is initiated, sensory information is needed to guide the finger to its precise destination. In addition to sight, the most important source of information comes from the "position sense," provided by the many sensory receptors located within the limbs (proprioception). Proprioception allows a person to touch his or her nose with a finger even with the eyes closed. The balance organs in the ears provide important information about posture. Both postural and proprioceptive information are processed by a structure at the rear of the brain, called the cerebellum. The cerebellum sends out electrical signals to modify movements as they progress, "sculpting" the barrage of voluntary commands into a tightly controlled, constantly evolving pattern. Cerebellar disorders cause inability to control the force, fine positioning, and speed of movements (ataxia). Disorders of the cerebellum may also impair the ability to judge distance, so that a person under- or overreaches the target (dysmetria). Tremor during voluntary movements can also result from cerebellar damage.

THE BASAL GANGLIA. Both the cerebellum and the motor cortex send information to a set of structures deep within the brain that helps control involuntary components of movement (basal ganglia). The basal ganglia send output messages to the motor cortex, helping to initiate movements, regulate repetitive or patterned movements, and control muscle tone.

Circuits within the basal ganglia are complex. Within this structure, some groups of cells begin the action of other basal ganglia components, and some groups of cells block the action. These complicated feedback circuits are not entirely understood. Disruptions of these circuits are known to cause several distinct movement disorders. A portion of the basal ganglia, called the *substantia nigra*, sends electrical signals that block output from another structure, the subthalamic nucleus. The subthalamic nucleus sends signals to the globus pallidus, which in turn blocks the thalamic nuclei. Finally, the thalamic nuclei send signals to the motor cortex. The substantia nigra then begins movement, and the globus pallidus blocks it.

This complicated circuit can be disrupted at several points. Loss of substantia nigra cells increases blocking of the thalamic nuclei and prevents them from sending signals to the motor cortex. Degeneration of these nerve cells, as in PD, results in lower production of dopamine and fewer connections with other nerve cells and muscles, leading to a loss of movement (motor activity).

In contrast, cell loss in early HD decreases the blocking of signals from the thalamic nuclei, causing more cortex stimulation and stronger, but uncontrolled, movements.

Disruptions in other portions of the basal ganglia are thought to cause tics, tremors, dystonia, and a variety of other movement disorders, although the exact mechanisms are not well understood.

Some movement disorders, including HD, are caused by inherited genetic defects and inherited ataxias. Some diseases that cause sustained muscle contraction limited to a particular muscle group (focal dystonia) are inherited, but others are caused by trauma. The cause of most cases of PD is unknown, although genes have been identified for some familial forms.

ANTAGONISTIC MUSCLE PAIRS. This picture of movement, however, is too simple. One important refinement to it comes from considering the role of opposing, or antagonistic, muscle pairs. Contraction of the bicep muscle, located on the top of the upper arm, pulls on the forearm to flex the elbow and bend the arm. Contraction of the triceps, located on the opposite side, extends the elbow and straightens the arm. Within the spine, these muscles are normally wired so that willed (voluntary) contraction of one is automatically accompanied by blocking of the other. In other words, the command to contract the biceps provokes another command within the spine to prevent contraction of the triceps. In this way, these antagonist muscles are kept from resisting one another. Spinal cord or brain injury can damage this control system and cause involuntary simultaneous contraction and spasticity, an increase in resistance to movement during motion.

While the peripheral mechanism, antagonistic muscle pairs, is certainly important, it is not the only one of concern with regard to movement disorders. Central pattern generators (CPGs) in the spinal cord are especially relevant because of their role in sensory processing. Filtration and processing of sensory input is accomplished locally, where the response of spinal pattern generator circuitry fits into continual movement, as necessary. Thus, although the brain receives much of the sensory input, the responses to spinal inputs are first the responsibility of the local spinal circuitry. Multi-segmental reflexes and anticipatory postural adjustments are as critical in the etiology of these syndromes.

Common conditions causing motor disorders

SPINAL CORD INJURY. Spinal cord injury (SCI) is very complex and can be very serious. An injury can affect the body in a multitude of ways depending on where the spinal cord (SC) is damaged. It is the largest nerve in the body and is composed of nerve fibers. These nerve fibers that manage the body's communication systems are responsible for its motor, sensory, and autonomic functions. They act as messenger between the brain and the rest of the body. The vertebral column—protective bone segments—surrounds the SC, perhaps because of its important in the nervous system. Approximately 18 in. (39 cm) long, the SC runs from the base of the brain, down the middle of the back, to the waist. Nerve fibers in the upper SC are upper motor neurons (UMNs). Spinal nerves branching off the SC that run up and down the neck and back are lower motor neurons (LMNs) and branch off between each vertebrae and go out to all part of the body. The lower spinal nerve fibers continue down

through the spinal canal to the sacrum (tailbone) at the end of the SC.

The spine is divided into four sections. At the top of the spinal column is the cervical spine. It is composed of eight cervical nerves and seven cervical vertebrae. Further down is the thoracic spine, which includes the chest and twelve thoracic vertebrae. The lumbar spine is below that and comprises five lumbar vertebrae. The bottom section is the sacral area, and there the bones fuse together.

When the SC is damaged by either a traumatic injury or from a disease, all nerves above the injury level still function normally. Those from the point of injury and below are damaged, and messages between the brain and parts of the body that could once be sent are no longer possible. The patient must undergo physical examination by the doctor to identify the exact location of injury to the spinal cord. Frequently, the physician will use a "pin-prick" test, which evaluates the patient's level of feeling (sensory level). X rays are also used to image the affected vertebrae. The patient's input is critical; he or she will be asked what parts of the body can be moved, and all major muscle groups will be tested (motor level) for strength. All of these tests are important, as they reveal what nerves and muscles are functioning. Each SCI is unique and is defined by its type and level. Its level will be judged by the lowest level on the SC after which there is absence of feeling and/or movement (motor level).

Loss of feeling and/or movement in the head, neck, shoulder, arms, and/or upper chest is termed "tetraplegia" and is injury at level C1 to T1. The cervical spine is the highest part of the spinal cord and is designated by the letter "C." The thoracic spine is next to the highest, and is designated by the letter "T." T2 to S5 is paraplegia. The higher on the vertebral column, the closer the SCI is to the brain. Therefore, someone with a T-8 (thoracic spine; eight of 12 thoracic vertebrae) level injury would have more feeling and movement than someone with a C-5 (cervical spine; five of seven cervical vertebrae) level of injury.

STROKE. During a stroke, brain tissue is destroyed. This is caused by some malfunction of the brain's blood vessels. There are two major classifications of stroke: hemorrhagic and ischemic. The most common type of stroke is ischemic, caused by the same kind of vascular disease as heart attack. Ischemic means that the blood flow to an area is insufficient; there is not enough oxygen to support the cells. The brain cells will cease to function if blood circulation is not restored quickly enough after a stroke. Cell death by lack of oxygen is termed "infarction." To be more specific, physicians often refer to this type of infarction as cerebral. Stroke is the third leading cause of disability and the fifth leading cause of death in the United States. Annually, 500,000 people suffer strokes; 150,000 die of them.

A hemorrhagic stroke happens with the rupture of a blood vessel. Bleeding occurs inside the skull. Usually, the cause is hypertension, or high blood pressure—but it can also be caused by trauma. An aneurysm (a sac formed by localized dilatation of the wall of an artery, a vein, or the heart) may also cause a hemorrhagic stroke. Whatever the origin of the stroke, bleeding can rip through the tender connections within the brain and ultimately compress brain cells until they die.

The extent of the damage due to stroke depends on the severity of the stroke and where in the brain the blood supply was suspended. Each area of the brain is served by specific blood vessels; if a blood vessel in the area that controls muscle movements become blocked, those muscles will be weak or paralyzed. The loss of function is greatest immediately after a stroke, but some function is usually regained. Some brain cells do die, while some injured cells may recover. Bleeding on the brain, such as from a head injury or brain aneurysm, can also cause brain cell death from lack of oxygen. Symptoms may resemble those of a stroke. The best prevention for a stroke is for the patient to discuss risk factors with a physician.

MULTIPLE SCLEROSIS. Multiple sclerosis (MS) is an autoimmune disorder, meaning it is caused by the body's own immune system. For unknown reasons, immune cells attack and destroy the myelin sheath that insulates neurons in the brain and spinal cord. This myelin sheath speeds and insulates the transmission of nerve impulses. The demyelinated areas appear as plaques, small round areas of gray neuron without the white myelin covering. The progression of symptoms in MS is correlated with development of new plaques in the portion of the brain or spinal cord controlling the affected areas.

MUSCULAR DYSTOPHY. Muscular dystrophy (MD) encompasses a number of progressive hereditary diseases that make muscles weaken and degenerate. It is not a contagious disease and there are a multitude of variations. Each type has its own pattern of heredity, onset age, and speed with which muscle is lost. Alterations in specific genes cause different types of disease. There is no prevention or cure for MD; however, because of research, there is reason for hope for a cure.

HUNTINGTON'S CHOREA. A genetically inherited disease, Huntington's chorea (HC) has neurological and psychotic characteristics. The usual onset is in the fourth or fifth decade, but early and late onset are also possible. Either neurological or psychotic changes can mark the beginning of the disease. Symptoms of neurological changes may vary but can begin with chorea—a series of movements that resemble dancing, with jerkiness and one part of the body moving to another. One might display clumsiness, jumpiness, and become fidgety. There may be movement in the face, particularly around the jaw, and walking may become difficult. It may be difficult to maintain posture. Paranoia, personality changes, and confusion may present, as well. It is also possible for dementia to occur.

Diagnosis of HC is dependent upon clinical symtomatology and MRI (magnetic brain imaging), as well as discovering family history of the disease. An MRI that reveals atrophy (shrinkage) of part of the basal ganglia, which is involved in movement and known as the caudate nucleus, is characteristic of HC.

CEREBRAL PALSY. In cerebral palsy (CP), abnormal development of or damage to motor areas in the brain disrupts the brain's ability to control movement and posture. The term "cerebral palsy" refers to a group of chronic disorders impairing control of movement that appear in the first few years of life and generally do not worsen over time. Symptoms differ from person to person and may change over time. Individuals with the disease may have difficulty with fine motor tasks (e.g., writing), and balance or walking. They may have involuntary movements. Cerebral palsy, which may be congenital (present at birth) or acquired after birth, results from brain injury that does not worsen over time. Possible causes of CP are developmental abnormalities of the brain, brain injury caused by low oxygen levels (asphyxia) or poor circulation, infection, and trauma to the fetus or newborn. Doctors encourage pregnant women to follow a program of regular prenatal care beginning early in pregnancy to help prevent CP.

DYSTONIAS. Dystonias are sustained muscle contractions that often cause twisting or repetitive movements and abnormal postures. Dystonias may be limited to one area (focal) or may affect the entire body (general). Focal dystonias may affect the neck (cervical dystonia or torticollis), the face (one-sided, or hemifacial spasm), contraction of the eyelid (blepharospasm), contraction of the mouth and jaw (oromandibular dystonia), simultaneous spasm of the chin and eyelid (Meige syndrome), the vocal cords (laryngeal dystonia), or the arms and legs (writer's and occupational cramps). Dystonia may be painful and incapacitating.

TREMORS. Uncontrollable (involuntary) shaking of body parts is known as tremors. Tremors may occur only when muscles are relaxed during actions, or when holding active postures.

MYASTHENIA GRAVIS. Myasthenia gravis (MG), a chronic autoimmune disease, is characterized by fluctuating degrees of weakness of the skeletal or voluntary muscles. Muscle weakness of increasing severity is the key symptom of this disorder; it worsens with activity and improves after periods of rest. It does not always include muscles that control facial expression, such as muscles of the eyes or those involved with talking, chewing, and swallowing, but can affect the muscles involved with breathing, the neck, and limb movements. A defect in the transmission of nerve impulses to muscles is responsible for MG. The symptoms of MG range in type and degree. It is not directly genetic, and it is not infectious. It can be controlled through medications that improve neuromuscular transmission, thereby improving muscle strength, or through medications that suppress the manufacture by the body of abnormal antibodies. Because of unpleasant, major side effects, these drugs must be used with caution and monitored carefully. Myasthenia gravis is caused by an autoimmune response attack on acetylcholine (neurotransmitter) receptors at muscular junctions.

PARKINSON'S DISEASE. The possibility of developing Parkinson's disease (PD), or parkinsonism, increases with age, with onset usually not earlier than 40 years of age. Approximately 500,000 people in the United States suffer from the disease, which affects both sexes equally. The cause of the most common form of PD (as well as related disorders) is not known—though genetic risk has been identified as a probable factor by the National Institutes of Health. Interestingly, the disorder is observed at the same rate in almost every part of the globe and is as common in the early twenty-first century as it was in late 1800s.

The two terms, Parkinson's disease (PD) and parkinsonism, are used interchangeably, as they both describe patients with the same symptoms. The four primary symptoms of PD are tremor or trembling, rigidity or stiffness of the limbs and trunk, bradykinesia (slowness of movement), and impaired balance and coordination.

There are a number of causes of parkinsonism, including degenerative neurologic disease, metabolic conditions, toxins, drugs, viral encephalitis (von Economo's disease), and related disorders that result from the loss of dopamine, a chemical messenger responsible for transmitting signals within the brain. When certain nerve cells (neurons) that produce dopamine die or become impaired, dopamine is depleted. The result is nerve cells that fire out of control. Individuals with PD are then unable to direct or control their movements in a normal manner. The disease, which is usually not inherited, is both chronic and progressive, with subtle early symptoms and gradual progression.

Management of a movement disorder begins with determining its cause. Physical and occupational therapy may help to compensate for lost control and strength. Pharmacologic therapy can help to compensate for some imbalances of the basal ganglionic circuit. For instance, levodopa (L-dopa), or related compounds, can substitute for the loss of dopamine-producing cells in PD. Conversely, blocking normal dopamine action may be used to treat some hyperkinetic disorders, including tics. Oral medications can also help to reduce overall muscle tone. Local injections of botulinum toxin (Botox) can selectively weaken overactive muscles in dystonia and spasticity. Destruction of peripheral nerves through injection of phenol can reduce spasticity. It should be noted that all of these treatments have some side effects.

Other movement disorders

Tic disorders are very quick, involuntary, rapid, non-rhythmic, and short-lived movements or sounds; tics can sometimes be controlled briefly. Tics are usually repeated movements. They commonly involve the motor systems and often involve the facial muscles, such as the eyelids or eyebrows. The most well-known tic disorder is Tourette syndrome (TS), an abnormal condition that causes uncontrollable facial grimaces and tics and arm and shoulder movements. Tourette syndrome is best known, perhaps, for uncontrollable vocal tics that include grunts, shouts, and use of obscene language (coprolalia). It is also known as Gilles de la Tourette syndrome. Tics are more common among males than females. As with Tourette syndrome, tics may be associated with head injury, stroke, carbon monoxide poisoning, and mental retardation.

Myoclonus is a sudden, shock-like muscle contraction. Myoclonic jerks may occur singly or repetitively. Unlike tics, myoclonus cannot be controlled even briefly.

Postural instability is the loss of ability to maintain upright posture caused by slow or absent righting reflexes (those that help to maintain balance).

Spasticity is a condition in which certain muscles are continuously contracted, causing stiffness or tightness of the muscles.

Flaccid paralysis is the loss of muscle tone of the paralyzed part and an accompanying absence of reflexes.

Botulinum toxin (Botox)—Any of a group of potent bacterial toxins or poisons produced by different strains of the bacterium *Clostridium botulinum*. The toxins cause muscle paralysis and thus force the relaxation of a muscle in spasm.

Cerebral palsy (CP)—A movement disorder caused by a permanent brain defect or an injury present at birth or shortly after. It is frequently associated with premature birth. Cerebral palsy is not progressive.

Computed tomography (CT)—An imaging technique in which cross-sectional x rays of the body are compiled to create a three-dimensional image of the body's internal structures.

Encephalopathy—An abnormality in the structure or function of tissues of the brain.

Fetal tissue transplantation (FTT)—A method of treating PD and other neurological diseases by grafting brain cells from human fetuses onto the basal ganglia. Human adults cannot grow new brain cells, but developing fetuses can. Grafting fetal tissue stimulates the growth of new brain cells in affected adult brains.

Huntington's chorea (HC)/disease (HD)—A rare, genetically inherited condition with both neurological and psychiatric manifestations that begins with either type of change. The chorea is progressive, and presents as jerky muscle movements and mental deterioration that ends in dementia. The symptoms of HC usually appear in patients in their 40s or 50s; however, early- or late-onset is possible. Huntington's chorea may also cause clumsiness, jumpiness, and fidgetiness, and facial movements—particularly around the jaw—may occur. It may become difficult to walk and can affect posture. Paranoia, confusion, or personality changes may be noted. A significant dementia develops as the disease progresses. There is no cure or effective treatment for the condition.

Levodopa (L-dopa)—A substance used in the treatment of PD. Levodopa can cross the blood-brain barrier that protects the brain. Once in the brain, it is converted to dopamine, and thus can replace the dopamine lost in PD.

Magnetic resonance imaging (MRI)—An imaging technique that uses a large circular magnet and

Diagnosis

A complete and thorough clinical examination should be performed. Diagnosis of movement disorders requires a careful medical history and a thorough physical and neurological examination. A thorough orthopedic exam may be important because patients with increased muscle tone may develop curvature of the spine (scoliosis), hip dislocation, and tendon shortening. During the neurologic exam, the doctor will observe the individual's posture, tone, symmetry, and reflexes.

Certain symptoms may indicate a movement disorder disease. Doctors will pay special attention to the rate of development of children with CP, particularly with regard to head size and head growth, since abnormalities in these areas may point to a brain problem. Eye problems, such as blurred or double vision, red-green color distortion, or blindness in one eye, may occur. When combined with muscle weakness in extremities and paresthesias (transitory abnormal sensory feeling such as numbness or prickling), MS may be suspected.

Diagnostic tests should be conducted. These include brain imaging studies, such as computed tomography

(CT) scan, positron emission tomography (PET), or MRI. Routine blood and urine analyses are performed. A lumbar puncture (spinal tap) may be necessary. Video recording of the abnormal movement is often used to analyze movement patterns and to track progress of the disorder and its management. Genetic testing is available for some forms of movement disorders. If MS is suspected, physicians may study the patient's cerebrospinal fluid and the antibody, immunoglobulin G.

Treatment

Ongoing clinical studies indicate that estrogen may have beneficial effects on controlling movement disorders, such as PD, chorea, dystonia, tics, and myoclonus.

Deep brain stimulation, which inactivates the thalamus or globus pallidus through electrical shocks, may be useful to ease tremor of the arm in individuals with ET and tremor due to MS. In PD, the procedure may improve arm speed and dexterity, reduce tremor, and block the involuntary movements (dyskinesia) associated with the medications used to treat the disease.

Surgical destruction, or inactivation of basal ganglionic circuits, has proven effective for PD, and is radio waves to generate signals from atoms in the body. These signals are used to construct images of internal structures.

Paraplegia—Paralysis of the lower half of the body involving both legs and usually due to disease or injury to the spinal cord.

Parkinson's disease (PD)—A slowly progressive disease that destroys nerve cells in the basal ganglia and thus causes loss of dopamine, a chemical that aids in transmission of nerve signals (neurotransmitter). Parkinsonism is characterized by shaking in resting muscles, a stooping posture, slurred speech, muscular stiffness, and weakness.

Positron emission tomography (PET)—A diagnostic technique in which computer-assisted x rays are used to track a radioactive substance inside a patient's body. Biochemical activity of the brain can be studied using PET.

Progressive supranuclear palsy—A rare disease that shows some of the same features of PD, but differs in several ways. People with progressive supranuclear palsy usually do not develop tremors, but

they have rigidity, bradykinesia (slow movements), and falls. The disorder gradually destroys nerve cells in the parts of the brain that control eye movements, breathing, and muscle coordination. The loss of nerve cells causes palsy (paralysis) that slowly gets worse as the disease progresses. The palsy affects the ability to move the eyes vertically (up and down) at first. Their eye movements then become even more restrictive (ophthalmoplegia). The ability to relax the muscles is lost, as is control over balance.

Tourette syndrome (TS)—An abnormal condition that causes uncontrollable facial grimaces and tics, and arm and shoulder movements. Tourette syndrome is best known, perhaps, for uncontrollable vocal tics that include grunts, shouts, and use of obscene language (coprolalia). Also known as Gilles de la Tourette syndrome.

Wilson's disease (WD)—An inborn defect of copper metabolism in which free copper may be deposited in a variety of areas of the body. Deposits in the brain can cause tremor and other symptoms of PD.

being tested for other movement disorders. Transplantation of fetal cells into the basal ganglia has produced mixed results in PD.

Health care team roles

Nursing and allied health professionals play a key role in educating individuals with movement disorders about their conditions and appropriate treatment options. Physical, speech, and occupational therapy are often essential to the rehabilitation of individuals with movement disorders. Psychological counseling may be helpful to the individual and to family members and close friends.

The patient who has had a stroke may be treated by doctors, therapists, and nurses who work to keep the patient's muscles strong, prevent muscular contractions, avoid the bedsores that can result from being in one position for too long, and teach the patient to walk and talk again. With SCI, expert nursing care is important to prevent complications from weakness and paralysis, including bedsores. Physical and occupational therapy help to preserve muscle

function and teach techniques to help the patient function despite lost functionality.

Prognosis

The prognosis for a patient with a movement disorder depends on the nature of the disorder. The age of onset has major implications in prognosis.

Prevention

Prevention depends on the specific disorder. With some diseases, certain preventive strategies can be particularly helpful. In the case of MS and stroke, for example, smoking cessation would drastically reduce the number of cases. Longtime smokers may face a much higher risk of both MS and stroke, according to researchers at Harvard University. In the case of MS, women who smoked at least one pack per day for at least 25 years had a greater chance of developing the disorder than nonsmokers.

A number of permanent cases of parkinsonism that presented in the early 1980s were caused by a contaminant found in some illicit street drugs. For the most part, cases of the disease induced by legal, prescribed drugs were only temporary: when the drug was stopped, the symptoms stopped, too. Permanent parkinsonism had only been the result of the contaminant found in the street drug.

In 1996, clinicians at the University of Hawaii found that patients with high blood levels of uric acid, a natural antioxidant, have a lower chance of developing parkinsonism and gout (acute inflammatory arthritis) than people with lower levels. The study concluded that people with high levels of the antioxidant uric acid may be more resistant to developing parkinsonism. This was also shown in 1991, when investigator Stanley Fahn of Columbia University found that parkinsonism patients who were administered large doses of oral vitamin C and synthetic vitamin E supplements (3000 mg and 3200 IU daily, respectively) delayed the progression of the disease. He concluded that it was likely that it was the vitamin C alone, or in combination with vitamin E that actively worked.

Preventive measures for certain movement disorders include:

• Parkinsonism (PD). Deprenyl (selegiline), administered early in the onset of the disorder, can slow progression of the disease. Antioxidants such as vitamin E and selenium may be of some benefit, as well.

• Spinal cord injury (SCI). Attention to following safety precautions may help to reduce the risk of SCI. The most frequent causes of SCI are motor vehicle crashes, falls, violence, and sports and recreation, especially diving. Proper protective equipment should be used if an injury is possible, and appropriate safety measures should be practiced. Depth of water should be checked and obstructions should be noted before diving. When in an automobile, seat belts should always be used.

• Stroke. Major risk factors include high blood pressure, high cholesterol level, smoking, and diabetes. Drugs, such as aspirin (half of an adult tablet or one children's tablet daily), can be taken to reduce the tendency of blood platelets (responsible for the clotting of blood) to form dangerous blood clots, a major cause of stroke. When stronger drugs are needed, a doctor may prescribe anticoagulants, such as heparin or warfarin (Coumadin). Research suggested that paralysis and other symptoms may be prevented or reversed if certain drugs that break up clots are given within three hours of the onset of a stroke.

Resources

BOOKS

Bradley, W., et al. *Neurology in Clinical Practice*. 5th ed. Philadelphia: Butterworth-Heinemann, 2008.

Goetz, C.G. *Goetz's Textbook of Clinical Neurology*. 3rd ed. Philadelphia: Saunders, 2007.

PERIODICALS

Mostile, G. "Alcohol in essential tremor and other movement disorders." *Movement Disorders* 2 (2010): 2274–84.

WEBSITES

"Huntington's diease." Mayo Clinic. http://www.mayoclinic.com/health/huntingtons-disease/DS00401 (accessed August 26, 2011).

"Multiple Sclerosis." PubMed Health. http://www.ncbi.nlm.nih.gov/pubmedhealth/PMH0001747/ (accessed August 26, 2011).

ORGANIZATIONS

American Spinal Injury Association, 2020 Peachtree Road, NW, Atlanta, GA 30309, (404) 355-9772, Fax: (404) 355-1826, ASIA_office@shepherd.org, http://www.asia-spinalinjury.org.

Movement Disorder Society, 555 East Wells Street, Suite 1100, Milwaukee, WI 53202-3823, (414) 276-2145, Fax: (414) 276-3349, info@movement disorders.org, http://www.movementdisorders.org.

Muscular Dystrophy Association, 3300 East Sunrise Drive, Tucson, AZ, 85718-3208, (520) 529-2000, (800) 572-1717, Fax: (520) 529-5300, mda@mdausa.org, http://www.mda.org.

Myasthenia Gravis Foundation of America, 355 Lexington Avenue, 15th Floor, New York, NY 10017, Fax: (212) 370-9047, (800) 541-5454, http://www. myasthenia.org.

National Institute of Neurological Disorders and Stroke (NINDS), P.O. Box 5801, Bethesda, MD 20824, (301) 496-5751, (800) 352-9424, http://www.ninds.nih.gov.

National Spinal Cord Injury Association, 75-20 Astoria Boulevard, Suite 120, Jackson Heights, NY 11370, (718) 512-0010, (800) 962-9629, Fax: (866) 387-2196, info@spinalcord.org, http://www. spinalcord.org.

National Spinal Cord Injury Statistical Center, 515 Spain Rehab Center, 1717 6th Avenue South, Birmingham, AL 35233, (205) 934-5049, Fax: (205) 974-2709, nscisc@uab.edu, https://www.nscisc. uab.edu.

Paralyzed Veterans of America, 801 18th Street NW, Washington, DC 20006-3517, (800) 424-8200, info@pva.org, http://www.pva.org.

Worldwide Education and Awareness for Movement Disorders (WE MOVE), 5731 Mosholu Avenue, Bronx, NY 10471, (347) 843-6132, Fax: (718) 601-5112, wemove@wemove.org, http://www. wemove.org.

Randi B. Jenkins
Rosalyn Carson-DeWitt, MD

Moyamoya disease

Definition

Moyamoya disease is a rare disorder of blood vessels in the brain known as internal carotid arteries (ICA). The condition is characterized by stenosis (narrowing) or occlusion (blockage) of one or both ICA with subsequent formation of an abnormal network of blood vessels adjacent to the ICA.

Description

Moyamoya disease was first described in Japan in 1955. The term *moyamoya*, a Japanese word that means "puff of smoke," describes the appearance of the abnormal vessels that form adjacent to the internal carotid arteries. Alternate names for the disorder are spontaneous occlusion of the circle of Willis and basal occlusive disease with telangiectasia.

Moyamoya disease can occur in children (juvenile type) or in adults (adult type). Children tend to be less than age 10 and adults are usually between age 30 and 49. Affected individuals typically present with signs of stroke or other types of cerebral ischemia (decreased blood flow to an area of the brain due to obstruction in an artery), cerebral hemorrhage (bleeding), or seizures (mainly in children). Symptoms in an affected child or adult may include disturbed consciousness, speech deficits, sensory and cognitive impairment, involuntary movements, or vision problems. Options for treatment for people with moyamoya disease consist of medications and brain surgery. Without treatment, repeated strokes, transient ischemic attacks, brain hemorrhages, or seizures can lead to serious cognitive impairment, physical disability, or death.

Demographics

Moyamoya disease occurs worldwide and is most prevalent in Asia, and especially in Japan. According to a report in 1998, more than 6,000 cases had been described. The disease occurs in about one in a million people per year. Estimates of disease incidence in Japan are as much as ten times greater. Slightly more females than males are affected. The male-to-female ratio has been reported to be around 2:3. Approximately 10% of cases of moyamoya disease are familial.

Causes and symptoms

Causes

The cause of moyamoya disease is unknown. Possible explanations for the disorder include injuries to the brain, infection, multifactorial inheritance, genetic factors, or other causes. For example, moyamoya disease has been associated with meningitis; radiation therapy to the skull in children; and genetic conditions such as Down syndrome, neurofibromatosis, and sickle cell anemia. Also, there have been reports linking a region on chromosome 3 (MYM1) and a region on chromosome 17 (MYM2) to moyamoya disease in some families.

Symptoms

The initial symptoms of moyamoya disease are somewhat different in children and adults. In children, there is ischemia due to stenosis and occlusion of the circle of Willis, a ring of arteries at the base of the brain. In children, the disease tends to cause repeated "ministrokes" known as transient ischemic attacks (TIAs) or, less often, seizures. The TIAs usually manifest as weakness of one side of the body (hemiparesis), speech disturbances, and sensory deficits. TIAs may be made worse by hyperventilation, such as with intense crying. Involuntary movements may occur. Mental retardation may be present.

Adults with moyamoya disease typically have bleeding in the brain (cerebral hemorrhage) or strokes. cerebral hemorrhage occurs as a result of breakdown of the coexisting blood vessels that formed earlier in life due to stenosis or occlusion of the ICA. The cerebral hemorrhages are commonly located in the thalamus, basal ganglia, or deep white matter of the brain. Symptoms can include disturbance of consciousness and/or hemiparesis. Adult patients with moyamoya disease may go on to have further hemorrhages and strokes that can result in significant and irreversible brain damage.

Diagnosis

A diagnosis of moyamoya disease is based on findings from neuroradiologic studies and on clinical signs consistent with this diagnosis. Neuroradiologic studies used to establish the diagnosis of moyamoya disease include cerebral angiography, magnetic resonance imaging (MRI), magnetic resonance angiography (MRA), and computed tomography (CT) scan. Cerebral angiography is the most common means of confirming a diagnosis of moyamoya disease. MRI and MRA, which are less invasive procedures, may be used instead of cerebral angiography. CT scan findings tend to be non-specific and not as useful as CA, MRI, and MRA in making the diagnosis.

Characteristic brain findings in moyamoya disease include: narrowing or occlusion of the end portion of one or both internal carotid arteries, an abnormal network or blood vessels at the base of the brain, and presence of these findings on both sides of the brain. In about 10% of cases, cerebral aneurysms may also be found. Nuclear medicine studies such as Xenon-enhanced CT, positron emission tomography (PET), or single photon emission computed tomography (SPECT) may be performed in order to evaluate cerebral blood flow (CBF) patterns. The information obtained from CBF studies helps the neurologist and/or neurosurgeon to devise a treatment plan.

Treatment

There is no cure for moyamoya disease. Early treatment is important to avoid mental and physical impairment. Treatment options include medications and surgical revascularization.

Medications. Individuals having TIAs and stroke may be given antiplatelet drugs, vasodilators, or anticoagulants to help prevent future attacks. Steroid therapy may be prescribed for a person who has involuntary movements. For a patient with a cerebral hemorrhage, treatment may include management of hypertension, if present.

Surgery. The purpose of revascularization surgery in moyamoya disease is to augment or redirect blood flow in the brain. Surgical revascularization has been reported to improve cerebral blood flow, to reduce ischemic attacks, and, in children, to increase IQ. The optimal method of surgery depends on the patient's history and clinical status. There are various direct and indirect methods of restoring blood supply in the brain. Examples of direct bypass surgery include techniques known as superficial temporal artery to middle cerebral artery bypass, and extracranial-intracranial bypass to anterior or posterior cerebral artery. Examples of indirect bypass surgery include techniques known as encephaloduroarteriosynangiosis, encephalomyosynangiosis, and encephaloarteriosynangiosis.

Treatment team

Management of moyamoya disease requires a multidisciplinary approach. In addition to the patient's primary health care professionals, medical professionals involved in the care of patients with moyamoya disease generally include specialists in neurology, neurosurgery, neuroradiology, and anesthesiology. Specialists in orthopedic surgery, ophthalmology, rehabilitation, physical therapy, occupational therapy, speech therapy, and mental health may also be involved in the care of affected

individuals. Psychological counseling and contact with other affected patients may assist families in coping with this condition, especially given it's rarity.

Recovery and rehabilitation

The potential for rehabilitation in moyamoya disease depends in part on the degree of impairment caused by complications such as strokes, cerebral hemorrhages, and seizures. Interventions such as physical, occupational, and speech therapy may be recommended for management of problems such as hemiparesis, speech problems, and sensory deficits. Some patients may require assistance with daily living. In cases in which there is significant disability, consideration may be given to in-home nursing care or placement in a residential care facility that can provide 24-hour care and support services.

Clinical trials

There are no clinical trials specifically for patients with moyamoya disease. As more is learned about the causes of moyamoya disease, it is hoped that novel therapies will be developed. Current information about clinical trials can be found at ClinicalTrials.gov.

Prognosis

The prognosis for moyamoya disease is not well defined. The prognosis depends in part on the extent of brain injury present at the time of diagnosis and the success of treatment. For example, a person who had a major stroke or cerebral hemorrhage may already be permanently impaired, both physically and mentally. Reports of clinical outcome after treatment are mixed. Some individuals experience improvement of symptoms while others continue to show progressive decline. Moyamoya disease tends to be more progressive in children than in adults. In those patients who do not stabilize clinically, significant disability or death may occur.

Special concerns

Children with moyamoya disease may have learning disabilities or mental retardation. They may also experience physical disabilities that impact academic performance. Such children may be eligible to have an Individual Education Plan (IEP). An IEP provides a framework from which administrators, teachers, and parents can meet the educational needs of a child with special learning needs. Depending upon severity of

KEY TERMS

Stroke—Interruption of blood flow to a part of the brain with consequent brain damage. A stroke may be caused by a blood clot or by hemorrhage due to a burst blood vessel. Also known as a cerebrovascular accident.

Transient ischemic attacks—A brief interruption of the blood supply to part of the brain that causes a temporary impairment of vision, speech, or movement. Usually, the episode lasts for just a few moments, but it may be a warning sign for a full-scale stroke.

symptoms and the degree of learning difficulties, some children with moyamoya disease may be best served by special education classes or a private educational setting.

Resources

BOOKS

Cho, Byung-Kyu, and Teiji Tominaga, eds. *Moyamoya Disease Update*. New York: Springer, 2010.

PERIODICALS

Araki, Yoshio, et al. "Identification of novel biomarker candidates by proteomic analysis of cerebrospinal fluid from patients with moyamoya disease using SELDI-TOF-MS." *BMC Neurology* 10 (2010): 112.

Cece, Hasan, et al. "Axillary brachial plexus blockade in moyamoya disease?" *Indian Journal of Anaesthesia* 55.2 (2011): 160.

Chiapparini, Luisa, et al. "Paediatric stroke: review of the literature and possible treatment options, including endovascular approach." *Stroke Research and Treatment* (2011).

Cugati, Goutham, et al. "Multiple burr hole surgery as a treatment modality for pediatric moyamoya disease." *Journal of Pediatric Neurosciences* 5.2 (2010): 115.

WEBSITES

National Institute of Neurological Disorders and Stroke (NINDS). "Moyamoya Disease Information Page." http://www.ninds.nih.gov/health_and_medical/disorders/moyamoya.htm (accessed August 30, 2011).

Online Mendelian Inheritance In Man (OMIM). "Moyamoya Disease 1." http://omim.org/entry/252350 (accessed August 30, 2011).

ORGANIZATIONS

Children's Hemiplegia and Stroke Association (CHASA). 4101 West Green Oaks Blvd., PMB #149, Arlington, TX 76016. Phone: (817) 492-4325. Tollfree Email: info5@chasa.org. http://www.hemikids.org.National Stroke Association. 9707 East Easter Lane, Englewood, CO

80112-3747. Phone: (303) 649-9299. Fax:(303) 649-1328. Tollfree phone: 800-STROKES (787-6537). Email: info@stroke.org. http://www.stroke.org.

Families with Moyamoya Support Network. 4900 McGowan Street SE, Cedar Rapids, IA 52403.

National Stroke Association. 9707 East Easter Lane, Englewood, CO 80112-3747. Phone: (303) 649-9299. Fax: (303) 649-1328. Tollfree phone: 800-STROKES (787-6537). Email: info@stroke.org. http://www.stroke.org.

Dawn J. Cardeiro, MS, CGC

Mucopolysaccharidoses

Definition

Mucopolysaccharidosis (MPS) is a general term for a number of inherited diseases that are caused by the accumulation of mucopolysaccharides, resulting in problems with an individual's development. With each condition, mucopolysaccharides accumulate in the cells and tissues of the body because of a deficiency of a specific enzyme. The specific enzyme that is deficient or absent is what distinguishes one type of MPS from another. However, before these enzymes were identified, the MPS disorders were diagnosed by the signs and symptoms that an individual expressed. The discovery of these enzymes resulted in a reclassification of some of the MPS disorders. These conditions are often referred to as MPS I, MPS II, MPS III, MPS IV, MPS VI, MPS VII, and MPS IX. However, these conditions are also referred to by their original names, which are Hurler, Hurler-Scheie, Scheie (all MPS I), Hunter (MPS II), Sanfilippo (MPS III), Morquio (MPS IV), Maroteaux-Lamy (MPS VI), Sly (MPS VII), and Hyaluronidase deficiency (MPS IX).

Description

Mucopolysaccharides are long chains of sugar molecules that are essential for building bones, cartilage, skin, tendons, and other tissues in the body. Normally, the human body continuously breaks down and builds mucopolysaccharides. Another name for mucopolysaccharides is glycosaminoglycans (GAGs). There are many different types of GAGs and specific GAGs are unable to be broken down in each of the MPS conditions. There are several enzymes involved in breaking down each GAG and a deficiency or absence of any of the essential enzymes can cause the GAG to not be broken down completely and result in its accumulation in the tissues and organs in the body. In some

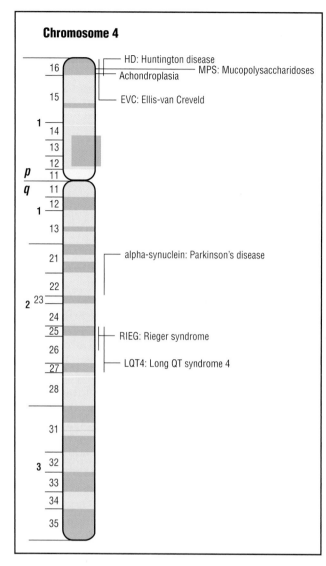

Chromosome 4

HD: Huntington disease
MPS: Mucopolysaccharidoses
Achondroplasia
EVC: Ellis-van Creveld

alpha-synuclein: Parkinson's disease

RIEG: Rieger syndrome
LQT4: Long QT syndrome 4

Mucopolysaccharidoses, on chromosome 4. *(Illustration by Argosy, Inc. Reproduced by permission of Gale, a part of Cengage Learning.)*

MPS conditions, in addition to the GAG being stored in the body, some of the incompletely broken down GAGs can leave the body in urine. When too much GAG is stored, organs and tissues can be damaged or not function properly.

Genetic profile

Except for MPS II, the MPS conditions are inherited in an autosomal recessive manner. MPS conditions occur when both of an individual's genes that produce the specific enzyme contain a mutation, causing them to not work properly. When both genes do not work properly, either none or a reduced amount of the enzyme is produced. An individual with an autosomal

recessive condition inherits one of those non-working genes from each parent. These parents are called "carriers" of the condition. When two people are known carriers for an autosomal recessive condition, they have a 25% chance with each pregnancy to have a child affected with the disease. Some individuals with MPS do have children of their own. Children of parents who have an autosomal recessive condition are all carriers of that condition. These children are not at risk to develop the condition unless the other parent is a carrier or affected with the same autosomal recessive condition.

Unlike the other MPS conditions, MPS II is inherited in an X-linked recessive manner. This means that the gene causing the condition is located on the X chromosome, one of the two sex chromosomes. Since a male has only one X chromosome, he will have the disease if the X chromosome inherited from his mother carries the defective gene. Females, because they have two X chromosomes, are called "carriers" of the condition if only one of their X chromosomes has the gene that causes the condition, while the other X chromosome does not.

Causes and symptoms

Each type of MPS is caused by a deficiency of one of the enzymes involved in breaking down GAGs. It is the accumulation of the GAGs in the tissues and organs in the body that cause the wide array of symptoms characteristic of the MPS conditions. The accumulating material is stored in cellular structures called lysosomes, and these disorders are also known as lysosomal storage diseases.

MPS I

MPS I is caused by a deficiency of the enzyme alpha-L-iduronidase. Three conditions, Hurler, Hurler-Scheie, and Scheie syndromes, are caused by a deficiency of this enzyme. Initially, these three conditions were felt to be separate because each was associated with different physical symptoms and prognoses. However, once the underlying cause of these conditions was identified, it was realized that these three conditions were all variants of the same disorder. The gene involved with MPS I is located on chromosome 4p16.3.

MPS I H (HURLER SYNDROME). It has been estimated that approximately one baby in 100,000 will be born with Hurler syndrome. Individuals with Hurler syndrome tend to have the most severe form of MPS I. Symptoms of Hurler syndrome are often evident within the first year or two after birth. Often these infants begin to develop as expected, but then reach a point where they begin to lose the skills that they have learned. Many of these infants may initially grow faster than expected, but their growth slows and typically stops by age three. Facial features also begin to appear "coarse." They develop a short nose, flatter face, thicker skin, and a protruding tongue. Additionally, their heads become larger and they develop more hair on their bodies with the hair becoming coarser. Their bones are also affected, with these children usually developing joint contractures (stiff joints), kyphosis (a specific type of curve to the spine), and broad hands with short fingers. Many of these children experience breathing difficulties, and respiratory infections are common. Other common problems include heart valve dysfunction, thickening of the heart muscle (cardiomyopathy), enlarged spleen and liver, clouding of the cornea, **hearing loss**, and **carpal tunnel syndrome**. These children typically do not live past age 12.

MPS I H/S (HURLER-SCHEIE SYNDROME). Hurler-Scheie syndrome is believed to be the intermediate form of MPS I, meaning that the symptoms are not as severe as those in individuals who have MPS I H but not as mild as those in MPS I S. Approximately one baby in 115,000 is born with Hurler-Scheie syndrome. These individuals tend to be shorter than expected, and they can have normal intelligence, however, some individuals with MPS I H/S experience learning difficulties. These individuals may develop some of the same physical features as those with Hurler syndrome, but usually they are not as severe. The prognosis for children with MPS I H/S is variable with some individuals dying during childhood, while others live to adulthood.

MPS I S (SCHEIE SYNDROME). Scheie syndrome is considered the mild form of MPS I. It is estimated that approximately one baby in 500,000 will be born with Scheie syndrome. Individuals with MPS I S usually have normal intelligence, but there have been some reports of individuals with MPS I S developing psychiatric problems. Common physical problems include corneal clouding, heart abnormalities, and orthopedic difficulties involving their hands and back. Individuals with MPS I S do not develop the facial features seen with MPS I H and usually these individuals have a normal life span.

MPS II (HUNTER SYNDROME). Hunter syndrome is caused by a deficiency of the enzyme iduronate-2-sulphatase. All individuals with Hunter syndrome are male, because the gene that causes the condition is located on the X chromosome, specifically Xq28. Like many MPS conditions, Hunter syndrome is divided into two groups, mild and severe. It has been estimated that approximately 1 in 110,000 males are born with Hunter syndrome, with the severe form being three times more common than the mild form. The severe form is felt to be associated with progressive **mental retardation** and physical disability, with most individuals dying before age 15. In the milder form, most of these individuals live to adulthood and have normal intelligence or only mild mental impairments. Males with the mild form of Hunter syndrome develop physical differences similar to the males with the severe form, but not as quickly. Men with mild Hunter syndrome can have a normal life span and some have had children. Most males with Hunter syndrome develop joint stiffness, chronic diarrhea, enlarged liver and spleen, heart valve problems, hearing loss, kyphosis, and tend to be shorter than expected. These symptoms tend to progress at a different rate depending on if an individual has the mild or severe form of MPS II.

MPS III (SANFILIPPO SYNDROME). MPS III, like the other MPS conditions, was initially diagnosed by the individual having certain physical characteristics. It was later discovered that the physical symptoms associated with Sanfilippo syndrome could be caused by a deficiency in one of four enzymes. Each type of MPS III is now subdivided into four groups, labeled A through D, based on the specific enzyme that is deficient. All four of these enzymes are involved in breaking down the same GAG, heparan sulfate. Heparan sulfate is mainly found in the **central nervous system** and accumulates in the brain when it cannot be broken down because one of those four enzymes is deficient or missing.

MPS III is a variable condition with symptoms beginning to appear between two and six years of age. Because of the accumulation of heparan sulfate in the central nervous system, the central nervous system is severely affected. In MPS III, signs that the central nervous system is degenerating usually are evident in most individuals between ages six and 10. Many children with MPS III will develop seizures, sleeplessness, thicker skin, joint contractures, enlarged tongues, cardiomyopathy, behavior problems, and mental retardation. The life expectancy in MPS III is also variable. On average, individuals with MPS III live until they are teenagers, with some living longer and others not that long.

MPS IIIA (SANFILIPPO SYNDROME TYPE A). MPS IIIA is caused by a deficiency of the enzyme heparan N-sulfatase. Type IIIA is felt to be the most severe of the four types, in which symptoms appear and death occurs at an earlier age. A study in British Columbia estimated that one in 324,617 live births is born with

MPS IIIA. MPS IIIA is the most common of the four types in Northwestern Europe. The gene that causes MPS IIIA is located on the long arm of chromosome 17 (location 17q25).

MPS IIIB (SANFILIPPO SYNDROME TYPE B). MPS IIIB is due to a deficiency in N-acetyl-alpha-D-glucosaminidase (NAG). This type of MPS III is not felt to be as severe as Type IIIA and the characteristics vary. Type IIIB is the most common of the four in southeastern Europe. The gene associated with MPS IIIB is also located on the long arm of chromosome 17 (location 17q21).

MPS IIIC (SANFILIPPO SYNDROME TYPE C). A deficiency in the enzyme acetyl-CoA-alpha-glucosaminide acetyltransferase causes MPS IIIC. This is considered a rare form of MPS III. The gene involved in MPS IIIC is believed to be located on chromosome 14.

MPS IIID (SANFILIPPO SYNDROME TYPE D). MPS IIID is caused by a deficiency in the enzyme N-acetylglucosamine-6-sulfatase. This form of MPS III is also rare. The gene involved in MPS IIID is located on the long arm of chromosome 12 (location 12q14).

MPS IV (MORQUIO SYNDROME). As with several of the MPS disorders, Morquio syndrome was diagnosed by the presence of particular signs and symptoms. However, it is now known that the deficiency of two different enzymes can cause the characteristics of MPS IV. These two types of MPS IV are called MPS IV A and MPS IV B. MPS IV is also variable in its severity. The intelligence of individuals with MPS IV is often completely normal. In individuals with a severe form, skeletal abnormalities can be extreme and include dwarfism, kyphosis (backward-curved spine), prominent breastbone, flat feet, and knock-knees. One of the earliest symptoms seen in this condition usually is a difference in the way the child walks. In individuals with a mild form of MPS IV, limb stiffness and joint pain are the primary symptoms. MPS IV is one of the rarest MPS disorders, with approximately one baby in 300,000 born with this condition.

MPS IV A (MORQUIO SYNDROME TYPE A). MPS IV A is the "classic" or the severe form of the condition and is caused by a deficiency in the enzyme galactosamine-6-sulphatase. The gene involved with MPS IV A is located on the long arm of chromosome 16 (location 16q24.3).

MPS IV B (MORQUIO SYNDROME TYPE B). MPS IV B is considered the milder form of the condition. The enzyme, beta-galactosidase, is deficient in MPS IV B. The location of the gene that produces beta-galactosidase is located on the short arm of chromosome 3 (location 3p21).

MPS VI (MAROTEAUX-LAMY SYNDROME). MPS VI, which is another rare form of MPS, is caused by a deficiency of the enzyme N-acetylglucosamine-4-sulphatase. This condition is also variable; individuals may have a mild or severe form of the condition. Typically, the nervous system or intelligence of an individual with MPS VI is not affected. Individuals with a more severe form of MPS VI can have airway obstruction, develop hydrocephalus (extra fluid accumulating in the brain) and have bone changes. Additionally, individuals with a severe form of MPS VI are more likely to die while in their teens. With a milder form of the condition, individuals tend to be shorter than expected for their age, develop corneal clouding, and live longer. The gene involved in MPS VI is believed to be located on the long arm of chromosome 5 (approximate location 5q11-13).

MPS VII (SLY SYNDROME). MPS VII is an extremely rare form of MPS and is caused by a deficiency of the enzyme beta-glucuronidase. It is also highly variable, but symptoms are generally similar to those seen in individuals with Hurler syndrome. The gene that causes MPS VII is located on the long arm of chromosome 7 (location 7q21).

MPS IX (HYALURONIDASE DEFICIENCY). MPS IX is a condition that was first described in 1996 and has been grouped with the other MPS conditions by some researchers. MPS IX is caused by the deficiency of the enzyme hyaluronidase. In the few individuals described with this condition, the symptoms are variable, but some develop soft-tissue masses (growths under the skin). Also, these individuals are shorter than expected for their age. The gene involved in MPS IX is believed to be located on the short arm of chromosome 3 (possibly 3p21.3-21.2)

Many individuals with an MPS condition have problems with airway constriction. This constriction may be so serious as to create significant difficulties in administering general anesthesia. Therefore, it is recommended that surgical procedures be performed under local anesthesia whenever possible.

Diagnosis

While a diagnosis for each type of MPS can be made on the basis of the physical signs described above, several of the conditions have similar features. Therefore, enzyme analysis is used to determine the specific MPS disorder. Enzyme analysis usually cannot accurately determine if an individual is a carrier for a MPS condition. This is because the enzyme levels in individuals who are not carriers overlap the enzyme levels seen in

KEY TERMS

Cardiomyopathy—A thickening of the heart muscle.

Enzyme—A protein that catalyzes a biochemical reaction or change without changing its own structure or function.

Joint contractures—Stiffness of the joints that prevents full extension.

Kyphosis—An abnormal outward curvature of the spine, with a hump at the upper back.

Lysosome—Membrane-enclosed compartment in cells, containing many hydrolytic enzymes; where large molecules and cellular components are broken down.

Mucopolysaccharide—A complex molecule made of smaller sugar molecules strung together to form a chain. Found in mucous secretions and intercellular spaces.

Recessive gene—A type of gene that is not expressed as a trait unless inherited from both parents.

X-linked gene—A gene carried on the X chromosome, one of the two sex chromosomes.

those individuals who are carrier for a MPS. With many of the MPS conditions, several mutations have been found in each gene involved that can cause symptoms of each condition. If the specific mutation is known in a family, DNA analysis may be possible.

Once a couple has had a child with an MPS condition, prenatal diagnosis is available to them to help determine if a fetus is affected with the same MPS as their other child. This can be accomplished through testing samples using procedures such as an amniocentesis or chorionic villus sampling (CVS). Each of these procedures has its own risks, benefits, and limitations.

Treatment

There is no cure for mucopolysaccharidosis. There are several types of experimental therapies that are being investigated. Typically, treatment involves trying to relieve some of the symptoms. For MPS I and VI, bone marrow transplantation has been attempted as a treatment option. In those conditions, bone marrow transplantation has sometimes been found to help slow down the progression or reverse some of symptoms of the disorder in some children. The benefits of a bone marrow transplantation are more likely to be noticed when performed on children under two years

of age. However it is not certain that a bone marrow transplant can prevent further damage to certain organs and tissues, including the brain. Furthermore, bone marrow transplantation is not felt to be helpful in some MPS disorders, and there are risks, benefits, and limitations with this procedure. In 2000, ten individuals with MPS I received recombinant human alpha-L-iduronidase every week for one year. Those individuals showed an improvement with some of their symptoms. Additionally, there is ongoing research involving gene replacement therapy (the insertion of normal copies of a gene into the cells of patients whose gene copies are defective).

Prevention

No specific preventive measures are available for genetic diseases of this type. For some of the MPS diseases, biochemical tests are available that will identify healthy individuals who are carriers of the defective gene, allowing them to make informed reproductive decisions. Prenatal diagnosis is also available for all MPS disease to detect affected fetuses.

Resources

PERIODICALS

Clark, Lorne A. "Laronidase for the treatment of mucopolysaccharidosis type I." *Expert Review of Endocrinology & Metabolism* 6.6 (2011): 755.

Colland, Vivian, et al. "Cognitive development in patients with Mucopolysaccharidosis type III (Sanfilippo syndrome)." *Orphanet Journal of Rare Diseases* 6 (2011): 43.

OTHER

"Mucopolysaccharidoses." Genetics Home Reference. http://ghr.nlm.nih.gov/search?query = Mucopoly saccharidoses&show = conditions (accessed October 24, 2011).

"Mucopolysaccharidoses Information Page." National Institute of Neurological Disorders and Stroke (NINDS) (June 22, 2011). http://www.ninds.nih.gov/disorders/mucopolysaccharidoses/mucopolysaccharidoses.htm (accessed October 24, 2011).

ORGANIZATIONS

Canadian Society for Mucopolysaccharide and Related Diseases. PO Box 64714, Unionville, ONT L3R-OM9. Canada (905) 479-8701 or (800) 667-1846. http://www.mpssociety.ca.

Children Living with Inherited Metabolic Diseases. The Quadrangle, Crewe Hall, Weston Rd., Crewe, Cheshire, CW1-6UR. UK 127 025 0221. Fax: 0870-7700-327. http://www.climb.org.uk.

Metabolic Information Network. PO Box 670847, Dallas, TX 75367-0847. (214) 696-2188 or (800) 945-2188.

National MPS Society. 102 Aspen Dr., Downingtown, PA 19335. (610) 942-0100. Fax: (610) 942-7188. info@ mpssociety.org. http://www.mpssociety.org.

National Organization for Rare Disorders (NORD). PO Box 8923, New Fairfield, CT 06812-8923. (203) 746-6518 or (800) 999-6673. Fax: (203) 746-6481. http:// www.rarediseases.org.

Society for Mucopolysaccharide Diseases. 46 Woodside Rd., Amersham, Buckinghamshire, HP6 6AJ. UK +44 (01494) 434156. http://www.mpssociety.co.uk.

Zain Hansen MPS Foundation. 23400 Henderson Rd., Covelo, CA 95420. (800) 767-3121.

Sharon A. Aufox, MS, CGC

Multi-infarct dementia

Definition

Multi-infarct **dementia** is one form of dementia that occurs when small blood vessels in the brain are blocked by blood clots or fatty deposits. The blockage interrupts the flow of blood to regions of the brain (a stroke), which, if sustained, causes the death of cells in numerous areas of the brain. Another form of multi-infarct dementia is inherited.

Description

Blockage or narrowing of small blood vessels by blood clots or by deposits of fat can impede the flow of blood through the vessel. Deprivation of the essential blood is catastrophic for the regions that are supplied by the vessels. In the brain, such vessel blockage can cause the death of brain cells. This event is also called a stroke. The stroke-related cell death affects the functioning of the brain.

Multi-infarct dementia is the most common form of dementia (the loss of cognitive brain due to disease or injury) due to changes in blood vessels. **Alzheimer's disease** is the most common of these so-called vascular dementias. The term multi-infarct is used because there are many areas in the brain where cell damage or death occurs. Besides dementia, multi-infarct dementia can cause stroke, headaches of migraine-like intensity, and behavioral disturbances.

An inherited form of multi-infarct dementia is designated as CADASIL, which is an acronym for cerebral autosomal dominant arteriopathy with subcortical infarcts and leukoencephalopathy.

Demographics

Multi-infarct dementia usually begins between the ages of 60–75 years. For as-yet-undetermined reasons, it affects men more than women. Multi-infarct dementia is the second most common cause of dementia in older people after Alzheimer's disease, accounting for up to 20% of all progressively worsening dementias.

CADASIL occurs in young male and female adults. It has been diagnosed in Americans, Africans, and Asians, and may occur in other groups.

Causes and symptoms

The root cause of multi-infarct dementia is usually small blood clots that lodge in blood vessels in the brain, which results in the death of brain cells. Over time, the series of small strokes (also known as ministrokes, transient ischemic attacks, or TIAs) magnifies the brain cell damage. Blood clots can result from an elevated blood pressure. Indeed, it is uncommon for someone affected with multi-infarct dementia not to have a history of high blood pressure.

There are a variety of symptoms caused by the brain cell loss. These include mental confusion, difficulty retaining information even for a short time, loss of recognition of surroundings that are familiar (which can lead to getting lost in previously familiar territory), loss of control of urination and defecation, moving with a rapid shuffling motion, difficulty in following instructions, rapid swings in emotion, and difficulty performing tasks that were previously routine. These symptoms appear in a stepwise manner, from less to more severe. As well, the initial symptoms can be so slight as to be unrecognized, disregarded, or rationalized as being due to other causes such as a temporarily stressful period. These early problems include a mild **weakness** in an arm or a leg, slurred speech, or **dizziness** that only lasts for a few days. As more blood vessels become blocked with the occurrence of more strokes, the more severe symptoms associated with mental decline become apparent.

CADASIL is characterized by a series of strokes, which is thought to be triggered by genetically determined deficiencies of small cerebral arteries. The defects affect blood flow to the brain in a similar fashion as occurs in multi-infarct dementia. The symptoms associated with CADASIL range from migraines to a slowly progressing series of symptoms that are similar to the symptoms that develop in multi-infarct dementia.

Diagnosis

Multi-infarct dementia is diagnosed based on the history of symptoms, especially of high blood pressure and strokes. A physician will look for several features during the examination, which include arm or leg weakness, speech difficulties, or dizziness. Tests that can be performed in the doctor's office include taking a blood pressure reading, recording heartbeat (an electroencephalogram, or EEG), and obtaining blood for laboratory analysis. Ultrasound studies of the carotid artery may also be performed.

Diagnosis most often involves the non-destructive imaging of the brain by means of computed tomography (CT) or magnetic resonance imaging (MRI) to reveal blood clots or the characteristic damaged regions of the brain.

Diagnosis can also be aided by an examination by a psychologist or a psychiatrist to test a person's degree of mental reasoning, ability to learn and retain new information, and attention span. Symptoms can be similar to those of Alzheimer's disease, which can complicate and delay the diagnosis of both disorders. Indeed, a person can have both disorders at the same time, as their causes are different.

Treatment team

A person with multi-infarct dementia can benefit from a support network that includes a family physician, neurologist, pharmacist, nurses, and supportive family members and other care givers. Community resources are also important, such as assisted living facilities, adult day or **respite** care centers, and local agencies on aging.

Treatment

There is no specific treatment for multi-infarct dementia, as the damage to the brain cells cannot be reversed. Treatment typically involves trying to limit further deterioration. This focuses on establishing and/or maintaining a lower blood pressure, which lessens the tendency of blood clot formation. Those people who are diabetic will be treated for this condition, as diabetes can contribute to stroke. Other factors that can be involved in lessening blood pressure include maintaining a target cholesterol level, exercise, avoiding smoking, and moderation in alcohol consumption.

Aspirin is known to reduce the tendency of the blood to clot. Some physicians will prescribe aspirin or similarly acting drugs for this purpose. As well, those

with high cholesterol may benefit from a diet change and/or the use of cholesterol-lowering drugs such as statins. In some people, surgery that removes blockages in the main blood vessel to the brain (the carotid artery) can be done. Other surgical treatments that increase blood flow through vessels are angioplasty and stenting to increase arterial flow to the brain.

Recovery and rehabilitation

As damage to the brain cannot be reversed, the focus for a person with multi-infarct dementia is placed upon prevention of further brain tissue injury and maintaining optimum independent functioning.

Clinical trials

There are no clinical trials underway or in the process of recruiting patients for either multi-infarct dementia or CADASIL. However, research is being funded by agencies such as the National Institute of Neurological Disorders and Stroke and is aimed at understanding the development of dementia. The hope is that the diagnosis of dementias will be improved. Ultimately, the goal is to reverse or prevent the disorder. Information on current relevant clinical trials can be found at ClinicalTrials.gov.

Prognosis

The outlook for people with multi-infarct dementia is poor. While some improvement in mental faculty may occur, this is typically of short-term duration. Over time, mental decline is inevitable and marked.

Special concerns

A person with multi-infarct dementia is often reliant on family and friends for daily care and support. Family and caregivers can help by stimulating a person's mental activity and prompting the individual to recall past experiences. Eventually, around-the-clock care may become necessary to provide a safe and stimulating environment.

Resources

BOOKS

Bourgeois, Michelle S., and Ellen Hickey. *Dementia: From Diagnosis to Management—A Functional Approach.* Psychology Press: 2009.

Hughes, Julian C. *Alzheimer's and other Dementias.* Oxford University Press: 2011.

WEBSITES

"Multi-infarct dementia." MedlinePlus Medical Encyclopedia (March 22, 2010). http://www.nlm.nih.gov/medlineplus/ency/article/000746.htm (accessed October 24, 2011).

"Multi-Infarct Dementia Information Page." National Institute of Neurological Disorders and Stroke (NINDS) (November 19, 2010). http://www.ninds.nih.gov/disorders/multi_infarct_dementia/multi_infarct_dementia.htm (accessed October 24, 2011).

ORGANIZATIONS

National Institute for Neurological Diseases and Stroke. P.O. Box 5801, Bethesda, MD 20824. Phone: (301) 496-5751. Tollfree phone: (800) 352-9424. http://www.ninds/nih.gov.

National Institute of Mental Health (NIMH). 6001 Executive Blvd. Rm. 8184, MSC 9663, Bethesda, MD 20892-9663. Phone: (301) 443-4513. Fax: (301) 443-4279. Tollfree phone: (866) 615-6464. Email: nimhinfo@nih.gov. http://www.nimh.nih.gov.

National Institute on Aging (NIA). 31 Center Drive, Rm. 5C27 MSC 2292, Bethesda, MD 20892-2292. Phone: (301) 496-1752. Tollfree phone: (800) 222-2225. Email: niainfo@nih.gov. http://www.nia.nih.gov.

Brian Douglas Hoyle, PhD

Multifocal motor neuropathy

Definition

Multifocal motor neuropathy is a rare condition in which the muscles in the body become progressively weaker over months to years.

Description

Multifocal motor neuropathy is often mistaken for the more catastrophic, inevitably fatal condition called **amyotrophic lateral sclerosis** (ALS). Unlike ALS, however, multifocal motor neuropathy can be treated; therefore, distinguishing between these two conditions is crucial.

Demographics

Multifocal motor neuropathy is a very rare condition, affecting only about 1 per 100,000 people in the population. Men are about three times as likely to be affected as women. Most patients are between the ages of 30 and 50 when symptoms are noted, with the average age of onset being 40 years.

Causes and symptoms

Multifocal motor neuropathy is thought to result from an autoimmune disorder; that is, the body's immune system accidentally misidentifies markers on the body's own nerve cells as foreign. The immune system then begins to produce cells that attack and injure or destroy either the nerve cells or the myelin sheath wrapped around the nerve cells. Because the myelin sheath allows messages to be conducted down a nerve quickly, injury to the sheath or to the nerve itself results in slowed or faulty nerve conduction.

Symptoms of multifocal motor neuropathy usually begin with gradually progressive **weakness** of the hands. Leg and foot weakness may follow, as well as decreased muscle volume (called muscle wasting), muscle cramps, and involuntary twitching and cramping of muscles. The weakness is asymmetric; that is, a muscle group on only one side of the body may be affected. Over time, numbness or tingling of affected areas may occur, although sensation is not lost.

Diagnosis

Diagnosis of multifocal motor neuropathy usually requires both a careful physical examination, as well as electromyographic (EMG) testing. Physical examination will reveal weakness and decreased muscle size, abnormal reflexes, muscle twitches, and totally normal sensation. EMG involves inserting a needle electrode into a muscle and measuring the electrical activity within the muscle at rest and during use. A characteristic pattern of abnormal nerve conduction and muscle contraction will be noted on EMG.

Blood tests will usually reveal the presence of antibodies (immune cells) directed against ganglioside, a component of nerve cells.

Treatment team

Patients with multifocal motor neuropathy are usually cared for by neurologists.

Treatment

Treatment for multifocal motor neuropathy involves using intravenous immunoglobulin (IVIg) to dampen down the immune system's overactivity. If IVIg is not successful, then the immunosuppressant drug cyclophosphamide may be administered.

In very mild, early cases, treatment may not be necessary. If the condition progresses or prompts serious disability, treatment may be necessary. Treatment may then be required intermittently, if the condition progresses again.

Prognosis

Muscle strength usually begins to improve within three to six weeks of the initiation of treatment. Early treatment of multifocal motor neuropathy usually results in sufficient symptom resolution to prevent any permanent disability. Over many years, however, many patients will note a continued, slow progression of muscle weakness.

Resources

BOOKS

Cohen, Jeffrey A., and Justin Mowchun, Jon Grudem. *Peripheral Nerve and Muscle Disease (What Do I Do Now?)*. Oxford University Press: 2009.

Dyck, Peter James, et al. *Companion to Peripheral Neuropathy: Illustrated Cases and New Developments*. Saunders: 2010.

Herskovitz, Steven, and Stephen Scelsa, Herbert Schaumburg. *Peripheral Neuropathies in Clinical Practice*. Oxford University Press: 2010.

WEBSITES

"Multifocal Motor Neuropathy Information Page." National Institute of Neurological Disorders and Stroke (NINDS) (February 13, 2007). http://www.ninds.nih.gov/disorders/multifocal_neuropathy/multifocal_neuropathy.htm (accessed October 24, 2011).

Rosalyn Carson-DeWitt, MD

Multiple Sclerosis

Definition

Multiple sclerosis (MS) is a chronic autoimmune disorder affecting movement, sensation, and bodily functions. It is caused by destruction of the myelin insulation covering nerve fibers (neurons) in the **central nervous system** (brain and spinal cord).

Demographics

As of 2011, approximately 400,000 people in the United States have been diagnosed with MS, with 10,000 new cases being diagnosed each year. Worldwide, MS affects between 1.5 and 2.5 million people. Most people have their first symptoms between the ages of 20 and 40; symptoms rarely begin before age 15 or after age 60. The mean age range is 29–33 years. Women are almost twice as likely to get MS as men, especially in their early years. People of northern European ancestry are more likely to be affected than people of other backgrounds, and MS rates are higher in the United States, Canada, and Northern Europe than other parts of the world. The disorder is unknown among certain native peoples such as the Inuit (native people of the Arctic) and Maori (native people of New Zealand).

Description

Multiple sclerosis is a slowly progressive disease of the central nervous system (CNS), which is comprised of the brain and spinal cord. In 1868, French physician Jean-Martin Charcot (1825–1893) provided the first detailed clinical description of the disease. Today researchers know that MS is an autoimmune disorder that causes the destruction of myelin, the insulating material that surrounds nerve fibers (neurons). Myelin helps electrical signals pass quickly and smoothly between the brain and the rest of the body. When the myelin layer is destroyed, nerve messages are sent more slowly and less efficiently. Patches of scar tissue, called plaques, form over the affected areas, further disrupting nerve communication. The symptoms of MS occur when the brain and spinal cord nerves no longer communicate properly with other parts of the body. MS causes a wide variety of symptoms and can affect vision, balance, strength, sensation, coordination, and bodily functions.

Risk factors

The risk of developing MS is slightly higher if another family member is affected, suggesting the

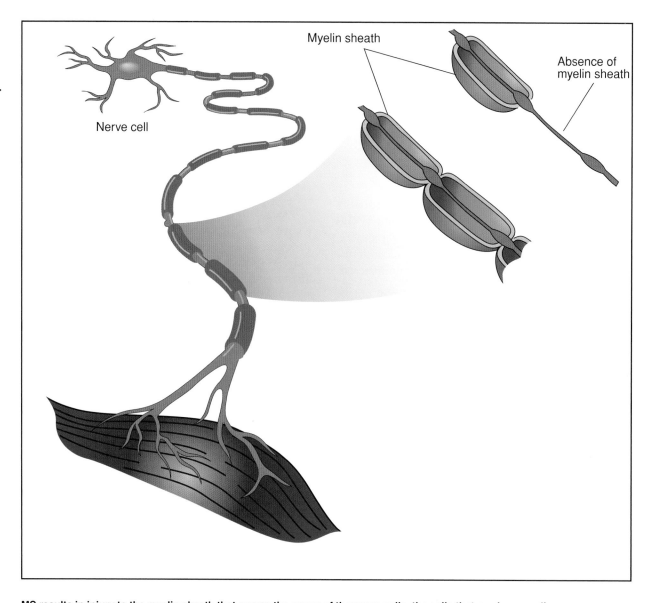

Myelin sheath

Absence of
myelin sheath

Nerve cell

MS results in injury to the myelin sheath that covers the axons of the nerve cells, the cells that produce myelin (oligodendrocytes), and, to a lesser extent, the axons and nerve cells themselves. *(Illustration by Electronic Illustrators Group. Reproduced by permission of Gale, a part of Cengage Learning.)*

influence of genetic factors. If one person in a family has MS, then that person's close family relatives (parents, children, siblings) have about a 5% greater chance of developing MS than people who do not have family members with the disorder. In addition, the higher prevalence of MS among people of northern European background suggests some genetic susceptibility.

Causes and symptoms

Causes

Multiple sclerosis is an autoimmune disorder, meaning it is caused by the body's own immune system.

For unknown reasons, immune cells attack and destroy the myelin sheath that insulates neurons in the brain and spinal cord. This myelin sheath speeds transmission of nerve impulses and prevents electrical activity in one cell from short-circuiting to another cell. Disruption of communication between the brain and other parts of the body prevents normal passage of sensations and control messages, leading to the symptoms of MS. The demyelinated areas appear as plaques, small round areas of gray neuron without the white myelin covering. The progression of symptoms in MS is correlated with development of new plaques in the portion of the brain or spinal cord controlling the affected areas. Because there appears to be no pattern in the appearance of new plaques, the progression of MS can be unpredictable.

Despite considerable research, the trigger for this autoimmune destruction is still unknown. At various times, evidence has pointed to genes, environmental factors, viruses, or a combination of these.

The fact that the risk of developing MS is slightly higher if another family member is affected, suggests that there is a genetic susceptibility to the disease.

The role of an environmental factor is suggested by studies of the effect of migration on the risk of developing MS. Age plays an important role in determining this change in risk—young people in low-risk groups who move into countries with higher MS rates display the risk rates of their new surroundings, while older migrants retain the risk rate of their original home country. One interpretation of these studies is that an environmental factor, either protective or harmful, is acquired in early life; the risk of disorder later in life reflects the effects of the early environment.

These same data can be used to support the involvement of a slow-acting virus, one that is acquired early in life but begins its destructive effects much later. Slow viruses are known to cause other disorders, including **AIDS**. In addition, viruses have been implicated in other autoimmune disorders. Many claims have been made for the role of viruses, slow or otherwise, as the trigger for MS, but as of 2011 no strong candidate has emerged.

How a virus could trigger the autoimmune reaction is also unclear. There are two main models of virally induced autoimmunity. The first suggests the immune system is actually attacking a virus (one too well-hidden for detection in the laboratory), and the myelin damage is an unintentional consequence of fighting the infection. The second model suggests the immune system mistakes myelin for a viral protein, one it encountered during a prior infection. Primed for the attack, it destroys myelin because it resembles the previously-recognized viral invader.

Either of these models allows a role for genetic factors, since certain genes can increase the likelihood of autoimmunity, and it seems likely that more than one gene is involved in a person's susceptibility to MS. Environmental factors as well might change the sensitivity of the immune system or interact with myelin to provide the trigger for the secondary immune response. Possible environmental triggers that have been invoked in MS include viral infection, trauma, electrical injury, and chemical exposure, although controlled studies do not support a causative role.

Symptoms

MS is a diverse disease. No two affected persons are the same and each will experience different combinations of symptoms with differing severity. The symptoms of MS may occur in one of three patterns:

- The most common pattern is the relapsing-remitting pattern, in which there are clearly defined symptomatic attacks lasting 24 hours or more, followed by complete or almost complete improvement. The period between attacks may be a year or more at the beginning of the disorder but may shrink to several months later on. About three-quarters of all people diagnosed with MS have this version of the disorder. This pattern is especially common in younger people who develop MS.

- In the primary progressive pattern, the disorder progresses without remission or with only occasional plateaus or slight improvements. This pattern is more common in older people. About 10% of people with the disorder have this pattern.

- In the secondary progressive pattern, the person with MS begins with relapses and remissions, followed by more steady progression of symptoms. In some people, what begins as a relapsing-remitting pattern develops into a secondary progressive pattern.

Between 10–20% of people have a benign type of MS, meaning their symptoms progress very little over the course of their lives.

Because plaques may form in any part of the central nervous system, the symptoms of MS vary widely from person-to-person and from stage-to-stage of the disorder. Initial symptoms often include:

- muscle weakness, causing difficulty walking
- loss of coordination or balance
- numbness, "pins and needles," (paresthesias) or other abnormal sensations
- visual disturbances, including blurred or double vision

Later symptoms may include:

- fatigue
- muscle spasticity and stiffness
- tremors
- paralysis
- pain
- vertigo
- speech or swallowing difficulty
- loss of bowel and bladder control
- incontinence
- constipation
- sexual dysfunction
- cognitive changes

Weakness in one or both legs is common and may be the first symptom noticed by a person with MS. Muscle **spasticity**, where muscles are excessive and continuously contracted, is also common and may be more disabling than weakness.

Double vision or eye **tremor** (nystagmus) may result from involvement of the nerve pathways controlling movement of the eye muscles. **Visual disturbances** result from involvement of the optic nerves (optic neuritis) and may include development of blind spots in one or both eyes, changes in color vision, or blindness. Optic neuritis usually involves only one eye at a time and is often associated with movement of the effected eye.

More than half of all people affected by MS have pain during the course of their disorder, and many experience chronic pain, including pain from spasticity. Acute pain occurs in about 10% of cases. This pain may be a sharp, stabbing pain especially in the face, neck, or down the back. Facial numbness and weakness are also common.

Cognitive changes, including memory disturbances, **depression**, and personality changes, are found in people affected by MS, although it is not entirely clear whether these changes are due primarily to the disorder or to the psychological reaction to it. Depression may be severe enough to require treatment in up to 25% of those with MS. A smaller number of people experience disorder-related euphoria, or abnormally elevated mood, usually after a long disorder duration and in combination with other psychological changes.

Symptoms of MS may be worsened by heat or increased body temperature, including fever, intense physical activity, or exposure to sun, hot baths, or showers.

Diagnosis

There is no single test that confirms the diagnosis of MS, and there are a number of other disorders with similar symptoms. While one person's diagnosis may be immediately suggested by symptoms and history, another's may not be confirmed without multiple tests and prolonged observation. The distribution of symptoms is important: MS affects multiple areas of the body over time. The pattern of symptoms is also critical, especially as evidence of the relapsing-remitting pattern, so a detailed medical history is one of the most important parts of the diagnostic process.

A thorough search to exclude other causes of a patient's symptoms is especially important if any of the following features are present:

• family history of neurologic disorder

KEY TERMS

Clinical trial—All new drugs undergo clinical trials before approval. Clinical trials are carefully conducted tests in which effectiveness and side effects are studied, with the placebo effect eliminated.

Evoked potentials—Tests that measure the brain's electrical response to stimulation of sensory organs (eyes or ears) or peripheral nerves (skin). These tests may help confirm the diagnosis of MS.

Myelin—A layer of insulation that surrounds the nerve fibers in the brain and spinal cord.

Plaque—Patches of scar tissue that form where the layer of myelin covering the nerve fibers is destroyed by the MS disorder process.

Primary progressive—A pattern of symptoms of MS in which the disorder progresses without remission or with occasional plateaus or slight improvements.

Relapsing-remitting—A pattern of symptoms of MS in which symptomatic attacks occur that last 24 hours or more, followed by complete or almost complete improvement.

Secondary progressive—A pattern of symptoms of MS in which there are relapses and remissions, followed by more steady progression of symptoms.

• symptoms and findings attributable to a single anatomic location

• persistent back pain

• age of onset over 60 or under 15 years of age

• progressively worsening disorder

Tests

In addition to the medical history and a standard neurological exam, several lab tests are used to help confirm or rule out a diagnosis of MS:

• Magnetic resonance imaging (MRI) can reveal plaques on the brain and spinal cord. Gadolinium enhancement can distinguish between old and new plaques, allowing a correlation of new plaques with new symptoms. Plaques may be seen in several other disorders as well, including encephalomyelitis, neurosarcoidosis, and cerebral lupus. Plaques on MRI may be difficult to distinguish from small strokes, areas of decreased blood flow, or changes seen with trauma or normal aging.

• A lumbar puncture, or spinal tap, is done to measure levels of immune system proteins, which are usually

---

elevated in the cerebrospinal fluid of a person with MS. This test may not be necessary if other tests are diagnostic.

- Evoked potential tests are electrical tests of conduction speed in the nerves that can reveal reduced speeds consistent with the damage caused by plaques. These tests may be done with small electrical charges applied to the skin (somatosensory evoked potential), with light patterns flashed on the eyes (visual evoked potential), or with sounds presented to the ears (auditory evoked potential).

The clinician making the diagnosis, usually a neurologist, may classify the disorder as "definite MS," meaning the symptoms and test results all point toward MS as the cause. "Probable MS" and "possible MS" reflect less certainty and may require more time to pass to observe the progression of the disorder and the distribution of symptoms.

Treatment

There is no known cure for MS. Nevertheless, several drugs may slow progression of the disorder and moderate some symptoms in many patients, especially if started early.

Multiple sclerosis causes a wide variety of symptoms, and the treatments for these are equally diverse. Most symptoms can be treated and complications avoided with good care and attention from medical professionals. Good health and nutrition remain important preventive measures. Vaccination against influenza can prevent respiratory complications. Preventing complications such as pneumonia, bedsores, injuries from **falls**, or urinary infection requires attention to the primary problems that may cause them. Shortened life spans with MS are almost always due to complications rather than primary symptoms themselves.

Drugs

Drug treatment must be individualized. Not all drugs are appropriate for all patients. In the United States, as of 2011, MS was most often treated with four drugs known as the ABCR drugs. These drugs are interferon beta-1a (Avonex), interferon beta-1b (Betaseron and Rebif), and glatiramer acetate (Copaxone). These drugs, on average, reduce relapses in the relapsing-remitting form of MS by about one-third. Different measurements from tests of each have demonstrated other benefits as well: Avonex may slow the progress of physical impairment, Betaseron and Rebif may reduce the severity of symptoms, and Copaxone may decrease disability. All four drugs are administered by injection, some into muscle (IM), and some under the skin (SC).

Some controversy exists on the most effective dose and the frequency with which these drugs should be administered.

Although the ABCR drugs reduce relapses and may keep patients in relatively good health for the short-term, their long-term success has not been proven, and they do not work well for patients who have reached a steadily progressive stage of MS. Individuals with progressive forms of MS may be treated with mitoxantrone (Novantrone), cyclophosphamide (Cytoxan, Neosar), azathioprine (Imuran), or methotrexate (Rheumatrex). All these drugs suppress the immune system. None is ideal, and all have potentially serious side effects. Corticosteroid drugs such as methylprednisolone (Medrol) also may be used to reduce inflammation. Long-term use of corticosteroids also causes serious side effects.

Two disease modifying agents, fingolimod (Gilenya) and natalizumab (Tysabri), are effective in keeping white blood cells in the lymph system thus, preventing these cells from crossing the blood-brain barrier into the central nervous system which in turn, reduces inflammation and damage to nerve cells.

Training in bowel and bladder care may be needed to prevent or compensate for incontinence. If the urge to urinate becomes great before the bladder is full, some drugs may be helpful, including propantheline bromide (Probanthine), oxybutynin chloride (Ditropan), or imipramine (Tofranil). Baclofen (Lioresal) may relax the sphincter muscle, allowing full emptying. Intermittent catheterization is effective in controlling bladder dysfunction. In this technique, a catheter is used to periodically empty the bladder.

Spasticity can be treated with oral medications, including baclofen and **diazepam** (Valium), or by injection with **botulinum toxin** (Botox). Spasticity relief may also bring relief from chronic pain. More acute types of pain may respond to **carbamazepine** (Tegretol) or diphenylhydantoin (Dilantin). Low **back pain** is common from increased use of the back muscles to compensate for weakened legs. Physical therapy and over-the-counter pain relievers may help.

Fatigue may be partially avoidable with changes in the daily routine to allow more frequent rests. **Amantadine** (Symmetrel) and **Modafinil** (Provigil), although not specifically approved for use with MS, are often used to treat fatigue and improve alertness. Pemoline (Cylert), a drug formerly used to treat fatigue in MS patients, was withdrawn from sale in the United States in October 2005 because of potentially fatal liver complications. Visual disturbances often respond to corticosteroids. Other symptoms that may be treated with drugs include seizures, **vertigo**, and tremor.

Treatment for significant acute exacerbations include the use of steroids such as methyl-prednisolone (Medrol), administered in high doses for a number of days, then tapering to lower doses for a number of weeks.

Clinical trials of new drugs and drug combinations to treat MS are ongoing. Individuals with MS who wish to participate in the trial of an experimental therapy can find a list of clinical trials currently enrolling volunteers at http://clinicaltrials.gov. There is no cost to the patient to participate in a clinical trial.

Other drugs used for the treatment or management of symptoms associated with MS include:

Bladder dysfunction:

- tolterodine (Detrol)
- darifenacin (Enablex)
- tamsulosin (Flomax)
- terazosin (Hytrin)
- prazosin (Minipress)
- oxybutynin (Oxytrol)
- trospium chloride (Sanctura)
- solifenacin succinate (Vesicare)

Constipation:

- docusate (Colace)
- bisacodyl (Dulcolax)
- sodium phosphate (Fleet Enema)
- psyllium (Metamucil)

Depression and fatigue:

- venlafaxine (Effexor)
- paroxetine (Paxil)
- bupropion (Wellbutrin)
- sertraline (Zoloft)
- duloxetine hydrochloride (Cymbalta)
- fluoxetine (Prozac)

Dizziness:

- meclizine (Antivert)

Erectile dysfunction:

- tadalafil (Cialis)
- vardenafil (Levitra)
- alprostadil (Prostin VR)
- sildenafil (Viagra)

Itching:

- hydroxazyne (Atarax)

Pain:

- gabapentin (Neurontin)

- nortriptyline (Pamelor)
- amitriptyline (Elavil)

Spasticity:

- dantrolene (Dantrium)
- tizanidine (Zanaflex)

Urinary frequency:

- desmopressin (DDAVP)

Urinary tract infections:

- sulfamethoxazole (Bacrim, Septra)
- ciprofloxacin (Cipro)
- nitrofurantoin (Macrodantin)
- methenamine (Hiprex)
- vphenazopyridine (Pyridium)

Tremor:

- isoniazid (Laniazid, Nydrazid)
- clonazepam (Klonopin)

Walking:

- dalfampride (Ampyra)

Rehabilitative therapy

Physical therapy helps the person with MS to strengthen and retrain affected muscles, maintain range of motion, prevent muscle stiffening, learn to use assistive devices such as canes and walkers, and to learn safer and more energy-efficient ways of moving, sitting, and transferring. Exercise and stretching programs are usually designed by the physical therapist and taught to the patient and caregivers for use at home. Exercise is an important part of maintaining function for the person with MS. Swimming is often recommended, not only for its low-impact workout, but also because it allows strenuous activity without overheating.

Occupational therapy helps the person with MS adapt to her environment and adapt the environment to her. The occupational therapist suggests alternate strategies and assistive devices for activities of daily living, such as dressing, feeding, and washing, and evaluates the home and work environment for safety and efficiency improvements that may be made.

Alternative therapies

Bee venom has been suggested as a treatment for MS, but no studies or objective reports support this claim.

In several studies, marijuana has been shown to have variable effects on the symptoms of MS. Improvements have been documented for tremor, pain, and spasticity, and worsening for posture and balance. Side effects have included weakness, dizziness, relaxation, and incoordination, as well as euphoria.

Some studies support the value of high doses of vitamins, minerals, and other dietary supplements for controlling disorder progression or improving symptoms. Alpha-linoleic and linoleic acids, as well as selenium and vitamin E, have shown effectiveness in the treatment of MS. Selenium and vitamin E act as antioxidants. In addition, a diet low in saturated fats, maintained over a long period, may retard the disorder process.

Studies have also shown that t'ai chi can be an effective therapy for MS because it works to improve balance and increase strength.

There are conflicting views about the herb Echinacea and its benefit to MS. Some alternative practitioners recommend Echinacea for people with MS; however, Echinacea appears to stimulate different parts of the immune system, particularly immune cells known as macrophages. In MS these cells are very active already and further stimulation could worsen the disorder.

Prognosis

It is difficult to predict how MS will progress in any one person. Most people with MS will be able to continue to walk and function at their work for many years after their diagnosis. The factors associated with the mildest course of MS are being female, having the relapsing-remitting form, having the first symptoms at a younger age, having longer periods of remission between relapses, and initial symptoms of decreased sensation or vision rather than of weakness or incoordination.

Fewer than 5% of people with MS have a severe progressive form, leading to death from complications within five years. At the other extreme, 10–20% have a benign form, with a very slow or no progression of their symptoms. Studies have shown that about seven out of ten people with MS are still alive 25 years after their diagnosis, compared to about nine out of ten people of similar age without disorder. On average, MS shortens the lives of affected women by about six years, and men by 11 years. Suicide is a significant cause of death in MS, especially in younger patients. Suicide is completed 7.5 times more often in patients with MS than in those without the disorder.

The degree of disability a person experiences five years after onset is, on average, about three-quarters of the expected disability at 10–15 years. A benign course for the first five years usually indicates the disorder will not cause marked disability.

QUESTIONS TO ASK YOUR DOCTOR

- What are the indications that I may have multiple sclerosis?
- What symptom pattern for multiple sclerosis do I have?
- What diagnostic tests are needed for a thorough assessment?
- Can you estimate how rapidly my symptoms will progress?
- What treatment options do you recommend for me?
- What kind of changes can I expect to see with the medications you have prescribed for me?
- What are the side effects associated with the medications you have prescribed for me?
- Will medications for multiple sclerosis interact with my current medications?
- What kind of specialists should I contact?
- What tests or evaluation techniques will you perform to see if treatment has been beneficial for me?
- What changes in my health can I expect to see as my condition progresses?
- What physical or psychological limitations do you foresee?
- Will physical, occupational, or speech therapy benefit me?
- Does having multiple sclerosis put me at risk for other health conditions?
- How can my quality of life be improved?
- What research is being done to learn more about multiple sclerosis?
- What symptoms or adverse effects are important enough that I should seek immediate treatment?
- Can you recommend an organization that will provide me with additional information about multiple sclerosis?
- Can you refer me to a qualified person who can make an assessment of my home and recommend changes to make it safer and easier for me to get around?
- Can you recommend any support groups for me and my family?

Prevention

There is no known way to prevent MS. Until the cause of the disorder is discovered, this is unlikely to change. Good nutrition, adequate rest, avoidance of stress, heat, and extreme physical exertion, and good bladder hygiene may improve quality of life and reduce symptoms.

Resources

BOOKS

Bennett, Robin L. *The Practical Guide to the Genetic Family History*. 2nd ed. New York: Wiley-Blackwell, 2010.

Blackstone, Margaret. *The First Year: Multiple Sclerosis: An Essential Guide for the Newly Diagnosed*. New York: Marlowe, 2007.

Ferri, Fred F., editor. *Ferri's Clinical Advisor: Instant Diagnosis and Treatment*. St. Louis: Mosby, 2007.

Goetz, Christopher G., ed. *Textbook of Clinical Neurology*. Philadelphia: Saunders, 2007.

Nussbaum, Robert L., Roderick R. McInnes, and Huntington F. Willard. *Genetics in Medicine*. Philadelphia: Saunders, 2007.

Ruggieri, Martino, Luigi Grimaldi, and Agata Polizzi, eds. *Multiple Sclerosis in Childhood and Other Immune-Mediated Disorders of the Central Nervous System in Children*. New York: Springer, 2011.

WEBSITES

Clinical Trials Website. http://www.clinicaltrials.gov/ct/action/GetStudy (accessed July 17, 2011).

"Medications Used in MS by Chemical Name." National Multiple Sclerosis Society. http://www.nationalmssociety.org/about-multiple-sclerosis/what-we-know-about-ms/treatments/medications-by-chemical-name/index.aspx (accessed July 17, 2011).

"Multiple Sclerosis." Medline Plus. http://www.nlm.nih.gov/medlineplus/multiplesclerosis.html (accessed July 17, 2011).

"So You Have Multiple Sclerosis... What's Next?" Accelerated Cure Project for Multiple Sclerosis. http://www.acceleratedcure.org/downloads/bcp-ms-whatsnext.pdf (accessed July 17, 2011).

ORGANIZATIONS

American Academy of Neurology (AAN), 1080 Montreal Avenue, St. Paul, MN 55116, (651) 695-2717, Fax: (651) 695-2791, (800) 879-1960, memberservices@aan.com, http://www.aan.com.

American Academy of Physical Medicine and Rehabilitation, 9700 West Bryn Mawr Avenue, Suite 200, Rosemont, IL 60018-5701, (847) 737-6000, Fax: (847) 737-6001, info@aapmr.org, http://www. aapmr.org.

American Neurological Association, 5841 Cedar Lake Road, Suite 204, Minneapolis, MN 55416, (952) 545-6284, http://www.aneuroa.org.

American Physical Therapy Association, 1111 North Fairfax Street, Alexandria, VA 22314-1488, (800) 999-APTA (2782), (703) 684-APTA (2782), http://www.apta.org.

Genetic and Rare Diseases Information Center (GARD), P.O. Box 8126, Gaithersburg, MD 20898-8126, (301) 251-4925, Fax: (301) 251-4911, (888) 205-2311, http://rarediseases.info.nih.gov/GARD/Default.aspx.

Multiple Sclerosis Association of America, 706 Haddonfield Road, Cherry Hill, NJ 08002, (856) 488-4500, Fax: (856) 661-9797, (800) 532-7667, msaa@msaa. com, http://www.msaa.com.

Multiple Sclerosis Foundation, 6520 North Andrews Avenue, Fort Lauderdale, FL 33309-2130, (954) 776-6805, Fax: (954) 351-0630, (888) MSFOCUS, support@msfocus.org, http://www.msfocus.org.

National Institute of Neurological Disorders and Stroke (NINDS), P.O. Box 5801, Bethesda, MD 20824, (301) 496-5751, (800) 352-9424, http://www.ninds.nih.gov.

National Institutes of Health (NIH), 9000 Rockville Pike, Bethesda, MD 20892, (301) 496-4000, NIHinfo@od.nih.gov, http://www.nih.gov/index.html.

National Multiple Sclerosis Society, 733 Third Avenue, New York, NY 10017, (800) 344-4867, http://www.nmss.org.

National Organization for Rare Disorders (NORD), 55 Kenosia Avenue, P.O. Box 1968, Danbury, CT 06813-1968, (203) 744-0100, (800) 999-6673, http://www.rarediseases.org.

U.S. National Library of Medicine, 8600 Rockville Pike, Bethesda, MD, 20894, (301) 594-5983, (888) 346-3656, Fax: (301) 402-1384, custserv@nlm. nih.gov, http://www.nlm.nih.gov.

Tish Davidson, AM
Genevieve T. Slomski, Ph
Laura Jean Cataldo, RN, Ed

Multiple system atrophy

Definition

Multiple system atrophy (MSA) is a neurodegenerative disease characterized by parkinsonism, cerebellar dysfunction, and autonomic disturbances.

Description

MSA causes a wide range of symptoms, in keeping with its name of "multiple system" atrophy. Parkinsonian symptoms include **tremor**, rigidity and slowed movements; cerebellar symptoms include incoordination and unsteady gait; and autonomic symptoms include **orthostatic hypotension** (drop in blood pressure upon standing) and urinary incontinence. Because of this wide variety of symptoms, it was originally thought of as three distinct diseases: **striatonigral degeneration** (parkinsonian symptoms), **olivopontocerebellar atrophy** (cerebellar symptoms) and Shy-Drager syndrome (autonomic symptoms). Further study showed the overlap among these conditions was best explained by considering them as a single disease with symptoms clustered into three groups. Historically, confusion about the disease was made even worse because olivopontocerebellar atrophy is also the name of an unrelated genetically inherited disease. It is hoped that widespread use of the name MSA will clear up some of this confusion.

Demographics

Because MSA is often misdiagnosed, figures on its prevalence are not known with certainty. It is estimated there are between 25,000 and 100,000 people in the United States with MSA. Onset is usually in the early fifties, and men are slightly more likely to be affected than women.

Causes and symptoms

The cause or causes of MSA are unknown. No genes have been found for MSA. Some evidence indicates that toxins may be responsible, but no specific agents have been identified. The brains of MSA patients reveal that cells called glia undergo characteristic changes. Glia are supportive cells for neurons, brain cells that conduct electrical signals. In MSA, glia develop tangles of proteins within them, called glial cytoplasmic inclusions. It is not known whether these actually cause MSA or are caused by some other problem that is the real culprit.

The symptoms of MSA fall into three separate areas: parkinsonism, cerebellar symptoms, and autonomic disturbances. The distribution and severity of individual symptoms varies among patients. MSA is a progressive disease, and symptoms worsen over time.

Parkinsonism is the initial symptom in almost half of all patients. The classic symptoms of Parkinson's disease—tremor, stiffness or rigidity, and slowed movements—are seen in MSA, although tremor is not as common and is jerkier that the tremor of PD.

Cerebellar symptoms are the initial feature in very few MSA patients but occur in about half of patients at some point during the disease. The **cerebellum** is an important center for coordination, and degeneration of the cerebellum in MSA leads to loss of balance, incoordination in the limbs, and loss of smooth eye movements. A person with cerebellar dysfunction in MSA typically walks with a wide stance to improve stability and may lose the hand-eye coordination that makes so many simple activities possible.

Autonomic symptoms refer to those involving the autonomic nervous system. The autonomic nervous system controls a variety of "automatic" body functions, including blood pressure, heart rate, sweating, and bladder function. Autonomic symptoms are the initial complaint in half or more of all MSA patients. The most common initial problem is urinary dysfunction in women, and erectile dysfunction in men. Urinary dysfunction may be incontinence, or inability to void the bladder. Other autonomic symptoms include lack of sweating, constipation, and fecal incontinence.

Orthostatic hypotension is a common autonomic symptom. It refers to a significant drop in blood pressure shortly after standing. It can cause **dizziness**, lightheadedness, **fainting**, **weakness**, **fatigue**, yawning, slurred speech, headache, neck ache, cognitive impairment, and blurred vision.

Other symptoms may also occur in MSA. These may include:

- vocal cord paralysis, leading to hoarseness
- swallowing difficulty
- sleep apnea
- spasticity
- myoclonus
- Raynaud's phenomenon (cold extremities)

Diagnosis

The diagnosis of MSA is difficult, because it is easily mistaken in its earlier stages for **Parkinson's disease**, which is much more common. Autonomic disturbance also occurs in PD but is much more pronounced in MSA. MSA is the more likely diagnostic choice when disease progression is rapid and when the patient responds mildly or poorly to levodopa, the mainstay of PD treatment. Some centers use **electromyography** of the anal sphincter (the muscles surrounding the anus) in order to confirm the diagnosis of MSA. Abnormal results indicate MSA rather than PD, although this method is not universally recognized as valid.

Neuroimaging may be used to rule out other causes of similar symptoms, such as lesions in the brain or normal pressure hydrocephalus.

Treatment team

The treatment team includes the neurologist, possibly a movement disorders specialist, a urologist, and a speech/language pathologist.

Treatment

There are no treatments that halt or slow the degeneration of brain cells that causes MSA. Treatment is aimed at relieving symptoms.

Treatment of parkinsonian symptoms is attempted with standard PD drugs, namely levodopa and the dopamine agonists. Unfortunately, these are rarely as effective in MSA as they are in PD, although about one third of patients have at least a moderate response. In the best case, treatment relieves stiffness, tremor and slowed movements, allowing increased activities of daily living.

Orthostatic hypotension is treated with medications to increase retention of fluids (fludrocortisone), compressive stockings to keep blood from pooling in the legs, increasing fluids, and increasing salt intake. Midodrine, a drug that helps maintain blood pressure, is often prescribed.

A urologist may be needed to define the type of urinary dysfunction the patient has and to manage treatment. A bedside commode or condom catheter may be helpful for urge incontinence or inability to hold urine once the urge to urinate occurs. If incomplete voiding is the problem, intermittent catheterization may be needed. Detrusor hyperreflexia, in which the bladder muscle undergoes spasms, may be treated with drugs to reduce these spasms.

Male erectile dysfunction may be treated with sildenafil or other medications.

Anhidrosis, or lack of sweating, can be dangerous in an active patient, because of the risk of overheating. Awareness of the problem and avoidance of prolonged exercise are helpful.

Gait **ataxia** may require a mobility aid, such as a cane, walker, or eventually a wheelchair.

Speech and swallowing problems are dealt with by a speech/language pathologist, who may work with the patient to develop swallowing strategies, and instruct in the use of assistive communication devices. Sleep apnea may be treated with continuous positive airway pressure ventilation.

Clinical trials

Clinical trials for MSA are usually directed toward better diagnosis or symptomatic treatment. Until researchers develop a better understanding of the causes of the disease, little progress can be expected in development of treatments to slow its progression.

KEY TERMS

Atrophy—The progressive wasting and loss of function of any part of the body.

Cerebellum—The part of the brain involved in the coordination of movement, walking, and balance.

Neurodegeneration—The deterioration of nerve tissues.

Prognosis

The average survival after diagnosis is 9–10 years. Death usually occurs from pneumonia or suddenly from insufficient respiration, due to degeneration of the respiratory centers in the brain.

Resources

PERIODICALS

Hardy, Joanne. "Multiple system atrophy: pathophysiology, treatment and nursing care." *Nursing Standard* 22.22 (2008): 50.

WEBSITES

"Multiple System Atrophy Information Page." National Institute of Neurological Disorders and Stroke (NINDS) (August 10, 2011). http://www.ninds.nih. gov/disorders/ msa/msa.htm (accessed October 24, 2011).

Richard Robinson

Muscle-nerve biopsy *see* **Biopsy**

Muscular dystrophy

Definition

Muscular dystrophy (MD) is the name for a group of inherited disorders in which strength and muscle bulk gradually decline. Nine types of muscular dystrophies are generally recognized:

- Duchenne muscular dystrophy (DMD)
- Becker muscular dystrophy (BMD)
- Myotonic dystrophy (also known as Steinert's disease)
- Emery-Dreifuss muscular dystrophy (EDMD)
- Limb-girdle muscular dystrophy (LGMD)
- Facioscapulohumeral muscular dystrophy (FSH) or Landouzy-Dejerine disease
- Oculopharyngeal muscular dystrophy (OPMD)
- Distal muscular dystrophy (DD)
- Congenital muscular dystrophy (CMD)

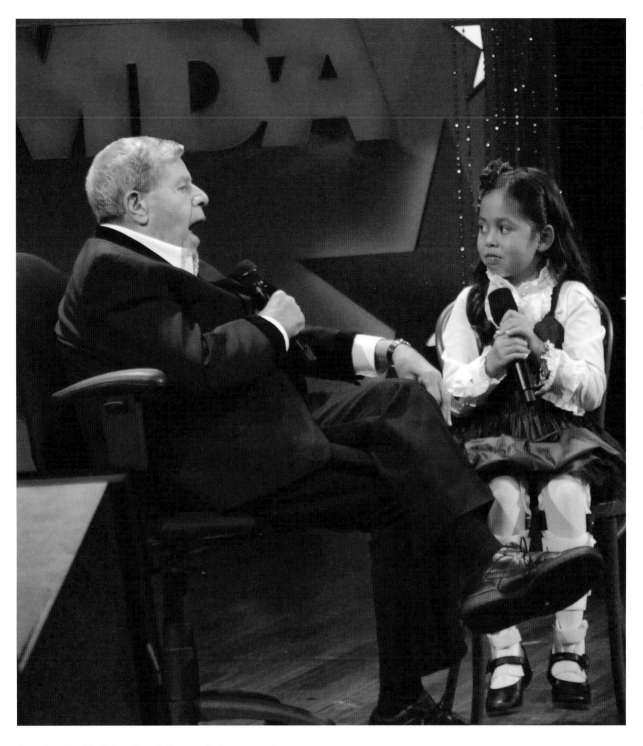

Jerry Lewis with Abbey Umali. *(www.splashnews.com)*

Demographics

According to National Institute for Neurological Disorders and Stroke (NINDS), MD occurs worldwide, and affects all races. Its incidence varies, as some types are more common than others.

- Mystotonic dystrophy is the most common form of MD in the United States. If affects more than 30,000 people.
- FSH affects approximately 13,000 Americans.
- Approximately 8,000 boys and young men in the United States have DMD, which occurs in about 1 in every 3,500 male births.

- BMD occurs in about 1 in 30,000 male births.
- The highest prevalence of LGMD is in a small mountainous Basque province in northern Spain, where the condition affects 69 persons per million. The number of Americans with LGMS may be in the low thousands.
- OPMD is most common among French Canadian families in Quebec and in Spanish-American families in the American Southwest.
- DD is most common in Sweden.
- A subtype of CMD called Fukuyama CMD is most common in Japan.
- Fewer than 300 cases of EDMD have been identified.

Description

The muscular dystrophies include:

- Duchenne muscular dystrophy (DMD): DMD affects young boys, causing progressive muscle weakness, usually beginning in the legs. It is a severe form of muscular dystrophy.
- *Becker muscular dystrophy (BMD)*: BMD affects older boys and young men, following a milder course than DMD.
- *Emery-Dreifuss muscular dystrophy (EDMD)*: EDMD affects both males and females because it can be inherited as an autosomal dominant or recessive disorder. Symptoms include contractures and weakness in the calves, weakness in the shoulders and upper arms, and problems in the way electrical impulses travel through the heart to make it beat (heart conduction defects).
- *Limb-girdle muscular dystrophy (LGMD)*: LGMD begins in late childhood to early adulthood and affects both men and women, causing weakness in the muscles around the hips and shoulders and weakness in the limbs. It is the most variable of the muscular dystrophies, and there are several different forms of the condition now recognized. Many people with suspected LGMD have probably been misdiagnosed in the past; therefore, the prevalence of the condition is difficult to estimate.
- *Facioscapulohumeral muscular dystrophy (FSH)*: FSH, also known as Landouzy-Dejerine condition, begins in late childhood to early adulthood and affects both men and women, causing weakness in the muscles of the face, shoulders, and upper arms. The hips and legs may also be affected.
- **Myotonic dystrophy**: Also known as Steinert's disease, it affects both men and women, causing generalized weakness first seen in the face, feet, and hands. It is accompanied by the inability to relax the affected muscles (myotonia). Symptoms may begin from birth through adulthood.
- *Oculopharyngeal muscular dystrophy (OPMD)*: OPMD affects adults of both sexes, causing weakness in the eye muscles and throat.
- *Distal muscular dystrophy (DD)*: DD is a group of rare muscle diseases that have weakness and wasting of the distal (farthest from the center) muscles of the forearms, hands, lower legs, and feet in common. In general, the DDs are less severe, progress more slowly, and involve fewer muscles than the other dystrophies. DD usually begins in middle age or later, causing weakness in the muscles of the feet and hands.
- *Congenital muscular dystrophy (CMD)*: CMD is a rare group of muscular dystrophies that have in common the presence of muscle weakness at birth (congenital) and abnormal muscle biopsies. CMD results in generalized weakness and usually progresses slowly.

Risk factors

The nine forms of muscular dystrophy are inherited. Therefore, people with a family history of MD are at increased risk.

Causes and symptoms

The muscular dystrophies are genetic conditions, meaning they are caused by alterations in genes. Parents pass along genes to their children, providing them with a complete set of instructions for making their own proteins.

Because both parents contribute genetic material to their offspring, each child carries two copies of almost every gene, one from each parent. For some conditions to occur, both copies must be altered. Such conditions are called autosomal recessive conditions. Some forms of LGMD and DD exhibit this pattern of inheritance, as does CMD. A person with only one altered copy, called a carrier, will not have the condition, but may pass the altered gene on to his children. When two carriers have children, the chances of having a child with the condition is one in four for each pregnancy.

Other conditions occur when only one altered gene copy is present. Such conditions are called autosomal dominant conditions. DM, FSH, and OPMD exhibit this pattern of inheritance, as do some forms of DD and LGMD. When a person affected by the condition has a child with someone not affected, the chances of having an affected child is one in two.

Because of chromosomal differences between the sexes, some genes are not present in two copies. The chromosomes that determine whether a person is male or female are called the X and Y chromosomes. A person with two X chromosomes is female, while a person with one X and one Y is male. While the X chromosome carries many genes, the Y chromosome carries almost none. Therefore, a male has only one copy of each gene on the X chromosome, and if it is altered, he will have the condition that alteration causes. Such conditions are said to be X-linked. X-linked conditions include DMD, BMD, and EDMD. Women are not usually affected by X-linked conditions, because they will likely have one unaltered copy as well as the altered one. Some female carriers of DMD have a mild form of the condition, probably because their one unaltered gene copy is shut down in some of their cells.

Women carriers of X-linked conditions have a one in two chance of passing the altered gene on to each child born. Daughters who inherit the altered gene will be carriers. A son born without the altered gene will be free of the condition and cannot pass it on to his children. A son born with the altered gene will have the condition. He will pass the altered gene on to each of his daughters, who will then be carriers, but to none of his sons (because they inherit his Y chromosome).

Not all genetic alterations are inherited. Up to one-third of DMD cases result from new mutations that occur as eggs are formed within the mother. New mutations are less common in other forms of muscular dystrophy.

Several of the muscular dystrophies, including DMD, BMD, CMD, and most forms of LGMD, are due to alterations in the genes for a complex of muscle proteins. This complex spans the muscle cell membrane (a thin sheath that surrounds each muscle cell) to unite a fibrous network on the interior of the cell with a fibrous network on the outside. Theory holds that by linking these two networks, the complex acts as a "shock absorber," redistributing and evening out the forces generated by contraction of the muscle, thereby preventing rupture of the muscle membrane. Alterations in the proteins of the complex lead to deterioration of the muscle during normal contraction and relaxation cycles. Symptoms of these conditions set in as the muscle gradually exhausts its ability to repair itself.

Both DMD and BMD are caused by alterations in the gene for the protein called dystrophin. The alteration leading to DMD prevents the formation of any dystrophin, while that of BMD allows some protein to be made, accounting for the differences in severity and age of onset between the two conditions. Differences among the other muscular dystrophies in terms of the muscles involved and the ages of onset are less easily explained.

A number of genes have been found to cause LGMD. A majority of the more severe autosomal recessive types of LGMD with childhood-onset are caused by alterations in the genes responsible for making proteins called sarcoglycans. The sarcoglycans are a complex of proteins that are normally located in the muscle cell membrane along with dystrophin. Loss of these proteins causes the muscle cell membrane to lose some of its shock absorber qualities. The genes responsible include LGMD2D on chromosome 17, which codes for the alpha-sarcoglycan protein; LGMD2E on chromosome 4, which codes for the beta-sarcoglycan protein; LGMD2C on chromosome 13, which codes for the gamma-sarcoglycan protein; and LGMD2F on chromosome 5, which codes for the delta-sarcoglycan protein. Some cases of autosomal recessive LGMD are caused by an alteration in a gene, LGMD2A, on chromosome 15, which codes for a muscle enzyme, calpain 3. The relationship between this alteration and the symptoms of the condition is unclear. Alterations in a gene called LGMD2B on chromosome 2 that codes for the dysferlin protein, is also responsible for a minority of autosomal recessive LGMD cases. The exact role of dysferlin is not known. Finally, alterations in the LGMD2G gene on chromosome 17 which codes for a protein, telethonin, is responsible for autosomal recessive LGMD in two reported families. The exact role of telethonin is not known. Some families with autosomal recessive LGMD are not accounted for by alterations in any of the above mentioned genes, indicating that there are as yet undiscovered genes which can cause LGMD. The autosomal dominant LGMD genes have mostly been described in single families. These types of LGMD are considered quite rare.

The causes of the other muscular dystrophies are not as well understood.

- EDMD is due to alterations in the genes that produce lamin A, lamin C, or emerin, three proteins that are found in the membrane of a cell's nucleus but whose exact function is unknown.

- Myotonic dystrophy is caused by alterations in a gene on chromosome 19 or chromosome 3. On chromosome 19, this alteration affects the genes for an enzyme called myotonin protein kinase that may control the flow of charged particles within muscle cells. This gene alteration is called a triple repeat, meaning it contains extra triplets of **DNA** code. It is possible that this alteration affects nearby genes as well and that the widespread symptoms of myotonic dystrophy are due to a range of genetic disruptions.

- The gene for OPMD appears to also be altered with a triple repeat. The function of the affected protein may involve translation of genetic messages in a cell's nucleus.

- The gene(s) for FSH is located on the long arm of chromosome 4 at gene location 4q35. Nearly all cases of FSH are associated with a deletion (missing piece) of genetic material in this region. Researchers are investigating the molecular connection of this deletion and FSH. It is not yet certain whether the deleted material contains an active gene or changes the regulation or activity of a nearby FSH gene. A small number of FSH cases are not linked to chromosome 4. Their linkage to any other chromosome or genetic feature is under investigation.

- The gene(s) responsible for DD have not yet been found.

- About 50% of individuals with CMD have their condition as a result of deficiency in a protein called merosin, which is made by a gene called laminin. The merosin protein usually lies outside muscle cells and links them to the surrounding tissue. When merosin is not produced, the muscle fibers degenerate soon after birth. A second gene called integrin is responsible for CMD in a few individuals but alterations in this gene are a rare cause of CMD. The gene responsible for Fukuyama CMD is FCMD, and it is responsible for making a protein called fukutin whose function is not clear.

All of the muscular dystrophies are marked by muscle weakness as the major symptom. The distribution of symptoms, age of onset, and progression differ significantly. Pain is sometimes a symptom of each, usually due to the effects of weakness on joint position.

DUCHENNE MUSCULAR DYSTROPHY (DMD). A boy with Duchenne muscular dystrophy usually begins to show symptoms as a preschooler. The legs are affected first, making walking difficult and causing balance problems. Most patients walk three to six months later than expected and have difficulty running. Later on, a boy with DMD will push his hands against his knees to rise to a standing position, to compensate for leg weakness. About the same time, his calves will begin to enlarge, though with fibrous tissue rather than with muscle, and feel firm and rubbery; this condition gives DMD one of its alternate names, pseudohypertrophic muscular dystrophy. He will widen his stance to maintain balance and walk with a waddling gait to advance his weakened legs. Contractures (permanent muscle tightening) usually begin by age five or six, most severely in the calf muscles. This pulls the foot down and back, forcing the boy to walk on tip-toes and further decreases balance. Climbing stairs and rising unaided may become impossible by age nine or ten, and most boys use a wheelchair for mobility by the age of 12. Weakening of the trunk muscles around this age often leads to **scoliosis** (a side-to-side spine curvature) and kyphosis (a front-to-back curvature).

The most serious weakness of DMD is weakness of the diaphragm, the sheet of muscles at the top of the abdomen that perform the main work of breathing and coughing. Diaphragm weakness leads to reduced energy and stamina and increased lung infection because of the inability to cough effectively. Young men with DMD often live into their twenties and beyond, provided they have mechanical ventilation assistance and good respiratory hygiene.

Among males with DMD, the incidence of cardiomyopathy (weakness of the heart muscle) increases steadily in teenage years. Almost all patients have cardiomyopathy after 18 years of age. It has also been shown that carrier females are at increased risk for cardiomyopathy and should also be screened.

About one-third of males with DMD experience specific learning disabilities, including difficulty learning by ear rather than by sight and difficulty paying attention to long lists of instructions. Individualized educational programs usually compensate well for these disabilities.

BECKER MUSCULAR DYSTROPHY (BMD). The symptoms of BMD usually appear in late childhood to early adulthood. Though the progression of symptoms may parallel that of DMD, the symptoms are usually milder and the course more variable. The same pattern of leg weakness, unsteadiness, and contractures occur later for the young man with BMD, often allowing independent walking into the twenties or early thirties. Scoliosis may occur but is usually milder and progresses more slowly. Cardiomyopathy occurs more commonly in BMD. Problems may include irregular heartbeats (arrhythmias) and congestive heart failure. Symptoms may include fatigue, shortness of breath, chest pain, and dizziness. Respiratory weakness also occurs and may lead to the need for mechanical ventilation.

EMERY-DREIFUSS MUSCULAR DYSTROPHY (EDMD). This type of muscular dystrophy usually begins in early childhood, often with contractures preceding muscle weakness. Weakness affects the shoulder and upper arm initially, along with the calf muscles, leading to foot-drop. Most men with EDMD survive into middle age, although an abnormality in the heart's rhythm (heart block) may be fatal if not treated with a pacemaker.

LIMB-GIRDLE MUSCULAR DYSTROPHY (LGMD). While there are several genes that cause the various types of LGMD, two major clinical forms of LGMD are usually recognized. A severe childhood form is similar in appearance to DMD but is inherited as an autosomal recessive trait. Symptoms of adult-onset LGMD usually appear in a person's teens or twenties and are marked by progressive weakness and wasting of the muscles closest to the trunk. Contractures may occur, and the ability to walk is usually lost about 20 years after onset. Some people with LGMD develop respiratory weakness that requires use of a ventilator. Life-span may be somewhat shortened. Autosomal dominant forms usually occur later in life and progress relatively slowly.

FACIOSCAPULOHUMERAL MUSCULAR DYSTROPHY (FSH). FSH varies in its severity and age of onset, even among members of the same family. Symptoms most commonly begin in the teens or early twenties, though infant or childhood onset is possible. Symptoms tend to be more severe in those with earlier onset. The condition is named for the regions of the body most severely affected by the condition: muscles of the face (facio-), shoulders (scapulo-), and upper arms (humeral). Hips and legs may be affected as well. Children with FSH may develop partial or complete deafness.

The first symptom noticed is often difficulty lifting objects above the shoulders. The weakness may be greater on one side than the other. Shoulder weakness also causes the shoulder blades to jut backward, called scapular winging. Muscles in the upper arm often lose bulk sooner than those of the forearm, giving a "Popeye" appearance to the arms. Facial weakness may lead to loss of facial expression, difficulty closing the eyes completely, and inability to drink through a straw, blow up a balloon, or whistle. A person with FSH may not be able to wrinkle their forehead. Contracture of the calf muscles may cause foot-drop, leading to frequent tripping over curbs or rough spots. People with earlier onset often require a wheelchair for mobility, while those with later onset rarely do.

MYOTONIC DYSTROPHY. Symptoms of myotonic dystrophy include facial weakness and a slack jaw, drooping eyelids (ptosis), and muscle wasting in the forearms and calves. A person with myotonic dystrophy has difficulty relaxing his grasp, especially if the object is cold. Myotonic dystrophy affects heart muscle, causing arrhythmias and heart block, and the muscles of the digestive system, leading to motility disorders and constipation. Other body systems are affected as well; myotonic dystrophy may cause cataracts, retinal degeneration, mental deficiency, frontal balding, skin disorders, testicular atrophy, sleep apnea, and insulin resistance. An increased need or desire for sleep is common, as is diminished motivation. The condition is extremely variable; some individuals show profound weakness as a newborn (congenital myotonic dystrophy), others show mental retardation in childhood, many show characteristic facial features and muscle wasting in adulthood, while the most mildly affected individuals show only cataracts in middle age with no other symptoms. Individuals with a severe form of mytonic dystropy typically have severe

disabilities within 20 years of onset, although most do not require a wheelchair even late in life.

OCULOPHARYNGEAL MUSCULAR DYSTROPHY (OPMD). OPMD usually begins in a person's thirties or forties, with weakness in the muscles controlling the eyes and throat. Symptoms include drooping eyelids and difficulty swallowing (dysphagia). Weakness progresses to other muscles of the face, neck, and occasionally the upper limbs. Swallowing difficulty may cause aspiration or the introduction of food or saliva into the airways. Pneumonia may follow.

DISTAL MUSCULAR DYSTROPHY (DD). DD usually begins in the twenties or thirties, with weakness in the hands, forearms, and lower legs. Difficulty with fine movements such as typing or fastening buttons may be the first symptoms. Symptoms progress slowly, and the condition usually does not affect life span.

CONGENITAL MUSCULAR DYSTROPHY (CMD). CMD is marked by severe muscle weakness from birth, with infants displaying "floppiness" and very poor muscle tone, and they often have trouble moving their limbs or head against gravity. Mental function is normal but some are never able to walk. They may live into young adulthood or beyond. In contrast, children with Fukuyama CMD are rarely able to walk and have severe mental retardation. Most children with this type of CMD die in childhood.

Diagnosis

For most forms of muscular dystrophy, accurate diagnosis is not difficult when done by someone familiar with the range of conditions. There are exceptions, however. Even with a muscle biopsy, it may be difficult to distinguish between FSH and another muscle condition, polymyositis. Childhood-onset LGMD is often mistaken for the much more common DMD, especially when it occurs in boys. BMD with an early onset appears very similar to DMD, and a genetic test may be needed to accurately distinguish them. The muscular dystrophies may be confused with conditions involving the motor neurons, such as **spinal muscular atrophy**; conditions of the neuromuscular junction, such as **myasthenia gravis**; and other muscle conditions, as all involve generalized weakness of varying distribution.

Examination

The diagnosis of muscular dystrophy involves a careful medical history and a thorough physical exam to determine the distribution of symptoms and to rule out other causes. Family history may give important clues, since all the muscular dystrophies are genetic conditions (though no family history will be evident in

Amniocentesis—A procedure performed at 16–18 weeks of pregnancy in which a needle is inserted through a woman's abdomen into her uterus to draw out a small sample of the amniotic fluid from around the fetus. Either the fluid itself or cells from the fluid can be used for a variety of tests to obtain information about genetic disorders and other medical conditions in the fetus.

Autosomal dominant—A pattern of genetic inheritance where only one abnormal gene is needed to display the trait or disease.

Autosomal recessive—A pattern of genetic inheritance where two abnormal genes are needed to display the trait or disease.

Becker muscular dystrophy (BMD)—A type of muscular dystrophy that affects older boys and men, and usually follows a milder course than Duchenne muscular dystrophy.

Chorionic villus sampling (CVS)—A procedure used for prenatal diagnosis at 10–12 weeks gestation. Under ultrasound guidance a needle is inserted either through the mother's vagina or abdominal wall and a sample of cells is collected from around the fetus. These cells are then tested for chromosome abnormalities or other genetic diseases.

Contracture—A tightening of muscles that prevents normal movement of the associated limb or other body part.

Distal muscular dystrophy (DD)—A form of muscular dystrophy that usually begins in middle age or later, causing weakness in the muscles of the feet and hands.

Duchenne muscular dystrophy (DMD)—The most severe form of muscular dystrophy, DMD usually affects young boys and causes progressive muscle weakness, usually beginning in the legs.

Dystrophin—A protein that helps muscle tissue repair itself. Both Duchenne muscular dystrophy and Becker muscular dystrophy are caused by flaws in the gene that instructs the body how to make this protein.

Facioscapulohumeral muscular dystrophy (FSH)—This form of muscular dystrophy, also known as Landouzy-Dejerine condition, begins in late childhood to early adulthood and affects both men and women, causing weakness in the muscles of the face, shoulders, and upper arms.

Limb-girdle muscular dystrophy (LGMD)—Form of muscular dystrophy that begins in late childhood to early adulthood and affects both men and women, causing weakness in the muscles around the hips and shoulders.

Myotonic dystrophy—A form of muscular dystrophy, also known as Steinert's condition, characterized by delay in the ability to relax muscles after forceful contraction, wasting of muscles, as well as other abnormalities.

Oculopharyngeal muscular dystrophy (OPMD)—Form of muscular dystrophy affecting adults of both sexes, and causing weakness in the eye muscles and throat.

the event of new mutations; in autosomal recessive inheritance, the family history may also be negative).

Tests

Lab tests may include:

- Blood level of the muscle enzyme creatine kinase (CK). CK levels rise in the blood due to muscle damage, and may be seen in some conditions even before symptoms appear.

- Muscle biopsy, in which a small piece of muscle tissue is removed for microscopic examination. Changes in the structure of muscle cells and presence of fibrous tissue or other aberrant structures are characteristic of different forms of muscular dystrophy. The muscle tissue can also be stained to detect the presence or absence of particular proteins, including dystrophin.

- Electromyogram (EMG). This electrical test is used to examine the response of the muscles to stimulation. Decreased response is seen in muscular dystrophy. Other characteristic changes are seen in DM.

- Genetic tests. Several of the muscular dystrophies can be positively identified by testing for the presence of the altered gene involved. Accurate genetic tests are available for DMD, BMD, DM, several forms of LGMD, and EDMD. **Genetic testing** for some of these conditions in future pregnancies of an affected individual or parents of an affected individual can be done before birth through **amniocentesis** or chorionic villus sampling. Prenatal testing can only be undertaken after the diagnosis in the affected individual has been genetically confirmed and the couple has been counseled regarding the risks of recurrence.

• Other specific tests as necessary. For EDMD, DMD and BMD, for example, an electrocardiogram may be needed to test heart function, and hearing tests are performed for children with FSH.

Prenatal diagnosis (testing of the baby while in the womb) can be done for those types of muscular dystrophy where the specific disease-causing gene alteration has been identified in a previously affected family member. Prenatal diagnosis can be done utilizing DNA extracted from tissue obtained by chorionic villus sampling or amniocentesis.

Treatment

There is no specific treatment that can stop or reverse any form of muscular dystrophy. MD management is focused on improving muscle and joint function, and slowing muscle deterioration. Treatment also seeks to prevent the complications of weakness, including decreased mobility and dexterity, contractures, scoliosis, heart alterations, and respiratory insufficiency.

Traditional

Physical therapy, regular stretching in particular, is used to maintain the range of motion of affected muscles and to prevent or delay contractures. Braces are used as well, especially on the ankles and feet to prevent tip-toeing. Full-leg braces may be used in children with DMD to prolong the period of independent walking. Strengthening other muscle groups to compensate for weakness may be possible if the affected muscles are few and isolated, as in the earlier stages of the milder muscular dystrophies. Regular, nonstrenuous exercise helps maintain general good health. Strenuous exercise is usually not recommended, since it may damage muscles further.

Occupational therapy also provides techniques and tools to compensate for the loss of strength and dexterity. Strategies may include modifications in the home, adaptive utensils and dressing aids, compensatory movements and positioning, wheelchair accessories, or communication aids.

Good nutrition helps to promote general health in all the muscular dystrophies. No special diet or supplement has been shown to be of use in any of the conditions. The weakness in the throat muscles seen especially in OPMD and later DMD may necessitate the use of a gastrostomy tube, inserted in the stomach to provide nutrition directly.

Drugs

For DMD, prednisone, a corticosteroid, has been shown to delay the progression of disease somewhat, for reasons that are still unclear. Some have reported improvement in strength and function in patients treated with a single dose. Improvement begins within ten days and plateaus after three months. Long-term benefit has not been demonstrated. Prednisone is also prescribed for BMD, though no controlled studies have tested its benefit.

Anticonvulsants, also known as antiepileptics, are also prescribed to control seizures and some muscle activity. Commonly used oral anticonvulsants include carbamazepine, phenytoin, clonazepam, gabapentin, topiramate, and felbamate. Respiratory infections are usually treated with antibiotics.

Alternative

When contractures become more pronounced, tenotomy surgery may be performed. In this operation, the tendon of the contractured muscle is cut, and the limb is braced in its normal resting position while the tendon regrows. In FSH, surgical fixation of the scapula can help compensate for shoulder weakness. For a person with OPMD, surgical lifting of the eyelids may help compensate for weakened muscular control. For a person with DM, sleep apnea may be treated surgically to maintain an open airway. Scoliosis surgery is often needed in boys with DMD, but much less often in other muscular dystrophies. Surgery is recommended at a much lower degree of curvature for DMD than for scoliosis due to other conditions, since the decline in respiratory function in DMD makes surgery at a later time dangerous. In this surgery, the vertebrae are fused together to maintain the spine in the upright position. Steel rods are inserted at the time of operation to keep the spine rigid while the bones grow together.

When any type of surgery is performed in patients with muscular dystrophy, anesthesia must be carefully selected. People with MD are susceptible to a severe reaction, known as malignant hyperthermia, when given halothane anesthetic.

The arrhythmias of EDMD and BMD may be treatable with antiarrhythmia drugs. A pacemaker may be implanted if these do not provide adequate control. Heart transplants are increasingly common for men with BMD. A complete cardiac evaluation is recommended at least once in all carrier females of DMD and EDMD.

People who develop weakness of the diaphragm or other ventilatory muscles may require a mechanical ventilator to continue breathing deeply enough. Air may be administered through a nasal mask or mouthpiece or through a tracheostomy tube, which is inserted through a surgical incision through the neck and into the windpipe. Most people with muscular dystrophy do not need a tracheostomy, although some may prefer it to continual use of a mask or mouthpiece. Supplemental oxygen is not needed. Good hygiene of the lungs is critical for health and long-term survival of a person with weakened ventilatory muscles. Assisted cough techniques provide the strength needed to clear the airways of secretions; an assisted cough machine is also available and provides excellent results.

Clinical trials for the treatment of muscular dystrophies are currently sponsored by the National Institutes of Health (NIH) and other agencies. Researchers are investigating the following many aspects of MD:

• evaluation of whether a high-dose weekly course of prednisone therapy is safer than and at least as effective as daily dose therapy for people with DMD

• efficacy of carvedilol on cardiac dysfunction in DMD

• evaluation of the safety and efficacy of antisense oligonucleotides in Duchenne muscular dystrophy

• possible use of human stem cells to treat MD

• electrostimulation of shoulder girdle and quadriceps muscles in FSH patients

Clinical trial information is constantly updated by NIH and the most recent information on muscular dystrophy trials can be found online.

Prognosis

The expected life span for a male with DMD has increased significantly in the past two decades. Most young men will live into their early or mid-twenties. Respiratory infections become an increasing problem as their breathing becomes weaker, and these infections are usually the cause of death.

The course of the other muscular dystrophies is more variable; expected life spans and degrees of disability are hard to predict but may be related to age of onset and initial symptoms. Prediction is made more difficult because, as new genes are discovered, it is becoming clear that several of the dystrophies are not uniform disorders but rather symptom groups caused by different genes.

People with dystrophies with significant heart involvement (BMD, EDMD, myotonic dystrophy) may nonetheless have almost normal life spans, provided that cardiac complications are monitored and treated aggressively. The respiratory involvement of BMD and LGMD similarly require careful and prompt treatment.

QUESTIONS TO ASK YOUR DOCTOR

• What type of MD was diagnosed?

• How does MD affect muscles?

• What does the treatment plan involve?

• What are the side effects of prescribed medications?

• Why should my child wear night splints for the ankles and when should they start?

• What are the features of a good splint?

• What is the prognosis?

Prevention

There is no way to prevent any of the muscular dystrophies in a person who has the genes responsible for these disorders. Individuals with muscular dystrophy and their families may benefit from genetic counseling for information on the condition and recurrence risks for future pregnancies.

Resources

BOOKS

Abramovitz, Melissa. *Muscular Dystrophy (Diseases and Disorders)*. San Diego, CA: Lucent Books, 2008.

Emery, Alan. *Muscular Dystrophy: The Facts*. New York: Oxford University Press, 2008.

PERIODICALS

Davidson, Z. E., and H. Truby "A review of nutrition in Duchenne muscular dystrophy." *Journal of Human Nutrition and Dietetics* 22, no. 5 (2009): 383–93.

Farini, A., et al. "Cell based therapy for Duchenne muscular dystrophy." *Journal of Cell Physiology* 221, no. 3 (2009): 526–34.

Meregalli, M., et al. "Stem cell therapies to treat muscular dystrophy: progress to date." *BioDrugs* 24, no. 4 (2010): 237–47.

Muir, L. A., and J. S. Chamberlain. "Emerging strategies for cell and gene therapy of the muscular dystrophies." *Expert Reviews in Molecular Medicine* 11 (2009): e18.

Quattrocelli, M., et al. "Cell therapy strategies and improvements for muscular dystrophy." *Cell death and differentiation* 17, no. 8 (2010): 1222–29.

OTHER

"Becker Muscular Dystrophy (BMD)." *MDA*. Information Page. http://www.mda.org/disease/bmd.html (accessed December 12, 2009).

"Congenital Muscular Dystrophy (CMD)." *MDA*. Information Page. http://www.mda.org/disease/cmd.html (accessed December 12, 2009).

"Duchenne Muscular Dystrophy (DMD)." *MDA*. Information Page. http://www.mda.org/disease/dmd.html (accessed December 12, 2009).

"Emery-Dreifuss Muscular Dystrophy (EDMD)." *MDA*. Information Page. http://www.mda.org/disease/edmd.html (accessed December 12, 2009).

"Limb-Girdle Muscular Dystrophy (LGMD)." *MDA*. Information Page. http://www.mda.org/disease/lgmd.html (accessed December 12, 2009).

"Muscular Dystrophy." *NINDS*. Information Page. http://www.ninds.nih.gov/disorders/md/md.htm (accessed December 12, 2009).

"Myotonic Muscular Dystrophy (MMD)." *MDA*. Information Page. http://www.mda.org/disease/dm.html (accessed December 12, 2009).

ORGANIZATIONS

Centers for Disease Control and Prevention, 1600 Clifton Road, Atlanta, GA 30333, (800) 232-4636, cdcinfo@cdc.gov, http://www.cdc.gov.

Facioscapulohumeral Muscular Dystrophy (FSH) Society, 64 Grove Street, Watertown, MA 02472, (617) 658-7877, Fax: (617) 658-7879, info@fshsociety.org, http://www.fshsociety.org.

Muscular Dystrophy Association (MDA), 3300 East Sunrise Drive, Tucson, AZ 85718, (800) 572-1717, http://www.mda.org.

Muscular Dystrophy Canada, 2345 Yonge St., Suite 900, Toronto ON, Canada M4P 2E5, (866) MUSCLE-8, Fax: (416) 488-7523, info@muscle.ca, http://www.muscle.ca.

Muscular Dystrophy Family Foundation, 7220 U.S. 31 South, Indianapolis, IN 46227, (317) 923-MDFF, (800) 544-1213, Fax: (317) 923-6334, http://www.mdff.org.

National Institute of Arthritis and Musculoskeletal and Skin Diseases (NIAMS), 1 AMS Circle, Bethesda, MD 20892-3675, (301) 495-2966, (877) (877) 22-NIAMS, Fax: (301) 718-6366, NIAMSinfo@mail.nih.gov, http://www.niams.nih.gov.

National Institute of Child Health and Human Development (NICHD), P.O. Box 3006, Rockville, MD 20846, (800) 370-2943, Fax: (866) (301) 496-7101, NICHDInformationResearchCenter@mail.nih.gov, http://www.nichd.nih.gov.

National Institute of Neurological Disorders and Stroke (NINDS), PO Box 5801, Bethesda, MD 20824, (301) 496-5751, (800) 352-9424, http://www.ninds.nih.gov.

Nada Quercia, Msc, CCGC
Monique Laberge, PhD
Fran Hodgkins

Myasthenia gravis

Definition

Myasthenia gravis is an autoimmune disease that causes muscle **weakness**.

Demographics

About 30,000 people in the United States are affected by MG. The prevalence in the United States is estimated at 20 cases per 100,000. The disease occurs in all ethnic groups and in both genders. It can occur at any age but is most common in women who are in their late teens and early twenties and in men in their sixties and seventies.

Description

Myasthenia gravis (MG) affects the neuromuscular junction, interrupting the communication between nerve and muscle and thereby causing weakness. A person with MG may have difficulty moving their eyes, walking, speaking clearly, swallowing, and even breathing, depending on the severity and distribution of weakness. Increased weakness with exertion, and improvement with rest, is a characteristic feature of MG.

Causes and symptoms

Myasthenia gravis is an autoimmune disease, meaning it is caused by the body's own immune system. In MG, the immune system attacks a receptor on the surface of muscle cells. This prevents the muscle from receiving the nerve impulses that normally make it respond. MG affects "voluntary" muscles, which are those muscles under conscious control responsible for movement. It does not affect heart muscle or the "smooth" muscle found in the digestive system and other internal organs.

A muscle is stimulated to contract when the nerve cell controlling it releases acetylcholine molecules onto its surface. The acetylcholine lands on a muscle protein called the acetylcholine receptor. This leads to rapid chemical changes in the muscle which cause it to contract. Acetylcholine is then broken down by acetylcholinesterase enzyme, to prevent further stimulation.

In MG, immune cells create antibodies against the acetylcholine receptor. Antibodies are proteins normally involved in fighting infection. When these antibodies attach to the receptor, they prevent it from receiving acetylcholine, decreasing the ability of the muscle to respond to stimulation.

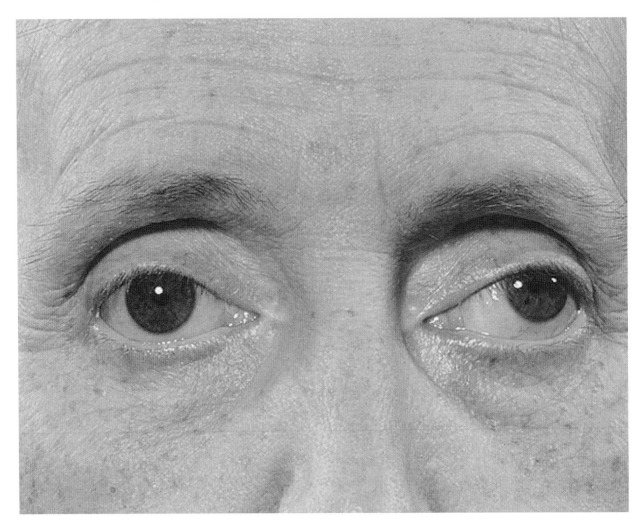

Although myasthenia gravis may affect any voluntary muscle, muscles that control eye and eyelid movement, facial expression, and swallowing are most frequently affected. *(© Custom Medical Stock Photo, Inc. Reproduced by permission.)*

Why the immune system creates these self-reactive "autoantibodies" is unknown, although there are several hypotheses:

- During fetal development, the immune system generates many B cells that can make autoantibodies, but B cells that could harm the body's own tissues are screened out and destroyed before birth. It is possible that the stage is set for MG when some of these cells escape detection.

- Genes controlling other parts of the immune system, called MHC genes, appear to influence how susceptible a person is to developing autoimmune disease.

- Infection may trigger some cases of MG. When activated, the immune system may mistake portions of the acetylcholine receptor for portions of an invading virus, though no candidate virus has yet been identified conclusively.

- About 10% of those with MG also have thymomas, or benign tumors of the thymus gland. The thymus is a principal organ of the immune system, and researchers speculate that thymic irregularities are involved in the progression of MG.

Some or all of these factors (developmental, genetic, infectious, and thymic) may interact to create the autoimmune reaction.

The earliest symptoms of MG often result from weakness of the extraocular muscles, which control eye movements. Symptoms involving the eye (ocular symptoms) include double vision (diplopia), especially when not gazing straight ahead, and difficulty raising the eyelids (ptosis). Individuals with ptosis may need to tilt their head back to see. Eye-related symptoms remain the only symptoms for about 15% of MG patients. Another common early symptom is difficulty chewing and swallowing, due to weakness in the bulbar muscles, which are in the mouth and throat. Choking becomes more likely, especially with food that requires extensive chewing.

Weakness usually becomes more widespread within several months of the first symptoms, reaching their maximum within a year in two-thirds of patients. Weakness may involve muscles of the arms, legs, neck, trunk, and face, and affect the ability to lift objects, walk, hold the head up, and speak.

Symptoms of MG become worse upon exertion and better with rest. Heat, including heat from the sun, hot showers, and hot drinks, may increase weakness. Infection and stress may worsen symptoms. Symptoms may vary from day to day and month to month, with intervals of no weakness interspersed with a progressive decline in strength.

"Myasthenic crisis" may occur, in which the breathing muscles become too weak to provide adequate respiration. Symptoms include weak and shallow breathing, shortness of breath, pale or bluish skin color, and a racing heart. Myasthenic crisis is an emergency condition requiring immediate treatment. In patients treated with anticholinesterase agents, myasthenic crisis must be differentiated from cholinergic crisis related to overmedication.

Pregnancy worsens MG in about one-third of women, has no effect in one third, and improves symptoms in another third. About 12% of infants born to women with MG have "neonatal myasthenia," a temporary but potentially life-threatening condition. It is caused by the transfer of maternal antibodies into the fetal circulation just before birth. Symptoms include weakness, floppiness, feeble cry, and difficulty feeding. The infant may have difficulty breathing, requiring the use of a ventilator. Neonatal myasthenia usually clears up within a month.

Some myasthenia gravis variants may be observed and associated with the use of certain drugs. The drug-induced symptoms may be associated with the administration of certain antibiotics, anti-rheumatics, and neuromuscular drugs. The development of myasthenic signs are usually within days of drug use and rapidly disappear after drug withdrawal. It is thought that patients who present with myasthenia gravis variants most likely have an underlying pre-existing disorder related to neuromuscular transmission.

Diagnosis

Myasthenia gravis is often diagnosed accurately by a careful medical history and a neuromuscular exam, but several tests are used to confirm the

---

KEY TERMS

Antibody—An immune protein normally used by the body for combating infection and which is made by B cells.

Autoantibody—An antibody that reacts against part of the self.

Autoimmune disease—A disease caused by a reaction of the body's immune system.

Bulbar muscles—Muscles that control chewing, swallowing, and speaking.

Neuromuscular junction—The site at which nerve impulses are transmitted to muscles.

Pyridostigmine bromide (Mestinon)—An anticholinesterase drug used in treating myasthenia gravis.

Tensilon test—A test for diagnosing myasthenia gravis. Tensilon is injected into a vein and, and in individuals who have MG, their muscle strength will improve for about five minutes.

Thymus gland—A small gland located just above the heart, involved in immune system development.

---

diagnosis. Other conditions causing worsening of bulbar and skeletal muscles must be considered, including drug-induced myasthenia, thyroid disease, **Lambert-Eaton myasthenic syndrome**, **botulism**, and inherited muscular dystrophies.

MG causes characteristic changes in the electrical responses of muscles that may be observed with an electromyogram, which measures muscular response to electrical stimulation. Repetitive nerve stimulation leads to reduction in the height of the measured muscle response, reflecting the muscle's tendency to become fatigued.

Blood tests may confirm the presence of the antibody to the acetylcholine receptor, though up to one-fourth of MG patients will not have detectable levels. A chest x ray or chest computed tomography (CT) scan may be performed to look for thymoma.

Treatment

While there is no cure for myasthenia gravis, there are a number of treatments that effectively control symptoms in most people.

Edrophonium (Tensilon) blocks the action of acetylcholinesterase, prolonging the effect of acetylcholine and increasing strength. An injection of edrophonium rapidly leads to a marked improvement in most people with MG. An alternate drug, neostigmine, may also be used.

Pyridostigmine (Mestinon) is usually the first drug tried. Like edrophonium, pyridostigmine blocks acetyl-cholinesterase. It is longer-acting, taken by mouth, and well-tolerated. Loss of responsiveness and disease progression combine to eventually make pyridostigmine ineffective in tolerable doses in many patients.

Thymectomy, or surgical removal of the thymus gland, has increasingly become standard treatment for MG. Up to 85% of people with MG improve after thymectomy, with complete remission eventually seen in about 30%. The improvement may take months or even several years to fully develop. Thymectomy is not usually recommended for children with MG, since the thymus continues to play an important immune role throughout childhood.

Immune-suppressing drugs are used to treat MG if response to pyridostigmine and thymectomy are not adequate. Drugs include corticosteroids such as prednisone and the non-steroids azathioprine (Imuran) and cyclosporine (Sandimmune). These drugs help suppress the abnormal immune system functioning associated with MS.

Plasma exchange (called plasmapheresis) may be performed to treat myasthenic crisis or to improve very weak patients before thymectomy. In this procedure, blood plasma is removed and replaced with purified plasma free of autoantibodies. Improvement in muscle strength may be apparent, but it is usually short-lived. The procedure can produce a temporary improvement in symptoms but is considered quite costly for extensive, long-term treatment. Another blood treatment, intravenous immunoglobulin therapy, is also used for myasthenic crisis. In this procedure, large quantities of purified immune proteins (immunoglobulins) are injected. For unknown reasons, this leads to symptomatic improvement in up to 85% of patients. It is also considered costly for long-term treatment.

People with weakness of the bulbar muscles may need to eat softer foods that are easier to chew and swallow. In more severe cases, it may be necessary to obtain nutrition through a feeding tube placed into the stomach (gastrostomy tube).

Clinical trials

Clinical trials of new drugs and drug combinations to treat myasthenia gravis are ongoing. Individuals with myasthenia gravis who wish to participate in the trial of an experimental therapy can find a list of clinical trials currently enrolling volunteers at

QUESTIONS TO ASK YOUR DOCTOR

- What are the indications that I may have myasthenia gravis?
- What diagnostic tests are needed for a thorough assessment?
- Can you estimate how rapidly my symptoms will progress?
- What treatment options do you recommend for me?
- What kind of changes can I expect to see with the medications you have prescribed for me?
- What are the side effects associated with the medications you have prescribed for me?
- Will medications for myasthenia gravis interact with my current medications?
- What kind of specialists should I contact?
- If surgery is needed, what kind of surgical specialist should I contact?
- What tests or evaluation techniques will you perform to see if treatment has been beneficial for me?
- What changes in my health can I expect to see as my condition progresses?
- What physical or psychological limitations do you foresee?
- Will physical, occupational, or speech therapy benefit me?
- Does having myasthenia gravis put me at risk for other health conditions?
- How can my quality of life be improved?
- What research is being done to learn more about myasthenia gravis?
- What symptoms or adverse effects are important enough that I should seek immediate treatment?
- Can you recommend an organization that will provide me with additional information about myasthenia gravis?
- Can you refer me to a qualified person who can make an assessment of my home and recommend changes to make it safer and easier for me to get around?
- Can you recommend any support groups for me and my family?

http://clinicaltrials.gov. There is no cost to the patient to participate in a clinical trial.

Prognosis

Most people with MG can be treated successfully enough to prevent their condition from becoming debilitating; however, in some cases, symptoms may worsen even with vigorous treatment, leading to generalized weakness and disability. MG rarely causes early death except from myasthenic crisis.

Prevention

There is no known way to prevent myasthenia gravis. Thymectomy improves symptoms significantly in many patients, and relieves them entirely in some. Avoiding heat can help minimize symptoms.

Some drugs should be avoided by people with MG because they interfere with normal neuromuscular function.

Drugs to be avoided or used with caution include:

- many types of antibiotics, including erythromycin, streptomycin, and ampicillin
- some cardiovascular drugs, including Verapamil, betaxolol, and propranolol
- some drugs used in psychiatric conditions, including chlorpromazine, clozapine, and lithium

Many other drugs may worsen symptoms as well, so patients should check with the doctor who treats their MG before taking any new drugs.

A Medic-Alert card or bracelet provides an important source of information to emergency providers about the special situation of a person with MG. They are available from health care providers.

Resources

BOOKS

Benatat, Michael. *Neuromuscular Disease: Evidence and Analysis in Clinical Neurology*. Totowa, NJ: Humana, 2010.

Bennett, Robin L. *The Practical Guide to the Genetic Family History*. 2nd ed. New York: Wiley-Blackwell, 2010.

"Chapter 45: Electrophysiologic Testing and Laboratory Aids in the Diagnosis of Neuromuscular Disease." In *Adams and Victor's Principles of Neurology*, edited by Maurice Victor and Raymond D. Adams. New York: McGraw-Hill, 2009.

"Chapter 48: Principles of Clinical Myology: Diagnosis and Classification of Muscle Diseases-General Considerations." In *Adams and Victor's Principles of Neurology*, edited by Maurice Victor and Raymond D. Adams. New York: McGraw-Hill, 2009.

Jenkinson, Crispin, Michele Peters, and Mark B. Bromberg, eds. *Quality of Life Measurement in Neurodegenerative and Related Conditions*. New York: Cambridge University Press, 2011.

Kaminski, Henry J., ed. *Myasthenia Gravis and Related Disorders*. 2nd ed. Totowa, NJ: Humana, 2011.

Monaghan, Gerri, and Brian Monaghan. *When a Loved One Falls Ill: How to Be an Effective Patient Advocate*. New York: Workman, 2011.

Sayadi, Roya, and Joel Herskowitz. *Swallow Safely: How Swallowing Problems Threaten the Elderly and Others. A Caregiver's Guide to Recognition, Treatment, and Prevention*. Natick, MA: Inside/ Outside, 2010.

WEBSITES

Clinical Trials Website. http://www.clinicaltrials.gov/ct/ action/GetStudy (accessed July 17, 2011).

"Myasthenia Gravis." MedlinePlus. http://www.nlm.nih. gov/medlineplus/myastheniagravis.html (accessed July 17, 2011).

"Myasthenia Gravis Center." University of Maryland Medical Center. http://www.umm.edu/mg/?gclid = CNjHjrLdl6kCFVJ25Qod_xbNsg (accessed July 17, 2011).

ORGANIZATIONS

American Academy of Physical Medicine and Rehabilitation, 9700 West Bryn Mawr Avenue, Suite 200, Rosemont, IL 60018-5701, (847) 737-6000, Fax: (847) 737-6001, info@aapmr.org, http://www. aapmr.org.

American Physical Therapy Association, 1111 North Fairfax Street, Alexandria, VA 22314-1488, (800) 999-APTA (2782), (703) 684-APTA (2782), http:// www.apta.org.

Family Caregiver Alliance, 180 Montgomery Street, Suite 900, San Francisco, CA 94104, (415) 434-3388, (800) 445-8106, http://www.caregiver.org.

Genetic and Rare Diseases Information Center (GARD), P.O. Box 8126, Gaithersburg, MD 20898-8126, (301) 251-4925, Fax: (301) 251-4911, (888) 205-2311, http://rarediseases.info.nih.gov/GARD/ Default.aspx.

Myasthenia Gravis Foundation of America, 355 Lexington Avenue, 15th Floor, New York, NY 10017, Fax: (212) 370-9047, (800) 541-5454, http://www.myasthenia.org.

National Institute of Neurological Disorders and Stroke (NINDS), P.O. Box 5801, Bethesda, MD 20824, (301) 496-5751, (800) 352-9424, http://www.ninds. nih.gov.

National Institutes of Health (NIH), 9000 Rockville Pike, Bethesda, MD 20892, (301) 496-4000, NIHinfo@od.nih.gov, http://www.nih.gov/ index.html.

National Organization for Rare Disorders (NORD), 55 Kenosia Avenue, P.O. Box 1968, Danbury, CT 06813-1968, (203) 744-0100, (800) 999-6673, http:// www.rarediseases.org.

U.S. National Library of Medicine, 8600 Rockville Pike, Bethesda, MD 20894, (301) 594-5983, (888) 346-3656, Fax: (301) 402-1384, custserv@nlm. nih.gov, http://www.nlm.nih.gov.

Richard Robinson
Laura Jean Cataldo, RN, Ed

Myelinoclastic diffuse sclerosis *see* **Schilder's disease**

Myoclonic encephalopathy of infants *see* **Opsoclonus myoclonus**

Myoclonus

Definition

Myoclonus is a brief, rapid, shock-like jerking movement.

Description

Myoclonus can be a symptom of a separate disorder or can be the only or primary neurological finding, in which case it is termed "essential myoclonus." Myoclonus may occur in epilepsy or following many different types of brain injury, such as lack of oxygen, stroke, trauma, or poisoning. Myoclonus can occur in one or more limbs or may be generalized, involving much of the body.

Demographics

Because myoclonus is so often part of another disorder, the prevalence of myoclonus is not known with certainty. One study indicates that the prevalence of all types of myoclonus may be approximately 10 per 100,000 population.

Causes and symptoms

Myoclonus can be a symptom of a very wide variety of disorders. A partial list includes:

- epilepsy (several types)
- Tay-Sachs disease and other storage diseases
- Spinocerebellar degenerative diseases
- Hallervorden-Spatz syndrome
- Huntington's disease
- Multiple system atrophy

- corticobasal degeneration
- Creutzfeldt-Jakob disease
- Brain infections, including HIV
- Focal brain damage, including from stroke or tumor
- Heat stroke
- Electrical shock
- Hypoxia (oxygen deprivation)
- toxins and drugs

Myoclonus also occurs normally, as a person falls asleep or while sleeping. This type of myoclonus is not associated with disease.

Diagnosis

The diagnosis of myoclonus is not difficult and depends on careful patient description of the symptoms. Much more effort is devoted to determining the underlying cause. Blood tests, neuroimaging studies, genetic tests, electroencephalography (EEG) and other types of studies may be performed in order to determine the underlying disorder.

Treatment team

Myoclonus is treated by a neurologist.

Treatment

If an underlying disorder can be identified, this is treated with the expectation that successful treatment may diminish the myoclonus. In many cases this is not possible, however. Alternatively, the underlying disorder may be discovered but cannot be treated. Such is the case with hypoxic myoclonus or damage done by a stroke or trauma.

Several medications can be used to reduce the severity or frequency of the myoclonus. **Valproic acid** and clonazepam are the two most widely used drugs. Anticholinergic drugs, such as benztropine or trihexyphenidyl, may be useful. Anticonvulsants may be helpful, as may **benzodiazepines**, depending on the type of myoclonus. **Deep brain stimulation** has been reported to help at least one patient. **Botulinum toxin** injection may be useful in focal myoclonus.

Recovery and rehabilitation

Treatment of myoclonus is rarely entirely successful. The patient is likely to have some residual myoclonus even with the most successful treatments. Nonetheless, treatment may reduce frequency and severity, allowing more normal function.

Prognosis

Myoclonus is not a life-threatening disorder but may continue to have a significant impact on quality of life and activities of daily living.

Resources

WEBSITES

Myoclonus Research Foundation. http://www.myoclonus.com/index.htm.
WE MOVE. www.wemove.org.

Richard Robinson

Myofibrillar myopathy

Definition

Myofibrillar myopathies (MFMs) are a group of skeletal muscle diseases that are frequently associated with involvement of the heart muscle. Myofibrillar myopathies can be hereditary or occur sporadically (spontaneously). The hallmark of myofibrillar disease is the abnormal accumulation of the protein desmin in the muscles, causing progressive **weakness**.

Description

The term myofibrillar **myopathy** was proposed in 1996 as a broad term for an abnormal pattern of muscle deterioration associated with the excess accumulation of multiple proteins that include desmin. Desmin, the main muscle intermediate fiber of the cytoskeleton (the fibrous network that provides structure for the cell), is a protein in cardiac, skeletal and smooth muscles. This protein interacts with other proteins to form a network that maintains the structure of the cell.

The main features of myofibrillar myopathies include shoulder and hip muscle deterioration, often called "limb-girdle" myopathy, along with weakness of muscles farther away from the center of the body, called distal muscle weakness. The muscles involved often include the heart, and complications such as conduction blocks, arrhythmias, and congestive heart failure are often experienced.

Most persons with myofibrillar myopathy develop the disorder due to an autosomal dominant or autosomal recessive inheritance pattern, which means that males and females are equally affected, and there is a 50% chance of passing on the disorder in each pregnancy. In an autosomal recessive inheritance pattern,

the affected gene is recessive and one parent is its carrier. The risk of a child being affected with myofibrillar myopathy in an autosomal recessive inheritance pattern is 25% for each pregnancy. A lesser number of myofibrillar myopathy cases are sporadic, meaning no inheritance pattern can be found.

The pattern of weakness in this condition is often similar to patients with the other limb-girdle muscular dystrophies, but some patients have more weakness in the hands and ankles in addition to the more typical shoulder and hip weakness. Myofibrillar myopathy, like limb-girdle muscular dystrophy, slowly worsens over time, but the rate of progression is variable and some affected persons remain functional for many years.

Desmin-related myopathy (DRM) is a subgroup of myofibrillar myopathy and is the most clearly recognized type among this group. DRM was originally described as a skeletal and cardiac myopathy characterized by abnormal accumulation of desmin within muscle fibers. This definition focused attention on desmin as a key molecule associated with a diverse group of clinically and pathologically related disorders.

Demographics

The true incidence of myofibrillar myopathy is unknown, but it is very rare. Both sexes are affected equally in MFM since inheritance is usually autosomal recessive or autosomal dominant.

Causes and symptoms

Causes

Two gene mutations have been described in myofibrillar myopathy. Mutations on chromosome 2 in the gene for desmin are transmitted in an autosomal-dominant or recessive inheritance pattern. Mutations on chromosome 11 in the gene for αBC (alpha-B-crystallin) are transmitted in an autosomal-dominant inheritance pattern, which can also cause a desmin storage myopathy.

Defects in the function of desmin, as well as in other proteins, cause fragility of the myofibrils, structures in muscles that help them contract. In the heart, normal desmin protects the structural integrity of myofibrils during repeated muscle contractures over time. When desmin accumulates in abnormal amounts and locations of the heart muscle cell, myofibrils degrade and lose their ability to contract efficiently, resulting in weakness and inefficient pumping ability of the heart.

Symptoms

Myofibrillar myopathy becomes apparent in early to middle adulthood when muscle weakness in the lower extremities and gait (manner of walking) disturbances develop. The myopathy slowly progresses to also involve respiratory, facial, and heart muscles. Occasionally, this pattern is reversed and the heart muscle shows weakness before the skeletal muscles. Symptoms of alterations in the heart include abnormal rhythms that may cause **fainting** or, rarely, sudden death.

Diagnosis

Diagnostic difficulties arise from the fact that the disease has many variations: in some cases, myofibrillar myopathy is a relentlessly progressive skeletal disorder with no signs of cardiac involvement, while in others, cardiomyopathy (weak heart muscle action) is the leading or even exclusive feature. Respiratory muscle insufficiency may also be a major factor in myofibrillar myopathy and is a leading cause of death.

Most of the known genetic mutations responsible for myofibrillar myopathy are autosomal dominant, but some are autosomal recessive. A significant number of the mutations also occur spontaneously without inheritance pattern. For this reason, genetic testing is critical for establishing an accurate diagnosis. The true prevalence of myofibrillar myopathy may be assessed only when most or all persons with characteristic symptoms are tested genetically.

Electromyography (EMG) and nerve conduction studies (NCSs) should be performed in all persons in whom a myofibrillar myopathy is suspected. EMG and NCSs are important to exclude causes of weakness that result from nerve malfunction, including peripheral nerve disorders. Because electromyography involves inserting a needle into a muscle, it is becoming less favored in investigating muscle weakness in children, but it still has an important role in the diagnosis of the adult disease. In myofibrillar myopathy, **nerve conduction study** findings are normal and EMG findings are either normal or show typical patterns of myopathies.

Muscle **biopsy** is an important part of the diagnostic approach because it shows myofibrillar myopathy's histologic features (i.e., its organization and effect on tissue structure). In the typical diagnostic sequence, muscle biopsy is done first, then genetic studies are pursued.

Treatment team

The treatment team of hereditary muscle diseases, depending on the needs of a particular patient, includes a neurologist, pulmonologist, cardiologist, orthopedic surgeon, physiatrist, physical therapist, orthotist, and genetic counselors.

Because the diagnosis of hereditary myopathy is often difficult, interpretation of muscle biopsy, laboratory tests, and electrodiagnostic studies should be performed by a clinician experienced in the diagnosis and treatment of neuromuscular diseases.

Treatment

No specific treatment is available for any of the myofibrillar myopathies, but aggressive supportive care is essential to preserve muscle activity, to allow for maximal functional ability, and to prolong life expectancy.

The primary concerns are preventing and correcting skeletal abnormalities (e.g., scoliosis, foot deformities, and contractures) and maintaining ambulation. Aggressive use of passive stretching, bracing, and orthopedic procedures allows the affected person to remain independent for as long as possible.

Complications with the heart and lungs are the other chief concern. Early intervention to treat cardiac and respiratory insufficiency, at times requiring intermittent positive pressure ventilation (BiPAP/CPAP), can help improve function and prolong life expectancy.

Orthopedic surgery may be needed to help correct or prevent contractures (rigid muscles near joints), foot deformities, and scoliosis.

While no dietary restrictions are indicated for persons with myopathies, the diet should be tailored to the caloric needs of the patient. This may include restricting calories, especially in children with minimal mobility.

Recovery and rehabilitation

To date, there is no known treatment, medicine, or surgery that will cure MFM or stop the muscles from weakening. The goal is to prevent deformity and allow the patient to function as independently as possible. Since myofibrillar myopathy is a life-long condition that is not correctable, management includes focusing on preventing or minimizing deformities and maximizing the patient's functional ability at home and in the community.

In general, patients are given supportive care, together with leg braces and physical therapy, to maximize their ability to function in daily life. Stretching limbs to avoid tightened tendons and muscles is particularly important.

KEY TERMS

Cardiomyopathy—A disease of the heart muscle that leads to generalized deterioration of the muscle and its pumping ability.

Cytoskeleton—A network of filaments that give structure and shape to the cell.

Desmin—A protein that provides part of the structure to heart, skeletal, and smooth muscle cells.

Limb-girdle myopathy—A muscular dystrophy-type disorder characterized by weakness in the muscles of the shoulders trunk, and pelvic girdle, often progressing to respiratory or cardiac failure.

Myopathy—A disorder of the muscles.

Clinical Trials

There are no clinical trials recruiting participants specific for myofibrillar myopathy.

Prognosis

Myofibrillar myopathies are among a large group of related, but distinct diseases. In general, it is expected that there will be slow progression of weakness, which worsens in affected muscles then spreads and progresses with time.

Heart muscle weakness and the tendency to have abnormal electrical activity of the heart can increase the risk of palpitations, fainting, and sudden death. Most patients with this group of diseases live into adulthood but do not reach their full life expectancy.

Special concerns

Genetic counseling is often helpful to assist patients with family-planning decisions.

Vigorous physical activity is often impossible (or impractical) for patients with significant weakness, but activities like swimming, water aerobics, and low-resistance exercise equipment are often tolerated very well. The goal of these activities should be to increase the number of calories burned but not to build strength.

Maintaining ambulation and functional ability with the aggressive use of physical therapy and bracing is highly recommended. Children and young adults are often encouraged to continue with school in regular classes, with modifications designed to meet their specific physical needs.

Resources within the community may be explored. Educational institutions have resources that may be used. Adaptive physical education programs and disabled student services are generally available for qualified individuals. Access and mobility concerns in the community invariably touch upon the adjustment issues faced by individuals with a progressive disability.

Resources

BOOKS

Amato, Anthony, and James Russell. *Neuromuscular Disorders*. McGraw-Hill Professional: 2008.

Rolak, Loren A. *Neurology Secrets*, 5th Edition. Mosby: 2010.

PERIODICALS

Selcen, D., et al. "Myofibrillar Myopathy: Clinical, Morphological and Genetic Studies in 63 Patients." *Brain* 127 (2004): 439–51.

WEBSITES

"Myofibrillar Myopathy." GeneReviews: NCBI Bookshelf. http://www.ncbi.nlm.nih.gov/books/NBK1499/ (accessed October 24, 2011).

"Myofibrillar myopathy." Genetics Home Reference (January 2011). http://ghr.nlm.nih.gov/condition/myofibrillar-myopathy (accessed October 24, 2011).

"Myofibrillar myopathy." OMIM: Genetic disorder catalog, Genetics Home Reference (January 2011). http://ghr.nlm.nih.gov/condition/myofibrillar-myopathy/show/OMIM (accessed October 24, 2011).

ORGANIZATIONS

American Heart Association. 7272 Greenville Avenue, Dallas, TX 75231-4596. Phone: (214) 373-6300. Fax: (214) 373-0268. Tollfree phone: (800) 242-8721. Email: inquire@heart.org. http://www.americanheart.org.

Muscular Dystrophy Association. 3300 East Sunrise Drive, Tucson, AZ 85718-3208. Phone: (520) 529-2000. Fax: (520) 529-5300. Tollfree phone: (800) 572-1717. Email: mda@mdausa.org. http://www.mdausa.org/.

National Institute of Arthritis and Musculoskeletal and Skin Diseases (NIAMS). Bldg. 31, Rm. 4C05, Bethesda, MD 20892-2350. Phone: (301) 496-8188. Tollfree phone: (877) 22-NIAMS (226-4267). Email: NIAMSInfo@mail.nih.gov. http://www.nih.gov/niams.

Francisco de Paula Careta
Iuri Drumond Louro, MD, PhD

Myopathy

Definition

Myopathy is a general term referring to any skeletal muscle disease or neuromuscular disorder. Myopathy can be acquired or inherited and occur at birth or later in life. Myopathies can result from endocrine disorders, metabolic disorders, muscle infection or inflammation, drugs, and mutations in genes.

Description

Skeletal muscle diseases, or myopathies, are disorders with structural changes or functional impairment of the muscle. These conditions can be differentiated from other diseases of the motor unit by characteristic clinical and laboratory findings. The main symptom is muscle **weakness** that can be either intermittent or persistent. Different myopathies types exist with different associated causes. The main types include congenital myopathy, muscular dystrophy, **inflammatory myopathy**, and drug-induced myopathy.

Congenital Myopathy (CM) is a term used for muscle disorders present at birth. According to this definition, the CMs could include hundreds of distinct neuromuscular syndromes and disorders. In general, this disease causes loss of muscle tone and muscle weakness in infancy and delayed motor skills, such as walking, later in childhood. Four distinct disorders are classified as CMs: central core disease, nemaline rod myopathy, centronuclear (myotubular) myopathy, and multicore myopathy.

Muscular Dystrophy (MD) refers to a group of genetic diseases characterized by progressive weakness and degeneration of the skeletal or voluntary muscles that control movement. The muscles of the heart and some other involuntary muscles are also affected in some forms of MD, and a few forms involve other organs as well. The major forms of MD are myotonic, Duchenne, Becker, limb-girdle, facioscapulohumeral, congenital, oculopharyngeal, distal and Emery-Dreifuss.

Inflammatory Myopathies (IM) are a group of muscle diseases involving the inflammation and degeneration of skeletal muscle tissues. They are thought to be autoimmune disorders. In IMs, inflammatory cells surround, invade, and destroy normal muscle fibers as though they were defective or foreign to the body. This eventually results in discernible muscle weakness. This muscle weakness is usually symmetrical and develops slowly over weeks to months or even years. The IMs include **dermatomyositis**, **polymyositis**, and **inclusion body myositis**.

Drug-induced Myopathy (DIM) is a muscle disease caused by toxic substances that produce muscle damage. The toxic substances may act directly on muscle cells, but muscle damage can also be secondary to electrolyte disturbances, excessive energy requirements, or the inadequate delivery of oxygen and nutrients due to muscle compression. Drug use may also result in development of an immunologic reaction directed against the muscle. Muscle damage can be generalized or local, as occurs when a drug is injected into a muscle.

Demographics

Worldwide, CMs account for about 14% of all myopathies. Central core disease accounts for 16% of cases; nemaline rod myopathy for 20%; centronuclear myopathy for 14%; and multicore myopathy for 10%. Prevalence of MD is higher in males. In the United States, Duchenne and Becker MD occur in approximately 1 in 3,300 boys. Overall incidence of MD is about 63 per 1 million people.

Worldwide incidence of IM is about 5–10 per 100,000 people. These disorders are more common in women. Incidence and prevalence of DIM are unknown. Myopathy caused by corticosteroids is the most common disorder, and it is more common in women.

Causes and symptoms

Causes

CMs and MDs are caused by a genetic defect. In both conditions, mutations have been identified in genes that encode for muscle proteins. The loss or dysfunction of these proteins presumably leads to the specific morphological feature in the muscle and to clinically noticeable muscle disease. For example, in Becker dystrophy, there is a less-active form of dystrophin (a protein involved in the complex interactions of the muscle membrane and extracellular environment) that may not be effective a gateway regulator, allowing some leakage of intracellular substances, resulting in the myopathy.

The causes of IM are not known. An autoimmune process is likely, as these conditions are often associated with other **autoimmune diseases** and because they respond to immunosuppressive medication. Muscle **biopsy** typically shows changes attributed to destruction by infiltrating lymphocytes (white blood cells).

In DIMs, there are a number of causative agents. Drugs such as lipid-lowering agents (statins, clofibrate and gemfibrizol), agents that cause hypokalemia (diuretics, theophylline, amphotericin B), lithium, succinylcholine, antibiotics (trimethoprim, isoniazid), anticonvulsants (**valproic acid**, lamotrigine, prolonged propofol infusion), vasopressin, colchicine, episilon, aminocaproic acid, high dose alfa-interferon and illicit drugs (cocaine, heroin, phencyclidine, amphetamines) are possible myopathy inducers.

Symptoms

Although symptoms depend on the type of myopathy, some generalizations can be made. Skeletal muscle weakness is the hallmark of most myopathies. In most myopathies, weakness occurs primarily in the muscles of the shoulders, upper arms, thighs, and pelvis (proximal muscles). In some cases, the distal muscles of the hands and feet may be involved during advanced stages of the disease. Other typical symptoms of muscle disease include the following:

- muscle aching
- muscle cramping
- muscle pain
- muscle stiffness
- muscle tenderness
- muscle tightness

Initially, individuals may feel fatigued during very light physical activity. Walking and climbing stairs may be difficult because of weakness in the pelvic and leg muscles that stabilize the trunk. Patients often find it difficult to rise from a chair. As the myopathy progresses, there may be muscle wasting.

Diagnosis

Generally, diagnosis involves several outpatient tests to determine the type of myopathy. Sometimes it is necessary to wait until the disease progresses to a point at which the syndrome can be identified.

A blood serum enzyme test measures how much muscle protein is circulating in the blood. Usually, this is helpful only at the early stages of the disease, when the sudden increase of muscle protein in the blood is conspicuous. Antibodies found in the blood might indicate an IM. DNA may be collected to evaluate whether one of the known genetic defects is present.

An electromyogram (EMG) measures the electrical activity of the muscle. It involves placing a tiny needle into the muscle and recording the muscular activity on a TV monitor (oscilloscope). This helps identify which muscles are weakened.

A muscle tissue biopsy involves surgically removing a very small amount of tissue to be examined under the microscope and analyzed for abnormalities.

Treatment team

A multidisciplinary team is involved in the treatment of myopathy patients. This team may include a neurologist, a rheumatologist, an orthopedic surgeon, a pulmonologist, a cardiologist, an orthopedist, a dermatologist, and a genetic counselor. It can also include physical and occupational therapists.

Treatment

Treatment depends on the cause, and goals are to slow progression of the disease and relieve symptoms.

Treatments range from drug therapy for MD and IM, to simply avoiding situations that work the muscles too hard. Some physicians recommend that patients keep their weight down (a lighter body demands less work from the muscles) and avoid overexerting their muscles. For MD, the corticosteroids deflazacort and prednisone seem to be the most effective medications. Calcium supplements and antidepressants may be prescribed to counteract the side effects. The IM is usually treated with drugs that suppress the action of the immune system such as methotrexate, cyclosporine, and azathioprine, all of which have potentially serious side effects. For CM, treatment involves supportive measures to help patients cope with the symptoms.

Recovery and rehabilitation

Physical therapy can prevent weakening in patient's healthy muscles; however, it cannot restore already weakened muscles. Occupational and respiratory therapy help patients learn how to use special equipment that can improve a person's quality of life.

Clinical trials

Updated information on clinical trials can be found on the National Institutes of Health clinical trials website at www.clinicaltrials.gov.

Prognosis

The prognosis for persons with myopathy varies. Some individuals have a normal life span and little or no disability. In others, however, the disorder may be progressive, severely disabling, life threatening, or fatal. If the underlying cause of the disorder can be treated successfully, the prognosis is usually good. Progressive myopathies that develop later in life usually have a better prognosis than conditions that develop during childhood. Persons with Duchenne MD rarely live beyond their middle to late 20s, and persons with Becker MD may live until middle age.

Special concerns

If the cardiac muscle is affected in later disease stages, abnormal heart rhythms or heart muscle insufficiency (cardiomyopathy) may develop. Cardiomyopathy patients are at risk for congestive heart failure.

When muscles involved in breathing weaken, there may be significant breathing difficulties and increased risk for pneumonia, flu, and other respiratory infections. In severe cases, patients may require a respirator.

KEY TERMS

Autoimmune disorder—A large group of diseases characterized by abnormal functioning of the immune system that produces antibodies against its own tissues.

Congenital—Present at birth.

Myopathy—Disease of the muscle, most often associated with weakness.

When swallowing muscles are affected, persons are at increased risk for choking and malnutrition.

Resources

BOOKS

Kagen, Lawrence J., ed. *The Inflammatory Myopathies.* Humana Press: 2009.

Mastaglia, Frank L., and David Hilton-Jones, eds. *Myopathies and Muscle Diseases: Handbook of Clinical Neurology. Elsevier: 2007.*

WEBSITES

"Muscle Disorders." MedlinePlus. (September 29, 2011). http://www.nlm.nih.gov/medlineplus/muscledisorders. html (accessed October 24, 2011).

"Myopathies, Structural, Congenital." Genetics Home Reference (October 17, 2011). http://ghr.nlm.nih.gov/ conditionGroup/myopathies-structural-congenital (accessed October 24, 2011).

"Myopathy Information Page." National Institute of Neurological Disorders and Stroke (NINDS) (September 9, 2011). http://www.ninds.nih.gov/disorders/myopathy/ myopathy.htm (accessed October 24, 2011).

ORGANIZATIONS

Muscular Dystrophy Association. 3300 East Sunrise Drive, Tucson, AZ 85718-3208. Phone: (520) 529-2000. Fax: (520) 529-5300. Tollfree phone: (800) 572-1717. Email: mda@mdausa.org. http://www. mdausa.org.

National Institute of Arthritis and Musculoskeletal and Skin Diseases: National Institutes of Health. Bldg. 31, Rm. 4C05, Bethesda, MD 20892-2350. Phone: (301) 496-8188. Tollfree phone: (877)22-NIAMS (226-4267). Email: NIAMSInfo@mail.nih.gov. http://www.nih. gov/niams.

Muscular Dystrophy Association. 3300 East Sunrise Drive, Tucson, AZ 85718-3208. Phone: (520) 529-2000. Fax: (520) 529-5300. Tollfree phone: (800) 572-1717. Email: mda@mdausa.org. http://www.mdausa.org.

Greiciane Gaburro Paneto
Iuri Drumond Louro

Myotonic dystrophy

Definition

Myotonic dystrophy is a progressive disease in which the muscles are weak and are slow to relax after contraction.

Description

Myotonic dystrophy (DM), also called dystrophia myotonica, myotonia atrophica, or Steinert's disease, is a common form of muscular dystrophy. DM is an inherited disease, affecting males and females approximately equally. About 30,000 people in the United States are affected. Symptoms may appear at any time from infancy to adulthood. DM causes general **weakness**, usually beginning in the muscles of the hands, feet, neck, or face. It slowly progresses to involve other muscle groups, including the heart. DM affects a wide variety of other organ systems as well.

A severe form of DM, congenital myotonic dystrophy or Thomsen's disease, may appear in newborns of mothers who have DM. Congenital means that the condition is present from birth. The incidence of congenital myotonic dystrophy is thought to be about 1:20,000.

DM occurs in about 1 per 7,000–8,000 people and has been described in people from all over the world.

Causes and symptoms

The most common type of DM is called DM1 and is caused by a mutation in a gene called myotonic dystrophy protein kinase (DMPK). The DMPK gene is located on chromosome 19q. When there is a mutation in this gene, a person develops DM1. The specific mutation that causes DM1 is called a trinucleotide repeat expansion.

Some families with symptoms of DM do not have a mutation in the DMPK gene. Scientists have found that the DM in many of these families is caused by a mutation in a gene on chromosome 3. These families are said to have DM2.

Congenital myotonic dystrophy has been linked to a region on chromosome 7 that contains a muscle chloride channel gene.

Trinucleotide repeats

In the DMPK gene, there is a section of the genetic code called a CTG repeat. The letters stand for three nucleotides (complex organic molecules) known as cytosine, thymine, and guanine, and are repeated a certain number of times. In people who have DM1, this sequence of nucleotides is repeated too many times—more than the normal number of 37 times—and thus this section of the gene is too big. This enlarged section of the gene is called a trinucleotide repeat expansion.

People who have repeat numbers in the normal range will not develop DM1 and cannot pass it to their children. Having more than 50 repeats causes DM1. People who have 38–49 repeats have a premutation and will not develop DM1 but can pass DM1 onto their children. Having repeats numbers greater than 1,000 causes congenital myotonic dystrophy.

In general, the more repeats in the affected range that someone has, the earlier the age of onset of symptoms and the more severe the symptoms. However, this is a general rule. It is not possible to look at a person's repeat number and predict at what age that person will begin to have symptoms or how that condition will progress.

Exactly how the trinucleotide repeat expansion causes myotonia, the inability to relax muscles, is not yet understood. The disease somehow blocks the flow of electrical impulses across the muscle cell membrane. Without proper flow of charged particles, the muscle cannot return to its relaxed state after it has contracted.

DM2 is caused by a CCTG (cytosine-cytosine-thymine-guanine) expansion on chromosome 3 at locus 3q21, but it is not known how this repeat affects muscle cell function.

Anticipation

Sometimes when a person who has repeat numbers in the affected or premutation range has children, the expansion grows larger. This is called anticipation. A larger expansion can result in an earlier age of onset in children than in their affected parent. Anticipation happens more often when a mother passes DM1 onto her children than when it is passed from the father. Occasionally repeat sizes stay the same or even get smaller when they are passed to a person's children.

Inheritance

DM is inherited through autosomal dominant inheritance. This means that equal numbers of males and females are affected. It also means that only one gene in the pair needs to have the mutation in order for a person to be affected. Since individuals only passes one copy of each gene onto their children, there is a 50% or one in two chance that persons who have DM will pass it onto each of their children. This percentage is not changed by results of other pregnancies. A person with a premutation also has a 50%, or one in two, chance of passing the altered gene on to each child. However, whether the child develops. DM1 depends on whether the trinucleotide repeat becomes further expanded. Individuals who have repeat numbers in the normal range cannot pass DM1 onto their children.

There is a range in the severity of symptoms in DM and not everyone will have all of the symptoms listed here.

Myotonic dystrophy causes weakness and delayed muscle relaxation called myotonia. Symptoms of DM include facial weakness and a slack jaw, drooping eyelids called ptosis, and muscle wasting in the forearms and calves. Individuals with DM have difficulty relaxing their grasp, especially in the cold. DM affects the heart muscle, causing irregularities in the heartbeat. It also affects the muscles of the digestive system, causing constipation and other digestive problems. DM may cause cataracts, retinal degeneration, low IQ, frontal balding, skin disorders, atrophy of the testicles, and diabetes. It can also cause sleep apnea—a condition in which normal breathing is interrupted during sleep. DM increases the need for sleep and decreases motivation. Severe disabilities do not set in until about 20 years after symptoms begin. Most people with myotonic dystrophy maintain the ability to walk, even late in life.

A severe form of DM, congenital myotonic dystrophy, may appear in newborns of mothers who have DM1. Congenital myotonic dystrophy is marked by severe weakness, poor sucking and swallowing responses, respiratory difficulty, delayed motor development, and **mental retardation**. Death in infancy is common in this type.

Some people who have a trinucleotide repeat expansion in their DMPK gene do not have symptoms or have very mild symptoms that go unnoticed. It is not unusual for a woman to be diagnosed with DM after she has an infant with congenital myotonic dystrophy.

Predictive testing

It is possible to test individuals who are at risk for developing DM1 before they are showing symptoms to see whether they inherited an expanded trinucleotide repeat. This is called predictive testing. Predictive testing cannot determine the age of onset that someone will begin to have symptoms or the course of the disease.

Diagnosis

Diagnosis of DM is not difficult once the disease is considered. However, the true problem may be masked because symptoms can begin at any age, can be mild or severe, and can occur with a wide variety of associated complaints. Diagnosis of DM begins with a careful medical history and a thorough physical exam to determine the distribution of symptoms and to rule out other causes. A family history of DM or unexplained weakness helps to establish the diagnosis.

A definitive diagnosis of DM1 is done by genetic testing, usually by taking a small amount of blood. The DNA in the blood cells is examined and the number of repeats in the DMPK gene is determined. Various other tests may be done to help establish the diagnosis, but only rarely would other testing be needed. An electromyogram (EMG) is a test is used to examine the response of the muscles to stimulation. Characteristic changes are seen in DM that help distinguish it from other muscle diseases. Removing a small piece of muscle tissue for microscopic examination is called a muscle **biopsy**. DM is marked by characteristic changes in the structure of muscle cells that can be seen on a muscle biopsy. An electrocardiogram could be performed to detect characteristic abnormalities in heart rhythm associated with DM. These symptoms often appear later in the course of the disease.

Prenatal testing

Testing a pregnancy to determine whether an unborn child is affected is possible if genetic testing in a family has identified a DMPK mutation. This can be done at 10–12 weeks gestation by a procedure called chorionic villus sampling (CVS) that involves removing a tiny piece of the placenta and analyzing DNA from its cells. It can also be done by amniocentesis after 14 weeks gestation by removing a small amount of the amniotic fluid surrounding the baby and analyzing the cells in the fluid. Each of these procedures has a small risk of miscarriage associated with it, and those who are interested in learning more should check with their doctor or genetic counselor.

There is also another procedure called preimplantation diagnosis that allows a couple to have a child that is unaffected with the genetic condition in their family. This procedure is experimental and not widely available. Those interested in learning more about this procedure should check with their doctor or genetic counselor.

A group of researchers in Houston, Texas, reported in 2004 that they have successfully developed a

> **KEY TERMS**
>
> **Electrocardiogram (ECG, EKG)**—A test that uses electrodes attached to the chest with an adhesive gel to transmit the electrical impulses of the heart muscle to a recording device.
>
> **Electromyography (EMG)**—A test that uses electrodes to record the electrical activity of muscle. The information gathered is used to diagnose neuromuscular disorders.
>
> **Muscular dystrophy**—A group of inherited diseases characterized by progressive wasting of the muscles.
>
> **Nucleotide**—Any of a group of organic molecules that link together to form the building blocks of DNA or RNA.
>
> **Sleep apnea**—Temporary cessation of breathing while sleeping.
>
> **Trinucleotide repeat expansion**—A sequence of three nucleotides that is repeated too many times in a section of a gene.

technique for detecting the CCTG expansion that causes DM2 and estimating the size of the repeat expansion.

Treatment

Myotonic dystrophy cannot be cured, and no treatment can delay its progression. As of the early 2000s there is no standardized treatment for these disorders because the precise reasons for muscle weakness are not yet fully understood. However, many of the symptoms can be treated. Physical therapy can help preserve or increase strength and flexibility in muscles. Ankle and wrist braces can be used to support weakened limbs. Occupational therapy is used to develop tools and techniques to compensate for loss of strength and dexterity. A speech-language pathologist can provide retraining for weakness in the muscles controlling speech and swallowing.

Irregularities in the heartbeat may be treated with medication or a pacemaker. A yearly electrocardiogram is usually recommended to monitor the heartbeat. Diabetes mellitus in DM is treated in the same way that it is in the general population. A high-fiber diet can help prevent constipation. Sleep apnea may be treated with surgical procedures to open the airways or with nighttime ventilation. Treatment of sleep apnea may reduce drowsiness. Lens replacement surgery is available when cataracts develop. Pregnant women should be followed by an obstetrician familiar with the particular problems of DM because complications can occur during pregnancy, labor, and delivery.

Wearing a medical bracelet is advisable. Some emergency medications may have dangerous effects on the heart rhythm in a person with DM. Adverse reactions to general anesthesia may also occur.

Prognosis

The course of myotonic dystrophy varies. When symptoms appear earlier in life, disability tends to become more severe. Occasionally people with DM may require a wheelchair later in life. Children with congenital DM usually require special educational programs and physical and occupational therapy. For both types of DM, respiratory infections pose a danger when weakness becomes severe.

Resources

BOOKS

Harper, Peter. *Myotonic Dystrophy*. Oxford University Press: 2009.

PERIODICALS

Anand, Raktima, et al. "Myotonic Dystrophy: An Anaesthetic Dilemma." *Indian Journal of Anaesthesia* 53.6 (2009): 688.

Cup, Edith HC., et al. "Living with myotonic dystrophy; what can be learned from couples? a qualitative study." *BMC Neurology* 11 (2011): 86.

Ficek, Andrej, Ludevit Kadasi, and Jan Radvansky. "Repeat-primed polymerase chain reaction in myotonic dystrophy type 2 testing." *Genetic Testing and Molecular Biomarkers* 15.3 (2011): 133.

Jensen, Christer, et al. "Depression in Myotonic Dystrophy type 1: clinical and neuronal correlates." *Behavioral and Brain Functions* 6 (2010): 25.

Kadasi, Ludevit, and Jan Radvansky. "The expanding world of myotonic dystrophies: how can they be detected?" *Genetic Testing and Molecular Biomarkers* 14.6 (2010): 733.

OTHER

Gene Clinics. http://www.geneclinics.org.

Myotonic Dystrophy. http://www.umd.necker.fr/myotonic_dystrophy.html.

NCBI Genes and Disease. http://www.ncbi.nlm. nih.gov/disease/Myotonic.html.

ORGANIZATIONS

Muscular Dystrophy Association. 3300 East Sunrise Dr., Tucson, AZ 85718. (520) 529-2000 or (800) 572-1717. http://www.mdausa.org.

Karen M. Krajewski, M, C
Rebecca J. Frey, PhD

N

Narcolepsy

Definition

Narcolepsy is a neurological disorder marked by excessive daytime sleepiness, uncontrollable sleep attacks, and cataplexy (a sudden loss of muscle tone, usually lasting up to half an hour).

Demographics

According to the National Institute for Neurological Disorders and Stroke (NINDS), narcolepsy is an underrecognized and underdiagnosed condition in the United States. The exact prevalence is not known, but it is estimated to affect about one in every 2,000 Americans. The disorder occurs worldwide in every racial and ethnic group, affecting males and females equally. However, prevalence varies among populations. For example, narcolepsy is less prevalent in Israel (about one per 500,000) but considerably more prevalent in Japan (about one per 600).

Description

Narcolepsy is the second-leading cause of excessive daytime sleepiness (after obstructive sleep apnea). Persistent sleepiness and sleep attacks are the hallmarks of this condition. The sleepiness has been compared to the feeling of trying to stay awake after not sleeping for two or three days.

People with narcolepsy fall asleep suddenly— anywhere, at any time, maybe even in the middle of a conversation. These sleep attacks can last from a few seconds to more than an hour. Depending on where they occur, they may be mildly inconvenient or even dangerous to the individual. Some people continue to function outwardly during the sleep episodes, such as talking or putting things away. But when they wake up, they have no memory of the event.

Narcolepsy is related to the deep, dreaming part of sleep known as rapid eye movement (REM) sleep. Normally when people fall asleep, they experience 90 minutes of non-REM sleep, which is then followed by REM sleep. People with narcolepsy, however, enter REM sleep immediately. In addition, REM sleep occurs inappropriately throughout the day.

Risk factors

According to the NINDS, close relatives of people with narcolepsy have a statistically higher risk of developing the condition than do members of the general population.

Causes and symptoms

Narcolepsy sometimes runs in families, but most cases are sporadic, meaning that the disorder occurs independently in individuals without strong evidence of being inherited. Some researchers, therefore, believe that the inheritance of narcolepsy is similar to that of heart disease. In heart disease, several genes play a role in being susceptible to the disorder, but it usually does not develop without an environmental trigger of some sort. Other factors, such as infection, immune system deficiencies, trauma, hormonal changes, and stress may also play a role in the development of the disease.

The immediate cause of narcolepsy remains unknown, but medical researchers have made considerable progress in understanding the disorder and in identifying genes strongly associated with it. Abnormalities in various parts of the brain involved in regulating REM sleep were also discovered. Narcolepsy is now known to have one of the tightest associations with a specific HLA allele. The HLA gene family provides instructions for making a group of related proteins known as the human leukocyte antigen (HLA) complex. The HLA complex helps the immune system distinguish the body's own proteins from proteins made by foreign invaders such as viruses and bacteria. From 88% to 98% of patients affected by narcolepsy

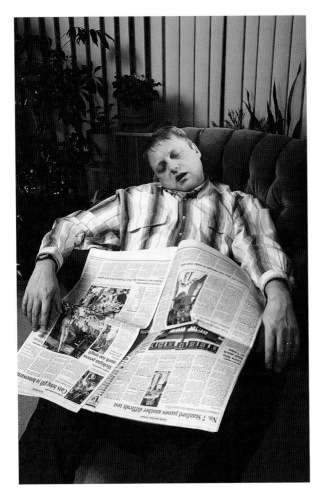

A narcoleptic has lost consciousness while reading the paper. (© *Custom Medical Stock Photo, Inc. Reproduced by permission.*)

have been shown to be HLA DQB1*0602 positive. This allele strongly increases the susceptibility for cataplexy although 41% of patients without cataplexy are carriers. DRB1 and DQB1 genes have been sequenced in narcolepsy patients but no mutation has been identified. This suggests that these genes strongly confer susceptibility to narcolepsy without their function being defective. It is accordingly believed that non-HLA genes may also be involved in susceptibility to narcolepsy.

While the symptoms of narcolepsy usually appear during the teens or 20s, the disease may not be diagnosed for many years. The most common major symptom is excessive daytime sleepiness (EDS), an overwhelming feeling of **fatigue**. After several months or years, cataplexy and other symptoms appear.

Cataplexy is the most dramatic symptom of narcolepsy. It affects 75% of people with the disorder.

During attacks, the knees buckle and the neck muscles go slack. In extreme cases, the person may become paralyzed and fall to the floor. This loss of muscle tone is temporary, lasting from a few seconds to half an hour, but frightening. The attacks can occur at any time but are often triggered by strong emotions, such as anger, joy, or surprise.

Other symptoms of narcolepsy include:

- Sleep attacks: short, uncontrollable sleep episodes throughout the day
- Sleep paralysis: a frightening inability to move shortly after awakening or dozing off
- Auditory or visual hallucinations: intense, sometimes terrifying experiences at the beginning or end of a sleep period
- Disturbed nighttime sleep: tossing and turning, nightmares, and frequent awakenings during the night

Diagnosis

Examination

In most patients, narcolepsy is not diagnosed until 10 to 15 years after the first symptoms appear. This is due to the disorder not being familiar to most of the general public. The disorder is suspected when a person reports experiencing both excessive daytime

QUESTIONS TO ASK YOUR DOCTOR

- What can be done to control excessive sleepiness during the day?
- What medications can help control symptoms?
- How efficient is sodium oxybate for treatment of cataplexy?
- What are the side effects?
- What lifestyle adjustments can help cope with the disorder?

sleepiness and cataplexy. Diagnosis is established on the basis of a clinical examination and comprehensive medical history.

Tests

Laboratory tests, however, are required to confirm a diagnosis. These may include an overnight polysomnogram—a test in which sleep is monitored with electrocardiography, video, and respiratory parameters. A Multiple Sleep Latency Test, which measures sleep latency (onset) and how quickly REM sleep occurs, may be used. People who have narcolepsy usually fall asleep in less than five minutes.

If a diagnosis is in question, a genetic blood test can reveal the existence of certain substances in people who have a tendency to develop narcolepsy. Positive test results suggest, but do not prove, the existence of narcolepsy.

Treatment

Traditional

There is no cure for narcolepsy. It is not progressive, and it is not fatal, but it is chronic. The symptoms can be managed with medication or lifestyle adjustment.

Drugs

Amphetamine–like stimulant drugs are often prescribed to control drowsiness and EDS attacks. Patients who do not like taking high doses of stimulants may choose to take smaller doses and "manage" their lifestyles, such as by napping every couple of hours, to relieve daytime sleepiness. Antidepressants are often effective in treating symptoms of abnormal REM sleep. In 2002, the FDA approved Xyrem (**sodium oxybate** or gamma hydroxybutyrate, also

known as GHB) for treating people with narcolepsy who experience episodes of cataplexy.

Prognosis

Narcolepsy is not a degenerative disease, and patients do not develop other neurologic symptoms. However, narcolepsy can interfere with a person's ability to work, play, drive, and perform other daily activities. In severe cases, the disorder prevents people from living a normal life, leading to **depression** and a loss of independence.

Prevention

Narcolepsy cannot be prevented.

Resources

BOOKS

Goswami, Meeta, et al., eds. *Narcolepsy: A Clinical Guide.* New York: Springer, 2009.

ICON Health Publications. *Narcolepsy—A Medical Dictionary, Bibliography, and Annotated Research Guide to Internet References.* San Diego, CA: Author, 2004.

Lee–Chiong, Teofilo L. *Sleep Medicine Essentials.* New York: Wiley-Blackwell, 2009.

McBrewster, John, et al, eds. *Rapid eye movement (sleep): Sleep (non–human), Polysomnogram, Sleep disorder, PGO waves, Dream, Narcolepsy, Parasomnia, Lucid dream.* Beau Bassin, Mauritius: Alphascript, 2009.

Parker, James and Philip Parker, eds. *The Official Patient's Sourcebook on Narcolepsy.* San Diego, CA: ICON Health Publications, 2002.

PERIODICALS

Arias-Carrión, O., and E. Murillo-Rodríguez. "Cell transplantation: a future therapy for narcolepsy?" *CNS & Neurological Disorders Drug Targets* 8, no. 4 (2009): 309–14.

Black, J., et al. "The nightly administration of sodium oxybate results in significant reduction in the nocturnal sleep disruption of patients with narcolepsy." *Sleep Medicine* 10, no. 8 (2009): 829–35.

Caylak, E. "The genetics of sleep disorders in humans: narcolepsy, restless legs syndrome, and obstructive sleep apnea syndrome." *American Journal of Medical Genetics. Part A* 149A, no. 11 (2009): 2612–26.

Didato, G., and L. Nobili. "Treatment of narcolepsy." *Expert Review of Neurotherapeutics* 9, no. 6 (2009): 897–910.

Kroeger, K., and L. de Lecea. "The hypocretins and their role in narcolepsy." *CNS & Neurological Disorders Drug Targets* 8, no. 4 (2009): 271–280.

Todman, D. "Narcolepsy." *European Neurology* 61, no. 4 (2009): 255.

Undurraga, J., et al. "Treatment of narcolepsy complicated by psychotic symptoms." *Psychosomatics* 50, no. 4 (July/August 2009): 427–28.

Vernet, C., and I. Arnulf. "Narcolepsy with long sleep time: a specific entity?" *Sleep* 32, no. 9 (2009): 1229–35.

Wang, W., et al. "Two patients with narcolepsy treated by hypnotic psychotherapy." *Sleep Medicine* 10, no. 10 (2009): 1167.

OTHER

"Do I Have Narcolepsy?" *Narcolepsy Network*. Information Page. http://www.narcolepsynetwork.org/?page_id = 7 (accessed November 14, 2009).

"Narcolepsy." *Medline Plus*. Encyclopedia. http://www.nlm.nih.gov/medlineplus/ency/article/000802.htm (accessed November 14, 2009).

"Narcolepsy and Sleep." *National Sleep Foundation*. Information Page. http://www.sleepfoundation.org/article/sleep-related-problems/narcolepsy-and-sleep (accessed November 14, 2009).

"Narcolepsy Fact Sheet." *NINDS*. Information Page. http://www.ninds.nih.gov/disorders/narcolepsy/detail_narcolepsy.htm (accessed November 14, 2009).

ORGANIZATIONS

Narcolepsy Network, Inc., 110 Ripple Lane, North Kingstown, RI 02852, (401) 667-2523, (888) 292-6522, Fax: (401) 633-6567, narnet@narcolepsynetwork.org, http://www.narcolepsynetwork.org.

National Heart, Lung, and Blood Institute (NHLBI), Building 31, Room 5A52, 31 Center Drive MSC 2486, Bethesda, MD 20892, (301) 592-8573, Fax: (240) 629-3246, nhlbiinfo@nhlbi.nih.gov, http://www.nhlbi.nih.gov.

National Institute of Neurological Disorders and Stroke (NINDS), PO Box 5801, Bethesda, MD 20824, (301) 496-5751, (800) 352-9424, http://www.ninds.nih.gov.

National Sleep Foundation, 1522 K Street NW, Suite 500, Washington, DC 20005, (202) 347-3471, Fax: (202) 347-3472, nsf@sleepfoundation.org, http://www.sleepfoundation.org.

Michelle Lee Brandt
Monique Laberge, PhD

Neostigmine *see* **Cholinergic stimulants**

Nerve compression

Definition

Nerve compression is the restriction in the space around a nerve that can occur due to several reasons. Functioning of the nerve is compromised.

Description

There are a variety of circumstances that cause nerve compression. Despite this variety, the resulting damage to the nerve produces a similar diminished functioning of the nerve.

Demographics

The incidence of brachial plexus palsy, usually a result of birth injury to the nerves that conduct signals from the spine to the shoulder and resulting in a limp or paralyzed arm, is low, on the order of one to two births out of every 1,000. Brachial plexus palsy is associated with a difficult labor, especially compression on the baby's shoulders. Intervention or assistance during labor can lessen the chance of the physical trauma that causes the nerve damage. However, the condition cannot be totally eliminated, especially in times where an emergency response is needed to speed the birth of a fetus in distress.

Meralgia parasthetica, a condition involving compression of the lateral femoral cutaneous nerve, results in paresthesia, or tingling, numbness, and burning pain in the outer side of the thigh. Meraglia parasthetica has traditionally affected men more than women. The condition is not rare, but its overall prevalence is unknown. **Meralgia paresthetica** may occur after abdominal surgery or significant weight gain, in military members who often march, soccer players, or for no apparent reason in the general population. Other nerve compression maladies such as **carpal tunnel syndrome** can be quite common.

Causes and symptoms

There are a variety of conditions that lead to nerve compression, according to the affected nerve.

Carpal tunnel syndrome

In carpal tunnel syndrome, the nerves that pass through the wrist are pinched due to the enlargement of local tendons and ligaments. The enlargement occurs due to inflammation, which can be associated with the strain of performing a repetitive task such as typing. Carpal tunnel syndrome is also associated with maladies like diabetes, and with the restricted space that can develop in the wrist as weight is gained during pregnancy or in someone who is obese. The enlargement of the tendons and ligaments restricts the space available for the nerves that reach to the finger and also for the muscle that connects to the base of the thumb. As a consequence, the ability of the nerve to properly transmit impulses to the muscles in the fingers and thumb is affected.

The initial symptoms of carpal tunnel syndrome tend to be felt at night because the hand is at rest. The symptoms can be a burning or a tingling numbness in the fingers, in particular the thumb, along with the index and middle fingers. As well, the reduced transmission of nerve impulses to the muscles decrease muscle strength. It can become difficult to grip an object or make a fist.

Thoracic outlet syndrome

In **thoracic outlet syndrome**, nerve compression can occur as a result of stresses on the neck and shoulders that cause these areas to impinge on local nerves. While the underlying cause of the syndrome is not clear, there seems to be an association between thoracic outlet syndrome and physical labor, in particular the repeated lifting of heavy objects onto the shoulders, causing the shoulders to pull back and down. Reaching for objects that are positioned above shoulder level can also be irritating to muscles in the shoulders and the upper arms. Swelling and inflammation of the muscles can compress nerves between the neck and shoulders.

The symptoms of thoracic outlet syndrome include **weakness** of the arms, pain, and numbness of the arms and fingers. In more extreme cases, the sense of touch and ability to sense temperature changes can be lost in the fingers.

Brachial plexus palsy

"Palsy" is a term meaning the inability to purposely move a body part. Brachial plexus palsy refers to paralysis that is associated with compression and tearing of a group of nerves called the brachial plexus. These nerves are a connection between the spinal cord and the nerves that run into the arms neck, and shoulders. The nerves can become compressed and even torn when the neck is stretched. This can occur in an infant born following a difficult delivery, such as can occur if the baby is large or in a breech position or if the period of labor is long. In these situations, the baby's neck can be abnormally flexed. The abnormal position damages the brachial plexus nerves.

The brachial plexus affects certain segments of the spinal cord. (When viewed in a X-ray, the spinal cord is reminiscent of Lego blocks stacked on each other. Each 'block' represents a segment.) Typically, brachial nerves that originate from upper segments of the spinal column (segments C5 and C6) are affected. This condition is also called Erb's palsy. Less commonly, nerves associated with lower segments (C7 and T1) can

be deranged. This condition is called Klumke's paralysis. In some cases, all the nerves of the brachial plexus can be affected.

The causes of nerve damage can also involve injuries to the shoulder, arm, and the collarbone (clavicle). The main symptom of brachial plexus palsy, paralysis in an arm, is evident immediately after birth. A newborn will lie with the affected arm by its side, with the elbow extended. While the other arm will be capable of a normal range of motion, the affected arm will be immobile.

Meralgia paresthetica

This painful condition is due to the pinching of the lateral femoral cutaneous nerve as the nerve exits the pelvis. The nerve can become pinched as the position of the pelvic region changes due to weight gain, injury, pregnancy, or extended periods of standing of walking (i.e., military marching). The affected nerve becomes compressed as it crosses a region of the pelvis called the iliac crest. As well, the nerve can be rubbed during the pelvic motions that occur with walking. This friction increases the nerve damage.

Individuals with meralgia paresthetica experiences an ache, numbness, tingling, or burning sensations in their thigh. The ache can be mild or severe and generally eases during rest and returns with resumption of activity.

Cubital tunnel syndrome

This syndrome results from pressure that compresses the ulnar nerve. The ulnar nerve is one of the main nerves of the hand, which connects the muscles of the forearm and hand with the spinal cord. The nerve passes across the back of the elbow behind a bump called the medial epicondyle. The sensation that is described as the funny bone is actually the transient sensation that occurs when the ulnar nerve is compressed in a bump.

Cubital tunnel syndrome is a more protracted form of the nerve compression. It results from the stretching or pushing of the nerve against the medial epicondyle when the elbow is bent. The condition is aggravated over time by the bending of the elbow. Symptoms of cubital tunnel syndrome are typically a numb feeling in the ring finger and small finger, weakness in muscles of the hand and forearm, and elbow pain. Without intervention, more serious nerve damage can occur.

Diagnosis

Carpal tunnel syndrome is diagnosed based on the pattern of the symptoms, the location of the symptoms, and a history of repetitive activity that might predispose to the syndrome. Similarly, thoracic outlet syndrome is diagnosed by the location of the symptoms and a person's work history (i.e., a job involving a lot of lifting).

The diagnosis of brachial plexus palsy is prominently based on the visual observation of the motion difficulties experienced by the newborn. X rays may be taken to discount any other injuries such as fractures of the spine, clavicle (collarbone), humerus (the large bone in the upper arm), or a dislocation of the shoulder.

Meralgia paresthetica is diagnosed by the nature of the symptoms and the occupation of the person. For example, hip and thigh pain in a soldier can alert a clinician to the possibility of this malady. As well, people usually experience tenderness in a specific spot over a ligament in the hip, and symptoms can be made worse by extending the hip in the Nachlas test.

Diagnosis of meralgia paresthetica needs to rule out other maladies to the pelvis and spine, as well as diabetes mellitus. For example, damage to spinal discs will impair reflexes, while reflexes are normal in meralgia paresthetica.

Cubital tunnel syndrome is diagnosed by the type and location of the symptoms.

Treatment team

Treatment often involves involve the family physician, family members, and physical and occupational therapists. In severe cases, a surgeon may be consulted for many types of nerve compression

Treatment

Carpal tunnel syndrome responds to immobilization of the affected area. Often, a person will wear a splint that keeps the wrist from flexing. This reduces the strain and pressure on the nerves. Another option is to administer anti-inflammatory drugs or injections of cortisone. These compounds help reduce the swelling in the wrist. In a small number of cases of carpal tunnel syndrome, surgery can be a useful option. The ligament that connects to the bottom of the wrist is cut.

Persons with thoracic outlet syndrome are put on a planned program of exercise therapy designed to relieve the inflammation. Avoiding the repetitive activities that caused the muscle inflammation, at least temporarily, is a must. Re design of the workplace so that heavy objects do not have to be placed above shoulder level can be a wise strategy. Anti-inflammatory drugs may be prescribed. Finally, if these efforts have not produced a satisfactory response, surgery may be an option.

Treatment for brachial plexus palsy consists of physical therapy that relieves the strain on the affected nerves. The therapy usually involves a gentle range of motions and the use of electrical stimulation of the muscles that are associated with the damaged nerves. Keeping the muscles supple and strong is an important part of the treatment. When a nerve has been more seriously damaged, surgery may be necessary to repair the tear or other damage. This is usually evident within three months of birth. Surgery can involve the grafting of a new section of nerve to replace the damaged and now-defective region of the original nerve.

Treatment for meralgia paresthetica can involve relief of the stress on the pelvis through weight loss or modifying the activity that causes the stress. Treatment for cubital tunnel syndrome can involve the use of medications that reduce inflammation. These include non-steroidal anti-inflammatory medications such as aspirin and ibuprofen. Some people gain relief by wearing a special brace while sleeping that prevents the elbow from bending.

Recovery and rehabilitation

Rehabilitation and recovery from carpal tunnel syndrome can be complete for some people. Avoiding the activity that inflamed the wrist can help ensure that the inflammation and nerve injury does not reoccur. Other people do recover, but more slowly. For others, the syndrome becomes a chronic concern.

Recovery from brachial plexus palsy ranges from limited to complete. Most recovery occurs by two years of age. The Erb's type of palsy is a milder form, and recovery can occur in 3–4 months. With the more serious Klumke's paralysis, 18–24 months of physical therapy can be required to achieve significant improvement.

Clinical trials

Rather than specific clinical trials, research is ongoing to better understand the triggers for the various nerve compression syndromes, and to find better and more efficient rehabilitation techniques. In the United States, organizations, including the National Institute of Arthritis and Musculoskeletal and Skin Diseases, fund such research.

Prognosis

For carpal tunnel syndrome, the outlook for many people is quite good. Once the inflammation has been dealt with, avoiding the cause of the irritation can prevent a reoccurrence of the trouble. However, for about 1% of those with carpal tunnel syndrome, permanent injury develops.

The prognosis for brachial plexus palsy varies upon the nature of the nerve damage. Some cases resolve quickly and completely without intervention, others require extended time and therapy, and in the worst cases, impaired use of an arm can be permanent.

Meralgia paresthetica due to pregnancy, obesity, and diabetes may resolve completely when the condition is properly treated. Other mechanically related causes of the malady can be less successfully treated. In the latter case, modification of lifestyle may be needed.

Most people with cubital tunnel syndrome respond well to conservative treatment, although surgery is necessary for some. For those resulting to surgery, permanent elbow numbness may result.

Resources

OTHER

"Cubital Tunnel Syndrome." *e-hand.com*. http://www.e-hand.com/hw/hw007.htm (May 4, 2004).

"Meralgia Paresthetica." *eMedicine.com*. http://www.emedicine.com/neuro/topic590.htm (May 6, 2004).

"NINDS Carpal Tunnel Syndrome Information Page." National Institute of Neurological Diseases and Stroke. http://www.ninds.nih.gov/health_and_medical/disorders/carpal_doc.htm (May 6, 2004).

"What is thoracic outlet syndrome?" *Canadian Centre for Occupational Health and Safety*.http://www.ccohs.ca/oshanswers/diseases/thoracic.html (May 6, 2004).

ORGANIZATIONS

American Chronic Pain Association (ACPA). P.O. Box 850, Rocklin, CA 95677-0850. Phone: (916) 632-0922. Fax: (916) 632-3208. Tollfree phone: (800) 533-3231. Email: ACPA@pacbell.net. http://www.theacpa.org.

National Institute for Neurological Diseases and Stroke. P.O. Box 5801, Bethesda, MD 20824. Phone: (301) 496-5751. Tollfree phone: (800) 352-9424. http://www.ninds/nih.gov.

National Chronic Pain Outreach Organization (NCPOA). P.O. Box 274, Millboro, VA 24460. Phone: (540) 862-9437. Fax: (540) 862-9485. Tollfree Email: ncpoa@cfw.org. http://www.chronicpain.org.

National Institute of Arthritis and Musculoskeletal and Skin Diseases (NIAMS). 31 Centre Dr., Rm. 4Co2 MSC 2350, Bethesda, MD 20892-2350. Phone: (301) 496-8190. Tollfree phone: (877) 226-4267. Email: info@mail.nih.gov.http://www.niams.nih.gov.

Brian Douglas Hoyle, Ph

Nerve conduction study

Definition

A nerve conduction study is a test that measures the movement of an impulse through a nerve after the deliberate stimulation of the nerve.

Purpose

The ability of a nerve to swiftly and properly transmit an impulse down its length and to pass on the impulse to the adjacent nerve or to a connection muscle in which it is embedded is vital to the performance of many activities in the body.

When proper functioning of nerves does not occur, as can happen due to accidents, infections, or progressive and genetically based diseases, the proper treatment depends on an understanding of the nature of the problem. The nerve conduction study is one tool that a clinician can use to assess nerve function. Often, the nerve conduction study is performed in concert with a test called an electromyogram. Together, these tests, along with other procedures that comprise what is known as electrodiagnostic testing, provide vital information on the functioning of nerves and muscles.

Description

Nerve cells consist of a body, with branches at one end. The branches are called axons. The axons are positioned near an adjacent nerve or a muscle. Nerve impulses pass from the axons of one nerve to the next nerve or muscle. The impulse transmission speed can be reduced in damaged nerves.

Surrounding a nerve is a tough protective coat of a material called myelin. Nerve damage can involve damage or loss of myelin, damage to the nerve body, or damage to the axon region. The nerve conduction study, which was devised in the 1960s, can detect the loss of nerve function dues to these injuries, and, from the nature of the nerve signal pattern that is produced, offer clues as to the nature of the problem.

The nature of the nerve damage determines the pattern of signal transmission. For example, in a normal nerve cell, sensors placed at either end of the cell will register the same signal pattern. But in a nerve cell that is blocked somewhere along its length, these sensors will register different signal patterns. In another example, in a nerve cell in which transmission is not completely blocked, the signal pattern at the axon may be similar in shape but reduced in intensity to that of the originating signal, because not as much of the signal is completing the journey down the nerve cell.

Diseases of the nerve itself mainly affect the size of the responses (amplitudes); diseases of the myelin mainly affect the speed of the responses.

Nerve conduction studies are now routine and can be done in virtually any hospital equipped with the appropriate machine and staffed with a qualified examiner. The nerve conduction study utilizes a computer, computer monitor, amplifier, loudspeaker, electrical stimulator, and filters. These filters are mathematical filters that can distinguish random, background electrical signals from the signal produced by an activated nerve. When the study is done, small electrodes are placed on the skin over the muscles being tested. Generally, these muscles are located in the arms or legs. Some of the electrodes are designed to record the electrical signal that passes by them. Other electrodes (reference electrodes) are designed to monitor the quality of the signals to make sure that the test is operating properly. If monitoring of the test is not done, then the results obtained are meaningless.

After the electrodes are in place, a small electrical current can be applied to the skin. The electrical stimulation is usually done at several points along the nerve, not just at a single point. This is done because conduction of an impulse through a nerve is not uniform. Some regions of a nerve conduct more slowly than other regions. By positioning the stimulating electrodes at several sites, a more accurate overall measurement of conduction velocity is obtained.

The electrical current activates nerves in the vicinity, including those associated with the particular muscle. The nerves are stimulated to produce a signal. This is known as the "firing" of the nerve. The nerve signal, which it also electric, can be detected by some of the electrodes and conveyed to the computer for analysis.

The analysis of the nerve signal involves the study of the movement of the signal through the nerve and from the nerve to the adjacent muscle. Using characteristics such as the speed of the impulse and the shape, wavelength, and height of the signal wave, an examiner can assess whether the nerve is functional or defective.

Risks

A nerve conduction study can be done quite quickly. A person will experience some discomfort from the series of small electrical shocks that are felt. Otherwise, no damage or residual effects occur.

Normal results

Analysis of the results of a nerve conduction study

Under normal circumstances, the movement of the electrical impulse down the length of a nerve is very fast, on the order of 115–197 ft/sec (35–60 m/sec).

A number of aspects of the nerve impulse are measured in nerve conduction studies. The first aspect (or parameter) is known as latency. Latency is the time between the stimulus (the applied electrical current) and the response (the firing of the nerve). In damaged nerves, latency is typically increased.

Another parameter is known as the amplitude. Electrical signals are waves. The distance from the crest of one wave to the bottom of the trough of the adjacent wave is the amplitude. Impulses in damaged nerves can have an abnormal amplitude or may show different amplitudes in the undamaged and damaged sections of the same nerve.

The area under a wave can also vary if not all muscle fibers are being stimulated by a nerve or if the muscle fibers are not all reacting to a nerve impulse at the same time. The speed of a nerve impulse (the conduction velocity) can be also be determined and compared to data produced by a normally functioning nerve.

A number of other, more technically complex parameters can also be recorded and analyzed. A skilled examiner can tell from the appearance of the impulse waves on the computer monitor whether a nerve or muscle is functioning normally and can even begin to gauge the nature of a problem. Examples of maladies that can be partially diagnosed using the nerve conduction study include **Guillain-Barré syndrome**, **amyotrophic lateral sclerosis** (ALS, or Lou Gehrig's disease, Charcot's disease), and **multifocal motor neuropathy**.

Conditions affecting the nerve conduction study

The nerve conduction study does not produce uniform results from person to person. Various factors affect the transmission of a nerve impulse and the detected signal.

Temperature affects the speed of impulse movement. Signals move more slowly at lower temperatures, due to the tighter packing of the molecules of the nerve. This variable can be minimized during the nerve conduction study by maintaining the skin temperature at 80–85° Fahrenheit (27–29° Celcius). Use of a controlled temperature also allows study runs done at different times to be more comparable, which can be very useful in evaluating whether muscle or nerve problems are worsening or getting better.

The speed of nerve impulse transmission changes as the body ages. In infants, the transmission speed is only about half that seen in adults. By age five, most people have attained the adult velocity. A gradual decline in conduction velocity begins as people reach their 20s and continues for the remainder of life. Another factor that influences conduction velocity is the length of the nerve itself. An impulse that has to travel a longer distance will take longer. Some nerves are naturally longer than others. Measurement of nerve conduction takes into account the length of the target nerve.

Resources

OTHER

"Electromyography (EMG) and Nerve Conduction Studies." *WebMD*. May 1, 2004 (June 2, 2004). http://my.webmd.com/hw/health_guide_atoz/hw213852.asp.

"Nerve conduction velocity." *Medline Plus*. National Library of Medicine. May 3, 2004 (June 2, 2004). http://www.nlm.nih.gov/medlineplus/print/ency/article/003927.htm.

"Nerve Conduction Velocity Test." *MedicineNet.com*. May 1, 2004 (June 2, 2004). http://www.medicinenet.com/Nerve_Conduction_Velocity_Test/article.htm.

Brian Douglas Hoyle, PhD

Neurocysticercosis

Description

Neurocysticercosis (NCC) is a medical condition in which a patient has accidentally ingested the eggs of the pork tapeworm (*Taenia solium*), and the resultant larvae have invaded the nervous system. The pork tapeworm eggs pass through the host by the fecal-oral route via contaminated food or water or through food infected with larval cysts. It has a complex life cycle involving both humans and pigs. The eggs are spread through infected feces, are spread in the soil, and ingested by pigs. Within the pig the eggs hatch and an early mobile stage of the organism migrates through the intestinal wall to the bloodstream and into the muscle tissue of the pig. Here they form cysticerci, which are cysts of larvae that may survive in the pig musculature for years. Humans ingest raw or undercooked infected meat and acquire the pork tapeworm larvae. The larval cysticerci come out of their cysts and develop into adult tapeworms in the human intestines over about a two month time span. They do not migrate from the intestines to the rest of the body in this phase.

Once the worm is in the adult stage it can survive for years in the human intestine, at a length of two to seven meters. The adult tapeworm head, called the scolex, has suckers and hooks that allow it to latch on to human tissue. The adult produces approximately one thousand proglottids, which are hermaphroditic body segments containing both male and female reproductive capacity that can function as independent organisms. The proglottids mature, are detached, migrate to the anus, and are passed in the feces at a rate of approximately six per day.

After leaving the human host they may then produce up to fifty thousand eggs per proglottid. Ingestion of either the eggs or the proglottids from contaminated soil or the cysticerci from poorly cooked infected meat starts the lifecycle process again. Cysticerci may only form in the muscle or other tissues in humans who have ingested the eggs of the tapeworm, who are then diagnosed with cysticercosis. When cysticerci form in the **central nervous system**, which is the brain and spinal cord, the diagnosis is made for NCC.

Demographic

NCC is the most common parasitic disease of the nervous system, producing seizures and headache in many patients. Approximately 2.5 million people worldwide carry the adult tapeworm, and many more are infected with cysticerci. It is considered the main cause of adult onset seizures in developing countries. Historically a disease more common in developing countries, NCC is becoming a growing problem in industrialized countries because of the immigration of human tapeworm carriers from areas of endemic disease. NCC is endemic in Mexico, Central and South America, sub-Saharan Africa, the Indian subcontinent, Indonesia, and China. The highest rates of tapeworm infection are found in parts of Latin America, Asia, and Africa that have poor sanitation and free-range pigs raised with access to human feces. Immigrants to the United States have the highest rates in California, Texas, and New Mexico, and it is a major cause of morbidity in the Hispanic population. The subcutaneous (under the skin) form of cysticercosis is more common in Asian populations. The peak incidence is in people in their thirties and forties, but NCC can occur at any age.

Causes

There is a distinction between acquiring the pork tapeworm and acquiring any form of cysticercosis, including NCC. Humans must ingest the eggs to accommodate the lifecycle stage of the pork tapeworm that will migrate from the intestines to the other tissues and form cysts; however, in addition to egg ingestion the tapeworm itself may be ingested and acquired in multiple lifecycle stages. Humans may get the tapeworm by ingesting the larval cysts in the meat of infected pigs as well as by ingesting eggs or proglottids from a contaminated environment. Since the adult tapeworm proglottids do not release eggs until excreted in human feces, infection with the adult tapeworm does not mean the patient will have cysticercosis in the brain or elsewhere. Ingestion of any of the other forms other than the eggs (proglottids and cysticerci) will result in tapeworm infection alone.

Pork tapeworm eggs can be acquired via fecal-oral contact with human carriers of the adult tapeworm. This usually requires the presence of a tapeworm carrier in the immediate household or the ingestion of contaminated food prepared by carriers without proper hygiene. People living in the same household with a tapeworm carrier have a much higher risk of getting cysticercosis than others. Cases of autoingestion, in which persons with the adult tapeworm may accidentally ingest eggs into their intestine via fecal-oral contact, have been reported. Using the bathroom, not washing the hands, and then touching contaminated fingers to the mouth is one way in which this may inadvertently happen. Ingestion of infected pork that is raw or undercooked is a major route of tapeworm infection but is not the route by which humans develop NCC.

Symptoms

NCC is a disease that takes many forms and may not have any symptoms at all in some patients. Patients that do have symptoms vary greatly in type of symptoms and severity. This high degree of variability is due to differences in the exact location of the cysts (also called lesions in this context) in the brain or spinal cord, the number of lesions, and the severity of the immune response of the human host. Some of the most common symptoms are the development of headaches, **dizziness**, and seizures. The adult onset seizures of NCC, also termed acquired epilepsy, occur in approximately 70% of patients. It is the most common presenting symptom that indicates a possible NCC diagnosis. Headaches from NCC may mimic migraines, with associated nausea and vomiting. If the flow of cerebrospinal fluid (CSF), the fluid bathing the brain, is obstructed by the location of the cystic lesion, increased brain pressure—known as intracranial hypertension—may occur. It is also possible for cystic lesions to block blood vessels that are a major part of the oxygen supply to parts of the brain and cause a stroke. Strokes or lesions in the area of the brain involved in motor coordination may cause disturbances in gait or balance. If the cystic lesion impacts certain nerves of the head known as cranial nerves, they may have an effect on the visual system as well, causing symptoms such as double or blurry vision. Spinal NCC is very rare but may produce symptoms of **weakness** or numbness and tingling in the extremities whose nerve roots lie at the same level as the lesion in the spinal cord. NCC is a serious disease that may become fatal if not treated properly.

Diagnosis

The diagnosis of NCC involves multiple tests and modalities. To understand diagnosis, it is important to understand what happens to the cysticerci once they are lodged in the nervous system. The cysticerci goes through different stages of involution (degenerative changes) while in the brain, only remaining alive for a finite period of time. The first stage is the vesicular stage, in which there is a functional live parasite and a mild inflammatory reaction in the surrounding brain tissue. The second stage is the colloidal stage, where the scolex remains in the cyst but the rest of the larva degenerates. This stage causes a more severe inflammatory reaction that can be seen on neuroimaging studies. The third stage is the granular stage where even the scolex is degenerating and the brain is forming a protective barrier around the cyst to wall it off from the rest of the brain. The fourth and last stage is the calcified stage, where the parasite has fully degenerated into a calcified nodule and is completely walled off by protective brain tissue. Both CT scan and MRI are used as neuroimaging tools to diagnose NCC, but which test is best and what is seen on these imaging studies depends on the stage of the cystic lesion and may greatly vary in appearance.

If the neuroimaging technique used does not give a definitive diagnosis, the CSF may be analyzed. Specifically those patients with new onset seizures (patients who do not have a previous history of a disease that causes seizures) or patients who have a new localized alteration in their nervous system function may have this analysis. Depending on where the cysticercus is located, the results may be normal or abnormal in a patient with NCC. Specific findings include alterations in glucose or protein of the CSF, or in the types and proportions of immune cells.

Stool samples may or may not be useful in adding information to a NCC case. Tapeworm infection and NCC do not coexist in many patients. Stool samples only tell which patients have an infection with an adult tapeworm, not which patients have NCC. Measuring the stool of family members may help in identifying the source of infection for the patient with NCC in some cases.

Treatment and Prognosis

Treatment of NCC is based on which stage the cystic lesions are in, particularly whether there are still viable live parasite larvae present in the cysts. Treatment also depends on where the cysts are located and what problems they are causing for the patient. If the parasite is still alive, efforts may be made to eradicate the parasite in the body with antiparasitic medications. Corticosteroid medications may need to be added to keep down robust immune responses that lead to inflammation and tissue damage before using antiparasitics in some patients. The antiparasitic medications may decrease the incidence of seizures in patients with live parasites in their cysticerci. If the cystic lesions no longer contain live parasites, treatment involves management of symptoms such as seizures with anticonvulsant medications. Some cases with severe complications in blockage of the CSF or compression of structures in the brain may require brain surgery for relief of symptoms and patient survival. In some cases, NCC can be fatal, so appropriate treatment is critical.

Antiparasitic Medications for NCC

Antiparasitic medications may be used in an attempt to reduce or eliminate the live parasite from the human host (hasten the resolution of active cysts containing live parasite), as well as to reduce medical complications and symptoms such as seizures. The two main antiparasitic medications used are praziquantel (Biltricide) and albendazole (Albenza). The potential risk of treatment with antiparasitics is worsening of the neurologic symptoms due to increased inflammation around the degenerating cyst. This is especially a problem in patients with many cystic lesions that will all increase inflammation upon treatment. The impact of inflammation can lead to disability or death in some cases. To prevent this,

corticosteroids are given at the same time as the antiparasitics to reduce the immune response and inflammation. Praziquantel specifically acts to destroy the scolex of live parasites, paralyze their musculature, and destroy their bodies. Praziquantel interacts with some types of anticonvulsants and its effectiveness may be weakened if administered in the same time frame as some of these drugs. Albendazole inhibits tapeworm energy production, and also acts to paralyze and destroy the parasite. It does not interact with anticonvulsants in the same manner and for this reason is generally preferred over praziquantel. How many days of therapy with antiparasitics are required depends on the type of NCC in question.

Antiseizure Medications for NCC

Seizure control is an important part of NCC management in patients who have developed seizures or are high risk for the development of seizures due to the number, type, or location of cystic lesions. Antiseizure medications commonly used in NCC include phenytoin (Dilantin) and **carbamazepine** (Tegretol). Phenytoin has a mechanism of action that involves

QUESTIONS TO ASK YOUR DOCTOR

- How could I have gotten neurocysticercosis, and how do I prevent getting it again?
- Should any of my family members be tested for pork tapeworm infection?
- Where are my neurocysticercosis lesions?
- Do I need surgery?
- Do I need any medication?
- Will this medication interact with any of my other prescription medications?
- Are there any over-the-counter medications I should not take with this medicine?
- Will this medicine interact with any of my herbal supplements?
- Can I drink alcoholic beverages in the same time frame as taking this medication?
- With the information we have now, how long should I expect to take medication?

modulation of sodium and calcium ion flow in the brain, which has an impact on the formation of seizures. Carbamazepine has a mechanism of action that reduces the neuronal signaling involved in seizure spread. Neither type of antiseizure medication can be used at the same time as the antiparasitic medication praziquantel. How long antiseizure medication is given depends on the type of cystic lesion, location, and whether seizures are recurrent. Treatment may continue for six months to a year after the cystic lesions have reached advanced degenerative stages. If seizures recur after a trial period off of antiseizure medication, the therapy may be instituted long-term.

Prognosis for NCC

In many patients with NCC, the prognosis is good. Patients who are experiencing seizures with active, live cysticerci seem to improve after treatment with antiparasitic and anti-inflammatory drugs. While duration of treatment is difficult to define and may be extended, seizure control is generally good with antiseizure medication. Patients with complications requiring brain surgery or with chronic inflammation of the membranes covering the brain due to the cystic lesions have a poorer prognosis than those less complicated medical NCC conditions. Patients who develop chronic epilepsy from the lesions will require life changes to accommodate their new condition. Many other patients will have seizures and other problems associated with NCC resolve with treatment.

Resources

BOOKS

Abd El Bagi, Mohamed E. and Jean C. Tamraz, Maurice C. Haddad, eds. *Imaging of Parasitic Diseases*. New York: Springer, 2010.

Brunton, Laurence, Bruce A. Chabner, and Bjorn Knollman. *Goodman & Gilman's The Pharmacological Basis of Therapeutics*. 12th ed. New York: McGraw-Hill Professional, 2010.

World Health Organization. *Working to Overcome the Global Impact of Neglected Tropical Diseases: First WHO Report on Neglected Tropical Diseases 2010*. Geneva: Author, 2011.

PERIODICALS

Auer, Herbert, et al. "A cross-sectional study of people with epilepsy and neurocysticercosis in tanzania: clinical characteristics and diagnostic approaches." *PLoS Neglected Tropical Diseases* 5.6 (2011).

Budke, Christine M., et al. "Clinical manifestations associated with neurocysticercosis: a systematic review." *PLoS Neglected Tropical Diseases* 5.5 (2011).

Dewan, Pooja, et al. "Uncommon presentation of neurocysticercosis." *South African Journal of Child Health* 5.2 (2011): 58+.

Nanda, Smiti, Savita R. Singhal, and Suresh K. Singhal. "Neurocysticercosis as an important differential of seizures in pregnancy: two case reports." *Journal of Medical Case Reports* 5 (2011): 206.

WEBSITES

Epocrates. https://online.epocrates.com/ (accessed July 17, 2011).

"Parasites—Cysticercosis." Centers for Disease Control and Prevention (CDC). http://www.cdc.gov/parasites/cysticercosis/ (accessed July 17, 2011).

"Tapeword Infection." MayoClinic.com. http://www.mayoclinic.com/health/tapeworm/DS00659/DSECTION=complications (accessed July 17, 2011).

White, A. Clinton, Jr. "Treatment of Cysticercosis." UpTo Date. http://www.uptodate.com/contents/treatment-of-cysticercosis (accessed July 17, 2011).

Zafar, Mohammed J. "Neurocysticercosis." Medscape Reference. http://emedicine.medscape.com/article/1168656-overview (accessed July 17, 2011).

ORGANIZATIONS

Centers of Disease Control and Prevention (CDC), 1600 Clifton Road, Atlanta, GA 30333, (800) CDC-INFO, cdcinfo@cdc.gov, http://www.cdc.gov.

Maria Eve Basile, PhD

Neurodegeneration with brain iron accumulation *see* Pantothenate kinase-associated neurodegeneration

Neurofibromatosis

Definition

Neurofibromatosis (NF), or von Recklinghausen disease, is a genetic disease in which patients develop multiple soft tumors (neurofibromas). These tumors occur under the skin and throughout the nervous system.

Description

Neural crest cells are primitive cells that exist during fetal development. These cells eventually turn into the following:

- cells that form nerves throughout the brain, spinal cord, and body
- cells that serve as coverings around the nerves that course through the body
- pigment cells, which provide color to structures
- the meninges, the thin, membranous coverings of the brain and spinal cord
- cells that ultimately develop into the bony structures of the head and neck

In neurofibromatosis, a genetic defect causes these neural crest cells to develop abnormally. This results in numerous tumors and malformations of the nerves, bones, and skin.

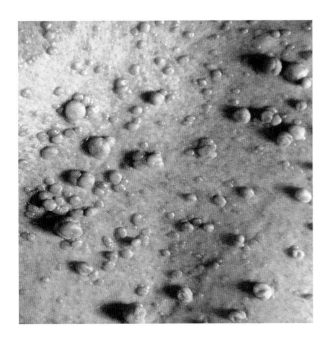

Neurofibromas are large and small smooth, round, protruding growths scattered across this patient's back.
(© Custom Medical Stock Photo, Inc. Reproduced by permission.)

Neurofibromatosis occurs in about one of every 4,000 births. Two types of NF exist: NF-1 (90% of all cases), and NF-2 (10% of all cases).

Causes and symptoms

Both forms of neurofibromatosis are caused by a defective gene. NF-1 is due to a defect on chromosome 17; NF-2 results from a defect on chromosome 22. Both of these disorders are inherited in a dominant fashion. This means that anybody who receives just one defective gene will have the disease. However, a family pattern of NF is only evident for about half of all cases of NF. The other cases of NF occur due to a spontaneous mutation (a permanent change in the structure of a specific gene). Once such a spontaneous mutation has been established in an individual, however, it is then possible to be passed on to any offspring. The chance of a person with NF passing on the NF gene to a child is 50%.

NF-1 has a number of possible signs and can be diagnosed if any two of the following are present:

- The presence of café-au-lait (French for coffee-with-milk) spots. These are patches of tan or light brown skin, usually about 5-15 mm in diameter. Nearly all patients with NF-1 will display these spots.
- Multiple freckles in the armpit or groin area
- Ninty percent of patients with NF-1 have tiny tumors called Lisch nodules in the iris (colored area) of the eye.
- Neurofibromas. These soft tumors are the hallmark of NF-1. They occur under the skin, often located along nerves or within the gastrointestinal tract. Neurofibromas are small and rubbery, and the skin overlying them may be somewhat purple.
- Skeletal deformities, such as a twisted spine (scoliosis), curved spine (humpback), or bowed legs
- Tumors along the optic nerve, which cause vision disturbance in about 20% of patients
- The presence of NF-1 in a patient's parent, child, or sibling

There are very high rates of speech impairment, learning disabilities, and attention deficit disorder in children with NF-1. Other complications include the development of a seizure disorder, or the abnormal accumulation of fluid within the brain (hydrocephalus). A number of cancers are more common in patients with NF-1. These include a variety of types of malignant **brain tumors**, as well as leukemia, and cancerous tumors of certain muscles (rhabdomyosarcoma), the adrenal glands (pheochromocytoma), or the kidneys (Wilms' tumor).

KEY TERMS

Chromosome—A structure within the nucleus of every cell, which contains genetic information governing the organism's development.

Mutation—A permanent change to the genetic code of an organism. Once established, a mutation can be passed on to offspring.

Neurofibroma—A soft tumor usually located on a nerve.

Tumor—An abnormally multiplying mass of cells.

Patients with NF-2 do not necessarily have the same characteristic skin symptoms (café-au-lait spots, freckling, and neurofibromas of the skin) that appear in NF-1. The characteristic symptoms of NF-2 are due to tumors along the acoustic nerve. Interfering with the function of this nerve results in the loss of hearing, and the tumor may spread to neighboring nervous system structures, causing **weakness** of the muscles of the face, headache, **dizziness**, poor balance, and uncoordinated walking. Cloudy areas on the lens of the eye (called cataracts) frequently develop at an unusually early age. As in NF-1, the chance of brain tumors developing is unusually high.

Diagnosis

Diagnosis is based on the symptoms outlined above. Diagnosis of NF-1 requires that at least two of the listed signs are present. Diagnosis of NF-2 requires the presence of either a mass on the acoustic nerve or another distinctive nervous system tumor. An important diagnostic clue for either NF-1 or NF-2 is the presence of the disorder in a patient's parent, child, or sibling.

Monitoring the progression of neurofibromatosis involves careful testing of vision and hearing. X-ray studies of the bones are frequently done to watch for the development of deformities. CT scans and MRI scans are performed to track the development/progression of tumors in the brain and along the nerves. Auditory evoked potentials (the electric response evoked in the cerebral cortex by stimulation of the acoustic nerve) may be helpful to determine involvement of the acoustic nerve, and EEG (electroencephalogram, a record of electrical currents in the brain) may be needed for patients with suspected seizures.

Treatment

There are no available treatments for the disorders that underlie either type of neurofibromatosis. To some extent, the symptoms of NF-1 and NF-2 can be treated individually. Skin tumors can be surgically removed. Some brain tumors and tumors along the nerves can be surgically removed or treated with drugs (chemotherapy) or x-ray treatments (radiation therapy). Twisting or curving of the spine and bowed legs may require surgical treatment or the wearing of a special brace.

Prognosis

Prognosis varies depending on the types of tumors which an individual develops. As tumors grow, they begin to destroy surrounding nerves and structures. Ultimately, this destruction can result in blindness, deafness, increasingly poor balance, and increasing difficulty with the coordination necessary for walking. Deformities of the bones and spine can also interfere with walking and movement. When cancers develop, prognosis worsens according to the specific type of cancer.

Prevention

There is no known way to prevent the approximately 50% of all NF cases that occur due to a spontaneous change in the genes (mutation). New cases of inherited NF can be prevented with careful genetic counseling. Individuals with NF can be made to understand that each of their offspring has a 50% chance of also having NF. When a parent has NF, and the specific genetic defect causing the parent's disease has been identified, tests can be performed on the fetus (developing baby) during pregnancy. Amniocentesis or chorionic villus sampling are two techniques that allow small amounts of the baby's cells to be removed for examination. The tissue can then be examined for the presence of the parent's genetic defect. Some families choose to use this information in order to prepare for the arrival of a child with a serious medical problem. Other families may choose not to continue the pregnancy.

Resources

ORGANIZATIONS

March of Dimes Birth Defects Foundation. 1275 Mamaroneck Ave., White Plains, NY 10605. (914) 428-7100. resourcecenter@modimes.org. http://www.modimes.org.

National Neurofibromatosis Foundation, Inc. 95 Pine St., 16th Floor, New York, NY 10005. (800) 323-7938. http://nf.org.

Neurofibromatosis, Inc. 8855 Annapolis Rd., No.110, Lanham, MD 20706-2924. (800) 942-6825.

Rosalyn Carson-DeWitt, MD

Neuroleptic malignant syndrome

Definition

Neuroleptic malignant syndrome is a rare, potentially life-threatening disorder that is usually precipitated by the use of medications that block the neurotransmitter called dopamine. Most often, the drugs involved are those that treat psychosis, called neuroleptic medications. The syndrome results in dysfunction of the autonomic nervous system, the branch of the nervous system responsible for regulating such involuntary actions as heart rate, blood pressure, digestion, and sweating. Muscle tone, body temperature, and consciousness are also severely affected.

Description

Most cases of neuroleptic malignant syndrome develop 4–14 days of the initiation of a new drug or an increase in dose. However, the syndrome can begin as soon as hours after the first dose or as long as years after medication initiation.

A variety of factors may increase an individual's risk of developing this condition:

• High environmental temperatures

• Dehydration

• Agitation or catatonia in a patient

• High initial dose or rapid dose increase of neuroleptic, and use of high-potency or intramuscular, long-acting (depot) preparations

• Simultaneous use of more than one causative agent

• Sudden discontinuation of medications for Parkinson's disease

• Past history of organic brain syndromes, depression, or bipolar disorder

• Past episode of neuromuscular malignant syndrome (risk of recurrence may be as high as 30%)

Because of heightened awareness of this syndrome and improved monitoring for its development, mortality rates have dropped from 20–30% to 5–11.6%.

Demographics

Neuroleptic malignant syndrome is thought to affect about 0.02–12.2% of all patients using neuroleptic medications. Because more men than women take neuroleptic medications, the male-to-female ratio is about 2:1.

Causes and symptoms

Neuroleptic malignant syndrome occurs due to interference with dopamine activity in the **central nervous system**, either by depletion of available reserves of dopamine or by blockade of receptors that dopamine usually stimulates.

Neuroleptic malignant syndrome most commonly affects patients who are using neuroleptic or antipsychotic medications, including prochlorperazine (Compazine), promethazine (Phenergan), olanzapine (Zyprexa), clozapine (Clozaril), and risperidone (Risperdal) . Other medications that block dopamine may also precipitate the syndrome, including metoclopramide (Reglan), amoxapine (Ascendin), and lithium. Too-fast withdrawal of drugs used to treat Parkinson's disease (levodopa, bromocriptine, and **amantadine**) can also precipitate neuroleptic malignant syndrome.

Symptoms of the disorder include:

• Extremely high body temperature (hyperthermia), ranging from 38.6° to 42.3° C or 101° to 108° F

• Heavy sweating

• Fast heart rate (tachydardia)

• Fast respiratory rate (tachypnea)

• Rapidly fluctuating blood pressure

• Impaired consciousness

• Tremor

• Rigid, stiff muscles (termed "lead pipe rigidity")

• Catatonia (a fixed stuporous state)

Without relatively immediate, aggressive treatment, **coma** and complete respiratory and cardiovascular collapse will take place, followed by death.

Diagnosis

Diagnosis requires a high level of suspicion when characteristic symptoms appear in a patient treated with agents known to cause neuroleptic malignant syndrome.

The usual diagnostic criteria for neuroleptic malignant syndrome includes the presence of hyperthermia (temperature over 38° C or 101° F) with no other assignable cause, muscle rigidity, and at least five of the following signs or symptoms: impaired mental status, **tremor**, fast heart rate, fast respiratory rate, loss of bladder or bowel control, fluctuating blood pressure, metabolic acidosis, fluctuating blood pressure, excess blood acidity (metabolic acidosis), increased blood levels of creatanine phosphokinase (normally found in muscles and released into the bloodstream due to muscle damage), heavy sweating, drooling, or increased white blood cell count (leukocytosis).

KEY TERMS

Autonomic nervous system—The divisions of the nervous system that control involuntary functions, such as breathing, heart rate, blood pressure, digestion, glands, smooth muscle.

Bipolar disorder—A psychiatric illness characterized by both recurrent depression and recurrent mania (abnormally high energy, agitation, irritability).

Catatonia—A fixed, motionless stupor.

Creatanine phosphokinase—A chemical normally found in the muscle fibers and released into the bloodstream when the muscles undergo damage and breakdown.

Depot—A type of drug preparation and administration that involves the slow, gradual release from an area of the body where the drug has been injected.

Depression—A psychiatric disorder in which the mood is low for a prolonged period of time, and feelings of hopelessness and inadequacy interfere with normal functioning.

Dopamine—A brain neurotransmitter involved in movement.

Hyperthermia—Elevated body temperature.

Leukocytosis—An elevated white blood cell count.

Metabolic acidosis—Overly acidic condition of the blood.

Neuroleptic—Referring to a type of drug used to treat psychosis.

Neurotransmitter—A chemical that transmits information in the nervous system.

Organic brain syndrome—A brain disorder that is caused by defective structure or abnormal functioning of the brain.

Parkinson's disease—A disease caused by deficient dopamine in the brain and resulting in a progressively severe movement disorder (tremor, weakness, difficulty walking, muscle rigidity, fixed facial expression).

Receptor—An area on the cell membrane where a specific chemical can bind in order to either activate or inhibit certain cellular functions.

Tachycardia—Elevated heart rate.

Tachypnea—Elevated breathing rate.

Treatment team

Neuroleptic malignant syndrome usually requires treatment in an intensive care unit, with appropriate specialists, including intensivists, pulmonologists, cardiologists, psychiatrists.

Treatment

Treatment must be aggressive. Supportive treatment should include hydration with fluids, cooling, and supplemental oxygen. Causative medications should be immediately discontinued, and medications that restore dopamine levels (bromocriptine, amantadine) administered. Dantrolene can be given to more quickly resolve muscle rigidity and hyperthermia. **Benzodiazepines**, such as lorazepam, may help agitated patients and may also help relax rigid muscles. Benzodiazepines may also aid in the reversal of catatonia. In severe or intractable cases of catatonia or psychosis that remains after other symptoms of neuroleptic malignant syndrome have resolved, electroconvulsive therapy may be required.

Prognosis

With quick identification of the syndrome and immediate supportive treatment, the majority of patients recover fully, although mortality rates are still significant. Signs that may warn of a poor prognosis include temperature over 104° F and kidney failure. In patients whose syndrome was precipitated by the use of oral medications, symptoms may last for 7–10 days. In patients whose syndrome was precipitated by the use of long-acting, intramuscular preparation, symptoms may continue as long as 21 days.

Special concerns

Patients with a history of neuroleptic malignant syndrome are also at increased risk for a similar malignant hyperthermia syndrome that is precipitated by the administration of surgical anesthetics.

Resources

BOOKS

Saper, Clifford B. "Autonomic disorders and their management." In *Cecil Textbook of Medicine*, edited by Lee Goldman. Philadelphia: W. B. Saunders, 2003.

Kompoliti, Katie, and Stacy S. Horn. "Drug-induced and iatrogenic neurological disorders." In *Ferri's Clinical Advisor: Instant Diagnosis and Treatment*, edited by Fred F. Ferri. St. Louis: Mosby, 2004.

Olson, William H. "Neuroleptic malignant syndrome." In *Nelson Textbook of Pediatrics,* edited by Richard E. Behrman, et al. Philadelphia: W. B. Saunders, 2004.

WEBSITES

National Institute of Neurological Disorders and Stroke (NINDS). *NINDS Neuroleptic Malignant Syndrome Information Page.* January 23, 2002. http://www.ninds. nih.gov/health_and_medical/disorders/neuroleptic_ syndrome.htm (June 4, 2004).

ORGANIZATIONS

Neuroleptic Malignant Syndrome Information Service. PO Box 1069 11 East State Street, Sherburne, NY 13460. Phone: (607) 674-7920. Fax: (607) 674-7910. Tollfree phone: (888) 667-8367. Email: gillesan@exchange.nih. gov, info@nmsis.org. http://www.nmsis.org/index. shtml.

Rosalyn Carson-DeWitt, MD

Neurological emergencies

Definition

Neurological emergencies are treatable disorders of or injuries to the **central nervous system** in which the patient is at risk of irreversible damage or death if treatment is delayed.

Description

Neurological emergencies include a range of different conditions ranging from traumatic injury to the brain or spinal column, generalized **weakness**, and cerebrovascular disorders (stroke, transient ischemic attacks) to seizures, infections of the central nervous system (**meningitis, encephalitis**), and autoimmune disorders (**myasthenia gravis, Guillain-Barré syndrome**). The specific symptoms vary.

Demographics

Neurological emergencies are common occurrences in the United States and Canada. According to the National Institutes of Health (NIH), 1.1 million Americans annually suffer an emergency affecting the central nervous system—one emergency every 28 seconds. The most common causes of these emergencies are strokes, seizures, motor vehicle accidents, **falls**, or severe blows to the head. About 250,000 people in the United States die each year from neurological emergencies, and many of the survivors lose their ability to live independently.

Specific neurological emergencies

The conditions or disorders most commonly considered neurological emergencies include:

• Coma. Coma is defined as a state of unconsciousness lasting longer than six hours, in which the person cannot be awakened; does not respond to light, sound, or painful stimuli; and does not initiate voluntary actions. Coma can result from a variety of disorders and conditions, including stroke, lack of oxygen, hypoglycemia (low blood sugar), head trauma, a brain tumor, or drug intoxication.

• Acute stroke. Stroke is a neurological emergency that occurs when blood flow is interrupted to part of the brain. Without blood to supply oxygen and nutrients and to remove waste products, brain cells quickly begin to die. Depending on the region of the brain affected, a stroke may cause paralysis, speech impairment, loss of memory and reasoning ability, coma, or death. A stroke also is sometimes called a brain attack or a cerebrovascular accident (CVA).

• Seizures and status epilepticus. Status epilepticus (SE) is a potentially life-threatening persistent seizure. The Epilepsy Foundation defines it as "More than 30 minutes of continuous seizure activity or two or more sequential seizures without full recovery of consciousness between seizures." Emergency department physicians generally treat any seizure lasting 10 minutes or longer as a case of SE.

• Subarachnoid hemorrhage. Subarachnoid hemorrhage (SAH) is a neurological emergency caused by bleeding into the space between the middle of the three layers of membrane covering the brain (the arachnoid mater) and the innermost layer (the pia mater). SAH may result from the rupture of an aneurysm in the brain or from a head injury. It is characterized by a sudden intense "thunderclap" headache, vomiting, confusion, and sometimes seizures, and accounts for about 7% of all strokes.

• Traumatic injury to the brain or spinal cord. A head injury is defined as any alteration in mental or physical functioning related to a blow to the head. It is not necessary for the person to lose consciousness; however, loss of consciousness generally indicates a more severe injury.

• Cerebral infections. Infections of the brain and spinal cord include prion diseases, meningitis (inflammation of the tissues covering the brain and spinal cord due to infection), and encephalitis (inflammation of the brain itself). Encephalitis and meningitis are most often caused by viruses, but meningitis can also be caused by bacterial or fungal infections.

Bacterial meningitis is generally a more serious infection than viral meningitis.

- Acute compression of the spinal cord. Compression of the spinal cord is a neurological emergency that can be caused by a tumor pressing on the spinal cord, by bone fragments from a fractured vertebra, by a ruptured spinal disk, or by an abscess (a collection of pus in a body cavity). The person may experience severe back pain, paralysis of the limbs or decreased sensation below the level of the compression, urinary or fecal incontinence, painless urinary retention (inability to empty the bladder), or intermittent shooting electrical sensations.

- Neuromuscular paralysis of the respiratory system. The most common causes of this type of disorder are Guillain-Barré syndrome (GBS), a progressive auto-immune disorder of the nervous system often triggered by an acute infection, and myasthenia gravis (MG), an autoimmune neuromuscular disorder. The patient with MG may have difficulty breathing, swallowing, seeing, walking, or holding up the head. A person with GBS may experience abnormal tingling sensations, choking, or difficulty breathing.

- Altered mental status. Altered mental status, also known as altered level of consciousness, refers to any state of alertness that is less than normal. The various levels of altered consciousness are confusion, delirium, sleepiness, stupor, and coma. Altered mental status can have a variety of causes, including insufficient supply of oxygen to the brain, exposure to toxins, excessive fluid pressure within the skull, high fever, various infections, and drug or alcohol withdrawal.

- Acute generalized weakness.

- Syncope. Syncope (pronounced SINK-uh-pee) is a temporary loss of consciousness followed by loss of postural tone and spontaneous recovery. The affected person will typically have cool extremities, a weak pulse, and shallow breathing. Most cases of syncope result from insufficient blood flow to the brain, and most causes of syncope are benign. They include postural hypotension (sudden drop in blood pressure from standing up too quickly), prolonged standing, situational (having blood drawn or being in an emotionally distressing situation), pregnancy, heat exposure, anemia, migraine headaches, side effects of certain drugs, and some psychiatric disorders. Causes of syncope that are potentially dangerous include abnormal heart rhythms, aortic stenosis, cardiomyopathy (deterioration of the heart muscle), pulmonary embolism, or an aortic dissection (tear in the inner wall of the aorta).

Some neurologists also define the following disorders as neurological emergencies:

- acute visual loss or double vision
- psychogenic neurological syndromes/behavior disturbances
- movement disorders
- transient ischemic attack (TIA), which has the same symptoms as a full-blown stroke but goes away in a few minutes or hours, leaving no permanent effects. It is, however, a warning sign—an indication that the person is at risk of a major stroke and should see a doctor right away.

Treatment team

The treatment team in a neurological emergency may include emergency medical technicians (EMTs) if the emergency has resulted from a motor vehicle accident, fall, or other accident in the home, or an emergency in a public place requiring transport to the hospital. Most people with neurological emergencies will be seen first in the emergency department by specialists in emergency medicine, which has been a recognized specialty in the United States since 1979.

The emergency medical staff will consult other specialists according to the nature of the patient's injuries or overall neurological condition. These may include neurologists, anesthesiologists, orthopedic surgeons, oral surgeons, ophthalmologists, trauma surgeons, psychiatrists, cardiologists, and critical care specialists.

When to call 911

It can be difficult for people who are not medical professionals to know when a friend, relative, or stranger taken ill in a public place is having a neurological emergency and needs immediate help. The following are some general guidelines for knowing when to call 911.

- Seizures and status epilepticus—if the seizure lasts longer than 5 minutes, the person stops breathing, the seizure happened in the water, or the person appears to be injured in any way, call 911.

- Spinal cord injury—if the person has a visible head injury and is drifting in and out of consciousness; is lying with the neck or back twisted or oddly positioned; complains of pain in the neck or back; cannot move the neck; complains of weakness, numbness, or paralysis; cannot control the limbs, bladder, or bowels; and/or the injury to the head or neck was caused by significant force, call 911.

- Head injury—if the person is unconscious; is confused or disoriented either immediately or several hours after the blow on the head; if the injury was caused by a falling object or a criminal attack; if the person complains of a worsening headache, nausea, or vomiting; if the person is unsteady on their feet; if the person has loss of memory or sudden mood changes, call 911.

- Coma—call 911 at once if the person is unresponsive to light or painful stimuli (such as pinching), is breathing irregularly, and is not moving the limbs.

- Subarachnoid hemorrhage—about 50% of cases of SAH are fatal. Call 911 at once if the person complains of a sudden severe headache, loses consciousness, or has a seizure.

- Syncope—in most cases of syncope, the person will feel better as soon as they regain consciousness and remain quiet for 10–15 minutes. Call 911 if the syncope occurs together with signs of a seizure; if the person is known to have a heart condition; if the person has had several episodes of syncope in a brief period of time; or if the person has suffered an injury from falling as a result of the syncope.

- Encephalitis—call 911 if an adult or older child has high fever, altered consciousness, severe headache, muscle weakness or paralysis, seizures, hallucinations, or double vision. For infants or small children, call 911 if the soft spots in the skull (fontanelles) are bulging, the infant is feeding poorly, cries inconsolably, has a stiff body, or has nausea and vomiting.

- Meningitis—for an adult or older child, call 911 if the person has the classic signs of severe meningitis, including stiff neck, fever, severe headache, nausea and vomiting, and mental confusion. For infants or small children, call 911 if the soft spots in the skull (fontanelles) are bulging, the infant is feeding poorly, is excessively sleepy, cries inconsolably, cries even harder when picked up, has seizures, or has nausea and vomiting.

- Neuromuscular disorders—for myasthenia gravis, call 911 if the person has trouble breathing, holding up the head, seeing, walking, or swallowing. Guillain-Barré syndrome is a more serious and potentially fatal disorder. Call 911 if the person is choking on saliva, complains of tingling sensations that began in the feet and are moving up the body, tingling sensations that are getting worse, tingling that involves both hands and feet, or difficulty breathing.

- Spinal cord compression—call 911 if the person complains of severe back pain without a traumatic injury or occasional pain resembling an electric shock, is experiencing loss of sensation or decreased sensation in the limbs, cannot control their bowels or bladder, or cannot empty their bladder.

- Altered level of consciousness—in some cases it can be difficult to distinguish the symptoms of delirium from those of dementia. But if the person's confusion and difficulty paying attention has come on suddenly or goes up and down over the course of the day, is accompanied by high fever, or appears to be related to drug or alcohol abuse, call 911.

Stroke has five major signs or symptoms. The American Stroke Association has a quick symptom checklist called "Give Me 5" that can be used by a friend, relative, coworker, or bystander as well as by individuals who think they may be having a stroke:

- Walk: Is the person having trouble with balance or coordination?
- Talk: Is speech difficult or slurred? Is the person's face drooping?
- Reach: Is one side of the body weak or numb?
- See: Is vision partly or entirely lost?
- Feel: Does the person have a sudden severe headache with no obvious cause?If any of these symptoms are present, call 911.

Appropriate use of the 911 system

As of 2011, most people in the United States call 911 when they need to summon help for any emergency, medical or otherwise. Because of changes in communications technology, such as smartphones, wireless phones, text messaging and others that were not in existence when the 911 system first came into use in the 1960s, Congress formed the National 911 Office, currently part of the National Highway Traffic Safety Administration (NHTSA). The office conducted a public information campaign on the appropriate use of the 911 system.

Tips for making 911 calls in a neurological or other medical emergency:

- If a witness or bystander is not sure whether the situation is a true emergency, they should *call 911 and allow the call-taker to determine whether emergency help is needed.*

- The witness or bystander should be prepared to answer the call-taker's questions, such as the location of the emergency, the phone number being used to make the call, the nature of the emergency, the details of the person's injuries or symptoms, and any information they may have about the patient's general health.

- The witness or bystander should follow any instructions the call-taker gives them. Many 911 centers can tell people exactly what to do in a medical emergency until first responders arrive, such as providing step-by-step instructions regarding first aid or CPR.

- The witness or bystander should not hang up until the call-taker instructs them to do so.

KEY TERMS

Aneurysm—A pouchlike bulging of a blood vessel. Aneurysms can rupture, leading to stroke or subarachnoid hemorrhage.

Cerebrovascular—Referring to the blood vessels that supply the brain.

Coma—A state of deep unconsciousness lasting longer than six hours caused by disease, injury, drug overdose, or poison.

Confusion—In medicine, a condition in which a person is disoriented with respect to time, place, and personal identity, and generally does not function mentally at their normal level.

Delirium—Sometimes called acute confusional state, delirium is an altered state of consciousness marked by an acute onset, fluctuations over the course of the day, disorganized behavior, and difficulty paying attention. The person may also have hallucinations and delusions.

Encephalitis—The medical term for inflammation of the brain.

Guillain-Barré syndrome—An autoimmune disorder of the peripheral nervous system often triggered by an infection.

Meningitis—The medical term for inflammation of the meninges, the three layers of membranous tissue that cover the brain and spinal cord.

Myasthenia gravis—An autoimmune disorder of the neuromuscular system characterized by weakness and rapid fatigue of the voluntary muscles.

Status epilepticus—An acute prolonged brain seizure lasting 30 minutes or more.

Stupor—A decreased level of consciousness in which a person responds only to painful stimuli.

Subarachnoid hemorrhage—A disorder caused by bleeding between the second and the innermost of the three layers of membrane (meninges) covering the brain.

Syncope—Temporary loss of consciousness followed by loss of postural tone and spontaneous revival.

Transient ischemic attack (TIA)—A brief stroke lasting from a few minutes to 24 hours. TIAs are sometimes called mini-strokes.

QUESTIONS TO ASK YOUR DOCTOR

- How can I tell when someone is having a neurological emergency?

- Have you ever treated a patient in the office who was having a neurological emergency?

- What are some useful guidelines for calling 911?

- Is there any training for people who are not medical professionals that you would recommend for dealing better with these emergencies?

Clinical trials

The National Institutes of Health established the Neurological Emergencies Treatment Trials (NETT) in early 2007. NETT is a research consortium that involved 17 university-related meducal centers throughout the United States as of 2011. The purpose of NETT is to draw together neurologists, emergency physicians, orthopedic surgeons, trauma surgeons, and doctors from other disciplines to investigate better treatment options for neurological emergencies.

A distinctive feature of NETT clinical trials is that some may involve what is called exception from informed consent. In most clinical trials, those accepted to participate as subjects are given detailed information about the drugs or procedures used in the trial and possible complications or side effects. They are then asked to sign an informed consent document. People who are suffering a neurological emergency may be unconscious or otherwise unable to give informed consent for an investigational treatment. In some cases, a relative or guardian can give consent for the patient.

Federal law also provides for an exception to informed consent in the event that someone has a neurological emergency and no relative can be found. Physicians may administer an investigational treatment to the patient without informed consent *when no proven or effective treatment is available*. If a NETT clinical study will require exception from informed consent, the public must be informed and asked to submit comments before the study can begin.

Resources

BOOKS

American Academy of Orthopaedic Surgeons and American College of Emergency Physicians. *Critical Care Transport*. Sudbury, MA: Jones and Bartlett, 2011.

Henry, Gregory L., Neal Little, et al. *Neurologic Emergencies*. 3rd ed. New York: McGraw-Hill, 2010.

Parvensky Barwell, Catherine A. *Emergency Medical Technician Manual*. Sudbury, MA: Jones and Bartlett, 2012.

Stone, C. Keith, and Roger L. Humphries, eds. *Current Diagnosis and Treatment: Emergency Medicine*. 6th ed. New York: McGraw-Hill, 2008.

PERIODICALS

Brandon, J., and G.J. Hill. "Altered Mental Status in a U.S. Army Special Forces Soldier." *Journal of Special Operations Medicine* 11 (Winter 2011): 27–29.

Brown, E.N., et al. "General Anesthesia, Sleep, and Coma." *New England Journal of Medicine* 363 (December 30, 2010): 2638–50.

D'Onofrio, G., et al. "NIH Roundtable on Opportunities to Advance Research on Neurologic and Psychiatric Emergencies." *Annals of Emergency Medicine* 56 (November 2010): 551–64.

Marcantonio, E.R. "Delirium." *Annals of Internal Medicine* 154 (2011): ITC61.

Martin, C.O., and M.M. Rymer. "Hemorrhagic Stroke: Aneurysmal Subarachnoid Hemorrhage." *Missouri Medicine* 108 (March-April 2011): 124–27.

Mateen, F.J. "Neurological Disorders in Complex Humanitarian Emergencies and Natural Disasters." *Annals of Neurology* 68 (September 2010): 282–94.

McMullen, J.T., et al. "Time-critical Neurological Emergencies: The Unfulfilled Role for Point-of-care Testing." *International Journal of Emergency Medicine* 18 (May 2010): 127–31.

Raza, S.S., et al. "21-year-old Man with Chest Pain, Respiratory Distress, and Altered Mental Status." *Mayo Clinic Proceedings* 86 (May 2011): e29–e32.

Stern, S. "Observing and Recording Neurological Dysfunction." *Emergency Nurse* 18 (March 2011): 28–31.

Wang, V.Y., et al. "Spine and Spinal Cord Emergencies: Vascular and Infectious Causes." *Meuroimaging Clinics of North America* 20 (November 2010): 639–50.

WEBSITES

Alagiakrishnan, Kannayiram. "Delirium." Medscape Reference. http://emedicine.medscape.com/article/288890-overview (accessed July 24, 2011).

Becske, Tibor. "Subarachnoid Hemorrhage." Medscape Reference. http://emedicine.medscape.com/article/1164341-overview (accessed July 24, 2011).

"Brain Aneurysm." Mayo Clinic. http://www.mayoclinic.com/health/brain-aneurysm/DS00582 (accessed July 24, 2011).

"Coma." Mayo Clinic. http://www.mayoclinic.com/health/coma/DS00724 (accessed July 24, 2011).

"Encephalitis." Mayo Clinic. http://www.mayoclinic.com/health/encephalitis/DS00226 (accessed July 24, 2011).

Olson, David A. "Head Injury." Medscape Reference. http://emedicine.medscape.com/article/1163653-overview (accessed July 24, 2011).

Razonable, Raymund R. "Meningitis." Medscape Reference. http://emedicine.medscape.com/article/232915-overview (accessed July 24, 2011).

Roth, Julie L. "Status Epilepticus." Medscape Reference. http://emedicine.medscape.com/article/1164462-overview (accessed July 24, 2011).

"What Is EMS?" Emergency Medical Services (EMS). http://www.ems.gov/emssystem/whatisems.html (accessed July 24, 2011).

"When to Call 911." 911.gov. http://www.911.gov/whencall.html (accessed July 24, 2011).

ORGANIZATIONS

American Academy of Neurology (AAN), 1080 Montreal Avenue, Saint Paul, MN 55116, (651) 695-2717, (800) 879-1960, Fax: (651) 695-2791, member services@aan.com, http://www.aan.com.

American College of Emergency Physicians (ACEP), P.O. Box 619911, Dallas, TX 75261-9911, (972) 550-0911, (800) 798-1822, Fax: (972) 580-2816, membership@acep.org, http://www.acep.org.

Foundation for Education and Research in Neurological Emergencies (FERNE), c/o UIC Dept of Emergency Medicine, 471 H, CME, (MC724), 808 South Wood Street, Chicago, IL 60612-7354, (312) 355-1651, Fax: (312) 355-1269, ferne@ferne.org, http://www.ferne.org.

National Highway Traffic Safety Administration (NHTSA), Office of Emergency Medical Services (EMS), 1200 New Jersey Avenue S.E., Washington, DC 20590, (202) 366-5440, Fax: (202) 366-7149, http://www.ems.gov.

National Institute of Neurological Disorders and Stroke (NINDS), P.O. Box 5801, Bethesda, MD 20824, (301) 496-5751, (800) 352-9424, http://www.ninds.nih.gov.

Neurological Emergencies Treatment Trials (NETT), University of Michigan Health System, Dept. of Emergency Medicine, 24 Frank Lloyd Wright Drive, Suite H3100, Ann Arbor, MI 48106, (734) 232-2142, Fax: (734) 232-2122, http://www.nett.umich.edu.

Society for Academic Emergency Medicine (SAEM), 2340 S. River Road, Suite 200, Des Plaines, IL 60018, (847) 813-9823, Fax: (847) 813-5450, http://www.saem.org.

Rebecca J. Frey, PhD

Neurologist

Definition

A neurologist is a physician who has undergone additional training to diagnose and treat disorders of the nervous system.

Description

The training a neurologist receives enables the individual to recognize nervous system malfunctions, to accurately diagnose the nature of the dysfunction (such as disease or injury), and to treat the malady. While many people associate a neurologist with treating brain injuries, this is just one facet of a neurologist's responsibility and expertise. Diseases of the spinal cord, nerves, and muscles that affect the operation of the nervous system can also be addressed by a neurologist.

The training that is necessary to become a neurologist begins with the traditional medical background. From there, the medical doctor or osteopath trains for several more years to acquire the expertise in the structure, functioning, and repair of the body's neurological structures, including the area of the brain called the cerebral cortex and how the various regions of the cortex contribute to the normal and abnormal functioning of the body.

Typically, a neurologist's educational path begins with premed studies at a university or college. These studies can last up to four years. Successful candidates enter medical school. Another four years of study is required for the degree of doctor of medicine (MD) or a doctor of osteopathy (OD). Following completion of the advanced degree, a one-year internship is usually undertaken in internal medicine; sometimes, internships in transitional programs that include pediatrics and emergency-room training are chosen. Finally, another training period of at least three years follows in a neurology residency program. The latter program provides specialty experience in a hospital and can include research. Postdoctoral fellowships lasting one year or more offer additional opportunities for specialization.

After completion of the more than decade-long training, medical doctors or osteopaths can become certified as neurologists through the American Board of Psychiatry and Neurology. Those with an osteopathy background can be certified through the American Board of Osteopathic Neurologists and Psychiatrists. Most neurologists belong to professional organizations such as the American Academy of Neurology (AAN), which is dedicated to setting practice standards, supporting research, providing continuing education, and promoting optimum care for persons with neurological disorders. Numerous professional publications specialize in neurology, including *Neurology Today*, *Neurology*, *Brain*, and *Archives of Neurology*.

Subspecialties in neurology include clinical neurophysiology, neurodevelopmental disabilities, pain medicine, vascular neurology, and neuromuscular medicine. The American Board of Psychiatry and Neurology hopes the number of fellows and programs in the latter two subspecialties grow.

A neurologist can sometimes be a patient's principal physician. Such is the case when the patient has a neurological problem such as Parkinson's or Alzheimer's disease or multiple sclerosis. As well, an important aspect of a neurologist's daily duties is to offer advice to other physicians on how to treat neurological problems. A family physician might consult a neurologist when caring for patients with stroke or severe headache.

When a neurologist examines a patient, details such as vision, physical strength and coordination, reflexes, and sensations such as touch and smell are probed to help determine if the medical problem is related to nervous system damage. More tests might be done to help determine the exact cause of the problem and how to treat the condition. Among the tests a neurologist may perform are computed axial tomography (CAT) scans, magnetic resonance imaging (MRI) and lumbar punctures. While neurologists can recommend surgery, they do not actually perform the surgery. That is the domain of the neurosurgeon.

One well-known neurologist is the English-born physician and writer Oliver Sacks (1933–). In addition to maintaining a clinical practice, Sacks has written numerous popular books that describe patients' experiences with neurological disorders and neurologists' experiences in treating them. Another notable neurologist was Alois Alzheimer (1864–1915). A German neurologist, he first observed and identified the symptoms of what is now known as Alzheimer's disease.

Resources

BOOKS

Blustein, Bonnie Ellen. *Preserve Your Love for Science: Life of William A. Hammond, American Neurologist*. Cambridge, UK: Cambridge University Press, 1991.

Restak, Richard. *The Brain Has a Mind of Its Own: Insights from a Practicing Neurologist*. Three Rivers, MI: Three Rivers, 1999.

Sacks, Oliver. *The Mind's Eye*. New York: Knopf, 2010.

WEBSITES

Gandey, Allison. "Future of neurology subspecialties in question." *Medscape Medical News*. http://www.medscape.com/viewarticle/729845 (accessed August 27, 2011).

"What Is a Neurologist?" Remedy's Health Communities. http://www.neurologychannel.com/neurologist/what-is-a-neurologist.shtml (accessed August 27, 2011).

ORGANIZATIONS

American Academy of Neurology (AAN), 1080 Montreal Avenue, Saint Paul, MN 55116, (651) 695-2717, (800) 879-1960, Fax: (651) 695-2791, memberservices@ aan.com, http://www.aan.com.

American Board of Psychiatry and Neurology (ABPN), 2150 E. Lake Cook Road, Suite 900, Buffalo Grove, IL 60089, (847) 229-6500, Fax: (847) 229-6600, questions@ abpn.com, http://www.abpn.com.

Brian Douglas Hoyle
Fran Hodgkins

Neuromuscular blockers

Definition

Neuromuscular blocking agents are a class of drugs primarily indicated for use as an adjunct to anesthesia. Neuromuscular blocking drugs relax skeletal muscles and induce paralysis.

Interest in neuromuscular blockers began in the nineteenth century, when British and German chemists and physicians began to experiment with curare, an arrow poison that had been used by various South American tribes to paralyze animals in the hunt. By the end of the nineteenth century it was known that curare does not kill animals and that they will recover if kept on artificial respiration; however, it was not until 1935 that the British researcher Harold King (1887–1956) successfully isolated tubocurarine, the active chemical in curare and established its chemical structure. Tubocurarine, also known as d-tubocurarine or DTC, was the first neuromuscular blocker used in surgery; it was introduced in the 1940s. DTC is used less often as of 2011 than blockers that were developed later; one of them, suxamethonium (also called succinylcholine) won its developer the Nobel Prize in Medicine in 1957.

Purpose

Neuromuscular blockers are indicated for a wide variety of uses in a hospital setting, from surgery to trauma care. In surgery, they are used to prepare patients for intubation before being placed on a ventilator and to suppress the patient's spontaneous breathing once on a ventilator.

Description

Neuromuscular blockers relax skeletal muscle tone by blocking transmission of key neurotransmitters through the neuron receptors at the neuromuscular junction (NMJ). They are divided into two major categories, depolarizing and non-depolarizing neuromuscular blockers, corresponding to the manner in which they exert their therapeutic effect. Depolarizing neuromuscular blocking agents, which are also called leptocurares, mimic the effects of the neurotransmitter acetylcholine (ACh) and change the interaction between ACh and neuron receptors. Depolarization refers to a change in the membrane of a cell when its electrical charge becomes either more positive or less negative. Blockade occurs when depolarizing neuromuscular blockers are used because the cell membranes surrounding the neuromuscular junction become unresponsive to typical ACh-receptor interaction.

By contrast, nondepolarizing neuromuscular blockers, also known as pachycurares, bind to receptors to prevent transmission of impulses through ACh neurotransmitters. The majority of neuromuscular blockers fall into this category.

Neuromuscular blockers are primarily used in a clinical or hospital setting. In the United States, they are known by several generic and brand names, including atracurium (Tracurium), cisatracurium (Nimbex), doxacurium (Neuromax), pancuronium (Pavulon), pipecuronium (Arduan), rocuronium (Zemeron), suxamethonium or succinylcholine (Anectine), tubocurarine, and vecuronium (Norcuron). According to the Food and Drug Administration (FDA), production of mivacurium (Mivacron), a nondepolarizing blocker, was discontinued by the manufacturer in June 2006 because of manufacturing and financial concerns.

A physician will decide which neuromuscular blocking agent or combination of neuromuscular blocker and other type of anesthesia is appropriate for an individual patient. During surgical anesthesia, neuromuscular blockers are administered after the induction of unconsciousness in order to avoid patient distress at the inability to purposefully move muscles. Neuromuscular blockers can be used on pediatric as well as adult patients; they are also used in veterinary medicine.

Recommended dosage

Neuromuscular blocking agents are most often administered though an intravenous (IV) infusion tube. Typically, the time in which the medicines begin to exert their effects and duration of action are more predictable when neuromuscular blocking agents are administered via IV. Dosages vary depending on the neuromuscular blocking agent used and the duration of action desired. The age, weight, and general health of an individual patient can also affect dosing requirements.

Depolarizing and non-depolarizing agents are grouped together into three categories based on the time in which they begin to exert their anesthetic effects, causing muscle relaxation or paralysis and desensitization, and the duration of those effects (duration of action). Short-acting neuromuscular blockers begin work within 30 seconds to 2.5 minutes and have a typical duration of action ranging 5–20 minutes. Short-acting agents include rocuronium and succinylcholine. Intermediate-acting agents exert their effects within 2–5 minutes and typically last for 20–60 minutes. Atracurium, cisatracurium, pancuronium, and vecuronium are intermediate-acting neuromuscular blockers. Long-acting neuromuscular blocking agents take effect within 2.5–6 minutes and last as long as 75–100 minutes. Doxacurium, pipecuronium, and tubocurarine are long-acting neuromuscular blocking agents.

The duration of action of any neuromuscular blocking agent can be prolonged by administering smaller supplemental (maintenance) doses via IV following the initial blockade-creating dose.

In 2008 the European Union approved the use of a drug called sugammadex (Bridion) to reverse the effects of rocuronium. Clinical trials indicate that sugammadex can reverse the effects of vecuronium and pancuronium as well as rocuronium. Sugamadex is the first of a new class of drugs called selective relaxant binding agents (SRBAs). The advantage of these new drugs is that they can reverse the action of neuromuscular blockers without the side effects of such other reversal agents as neostigmine.

Precautions

Each neuromuscular blocking agent has its own particular precautions, contraindications, and side effects; however, many precautions are common to all neuromuscular blockers. Neuromuscular blocking agents may not be suitable for persons with a history of lung diseases; malnutrition; stroke; increased intracranial pressure; increased intraocular (within the eye) pressure, as in glaucoma; liver or kidney disease; decreased renal function; diseases or disorders affecting the muscles; angina (chest pain); and irregular heartbeats and other heart problems. Neuromuscular blockers are not typically used on patients with recent severe burns, elevated potassium levels, or severe muscle trauma. There is an increased risk of seizure in patients with such seizure disorders as epilepsy.

Neuromuscular blockers can be administered to patients who have suffered a spinal cord injury resulting in **paraplegia** (paralysis) immediately following the injury. But further use of neuromuscular blockers is typically avoided 10–100 days after the initial trauma.

Patients who are obese or have increased plasma cholinesterase activity may exhibit increased resistance to neuromuscular blocking agents. Some **cholinergic stimulants** that act as **cholinesterase inhibitors**, including medications used in the treatment of **Alzheimer's disease**, may enhance neuromuscular blockade and prolong the duration of action of neuromuscular blockers.

With careful supervision, neuromuscular blocking agents can be used in pediatric patients. Rare but serious complications such as bradycardia (decreased heart rate) are more likely to develop in children than in adults.

Placental transfer (passing of the medication to the fetus) of neuromuscular blocking agents is minimal. Histamine release is associated with the neuromuscular blocking agents tubocurare and succinylcholine. Such complications as bronchospasm, decreased blood pressure, and blood clotting problems could arise in patients especially sensitive or susceptible to changes in histamine levels.

Although such cases are fortunately rare, neuromuscular blockers have been used in homicides. The journal *Anesthesiology* reported on two such cases in its March 2011 issue. The first case involved a nurse practitioner convicted in 2007 of killing her husband with rocuronium; the second involved an anesthesiologist found guilty of killing his wife and his lover's husband with injections of succinylcholine.

Side effects

In some patients, neuromuscular blockers may produce mild or moderate side effects. Anesthesiologists (specialists in administering anesthesia and treating pain) may notice a slight red flushing of the face as neuromuscular blockers are administered to the patient. After completion of the surgical procedure, headache, nausea, muscle soreness, and muscle **weakness** are the most frequently reported side effects attributed to neuromuscular blockers. Most of these side effects disappear or occur less frequently after a few hours or days.

With depolarizing neuromuscular blocking agents, fasciculations (involuntary muscle contractions) may occur before the onset of muscle relaxation or paralysis. Some patients report generalized muscle soreness or pain after taking a neuromuscular blocking agent that

KEY TERMS

Acetylcholine—The neurotransmitter (chemical that works in the brain to transmit nerve signals) involved in regulating muscles, memory, mood, and sleep.

Bradycardia—Slower than normal heart rate, usually defined as a resting heart rate of 60 beats per minute or less.

Depolarization—A change in a cell's membrane potential (the difference in voltage between the interior and exterior of the cell) in which it becomes more positive or less negative.

Fasciculations—Fine tremors of the muscles.

Intubation—The placement of a flexible tube into a patient's trachea (windpipe) to maintain an open airway or to administer certain drugs.

Neuromuscular junction—The junction between a nerve fiber and the muscle it supplies.

Neurotransmitter—Chemicals that allow the movement of information from one neuron across the gap between the adjacent neuron.

Selective relaxant binding agents (SRBAs)—A new class of drugs that can be used to reverse the effects of neuromuscular blockers. Sugammadex is the first drug in this category. It was discovered in Scotland in 2007.

causes fasciculations. Women and middle-aged patients reported this side effect more frequently.

Other uncommon side effects or complications associated with neuromuscular blockers can be serious or may indicate an allergic reaction. As neuromuscular blockers are most frequently used in trauma, surgical, and intensive hospital care, physicians may be able to counteract the following side effects or complications as they occur:

- bradycardia
- cessation of breathing
- severe bronchospasm
- prolonged numbness in the extremities
- extended paralysis
- jaw rigidity
- skeletal muscle atrophy or trauma
- impaired blood clotting
- severe decrease in blood pressure
- chest pain or irregular heartbeat

Interactions

Neuromuscular blocking agents may have negative interactions with some anticoagulants, anticonvulsants (especially those also indicated for use as skeletal muscle relaxants), antihistamines, antidepressants, antibiotics, pain killers (including nonprescription medications), and monoamine oxidase inhibitors (MAOIs; a class of antidepressant medications).

Cholinergic stimulants, some insecticides, diuretics (furosemide), local anesthetics, magnesium, antidepressants, anticonvulsants, aminoglycoside antibiotics, high estrogen levels, and metoclopramide (Reglan) may affect the duration of action of neuromuscular blocking agents.

Resources

BOOKS

Evers, Alex S., Mervyn Maze, and Evan D. Kharasch, eds. *Anesthetic Pharmacology*. 2nd ed. New York: Cambridge University Press, 2011.

Mashour, George A., and Ralph Lydic. *Neuroscientific Foundations of Anesthesiology*. New York: Oxford University Press, 2011.

PERIODICALS

Akha, A.S., et al. "Sugammadex: Cyclodextrins, Development of Selective Binding Agents, Pharmacology, Clinical Development, and Future Directions." *Anesthesiology Clinics* 28 (December 2010): 691–708.

Bennett, S., and W.E. Hurford. "When Should Sedation or Neuromuscular Blockade Be Used during Mechanical Ventilation?" *Respiratory Care* 56 (February 2011): 168–76.

Johnstone, R.E., et al. "Homicides Using Muscle Relaxants, Opioids, and Anesthetic Drugs: Anesthesiologist Assistance in Their Investigation and Prosecution." *Anesthesiology* 114 (March 2011): 713–16.

Meretoja, O.A. "Neuromuscular Block and Current Treatment Strategies for Its Reversal in Children." *Paediatric Anaesthesiology* 20 (July 2010): 591–604.

Porter, M.V., and M.S. Paleologos. "The Use of Rocuronium in a Patient with Cystic Fibrosis and End-stage Lung

Disease Made Safe by Sugammadex Reversal." *Anaesthesia and Intensive Care* 39 (March 2011): 299–302.

WEBSITES

"Death without Mercy." *48 Hours.* CBS News. http://www.cbsnews.com/video/watch/?id = 4280957n&tag = contentMain;contentBody (accessed July 17, 2011).
"Neuromuscular Blockers." GlobalRPh.com. http://www.globalrph.com/neuromuscular.htm (accessed July 17, 2011).
"PowerPoint on Neuromuscular Blockers Pharmacology: Mechanism of Action, Classification, Uses, Interactions and More." Pharmacology Corner. http://pharmacolo gycorner.com/powerpoint-on-neuromuscular-blockers-pharmacology-mechanism-of-action-classification-uses-interactions-and-more/ (accessed July 17, 2011).

ORGANIZATIONS

American Association of Nurse Anesthetists (AANA), 222 S. Prospect Avenue, Park Ridge, IL 60068, (847) 692-7050, Fax: (847) 692-6968, info@aana. com, http://www.aana.com.
American Society of Anesthesiologists (ASA), 520 N. Northwest Highway, Park Ridge, IL 60068-2573, (847) 825-5586, Fax: (847) 825-1692, communications@asahq.org, http://www.asahq.org.
U.S. Food and Drug Administration, 10903 New Hampshire Avenue, Silver Spring, MD 20993-0002, (888) 463-6332, http://www.fda.gov.

Adrienne Wilmoth Lerner
Rebecca J. Frey, PhD

Neuromyelitis optica *see* **Devic syndrome**
Neuronal ceroid lipofuscinosis *see* **Batten disease**

Neuronal migration disorders

Definition

Neuronal migration disorders are a diverse group of congenital brain abnormalities that arise specifically from defective formation of the central nervous system. During early brain development, neurons are born and move over large distances to reach their targets and thereby give rise to the different parts of the brain. The control of this process is highly orchestrated and dependent on the expression of various environmental and genetic factors that continue to be discovered in genetic studies of mice and humans. The critical role neuronal migration plays in brain development is evident from the variety of gross malformations that can occur when it goes wrong. Defective neuronal migration leads to a broad range of clinical syndromes, and most affected patients will have a combination of mental retardation and epilepsy.

Description

Neuronal migration disorders include lissencephaly as part of the agyria-pachygyria-band spectrum, cobblestone lissencephaly, periventricular heterotopia, and other variants such as Zellweger and Kallman syndrome. Patients may have only focal collections of abnormally located neurons known as heterotopias. The common factor in these disorders is a defect in neuronal migration, a key process in brain development that occurs during weeks 12 to 16 of gestation. Some disorders such as polymicrogyria and schizencephaly are presumably due to abnormal neuronal migration due to studies showing heterotopias in other parts of the brain, but the exact relationship is unclear. Early in brain development, neurons are born in specific locations in the brain and migrate to their final destinations to create distinct brain regions. Each step of this process, from starting, continuing, and stopping migration, is controlled by distinct molecular mechanisms that are regulated by the activity of genes. Defects in these genes lead to the various presentations of neuronal migration disorders seen in clinical practice.

Lissencephaly

Lissencephaly is the most extreme example of defective neuronal migration. In lissencephaly or agyria, neuronal migration fails globally, causing the brain to appear completely smooth and have abnormal layering in the cortex. Various genes have been associated with varying levels of severity of lissencephaly giving rise to a spectrum of disorders ranging from classical lissencephaly to milder forms such as double cortex syndrome or pachygyria. Classical or type I lissencephaly differs from type II or cobblestone lissencephaly. In cobblestone lissencephaly, the defect is presumably an overmigration of neurons past their targets, giving rise to the abnormally bumpy surface seen.

Periventricular heterotopia

Periventricular heterotopia is a disorder where neurons fail to begin the process of migration. Neurons are generated near the ventricular zone but do not start the process of migration to their destinations. Instead, they are stuck and collect around the ventricles, giving rise to the distinct appearance on brain imaging.

Other neuronal migration disorders

Zellweger syndrome is a disorder of neuronal migration that may consist of abnormally large folds (pachygyria) and heterotopias spread throughout the brain. It is thought to be due to a defect in peroxisome metabolism, a pathway by which cells break down waste products. The relationship between this metabolic defect and neuronal migration is unclear at this time. Kallman syndrome is a disorder where cells fail to migrate to the portion of the brain controlling smell as well as the hypothalamus, a region that controls hormone secretion. The mechanism underlying this disease is unclear.

Schizencephaly is grouped as a neuronal migration disorder although the exact etiology is unknown. Schizencephaly is an example of abnormal neuronal migration that may occur locally rather than globally. In schizencephaly, an early insult to the brain in the form of an infection, stroke, or genetic defect leads to abnormal migration of neurons in a portion of the brain and subsequent lack of developed brain tissue, giving rise to the characteristic brain clefts that define this syndrome. Schizencephaly may show a wide range of presentations, with bilateral clefts that vary in size and extent of involvement.

Polymicrogyria refers to an abnormal amount of small convolutions (gyri) in affected areas of the cerebral cortex and is believed to be a neuronal migration disorder, although the exact etiology is unknown.

Demographics

Neuronal migration disorders are rare overall, but the exact incidence is unknown. Patients may have very mild degrees of the different disorders and may not be diagnosed if they do not manifest symptoms, making the actual incidence difficult to determine.

Causes and symptoms

Causes

The majority of neuronal migration disorders seen in clinical practice are thought to be genetic in cause. Much of what is known about neuronal migration disorders to date has been discovered from intense research identifying the genes affected in individuals with these diseases. The widespread abnormal expression of defective genes leads to the global nature of the disorders, contrary to acquired developmental brain insults, which lead to more localized defects. Several genes have been implicated in causing the various disorders, and they continue to be identified. The most well characterized genes include DCX on the X chromosome, responsible for double cortex syndrome, and LIS1 on chromosome 17, the first gene identified for lissencephaly. Cobblestone lissencephaly is associated with abnormalities in fukutin, a gene responsible for Fukuyama Muscular Dystrophy, a syndrome consisting of muscle weakness and cobblestone lissencephaly. Periventricular heterotopia is associated with abnormalities of the filamin1 gene on the X chromosome. DCX, LIS1, and filamin1 are genes responsible for controlling the mechanics of cell movement during neuronal migration. Schizencephaly has been associated with abnormalities in EMX2, a transcription factor gene whose role in neuronal migration is as yet unidentified. Neuronal migration disorders can also be associated with early insults to the brain from infections or damage from stroke.

Symptoms

Most neuronal migration disorders show some combination of epilepsy, mental retardation, and abnormalities in head size, known as microcephaly. Some patients, such as those with small heterotopias, may have no symptoms at all since the severity of the defect is very mild. Patients may also have cerebral palsy or abnormalities in muscle tone. Depending on the severity of the malformation, the level of mental retardation may vary from mild to severe. Patients with lissencephaly are usually severely delayed, have failure to thrive, and are microcephalic. They may also have accompanying eye problems. Patients with double cortex syndrome or schizencephaly may have milder symptoms and may only present with seizures. Schizencephaly may have associated complications of increased fluid pressure in the brain, known as hydrocephalus. Periventricular heterotopia and polymicrogyria may present with only seizures. Some neuronal migration disorders such as lissencephaly may be part of a larger syndrome affecting other body parts such as the muscle, eyes, or face.

Diagnosis

Diagnosis is usually made by neuroimaging. CT scan or MRI of the brain will show the characteristic abnormality. MRI has better resolution and may detect polymicrogyria or small heterotopias more easily than CT. Genetic testing is available for patients with lissencephaly to identify whether the DCX or LIS1 gene is defective. Knowledge of the genes affected allows for counseling and family planning. Laboratory tests are not useful in diagnosis.

Treatment team

Management of neuronal migration disorders involves a pediatrician, pediatric neurologist and physical therapists. With symptoms of later onset, an adult neurologist may be involved in treating symptoms of seizures. Rehabilitation specialists may help in prescribing medications for cerebral palsy or increased muscle tone. A case manager may be involved in coordinating care and resources.

Treatment

There are no known cures for the various neuronal migration disorders at this time. The majority of treatments are directed towards symptoms caused by the malformed brain. Seizures may be treated with anticonvulsant medications. Refractory seizures may respond to neurosurgical removal of abnormal brain tissue. Neurosurgery may be required to relieve hydrocephalus, by placement of a shunt. Increased muscle tone may respond to injections of botulinum toxin or muscle relaxants. Patients may require feeding through a tube due to inability to swallow normally.

Recovery and rehabilitation

Due to the congenital nature of neuronal migration disorders, most patients do not recover from their symptoms. The course of disease tends to be static. Physical and occupational therapists may help treat symptoms of weakness or increased tone that limit mobility and daily hand use.

Clinical trials

Clinical trials are funded by the National Institutes of Health to identify genes responsible for neuronal migration disorders such as lissencephaly and schizencephaly. For contact information for the Walsh Lab Site, see Resources below. Information about current relevant clinical trials can be found at ClinicalTrials.gov.

Prognosis

There is no known cure for any of the neuronal migration disorders. Due to the congenital nature of the diseases, the symptoms tend to be static and do not improve. The prognosis varies for each individual depending on the extent of the defect and the accompanying neurologic deficits. Most individuals with severe malformations such as classical lissencephaly or bilateral schizencephaly will die at an early age due to failure to thrive or infections such as pneumonia. Their cognitive development stays at the 3 month level. Patients with milder forms such as unilateral schizencephaly, periventricular heterotopia, or subcortical band heterotopia may have mild mental retardation and seizures only and live a normal life span.

Special concerns

Educational and Social Needs

Due to developmental disability, children with neuronal migration disorders who survive beyond the age of two may benefit from special education programs. Various state and federal programs are available to help individuals and their families with meeting these needs.

Resources

BOOKS

Kinsman, Steven L., and Michael V. Johnston. "Congenital Anomalies of the Central Nervous System," Chapter 592. In *Nelson Textbook of Pediatrics,* 18th edition, edited by Richard E. Behrman, Robert M. Kliegman, and Hal B. Jenson. Philadelphia: Saunders 2007.

PERIODICALS

Agarwal, Sunil, and Namit Singhal. "Septal agenesis and lissencephaly with colpocephaly presenting as the 'Crown Sign'." *Journal of Pediatric Neurosciences* 5.2 (2010): 121.

Chang, YoonJeung, et al. "Dcx reexpression reduces subcortical band heterotopia and seizure threshold in an animal model of neuronal migration disorder." *Nature Medicine* 15.1 (2009): 84.

WEBSITES

"Cephalic Disorders Fact Sheet." National Institute of Neurological Disorders and Stroke (NINDS). http://www.ninds.nih.gov/disorders/cephalic_disorders/detail_cephalic_disorders.htm (accessed August 30, 2011).

ORGANIZATIONS

March of Dimes Birth Defects Foundation. 1275 Mamaroneck Avenue, White Plains, NY 10605. Phone: (914) 428-7100. Fax: (914) 428-8203. Tollfree phone: (888) MODIMES. Email: askus@marchofdimes.com. http://www.marchofdimes.com.

National Information Center for Children and Youth with Disabilities. P.O. Box 1492, Washington, DC 20013-1492. Phone: (202) 884-8200. Fax: (202) 884-8441. Tollfree phone: (800) 695-0285. Email: nichcy@aed.org. http://www.nichcy.org.

National Institute of Child Health and Human Development (NICHD). Bldg. 31, Rm. 2A32, Bethesda, MD 20892-2425. Phone: (301) 496-5133. (800) 370-2943. Email: NICHDClearinghouse@mail.nih.gov. http://www.nichd.nih.gov.

Walsh Lab Web Site. 4 Blackfan Circle, Boston, MA 02115. Phone: (617) 667-0813. Fax: (617) 667-0815. Email: cwalsh@bidmc.harvard.edu. http://walshlab.bidmc.harvard.edu/.

Peter T. Lin, MD

Neuropathologist

Definition

A pathologist is a medical doctor who is specialized in the study and diagnosis of the changes that are produced in the body by various diseases. A neuropathologist is a specialized pathologist, who is concerned with diseases of the **central nervous system** (the brain and spinal cord). Often a neuropathologist is concerned with the diagnosis of **brain tumors**.

A neuropathologist is also an expert in the various aspects of diseases of the nervous system and skeletal muscles. This range of disease includes degenerative diseases, infections, metabolic disorders, immunologic disorders, disorders of blood vessels, and physical injury. A neuropathologist functions as the primary consultant to neurologists and neurosurgeons.

Description

A neuropathologist is a medical doctor who has pursued specialized training. Aspects of this training include neurology, anatomy, cell biology, and biochemistry. Typically, a patient will not see a neuropathologist. Rather, the specialist works in the background, in the setting of the laboratory, to assist in the patient's diagnosis. In the path that leads to the diagnosis of a tumor, disease, or other malady, a neuropathologist typically becomes involved at the request of a neurologist. It is the neurologist who suspects a problem or seeks to confirm the presence of a tumor, based on tests such as magnetic resonance imaging (MRI) or a computerized assisted tomography (CAT) scan. The neurologist can obtain some of the tissue of concern in a procedure known as a **biopsy**, as well as obtaining fluid or cell samples.

It is this material that is sent to the pathology lab where the neuropathologist seeks to identify the nature of the problem. The diagnosis of brain and spinal cord related damage often involves a visual look at the samples using the extremely high magnification of the electron microscope. The neuropathologist can assess from the appearance of the sample whether the sample is unaffected or damaged. For example, in brain tissue obtained from a patient with suspected Alzheimer's disease, the neuropathologist will look for evidence of the presence of amyloid plaques, which are caused by abnormal folding of protein. As well, the neuropathologist will look for other diagnostic signs that support or do not support the suspected malady.

In the case of a tumor, part of a neuropathologist's responsibility is to identify the tumor and grade it as malignant or benign. This is no small task, as

there are literally hundreds of different types of tumors. The correct identification greatly aids the subsequent treatment process and the patient's prognosis.

The neuropathological analysis of a tumor is concerned mainly with two areas. The first is the origin of the tumor in the brain. Determining the tumor's origin aids in naming the tumor. Secondly, the neuropathologist determines if the tumor displays signs of rapid growth. The speed of growth of the tumor can be quantified as a grade. A result such as "grade three astrocytoma" is very informative to the neurologist. Even if the neuropathologist determines that a brain or spinal cord tumor is benign, the location of the tumor may still pose serious health risks, and this important determination is also usually made by the neuropathologist.

Another important tool that a neuropathologist uses to examine tissue samples is histology. The treatment of a thin section of a sample with specific compounds that will bind to and highlight (stain) regions of interest in the specimen allows the neuropathologist to determine if the stained regions are normal or abnormal in character. The histological stains can be applied to a section that has been sliced from the sample at room temperature or at a very low temperature. The use of frozen sections can help preserve structural detail in the specimen that might otherwise be changed at a higher temperature.

The assessment of a stained specimen by the neuropathologist is typically done by examining the material using a light microscope. This type of microscope does not magnify the specimen nearly as much as does the electron microscope. But such high-power magnification is not necessary to detect the cellular changes in the stained specimen. By carefully selecting the stain regimen, a skilled neuropathologist can reveal much detail about a specimen. Histological examinations can also be done much more quickly and easily than electron microscopic examinations. Saving time can be important in diagnosis and treatment, especially when dealing with brain tumors.

Finally, one of the consultative duties of neuropathologists can also be legal testimony. Their expert knowledge can be useful in court cases in which the mental state or functional ability of a person is an important consideration.

Resources

BOOKS

Nelson, James S. *Principles and Practice of Neuropathology.* New York: Oxford University Press, 2003.

OTHER

Department of Neurology, University of Debrecen, Hungary. *Neuroanatomy and Neuropathology on the Internet.* http://www.neuropat.dote.hu/ (February 10, 2004).

ORGANIZATIONS

American Association of Neuropathologists (AANP). 2085 Adelbert Rd, Cleveland, OH 44106. Phone: (216) 368–2488. Fax: (216) 368–8964. Email: aanp@cwru.edu. http://www.aanp-jnen.com.

Brian Douglas Hoyle, Ph

Neuropathy, hereditary *see* **Charcot-Marie-Tooth disorder**

Neuropsychological testing

Definition

Clinical neuropsychology is a field with historical origins in both psychology and neurology. The primary activity of neuropsychologists is assessment of brain functioning through structured and systematic behavioral observation. Neuropsychological tests are designed to examine a variety of cognitive abilities, including speed of information processing, attention, memory, language, and executive functions, which are necessary for goal-directed behavior. By testing a range of cognitive abilities and examining patterns of performance in different cognitive areas, neuropsychologists can make inferences about underlying brain function. Neuropsychological testing is an important component of the assessment and treatment of traumatic brain injury, dementia, neurological conditions, and psychiatric disorders. Neuropsychological testing is also an important tool for examining the effects of toxic substances and medical conditions on brain functioning.

Description

As early as the seventeenth century, scientists theorized about associations between regions of the brain and specific functions. The French philosopher René Descartes (1596–1650) believed the human soul could be localized to a specific brain structure, the pineal gland. In the eighteenth century, Franz Gall (1758–1828) advocated the theory that specific mental qualities such as spirituality or aggression were governed by discrete parts of the brain. In contrast, Pierre Flourens (1794–1867) contended that the brain was an integrated system that governed cognitive functioning in a holistic manner. Later discoveries indicated that brain function is both localized and integrated. Paul Broca (1824–1880) and Karl Wernicke (1848–1905) furthered understanding of localization and integration of function when they reported the loss of language abilities in patients with lesions to two regions in the left hemisphere of the brain.

The modern field of neuropsychology emerged in the twentieth century, combining theories based on anatomical observations of neurology with the techniques of psychology, including objective observation of behavior and the use of statistical analysis to differentiate functional abilities and define impairment. The famous Soviet neuropsychologist Alexander Luria (1902–1977) played a major role in defining neuropsychology as it is practiced today. Luria formulated two principle goals of neuropsychology: to localize brain lesions and analyze psychological activities arising from brain function through behavioral observation. American neuropsychologist Ralph Reitan (1922–) emphasized the importance of using standardized psychometric tests to guide systematic observations of brain-behavior relationships.

Before the introduction of neuroimaging techniques doctors lacked nonsurgical ways to observe the brain. Since clinicians lacked non-surgical methods for directly observing brain lesions or structural abnormalities in living patients, neuropsychological testing was the only way to determine which part of the brain was affected in a given patient. Neuropsychological tests can identify syndromes associated with problems in a particular area of the brain. For instance, a patient who performs well on tests of attention, memory, and language, but poorly on tests that require visual spatial skills such as copying a complex geometric figure or making designs with colored blocks may have dysfunction in the right parietal lobe, the region of the brain involved in complex processing of visual information. When a patient complains of problems with verbal communication after a stroke, separate tests that examine production and comprehension of language help neuropsychologists identify the location of the stroke in the left hemisphere. Neuropsychological tests can also be used as screening tests to see if more extensive diagnostic evaluation is appropriate. Neuropsychological screening of elderly people complaining of memory problems can help identify those at risk for dementia versus those experiencing normal age-related memory loss.

As neuropsychological testing came to play a less vital role in localization of brain dysfunction, clinical neuropsychologists found new uses for their skills and knowledge. By clarifying which cognitive abilities are impaired or preserved in patients with brain injury or illness, neuropsychologists can predict how well individuals will respond to different forms of treatment or rehabilitation. Although patterns of test scores illustrate profiles of cognitive strength and weakness, neuropsychologists can also learn a great deal about patients by observing how they approach a particular test. For example, two patients can complete a test in very different ways yet obtain similar scores. One patient may work slowly and methodically, making no errors, while another rushes through the test, making several errors but quickly correcting them. Some individuals persevere despite repeated failure on a series of test items, while others refuse to continue after a few failures. These differences might not be apparent in test scores but can help clinicians choose among rehabilitation and treatment approaches.

Performance on neuropsychological tests is usually evaluated through comparison to the average performance of large samples of normal individuals. Most tests include tables of these normal scores, often divided into groups based on demographic variables such as age and education that appear to affect cognitive functioning. This allows individuals to be compared to appropriate peers.

The typical neuropsychological examination evaluates sensation and perception, gross and fine motor skills, basic and complex attention, visual spatial skills, receptive and productive language abilities, recall and recognition memory, and executive functions such as cognitive flexibility and abstraction. Motivation and personality are often assessed as well, particularly when clients are seeking financial compensation for injuries, or cognitive complaints are not typical of the associated injury or illness.

Some neuropsychologists prefer to use fixed test batteries like the Halstead-Reitan Battery or the Luria-Nebraska Battery for all patients. These batteries include tests of a wide range of cognitive functions, and those who advocate their use believe that all functions must be assessed in each patient in order to avoid diagnostic bias

or failure to detect subtle problems; however, the more common approach is to use a flexible battery based on hypotheses generated through a clinical interview, observation of the patient, and review of medical records. While this approach is more prone to bias, it has the advantage of preventing unnecessary testing. Since patients often find neuropsycholgical testing stressful and fatiguing, and these factors can negatively influence performance, advocates of the flexible battery approach argue that tailoring test batteries to particular patients can provide more accurate information.

Resources

BOOKS

Bradley, W., et al. *Neurology in Clinical Practice.* 5th ed. Philadelphia: Butterworth-Heinemann, 2008.
Goetz, C.G. *Goetz's Textbook of Clinical Neurology.* 3rd ed. Philadelphia: Saunders, 2007.

PERIODICALS

Randolph, C. "Baseline neuropsychological testing in managing sport-related concussion: does it modify risk?" *Current Sports Medicine Reports* 10 (January 1, 2011): 21–26.
Reitan, R.M. "The use of serial testing in evaluating the need for comprehensive neuropsychological testing of adults." *Applied Neuropsychology* 15 (January 1, 2008): 21–32.

ORGANIZATIONS

American Psychological Association, Division 40, 750 First Street, N.E., , Washington, DC 20002-4242, http://www.div40.org.
International Neuropsychological Society, 700 Ackerman Road, Suite 625, Columbus, OH 43202, (614) 263-4200, Fax: (614) 263-4366, http://www.the-ins.org.
National Academy of Neuropsychology, 7555 East Hampden Avenue, Suite 525, Denver, CO 80231, (303) 691-3694, Fax: (303) 6915983, office@nanonline. org, http://nanonline.org.

Danielle Barry, M
Rosalyn Carson-DeWitt, MD

Neuroradiology

Definition

Neuroradiology is a subspecialty of diagnostic radiology that makes use of various diagnostic and interventional techniques to evaluate and treat conditions of the **central nervous system** (brain and spinal cord), spine, head, and neck.

Description

Historical background

Radiology as a medical specialty began with the discovery of x rays in 1895 by Wilhelm Roentgen (1845–1923), a German physicist who was awarded the first Nobel Prize in Physics for this discovery in 1901. The earliest radiological studies of the central nervous system were radiographs of the skull that were done to evaluate **brain tumors**. Ventriculography, a technique for improving radiographic visualization of structures inside the brain by injecting air into the ventricles of the brain through holes drilled in the skull, was developed in 1918 by Walter Dandy (1886–1946). Ventriculography was followed in 1927 by arteriography, which was a technique for studying the arteries of the brain by injecting a contrast material through a catheter inserted into the femoral artery in the thigh and threading upward until it reached the carotid artery. A series of radiographs were taken as the contrast material spread through the arteries of the brain. Arteriography was developed by Egas Moniz (1874–1955), a Portuguese neurologist. The first doctor hired as a full-time neuroradiologist was Cornelius Dyke (1900–1943), who took the specialized position at the Neurological Institute in New York City in 1930.

It was not until the 1960s that neuroradiology became a distinctive subspecialty within diagnostic radiology. Juan Taveras (1919–2002), a radiologist from the Dominican Republic who had joined the Neurological Institute, developed the first neuroradiology fellowship program sponsored by the National Institutes of Health (NIH) in 1960. A second fellowship program quickly followed at the Albert Einstein College of Medicine in the Bronx. In 1962, Taveras gathered a group of 14 neuroradiologists from Canada and the United States at a dinner meeting to form what is now the American Society of Neuroradiology (ASNR).

Taveras was also instrumental in recognizing the importance of the new imaging technologies that emerged in the 1970s, particularly CT scanning, which was developed at the Maida Vale Hospital in London in 1971 and brought to the United States in 1973, and magnetic resonance imaging (MRI), which came along in the late 1970s and early 1980s. These technologies not only allowed neuroradiologists to diagnose and treat disorders of the brain that could not be detected by the older techniques of radiography (such as **multiple sclerosis** and other disorders of the white matter of the brain), but they were also much less invasive and could be repeated as often as needed to monitor injuries to brain tissue caused by trauma,

infection, or metabolic disorders. CT and MRI also allowed neuroradiologists to start treatment much more rapidly, with improved outcomes for the patients. Further refinements of these technologies have allowed for such advances as direct imaging of the blood flow in the arteries of the brain without the need to inject contrast materials.

Current subspecialties

As of 2011, neuroradiology has developed some subspecialties of its own:

- Interventional neuroradiology. Interventional radiologists treat as well as diagnose various disorders of the central nervous system using minimally invasive techniques. This subspecialty is also known as neurointerventional surgery. Radiologists in this subspecialty frequently treat disorders of the blood vessels in the brain and take tissue biopsies.
- Pediatric neuroradiology. Pediatric neuroradiology is the subspecialty that diagnoses and treats disorders of the central nervous system in children.

Imaging modalities

Neuroradiologists have a range of imaging modalities available for use as of 2011:

- Conventional radiography.
- Computed tomography (CT) scans. Also known as computed axial tomography, CT is an imaging technique in which a computer synthesizes data from a large series of two-dimensional x-ray images taken around a single axis of rotation to generate a three-dimensional image of internal organs.
- Magnetic resonance imaging (MRI). MRI is an imaging technique, first used on humans in 1977, that aligns the magnetic nuclei (especially protons) of the patient in a strong uniform magnetic field. The nuclei absorb energy from tuned radio frequency pulses and emit radio frequency signals as their excitation decays. The signals are converted into a series of tomographic images; these images can be constructed because the protons in different tissues return to their equilibrium state at different rates. MRI is particularly useful for imaging tissues like those in the brain, which have little density contrast. Unlike CT scanning, MRI does not involve the use of radiation.
- Functional magnetic resonance imaging (fMRI). Functional magnetic resonance imaging is a refinement of MRI that allows radiologists to detect and measure metabolic changes taking place in a specific area of the brain. These changes are reflected in increased blood flow to active areas of the brain.

The differences in the rate of blood flow can be measured by evaluating the relative levels of oxygenated and deoxygenated hemoglobin in the blood flowing through the vessels. The magnetic resonance signal of blood differs according to the level of oxygenation.

- Ultrasound. Ultrasound is a diagnostic method that uses high-frequency sound waves to create images of the body's internal structures. The echoes of the sound waves are displayed in real time on a computer screen. Also known as sonography, ultrasound does not involve the use of radiation.

- Discography. Discography is a technique for investigating whether a disk in the spinal column is the source of the patient's back or neck pain by injecting a contrast material directly into the disk. It is usually followed by a CT scan.

- Positron emission tomography (PET). A PET scan is an imaging technique in which a radioactive tracer that emits subatomic particles called positrons is given to the patient. The concentrations of the tracer within body tissues are combined by computer analysis to form three-dimensional images. PET scans are typically used to evaluate the body's metabolic processes (the biochemical functioning of the organ or tissue). They are often done alongside CT or MRI scans, which yield information about the anatomy of the structures. To obtain this information about structure and function at the same time, most PET scans as of 2011 are performed with combined PET/CT machines.

- Single photon emission computed tomography (SPECT). SPECT is an imaging technique similar to CT scanning that uses gamma rays instead of x rays to create the image. A radioisotope that emits gamma rays is injected into the patient's bloodstream. It is selectively absorbed by the organ or structure to be imaged. A gamma camera is then rotated around the patient to capture the images. As of 2011 some manufacturers are making combined SPECT/CT units that can perform both types of scan at the same time.

Conditions diagnosed or treated

Neuroradiologists detect and treat disorders of the brain, head, neck, and spine. The imaging techniques used most often are CT and MRI imaging, with less frequent use of ultrasound and plain radiography. The conditions investigated and treated by neuroradiologists, and the procedures they employ, include the following:

- Abnormalities and disorders of the spine. These can be detected by myelography followed by a CT scan.

Myelography is a technique in which a contrast material is injected into the cerebrospinal fluid within the spinal cord and subjected to x rays. The technique can be used to detect herniated spinal disks, tumors of the spine, or narrowing of the spinal column.

- Biopsies of the skull, scalp, bone, or spine. Neuroradiologists use CT scanning and a fluoroscope to guide them while removing samples of tissue after administering a local anesthetic.

- Disorders of the arteries in the brain. Neuroradiologists use cerebral angiography to diagnose aneurysms (bulges or weakened areas in the arterial wall that may rupture); arteriovenous malformations; narrowing of the arteries in the brain caused by atherosclerosis; and identifying cerebral arteries that are feeding a brain tumor. Cerebral angiography can also be used to monitor the effectiveness of stent placement and other treatments.

- Disorders of the central nervous system. Neuroradiologists diagnose various CNS disorders by administering spinal taps, which involve injecting medications or contrast materials directly into the spinal cord.

Interventional neuroradiologists frequently treat disorders of the blood vessels in the head and neck. They are trained to perform the following procedures:

- Aneurysm coil embolization. Aneurysms are bulges or weak spots in a cerebral artery that can rupture and cause severe headache or even death. An interventional neuroradiologist can embolize (block off) an aneurysm by threading a catheter into the artery and inserting one or more platinum coils. The artery forms a blood clot (embolus) around the coils, sealing off the aneurysm and greatly reducing the risk of rupture. Embolization can also be used to treat congenital arteriovenous malformations (AVMs) and severe nosebleeds that do not respond to other therapies. In the case of nosebleeds, small particles of gelfoam may be used as well as platinum coils.

- Stroke therapy. After using a CT scan or CT angiography, an interventional radiologist can insert a catheter into the blocked cerebral blood vessel to deliver a clot-busting drug in patients who have reached the hospital within six hours after the stroke. They can also use various devices (e.g., Merci or Penumbra) to retrieve the clot from inside the vessel.

- Angioplasty and stent placement. Angioplasty is a procedure in which a blood vessel is reopened or restructured. An interventional neuroradiologist can perform an angioplasty by using an imaging technique to guide a balloon-tipped catheter into a blocked artery or vein to the point of blockage. The balloon is then inflated to reopen the vein, after which it is

Aneurysm—A localized blood-filled bulge or weak spot in the wall of a blood vessel.

Angiography—A technique for visualizing blood vessels by threading a catheter through a large vein in the patient's arm or leg, injecting a contrast material when the catheter reaches the desired location, and taking images by standard radiography or a CT scan. Angiography of the blood vessels in the brain is called cerebral angiography.

Angioplasty—A technique for mechanically widening a narrowed or blocked blood vessel by inserting a balloon catheter, inflating the balloon to crush the fatty deposits obstructing the blood vessel, and deflating the balloon and withdrawing the catheter.

Arteriovenous malformation (AVM)—An abnormal connection between veins and arteries, usually congenital. A cerebral AVM may result in epilepsy; severe headache; bleeding into the brain; difficulties with speech, movement or coordination; or hallucinations, memory problems, and confusion.

Congenital—Present at birth.

Contrast material—Any material introduced into the body that has a different opacity from soft tissue and can be used in radiography, magnetic resonance imaging, or CT scans to help the radiologist visualize internal body structures. Contrast materials are also known as contrast media or contrast agents.

Embolization—The deliberate introduction of a metal coil or gelatin sponge into a blood vessel to stop bleeding or to seal off a tumor or aneurysm.

Endovascular—Referring to any procedure or treatment performed within a blood vessel.

Interventional neuroradiology—The subspecialty of neuroradiology that involves treatment of patients utilizing minimally invasive interventional techniques as well as performing diagnostic imaging. It is also known as neurointerventional surgery.

Myelography—A technique for imaging abnormalities of the spinal cord and spinal nerves by injecting a contrast material into the cerebrospinal fluid inside the spinal cord and then making a radiographic image. A myelogram is usually followed by a CT scan.

Radiography—The use of x rays to create photographic records on specially sensitized plates or films.

Stent—A wire tube or tube-like device placed in a blood vessel to keep it permanently open.

Tomography—The general term for creating a three-dimensional image of an object by gathering a series of two-dimensional cross-sectional images and combining them using tomographic reconstruction software processed by a computer.

Vasospasm—A condition in which a major blood vessel goes into spasm and suddenly constricts, cutting off or restricting blood supply to an organ or body part. Vasospasm in a cerebral artery can lead to stroke.

Ventricle—Any of four hollow spaces in the human brain filled with cerebrospinal fluid.

---

deflated and the catheter removed. To ensure that the blood vessel remains open, the neuroradiologist may place a stent, which is a wire tube or other tube-like device inserted to keep the blood vessel open permanently.

• Treatment of head and neck tumors.

• Treatment of vasospasm. Vasospasm is a condition in which a blood vessel suddenly constricts, shutting off blood flow to a body part or organ. It can lead to stroke if it occurs in one of the arteries of the brain. An interventional neuroradiologist can confirm a diagnosis of vasospasm with an angiogram and then treat it by either balloon angioplasty or a dose of intra-arterial verapamil (Isoptin) or nimodipine (Nimotop).

Pediatric neuroradiologists diagnose and treat the following central nervous system disorders in fetuses, newborn infants, and young children:

• aneurysms and arteriovenous malformations in the brain

• disorders that affect the development of the brain in children

• responses of brain tumors to chemotherapy and radiation therapy

• epileptic seizures

Like adult interventional neuroradiologists, pediatric neuroradiologists can perform angioplasty, embolization, and other endovascular procedures that eliminate the need for invasive surgery.

Educational requirements and certification

To practice neuroradiology, a person must hold an M.D. or D.O. (doctor of osteopathy) degree from an accredited medical school and complete a year of internship, followed by four years of residency in radiology. At this point most candidates will take the board examination of either the American Board of Radiology (ACR) to earn an M.D., or the American Osteopathic Board of Radiology to earn a D.O.

Following board certification, the radiologist will enter a fellowship program approved by the Accreditation Council for Graduate Medical Education (ACGME) in order to specialize in neuroradiology. According to the ACGME, there are 85 accredited fellowship programs in neuroradiology for the academic year 2011–12, with 252 on-duty residents enrolled. Most fellowship programs are one year in length, although interventional neuroradiologists may take an additional year of training. After completing the fellowship and an additional year in practice, the neuroradiologist is eligible to take an examination for the Certificate of Added Qualification (CAQ) from the American Board of Radiology.

Safety concerns

The growing use of imaging techniques that use radiation (radiography, CT scans, **PET**, and SPECT) has led to concern about the possible long-term effects (particularly the increased risk of cancer) of exposure to radiation. This concern is particularly acute in patients whose conditions may require repeated x rays or CT imaging to monitor the effectiveness of therapy. It is important to keep in mind that people are exposed to background radiation from cosmic rays and radioactive materials in the earth in their everyday lives. The amount of background radiation varies somewhat with geographic location; people living on the high plateaus of the Four Corners region of the Southwest receive more radiation than those living in other parts of North America at sea level. In addition, frequent fliers receive additional small doses of cosmic rays during each airplane trip; however, on the whole, the dose of radiation from one chest x ray is about the same as that received from background radiation in ten days.

The long-term risks of developing cancer from CT scans of the central nervous system are considered low for one CT scan of the spine and very low for one CT scan of the head. Interventional neuroradiology, by contrast, makes much more extensive use of radiation than diagnostic neuroradiology, particularly for such complex procedures as balloon angioplasty and stent

QUESTIONS TO ASK YOUR DOCTOR

- Does my disorder require the specialized skills of a neuroradiologist?
- Will my treatment require repeated exposure to radiation?
- What are the risks and benefits involved in treatments like balloon angioplasty and stent placement?

placement, or embolization of AVMs. These procedures are often lifesaving, and the long-term risks of cancer from exposure to radiation are secondary. Patients should discuss with their doctors the risks and benefits of diagnostic imaging and treatments that require exposure to radiation. Ultrasound and MRI can be used for some interventional procedures, and these approaches do not involve radiation.

Resources

BOOKS

Castillo, Mauricio. *Neuroradiology Companion: Methods, Guidelines, and Imaging Fundamentals.* 4th ed. Philadelphia: Wolters Kluwer Health/Lippincott Williams amd Wilkins, 2011.

Faro, Scott H. *Functional Neuroradiology: Principles and Clinical Applications.* New York: Springer, 2011.

Krings, Timo, Sasikhan Geibprasert, and Karel G. ter Brugge. *Case-based Interventional Neuroradiology.* New York: Thieme, 2011.

PERIODICALS

Abruzzo, T.A., and M.K. Heran. "Neuroendovascular Therapies in Pediatric Interventional Radiology." *Techniques in Vascular and Interventional Radiology* 14 (March 2011): 50–56.

Cho, W.S., et al. "Intra-arterial Nimodipine Infusion for Cerebral Vasospasm in Patients with Aneurysmal Subarachnoid Hemorrhage." *Interventional Neuroradiology* 17 (June 2011): 169–78.

Currie, S., et al. "Endovascular Treatment of Intracranial Aneurysms: Review of Current Practice." *Postgraduate Medical Journal* 87 (January 2011): 41–50.

Fields, J.D., et al. "Drug eluting Stents for Symptomatic Intracranial and Vertebral Artery Stenosis." *Interventional Neuroradiology* 17 (June 2011): 241–47.

Hijaz, A., et al. "Imaging of Head Trauma." *Radiologic Clinics of North America* 49 (January 2011): 81–103.

Looby, S., and A. Flanders. "Spine Trauma." *Radiologic Clinics of North America* 49 (January 2011): 129–63.

Naggara, O.N., et al. "Endovascular Treatment of Intracranial Unruptured Aneurysms: Systematic Review and

Meta-analysis of the Literature on Safety and Efficacy." *Radiology* 256 (September 2010): 887–97.

Offiah, C., and E. Hall. "Post-treatment Imaging Appearances in Head and Neck Cancer Patients." *Clinical Radiology* 66 (January 2011): 13–24.

Prabhu, S.P. "The Role of Neuroimaging in Sport-related Concussion." *Clinics in Sports Medicine* 30 (January 2011): 103–14.

Schafer, J., et al. "Diffusion Magnetic Resonance Imaging in the Head and Neck." *Magnetic Resonance Imaging Clinics of North America* 19 (February 2011): 55–67.

WEBSITES

"Arteriovenous Malformations (AVMs)." Johns Hopkins Medicine, Neuroradiology Division. http://neuro radiology.rad.jhmi.edu/avm.html (accessed July 25, 2011).

"Myelography." Johns Hopkins Medicine, Neuroradiology Division. http://neuroradiology.rad.jhmi.edu/myelography.html (accessed July 25, 2011).

"Neuroradiology." Children's Hospital Boston. http://www.childrenshospital.org/clinicalservices/Site2121/mainpageS2121P0.html (accessed July 25, 2011).

"Radiation Exposure in X-ray and CT Examinations." Radiological Society of North America (RSNA). http://www.radiologyinfo.org/en/safety/index.cfm?pg=sfty_xray (accessed July 25, 2011).

Thiyagarajah, Aathi R. "Discography." Medscape Reference. http://emedicine.medscape.com/article/1145703-overview (accessed July 25, 2011).

"Your Radiologist Explains PET Scans." Radiological Society of North America (RSNA). http://www.radiologyinfo.org/en/photocat/gallery3.cfm?image=guibertea_PET_CT2.jpg&pg=pet&pid=1 (accessed July 25, 2011).

ORGANIZATIONS

American Academy of Neurology (AAN), 1080 Montreal Avenue, Saint Paul, MN 55116, (651) 695-2717, (800) 879-1960, Fax: (651) 695-2791, memberservices@aan.com, http://www.aan.com.

American College of Radiology (ACR), 1891 Preston White Drive, Reston, VA 20191, (703) 648-8900, (800) 227-5463, info@acr.org, http://www.acr.org.

American Society of Neuroradiology (ASNR), 2210 Midwest Road, Suite 207, Oak Brook, IL 60523, (630) 574-0220, Fax: (630) 574-0661, http://www.asnr.org.

Radiological Society of North America (RSNA), 820 Jorie Boulevard, Oak Brook, IL 60523-2251, (630) 571-2670, (800) 381-6660, Fax: (630) 571-7837, http://www.rsna.org.

Society of NeuroInterventional Surgery (SNIS), 3975 Fair Ridge Drive, Suite 200 North, Fairfax, VA 22033, (703) 691-2272, Fax: (703) 537-0650, http://www.snis online.org.

Rebecca J. Frey, PhD

Neurosarcoidosis

Definition

Neurosarcoidosis refers to an autoimmune disorder (involves formation of an inflammatory lesion called a granuloma) of unknown cause, which causes deposition of granulomas in the **central nervous system**.

Description

Sarcoidosis is a multisystem disease of unknown cause. It is thought that the disorder is caused by an inflammatory reaction in the body that forms a lesion called a granuloma. Neurosarcoidosis is characterized by formation of granulomas in the central nervous system. The granulomas consist of inflammatory cells (lymphocytes, mononuclear phagocytes) that function during inflammatory reactions. The disorder is often unrecognized since most patients do not exhibit symptoms. Typically the disease is diagnosed by routine chest x ray. If symptoms are present they usually include respiratory problems (shortness of breath, cough) since the lungs are affected most frequently.

Neurological Description

Patients can have a broad range of clinical signs and symptoms that typically could involve mononeuropathy, **peripheral neuropathy**, or central nervous system involvement. Mononeuropathy problems can include facial nerve palsy; impaired taste and smell; blindness (or other eye problems such as double vision, visual field defects, blurry vision, dry/sore eyes); or speech problems (impaired swollowing or hoarseness) patients can also develop **vertigo**, **weakness** of neck muscles, and tongue deviation and atrophy.

Peripheral Nerve Involvement

Neurosarcoidosis can cause damage to peripheral nerves that can affect motor nerves (responsible for movement of muscles) and sensory nerves (responsible for sensation.) Symptoms of sensory loss include loss of sensation and abnormal sensation (numb, painful, tingling sensations) over the thorax (chest) and the areas where stockings and gloves are usually worn. Motor neurosarcoidosis is characterized by weakness that can progress to immobility and joint stiffness.

Central nervous system (CNS) involvement can affect the pituitary gland, **cerebellum**, or cerebral cortex. The spinal cord is rarely involved. Signs and symptoms of CNS involvement can include polyuria, polydipsia, obesity, impotence, amenorrhea, confusion/

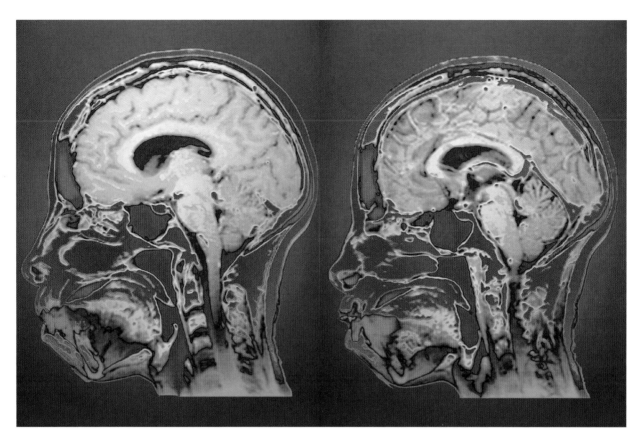

Cerebral MRIs of a 52-year-old patient with neurosarcoidosis. The MRIs show the presence of numerous granulomas in the meninges and cisterns. *(© ISM/Phototake. All rights reserved.)*

amnesia (short and long term memory), **meningitis**, and seizures (focal seizures).

Demographics

Sarcoid disorders are more prevalent in African Americans, and in the United States there seems to be a variable prevalence within different States. The prevalence is much higher in the southeastern United States among both Caucasian and African Americans. The prevalence is high in Puerto Rico, reaching approximately 175 cases per 100,000 persons. The frequency for neurological involvement for all cases of sarcoid disease is 5%. However, neurological involvement has been reported to occur in up to 5% to 16% of cases. Internationally the incidence of sarcoid varies widely. In Spain the incidence is low (0.04 per 100,000) whereas in Sweden the incidence is high representing 64 cases per 100,000 persons. Studies reveal the prevalence in London was 27 per 100,000 and 97 per 100,000 among Irish men. In the Caribbean, studies indicate that the prevalence is as high as 200 per 100,000 in men from the West Indies and 13% of individuals from Martinique.

There does not seem to be a racial predilection for the development of Sarcoid neuropathy. Sarcoid disease is uncommon in Chinese, Inuits, Southeast Asians, Canadian Indians, New Zealand Maoris, and native Japanese. Death from neurosarcoidosis is unusual. About 66% of patients with neurosarcoidosis have self-limited monophasic illness. Approximately 33% have a chronic remitting and relapsing course. Neurosarcoidosis commonly occurs in adults aged 25–50 years. Neurosarcoidosis is not common in children, but if it does occur, it affects children age 9–15 years. The clinical signs in children are different than adults. When neurosarcoidosis is present in children over 8 years, there is usually a triad of signs that includes arthritis, uveitis and cutaneous nodules. In children the rate of ocular (eye) problems occurs in approximately 100% of cases, which typically manifests as iritis and/or anterior vitreitis. For all cases, if the nervous system is involved, it usually occurs within 2 years of disease onset.

Causes and symptoms

The causes of sarcoid disease are not clear. Current evidence suggests that sarcoidosis is due to the abnormal proliferation (the cell multiplies quickly) of a certain cell called a T-helper cell (which functions to help immune cells attack a foreign substance.) The abnormal proliferation of T-helper cells is thought to result from an exaggerated response to a foreign substance or to self cells (a condition referred to as autoimmunity, in which, for unknown reasons, the bodies natural defense cells attack normal cells in organs).

During physical examination patients may exhibit weakness, absence of tendon reflexes, lack of sensation in a stocking and glove distribution, atrophy of muscles and focal mononueropathies that may affect the cranial nerves (causing problem with hearing, vision, smell, balance, or paralysis of facial muscles). Some patients may develop Heerfordt syndrome characterized by fever, uveitis, swelling of the parotid gland, and facial palsy.

Diagnosis

Blood analysis is essential since patients may have increased erythrocyte sedimentation rate (ESR), or anemia (hypochromic microcytic type). Blood analysis can provide information concerning multiple organs (kidney, liver, blood) and this is important since sarcoidosis is a multisystem disease (affects many different organs in the body). CT and MRI scans are important in assessing neurosarcoidosis. MRI is the imaging tool of choice in cases of neurosarcoidosis, because of the high quality images obtained. The presence of a mass or lesion in the CNS can be visualized by MRI images. To confirm the diagnosis it is necessary to take a **biopsy** of either muscle or nerve tissue. Examination of the tissue specimen with a microscope reveals the characteristic granuloma within tissues.

Treatment team

The effects of neurosarcoidosis can involve several symptoms from different organ systems. The treatment team consists of specialists who include neurologist, neurosurgeon, endocrinologist, rheumatologist, and pulmonologist.

Treatment

There is no definitive treatment, but corticosteroids remain the standard treatment. The most commonly used oral corticosteroid is prednisone which works to decrease inflammatory actions in the body that are responsible for granuloma formation. Doses are usually tapered down. Additionally, patients can be given immunosuppressant agents (i.e. cyclosporine), which can suppress autoimmune responses (which are responsible for granuloma formation). Surgery is rare and reserved in cases that require removal of a mass (space occupying lesion) in the brain.

KEY TERMS

Amenorrhea—The absence or abnormal stoppage of menstrual periods.

Anterior vitreitis—Inflammation of the corpus vitreum, which surrounds and fills the inner portion of the eyeball between the lens and the retina.

Atrophy—The progressive wasting and loss of function of any part of the body.

Iritis—Inflammation of the iris, the membrane in the pupil, the colored portion of the eye. It is characterized by photophobia, pain, and inflammatory congestion.

Mononeuropathy—Disorder involving a single nerve.

Pituitary gland—The most important of the endocrine glands (glands that release hormones directly into the bloodstream), the pituitary is located at the base of the brain. Sometimes referred to as the "master gland," it regulates and controls the activities of other endocrine glands and many body processes, including growth and reproductive function. Also called the hypophysis.

Polydipsia—Excessive thirst.

Polyuria—Excessive production and excretion of urine.

Uveitis—Inflammation of all or part the uvea. The uvea is a continuous layer of tissue which consists of the iris, the ciliary body, and the choroid. The uvea lies between the retina and sclera.

Vertigo—A feeling of dizziness together with a sensation of movement and a feeling of rotating in space.

Recovery and rehabilitation

Neurosarcoidosis is a slowly chronic disease with a progressive course, which is fatal in about 50% of patients. Follow-up visits with a neurologist every 3–6 months are advisable. During visits the neurologist will monitor progress and make recommendations.

Clinical trials

The National Heart, Lung and Blood Institute conducts clinical research trials with patients who have lung involvement (pulmonary sarcoidosis). Current information about relevant trials can be found at ClinicalTrials.gov.

Prognosis

Spontaneous resolution of neurosarcoidosis can occur but it is not common. Many patients with neurosarcoidosis have a slow chronic and progressive course with intermittent exacerbations. Neurosarcoidosis responds to steroid therapy, but long-term outcome of neurologic impairment is unknown.

Special concerns

Sarcoidosis is difficult to diagnosis and sometimes a delay can cause patients to get sicker before proper treatment is initiated. On rare occasions a patient may even die because the diagnosis is not suspected. Caution must be taken to exclude other diseases before a final diagnosis is made. Additionally, before corticosteroid therapy is initiated, the clinician must rule out an infectious cause.

Resources

BOOKS

Baughman, Robert. *Sarcoidosis (Lung Biology in Health and Disease)*. Informa Healthcare: 2005.
Khamashta, Munther A., and Manuel Ramos-Casals, eds. *Autoimmune Diseases: Acute and Complex Situations*. Springer: 2011.

WEBSITES

National Organization for Rare Disorders (NORD) http://www.rarediseases.org.

ORGANIZATIONS

Sarcoidosis Research Institute. 3475 Central Avenue, Memphis, TN 38111. Phone: (901) 766-6951. Fax: (901) 744-7294. Email: paula@sarcoidosisresearch.org. http://www.sarcoidosisresearch.org.

Laith Farid Gulli, MD
Nicole Mallory, MPA-C

Neurosurgery

Definition

Neurosurgery is the surgical specialty that deals with the diagnosis, treatment, and rehabilitation of disorders that affect the entire nervous system, including the **central nervous system** (brain and spinal cord) and the peripheral nerves.

Description

Neurosurgery is a complex specialty with a long history and a growing diversity of subspecialties. As of 2011, some neurosurgeons work by themselves as general neurosurgeons, but it is increasingly common for neurosurgeons in the subspecialties to be members of treatment teams.

Neurosurgery is a high-pressure specialty because many of the conditions treated by neurosurgeons—such as stroke, head trauma, spinal compression, and ruptured brain aneurysms—are life-threatening emergencies requiring inpatient treatment on short notice. In addition, while computer-assisted surgery and other technological advances have speeded up some neurosurgical procedures, improved the surgeon's ability to see and operate on very small structures in the brain, and shortened the patient's recovery time, other operations are still time-consuming and require a very high level of surgical skill. Some skull base procedures, for example, may take as long as 14 hours to complete and are not always successful.

Historical background

Humans have been performing surgical procedures involving the skull and the outer covering of the brain since prehistoric times. The oldest known surgical procedure, trepanation, is an operation in which a circular piece of bone is removed from the skull by a special saw-like instrument called a trephine or trepan. The operation is also known as trephination or trephining. Skulls of Cro-Magnon people estimated to be 40,000 years old have been discovered with circular holes as large as 2 inches in diameter, possibly to treat people suffering from psychotic disorders, epilepsy, or chronic migraine headaches. The procedure was refined in various ways in ancient Greece and Rome, the Middle Ages, the Renaissance, and the eighteenth and nineteenth centuries. Trepanations were done by premodern physicians to relieve pressure on brain tissue, not to perform surgery on the brain itself. Care was taken not to penetrate the dura mater, which is the outermost of the three **meninges** or membranes that lie beneath the skull and form a protective cover for the brain and spinal cord.

It was not until the late nineteenth century that three developments came together to make modern neurosurgery possible. The first was the theory of cerebral localization, which is the notion that such different functions as speech, vision, hearing, and control of voluntary movements are located (localized) in specific portions of the cerebral cortex. Although the theory of cerebral localization was first proposed in the mid-eighteenth century, it was not until the 1870s that studies of humans with speech loss and animals that had lost motor control demonstrated the validity of the theory. The other two major nineteenth-century developments that made successful neurosurgery possible were the introduction of antiseptic or aseptic surgery, which lowered the risk of infection following brain surgery, and the discovery of reliable general anesthesia.

Modern neurosurgery is generally considered to have begun after World War I (1914–18) with the work of Harvey Cushing (1869–1939), an American surgeon who pioneered the use of x-ray imaging to diagnose **brain tumors** as well as contributing to mapping the sensory areas of the cerebral cortex. Cushing founded the oldest professional society in neurosurgery, the American Association of Neurological Surgeons (AANS), in 1931. Other eminent neurosurgeons in this period were Walter Dandy (1886–1946), the founder of cerebrovascular neurosurgery, and Arthur Walker (1907–1996), a Canadian pioneer in epilepsy surgery. Advances in neurosurgery since the 1950s include pain management techniques, stereotactic surgery, and microsurgical procedures made possible by computers and improved imaging methods.

Current subspecialties

The AANS has official membership groups for the following subspecialties:

- Cerebrovascular neurosurgery. Cerebrovascular neurosurgeons diagnose and treat disorders of the veins and arteries that interfere with normal blood flow to the brain.
- Neurotrauma and critical care neurosurgery. This subspecialty deals with traumatic injuries to the brain and spinal cord, including sports-related injuries.
- Tumor neurosurgery. Also called neuro-oncology, tumor neurosurgery is the subspecialty that diagnoses and treats malignant tumors of the brain.
- Pediatric neurosurgery. Pediatric neurosurgery is the subspecialty that treats disorders of the central nervous system in children.
- Pain neurosurgery. Pain neurosurgery diagnoses and treats chronic pain syndromes involving the face, spine, and lower back.
- Spinal neurosurgery. Spinal neurosurgeons diagnose and treat disorders of the spine and spinal column, including cancerous tumors as well as traumatic injuries to the spine.
- Functional neurosurgery. Functional neurosurgery refers to the diagnosis and treatment of disorders of the brain that incapacitate patients, such as movement disorders like multiple sclerosis and Parkinson's disease.

The following are also considered neurosurgical subspecialties by some medical centers:

- Epilepsy surgery. Neurosurgeons who specialize in epilepsy surgery usually work together with other medical experts to treat complex seizure disorders that cannot be managed by medications alone.
- Endovascular neurosurgery. Endovascular neurosurgery is the subspecialty dealing with repair procedures carried out within the blood vessels. It is minimally invasive and is the preferred approach for treating patients who cannot undergo an open craniotomy.
- Neurointerventional surgery. Sometimes considered a subspecialty of neuroradiology, neurointerventional surgery uses minimally invasive interventional techniques as well as performing diagnostic imaging.
- Skull base surgery. Skull base surgery is a subspecialty that involves diagnosis and treatment of the complex and delicate nerves, blood vessels, and other structures in or close to the base of the skull.

Technologies and techniques

Neurosurgery has changed greatly since the 1990s because of technological advances that have facilitated the development of new treatment techniques as well as the emergence of subspecialties. Some of these technological advances are:

- The stereotactic method. Stereotactic surgery involves the use of a three-dimensional system of coordinates to locate small structures or lesions within the central nervous system and allow the surgeon to perform minimally invasive procedures. As of 2011, the stereotactic method typically involves computer-assisted surgery (CAS). CAS includes image guidance in diagnosis and preoperative planning, intraoperative feedback in real time, the use of robotics, neural prostheses (devices that are implanted in the tissues of the nervous system or the blood vessels that supply it to help restore function), and outcomes analysis.
- Computer navigational technology. Also known as neuronavigation, this advance began in the 1990s as an outgrowth of the stereotactic method. It refers to the set of computer-assisted technologies used by neurosurgeons to guide or "navigate" within the skull or spinal column during the actual surgical intervention.
- Programmable shunt devices. In general, a shunt in medicine is a hole or small passage, whether natural or artificial, that allows movement of fluid from one part of the body to another. The term is most often used to refer to mechanical tubelike devices inserted by neurosurgeons to pump excess cerebrospinal fluid through a long catheter into the abdominal cavity in

patients with hydrocephalus. The programmable shunt allows the surgeon to fine-tune the pressure setting of the device in the office after implantation without having to perform another surgical procedure, whereas the older fixed-pressure shunts required a second operation if the initial pressure setting was inaccurate or caused complications.

- Gamma knife radiosurgery. The gamma knife is a technique for delivering high doses of radiation to a precise location to shrink brain tumors without damaging nearby healthy tissue.

- Neurostimulation. Neurostimulation is an advanced technique for pain control that involves implanting electrodes on the spine or the motor cortex region of the brain. Using the electrodes to stimulate those areas can inhibit pain sensations.

- Operating microscopes. Operating microscopes are binocular microscopes used in surgery to provide a clear view of small and inaccessible parts of the body, improving the surgeon's hand/eye coordination and improving patient outcomes. Operating microscopes are used primarily to perform such microsurgical procedures as treating brain aneurysms, inserting stents in the arteries of the brain, removing small tumors, and completing the delicate maneuvers involved in skull base surgery.

Conditions diagnosed or treated

The various neurological subspecialties diagnose and treat the following disorders:

- Cerebrovascular neurosurgery: stroke, arteriovenous malformations (AVMs), and brain aneurysms. Cerebrovascular neurosurgeons may work together with endovascular neurosurgeons.

- Neurotrauma and critical care neurosurgery. Neurosurgeons in this subspecialty treat both blunt and penetrating injuries to the head and spine. They usually work together with critical care specialists for patients in intensive care units.

- Tumor neurosurgery. Neurosurgeons in this subspecialty often work together with radiation oncologists to treat brain cancers. They may use open craniotomies; minimally invasive neurosurgery performed through tiny burr holes in the skull or entry through the nose and sinus cavities, or gamma knife radiosurgery, which uses a concentrated beam of radiation rather than a scalpel to destroy tumors.

- Pediatric neurosurgery. In addition to treating traumatic injuries, tumors of the brain and spine, vascular malformations, and seizure disorders, pediatric neurosurgeons also treat children with hydrocephalus, a disorder in which there is an abnormal collection of cerebrospinal fluid in the ventricles (hollow areas) of the brain.

- Pain neurosurgery. Pain neurosurgery is used to treat chronic pain syndromes affecting the face, such as trigeminal neuralgia, and pain caused by disorders of the spine that do not respond to other methods of treatment. Pain surgery may involve neurostimulation, severing nerves that convey pain impulses, or removing blood vessels or other structures that are pressing on the nerves relaying pain signals. This latter technique is called decompression.

- Spinal neurosurgery. Spinal surgeons treat a range of different disorders, from congenital deformities to degenerative disorders of the spine and traumatic injuries. They may remove cancerous tumors and reconstruct bone destroyed during tumor removal; perform spinal fusion (union of two bony segments of the spine) or spinal stabilization; remove damaged spinal disks and replace them with artificial disks; correct deformities of the spine such as kyphosis and scoliosis; and treat fractures of the spine.

- Functional neurosurgery. Functional neurosurgeons use such techniques as deep brain stimulation (DBS) and drug delivery directly to the spine to treat Tourette syndrome, depression, tremor, dystonia, and obsessive-compulsive disorder (OCD) as well as movement disorders.

- Epilepsy surgery. Epilepsy surgery is generally performed only in patients who continue to have seizures in spite of anticonvulsant medications. This type of neurosurgery involves the placement of a grid of electrodes on the surface of the brain to identify the specific source of the abnormal electrical activity in the brain. When the focus of the seizure has been identified, the patient has a second operation in which that portion of the brain is removed. Another procedure that can be done in patients with poorly localized seizures is the implanting of an electrode to stimulate the left vagus nerve. The electrode is attached to a pulse generator implanted under the skin below the collarbone.

- Endovascular neurosurgery. Conditions treated by endovascular neurosurgeons include stroke, arteriovenous malformations, narrowing of the cerebral arteries, and aneurysms. Treatments include embolization of aneurysms, delivery of clot-dissolving medications in cases of stroke, placements of stents in narrowed arteries, and intracranial angioplasty (a method of improving blood flow through a narrowed artery by inserting a balloon-tipped catheter into the diseased section of the blood vessel,

Aneurysm—A localized blood-filled bulge or weak spot in the wall of a blood vessel.

Angioplasty—A technique for mechanically widening a narrowed or blocked blood vessel by inserting a balloon catheter, inflating the balloon to crush the fatty deposits obstructing the blood vessel, and deflating the balloon and withdrawing the catheter.

Arteriovenous malformation (AVM)—An abnormal connection between veins and arteries, usually congenital. A cerebral AVM may result in epilepsy; severe headache; bleeding into the brain; difficulties with speech, movement or coordination; or hallucinations, memory problems, and confusion.

Cerebral cortex—The outer layer of the cerebrum (forebrain), composed of gray matter and containing sensory, motor, and association areas.

Cerebrovascular—Referring to the blood vessels that supply the brain.

Congenital—Present at birth.

Craniotomy—Any surgical procedure in which a piece of bone is temporarily removed from the skull in order to gain access to the brain.

Dystonia—A neuromuscular disorder characterized by sustained muscle contractions that cause twisting and repetitive movements or abnormal body postures.

Embolization—The deliberate introduction of a metal coil or gelatin sponge into a blood vessel to stop bleeding or to seal off a tumor or aneurysm.

Endovascular—Referring to any procedure or treatment performed within a blood vessel.

Hydrocephalus—A condition marked by an abnormal accumulation of cerebrospinal fluid within the ventricles of the brain. Untreated hydrocephalus can lead to enlargement of the head, vision disorders, convulsions, mental disabilities, and even death.

Kyphosis—An abnormal curvature of the upper back that may result from osteoporosis, developmental disorders, arthritis, or trauma.

Neural prostheses—A general term for devices implanted in neurosurgery to help restore the structure or function of the central nervous system. They include stents, artificial spinal disks, platinum coils to treat aneurysms, vagus nerve stimulators, deep brain stimulators, and similar devices.

Scoliosis—A medical condition in which the spine is curved abnormally from side to side as well as from front to back. Scoliosis may be congenital, idiopathic (of unknown cause), or the result of a neuromuscular disorder.

Shunt—A channel through which blood or another body fluid is diverted from its normal path by surgical reconstruction or the insertion of a synthetic tube.

Stent—A wire tube or tube-like device placed in a blood vessel to keep it permanently open.

Trepanation—A surgical procedure in which a circular piece of bone is removed from the skull by a special saw-like instrument called a trephine or trepan. The operation is also known as trephination or trephining.

Trigeminal neuralgia—A disorder of the trigeminal nerve marked by episodes of intense facial pain that last from a few seconds to several minutes or hours.

Ventricle—Any of four hollow spaces in the human brain filled with cerebrospinal fluid.

expanding the balloon to widen the artery, and then withdrawing the catheter).

• Neurointerventional surgery. Sometimes considered a subspecialty of neuroradiology, neurointerventional surgery involves the treatment of patients by using minimally invasive interventional techniques as well as performing diagnostic imaging.

• Skull base surgery. Skull base surgery is a subspecialty that treats rare but potentially life-threatening disorders involving the lowermost portion of the skull. These disorders include cancerous tumors, infections, birth defects, and complicated traumatic injuries. Skull base disorders may affect the patient's sight, hearing, and balance. Some procedures require the neurosurgeon to approach the base of the skull through the nose, ear, or orbit of the eye in order to remove cancerous tumors of the head and neck or pituitary gland. A new approach to treating complex brain aneurysms located near the skull base involves a high-flow bypass technique that grafts a section of a large artery from the arm to bypass the damaged artery in the brain. Skull base surgery can also be used to treat facial pain and remove benign cysts from the base of the skull. Skull base surgery carries a higher risk of complications than other forms of neurosurgery.

- Am I likely to require specialized neurosurgical treatment for my condition?

- How many patients have you referred to neurosurgeons? Were the doctors subspecialists or general neurosurgeons?

- What were the outcomes?

Educational requirements and certification

Neurosurgery is one of the most demanding surgical specialties, requiring at least six years of training beyond the four years of medical school. Prior to 2009, candidates for board certification had to take a year's residency in general surgery before completing a specialized residency in neurosurgery. As of 2011, residents must complete a minimum of 72 months as a full-time resident enrolled in a program recognized by the American Board of Neurological Surgery (ABNS). The 72 months must include three months of clinical neurology and 42 months of core clinical neurosurgery—21 months must be taken in one institution as well as 12 months with senior resident responsibility. The aspiring neurosurgeon must then pass a primary written examination, followed by a three-hour oral examination that must be taken within five years of completing the residency.

Some neurosurgery residency programs are even longer. Neurosurgery programs can be approved by the ABNS for up to 84 months of training; 72 months for clinical and didactic education and 12 months for research or subspecialty training. The one-year subspecialty fellowship programs that are recognized by the ABNS as of 2011 include neuro-oncology, spinal surgery, epilepsy surgery, functional neurosurgery, cerebrovascular surgery, and pediatric neurosurgery. According to the Accreditation Council on Graduate Medical Education (ACGME), there are 101 accredited fellowship programs in neurosurgery in the United States and Canada for the academic year 2011–12, with 1,139 on-duty residents enrolled.

Resources

BOOKS

Barnett, Gene H., Robert J. Maciunas, and David W. Roberts, eds. *Computer-Assisted Neurosurgery*. New York: Taylor and Francis, 2006.

Benzil, Deborah L., and Karin M. Muraszko, eds. *Heart of a Lion, Hands of a Woman: What Women Neurosurgeons Do: Creativity in Honor of the 20th Anniversary of Women in Neurosurgery (WINS)*. Virginia Beach, VA: Donning, 2009.

Greenberg, Mark S., ed. *Handbook of Neurosurgery*. 7th ed. Tampa, FL: Greenberg Graphics, 2010.

Pickard, J.D., ed. *Advances and Technical Standards in Neurosurgery*. New York: Springer, 2011.

Shepherd, Gordon M. *Creating Modern Neuroscience: The Revolutionary 1950s*. New York: Oxford University Press, 2010.

PERIODICALS

Abdulrauf, S.I., et al. "Short Segment Internal Maxillary Artery to Middle Cerebral Artery Bypass: A Novel Technique for Extracranial-to-Intracranial Bypass." *Neurosurgery* 68 (March 2011): 804–08.

Cadotte, D.W., and M.G. Fehlings. "Spinal Cord Injury: A Systematic Review of Current Treatment Options." *Clinical Orthopaedics and Related Research* 469 (March 2011): 732–41.

Chakravarti, P.S., et al. "Microvascular Decompression Treatment for Trigeminal Neuralgia." *Journal of Craniofacial Surgery* 22 (May 2011): 894–98.

Chen, J.C., et al. "Frameless Image-guided Radiosurgery for Initial Treatment of Typical Trigeminal Neuralgia." *World Neurosurgery* 74 (October-November 2010): 538–43.

Duncan, J.S. "Epilepsy in 2010: Refinement of Optimal Medical and Surgical Treatments." *Nature Reviews. Neurology* 7 (February 2011): 72–74.

Elliott, R.E., et al. "Vagus Nerve Stimulation for Children with Treatment-resistant Epilepsy: A Consecutive Series of 141 Cases." *Journal of Neurosurgery. Pediatrics* 7 (May 2011): 491–500.

Gilliam, F.G., and B. Albertson. "Identifying Epilepsy Surgery Candidates in the Outpatient Clinic." *Epilepsy and Behavior* 20 (February 2011): 156–59.

Hadjipanavis, C.G., et al. "Current and Future Clinical Applications for Optical Imaging of Cancer: From Intraoperative Surgical Guidance to Cancer Screening." *Seminars in Oncology* 38 (February 2011): 109–18.

Muh, C.R., et al. "Clinical Problem Solving: Monster on the Hook—Case Problems in Neurosurgery." *Neurosurgery* 68 (March 2011): E874–82.

Shilpakar, S. "Subspecialties in Neurosurgery and Its Challenges in a Developing Country." *World Neurosurgery* 75 (March-April 2011): 335–37.

Xiong, Y., et al. "Neurorestorative Treatments for Traumatic Brain Injury." *Discovery Medicine* 10 (November 2010): 434–42.

WEBSITES

"Brain Tumor Surgery: Skull Base Neurosurgery at DMC." Detroit Medical Center (DMC). http://www.dmc.org/VideoLibrary/ShowVideo.aspx?Library=1&VideoID=93 (accessed July 25, 2011).

Chicago Tribune. "A Neurosurgeon Talks about His Job." YouTube. http://www.youtube.com/watch?v=eQ-F8or9shiQ&feature=related (accessed July 25, 2011).

"Harvey Cushing's 2000th Verified Brain Tumor Operation." Cyber Museum of Neurosurgery. http://www.neurosurgery.org/cybermuseum/leadershall/2KTumor.mov (accessed July 25, 2011).

"Patient Information: Anatomy of the Brain." American Association of Neurological Surgeons (AANS). http://www.aans.org/Patient%20Information/Conditions%20and%20Treatments/Anatomy%20of%20the%20Brain.aspx (accessed July 25, 2011).

"Primary Certification Process." American Board of Neurological Surgery (ABNS). http://www.abns.org/content/primary_certification_process.asp (accessed July 25, 2011).

"The Surgical Specialties: Neurological Surgery." American College of Surgeons (ACS). http://www.facs.org/residencysearch/specialties/neuro.html (accessed July 25, 2011).

ORGANIZATIONS

American Academy of Neurological Surgery (AAcNS), c/o Jude Sargent, Department of Neurosurgery, UCSF, 505 Parnassus Avenue, M-786, Box 0112, San Francisco, CA 94143-0112, (415) 353-3933, Fax: (415) 353-3910, judesargent@yahoo.com, http://americanacademyns.org.

American Academy of Neurology (AAN), 1080 Montreal Avenue, Saint Paul, MN 55116, (651) 695-2717, (800) 879-1960, Fax: (651) 695-2791, memberservices@aan.com, http://www.aan.com.

American Association of Neurological Surgeons (AANS), 5550 Meadowbrook Drive, Rolling Meadows, IL 60008-3852, (847) 378-0500, (888) 566-AANS, Fax: (847) 378-0600, http://www.aans.org.

Society of NeuroInterventional Surgery (SNIS), 3975 Fair Ridge Drive, Suite 200 North, Fairfax, VA 22033, (703) 691-2272, Fax: (703) 537-0650, http://www.snisonline.org.

Rebecca J. Frey, PhD

Neurotransmitters

Definition

Neurotransmitters are chemicals that allow the movement of information from one neuron across the gap between the adjacent neuron. The release of neurotransmitters from one area of a neuron and the recognition of the chemicals by a receptor site on the adjacent neuron causes an electrical reaction that facilitates the release of the neurotransmitter and its movement across the gap.

Description

The transmission of information from one neuron to another depends on the ability of the information to traverse the gap (also known as the synapse) between the terminal end of one neuron and the receptor end of an adjacent neuron. The transfer is accomplished by neurotransmitters.

In 1921, Austrian scientist Otto Loewi (1873–1961) discovered the first neurotransmitter. He named the compound *vagusstoff* as he was experimenting with the vagus nerve of frog hearts. Now, this compound is known as acetylcholine.

Neurotransmitters are manufactured in a region of a neuron known as the cell body. From there, they are transported to the terminal end of the neuron, where they are enclosed in small membrane-bound bags called vesicles (the sole exception is nitric oxide, which is not contained inside a vesicle, but is released from the neuron soon after being made). In response to an action potential signal, the neurotransmitters are released from the terminal area when the vesicle membrane fuses with the neuron membrane. The neurotransmitter chemical then diffuses across the synapse.

At the other side of the synapse, neurotransmitters encounter receptors. An individual receptor is a transmembrane protein, meaning part of the protein projects from both the inside and outside surfaces of the neuron membrane, with the rest of the protein spanning the membrane. A receptor may be capable of binding to a neurotransmitter, similar to the way a key fits into a lock. Not all neurotransmitters can bind to all receptors; there is selectivity within the binding process.

When a receptor site recognizes a neurotransmitter, the site is described as becoming activated. This can result in depolarization or hyperpolarization, which acts directly on the affected neurons, or the activation of another molecule (second messenger) that eventually alters the flow of information between neurons.

Depolarization stimulates the release of the neurotransmitter from the terminal end of the neuron. Hyperpolarization makes it less likely that this release will occur. This dual mechanism provides a means of control over when and how quickly information can pass from neuron to neuron. The binding of a neurotransmitter to a receptor triggers a biological effect; however, once the recognition process is complete, its ability to stimulate the biological effect is lost. The receptor is then ready to bind another neurotransmitter.

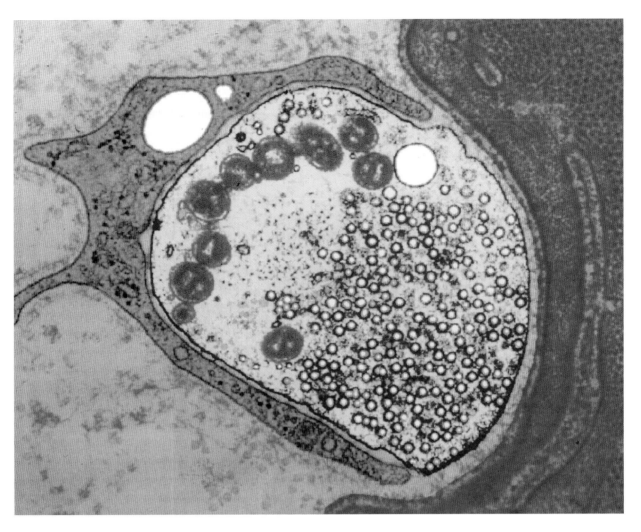

Nerve terminal synapses with muscle fiber (red). *(© Don Fawcett/Photo Researchers, Inc.)*

Neurotransmitters can also be inactivated by degradation by a specific enzyme (e.g., acetylcholinesterase degrades acetylcholine). Cells known as astrocytes can remove neurotransmitters from the receptor area. Finally, some neurotransmitters (norepinephrine, dopamine, and serotonin) can be reabsorbed into the terminal region of the neuron.

Since Loewi's discovery of acetylcholine, many neurotransmitters have been discovered, including the following partial list:

• Acetylcholine: Acetylcholine is particularly important in the stimulation of muscle tissue. After stimulation, acetylcholine degrades to acetate and choline, which are absorbed back into the first neuron to form another acetylcholine molecule. The poison curare blocks transmission of acetylcholine. Some nerve gases inhibit the breakdown of acetylcholine, producing a continuous stimulation of the receptor cells and spasms of muscles such as the heart.

• Epinephrine (Adrenaline) and Norepinephrine: These compounds are secreted principally from the adrenal gland. Secretion causes an increased heart rate and the enhanced production of glucose as a ready energy source (the "fight or flight" response).

• Dopamine: Dopamine facilitates critical brain functions and, when unusual quantities are present, abnormal dopamine neurotransmission may play a role in Parkinson's disease, certain addictions, and schizophrenia.

• Serotonin: Synthesized from the amino acid tryptophan, serotonin is assumed to play a biochemical role in mood and mood disorders, including anxiety, depression, and bipolar disorder.

• Aspartate: An amino acid that stimulates neurons in the central nervous system, particularly those that transfer information to the area of the brain called the cerebrum.

- Oxytocin: A short protein (peptide) that is released within the brain, ovary, and testes. The compound stimulates contractions during birth, the release of milk by mammary glands, and maternal behavior.

- Somatostatin: Another peptide, which is inhibitory to the secretion of growth hormone from the pituitary gland, of insulin, and of a variety of gastrointestinal hormones involved with nutrient absorption.

- Insulin: A peptide secreted by the pancreas that stimulates other cells to absorb glucose.

As exemplified above, neurotransmitters have different actions. In addition, some neurotransmitters have different effects depending upon the receptor to which they bind. For example, acetylcholine can be stimulatory when bound to one receptor and inhibitory when bound to another receptor.

Resources

BOOKS

Bradley, W., et al. *Neurology in Clinical Practice*. 5th ed. Philadelphia: Butterworth-Heinemann, 2008.

Goetz, C.G. *Goetz's Textbook of Clinical Neurology*. 3rd ed. Philadelphia: Saunders, 2007.

PERIODICALS

Nutt, D.J. "Relationship of neurotransmitters to the symptoms of major depressive disorder." *Journal of Clinical Psychiatry* 69 (January 1, 2008): 4–7.

Saudhof, T.C. "Neurotransmitter release." *Handook of Experimental Pharmacology* 29 (January 1, 2008): 1–21.

Brian Douglas Hoyle, PhD
Rosalyn Carson-DeWitt, MD

Nevus cavernosus *see* **Cerebral cavernous malformation**

Niemann-Pick Disease

Definition

Niemann-Pick Disease (NPD) is a term that defines a group of diseases that affect metabolism and which are caused by specific genetic mutations. Currently, there are three categories of Niemann-Pick diseases: type A (NPD-A): the acute infantile form; type B (NPD-B): a less common, chronic, non-neurological form; and type C (NPD-C): a biochemically and genetically distinct form of the disease.

Description

NPD-A is a debilitating neurodegenerative (progressive nervous system dysfunction) childhood disorder characterized by failure to thrive, enlarged liver, and progressive neurological deterioration, which generally leads to death by three years of age. In contrast, NPD-B patients have an enlarged liver, no neurological involvement, and often survive into adulthood. NPD-C, although similar in name to types A and B, is very different at the biochemical and genetic level. People with NPD-C are not able to metabolize cholesterol and other lipids properly within the cells. Consequently, excessive amounts of cholesterol accumulate in the liver and spleen. The vast majority of children with NPD-C die before age 20, and many before the age of 10. Later onset of

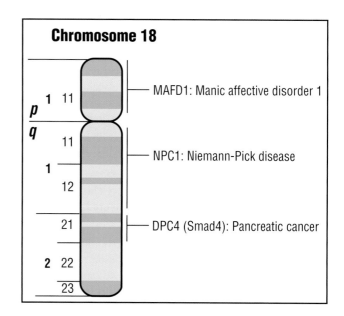

Niemann-Pick disease, on chromosome 18. *(Illustration by Argosy, Inc. Reproduced by permission of Gale, a part of Cengage Learning.)*

symptoms usually leads to a longer life span, although death usually occurs by age 40.

Demographics

Niemann-Pick disease types A and B NPD occur in many ethnic groups; however, they occur more frequently among individuals of Ashkenazi Jewish descent than in the general population. NPD-A occurs most frequently, and it accounts for about 85% of all cases of the disease. NPD-C affects an estimated 500 children in the United States.

Causes and symptoms

All forms of NPD are inherited autosomal recessive disorders, requiring the presence of an inherited genetic mutation in only one copy of the gene responsible for the disease. Both males and females are affected equally. Types A and B are both caused by the deficiency of a specific enzyme known as the acid sphingomyelinase (ASM). This enzyme is ordinarily found in special compartments within cells called lysosomes and is required to metabolize a certain lipid (fat). If ASM is absent or not functioning properly, this lipid cannot be metabolized and is accumulated within the cell, eventually causing cell death and the malfunction of major organs and systems.

NPD-C disease is a fatal, lipid storage disorder characterized by cholesterol accumulation in the liver, spleen, and **central nervous system**. Mutations in two independent genes result in the clinical features of this disease.

Symptoms of all forms of NPD are variable; no single symptom should be used to include or exclude NPD as a diagnosis. A person in the early stages of the disease may exhibit only a few of the symptoms and even in the later stages not all symptoms may be present.

NPD-A begins in the first few months of life. Symptoms normally include feeding difficulties, abdomen enlargement, progressive loss of early motor skills and cherry red spots in the eyes.

NPD-B is biochemically similar to type A, but the symptoms are more variable. Abdomen enlargement may be detected in early childhood, but there is almost no neurological involvement, such as loss of motor skills. Some patients may develop repeated respiratory infections.

NPD-C usually affects children of school age, but the disease may strike at any time from early infancy to adulthood. Symptoms commonly found are jaundice, spleen and/or liver enlargement, difficulties with upward and downward eye movements, gait (walking) unsteadiness, clumsiness, dystonia (difficulty in posturing of limbs), **dysarthria** (irregular speech), learning difficulties and progressive intellectual decline, sudden loss of muscle tone which may lead to **falls**, tremors accompanying movement, and, in some cases, seizures.

Diagnosis

The diagnosis of NPD-A and B is normally clinical, helped by measuring the ASM activity in the blood (white blood cells). While this test will identify affected individuals with the two mutated genes, it is not very reliable for detecting carriers, who have only one mutated gene.

NPD-C is diagnosed by taking a small skin **biopsy**, growing the cells (fibroblasts) in the laboratory, and studying their ability to transport and store cholesterol. Cholesterol transport in the cells is tested by measuring conversion of the cholesterol from one form to another. The storage of cholesterol is assessed by staining the cells with a compound that glows under ultraviolet light. It is important that both of these tests are performed, as reliance on one or the other may lead to the diagnosis being missed in some cases. NPD-C is often incorrectly diagnosed and misclassified as attention deficit disorder (ADD), learning disability, retardation, or delayed development.

Treatment team

The treatment team is normally composed of a nutritionist, a physical therapist and/or occupational therapist (walking and balance, motor skills and posturing), a neurologist (seizure medications and neurological assessments), a speech therapist, pulmonologist, a geneticist, a gastroenterologist, a psychologist, a social worker, and nurses.

Treatment

No specific definitive treatment is available for patients with any NPD type, and treatment is purely supportive. For NPD-C, a healthy, low-cholesterol diet is recommended. However, research into low-cholesterol diets and cholesterol-lowering drugs do not indicate that these halt the progress of the disease or change cholesterol metabolism at the cellular level.

Recovery and rehabilitation

All types of NPD require continuous family care and medical follow-up. Long-term survival and life quality will vary from patient to patient and seems to be directly related to the nature of the disease (genetic mutation) and the medical support provided.

KEY TERMS

Autosomal recessive—A pattern of inheritance in which both copies of an autosomal gene must be abnormal for a genetic condition or disease to occur. An autosomal gene is located on one of the autosomes or non-sex chromosomes. When both parents have one abnormal copy of the same gene, they have a 25% chance with each pregnancy that their offspring will have the disorder.

Hepatosplenomegaly—Enlargement of the liver and spleen.

Lipids—Organic compounds not soluble in water, but soluble in fat solvents such as alcohol. Lipids are stored in the body as energy reserves and are also important components of cell membranes. Commonly known as fats.

Clinical trials

Enzyme replacement has been tested in mice and shown to be effective for type NPD type B. It has also been used successfully in other storage diseases, such as Gaucher type I.

Laboratory studies of neurosteroids have shown encouraging results when tested on mice, but more work needs to be done before a clinical trial can be considered. Information on current clinical trials can be found at ClinicalTrials.gov.

Prognosis

Patients with NPD-A commonly die during infancy. NPD-B patients may live a few decades, but many require supplemental oxygen because of lung impairment. The life expectancy of patients with type C is variable. Some patients die in childhood while others, who appear to be less drastically affected, live into adulthood.

Special concerns

All types of NPD are autosomal recessive, which means that both parents carry one copy of the abnormal gene, without having any signs of the disease. When parents are carriers, in each pregnancy, there is a 25% risk of conceiving a child who is affected with the disease and a 50% risk that the child will be a carrier.

For NPD-A and B the ASM gene has been isolated and extensively studied. DNA testing and prenatal diagnosis is currently available. Research into treatment alternatives for these types has progressed rapidly since the early 1990s. Current research focuses on bone marrow transplantation, enzyme replacement therapy, and gene therapy. All of these therapies have had some success against NPD-B in a laboratory environment. Unfortunately, none of the potential therapies has been effective against NPD-A.

Resources

PERIODICALS

Madra, Moneek, and Stephen L Sturley. "Niemann-Pick type C pathogenesis and treatment: from statins to sugars." *Clinical Lipidology* June 2010: 387.

Vanier, Marie T. "Niemann-Pick disease type C." *Orphanet Journal of Rare Diseases* 5 (2010): 16.

OTHER

National Institute of Neurological Disorders and Stroke. *NINDS Niemann-Pick Disease Information Page.* http://www.ninds.nih.gov/health_and_medical/ disorders/niemann.doc.htm (January 4, 2003).

National Tay-Sachs & Allied Diseases Association (NTSAD). *Neimann-Pick Disease.* http://www.ntsad. org/pages/n-pick.htm (January 4, 2004).

ORGANIZATIONS

National Niemann-Pick Disease Foundation, Inc. PO Box 49, 415 Madison Ave, Ft. Atkinson, WI 53538. Phone: (920) 563-0930. Fax: (920) 563-0931. Tollfree phone: (877) 287-3672. Email: nnpdf @idcnet.com. http:// www.nnpdf.org.

Beatriz Alves Vianna
Iuri Drumond Louro

Nutritional deficiency *see* **Vitamin/ nutritional deficiency**

Occipital neuralgia

Definition

Occipital neuralgia is a persistent pain that is caused by an injury or irritation of the occipital nerves located in the back of the head.

Description

The greater and lesser occipital nerves run from the region where the spinal column meets the neck (the suboccipital region) up to the scalp at the back of the head. Trauma to these nerves can cause a pain that originates from the lower area of the neck between the shoulder blades.

Demographics

Although statistics indicating the frequency of persons with occipital neuralgia are unknown, the condition is more frequent in females than males.

Causes and symptoms

Occipital neuralgia is caused by an injury to the greater or lesser occipital nerves or some irritation of one or both of these nerves. The repeated contraction of the neck muscles is a potential cause. Spinal column compression, localized infection or inflammation, gout, diabetes, blood vessel inflammation, and frequent, lengthy periods of maintaining the head in a downward and forward position have also been associated with occipital neuralgia. Less frequently, the growth of a tumor can be a cause, as the tumor puts pressure on the occipital nerves.

The result of the nerve damage or irritation is pain, which is typically described as continuously aching or throbbing. Some people also have periodic jabs of pain in addition to the more constant discomfort. The level of pain can be intense, and similar to a migraine. This intense pain can cause nausea and vomiting.

The pain typically begins in the lower area of the neck and spreads upward in a "ram's horn" pattern on the side of the head. Ultimately, the entire scalp and forehead can be painful. The scalp is also often tender to the touch. Additionally, persons with occipital neuralgia may have difficulty rotating or flexing the neck, and pain may radiate to the shoulder. Pressure or pain may be felt behind the eyes, and eyes are sensitive to light, especially when headache is present.

Diagnosis

Diagnosis is based on the symptoms and especially on the location of the pain. Medical history is also useful. A history of muscle tension headaches over a long period of time is a good indicator that the current pain could be a neuralgic condition such as occipital neuralgia. While many people experience a tension headache due to the contraction of neck and facial muscles, few people experience the true neuralgic pain of occipital neuralgia. Nevertheless, physical and emotional tension can be contributing factors to the condition.

Treatment team

The treatment team typically is made up of someone capable of giving a massage and a family physician. A neurologist and pain specialist may also be consulted. In the rare cases that surgery is required, a neurosurgeon is also involved.

Treatment

Treatment usually consists in attempting to relieve the pain. This often involves a massage to relax the muscles in the area of the occipital nerves. Bed rest may relieve acute pain. In cases in which the nerve pain is suspected of being caused by a tumor, a more specialized examination is done using the techniques of nuclear imaging or computed tomography (CT). These techniques provide an image that can reveal a tumor. If present, the tumor can be removed surgically, which usually cures the condition.

In cases in which the pain is especially intense, as in a migraine type of pain, pain-relieving drugs and antidepressants can be taken. Other treatments involve the blocking of the impulses from the affected nerve by injection of compounds that block the functioning of the nerve. Steroids can also be injected at the site of the nerve to try to relieve inflammation. However, the usefulness and long-term effects of this form of steroid therapy are not clear.

In extreme cases where pain is frequent, the nerves can be severed at the point where they join the scalp. The person is pain-free, but sensation is permanently lost in the affected region of the head.

Recovery and rehabilitation

Recovery is usually complete after the bout of pain has subsided and the nerve damage has been repaired or lessened.

Clinical trials

There are no clinical trials in the United States that are directly concerned with occipital neuralgia. However, research is being funded through agencies such as the National Institute of Neurological Disorders and Stroke to find new treatments for pain and nerve damage and to uncover the biological processes that result in pain.

Prognosis

The periodic nature of mild occipital neuralgia usually does not interfere with daily life. The prognosis for persons with more severe occipital neuralgia is also good, as the pain is usually lessened or eliminated by treatment.

Resources

BOOKS

Parker, J. N., and P. M. Parker. *The Official Parent's Sourcebook on Occipital Neuralgia: A Revised and Updated Directory for the Internet Age.* San Diego: Icon Health, 2003.

OTHER

Loeser, J. D. "Occipital Neuralgia." *Facial Neuralgia Resources.* April 14, 2004 (June 2, 2004). http://www.facial-neuralgia.org/conditions/occipital.html.

"NINDS Occipital Neuralgia Information Page." *National Institute of Neurological Disorders and Stroke.* April 12, 2004 (June 2, 2004). http://www.ninds.nih.gov/health_and_medical/disorders/occipitalneuralgia.htm.

ORGANIZATIONS

National Institute for Neurological Diseases and Stroke (NINDS). 6001 Executive Boulevard, Bethesda, MD 20892. Phone: (301) 496-5751. Tollfree phone: (800) 352-9424. http://www.ninds.nih.gov.

National Institute of Arthritis and Musculoskeletal and Skin Diseases (NIAMS). 31 Center Dr., Rm. 4C02 MSC 2350, Bethesda, MD 20892-2350. Phone: (301) 496-8190. Tollfree phone: (877) 226-4267. Email: NIAMSinfo@mail.nih.gov. http://www.niams.nih.gov.

National Organization for Rare Disorders. 55 Kenosia Avenue, Danbury, CT 06813-1968. Phone: (203) 744-0100. Fax: (203) 798-2291. Tollfree phone: (800) 999-6673. Email: orphan@rarediseases.org. http://www.rarediseases.org.

Brian Douglas Hoyle

Occulocephalic reflex *see* **Visual disturbances; Traumatic brain injury**

Occult spinal dysraphism sequence *see* **Tethered spinal cord syndrome**

Olivopontocerebellar atrophy

Definition

Olivopontocerebellar atrophy (OPCA) comprises a group of disorders characterized by degeneration of three brain areas: the inferior olives, the pons, and the **cerebellum**. OPCA causes increasingly severe **ataxia** (loss of coordination) as well as other symptoms.

Description

Two distinct groups of diseases are called OPCA, leading to some confusion. Noninherited OPCA, also called sporadic OPCA, is now considered a form of **multiple system atrophy** (MSA). Hereditary OPCA, also called inherited OPCA and familial OPCA, is caused by inheritance of a defective gene, which is recognized in some forms but not in others.

Demographics

Hereditary OPCA affects approximately 10,000 people in the United States, with males affected approximately twice as often as females. The average age of onset is 28 years.

Causes and symptoms

By definition, hereditary OPCA is caused by the inheritance of a defective gene. Several genes have been identified. The two most common are known as SCA-1 and SCA-2 (SCA stands for **spinocerebellar ataxia**). These genes cause similar, though not identical, diseases. Besides these two genes, there are at least 20 other genetic forms of the disease. For reasons that are not understood, these gene defects cause degeneration (cell death) in specific parts of the brain, leading to the symptoms of the disorder. The cerebellum is a principal center for coordination, and its degeneration leads to loss of coordination.

The most common early symptom of OPCA is ataxia, or incoordination, which may be observed in an unsteady gait or over-reaching for an object with the hand. Other common symptoms include **dysarthria** (speech difficulty), dysphagia (swallowing difficulty), nystagmus (eye **tremor**), and abnormal movements such as jerking, twisting, or writhing. Symptoms worsen over time.

Diagnosis

An initial diagnosis of OPCA can be made with a careful neurological examination (testing of reflexes, balance, coordination, etc.), plus a magnetic resonance image (MRI) of the brain to look for atrophy (loss of tissue) in the characteristic brain regions. Genetic tests exist for SCA-1 and SCA-2 forms. Many other types of tests are possible, although they are usually done only to rule out other conditions with similar symptoms or to confirm the diagnosis in uncertain cases. Because the symptoms of OPCA can be so variable, especially at the beginning of the disease, it may be difficult to obtain a definite diagnosis early on.

Treatment team

The treatment team is likely to consist of a neurologist, physical therapist, occupational therapist, speech/language pathologist, genetic counselor, and nursing care specialist.

Treatment

There are no treatments that reverse or delay the progression of OPCA.

Very few medications have any beneficial effect on OPCA symptoms. In some patients, Levodopa, also prescribed for **Parkinson's disease**, may initially help. Some anti-tremor medications, including propranolol, may also slightly help. **Acetazolamide** may be useful in some forms of the disease.

Treatment of OPCA is primarily directed toward reducing the danger of ataxia and minimizing the impact of the disease on activities of daily living. Falling is the major danger early in the disease, and **assistive mobile devices** such as walkers and wheelchairs are often essential to prevent falling.

As the disease progresses, swallowing difficulties present the greatest danger. Softer foods and smaller mouthfuls are recommended. A speech-language pathologist can help devise swallowing strategies to lessen the risk of choking and can offer advice on assisted communication as well. Late in the disease, a feeding tube may be needed to maintain adequate nutrition.

Prognosis

The life expectancy after diagnosis is approximately 15 years, although this is an average and cannot be used to predict the lifespan of any individual person.

Special concerns

Because OPCA is an inherited disease with identified genetic causes, it is reasonable to have other family members tested for the genes to determine if they, too, are at risk. This information may help family members to make personal decisions about their future, including decisions about family planning.

Resources

WEBSITES

"Olivopontocerebellar atrophy." MedlinePlus Medical Encyclopedia (August 27, 2010). http://www.nlm.nih.gov/medlineplus/ency/article/000758.htm (accessed October 24, 2011).

"Olivopontocerebellar Atrophy Information Page." National Institute of Neurological Disorders and Stroke (NINDS) (August 16, 2011). http://www.ninds.nih.gov/disorders/opca/opca.htm (accessed October 24, 2011).

Richard Robinson

Opsoclonus myoclonus

Definition

Opsoclonus **myoclonus** is a syndrome in which the eyes dart involuntarily (opsoclonus or dancing eyes) and muscles throughout the body jerk or twitch involuntarily (myoclonus).

Description

Opsoclonus myoclonus is a very rare syndrome that strikes previously normal infants, children, or adults, often occurring in conjunction with certain cancerous tumors, viral infections, or medication use. Onset can be very sudden and dramatic, with a quick progression.

Demographics

Most children who develop opsoclonus myoclonus are under the age of two when they are diagnosed. Boys and girls are affected equally.

Causes and symptoms

Many cases of opsoclonus myoclonus follow a bout of a viral illness such as infection with influenza, Epstein-Barr or Coxsackie B viruses, or after St. Louis **encephalitis**. About half of all cases are associated with a cancerous tumor; a symptom that occurs due to cancer is termed a paraneoplastic syndrome. In children, the most common type of tumor that precipitates opsoclonus myoclonus is called neuroblastoma. Neuroblastoma can cause tumors in the brain, abdomen, or pelvic area. The cancerous cells develop from primitive nerve cells called neural crest cells. When opsoclonus myoclonus occurs in adults, it is usually associated with tumors in the lung, breast, thymus, lymph system, ovaries, uterus, or bladder. Rarely, opsoclonus myoclonus can occur after the use of certain medications such as intravenous phenytoin or **diazepam** or subsequent to an overdose of the antidepressant amitriptyline.

No one knows exactly why opsoclonus myoclonus occurs. It is postulated that the presence of a viral infection or tumor may kick off an immune system response. The immune system begins trying to produce cells that will fight the invaders, either viruses or cancer cells. However, the immune cells produced may accidentally also attack areas of the brain, producing the symptoms of opsoclonus myoclonus.

Patients with opsoclonus myoclonus all have both opsoclonus and myoclonus. They experience involuntary, rapid darting movements of their eyes, as well as lightning-quick jerking of the muscles in their faces, eyelids, arms, legs, hands, heads, and trunk. Many individuals with opsoclonus myoclonus also experience weak and floppy muscles and a **tremor**. The movement disorder symptoms are incapacitating enough to completely interfere with sitting or standing when they are at their most severe. Difficulties eating, sleeping, and speaking also occur. Other common symptoms include mood changes, rage, irritability, nervousness, anxiety, severe drowsiness, confusion, and decreased awareness and responsiveness.

Diagnosis

Diagnosis is primarily arrived at through identification of concurrent opsoclonus and myoclonus. Laboratory testing of blood and spinal fluid may reveal the presence of certain immune cells that could be responsible for attacking parts of the nervous system, such as autoantibodies. When opsoclonus myoclonus is diagnosed, a search for a causative condition such as tumor should be undertaken.

Treatment team

The treatment team will include a neurologist and neurosurgeon. A physical therapist, occupational therapist, and speech and language therapist may help an individual with opsoclonus myoclonus retain or regain as much functioning as possible.

Treatment

If opsoclonus myoclonus is due to the presence of a tumor, the first types of treatment will involve tumor removal and appropriate treatment of the cancer. Some adult cases of opsoclonus myoclonus resolve spontaneously, without specific treatment.

Treatment of the symptoms of opsoclonus myoclonus include clonzaepam or valproate. These may decrease the severity of both the opsoclonus and the myoclonus.

Other treatments for opsoclonus myoclonus include the administration of the pituitary hormone, called adrenocorticotropic hormone (ACTH). ACTH prompts the production of steroid hormones in the adrenal glands. When ACTH is given in high intravenous (IV) doses for about 20 weeks, the body produces large quantities of steroids, which can help quell any immune response that may be responsible for the opsoclonus myoclonus. Intravenous immunoglobulin treatment (IVIG), Azathioprine, and intravenous steroid treatments may also be given in an effort to suppress the immune system's response.

Two treatments that filter the blood in an effort to remove potentially damaging immune cells may also be attempted, although they are generally only able to be performed on adults. These include therapeutic apheresis and immunoadsorption. In these procedures, the patient's blood or plasma is processed to extract certain immune cells; the blood or plasma is then returned to the patient. These procedures may

KEY TERMS

Apheresis—A procedure in which the blood is removed and filtered in order to rid it of particular cells, then returned to the patient.

Autoantibodies—Antibodies that are directed against the body itself.

Immunoadsorption—A procedure that can remove harmful antibodies from the blood.

Myoclonus—Lightning-quick involuntary jerks and twitches of muscles.

Neuroblastoma—A malignant tumor of nerve cells that strikes children.

Opsoclonus—Often called "dancing eyes," this symptom involves involuntary, quick darting movements of the eyes in all directions.

Paraneoplastic syndrome—A cluster of symptoms that occur due to the presence of cancer in the body, but that may occur at a site quite remote from the location of the cancer.

need to be repeated five or six times, but improvement is often rapid and may last up to 2–3 months.

Prognosis

The prognosis for opsoclonus myoclonus is varied. The milder the case prior to treatment, the more likely full recovery may occur. When opsoclonus myoclonus is due to a viral illness, there is a higher possibility for resolution of symptoms than when the condition results from neuroblastoma. Furthermore, although the degree of myoclonus may decrease, there are still often some residual coordination problems, difficulties with learning, behavior and/or attention, and obsessive-compulsive disorder. Children with very severe cases of opsoclonus myoclonus are likely to continue to have severe problems and will probably never have normal intelligence or the ability to live independently.

Many children have flares of their symptoms or actual relapses of the disease when they suffer from viral illnesses, even years later. The treatments for such relapses are the same as for the initial illness.

Resources

BOOKS

Asha Das, Ramsis, K. Benjamin, and Fred H. Hochberg. "Metastatic Neoplasms and Paraneoplastic Syndromes." In *Textbook of Clinical Neurology*, edited by Christopher G. Goetz. Philadelphia: W. B. Saunders, 2003.

Al-Lozi, Muhammad, and Alan Pestronk. "Paraneoplastic Neurologic Syndromes." In *Harrison's Principles of Internal Medicine*, edited by Eugene Braunwald, et al. New York: McGraw-Hill Professional, 2001.

PERIODICALS

Dale, R. C. "Childhood Opsoclonus Myoclonus." *Lancet Neurology* 2, no. 5 (May 2003): 270.

Pranzatelli, M. R. "Screening for Autoantibodies in Children with Opsoclonus-Myoclonus-Ataxia." *Pediatric Neurology* 27 no. 5 (November 2002): 384–87.

Storey, Imogen, Alastair Denniston, and Sarah Denniston. "Dancing Eyes." *Hospital Medicine* 27, no. 5 (September 2003): 555–56.

Yiu, V. W. "Plasmapheresis as an Effective Treatment for Opsoclonus Myoclonus Syndrome." *Pediatric Neurology* 24 no. 1 (January 2001): 72–74.

ORGANIZATIONS

Opsoclonus-Myoclonus USA and International. SIU School of Medicine, 751 North Rutledge, Suite 3100, Springfield, IL 62702. Phone: (217) 545-7635. Fax: (217) 545-1903. Email: omsusa@siumed.edu. http://www.omsusa.org/index.htm.

Rosalyn Carson-DeWitt, MD

Organic voice tremor

Definition

Organic voice **tremor** is a neurogenic voice disorder of adulthood that most often occurs as a component of essential or hereditofamilial tremor; it may occur by itself, however. Organic voice tremor must be distinguished from other conditions, which also present with voice disturbances in the early stages. These include parkinsonism, cerebellar disease, thyrotoxicosis, and anxiety.

Description

Organic voice tremor is a disorder of voice production characterized by unsteadiness of pitch and loudness and quavering intonation. In some patients, it may result in rhythmic arrests of voicing that occur at a rate of 4-6 per second. Voice quality is characterized by harshness, vocal strain, abnormally low pitch, and voice stoppages. Laryngeal examination typically reveals vocal folds of normal appearance, with no evidence of aberrant innervation. The abnormal oscillations of the larynx occur as a result of vigorous up-and-down vertical movements that occur synchronously with the oscillation of the tremor. The quavering speech quality that characterizes organic voice tremor has been thought to include extralaryngeal influences arising from tremors in the diaphragm, lips, and tongue.

The origin of organic voice tremors has not been conclusively determined, though aging and occlusive arterial disease are thought to contribute significantly to the effects. Essential tremor occurs in persons with confirmed lesions in the brain stem, basal ganglia (e.g., putamen and lentiform nuclei) and within neural connections joining the red nucleus, dentate nucleus, and inferior olive. Vocal tremors usually coexist with tremors in the head and limbs but may be localized entirely within the larynx. Disturbed central innervation to the larynx is thought to disturb coordination between abductor and adductor groups of laryngeal muscles, which may affect the symmetry of vibration of the vocal folds and result in excess force of approximation or abruptness of vocal fold separation during conversational speech. Symptoms may be difficult to fully appreciate in conversational speech but become quite evident in sustained vowel production. This fact is significant for differential diagnosis of essential tremor from spasmodic dysphonia, a focal dystonia affecting voicing.

Demographics

Organic voice tremor is a condition that usually occurs in persons over age 50. Males and females appear to be affected equally. Specific incidence data are not available.

Causes and Symptoms

Causes

Organic voice tremor is thought to result from neural degeneration in one or more regions of the extrapyramidal system. It usually is part of a more general condition of tremor involving the head, neck, and limbs called essential tremor. For some individuals, these changes are inherited and may occur in several members of the same family, sometimes occurring in successive generations. These persons are said to have hereditofamilial tremor. When the onset of organic voice tremor is rapid, the etiology may result from occlusive vascular disease. When it is gradual, the etiology is likely related to progressive changes in several locations in the brainstem or basal ganglia.

Symptoms

Persons with organic voice tremor usually experience changes in voice slowly. In addition to changes in voice quality and reduced stability in pitch, loudness, and vocal flexibility, some patients may experience tremor in the pharynx, lips, and jaw. Some patients experience difficulties in initiating or maintaining voicing or experience sudden loss of voice during conversation. In addition to vocal tremor, some patients experience spasms in the diaphragm and expiratory musculature, which may contribute to instability within the vocal tract and add to the quavering property of the voice.

Diagnosis

Organic voice tremor is usually made by examination of a neurologist and speech-language pathologist. Detailed history and medical examination is essential to determine if disruptions in voice functioning are related to other neurological conditions such as parkinsonism, cerebellar disease, and systemic conditions such as thyrotoxicosis. Differential diagnosis needs to be made between organic voice tremor and spasmodic dysphonia, which is a focal dystonia. A complete laryngeal examination should be obtained from an otolaryngologist and include endoscopic and videostroboscopic examinations of the larynx. A battery of objective tests to assess the aerodynamic and acoustic properties of voice production should be obtained from a speech pathologist, who usually works with the otolaryngologist. In addition, neuromotor intactness of the speech mechanism (the motor speech examination) should be undertaken. In this examination attention is given to assessment of muscle strength, speed of movement, range of motion, accuracy of movement, motor steadiness, and muscle tone in the speech articulators, larynx, and resonatory systems.

Treatment Team

The treatment team for organic voice tremor consists of the neurologist, otolaryngologist, and the speech-language pathologist.

Treatment

There is no cure for organic voice tremor. Medications used to treat essential tremor have not emerged as a reliable treatment modality for organic voice tremor. Propranolol has been used to treat organic voice tremor, and it was found that voice tremor is more resistant to drug treatment than tremor in the hand. Some doctors have reported effective treatment of voice and hand tremors with clonazepan, and **diazepam. Botulinum Toxin** A (BOTOX) may be useful in treating some patients with organic voice tremor, in

Dysphonia—Disordered phonation or voice production.

Dystonia—Abnormalities of muscle tone involving involuntary twisting or distortions of the trunk or other body parts.

Endoscopy—A clinical technique using an instrument called an endoscope, used for visualization of structures within the body.

Extra-laryngeal—Actions of muscles outside the larynx, but usually in its vicinity, which influence its functioning.

Extrapyramidal system—Functional, rather than anatomical unit, comprising nuclei and nerve fibers that are chiefly involved with subconscious, automatic aspects of motor coordination but which also assist in regulation of postural and locomotor movements.

Hyperfunction—Term used to describe excess effort or strain involved in producing an action.

Innervation—Distribution or supply of nerves to a structure.

Neurogenic—Of neurological origin.

Otolaryngologist—A physician who specializes in medical and surgical treatment of disorders of the ear, nose, throat, and larynx.

Resonator—As used in regard to the human speech mechanism, the cavity extending from the vocal folds to the lips, which selectively amplifies and modifies the energies produced during speech and voice production. It is synonymous with the term "vocal tract."

Speech-language pathologist—A non-physician health care provider who evaluates and treats disorders of communication and swallowing.

Thyrotoxicosis—A condition caused by excess amounts of thyroid hormone.

Tremor—Involuntary rhythmic movements, which may be intermittent or constant, involving an entire muscle or only a circumscribed group of muscle bundles.

---

which vocal fold **spasticity** is a coexisting feature. Speech therapy may be useful in reducing laryngeal hyperfunction and in establishing improved respiratory support.

Recovery and Rehabilitation

Patients with organic voice tremor do not recover from the condition. They must learn to adapt or compensate for speech and voice deficits. Speech therapy may be useful in this regard.

Prognosis

Prognosis is very poor for clinically significant improvement of voice in those with organic voice tremor.

Resources

ORGANIZATIONS

American Speech-Language and Hearing Association. 10801 Rockville Pike, Rockville, MD 20852-3279. Phone: (301) 897-5700. www.asha.org.

National Spasmodic Dysphonia Association. One East Wacker Drive, Suite 2430, Chicago, IL 60601-1905. Tollfree phone: (800) 795-6732. Email: NSDA@ dysphonia.org. www.dysphonia.org.

Joel C. Kahane, PhD

O'Sullivan-McLeod syndrome *see* **Monomelic amyotrophy**

Orthostatic hypotension

Definition

Orthostatic hypotension refers to a reduction of blood pressure (systolic blood pressure that occurs when the heart contracts) of at least 20 mmHg or a diastolic pressure (pressure when the heart muscle relaxes) of at least 10 mmHg within 3 minutes of standing.

Description

Orthostatic hypotension is a decrease of blood pressure when standing, due to changes in the blood pressure regulation systems within the body. Normally in a healthy human there is an orthostatic pooling of venous blood in the abdomen and legs when shifting positions from the supine (lying on the back) to an erect position (standing up). This redistribution of blood flow is the result of normal physiological compensatory mechanisms built into body systems to prevent any adverse outcome (decrease in blood pressure, or hypotension) during positional change.

Compensatory mechanisms include sympathetic nervous system activation, parasympathetic inhibition, and an increase in heart rate and vascular resistance. These compensation responses restore cardiac output to vital organs and return blood pressure to normal.

Orthostatic hypotension can occur if a normal physiological mechanism becomes faulty, such as inadequate cardiovascular compensation when shifting positions (i.e., change from supine to erect position) or due to an excessive reduction in blood volume.

Elderly individuals are predisposed to orthostatic hypotension because of age-related changes; possible cardiovascular disease and the medications commonly taken by the elderly all predispose to potential changes in autonomic nervous system functions. Additionally, hypertension (present in 30% of individuals over 75 years of age), predisposes an individual to orthostatic hypotension, since hypertension reduces baroreflex sensitivity. Hypertension and the normal aging process (which typically causes blood vessel stiffness) decrease the sensitivity of specialized structures called baroreceptors, which function to maintain blood pressure by initiating compensatory mechanisms such as increasing the heart rate and vascular resistance.

Persons affected with symptomatic orthostatic hypotension have symptoms when tilting their head upward or when moving toward an erect position. Symptom severity varies among affected persons but can include blurred vision, lightheadedness, **weakness, vertigo**, tremulousness, and cognitive impairment. Symptoms can be relieved within one minute of lying down. Some individuals have orthostatic hypertension without symptoms.

Demographics

The demographics of orthostatic hypotension are different due to variables that include: the subjects position change, the specific population, and when measurements are taken. It is estimated that elderly in community living environments have prevalence rates of approximately 20% among individuals over 65 years of age and 30% in persons over 75 years of age. In frail elderly persons, the prevalence of orthostatic hypotension can be more than 50%. The disorder seems more prevalent among the elderly (especially if systolic blood pressure rises) with chronic diseases (e.g., hypertension and/or diabetes).

Causes and symptoms

Orthostatic hypotension can be caused by several different disorders that affect the entire body (systemic disorders), the **central nervous system** (consisting of the brain and spinal cord), and the autonomic nervous system (peripheral autonomic neuropathy), or as a result of taking certain medications that are commonly prescribed by clinicians. Systemic causes can include dehydration, prolonged immobility or an endocrine disorder called adrenal insufficiency. Diseases of the central nervous system that can cause orthostatic hypotension include multiple systems atrophy, **Parkinson's disease**, multiple strokes, brain stem lesions, and myelopathy.

Medications that can cause orthostatic hypotension include tricyclic antidepressants, antipsychotics, monoamine oxidase inhibitors, antihypertensives, diuretics, vasodilators, levodopa, beta-blockers (heart medications), and blood pressure medications that inhibit a chemical called angiotensin (angiotensin-converting-enzyme inhibitors, or ACE inhibitors). Disorders that cause peripheral autonomic neuropathy include diabetes mellitus, amyloidosis, **tabes dorsalis** (a late manifestations of syphilis infection), alcoholism, **nutritional deficiency**, pure autonomic failure, or paraneoplastic syndromes.

The most common symptoms of orthostatic hypotension are weakness, lightheadedness, cognitive impairment, blurred vision, vertigo, and tremulousness. Other symptoms that have been reported are headache, paracervical pain, lower **back pain**, syncope, palpitations, angina pectoris, unsteadiness, falling, and calf claudication.

Diagnosis

It is important that the clinician take numerous blood pressure measurements on different occasions since blood pressure can vary (e.g., postural hypotension, another disorder causing hypotension, is often worse in the morning when rising from bed). A detailed history and physical examination is important. The clinician should focus medical evaluation on autonomic symptoms and diseases. There are bedside tests that can determine autonomic (baroreceptor) response (i.e., Valsalva maneuver). Measurements of a chemical in blood called norepinephrine while lying down and for 5–10 minutes after standing can produce some useful information concerning deficits in autonomic nervous system functioning. Additionally, levels of another chemical in blood (vasopressin) during upright tilting, can help to distinguish if the cause is due to autonomic nervous system failure or as a result of multiple systems atrophy. Pure

Adrenal insufficiency—Problems with the adrenal glands that can be life threatening if not treated. Symptoms include sluggishness, weakness, weight loss, vomiting, darkening of the skin, and mental changes.

Amyloidosis—The accumulation of amyloid deposits in various organs and tissues in the body so that normal functioning is compromised. Primary amyloidosis usually occurs as a complication of multiple myeloma. Secondary amyloidosis occurs in patients suffering from chronic infections or inflammatory diseases such as tuberculosis, rheumatoid arthritis, and Crohn's disease.

Angina pectoris—Chest pain caused by an insufficient supply of oxygen and decreased blood flow to the heart muscle. Angina is frequently the first sign of coronary artery disease.

Autonomic nervous system—The part of the nervous system that controls so-called involuntary functions, such as heart rate, salivary gland secretion, respiratory function, and pupil dilation.

Baroreceptors—Sensors located in the blood vessels that detect the pressure of blood flowing through them. These sensors send messages to the nervous system as part of the physiological blood pressure regulation mechanism.

Brainstem—The stalk of the brain which connects the two cerebral hemispheres with the spinal cord. It is involved in controlling vital functions, movement, sensation, and nerves supplying the head and neck.

Claudication—Cramping or pain in a leg caused by poor blood circulation. This condition is frequently caused by hardening of the arteries (atherosclerosis). Intermittent claudication occurs only at certain times, usually after exercise, and is relieved by rest.

Diuretic drugs—A group of medications that increase the amount of urine produced and relieve excess fluid buildup in body tissues. Diuretics may be used in treating high blood pressure, lung disease, premenstrual syndrome, and other conditions.

Levodopa—A substance used in the treatment of Parkinson's disease. Levodopa can cross the blood-brain barrier that protects the brain. Once in the brain, it is converted to dopamine and thus can replace the dopamine lost in Parkinson's disease.

Mineralocorticoid—A steroid hormone, like aldosterone, that regulates the excretion of salt, potassium, and water.

Monoamine oxidase inhibitors—A class of antidepressants used to treat certain types of mental depression. Monoamine oxidase inhibitors are especially useful in treating people whose depression is combined with other problems such as anxiety, panic attacks, phobias, or the desire to sleep too much.

Myelopathy—A disorder in which the tissue of the spinal cord is diseased or damaged.

Parkinson's disease—A slowly progressive disease that destroys nerve cells in the basal ganglia, thus causing loss of dopamine, a chemical that aids in transmission of nerve signals (neurotransmitter). Parkinson's is characterized by shaking in resting muscles, a stooping posture, slurred speech, muscular stiffness, and weakness.

Syncope—A loss of consciousness over a short period of time, caused by a temporary lack of oxygen in the brain.

Valsalva maneuver—A strain against a closed airway combined with muscle tightening, such as happens when individuals hold their breath and try to move a heavy object. Most people perform this maneuver several times a day without adverse consequences, but it can be dangerous for anyone with cardiovascular disease. Pilots perform this maneuver to prevent blackouts during high-performance flying.

Vasodilator—Any drug that relaxes blood vessel walls.

Vertigo—A feeling of dizziness together with a sensation of movement and a feeling of rotating in space.

autonomic nervous system failure is characterized by increased vasopressin levels, whereas patients with multiple systems atrophy have no appreciable increase of vasopressin levels during head tilting.

Treatment team

The treatment team usually consists of a primary care practitioner (internist). In complicated cases, such as with severe orthostatic hypotension, a neurologist or a cardiovascular specialist may be consulted.

Treatment

Non-symptomatic orthostatic hypotension is a threat for **falls** or syncope and can be treated by preventive measures that include avoiding warm environments as well as straining, squatting, stooping, leaning forward, or crossing one's legs. Additionally, individuals affected with the non-symptomatic variation should increase salt intake, sleep in the head-up position, wear waist high compression stockings, and withdraw from drugs that are known to cause orthostatic hypotension as a side effect. Treatment for symptomatic orthostatic hypotension is important since it may be a manifestation of a new illness or as a result of medications.

Intervention can initially be non-pharmacologic (preventive measures and adjustments) or pharmacologic therapy. Non-pharmacologic intervention include a review of medications because elderly patients may be taking either over-the-counter or prescription drugs that can induce orthostatic hypotension. Persons affected should rise slowly to a standing position after a long period of sitting or lying down. They should avoid excessively hot environments (e.g., hot showers or central heating systems turned up high) as well as coughing, straining, or heavy lifting, since these events can precipitate episodes of orthostatic hypotension.

There are certain measures that can be taken to increase blood pressure and reduce symptoms associated with orthostatic hypotension. When standing up from a prone or supine position (lying down) or sitting position, do so slowly. Avoid crossed legs, squatting, or stooping forward as these decrease blood flow.

Pharmacological Treatment

One of the most commonly prescribed medications for treating orthostatic hypotension is fludrocortisone acetate. This chemical is a synthetic mineralocorticoid that expands circulatory volume. This drug can cause a decrease of an important body element called potassium, which is important for normal heart contraction. As a result, hypokalemia (a decrease in potassium in plasma), may occur. Elderly persons should be monitored for blood levels of potassium and cardiac status.

The drug midodrine is useful for cases of orthostatic hypotension caused by peripheral **autonomic dysfunction**. It is usually used in conjunction with fludrocortisone. Midodrine is not recommended for those with coronary or peripheral arterial disease. Other medications that may be helpful include clonidine or antihypertension medications.

In severe cases of autonomic nervous system deficits, a combination of medications may be indicated to provide brief periods of upright posture.

Recovery and rehabilitation

The recovery is variable and is dependent on the cause. Recovery varies according to the age and health status of the affected person, age-related complications, and co-morbidities (other existing disorders.)

QUESTIONS TO ASK YOUR DOCTOR

- What are the indications that I may have orthostatic hypotension?
- What diagnostic tests are needed for a thorough assessment?
- What treatment options do you recommend for me?
- What kind of changes can I expect to see with the medications you have prescribed for me?
- What are the side effects associated with the medications you have prescribed for me?
- Will medications for orthostatic hypotension interact with my current medications?
- What tests or evaluation techniques will you perform to see if treatment has been beneficial for me?
- Does having orthostatic hypotension put me at risk for other health conditions?
- What measures can be taken to prevent orthostatic hypotension?
- What symptoms or adverse effects are important enough that I should seek immediate treatment?

Clinical trials

Government sponsored research includes studies concerning treatment of orthostatic hypotension. Individuals with orthostatic hypotension who wish to participate in the trial of an experimental therapy can find a list of clinical trials currently enrolling volunteers at http://clinicaltrials.gov. There is no cost to the patient to participate in a clinical trial.

Prognosis

Careful evaluation and ongoing management is important for a positive outcome. Identifying the source of the hypotension is an important first step. Preventive measures, posture modification techniques, and avoidance of triggers can result in a significant reduction of falls, fractures, functional decline, and syncope.

Special concerns

Special attention should be given to medications that are prescribed, which may cause orthostatic hypotension as a side effect.

Resources

BOOKS

Aminoff, Michael J., ed. *Neurology and General Medicine*. 4th ed. New York: Churchill Livingstone, 2007.

Brignole, Michele, and David G. Benditt. *Syncope: An Evidence-Based Approach*. New York: Springer, 2011.

Brunton, Laurence, Bruce A. Chabner, and Bjorn Knollman. *Goodman & Gilman's The Pharmacological Basis of Therapeutics*. 12th ed. New York: McGraw-Hill Professional, 2010.

PERIODICALS

Cooke, J., and S. Carew, A. Costelloe, T. Sheehy, C. Quinn, D. Lyons. "The changing face of orthostatic and neurocardiogenic syncope with age." *QJM* 104, no. 8 (August 2011): 689–95.

Gugger, J.J. "Antipsychotic pharmacotherapy and orthostatic hypotension: identification and management." *CNS Drugs* 25, no. 8 (August 1, 2011): 659–71.

Ha, A.D., et al "The prevalence of symptomatic orthostatic hypotension in patients with Parkinson's disease and atypical parkinsonism." *Parkinsonism Relat Disord* (June 18, 2011).

Sharabi, Y., and D.S. Goldstein. "Mechanisms of orthostatic hypotension and supine hypertension in Parkinson disease." *J Neurol Sci* (July 13, 2011).

WEBSITES

Clinical Trials Website. http://www.clinicaltrials.gov/ct/action/GetStudy (accessed July 17, 2011).

Moses, Scott. "Orthostatic Hypotension." Family Practice Notebook. http://www.fpnotebook.com/CV/Exam/OrthstcHyptnsn.htm (accessed July 17, 2011).

ORGANIZATIONS

American Academy of Neurology (AAN), 1080 Montreal Avenue, Saint Paul, MN 55116, (651) 695-2717, (800) 879-1960, Fax: (651) 695-2791, memberservices@aan.com, http://www.aan.com.

American Heart Association, 7272 Greenville Avenue, Dallas, TX 75231, (800) 242-8721, http://www.heart.org.

American Neurological Association, 5841 Cedar Lake Road, Suite 204, Minneapolis, MN 55416, (952) 545-6284, http://www.aneuroa.org.

National Institute of Neurological Disorders and Stroke (NINDS), P.O. Box 5801, Bethesda, MD 20824, (301) 496-5751, (800) 352-9424, http://www.ninds.nih.gov.

National Institutes of Health (NIH), 9000 Rockville Pike, Bethesda, MD 20892, (301) 496-4000, NIHinfo@od.nih.gov, http://www.nih.gov/index.html.

U.S. National Library of Medicine, 8600 Rockville Pike, Bethesda, MD 20894, (301) 594-5983, (888) 346-3656, Fax: (301) 402-1384, custserv@ nlm.nih.gov, http://www.nlm.nih.gov.

Laith Farid Gulli, MD
Alfredo Mori, M
Laura Jean Cataldo, RN, Ed

Overactive bladder

Definition

An overactive bladder is a medical condition involving sudden, involuntary contraction of the muscle in the wall of the urinary bladder, called the detrusor muscle. This contraction causes an abrupt and hard-to-control need to urinate, referred to as urinary urgency. Overactive bladder is a form of urinary incontinence, which means there is an involuntary loss of urine from the bladder throughout the day and at inappropriate times. Patients report the sudden need to drop everything and run to the bathroom, as well as frequent urination at night, which can be very disruptive. Patients do not always arrive at a bathroom in time to accommodate this urge to urinate and also experience incontinence of urine while at work or social gatherings. The function of the bladder to store urine when the patient is not actively trying to void is dysfunctional, resulting in unintentional urine loss that can be embarrassing for patients and affect quality of daily life. Overactive bladder is most common in older adults but is not considered a normal part of aging and is treated as a medical disorder.

Demographics

The ability to hold urine depends on normal function of the bladder musculature, the kidneys, and the nervous system. While overactive bladder is not considered a normal part of aging, the risk of experiencing overactive bladder does increase with age. As individuals grow older they are both at increased risk of developing overactive bladder and more susceptible to diseases that may cause problems with bladder function, such as enlarged prostate and diabetes. Patients with an enlarged prostate are at greater risk of developing overactive bladder because an enlarged prostate obstructs bladder outflow and so alters functionality. Diabetes patients are more likely to have poor kidney function and high urine output, which contribute to problems with overactive bladder. Neurological disorders such as Parkinson's disease, stroke, and **multiple sclerosis** have been associated with overactive bladder. Bladder abnormalities such as bladder tumors, stones, inflammation, or infections are associated with the development of overactive bladder. Lifestyle choices that may reduce the risk of overactive bladder include regular exercise and limiting caffeine, alcohol, and carbonated drinks which irritate the bladder. Patients who follow these lifestyle parameters and maintain a healthy weight are at decreased risk for developing overactive

(Table by PreMediaGlobal. © 2012 Cengage Learning.)

bladder. Individuals who have an overactive bladder and are experiencing severe disruption of their life due to its effects are at increased risk for clinical **depression**.

Cause of Overactive Bladder

The function of the bladder is to fill with urine and then to be emptied. This requires a complex interaction between the kidneys, nerve impulses, and muscular activity. There are multiple points in this process that could be compromised and contribute to overactive bladder and urge incontinence.

Normal Bladder Function

The kidneys are responsible for filtering waste from the blood and producing urine. The urine then travels down a pair of tubes called the ureters from the kidneys to the bladder. The bladder fills with urine but holds the urine until it is time to void. During voiding, urine drains from the bladder through a section with an opening at the bottom (called the neck) and flows out of the body through a short tube called the urethra. In women, the urethral opening is located just above and separate from the vaginal opening, whereas in men the urethral opening is located at the tip of the penis.

While the bladder is filling with urine, it expands to accommodate the volume of fluid. When the bladder is approximately half full, nerve impulses begin to be sent to the brain to tell the brain the bladder is filling with urine. The need to urinate normally occurs when the bladder is approximately three-fourths full.

In order to release the urine it has been holding, the bladder relies on the specialized detrusor muscle, the pelvic floor muscles, and the urinary sphincter. During voiding, nerve signals coordinate the contraction or relaxation of these muscles for urination. The nerve signals cause the relaxation of the pelvic floor muscles and the urinary sphincter muscles. These are muscles surrounding the neck of the bladder and upper portion of the urethra that obstruct urine flow when contracted. They are normally contracted with a stronger pressure than that of the other bladder muscles and so hold urine inside until intentional voiding occurs. The relaxation of these muscles allows the urine to escape the bladder while the detrusor muscle of the bladder contracts, forcing urine out.

Abnormal Bladder Function

Often, overactive bladder symptoms occur because the detrusor muscle of the bladder involuntarily spasms and contracts due to inappropriate neuronal signaling, regardless of what volume of urine is present in the bladder. The contraction of the bladder muscles creates the sensation of urinary urgency or the urgent need to urinate. If the urinary sphincter remains constricted, it will prevent the bladder from leaking. In these cases patients will experience urgency and frequency of urination but will not necessarily lose urine unintentionally; however, if the urinary sphincter is overwhelmed by the detrusor muscle contraction, urge incontinence results. Overactive bladder is not the same disorder as stress incontinence, where a patient loses urine when coughing or exercising due to weakened pelvic floor and sphincter muscles. When overactive bladder occurs at the same time as stress incontinence in the same patient, the combined disorder is referred to as mixed incontinence.

Symptoms

Symptoms associated with overactive bladder include frequent urination, usually at least eight times per day. Awakening to urinate at night usually occurs at least twice. There is a sense of urinary urgency, and for many patients there is an involuntary loss of urine immediately following the urgent need to urinate (urge incontinence). Some individuals may also have what is called mixed incontinence, when both urge incontinence and stress incontinence occur. Stress incontinence is an involuntary loss of urine in response to the pressure caused by physical stressors such as coughing or laughing. Overactive bladder is distinct from stress incontinence but may occur in the same patient with mixed symptoms.

Although individuals with overactive bladder may be able to get to the bathroom in time when they experience urinary urgency, the frequency with which they must urinate both day and night is abnormal. The frequency combined with the need to suddenly rush to a bathroom is very disruptive for work and social activities. Overactive bladder can seriously impact the quality of life. For this reason, overactive bladder may cause significant social, psychological, occupational, and sexual problems.

Diagnosis

In the initial stages of an overactive bladder diagnosis, other medical issues that may be causing symptoms need to be ruled out. Medical history and a physical exam focusing on the abdomen and genitals are necessary. A urine test may be performed in order to rule out urinary tract infection or traces of blood. Once other more common causes of urinary urgency have been ruled out, more specialized testing may be performed to explore the possibility of overactive bladder.

Urodynamic tests are used to assess bladder function, including the ability to empty completely. This aspect of bladder function is assessed by measurement of the urine left in the bladder after voiding is complete. If the bladder cannot fully empty, it may be causing symptoms similar to overactive bladder. To assist in a diagnosis of overactive bladder, a technique known as cystometry is done to measure the pressure inside the bladder and assess bladder function. Two catheters are employed. The first enters the bladder and fills the bladder with water. The second catheter is attached to a pressure-measuring sensor and placed near the bladder in the vagina or rectum. Cystometry can identify involuntary muscle contractions, indicate the level of pressure that causes urge incontinence, and measure the pressure required for bladder voiding. Another technique known as **electromyography** examines the muscles of the bladder to assess the ability to coordinate impulses in the detrusor musculature of the bladder wall versus impulses in the urinary sphincter. If these muscles are not coordinated, the process of normal urination is compromised. A uroflowmeter is an apparatus into which the patient urinates to measure speed and volume of urination. A procedure known as cystoscopy may be performed to run a tiny lens up the urethra and check for abnormalities such as tumors. The bladder may be filled with a special dye that an x ray or ultrasound can take pictures of while voiding. All of these tests may help to provide detailed medical information and guide diagnosis and treatment.

KEY TERMS

Catheter—Tube inserted into a body cavity or blood vessel to allow drainage of fluids (as in a urinary catheter), injection of drugs, or insertion of a surgical instrument.

Detrusor—Muscle in the wall of the bladder that contracts to push urine out into the urethra.

Incontinence—A medical condition in which there is involuntary loss of urine from the bladder throughout the day and at inappropriate times.

Urinary sphincter—The muscles used to control the flow of urine out of the urinary bladder. When they are contracted, urine remains in the bladder, and when they are relaxed, urine is allowed to flow into the urethra and out of the body.

Urinary urgency—A strong desire to urinate that can be difficult to control.

Voiding—The act of urinating.

Treatment and Prognosis

Pelvic muscle rehabilitation is one treatment used to relieve the symptoms of overactive bladder. This treatment improves pelvic muscle tone and prevents leakage of urine at inappropriate times. Pelvic muscle rehabilitation includes doing Kegel exercises. Kegel exercises are sets of voluntary muscle contractions of the pelvic muscles and urinary sphincter, designed to improve their strength and help prevent urinary incontinence. Electrical stimulation of the muscles of the pelvic floor may also be performed in conjunction with Kegel exercises. Behavioral therapies such as scheduled bathroom appointments every two to three hours may help some people with the incontinence portion of the symptoms. Caffeine and alcohol should be avoided since they are drugs that increase the frequency of urination and irritate the bladder. Double voiding is a technique that involves emptying the bladder, waiting a few minutes, and then attempting to fully empty the bladder a second time. This technique may help people who have difficulty emptying their bladder completely during urination. At home intermittent catheterization may also improve bladder emptying and increase time periods of dryness. Patients who do this learn how to periodically insert a catheter into their bladder to empty it. Maintaining a healthy weight is also important for overactive bladder patients. Being overweight increases incidents of incontinence.

QUESTIONS TO ASK YOUR DOCTOR

- What is the cause of my overactive bladder?
- What lifestyle changes do I need to make?
- What behavioral therapy is available for me?
- Am I a candidate for prescription medication to treat overactive bladder?
- Will the prescribed medication interact with any of my other prescription medications?
- Are there any over the counter medications I should not take with this medicine?
- Will this medicine interact with any of my herbal supplements?

Medications that relax the bladder are used to alleviate symptoms of overactive bladder and reduce episodes of urge incontinence. These drugs include tolterodine (Detrol), oxybutynin (Ditropan), trospium (Sanctura), solifenacin (Vesicare), and darifenacin (Enablex). These medications act to block the nervous system signaling that leads to spasm and overactivity of the detrusor muscle. Common side effects include dry eyes, dry mouth, constipation, **fatigue**, and changes in vision. Less common but serious side effects include heat stroke and cardiac arrhythmias for some of the medications.

Surgery to treat overactive bladder is only used on severe cases that do not respond to other treatments. Surgery may be performed in order to improve the storage ability by increasing capacity of the bladder and reduce pressure. One type of surgical intervention is nerve stimulation of specific nerves involved in bladder function. Stimulation of the nerves of the bladder is analogous to stimulation of the heart by a pacemaker. A thin nerve stimulation wire attached to a small battery may be inserted under the skin. Additionally, augmentation cytoplasty is another, major type of surgery that is only used as a last resort treatment. A portion of the bladder is replaced with tissue from the bowel to decrease the number of involuntary contractions. After this procedure patients require catheterization for urination permanently.

The combination of behavioral therapy with medications offers a good prognosis. Up to 80% of cases are improved by treatment and have a better quality of life long term. Successful treatment greatly improves prognosis by providing improved sleep and resultant energy, improved social and job-related functioning, and decreased depression. Especially for the elderly, there is a decrease in hip fractures from **falls** due to nighttime trips to the bathroom, as well as a decrease in urinary tract infections, improving their prognosis significantly.

Resources

BOOKS

Blaivas, Jerry G., and Rajveer S. Purohit. *Diagnosis and Treatment of Overactive Bladder*. Oxford: Oxford University Press, 2011.

Brunton, Laurence, Bruce A. Chabner, and Bjorn Knollman. *Goodman & Gilman's The Pharmacological Basis of Therapeutics*. 12th ed. New York: McGraw-Hill Professional, 2010.

PERIODICALS

Banakhar, Mai, Magdy M. Hassouna, and Tariq F. Al-Shaiji. "Pelvic electrical neuromodulation for the treatment of overactive bladder symptoms." *Advances in Urology* (2011).

Schieszer, John. "Healthy habits may improve urinary, sexual function." *Renal & Urology News* (October 2010): 20.

Steele, Stephen S. "Moving beyond ineffective medication for OAB." *Canadian Urological Association Journal* 5.3 (2011): 206.

WEBSITES

DuBeau, Catherine E. "Treatment of Urinary Incontinence." UpToDate. http://www.uptodate.com/contents/treatment-of-urinary-incontinence?source = search_result&selectedTitle = 1%7E48 (accessed July 18, 2011).

Epocrates. https://online.epocrates.com/ (accessed July 18, 2011).

"Overactive Bladder." MayoClinic.com. http://www.mayoclinic.com/health/overactive-bladder/DS00827 (accessed July 18, 2011).

"Urge Incontinence." PubMed Health. http://www.ncbi.nlm.nih.gov/pubmedhealth/PMH0002250// (accessed July 18, 2011).

ORGANIZATIONS

American Urological Association, 1000 Corporate Boulevard, Linthicum, MD 21090, (410) 689-3700, (866) 746-4282, aua@auanet.org, http://www.auanet.org.

National Association for Continence (NAFC), P.O. Box 1019, Charleston, SC 29402-1019, (843) 377-0900, (800) BLADDER, Fax: (843) 377-0905, http://www.nafc.org.

Maria Basile, PhD

Overuse syndrome *see* **Repetitive motion disorders**

Oxazolindinediones

Definition

Oxazolindinediones are anticonvulsants, indicated for the treatment of absence seizures (sometimes called petit mal seizures) associated with epilepsy and other seizure disorders.

Purpose

Oxazolindinediones are thought to decrease abnormal activity and excitement within the **central nervous system** (CNS) that may trigger seizures. While oxazolindinediones is often effective in controlling petit mal seizures associated with epilepsy, there is no known cure for the disorder. If necessary, oxazolindinediones can be used in conjunction with other antiepileptic drugs (AEDs) that prevent or control other types of seizures.

Description

In the United States, oxazolindinediones are sold under the generic name trimethadione and the brand name Tridione.

Recommended dosage

Oxazolindinediones are taken orally and are available in tablet, chewable tablet, or suspension forms. Oxazolindinediones are appropriate for pediatric and adult patients. Physicians prescribe the medication in varying total daily dosages. Typically, the total daily dosage is administered in three to four divided doses.

When their patients are beginning a course of treatment that includes oxazolindinediones, most physicians will prescribe a carefully scheduled dosing regimen. The physician will determine the proper initial dosage and then gradually raise the patient's daily dosage over the course of several days or weeks until seizure control is achieved. Likewise, dosages are usually tapered down over time when ending treatment with oxazolindinediones.

It is important to not take a double dose of any anticonvulsant medication, including oxazolindinediones. If a daily dose is missed, it should be taken as soon as possible. However, if it is within four hours of the next scheduled dose, then the missed dose should be skipped.

Precautions

A physician should be consulted before taking oxazolindinediones with certain non-prescription medications. Patients should avoid alcohol and CNS depressants (medicines that can make one drowsy or less alert, such as antihistimines, sleep medications, and some pain medications) while taking oxazolindinediones or any other anticonvulsants, which can exacerbate the side effects of alcohol and other medications.

A course of treatment including oxazolindinediones may not be appropriate for persons with liver or kidney disease, anemia, eye disorders, mental illness, diabetes, high blood pressure, angina (chest pain), irregular heartbeats, or other heart problems. Periodic blood, urine, and liver function tests are advised for many patients (especially pediatric and elderly patients) using the medicine.

Persons taking oxazolindinediones should avoid prolonged exposure to sunlight and should wear protective clothing and sunscreen while outdoors. Oxazolindinediones may make skin sensitive to sunlight and prone to sunburn.

Before beginning treatment with oxazolindinediones, patients should notify their physician if they consume a large amount of alcohol, have a history of drug use, are pregnant, nursing, or plan on becoming pregnant. Anticonvulsant medications may increase the risk of some birth defects. Patients who become pregnant while taking oxazolindinediones should contact their physician.

Side effects

Patients should discuss with their physicians the risks and benefits of treatment with oxazolindinediones before taking the medication. Oxazolindinediones are usually well tolerated. However, in some patients, they may cause a variety of usually mild side effects. **Dizziness**, nausea, and drowsiness are the most frequently reported side effects of anticonvulsants. Possible side effects that do not usually require medical attention and may diminish with continued use of the medication include:

- unusual tiredness or weakness
- loss of appetite
- weight loss
- abdominal pain
- speech problems
- nausea
- diarrhea or constipation
- heartburn or indigestion
- dry mouth
- chills, joint aches, and other flu-like symptoms

KEY TERMS

Absence seizure—A type of generalized seizure in which the person may temporarily appear to be staring into space and/or have jerking or twitching muscles. Previously called a petit mal seizure.

Epilepsy—A disorder associated with disturbed electrical discharges in the central nervous system that cause seizures.

Seizure—A convulsion, or uncontrolled discharge of nerve cells, that may spread to other cells throughout the brain, resulting in abnormal body movements or behaviors.

If any symptoms persist or become too uncomfortable, the prescribing physician should be notified.

Other, uncommon side effects of oxazolindinediones can be serious or could indicate an allergic reaction. Patients who experience any of the following symptoms should contact a physician:

- purple spots on the skin
- jaundice (yellowing of the skin and eyes)
- bruising easily
- unusual bleeding
- dark urine, frequent urination, or burning sensation when urinating
- extreme mood or mental changes
- shakiness or unsteady walking
- severe unsteadiness or clumsiness
- excessive speech or language problems
- difficulty breathing
- chest pain
- faintness or loss of consciousness
- persistent, severe headaches
- persistent fever or pain

Interactions

Oxazolindinediones may have negative interactions with some antacids, heartburn or acid reflux prevention medications, anticoagulants, antihistamines, antidepressants, antibiotics, and monoamine oxidase inhibitors (MAOIs). Oxazolindinediones may be used in conjunction with other seizure prevention medications (anticonvulsants or anti-epileptic drugs) only if advised and monitored by a physician. Many anticonvulsants may decrease the effectiveness of oral contraceptives (birth control pills) or contraceptive injections or implants containing estrogen and progestins.

Resources

BOOKS

Devinsky, Orrin. *Epilepsy: Patient and Family Guide*, 2nd ed. Philadelphia: F. A. Davis, 2001.

Weaver, Donald F. *Epilepsy and Seizures: Everything You Need to Know*. Toronto: Firefly Books, 2001.

OTHER

"Trimethadione." *Medline Plus*. National Library of Medicine. May 6, 2004 (May 27, 2004). http://www.nlm.nih.gov/medlineplus/druginfo/medmaster/a601127.html.

"Trimethdione." *Yale New Haven Health Service Drug Guide*. May 6, 2004 (May 27, 2004). http://yalenewhavenhealth.org/Library/HealthGuide/DrugGuide/topic.asp?hwid = multumd00945a1.

ORGANIZATIONS

American Epilepsy Society. 342 North Main Street, West Hartford, CT 06117-2507. http://www.aesnet.org.

Epilepsy Foundation. 4351 Garden City Drive, Landover, MD 20785-7223. Tollfree phone: (800) 332-1000. http://www.epilepsyfoundation.org.

Adrienne Wilmoth Lerner

P

Pain

Definition

Pain is an unpleasant feeling that is conveyed to the brain by sensory neurons. The discomfort signals actual or potential injury to the body. However, pain is more than a sensation or the physical awareness of pain; it also includes perception, the subjective interpretation of the discomfort. Perception gives information on the pain's location, intensity, and something about its nature. The various conscious and unconscious responses to both sensation and perception, including the emotional response, add further definition to the overall concept of pain.

Description

Pain arises from any number of situations. Injury is a major cause, but pain may also arise from an illness. It may accompany a psychological condition, such as depression (psychophysiologic pain) or may even occur in the absence of a recognizable trigger.

Acute pain

Acute pain often results from tissue damage, such as a skin burn or broken bone. Acute pain can also be associated with headaches or muscle cramps. This type of pain usually goes away as the injury heals or the cause of the pain (stimulus) is removed.

To understand acute pain, it is necessary to understand the nerves that support it. Nerve cells, or neurons, perform many functions in the body. Although their general purpose, providing an interface between the brain and the body, remain constant, their capabilities vary widely. Certain types of neurons are capable of transmitting a pain signal to the brain.

As a group, these pain-sensing neurons are called nociceptors, and virtually every surface and organ of the body is wired with them. The central part of these cells is located in the spine, and they send threadlike projections to every part of the body. Nociceptors are classified according to the stimulus that prompts them to transmit a pain signal. Thermoreceptive nociceptors are stimulated by temperatures that are potentially tissue damaging. Mechanoreceptive nociceptors respond to a pressure stimulus that may cause injury. Polymodal nociceptors are the most sensitive and can respond to temperature and pressure. Polymodal nociceptors also respond to chemicals released by the cells in the area from which the pain originates.

Nerve cell endings, or receptors, are at the front end of pain sensation. A stimulus at this part of the nociceptor unleashes a cascade of neurotransmitters (chemicals that transmit information within the nervous system) in the spine. Each neurotransmitter has a purpose. For example, substance P relays the pain message to nerves leading to the spinal cord and brain. These neurotransmitters may also stimulate nerves leading back to the site of the injury. This response prompts cells in the injured area to release chemicals that not only trigger an immune response, but also influence the intensity and duration of the pain.

Chronic and abnormal pain

Chronic pain refers to pain that persists after an injury heals, cancer pain, pain related to a persistent or degenerative disease, and long-term pain from an unidentifiable cause. It is estimated that one in three people in the United States will experience chronic pain at some point in their lives. Of these people, approximately 50 million are either partially or completely disabled.

Chronic pain may be caused by the body's response to acute pain. In the presence of continued stimulation of nociceptors, changes occur within the nervous system. Changes at the molecular level are dramatic and may include alterations in genetic transcription of neurotransmitters and receptors. These changes may also occur in the absence of an identifiable cause; one of the frustrating aspects of chronic pain is that the stimulus may be unknown. Among the types of chronic pain that people live with are fibromyalgia, interstitial cystitis, and temporomandibular joint dysfunction.

Some types of pain arise from damage to the nerves themselves, known as neuropathic pain. Among such types of pain are allodynia, hyperalgesia, and phantom limb pain. Allodynia refers to a feeling of pain in response to a normally harmless stimulus. For example, some individuals who have suffered nerve damage as a result of viral infection experience unbearable pain from just the weight of their clothing. Hyperalgesia is somewhat related to allodynia in that the response to a painful stimulus is extreme. In this case, a mild pain stimulus, such as a pinprick, causes a maximum pain response. Phantom limb pain occurs after a limb is amputated; although an individual may be missing the limb, the nervous system continues to perceive pain originating from the area.

Causes and symptoms

Pain is the most common symptom of injury and disease, and the main reason people seek medical help. Descriptions can range in intensity from an milde ache to unbearable agony. Nociceptors have the ability to convey information to the brain that indicates the location, nature, and intensity of the pain. For example, stepping on a nail sends an information-packed message to the brain: The foot has experienced a puncture wound that hurts a lot.

Pain perception also varies depending on the location of the pain. The kinds of stimuli that cause a pain response on the skin include pricking, cutting, crushing, burning, and freezing. These same stimuli would not generate much of a response in the intestine. Intestinal pain arises from stimuli such as swelling, inflammation, and distension.

Diagnosis

Pain is considered in view of other symptoms and individual experiences. An observable injury, such as a broken bone, may be a clear indicator of the type of pain a person is suffering. Determining the specific cause of internal pain is more difficult. Other symptoms, such as fever or nausea, help narrow down the possibilities. In some cases, such as lower back pain, a specific cause may not be identifiable. Diagnosis of the disease causing a specific pain is further complicated by the fact that pain can be referred to (felt at) a skin site that does not seem to be connected to the site of the pain's origin. For example, pain arising from fluid

---

KEY TERMS

Acute pain—Pain in response to injury or another stimulus that resolves when the injury heals or the stimulus is removed.

Chronic pain—Pain that lasts beyond the term of an injury or painful stimulus. Can also refer to cancer pain, pain from a chronic or degenerative disease, and pain from an unidentified cause.

Neuron—A nerve cell.

Neurotransmitters—Chemicals within the nervous system that transmit information from or between nerve cells.

Nociceptor—A neuron that is capable of sensing pain.

Referred pain—Pain felt at a site different from the location of the injured or diseased part of the body. Referred pain is due to the fact that nerve signals from several areas of the body may "feed" the same nerve pathway leading to the spinal cord and brain.

Stimulus—A factor capable of eliciting a response in a nerve.

---

accumulating at the base of the lung may be referred to the shoulder.

Because pain is a subjective experience, it may be very difficult to communicate its exact quality and intensity to other people. There are no diagnostic tests that can determine the quality or intensity of an individual's pain. Therefore, a medical examination will include a lot of questions about where the pain is located, its intensity, and its nature. Questions are also directed at what kinds of things increase or relieve the pain, how long it has lasted, and whether there are any variations in it. An individual may be asked to use a pain scale to describe the pain. One such scale assigns a number to the pain intensity; for example, 0 may indicate no pain, and 10 may indicate the worst pain the person has ever experienced. Scales are modified for infants and children to accommodate their level of comprehension.

Treatment

There are many drugs aimed at preventing or treating pain. Nonopioid analgesics, narcotic analgesics, anticonvulsant drugs, and tricyclic antidepressants work by blocking the production, release, or uptake of neurotransmitters. Drugs from different classes may be combined to handle certain types of pain.

Nonopioid analgesics include common over-the-counter medications such as aspirin, acetaminophen (Tylenol), and ibuprofen (Advil). These are most often used for minor pain, but there are some prescription-strength medications in this class.

Opioid or narcotic analgesics are available only with a doctor's prescription and are used for more severe pain, such as that which results from cancer. These drugs include codeine, morphine, and methadone. Addiction to these painkillers is not as common as once thought. Many people who genuinely need these drugs for pain control typically do not become addicted, especially if they do not have a history of substance abuse. However, narcotic use is usually limited to patients thought to have a short life span (such as people with terminal cancer) or patients whose pain is only expected to last for a short time (such as people recovering from surgery).

Anticonvulsants, as well as antidepressant drugs, were initially developed to treat seizures and depression, respectively. However, these drugs also have pain-killing applications. Furthermore, since in cases of chronic or extreme pain, it is not unusual for an individual to suffer some degree of depression; antidepressants may serve a dual role. Commonly prescribed anticonvulsants for pain include gabapentin, phenytoin, carbamazepine, and clonazepam. Tricyclic antidepressants include doxepin, amitriptyline, and imipramine. Duloxetine is a mixed-mechanism reuptake inhibitor that has shown efficacy in fibromyalgia and diabetic neuropathic pain.

Intractable (unrelenting) pain may be treated by injections directly into or near the nerve that is transmitting the pain signal. These root blocks may also be useful in determining the site of pain generation. As the underlying mechanisms of abnormal pain are uncovered, other pain medications are being developed.

Drugs are not always effective in controlling pain. Surgical methods are used as a last resort if drugs and local anesthetics fail. The least destructive surgical procedure involves implanting a device that emits electrical signals. These signals disrupt the nerve and prevent it from transmitting the pain message. However, this method may not completely control pain and is not used frequently. Other surgical techniques involve destroying or severing the nerve, but the use of this technique is limited by side effects, including unpleasant numbness.

Two effective pain management treatments that have been used for generations are heat and cold. Both are used to treat acute and chronic pain. Ice is generally used to treat inflammation, especially acute

QUESTIONS FOR YOUR DOCTOR

- What is the source or cause of my pain?
- Do you understand my description of the pain?
- Should I see a specialist for the pain?
- Will medication reduce the pain?
- Are there non-medical ways of treating pain?

injuries to knees and other joints. Treatment usually lasts three to five days. Often it is used as part of the RICE regimen: rest, ice, compression, and elevation. Heat therapy is generally used for increasing tensile strength, increasing blood flow to the injured area, and helping muscles and tendons to relax. Sometimes ice is used in the early stages of an acute injury and then heat for the remainder of treatment. In recent years, scientists have identified heat and cold receptors in the body. This has allowed the development of medications, including patches, creams, and gels, that directly target these receptors, increasing the effectiveness of heat and cold treatments.

Alternative treatment

Both physical and psychological aspects of pain can be dealt with through alternative treatment. Some of the most popular treatment options include acupressure and acupuncture, massage, chiropractic, and relaxation techniques such as yoga, hypnosis, and meditation. Herbal therapies are gaining increased recognition as viable options; for example, capsaicin, the component that makes cayenne peppers spicy, is used in ointments to relieve the joint pain associated with arthritis. Contrast hydrotherapy can also be very beneficial for pain relief.

Lifestyles can be changed to incorporate a healthier diet and regular exercise. Regular exercise, aside from relieving stress, has been shown to increase endorphins, painkillers naturally produced in the body.

Prognosis

Successful pain treatment is highly dependent on successful resolution of the pain's cause. Acute pain will stop when an injury heals or when an underlying problem is treated successfully. Chronic pain and abnormal pain are more difficult to treat, and it may take longer to find a successful resolution. Some pain is intractable and will require extreme measures for relief.

Prevention

Pain is generally preventable only to the degree that the cause of the pain is preventable. For example, improved surgical procedures, such as those done through a thin tube called a laparascope, minimize post-operative pain. Anesthesia techniques for surgeries also continuously improve. Some disease and injuries are often unavoidable. However, pain from some surgeries and other medical procedures and continuing pain are preventable through drug treatments and alternative therapies.

Resources

BOOKS

Brady, Scott, and William Proctor. *Pain Free for Life: The 6-Week Cure for Chronic Pain—Without Surgery or Drugs.* Nashville, TN: Center Street, 2011.

Kassan, Stuart, et al. *Chronic Pain for Dummies.* Hoboken, NJ: For Dummies Press, 2008.

OTHER

"Pain." *Merck Manual for Health Care Professionals.* http://www.merckmanuals.com/professional/sec17/ch219/ch219a.html (accessed August 9, 2011).

ORGANIZATIONS

American Chronic Pain Association, P.O. Box 850, Rocklin, CA 95677-0850, (800) 533-3231, www.theacpa.org.

American Pain Society, 4700 W. Lake Ave., Glenview, IL 60025, (847) 375-4715, Fax: (847) 375-6479, www.ampainsoc.org.

Canadian Pain Society, 1143 Wentworth Street West, Suite 202, Oshawa, ON L1N 9K3, Canada, (905) 404-9545, Fax: (905) 404-3727, www.canadianpainsociety.ca.

Julia Barrett
Ken R. Wells
Fran Hodgkins

Pallidotomy

Definition

Pallidotomy is the destruction of a small region of the brain, the globus pallidus internus, in order to treat some of the symptoms of **Parkinson's disease**.

Purpose

The symptoms of Parkinson's disease (PD) include rigidity, slowed movements, and **tremor**, along with postural instability and a variety of non-motor symptoms (i.e., symptoms not involving movement). These symptoms are due to degeneration of a small portion of

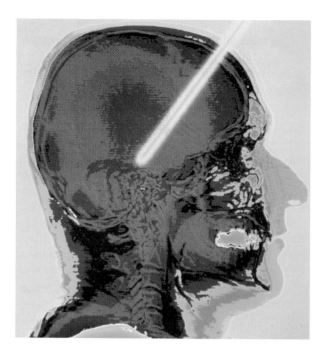

Pallidotomy is used to treat symptoms of Parkinson's disease by destroying a portion of the brain within the globus pallidus internus (GPi), which helps control voluntary movements. *(© John Greim/Photo Researchers, Inc.)*

the brain called the substantia nigra, the cells of which secrete the chemical dopamine that influences cells in another brain region called the globus pallidus internus (GPi). Together with other brain regions, these two structures take part in complex control loops that govern certain aspects of movement and, when substantia nigra cells degenerate, these loops are disrupted and movements become unregulated, producing the symptoms of Parkinson's disease.

The effects of dopamine on the brain can be mimicked by the drug levodopa; levodopa therapy is the mainstay of PD treatment in its early stages. Unfortunately, levodopa becomes less effective over time and also produces unwanted and uncontrolled movements called dyskinesias. This may occur after five to 10 years or more of successful levodopa treatment. Once a patient can no longer be treated effectively with levodopa, surgery is considered as a management option. Pallidotomy is one of the main surgical options for treatment of advanced PD.

The effect of dopamine on the cells of the GPi is to suppress them by preventing them from firing. Pallidotomy mimics this action by permanently destroying the GPi cells. It may seem odd that the treatment for degeneration of one brain area is to destroy another, but in the absence of dopamine, the GPi cells are overactive and, therefore, eliminating them is an appropriate treatment.

The GPi has two halves that control movements on opposites sides: right controls left, left controls right. Unilateral (one-sided) pallidotomy may be used if symptoms are markedly worse on one side or the other, or if the risks from bilateral (two-sided) pallidotomy are judged to be too great.

Demographics

Parkinson's disease affects approximately one million Americans. The peak incidence is approximately at age 62, but young-onset PD can occur as early as age 40. Because young-onset patients live with their disease for so many more years, they are more likely to become candidates for surgery than older-onset patients. In addition, younger patients tend to do better with surgery and suffer fewer adverse effects from the surgery. Approximately 5% of older PD patients receive one form or another of PD surgery; many more develop the symptoms for which surgery may be effective, but either develop them at an advanced age, making surgery inadvisable, or decide the risks of surgery are not worth the potential benefit, or do not choose surgery for some other reason.

Description

Pallidotomy requires the insertion of a long needle-like probe deep into the brain through a hole in the top of the skull. In order to precisely locate the GPi target and to ensure the probe is precisely placed in the target, a "stereotactic frame" is used. This device is a rigid frame attached to the patient's head, providing an immobile three-dimensional coordinate system, which can be used to precisely track the location of the GPi and the movement of the probe.

For unilateral pallidotomy, a single "burr hole" is made in the top of the skull; bilateral pallidotomy requires two holes. A strong topical anesthetic is used to numb the shaved area before this hole is drilled. Since there are no pain receptors in the brain, there is no need for deeper anesthetic. In addition, the patient must remain awake in order to report any sensory changes during the surgery. The lesion made in the GPi is very close to the optic tract that carries visual information from the eyes to the rear of the brain. Visual changes may indicate the probe is too close to this region.

Once the burr hole is made, the surgeon inserts a microelectrode probe, which is used to more precisely locate the GPi. Electrical stimulation of the brain through the electrode can help determine exactly which structure is being stimulated. This is harmless but may cause twitching, light flashes, or other sensations. A contrast dye may also be injected into the spinal fluid, which allows the surgeon to visualize the brain's structure using one or more imaging techniques. During the procedure, the patient will be asked to make various movements to assist in determining the location of the electrode.

When the proper target is located, the electrode tip is briefly heated, carefully destroying the surrounding tissue to about the size of a pearl. If bilateral pallidotomy is being performed, the localizing and lesioning will be repeated on the other side.

Diagnosis/Preparation

Pallidotomy is performed in patients with Parkinson's disease who are still responsive to levodopa but who have developed disabling drug treatment complications known as motor fluctuations, including rapid wearing off of drug effect, unpredictable "off states" (times of low levodopa levels in the blood), and disabling dyskinesias. Those who are very elderly, demented, or with other significant medical conditions that would be compromised by surgery are usually not candidates for pallidotomy.

The surgical candidate should discuss all the surgical options with the neurologist before deciding on pallidotomy. A full understanding of the risks and potential benefits must be understood before consenting to the surgery.

The patient will undergo a variety of medical tests, and one or more types of neuroimaging procedures, including magnetic resonance imaging (MRI), computed tomography (CT) scanning, **angiography** (imaging the brain's blood vessels), and ventriculography (imaging the brain's ventricles). On the day of the surgery, the stereotactic frame will be fixed to the patient's head. First, a local anesthetic is applied at the four sites where the frame's pins contact the head; there may nonetheless be some initial discomfort. A final MRI is done with the frame in place to help set the coordinates of the GPi in relation to the frame.

The patient will receive a mild sedative to ease the anxiety of the procedure.

Aftercare

The procedure requires several hours. Some centers perform pallidotomy as an outpatient procedure, sending the patient home the same day. Most centers keep the patient overnight or longer for observation. Patients will feel improved movement immediately. Medications may be adjusted somewhat to accommodate the changes in symptoms.

Risks

The key to successful outcome in pallidotomy is extremely precise placement of the electrode. While there are several controversies in the field of PD surgery, all experts agree that risks are reduced in procedures performed by the most experienced neurosurgeons.

Hemorrhage in the brain is a possible complication, as is infection. There are small but significant risks of damage to the optic tract, which can cause visual deficits. Speech impairments may also occur, including difficulty retrieving words and slurred speech. Some cognitively fragile patients may become even more impaired after surgery.

Normal results

Pallidotomy improves the motor ability of patients, especially during "off" periods. Studies show the procedure generally improves tremor, rigidity, and slowed movements by 25–60%. Dyskinesias typically improve by 75% or more. Improvements from unilateral pallidotomy are primarily on the side opposite the surgery. Balance does not improve nor do non-motor symptoms such as drooling, constipation, and **orthostatic hypotension** (lightheadedness on standing).

Morbidity and mortality rates

Among the best surgeons, the risk of serious morbidity or mortality is 1–2%. Hemorrhage may occur in 2–6%, visual field deficits in 0–6%, and **weakness** in 2–8%. Most patients gain weight after surgery.

Alternatives

Patients whose symptoms are well managed by drugs are not recommended for surgery, and significant effort will usually be made to adjust medications to control symptoms before surgery is considered.

Thalamotomy, surgery to the thalamus, was recommended in the past to control tremor. It is rarely performed today, and few centers would consider thalamotomy for any patient unless tremor was the only troubling and uncontrolled symptom.

Deep-brain stimulation (DBS) of the GPi is an alternative treatment in widespread use, as is DBS of another brain region, the subthalamic nucleus. Both procedures use permanemtly implanted, programmable electrodes to deliver a very small, continuous electric current to the target region. This has the same effect as a lesion, but is adjustable. DBS of the subthalamic nucleus typically produces better symtomatic

---

WHO PERFORMS THE PROCEDURE AND WHERE IS IT PERFORMED?

Pallidotomy is performed in the hospital by a neurosurgeon, in coordination with the patient's neurologist.

QUESTIONS TO ASK THE DOCTOR

- How many pallidotomies has the neurosurgeon performed?
- What is the surgeon's own rate of serious complications?
- Would deep brain stimulation of the subthalamic nucleus be appropriate for me?
- How will my medications change after the operation?

---

results that either DBS to the GPi or pallidotomy. However, both forms of DBS carry the risk of long-term complications from the implanted hardware, as well as other risks.

Resources

BOOKS

Goetz, C.G. *Goetz's Textbook of Clinical Neurology*, 3rd ed. Philadelphia: Saunders, 2007.

ORGANIZATIONS

National Parkinson's Disease Foundation. http://www.npf.org. WE MOVE. http://www.wemove.org.

Richard Robinson

PANDAS

Definition

PANDAS is the acronym for pediatric autoimmune neuropsychiatric disorders associated with streptococcal (strep) infections. PANDAS are rare childhood conditions characterized by the sudden development of obsessive-compulsive disorder (OCD) and/or **tics**, following a bacterial infection with group A beta-hemolytic *Streptococcus* (GAS or GABHS), such as a strep throat.

Description

Autoimmune disorders, such as PANDAS, develop when the body's immune system mistakenly responds to normal body constituents, or "self," as if they were foreign, or "non-self." When *Streptococcus* causes strep throat or, less commonly, scarlet fever or the skin disorder impetigo, antibodies are produced as part of the immune response. These antibodies specifically recognize and help eliminate the strep bacteria. PANDAS apparently develop when these same antibodies cross-react with normal proteins in the human brain.

It has been known since the 1950s that streptococcal infections can precipitate autoimmune disorders. The best-known example is rheumatic fever in children and young adults, in which antibodies produced to fight a strep infection mistakenly recognize and target the heart valves, joints, and/or parts of the brain. This is a result of molecular mimcry, in which proteins in the heart valves and other affected tissues are somehow similar to the proteins in the bacterial cell wall that are targeted by the antibodies. The antibodies trigger an immune response that damages these normal tissues, potentially causing heart disease, arthritis, and/or a brain disorder called Sydenham **chorea** (SD), characterized by abnormal movements.

In 1998, Susan E. Swedo and colleagues proposed that some cases of OCD in children might be a post-strep autoimmune reaction, similar to SD, for which they coined the acronym PANDAS. OCD is a neuropsychiatric condition characterized by obsessions and/or compulsions that monopolize thoughts and behaviors and cause anxiety and fear. PANDAS are also believed to involve tics or muscle spasms, especially in the face. PANDAS have been further implicated in a sudden worsening of symptoms in children with preexisting OCD or tic disorders, such as Tourette syndrome. Therefore, PANDAS are now sometimes classified as a subtype of OCD. Some researchers and physicians go further and attribute some cases of abrupt-onset attention-deficit/hyperactivity disorder (**ADHD**) and **autism** to PANDAS. Recurrent SD also has been associated with subsequent development of abrupt-onset OCD, tic disorders, ADHD, and autism.

Nevertheless, PANDAS remain a controversial diagnosis. Some researchers and physicians question whether there is any relationship between GAS and neuropsychiatric symptoms.

Demographics

By definition, PANDAS occur only in prepubescent children. They are thought to be relatively rare. Although most school-age children have strep throat at some point, very few develop subsequent neuropsychiatric disorders. Furthermore, although one in 100 teenagers suffer from OCD and one in 200 have tic disorders such as Tourette, very few of these cases can be attributed to PANDAS. Nevertheless, a small but increasing number of children are diagnosed with PANDAS, sometimes without having had a diagnosed strep infection.

Causes and symptoms

It is postulated that antibodies produced by the immune system in response to a cell wall protein of GABHS bacteria subsequently interact with proteins in the brain to cause PANDAS. The basal ganglia of the brain, which are involved in movement and behavior, are the suspected target of PANDAS. The basal ganglia, especially the caudate nucleus—one of the four basal ganglia in each hemisphere of the brain—are affected in SD as well. Children affected by PANDAS may have a genetic susceptibility to post-streptococcal autoimmune disorders.

The most common symptom of PANDAS is the abrupt and dramatic onset of OCD and/or tics in the weeks following a GABHS infection. In children with preexisting OCD or tic disorders, PANDAS may cause sudden worsening of symptoms. Typical symptoms of OCD include obsessive and irrational cleanliness, fears of contamination, and guilt feelings. OCD may involve extensive washing rituals, avoidance of people or situations, or strange movements. Tics may be motor or vocal. Whereas children with OCD or tic disorders from other causes often have symptoms that fluctuate in their severity over days or weeks, children with PANDAS tend to have episodes of severe symptoms. These severe symptoms may be associated with subtle abnormal movements that are similar to those of SD.

OCD and/or tics caused by PANDAS are often accompanied by other neurological or behavioral symptoms:

• ADHD symptoms, such as hyperactivity, inattention, or fidgetiness

• separation anxiety

• emotional changes, such as moodiness, irritability, or sadness

• sleep disturbances

• bedwetting or frequent daytime urination

• fine or gross motor changes, such as a deterioration of handwriting

• joint pain

KEY TERMS

Antibody—An immune system protein that recognizes and binds to a specific foreign protein.

Attention-deficit/hyperactivity disorder (ADHD)—Conditions characterized by age-inappropriate attention span, hyperactivity, and impulsive behavior.

Autism—A variable developmental disorder that includes an impaired ability to communicate and form normal social relationships.

Autoimmune disorders—Disorders caused when the immune system's antibodies or T cells attack the body's own molecules, cells, or tissues.

Basal ganglia—The four deeply imbedded masses of gray matter in each cerebral hemisphere, including the caudate nucleus and the amygdala.

Choreiform—Movements resembling chorea; spasmodic movements of the limb or facial muscles.

Cognitive-behavioral therapy (CBT)—A type of psychotherapy that involves recognizing and changing negative and self-defeating patterns of thinking and behavior.

Group A beta-hemolytic *Streptococcus* (GAS, GABHS)—Bacteria commonly found in the throat and on the skin, which most often cause no symptoms or a mild illness such as strep throat.

Intravenous immunoglobulins (IVIG)—Treatment with pooled antibodies from donor sera to treat autoimmune disorders or immune system deficiencies.

Neuropsychiatric disorder—A disorder with both neurological and psychiatric components.

Obsessive-compulsive disorder (OCD)—A psychoneurotic disorder characterized by obsessions and/or compulsions and anxiety or depression.

Selective serotonin reuptake inhibitor (SSRI)—A type of antidepressant, such as fluoxetine, that inhibits the inactivation of the neurotransmitter serotonin by blocking its reuptake by neurons.

Strep infection—An infection, such as strep throat, caused by the bacteria known as group A *Streptococcus*.

Sydenham chorea (SD)—Saint Vitus dance; an autoimmune neurological disorder of childhood resulting from a group A *Streptococcus* infection and characterized by abnormal involuntary movements.

Tic—Muscle spasms, especially of the face, or habitual unconscious quirks of behavior or speech.

Titer—The concentration of a specific antibody in blood serum.

Tourette syndrome—An inherited neuropsychiatric disorder characterized by involuntary muscle or vocal tics.

Diagnosis

Diagnosis of PANDAS remains poorly defined and controversial. Generally, two or three episodes of OCD or tics in association with a strep infection may suggest PANDAS. The clinical criteria for PANDAS diagnosis are:

- a child aged three years to puberty

- presence of OCD and/or a tic disorder

- sudden onset of severe symptoms, followed by alternating remission and episodes of severe symptoms

- a positive throat culture for strep, a history of scarlet fever, or an association between a strep infection and sudden onset or sudden worsening of OCD or tic symptoms

- association with other neurological movement abnormalities, such as hyperactivity, clumsiness, or choreiform (chorea-like) movements

Most clinics use rapid screens to diagnose strep infections; however, these screens can produce false negatives, so a full-plate strep culture may be required. Antibody titers—levels of specific antibodies—can be used to detect a recent, undiagnosed strep infection. The antistrepolysin O (ASO) titer rises 2–6 weeks after a strep infection and may remain elevated for 6–12 months. The antistreptococcal DNAase B titer rises 6–8 weeks after a strep infection, but the levels and persistence of anti-strep antibodies vary greatly among children and different laboratories have use normal values.

Treatment

Although PANDAS are sometimes treated with antibiotics, in general, antibiotics are recommended only if a rapid screen or throat culture is positive for strep. Otherwise PANDAS treatments are the same as for other types of OCD or tic disorders. OCD is usually treated with cognitive-behavioral therapy

QUESTIONS TO ASK YOUR DOCTOR

- Could my child's symptoms be caused by PANDAS?
- How will you test my child for a current or previous strep infection?
- Should my child be treated with antibiotics?
- What treatment do you recommend for my child's PANDAS symptoms?
- Will my child grow out of the PANDAS symptoms?

(CBT) and/or anti-obsessional medications. A selective serotonin reuptake inhibitor (SSRI), such as fluoxetine, in combination with CBT, appears to be the most effective treatment for OCD. Research indicates that either treatment alone is better than no treatment or a placebo. Mild or transient tics may not require treatment. Tics are sometimes treated with low dosages of stimulants used to treat ADHD or with a type of behavioral therapy called comprehensive behavioral intervention for tics (CBIT), previously called habit reversal therapy.

PANDAS have sometimes been treated with intravenous immunoglobulins (IVIG) or plasmapheresis or plasma exchange to inactivate the immune response; however, these treatments are not usually recommended except in the most severe cases because they are invasive procedures with associated risks and side effects.

Clinical trials

A phase III clinical trial was initiated by the U.S. National Institute of Mental Health in January 2011, to examine whether IVIG is an appropriate treatment for OCD and other PANDAS symptoms. The estimated completion date for the study is January 2016. Information about clinical trials can be found at ClinicalTrials.gov.

Prognosis

Antibiotic treatment that eradicates a strep infection usually resolves PANDAS symptoms. Otherwise, standard treatments for OCD and tic disorders are generally effective. In children with preexisting OCD, tic disorders, or ADHD, the increased symptom severity associated with PANDAS usually lasts for weeks to months before improving. Subsequent strep infections usually cause the abrupt return or worsening of symptoms.

Special concerns

Anecdotal evidence has sometimes extended PANDAS to include a variety of neuropsychiatric childhood disorders, despite a lack of scientific evidence. Some experts caution that overdiagnosis of PANDAS may contribute to the overuse of antibiotics, which has encouraged the spread of antibiotic-resistant bacteria. Although antibiotic treatment of confirmed strep infections can potentially prevent PANDAS, the use of antibiotics to prevent PANDAS in the absence of a confirmed strep infection is probably unwarranted.

Resources

BOOKS

Maloney, Beth Alison. *Saving Sammy: Curing the Boy Who Caught OCD*. New York: Crown, 2009.

WEBSITES

Brasic, James Robert. "Pediatric Obsessive-Compulsive Disorder." Medscape Reference. http://emedicine. medscape.com/article/1826591-overview (accessed July 18, 2011).

Celenia, Luz. "Personal Stories: Warrior Mom." International OCD Foundation. http://www.ocfoundation. org/ocdinkids/ocd_in_kids_parents.aspx?id = 1948&-terms = pandas (accessed July 18, 2011).

"A PANDAS Study is Currently Recruiting Patients." NIMH Pediatrics & Developmental Neuroscience Branch. http://intramural.nimh.nih.gov/pdn/web.htm (accessed July 18, 2011).

ORGANIZATIONS

American Academy of Neurology (AAN), 1080 Montreal Avenue, Saint Paul, MN 55116, (651) 695-2717, (800) 879-1960, Fax: (651) 695-2791, memberservices@aan. com, http://www.aan.com.

International OCD Foundation, P.O. Box 961029, Boston, MA 02196, (617) 973-5801, Fax: (617) 973-5803, info@ocfoundation.org, http://www.oc foundation.org.

National Institute of Mental Health (NIMH), 6001 Executive Boulevard, Room 8184, MSC 9663, Bethesda, MD 20892-9663, (301) 443-4513, (866) 615-6464, Fax: (301) 443-4279, nimhinfo@nih.gov, http://www.nimh.nih.gov/index.shtml.

Margaret Alic, PhD

Pantothenate kinase-associated neurodegeneration

Definition

Pantothenate kinase-associated neurodegeneration (PKAN), long known as Hallervorden-Spatz syndrome (HSS), is a very rare childhood neurodegenerative disorder that is associated with the accumulation of iron in the brain, which causes progressively worsening abnormal movements and **dementia**.

Description

In addition to its original name, Hallervorden-Spatz syndrome, pantothenate kinase-associated neurodegeneration has been called neurodegeneration with brain iron accumulation (NBIA). The name Hallervorden-Spatz is rapidly being discontinued by those who study and treat the disease, both because the new names indicate the nature of the underlying disorder and because Julius Hallervorden, who described the syndrome, was involved in a "selective euthanasia" program in Nazi Germany to kill intellectually disabled children.

Demographics

PKAN is so rare that there is no reliable information on its prevalence. It affects boys and girls equally. Typical age of onset is in middle childhood to early adolescence, although onset in early adulthood may occur.

Causes and symptoms

PKAN occurs due to mutation in the gene for pantothenate kinase 2 (PANK2), which is an enzyme, a type of protein that regulates a reaction inside a cell. PANK2 helps regulates the production of coenzyme A, an important intermediate in the production of energy within all cells. Mutations in the gene for PANK2 lead to loss of function of this enzyme, the consequence of which is accumulation of iron and the amino acid cysteine within brain cells. It is not yet known how this leads to the disease, but it is possible that cysteine interacts with iron, leading to buildup of other molecules within brain cells that puts stress on the cells and causes them to degenerate.

PKAN causes dystonia, a sustained posturing of lower limbs due to excessive muscle contraction. Leg dystonia leads to gait difficulties and other limitations of movement. Dystonia may also affect the upper limbs and the muscles of the face and neck. Abnormal movements may also include writhing or **tremor**. Ability to walk is usually lost within 15 years. **Dysarthria**, or impairment of the ability to speak, is common and is usually accompanied by swallowing difficulty. PKAN also causes progressive dementia, or impairment of normal intellectual function, although this is more variable among patients. PKAN may also cause a degenerative eye condition, retinitis pigmentosa.

An atypical form of PKAN has similar features, but with later age of onset and more variable and less severe symptoms. Speech difficulties tend to be more common in atypical patients. Atypical patients may or may not have a recognizable gene defect.

Diagnosis

Diagnosis of PKAN begins with a neurological exam, which is followed up by a magnetic resonance imaging (MRI) scan to reveal a characteristic signal from the affected portions of the brain. Genetic testing may be done to look for the mutation in the PKAN gene.

Treatment team

Treatment involves a pediatric neurologist, a speech-language pathologist, and physical and occupational therapists.

Treatment

There is no treatment that can halt or slow the degeneration of the brain that occurs in PKAN. The discovery of the gene defect may lead to a better understanding of the neurodegenerative process and thereby to better treatments.

Drug therapy for the movement disorders of PKAN is variably successful and becomes less so with time. Drugs used for **Parkinson's disease** such as levodopa may be beneficial in some patients. Trihexyphenidyl may be useful. Oral antispasticity medications, including **diazepam** and dantrolene, can help reduce muscle stiffness and **spasticity**. Intrathecal baclofen has been successful in several patients. A **pallidotomy**, a type of brain surgery that destroys part of the globus pallidus internus, a structure in the brain that regulates movements, has shown some success at relieving painful dystonia and returning some function to the affected limbs.

Speech impairment may be the most severe consequence of PKAN. Assistive communication devices such as computers or letter boards offer

KEY TERMS

Dystonia—Painful involuntary muscle cramps or spasms.

Enzyme—A protein that catalyzes a biochemical reaction without changing its own structure or function.

Neurodegeneration—The deterioration of nerve tissues.

the possibility of continued communication even as the disease progresses.

Clinical trials

PKAN is so rare there are few clinical trials. Some effort is underway to determine whether supplements with PANK2's normal products or related molecules may be effective.

Prognosis

The average duration of disease is 11 years. Death is usually caused by aspiration pneumonia, brought on by food inhaled into the airways.

Resources

BOOKS

The Official Patient's Sourcebook on Hallervorden-Spatz Disease: A Revised and Updated Directory for the Internet Age. San Diego: Icon Health, 2002.

WEBSITES

NBIA Disorders Association. http://www.hssa.org (April 27, 2004).

Richard Robinson

Papilledema *see* **Visual disturbances**

Paramyotonia congenita

Definition

Paramyotonia congenita is an inherited condition that causes stiffness and enlargement of muscles, particularly leg muscles.

Description

Paramyotonia congenita is passed on in families as an autosomal dominant trait. This means that males and females are affected equally; it also means that if one parent has the trait, the offspring have a 75% chance of also having the condition.

Demographics

Paramyotonia congenita is present from birth on. In some cases, the symptoms appear to grow more mild as the patient ages.

Causes and symptoms

Paramyotonia congenita is believed to be caused by a defect in the chloride channels of the muscles. As a result, the relaxation phase of the muscles is impaired, resulting in prolonged muscle contraction and stiffness. This "overuse" of the muscle results in the muscle becoming enlarged and bulky (muscle hypertrophy).

Symptoms of paramyotonia congenita include stiffness and enlargement of various muscle groups, particularly those in the legs. The muscle stiffness of paramyotonia congenita is often exacerbated by cold temperatures and inactivity and relieved by warmth and exercise.

Diagnosis

Electromyographic (EMG) testing involves placing a needle electrode into a muscle and measuring its electrical activity. EMG testing in paramyotonia congenita may reveal differences between electrical activity in a warm muscle and electrical activity in a cooled muscle. There are a number of genetic defects that are associated with the chloride channel defect of paramyotonia congenita, some of which can be revealed through genetic testing.

Treatment team

Paramyotonia congenita is diagnosed and treated by neurologists.

Treatment

Paramyotonia congenita is usually mild enough not to require any treatment at all. If muscle stiffness is truly problematic, quinine or anticonvulsant medications (such as phenytoin) may improve functioning.

Prognosis

Paramyotonia congenita has an excellent prognosis. Although annoying, it does not cause significant disability, and the patient usually learns to make lifestyle adjustments that prevent exacerbations (for example, dressing warmly and avoiding exposure to cold).

Resources

BOOKS

Brown, Robert H., and Jerry R. Mendell. "Muscular Dystrophies and Other Muscle Diseases." In *Harrison's Principles of Internal Medicine*, edited by Eugene Braunwald, et al. New York: McGraw-Hill Professional, 2001.

Rose, Michael, and Robert C. Griggs. "Hereditary Nondegenerative Neuromuscular Disease." In *Textbook of Clinical Neurology*, edited by Christopher G. Goetz. Philadelphia: W. B. Saunders, 2003.

WEBSITES

National Institute of Neurological Disorders and Stroke (NINDS). *NINDS Myotonia Congenita Information Page.* November 8, 2001. http://www.ninds.nih.gov/health_and_medical/disorders/myotoniacongenita.htm (June 3, 2004).

Rosalyn Carson-DeWitt, MD

Paraneoplastic syndromes

Description

Paraneoplastic syndromes are rare disorders caused by substances that are secreted by a benign tumor, a malignant (cancerous) tumor, or a malignant tumor's metastases. These syndromes are believed to be caused when cancer-fighting cells mistakenly attack normal, noncancerous nervous system cells.

The disturbances caused by paraneoplastic syndromes occur in body organs at sites that are distant or remote from the primary or metastatic tumors. Body systems that may be affected by paraneoplastic syndromes include neurological, endocrine, cutaneous, renal, hematologic, gastrointestinal, and other systems. The most common manifestations of paraneoplastic syndromes are cutaneous, neurologic, and endocrine disorders. An example of a cutaneous paraneoplastic disorder are telangiectasias, which can be caused by breast cancer and lymphomas. Lambert-Eaton myasthenic syndrome (LEMS, and also known as Eaton-Lambert syndrome) is a neurologic paraneoplastic syndrome that can be caused by a variety of tumors, including small cell lung cancer, lymphoma, breast, colon and other cancers. Syndrome of inappropriate antidiuretic hormone (SIADH) is an endocrine paraneoplastic syndrome, which is seen in as many as 40% of patients diagnosed with small cell lung cancer.

Approximately 15% of patients already have a paraneoplastic disorder at the time of initial diagnosis with cancer. As many as 50% of all cancer patients develop a paraneoplastic syndrome at some time during the course of their disease. Some clinicians categorize the anorexia, cachexia, and fever that occur as a result of cancer as metabolic paraneoplastic syndromes. Virtually all patients diagnosed with cancer are affected by at least one of these metabolic paraneoplastic syndromes.

Paraneoplastic syndromes can occur with any type of malignancy; however, they occur most frequently with lung cancer, specifically small-cell lung carcinoma. Other types of cancer that commonly cause paraneoplastic syndromes are breast cancer and stomach cancer. With the exception of Wilms' tumor and neuroblastoma, paraneoplastic syndromes do not usually occur in children diagnosed with cancer.

In general, paraneoplastic syndromes may be present in the patient before a diagnosis of cancer is made, or, as stated earlier, may be present at the time the patient is first diagnosed with cancer. Most paraneoplastic syndromes appear in the later stages of the disease. Frequently, the presence of a paraneoplastic syndrome is associated with a poor prognosis. Paraneoplastic syndromes are difficult to diagnose and are often misdiagnosed. Some paraneoplastic syndromes may be confused with metatastic disease or spread of the cancer. The presence of the syndrome may be the only indication that a patient has a malignancy or that a malignancy has recurred. Paraneoplastic syndromes may be useful as clinical indicators to evaluate the response of the primary cancer to the treatment. Resolution of the paraneoplastic syndrome can be correlated with tumor response to treatment. That is, if the paraneoplastic syndrome resolves, the tumor has usually responded to the treatment.

Causes

Paraneoplastic syndromes occur when the primary or original tumor secretes substances such as hormones, proteins, growth factors, cytokines, and antibodies. The substances are referred to as mediators. These mediators have effects at remote or

KEY TERMS

Anorexia—Loss of appetite.

Cachexia—Severe malnutrition, emaciation, muscle wasting, and debility associated with the inability to absorb the nutritional value of food eaten.

Cutaneous disorders—Disorders affecting the skin.

Hypokalemia—Decreased levels of the electrolyte potassium in the blood.

Hyponatremia—Decreased levels of the electrolyte sodium in the blood.

Metastasis—Tumors which originate from the primary or original tumor at distant locations in the body; secondary tumors.

Neurologic disorders—Disorders affecting the nervous system.

distant body organs, which are termed target organs. Mediators interfere with communication between cells in the body. This miscommunication results in abnormal or increased activity of the cell's normal function.

Treatment

There are usually two approaches taken in the treatment of paraneoplastic syndromes. The first step is treatment of the cancer that is causing the syndrome. This treatment can be surgery, administration of chemotherapy, biotherapy, radiation therapy, or a combination of these therapies. The next approach is to suppress the substance or mediator causing the paraneoplastic syndrome. Often treatment targeted to the underlying cancer and to the paraneoplastic syndrome occur at the same time; however, even with treatment, irreversible damage to the target organ can occur.

Selected Paraneoplastic Syndromes

LAMBERT-EATON MYASTHENIC SYNDROME. Lambert-Eaton myasthenic syndrome (LEMS or Eaton-Lambert syndrome) has been associated with a number of cancers, including small-cell lung cancer: more than half of the people who are diagnosed with LEMS develop small cell lung cancer. Potential mediators associated with paraneoplastic LEMS are antibodies that interfere with release of acetylcholine at the neuromuscular junction. This interference prevents the flow of calcium, which results in decreased or absent impulse transmission to muscle. The disruption in muscular impulse transmission leads to mild symptoms, including weakness in the legs and thighs, muscle aches, muscle stiffness, and muscle fatigue. Treatment of LEMS includes administration of corticosteroids, intravenous immunoglobulin, and plasmapheresis. For patients with cancer, treatment of the cancer comes first.

MYASTHENIA GRAVIS. Myasthenia gravis is the most common paraneoplastic syndrome found in patients who have a malignancy of the epithelial cells of the thymus (thymoma). MG is characterized by weakness of the skeletal muscles and fatigue. Thymoma is the underlying cause in 10–15% of myasthenia gravis cases. The antibodies attack the acetycholine receptors at the neuromuscular junctions of the skeletal muscles.

Systemic lupus erythematosis (SEL) may be found in patients who have lung cancer, breast cancer, ovarian or testicular cancer, or lymphoma. This disorder involves many immune disturbances. Treatment of SEL depends on the manifestations of the disorder, which can include musculoskeltal problems, fever, and cutaneous manifestations.

Resources

WEBSITES

"NINDS Paraneoplastic Syndromes Information Page." National Institute of Neurological Disorders and Stroke. http://www.ninds.nih.gov/disorders/paraneoplastic/paraneoplastic.htm (accessed August 27, 2011).

Santacroce, Luigi. "Paraneoplastic Syndromes Clinical Presentation." http://http://emedicine.medscape.com/article/280744-clinical (accessed August 27, 2011).

ORGANIZATIONS

American Autoimmune Related Diseases Association, 22100 Gratiot Avenue, Detroit, MI 48021-2227, (586) 776-3900, (800) 598-4668, Fax: (586) 776-3903, http://www.aarda.org.

American Cancer Society, 250 Williams Street, NW, Atlanta, GA 30303-1002, (800) 227-2345, www.cancer.org.

National Cancer Institute, 6116 Executive Boulevard, Suite 300, Bethesda, MD 20892-8322, (800) 422-6237, http://www.cancer.gov.

Melinda Granger Oberleitner, RN, DNS
Fran Hodgkins

Parkinson's disease

Definition

Parkinson's disease (PD) is a progressive degenerative brain disorder marked by tremors, rigidity, slow movements (bradykinesia), and posture instability. It occurs when cells in one of the movement-control centers of the brain begin to die for unknown reasons. PD was first described by British physician James Parkinson in the early 1817.

Demographics

About 1% of people over age 60 develop PD with an approximate prevalence of 120 cases per 100,000 population. The likelihood of developing PD increases with age, with an estimated 15% of those ages 65–74, and almost 30% of those ages 75–84 showing symptoms. Because PD is difficult to diagnose accurately, these numbers are only estimates. PD is about 1.5 times more common in men than in women. Average age of onset is 60 years; the disease is uncommon in people under age 40.

Description

Usually starting in a person's late fifties or early sixties, Parkinson's disease causes a progressive decline in movement control, affecting the ability to control initiation, speed, and smoothness of motion. Many cases of PD are the result of sporadic mutations. This means that there is a spontaneous and permanent change in nucleotide sequences (the building blocks of genes). Sporadic mutations also involve unknown environmental factors in combination with genetic defects. The abnormal gene (mutated gene) will form an altered end product or protein. This causes abnormalities in specific areas in the body where the protein is used. Some evidence suggests that there is also a genetic component that predisposes some people to develop the disease when exposed to certain (as yet undiscovered) environmental factors. Recent research (as of 2011) has linked PD with a gene that codes for a protein called alpha-synuclein. Researchers believe that a mutation in this gene results in abnormal folding of the alpha-synuclein protein. In itself, this is not the sole cause of PD. Further research is attempting to fully understand the relationship between the

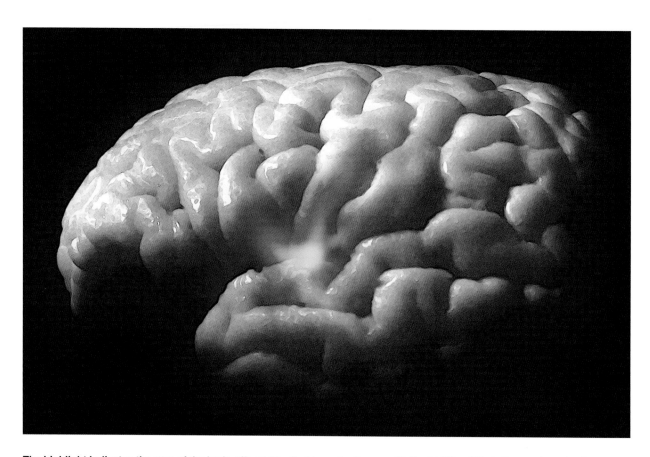

The highlight indicates the area of the brain affected by Parkinson's disease. *(© David Gifford/Photo Researchers, Inc.)*

build-up of this protein in Lewy bodies and nerve cell degeneration.

Risk factors

Age is the greatest risk factor for developing PD. Gender also is a risk factor, as men are more likely to be diagnosed with the disease. Family history can increase risk; people with a first-degree relative (parent, sibling, child) with PD have double the chance of developing the disease compared to people without PD in the immediate family.

Environmental factors that are suspected of increasing the chance of developing PD include exposure to pesticides and herbicides, living in a rural area or adjacent to an industrial plant or quarry, or drinking well water.

Smoking tobacco has consistently been shown to protect against the development of PD, as has caffeine consumption; however, other health risks of smoking far outweigh the potential protective effect.

Causes and symptoms

The immediate cause of PD is degeneration of brain cells in the area known as the substantia nigra, one of the movement control centers of the brain. Damage to this area leads to the cluster of symptoms known as parkinsonism. In PD, degenerating brain cells contain Lewy bodies, which are not found in healthy brain cells and which help to identify the disease. The cell death leading to parkinsonism may be caused by a number of conditions besides PD, including infection, trauma, and poisoning. Some drugs given for psychosis, such as haloperidol (Haldol) or chlorpromazine (Thorazine, Largactil), may cause parkinsonism. When no cause for nigral cell degeneration can be found, the disorder is called idiopathic parkinsonism, or Parkinson's disease. Parkinsonism may be seen in other degenerative conditions, known as the "parkinsonism plus" syndromes, such as **progressive supranuclear palsy**.

The substantia nigra, or "black substance," is one of the principal movement control centers in the brain. By releasing the neurotransmitter dopamine, it helps to refine movement patterns throughout the body. The dopamine released by nerve cells of substantia nigra stimulates another brain region, the corpus striatum. Without enough dopamine, the corpus striatum cannot control its target cells, and so on down the line. Ultimately, the neural patterns needed to control of walking, writing, reaching for objects, and other basic activities cannot be completed properly, and the symptoms of parkinsonism are the result.

Some known toxins can cause parkinsonism, most notoriously a chemical called MPTP, found as an impurity in some illegal drugs. Parkinsonian symptoms appear within hours of ingestion and are permanent. MPTP may exert its effects through generation of toxic molecular fragments called free radicals, and reducing free radicals has been a target of several experimental treatments for PD using antioxidants.

It is possible that early exposure to some as-yet-unidentified environmental toxin or virus leads to undetected nigral cell death, and PD then manifests as normal age-related decline, bringing the number of functioning nigral cells below the threshold needed for normal movement. It is also possible that, for genetic reasons, some people are simply born with fewer cells in their substantia nigra than others, and they develop PD as a consequence of normal decline.

Symptoms

The identifying symptoms of PD include:

- tremors, usually beginning in the hands, often occurring on one side before the other. The classic tremor of PD is called a "pill-rolling tremor," because the movement resembles rolling a pill between the thumb and forefinger. This tremor occurs at a frequency of about three per second.
- slow movements (bradykinesia), which may involve slowing down or stopping in the middle of familiar tasks such as walking, eating, or shaving. This may include freezing in place during movements (akinesia).
- muscle rigidity or stiffness, occurring with jerky movements replacing smooth motion.
- postural instability or balance difficulty occurs. This may lead to a rapid, shuffling gait (festination) to prevent falling.
- loss of facial expressions. In most cases, there is a "masked face," with little facial expression and decreased eye-blinking.

In addition, a wide range of other symptoms may often be seen, some beginning earlier than others:

- depression (reported in about half of all individuals with PD)
- speech changes, including rapid speech without inflection changes
- problems with sleep, including restlessness and nightmares
- emotional changes, including fear, irritability, and insecurity
- incontinence
- constipation

- handwriting changes, with letters becoming smaller across the page (micrographia)
- progressive problems with intellectual function (dementia)

Diagnosis

The diagnosis of Parkinson's disease can be difficult, It involves a careful medical history and a neurological exam to look for characteristic symptoms. There are no definitive tests for PD, although a variety of lab tests may be done to rule out other causes of symptoms, especially if only some of the identifying symptoms of PD are present. Tests for other causes of parkinsonism may include brain scans, blood tests, **lumbar puncture**, and x rays.

Treatment

There is no cure for Parkinson's disease. Treatment can be complicated and is based on the individual's age, level of impairment, cognitive function, and response to treatment.

Exercise, nutrition, and physical therapy

Regular, moderate exercise has been shown to improve motor function without an increase in medication for a person with PD. Exercise helps maintain range of motion in stiff muscles, improve circulation, and stimulate appetite. An exercise program designed by a physical therapist has the best chance of meeting the specific needs of the person with PD. A physical therapist may also suggest strategies for balance compensation and techniques to stimulate movement during slowdowns or freezes.

Good nutrition is important to maintenance of general health. A person with PD may lose some interest in food, especially if depressed, and may have nausea from the disease or from medications, especially those known as dopamine agonists. Slow movements may make it difficult to eat quickly, and delayed gastric emptying may lead to a feeling of fullness without having eaten much. Increasing fiber in the diet can improve constipation, soft foods can reduce the amount of needed chewing, and a prokinetic drug can increase the movement of food through the digestive system.

People with PD may need to limit the amount of protein in their diets. The main drug used to treat PD, levodopa (L-dopa), is an amino acid, and is absorbed by the digestive system by the same transporters that pick up other amino acids broken down from proteins in the diet. Limiting protein, under the direction of the physician or a nutritionist, can improve the absorption of levodopa.

KEY TERMS

AADC inhibitors—Drugs that block the amino acid decarboxylase; one type of enzyme that breaks down dopamine. Also called DC inhibitors, they include carbidopa and benserazide.

Akinesia—A loss of the ability to move; freezing in place.

Antioxidant—A molecule that prevents oxidation. In the body antioxidants attach to other molecules called free radicals and prevent the free radicals from causing damage to cell walls, DNA, and other parts of the cell.

Blood-brain barrier—An arrangement of cells within the blood vessels of the brain that prevents the passage of toxic substances, including infectious agents, from the blood and into the brain. It also makes it difficult for certain medications to pass into brain tissue.

Bradykinesia—Extremely slow movement.

COMT inhibitors—Drugs that block catechol-o-methyl transferase, an enzyme that breaks down dopamine. COMT inhibitors include entacapone and tolcapone.

Dopamine—A neurochemical made in the brain that is involved in many brain activities, including movement and emotion.

Dyskinesia—Impaired ability to make voluntary movements.

Free radical—A molecule with an unpaired electron that has a strong tendency to react with other molecules in DNA (genetic material), proteins, and lipids (fats), resulting in damage to cells. Free radicals are neutralized by antioxidants.

Idiopathic—Of unknown origin; without a known cause.

MAO-B inhibitors—Inhibitors of the enzyme monoamine oxidase B. MAO-B helps break down dopamine; inhibiting it prolongs the action of dopamine in the brain. Selegiline is an MAO-B inhibitor.

Orthostatic hypotension—A sudden decrease in blood pressure upon sitting up or standing. May be a side effect of several types of drugs.

Substantia nigra—One of the movement control centers of the brain.

No evidence indicates that vitamin or mineral supplements can have any effect on the disease other than in the improvement of the patient's general health. No antioxidants used to date have shown promise as a treatment except for selegiline, an MAO-B inhibitor that is discussed below. A large, carefully controlled study of vitamin E demonstrated that it could not halt disease progression; however, in a preliminary study, the antioxidant co-enzyme Q10 appeared to slow the progression of PD. As of 2011, co-enzyme Q10 remained under investigation with at least half a dozen clinical trials in progress.

Drugs

The pharmacological treatment of Parkinson's disease is complex. While there are a large number of drugs that can be effective, their effectiveness varies with the patient, disease progression, and the length of time the drug has been used. Dose-related side effects may preclude using the most effective dose, or require the introduction of a new drug to counteract them. Response to drug therapy is monitored and drugs may be adjusted in an attempt to find a treatment regimen that provides the most benefits with the fewest side effects. Research is ongoing in an effort to find drugs to treat PD. Individuals should consult their doctor about advances in drug therapy and clinical trials underway to test new PD drugs. As of 2011, multiple classes of drugs are used to treat PD.

DRUGS THAT REPLACE DOPAMINE. One drug that helps replace dopamine, levodopa, is the single most effective treatment for the symptoms of PD. Levodopa is a derivative of dopamine, and is converted into dopamine by the brain. It may be started when symptoms begin or when they become serious enough to interfere with work or daily living.

Levodopa therapy usually remains effective for five years or longer. Following this, many patients develop motor fluctuations, including peak-dose dyskinesias (abnormal movements such as **tics**, twisting, or restlessness), rapid loss of response after dosing (known as the "on-off" phenomenon), and unpredictable drug response. Higher doses may be tried, but often lead to an increase in dyskinesias. In addition, side effects of levodopa include nausea and vomiting and low blood pressure upon standing (**orthostatic hypotension**), which can cause **dizziness**. These effects may lessen after several weeks of therapy.

Dopamine is broken down by several enzyme systems in the brain and elsewhere in the body, and blocking these enzymes is a key strategy to prolonging the effect of dopamine. The two most commonly prescribed forms of levodopa contain a drug to inhibit the amino acid decarboxylase (an AADC inhibitor), one type of enzyme that breaks down dopamine.

Among these combination drugs are Sinemet and Parcopa (levodopa plus carbidopa), and Madopar (levodopa plus benzaseride; not marketed in the United States but available in some European countries). Controlled-release formulations also aid in prolonging the effective interval of an levodopa dose.

MAO-B INHIBITORS. The enzyme monoamine oxidase B (MAO-B) inhibitor selegiline (Eldepryl) may be given as add-on therapy for levodopa. Selegiline appears to have a neuroprotective effect, sparing nigral cells from damage by free radicals. Because of this, and the fact that it has few side effects, it is frequently prescribed early in the disease before levodopa is begun. Rasagiline (Azilect) is a second-generation MAO-B inhibitor with fewer potential side effects than selegiline.

ACETYLCHOLINESTERASE INHIBITORS. The cholinesterase inhibitor Exelon (rivastigmine) is a transdermal patch is used to treat **dementia** in mild to moderate PD.

DOPAMINE AGONISTS. Dopamine works by stimulating receptors on the surface of corpus striatum cells. Drugs that also stimulate these cells are called dopamine agonists, or DAs. DAs may be used before levodopa therapy, or added on to avoid requirements for higher levodopa doses late in the disease. DAs available in the United States as of 2011 include Apomorphine (Apokyn; a short-acting DA), bromocriptine (Parlodel), ropinirole (Requip), and pramipexole (Mirapex).

Other dopamine agonists in use elsewhere in the world include lisuride (Dopergine, Proclacam, Revanil) and apomorphine (Apokyn, Ixense, Spontane, Uprima). Side effects of all the DAs are similar to those of dopamine, plus confusion and hallucinations at higher doses. In 2007, the drug pergolide (Permax) was withdrawn from sale in the United States after studies showed it increased the risk of serious heart valve damage. It is still available in other countries.

ANTICHOLINERGIC DRUGS. Anticholinergics maintain dopamine balance as levels decrease, but the side effects of anticholinergics (dry mouth, constipation, confusion, and blurred vision) are usually too severe in older patients or in patients with dementia. In addition, anticholinergics rarely work for very long. They are often prescribed for younger patients who have predominant shaking. Trihexyphenidyl (Artane) is the drug most commonly prescribed.

N-METHYL-D-ASPARTIC ACID INHIBITORS. Amantadine (Symmetrel) is sometimes used as an early therapy before levodopa is begun, and as an add-on later in the disease. Its antiparkinson effects are mild and are not seen in many patients. Clozapine (Clozaril) is effective especially against psychiatric symptoms of late PD, including psychosis and hallucinations.

CATECHOL-O-METHYLTRANSFERASE (COMT) INHIBITORS. These drugs make more levodopa available for transport across the blood-brain barrier for a longer time. Entacapone (Comtan) often is used as an adjunct to levodopa when the patient is beginning to experience the on-off effect. Tolcapone (Tasmar) is a similar agent but has demonstrated the potential for inducing severe liver failure. As such, tolcapone is reserved for cases where all other adjunctive therapies have failed or are contraindicated.

Surgery

Two surgical procedures are used for treatment of PD that cannot be controlled adequately with drug therapy. In PD, a brain structure called the globus pallidus (GPi) receives excess stimulation from the corpus striatum. In a **pallidotomy**, the GPi is destroyed by heat, delivered by long thin needles inserted under anesthesia. Electrical stimulation of the GPi is another way to reduce its action. In this procedure, fine electrodes are inserted to deliver the stimulation, which may be adjusted or turned off as the response dictates. Other regions of the brain may also be stimulated by electrodes inserted elsewhere. In most patients, these procedures lead to significant improvement for some motor symptoms, including peak-dose dyskinesias. This allows the patient to receive more levodopa, since these dyskinesias are usually what cause an upper limit on the levodopa dose.

A third procedure, transplant of fetal nigral cells, is still highly experimental. Its benefits to date have been modest, although improvements in technique

COMMON QUESTIONS

- What can I do to help improve my quality of life while I am in the early stages of Parkinson's disease? Getting regular exercise and eating a healthy diet are two things that, although they will not stop the progression of PD, may help make activities of daily life easier to cope with. The doctor may prescribe physical therapy and the therapist may suggest specific exercises to be done at home. In addition, your doctor may prescribe drugs that have the potential to slow the progression of PD. Since about half of all people with PD experience depression, monitoring mental health and seeking treatment for depression, if needed, will help improve quality of life.

- What are the chances that my children will develop Parkinson's disease? The causes of PD are not known, but researchers suspect that there is both a genetic component and an environmental trigger that affect who gets PD. Children whose parents have PD have about twice the risk of developing the disease compared to children whose parents do not have PD, but the risk is still relatively low.

and patient selection may change that. Also, as of 2011, gene therapy was showing significant promise as a future treatment for PD. In one randomized double-blind phase 2 clinical trial completed in 2011, patients who received a gene transplant therapy called NLX-P101 showed a significant reduction in **tremor**, difficulty initiating movement, and muscle rigidity. Clinical trials of this therapy are continuing.

Alternative treatment

Currently, the best treatments for PD involve the use of conventional drugs such as levodopa. Alternative therapies, including **acupuncture**, massage, and yoga can help relieve some symptoms of the disease and loosen tight muscles. Alternative practitioners have also applied herbal and dietary therapies, including amino acid supplementation, antioxidant (vitamins A, C, E, selenium, and zinc) therapy, B vitamin supplementation, and calcium and magnesium supplementation, to the treatment of PD. People using these therapies in conjunction with conventional drugs should check with their doctor to avoid the possibility of adverse interactions. For example, vitamin B_6

(either as a supplement or from foods such as whole grains, bananas, beef, fish, liver, and potatoes) can interfere with the action of levodopa when the drug is taken without carbidopa.

Prognosis

Despite medical treatment, the symptoms of Parkinson's disease worsen over time and become less responsive to drug therapy. Late-stage psychiatric symptoms are often the most troubling, including difficulty sleeping, nightmares, intellectual impairment (dementia), hallucinations, and loss of contact with reality (psychosis).

Prevention

There is no known way to prevent Parkinson's disease.

Resources

BOOKS

Cram, David L., Steven H. Schechter, and Xiao-Ke Gao. *Understanding Parkinson's Disease: A Self-Help Guide.* 2nd ed. Omaha, NE: Addicus, 2009.

Lieberman, A.N. *The Muhammad Ali Parkinson Center: 100 Questions & Answers about Parkinson Disease.* 2nd ed. Sudbury, MA: Jones and Bartlett, 2011.

Pahwa, Rajesh, and Kelly E. Lyons. *Treatment Decisions in Parkinson's Disease.* New York : Oxford University Press, 2010.

Weiner, William J. *Parkinson's Disease: A Complete Guide for Patients and Families.* 2nd ed. Baltimore: Johns Hopkins University Press, 2007.

WEBSITES

American Academy of Family Physicians. "Parkinson's Disease." FamilyDoctor.org.http://familydoctor.org/online/famdocen/home/common/brain/disorders/187.html (accessed July 18, 2011).

Hauser, Robert A. "Parkinson Disease." Medscape Reference. http://emedicine.medscape.com/article/1831191-overview (accessed July 18, 2011).

"Parkinson's Disease." MedlinePlus. http://www.nlm.nih.gov/medlineplus/parkinsonsdisease.html (accessed July 18, 2011).

"Parkinson's Disease." WE MOVE. http://www.wemove.org/par (accessed July 18, 2011).

ORGANIZATIONS

American Parkinson Disease Association, 135 Parkinson Avenue, Staten Island, NY 10305, (718) 981-8001, (800) 223-2732, Fax: (718) 981-4399, adpa@adpapar kinson.org, http://www.apdaparkinson.org.

National Institute of Neurological Disorders and Stroke (NINDS), P.O. Box 5801, Bethesda, MD 20824, (301) 496-5751, (800) 352-9424, http://www.ninds.nih.gov.

National Parkinson Foundation, 1501 N.W. 9th Avenue/ Bob Hope Road, Miami, FL 33136-1494, (305) 243-6666, (800) 4PD-INFO (473-4636), Fax: (305) 243-6073, contact@parkinson.org, http://www.parkinson.org.

Parkinson's Disease Foundation, 1359 Broadway, Suite 1509, New York, NY 10018, (212) 923-4700, (800) 457-6676, Fax: (212) 923-4778, info@pdf. org, http://www.pdf.org.

Parkinson's Institute and Clinical Center, 675 Almanor Avenue, Sunnyvale, CA 94085, (408) 734-2800 , (800) 655-2273, info2@thepi.org, http://www.thepi.org.

Laith Farid Gulli, MD
Tish Davidson, AM

Paroxysmal hemicrania

Definition

Paroxysmal hemicrania (PH) is a rare form of headache. Paroxysmal hemicrania usually begins in adulthood, and affected persons experience severe throbbing, claw-like, or boring pain. The pain is usually on one side of the face, near or in the eye, temple, and occasionally reaching to the back of the neck. Red and tearing eyes, a drooping or swollen eyelid on the affected side of the face, and nasal congestion may accompany this pain. Persons experiencing the headache pain of paroxysmal hemicrania may also feel dull pain, soreness, or tenderness between attacks.

Description

Paroxysmal hemicrania syndromes have two forms: chronic, in which persons experience attacks on a daily basis for a year or more, and episodic, in which the headaches do not occur for months or years. Episodic paroxysmal hemicrania is four times more common than the chronic form.

Chronic paroxysmal hemicrania (CPH), also known as Sjaastad syndrome, is a primary headache disorder first described by the Norwegian neurologist Ottar Sjaastad in 1974. In 1976, Sjaastad proposed the term chronic paroxysmal hemicrania after observing two patients, who had daily, solitary, severe headache pain that remained on one side of the head. The main feature of chronic paroxysmal hemicrania is frequent attacks of strictly one-sided, severe pain localized in or around the eye or temple regions, lasting from 2–45 minutes in duration, and occurring 2–40 times per day.

Attacks of chronic paroxysmal hemicrania do not occur in recognizable time patterns. Episodic paroxysmal hemicrania (EPH), a more rare form of the disorder, is characterized by bouts of frequent, daily attacks with the same clinical features of CPH, but separated by relatively long periods without headache. Most episodic headaches in paroxysmal hemicrania occur at night or other recognizable time patterns.

Demographics

In the United States, CPH is a rare syndrome, but the number of diagnosed cases is increasing. The prevalence of CPH is not known, but it occurs more often than cluster headaches, a disorder that can sometimes be confused with CPH. Internationally, many cases of CPH have been described throughout the world, in different races and different countries.

Chronic paroxysmal hemicrania affects more women than men. In the past, because of female preponderance, CPH was considered a disease exclusive to women. However, CPH has been reported in increasing numbers of men. A study conducted in 1979 reported a female-to-male ratio of 7:1, but a review of 84 patients in 1989 reported a female-to-male ratio of 2.3:1. Chronic paroxysmal hemicrania can occur at any age, and the mean age of onset is 34 years.

Episodic paroxysmal hemicrania occurs in both sexes, with a slight female preponderance (1.3:1). The age of onset is variable; studies show EPH onset is 12–51 years.

Causes and symptoms

Causes

No definite cause of paroxysmal hemicrania is known. Persons who experience these headaches usually do not have additional neurological disorders, with the exception of **trigeminal neuralgia**, which has been observed in a small number of persons also having paroxysmal hemicrania. History of head or neck trauma is reported in about 20% of persons with paroxysmal hemicrania, but these findings are similar to **cluster headache** or migraine headaches. Occasionally, attacks may be provoked mechanically by bending or rotating the head and by applying external pressure against the back of the neck. There is no inheritable pattern or familial disposition known for paroxysmal hemicrania, and affected individuals do not have a higher incidence of other types of headaches, such as CH or migraine, than the general population.

Symptoms

Headache is the main symptom of both types of paroxysmal hemicrania. Chronic PH involves headaches that are one-sided, severe, affecting the eye or temple area, and lasting 2–45 minutes, occurring more than five times per day. Episodic paroxysmal hemicrania involves attacks of severe pain in the eye or temple area that last about 1–30 minutes, with a frequency of three or more events per day, and clear intervals between bouts of attacks that may last from months to years.

Both chronic and episodic paroxysmal hemicrania involve symptoms such as nasal congestion on the affected side, rhinorrhea (runny nose), and swelling of the eyelid on the affected side with tearing. Sweating, both on the forehead and generalized over the body, are also common.

Diagnosis

The diagnosis of paroxysmal hemicrania is based on a person's history and clinical symptoms. There are conditions involving underlying lesions in the brain (such as tumors or arteriovenous malformation) that can lead to symptoms similar to the headaches of paroxysmal hemicrania. Because of this, various tests of the brain are recommended to exclude structural abnormalities.

Laboratory studies such as routine blood tests can help identify metabolic and other causes of headache and facial pain. Imaging studies, including computed tomography (CT) scan or preferably **magnetic resonance imaging** (MRI) of the brain, may be needed to rule out structural disorders of the eye, ear, nose, neck, skull, and brain.

Testing the effectiveness of the drug indomethiacin may also be a useful tool in the assessment of one-sided headaches. The response to indomethacin is part of the criteria for a diagnosis of paroxysmal hemicrania. During two different periods, the drug is administered intramuscularly, and patterns of headache pain are evaluated. In paroxysmal hemicranias, indomethiacin relieves pain, prevents recurring pain, and/or decreases the frequency of pain. As the effects of indomethacin clear the body, the pain returns in its usual form and pattern.

Treatment team

A neurologist is the primary consultant for PH treatment. An ophthalmologist is also important to evaluate any eye disorders such as glaucoma.

Treatment

The nonsteroidal anti-inflammatory drug (NSAID) indomethacin often provides complete relief from symptoms. Other less effective NSAIDs, calcium-channel blocking drugs (such as verapamil) and corticosteroids, may be used to treat the disorder. Patients with both PH and trigeminal neuralgia (a condition of the fifth cranial nerve that causes sudden, severe pain typically felt on one side of the jaw or cheek) should receive separate treatment for each disorder.

Recovery and rehabilitation

When headaches are severe enough or frequent enough to interfere with a person's daily activities such as work, family life, and home responsibilities, a specially trained physical therapist can provide a variety of treatment and education services to manage or reduce headaches, including:

- exercises (stretching, strengthening and aerobic conditioning)
- safe sleep, standing and sitting postures
- performing daily activities safely
- relaxation

Clinical trials

There are no ongoing clinical trials specific to the study or treatment of paroxysmal hemicrania. The National Institute for Neurological Disorders and Stroke (NINDS), however, carries out multifaceted research on headaches and their causes.

Prognosis

Many patients experience complete relief or near-complete relief of symptoms following medical treatment for paroxysmal hemicrania. PH headaches may occur throughout life, but have also been known to go into remission or stop spontaneously.

Special concerns

Chronic paroxysmal hemicrania headaches have been reported to improve during pregnancy; however, they often recur after delivery. In some persons, menstruation lessens the headaches, while in others, headaches are worse during menstruation. Birth control pills do not seem to influence the frequency of attacks, and the effects of menopause on paroxysmal hemicrania are unknown.

Resources

BOOKS
Paulino, Joel, and Ceabert J. Griffith. *The Headache Sourcebook*. New York: McGraw-Hill/Contemporary Books, 2001.

PERIODICALS
Trucco, M., F. Maggioni, R. Badino, and G. Zanchin. "Chronic Paroxysmal Hemicrania, Hemicrania Continua and SUNCT Syndrome in Association with Other Pathologies: A Review." *Cephalalgia* 24 (2004): 173–84.

OTHER
"NINDS Paroxysmal Hemicrania Information Page." *National Institute of Neurological Disorders and Stroke*. May 8, 2004 (June 2, 2004). http://www.ninds.nih.gov/health_and_medical/disorders/paroxysmal_hemicrania.htm.

ORGANIZATIONS
American Council for Headache Education. 19 Mantua Road, Mt. Royal, NJ 08061. Phone: (856)423-0258. Fax: (856) 423-0082. Tollfree phone: (800) 255-ACHE (255-2243). Email: achehq@talley.com. http://www.achenet.org.
National Headache Foundation. 820 N. Orleans, Suite 217, Chicago, IL 60610-3132. Phone: (773) 388-6399. Fax: (773) 525-7357. Tollfree phone: (888) NHF-5552 (643-5552). Email: info@headaches.org. http://www.headaches.org.

Greiciane Gaburro Paneto
Iuri Drumond Louro, MD, PhD

Parsonage-Turner syndrome

Definition

Parsonage-Turner syndrome (PTS) is a rare syndrome of unknown cause, affecting mainly the lower motor neurons of the brachial plexus. The brachial plexus is a group of nerves that conduct signals from the spine to the shoulder, arm, and hand. PTS is usually characterized by the sudden onset of severe one-sided shoulder pain, followed by paralysis of the shoulder and lack of muscle control in the arm, wrist, or hand several days later. The syndrome can vary greatly in presentation and nerve involvement.

Description

PTS, also known as brachial plexus neuritis or neuralgic amyotrophy, is characterized by inflammation of a network of nerves that control and supply (innervate) the muscles of the chest, shoulders, and arms. Individuals with the condition first experience severe pain across the shoulder and upper arm. Within a few hours or days, **weakness**, wasting (atrophy), and paralysis may affect the muscles of the shoulder. Although individuals with the condition may experience paralysis of the affected areas for months or, in some cases, years, recovery is usually eventually complete.

Local pain around the shoulder girdle is the prevalent symptom of Parsonage-Turner syndrome. It is usually sudden and often severe, often awakening persons during the night. The pain worsens progressively for up to two days. Described as a constant, severe ache associated with tenderness of the muscles, the pain is not affected by coughing. However, it is accentuated by arm movements and muscular pressure, but almost unaltered by movements of the neck. The pain is commonly distributed across the back of the scapula (shoulder blade) and the tip of the shoulder. Pain often radiates down the outer side of the arm and up along the neck, and seldom spreads down as far as the outer side of the forearm, below the elbow. There is no exact correlation between the localization of the pain and the distribution of the subsequent muscle paralysis.

However, in general, pain radiating below the elbow is associated with involvement of the biceps or triceps, and radiation into the neck involves the sternocleidomastoid and trapezius muscles. Usually the severe pain lasts from a few hours to three weeks and then disappears rather suddenly; at the same time, muscular wasting and weakness are occurring. A less severe pain may persist considerably longer.

As the pain subsides, paralysis of some muscles of the shoulder girdle, and often of the arm, develops. Usually, muscle weakness appears suddenly, but sometimes gradually increases over two or three days, or up to one week in rare cases. The paralysis involves limpness and rapid wasting of the affected muscles. Tendon reflexes might be affected, depending on the severity and extent of muscular paralysis and wasting.

Weakened reflexes are frequently encountered, and fasciculations (fine tremors) occasionally occur.

Demographics

In the United States, the incidence is approximately 1.64 cases per 100,000 people per year. Internationally, PTS has been described in many countries around the world, although specific rates of incidence have not been reported. There is a male predominance in PTS with a male-to-female ratio ranging from 2:1–4:1. Individuals as young as three months or as old as 74 years can be affected with PTS; however, the prevalence is highest in young to middle-aged adults. When a child develops Parsonage-Turner syndrome, hereditary PTS should be considered.

Causes and symptoms

The exact cause of PTS is unknown, but the condition has been linked to many previous events or illnesses:

- viral infection (particularly of the upper respiratory tract)
- bacterial infection (e.g., pneumonia, diphtheria, typhoid)
- parasitic infestation
- surgery
- trauma (not related to shoulder)
- vaccinations (e.g., influenza; tetanus; diphtheria, tetanus toxoids, pertussis; smallpox; swine flu)
- childbirth
- miscellaneous medical investigative procedures (e.g., lumbar puncture, administration of radiologic dye)
- systemic illness (e.g., polyarteritis nodosa, lymphoma, systemic lupus erythematosus, temporal arteritis, Ehlers-Danlos syndrome)

In addition to these possible causes, a rare hereditary form of PTS has been localized to a defect on chromosome 17 and should be considered a distinct disorder. This form of the disorder occurs in a younger age group, affects males and females equally (autosomal-dominant inheritance), and is characterized by recurrent attacks that often cause pain on both sides of the body.

Acute pain in the shoulder girdle or arm is almost always the first symptom. Shortly thereafter, muscle weakness and wasting in the shoulder girdle and arm occur. The pain, which may be extraordinarily severe for a short time, eventually abates.

Diagnosis

PTS is a clinical syndrome; therefore, diagnosis is made by exclusion. Other disorders of the upper extremity or cervical spine have to be excluded, including abnormalities of the rotator cuff, acute calcific tendinitis, adhesive capsulitis, cervical **radiculopathy**, peripheral **nerve compression**, acute **poliomyelitis**, and **amyotrophic lateral sclerosis** (ALS). PTS may sometimes be confused with peripheral nerve compression or traction injury of the brachial plexus. Affected persons, however, do not experience the acute intense pain associated with PTS, and the loss of strength occurs simultaneously with the sensory changes.

In PTS, x rays of the cervical spine and shoulder show normal findings compatible with the patient's age. Nerve conduction studies and **electromyography** (EMG) are helpful in localizing the lesion. Three to four weeks after the onset of pain, EMG studies show changes consistent with PTS. Arthrography or ultrasound may be useful to rule out a tear of the rotator cuff. MRI may reveal muscles changes associated with PTS.

Treatment team

A specialist in neuromuscular disease may be consulted to confirm diagnosis and evaluate any potentially underlying causes. An orthopedic surgeon is important when nerve grafting or tendon transfer is necessary. Physical and occupational therapists may be asked to provide a comprehensive rehabilitation program.

Treatment

No specific treatment has yet been proved efficient in PTS. In the early stages, pain may require treatment. Common analgesic drugs are usually sufficient. Usually, steroidal medications do not relieve the pain or improve muscle function in PTS. Rest is recommended, and immobilization of the affected upper extremity may be helpful in relieving the pain and in preventing stretching of the affected muscles.

As pain subsides, physical therapy is recommended. Passive range of motion exercises of the shoulder and elbow are suggested to maintain full range of motion.

Surgical stabilization of the scapula to the thorax, or tendon transfers have been performed with benefit in persons with PTS who experience continuing pain and muscle weakness.

Recovery and rehabilitation

Physical therapy should focus on the maintenance of full range of motion (ROM) in the shoulder and other

KEY TERMS

Atrophy—Degeneration or wasting of tissues.

Brachial plexus—A group of nerves that exit the cervical (neck) and upper thoracic (chest) spinal column to provide muscle control to the shoulder, arms, and hands.

Scapula—The bone also known as the shoulder blade.

Trapezius—Muscle of the upper back that rotates the shoulder blade, raises the shoulder, and flexes the arm.

Triceps—Muscle of the back of the upper arm, primarily responsible for extending the elbow.

affected joints. Passive range of motion (PROM) and active range of motion (AROM) exercises should begin as soon as the pain has been controlled adequately, followed by regional conditioning of the affected areas. Strengthening of the rotator cuff muscles and scapular stabilization may be indicated. Passive modalities (e.g., heat, cold, transcutaneous electrical nerve stimulation) may be useful as adjunct pain relievers.

Another type of rehabilitation therapy in PTS is occupational therapy. Functional conditioning of the upper extremity may be helpful. Assistive devices and orthotics (such as splints or devices for grasping and reaching) may be used, depending on the particular disabilities present.

Clinical trials

In 2011, there were no clinical trials specific for PTS. Information on relevant current clinical trials can be found at ClinicalTrials.gov.

Prognosis

The overall prognosis for persons with PTS is good, as recovery of strength and sensation usually begins spontaneously as early as one month after the onset of symptoms. Almost 75% of persons with PTS experience complete recovery within two years. However, the period of time for complete recovery is variable, ranging from six months to five years. It seems that the delay in recovering strength depends on the severity and duration of pain, weakness, or both. Furthermore, patients with involvement of upper trunk lesions have the most rapid recovery. Although not very common, relapse might occur within a few months to several years after full recovery. In general, complete restoration of normal strength and function usually occurs within five years.

Resources

BOOKS

Liverson, Jay Allan. *Peripheral Neurology: Case Studies.* Oxford, UK: Oxford University Press, 2000.

PERIODICALS

Simon, J. P. A., and G. Fabry. "Parsonage-Turner Syndrome after Total-Hip Arthroplasty." *Journal of Arthroplasty* 16 (2001): 518–20.

OTHER

"Parsonage-Turner Syndrome" *Yale New Haven Health.* May 6, 2004 (June 2, 2004). http://yalenewhavenhealth. org/library/healthguide/IllnessConditions/topic.asp? hwid = nord726.

ORGANIZATIONS

American Autoimmune Related Diseases Association. 22100 Gratiot Avenue, Eastpointe, MI 48021. Phone: (586) 776-3900. Email: aarda@aarda.org. http://www. aarda.org/.

NIH/National Arthritis and Musculoskeletal and Skin Diseases Information Clearinghouse. 1 AMS Circle, Bethesda, MD 20892-3675. Phone: (301) 495-4484. Tollfree phone: (877) 226-4267. Email: niamsinfo@mail. nih.gov. http://www.niams.nih.gov.

Greiciane Gaburro Paneto
Iuri Drumond Louro

Pellegra *see* **Vitamin/nutritional deficiency**

Pemoline *see* **Central nervous system stimulants**

Perineural cysts

Definition

Perineural cysts (also called Tarlov cysts) are abnormal fluid-filled sacs located in the sacrum, the base of the spine.

Description

Perineural cysts appear to be dilated or ballooned areas of the sheaths that cover nerve roots exiting from the sacral area of the spine. The spaces or cysts created by the dilated sheaths are directly connected to the subarachnoid area of the spinal column, the area through which cerebrospinal fluid flows. Many people have perineural cysts but no symptoms at all; in fact, the majority of people with these cysts are completely unaware of their existence. However, when conditions cause these perineural cysts to fill with cerebrospinal fluid and expand, they can begin to compress important neighboring nerve fibers, resulting in a variety of symptoms, including pain, **weakness**, and abnormal sensation.

Demographics

More women than men develop perineural cysts.

Causes and symptoms

A variety of conditions that can increase the flow of cerebrospinal fluid may cause perineural cysts to expand, creating symptoms. Such conditions include traumatic injury, shock, or certain forms of exertion (such as heavy lifting) or exercise. Prolonged sitting or standing may cause cysts to fill and retain fluid. Other research suggests that herpes simplex virus can cause the body chemistry to become more alkaline, which predisposes the cerebrospinal fluid to fill the perineural cysts, thus prompting the advent of symptoms.

The symptoms of expanding perineural cysts occur due to compression of nerve roots that exit from the sacral area. Symptoms may include **back pain** and sciatica, a syndrome of symptoms that occur due to compression or inflammation of the sciatic nerve. Sciatica results in burning, tingling, numbness, stinging, or electric shock sensations in the lower back, buttocks, thigh, and down the leg to below the knee. Severe sciatica may also result in weakness of the leg or foot. Other more severe symptoms of perineural cysts include loss of bladder control and problems with sexual functioning.

Diagnosis

Because most perineural cysts do not cause symptoms, most perineural cysts are never diagnosed. When symptoms do develop that are suggestive of perineural cysts, MRI will usually demonstrate their presence, and CT myelography (a test in which dye is injected into the spine) may demonstrate the cerebrospinal fluid flow between the spinal subarachnoid area and the cyst.

Treatment team

Neurologists and neurosurgeons usually treat individuals with perineural cysts. A urologist may be called in to consult with individuals whose cysts are interfering with bladder or sexual functioning.

KEY TERMS

Cerebrospinal fluid—A fluid that bathes the brain and the spinal cord.

Cyst—A fluid-filled sac.

Sacrum—An area in the lower back, below the lumbar region.

Subarachnoid—The space underneath the layer of meningeal membrane called the arachnoid.

Treatment

Although using a needle to drain fluid from perineural cysts can temporarily relieve their accompanying symptoms, eventually the cysts will refill with cerebrospinal fluid and the symptoms will recur. Similarly, steroid injections can provide short-term pain relief. Pain may also be temporarily controlled by injecting the cysts with fibrin glue (a substance produced from blood chemicals involved in the clotting mechanism). Using diet or dietary supplements to decrease the body's alkalinity may prevent perineural cysts from filling with more fluid. Medications used to treat chronic nerve-related pain (such as anticonvulsants and antidepressants) may be helpful.

When pain is intractable, despite a variety of interventions, or when weakness or other neurological symptoms become severe, surgery to remove the cysts may be necessary. This is the only permanent treatment for perineural cysts; once removed, they very rarely recur.

Prognosis

Most individuals with perineural cysts have no symptoms whatsoever. Those who do have symptoms run a risk of neurological damage if the cysts continue to compress nerve structures over time. Individuals who undergo **neurosurgery** to remove the cysts usually have an excellent outcome, with no cyst recurrence.

Resources

BOOKS

Braunwald, Eugene, et al., eds. *Harrison's Principles of Internal Medicine.* New York: McGraw-Hill Professional, 2001.

Goetz, Christopher G., ed. *Textbook of Clinical Neurology.* Philadelphia: W. B. Saunders, 2003.

Goldman, Lee, et al., eds. *Cecil Textbook of Internal Medicine.* Philadelphia: W. B. Saunders, 2000.

PERIODICALS

Acosta, Frank L., et al. "Diagnosis and Management of Sacral Tarlov cysts." *Neurosurgical Focus* 15, no. 2 (August 2003). Available online at http://www.aans.org/education/journal/neurosurgical/aug03/15-2-15.pdf (June 3, 2004).

Voyadzis, J. M., et al. "Tarlov cysts: a study of 10 cases with review of the literature." *Journal of Neurosurgery* 95 (July 2001): 25–32.

WEBSITES

National Institute of Neurological Disorders and Stroke (NINDS). *NINDS Tarlov Cysts Information Page.* July 10, 2003. http://www.ninds.nih.gov/health_and_medical/disorders/tarlov_cysts.htm (June 3, 2004).

Tarlov Cyst Support Group. http://www.tarlovcyst.net/ (June 3, 2004).

Rosalyn Carson-DeWitt, MD

Periodic paralysis

Definition

Periodic paralysis (PP) is the name for several rare, inherited muscle disorders marked by temporary weakness, especially following rest, sleep, or exercise.

Description

Periodic paralysis disorders are genetic disorders that affect muscle strength. There are two major forms, hypokalemic and hyperkalemic, each caused by defects in different genes.

In hypokalemic PP, the level of potassium in the blood falls in the early stages of a paralytic attack, while in hyperkalemic PP, it rises slightly or is normal. (The root of both words, "kali," refers to potassium.) Hyperkalemic PP is also called potassium-sensitive PP.

Causes and symptoms

Causes

Both forms of PP are caused by inheritance of defective genes. Both genes are dominant, meaning that only one copy of the defective gene is needed for a person to develop the disease. A parent with the gene has a 50% chance of passing it along to each offspring, and the likelihood of passing it on is unaffected by the results of previous pregnancies.

The gene for hypokalemic PP (a type of channelopathy) is present equally in both sexes but leads to noticeable symptoms more often in men than in women. The normal gene is responsible for a muscle protein controlling the flow of calcium during muscle contraction.

The gene for hyperkalemic PP affects virtually all who inherit it, with no difference in male versus female expression. The normal gene is responsible for a muscle protein controlling the flow of sodium during muscle contraction.

Symptoms

The attacks of weakness in hypokalemic PP usually begin in late childhood or early adolescence and often become less frequent during middle age. The majority of patients develop symptoms before age 16. Since they begin in the school years, the symptoms of hypokalemic PP are often first seen during physical education classes or after-school sports and may be mistaken for laziness or lack of interest on the part of the child.

Attacks are most commonly brought on by the following:

• strenuous exercise followed by a short period of rest
• large meals, especially ones rich in carbohydrates or salt
• emotional stress
• alcohol use
• infection
• pregnancy

The weakness from a particular attack may last from several hours to as long as several days and may be localized to a particular limb or might involve the entire body.

The attacks of weakness of hyperkalemic PP usually begin in infancy or early childhood and may become less severe later in life. As in the hypokalemic form, attacks are brought on by stress, pregnancy, and exercise followed by rest. In contrast, though, hyperkalemic attacks are not associated with a heavy meal but rather with missing a meal, with high potassium intake, or use of glucocorticoid drugs such as prednisone. (Glucocorticoids are a group of steroids that regulate metabolism and affect muscle tone.)

Weakness usually lasts less than three hours, and often persists for only several minutes. The attacks are usually less severe but more frequent than those of the hypokalemic form. Weakness usually progresses from the lower limbs to the upper and may involve the facial muscles as well.

Diagnosis

Diagnosis of either form of PP begins with a careful medical history and a complete physical and neurological exam. A family medical history may reveal other affected relatives. Blood and urine tests done at the onset of an attack show whether there are elevated or depressed levels of potassium. Electrical tests of muscle and a muscle biopsy show characteristic changes.

Challenge tests, to aid in diagnosis, differ for the two forms. In hypokalemic PP, an attack of weakness can be brought on by administration of glucose and insulin, with exercise if necessary. An attack of hyperkalemic PP can be induced with administration of potassium after exercise during fasting. These tests are potentially hazardous and require careful monitoring.

Genetic tests are available at some research centers and are usually recommended for patients with a known family history. The number of different possible mutations leading to each form is too great to allow a single comprehensive test for either form, thus limiting the usefulness of genetic testing.

Treatment

Severe respiratory weakness from hypokalemic PP may require intensive care to ensure adequate ventilation. Potassium chloride may be given by mouth or intravenously to normalize blood levels.

Attacks requiring treatment are much less common in hyperkalemic PP. Glucose and insulin may be prescribed. Eating carbohydrates may also relieve attacks.

Prognosis

Most patients learn to prevent their attacks well enough that no significant deterioration in the quality of life occurs; however, strenuous exercise must be avoided. Attacks often lessen in severity and frequency during middle age. Frequent or severe attacks increase the likelihood of permanent residual weakness, a risk in both forms of periodic paralysis.

Prevention

There is no way to prevent the occurrence of either disease in a person with the gene for the disease. The likelihood of an attack of either form of PP may be lessened by avoiding the triggers (the events or combinations of circumstances which cause an attack) for each.

Hypokalemic PP attacks may be prevented with use of acetazolamide (or another carbonic anhydrase inhibitor drug) or a diuretic to help retain potassium in the bloodstream. These attacks may also be prevented by avoiding such triggers as salty food, large meals, a high-carbohydrate diet, and strenuous exercise.

Attacks of hyperkalemic PP may be prevented with frequent small meals high in carbohydrates and the avoidance of foods high in potassium such as orange juice or bananas. Acetazolamide or thiazide (a diuretic) may be prescribed.

Resources

BOOKS

Bradley, W., et al. *Neurology in Clinical Practice*. 5th ed. Philadelphia: Butterworth-Heinemann, 2008.

Goetz, C.G. *Goetz's Textbook of Clinical Neurology*. 3rd ed. Philadelphia: Saunders, 2007.

PERIODICALS

Fontaine, B. "Periodic paralysis." *Advanced Genetics* 63 (January 1, 2008): 3–23.

Finsterer, J. "Primary periodic paralyses." *Acta Neurologica Scandinavia* 2117 (April 1, 2009): 145–58.

ORGANIZATIONS

Muscular Dystrophy Association, 3300 East Sunrise Drive, Tucson, AZ 85718-3208, (520) 529-2000, (800) 572-1717, Fax: (520) 529-5300, mda@mdausa.org, http://www.mda.org.

Periodic Paralysis Association, 155 West 68th St., Suite 1732, New York, NY 10023, (407) 339-9499, http://www.periodicparalysis.org.

Richard Robinson
Rosalyn Carson-DeWitt, MD

Peripheral nervous system

Definition

The peripheral nervous system (PNS) consists of all parts of the nervous system, except the brain and spinal cord, which are the components of the **central nervous system** (CNS). The peripheral nervous system connects the central nervous system to the remainder of the body and is the conduit through which neural signals are transmitted to and from the central nervous system. Within the peripheral nervous system, sensory neurons transmit impulses to the CNS from sensory receptors. A system of motor neurons transmit neural signals from the CNS to effectors (glands, organs, and muscles).

Description

The peripheral nervous system is composed of nerve fibers that provide the cellular pathways for the various signals on which the proper operation of the nervous system relies. There are two types of neurons operating in the PNS. The first is the sensory neurons that run from the myriad of sensory receptors throughout the body. Sensory receptors provide the connection between the stimulus such as heat, cold, and pain and the CNS. The PNS consists of motor neurons, as well. These neurons connect the CNS to various muscles and glands throughout the body. These muscles and glands are also known as effectors, meaning they are the places where the responses to the stimuli are translated into action.

The peripheral nervous system is subdivided into two subsystems: the sensory-somatic nervous system and the autonomic nervous system.

The sensory-somatic nervous system

The sensory-somatic nervous system is the sensory gateway between the environment outside of the body and the central nervous system. Responses tend to be conscious.

The sensory nervous system comprises 12 pairs of cranial nerves and 31 pairs of spinal nerves. Some pairs are exclusively sensory neurons such as the pairs involved in smell, vision, hearing, and balance. Other pairs are strictly made up of motor neurons, such as those involved in the movement of the eyeballs, swallowing, and movement of the head and shoulders. Still other pairs consist of a sensory and a motor neuron working in tandem such as those involved in taste and other aspects of swallowing. All of the spinal neuron pairs are mixed: they contain both sensory and motor neurons. This allows the spinal neurons to properly function as the conduit of transmission of the signals of the stimuli and the subsequent response.

The autonomic nervous system

The autonomic nervous system (ANS) consists of three subsystems: the sympathetic nervous system, the parasympathetic nervous system, and the enteric nervous system. The ANS regulates the activities of cardiac muscle, smooth muscle, endocrine glands, and exocrine glands. The ANS functions involuntarily (i.e., reflexively) in an automatic manner without conscious control. Accordingly, the ANS is the mediator of visceral reflex arcs.

In contrast to the somatic nervous system that always acts to excite muscles groups, the autonomic nervous systems can act to excite or inhibit innervated tissue. The autonomic nervous system achieves this ability to excite or inhibit activity via a dual innervation of target tissues and organs. Most target organs and tissues are innervated by neural fibers from both the parasympathetic and sympathetic systems. The systems can act to stimulate organs and tissues in opposite ways (antagonistically). For example, parasympathetic stimulation acts to decrease heart rate. In contrast, sympathetic stimulation results in increased heart rate. The systems can also act in concert to stimulate activity (e.g., both increase the production of saliva by salivary glands, but parasympathetic stimulation results in watery as opposed to viscous or thick saliva). The ANS achieves this control via two divisions of the ANS, the sympathetic nervous system and the parasympathetic nervous system.

The autonomic nervous system also differs from the somatic nervous system in the types of tissue innervated and controlled. The somatic nervous system regulates skeletal muscle tissue, while the ANS services smooth muscle, cardiac muscle, and glandular tissue.

Although the sympathetic systems share a number of common features (i.e., both contain myelinated preganglionic nerve fibers that usually connect with unmyelinated postganglionic fibers via a cluster of neural cells termed ganglia), the classification of the parasympathetic and the sympathetic systems of the ANS is based both on anatomical and physiological differences between the two subdivisions.

The sympathetic nervous system

The nerve fibers of the sympathetic system innervate smooth muscle, cardiac muscle, and glandular tissue. In general, stimulation via sympathetic fibers increases activity and metabolic rate. Accordingly, sympathetic system stimulation is a critical component of the fight or flight response.

The cell bodies of sympathetic fibers traveling toward the ganglia (preganglionic fibers) are located in the thoracic and lumbar spinal nerves. These thoraco-lumbar fibers then travel only a short distance within the spinal nerve (composed of an independent mixture of fiber types) before leaving the nerve as myelinated white fibers that synapse with the sympathetic ganglia that lie close to the side of the vertebral column. The sympathetic ganglia lie in chains that line both the right and left sides of the vertebral column, from the cervical to the sacral region. Portions of the sympathetic preganglionic fibers do not travel to the vertebral ganglionic chains, but travel instead to specialized cervical or abdominal ganglia. Other variations are also possible. For example, preganglionic fibers can synapse directly with cells in the adrenal medulla.

In contrast to the parasympathetic system, the preganglionic fibers of the sympathetic nervous system are usually short, and the sympathetic postganglionic fibers are long fibers that must travel to the target tissue. The sympathetic postganglionic fibers usually travel back to the spinal nerve via unmyelinated or gray rami before continuing to the target effector organs.

With regard to specific target organs and tissues, sympathetic stimulation of the pupil dilates the pupil. The dilation allows more light to enter the eye and acts to increase acuity in depth and peripheral perception.

Sympathetic stimulation acts to increase heart rate and increase the force of atrial and ventricular contractions. Sympathetic stimulation also increases the conduction velocity of cardiac muscle fibers. Sympathetic stimulation also causes a dilation of systemic arterial blood vessels, resulting in greater oxygen delivery.

Sympathetic stimulation of the lungs and smooth muscle surrounding the bronchi results in bronchial muscle relaxation. The relaxation allows the bronchi to expand to their full volumetric capacity and thereby allow greater volumes of air passage during respiration. The increased availability of oxygen, and increased venting of carbon dioxide are necessary to sustain vigorous muscular activity. Sympathetic stimulation can also result in increased activity by glands that control bronchial secretions.

Sympathetic stimulation of the liver increases glycogenolysis and lipolysis to make energy more available to metabolic processes. Constriction of gastrointestinal sphincters (smooth muscle valves or constrictions), and a general decrease in gastrointestinal motility assure that blood and oxygen needed for more urgent needs (such as fight or flight) are not wasted on digestive system processes that can be deferred for short periods. The fight or flight response is a physical response; a strong stimulus or emergency release of a chemical called noradrenaline (also called norepinephrine) alternately stimulates or inhibits the functioning of a myriad of glands and muscles. Examples include the acceleration of the heartbeat, raising of blood pressure, shrinkage of the pupils of the eyes, and the redirection of blood away from the skin to muscles, brain, and the heart.

Sympathetic stimulation results in renin secretion by the kidneys and causes a relaxation of the bladder. Accompanied by a constriction of the bladder sphincter, sympathetic stimulation tends to decrease urination and promote fluid retention.

Acetylcholine is the neurotransmitter most often found in the sympathetic preganglionic synapse. Although there are exceptions (e.g., sweat glands utilize acetylcholine), epinephrine (noradrenaline) is the most common neurotransmitter found in postganglionic synapses.

The parasympathetic nervous system

Parasympathetic fibers innervate smooth muscle, cardiac muscle, and glandular tissue. In general, stimulation via parasympathetic fibers slows activity and results in a lowering of metabolic rate and a concordant conservation of energy. Accordingly, the parasympathetic nervous subsystem operates to return the body to its normal levels of function following the sudden alteration by the sympathetic nervous subsystem; the so-called "rest and digest" state. Examples include the restoration of resting heartbeat, blood pressure, pupil diameter, and flow of blood to the skin.

The preganglionic fibers of the parasympathetic system derive from the neural cell bodies of the motor nuclei of the occulomotor (cranial nerve: III), facial (VII), glossopharyngeal (IX), and vagal (X) cranial nerves. There are also contributions from cells in the sacral segments of the spinal cord. These cranio-sacral fibers generally travel to a ganglion that is located near or within the target tissue. Because of the proximity of the ganglia to the target tissue or organ, the postganglionic fibers are much shorter.

Parasympathetic stimulation of the pupil from fibers derived from the occulomotor (cranial nerve: III), facial (VII), and glossopharyngeal (IX) nerves constricts or narrows the pupil. This reflexive action is an important safeguard against bright light that could otherwise damage the retina. Parasympathetic stimulation also results in increased lacrimal gland secretions (tears) that protect, moisten, and clean the eye.

The vagus nerve (cranial nerve: X) carries fibers to the heart, lungs, stomach, upper intestine, and ureter. Fibers derived from the sacrum innervate reproductive organs, portions of the colon, bladder, and rectum.

With regard to specific target organs and tissues, parasympathetic stimulation acts to decrease heart rate and decrease the force of contraction. Parasympathetic stimulation also reduces the conduction velocity of cardiac muscle fibers.

Parasympathetic stimulation of the lungs and smooth muscle surrounding the bronchi results in bronchial constriction or tightening. Parasympathetic stimulation can also result in increased activity by glands that control bronchial secretions.

Parasympathetic stimulation usually causes a dilation of arterial blood vessels, increased glycogen synthesis within the liver, a relaxation of gastrointestinal sphincters (smooth muscle valves or constrictions), and a general increase in gastrointestinal motility (the contractions of the intestines that help food move through the system).

Parasympathetic stimulation results in a contracting spasm of the bladder. Accompanied by a relaxation of the sphincter, parasympathetic stimulation tends to promote urination.

The chemical most commonly found in both pre- and postganglionic synapses in the parasympathetic system is the neurotransmitter acetylcholine.

The enteric nervous system

The enteric nervous system is made up of nerve fibers that supply the viscera of the body: the gastrointestinal tract, pancreas, and gallbladder.

Regulation of the autonomic nervous system

The involuntary ANS is controlled in the hypothalamus, while the somatic system is regulated by other regions of the brain (cortex). In contrast, the somatic nervous system may control motor functions by neural pathways that contain only a single axon that innervates an effector (i.e., target) muscle. The ANS comprises pathways that must contain at least two axons separated by a ganglia that lies in the path between the axons.

ANS reflex arcs are stimulated by input from sensory or visceral receptors. The signals are processed in the hypothalamus (or regions of the spinal cord) and target effector control is then regulated via myelinated preganglionic neurons (cranial and spinal nerves that also contain somatic nervous system neurons). Ultimately, the preganglionic neurons terminate in a neural ganglion. Direct effector control is then regulated via unmyelinated postganglionic neurons.

The principal neurotransmitters in ANS synapses are acetylcholine and norepinephrine.

General PNS disorders

General PNS disorders include loss of sensation or hyperesthesia (abnormal or pathological sensitivity). Sensations such as prickling or tingling without observable stimulus (paresthesia) or burning sensations are also abnormal.

Stabbing or throbbing pains are often due to neuralgia (e.g., **trigeminal neuralgia**; also known as tic douloureux). Neuritis (an inflammation of the nerve) can be caused by a number of factors, including trauma, infection (both bacterial and viral), or chemical injury.

Resources

BOOKS

Goldman, Cecil. *Textbook of Medicine*, 21st ed. New York: W. B. Saunders, 2000.

Hall, John E. *Guyton and Hall Textbook of Medical Physiology*, 12th ed. New York: W. B. Saunders, 2011.

Tortora, G. J., and S. R. Grabowski. *Principles of Anatomy and Physiology*, 9th ed. New York: John Wiley Sons, 2000.

Brian Hoyle
Paul Arthur

Peripheral neuropathy

Definition

The term peripheral neuropathy encompasses a wide range of disorders in which the nerves outside of the brain and spinal cord—peripheral nerves—have been damaged. Peripheral neuropathy may also be referred to as peripheral neuritis, or if many nerves are involved, the terms polyneuropathy or polyneuritis may be used.

Demographics

Leprosy is extremely rare in the United States, where diabetes is the most commonly known cause of peripheral neuropathy. It has been estimated that upwards of 20 million Americans suffer from peripheral neuropathy and more than 17 million people in the United States and Europe have diabetes-related polyneuropathy. Many neuropathies are idiopathic, meaning that no known cause can be found. The

most common of the inherited peripheral neuropathies in the United States is Charcot-Marie-Tooth disease, which affects approximately 125,000 persons.

Description

Peripheral neuropathy is a widespread disorder, and there are many underlying causes. Some of these causes are common, such as diabetes, and others are extremely rare, such as acrylamide poisoning and certain inherited disorders. The most common worldwide cause of peripheral neuropathy is leprosy. Leprosy is caused by the bacterium *Mycobacterium leprae*, which attacks the peripheral nerves of affected people. According to statistics gathered by the World Health Organization, an estimated 1.15 million people have leprosy worldwide.

Another of the better known peripheral neuropathies is **Guillain-Barré syndrome**, which arises from complications associated with viral illnesses, such as cytomegalovirus, Epstein-Barr virus, and human immunodeficiency virus (HIV), or bacterial infection, including *Campylobacter jejuni* and **Lyme disease**. The worldwide incidence rate is approximately 1.7 cases per 100,000 people annually. Other well-known causes of peripheral neuropathies include chronic alcoholism, infection of the varicella-zoster virus, **botulism**, and **poliomyelitis**. Peripheral neuropathy may develop as a primary symptom, or it may be due to another disease. For example, peripheral neuropathy is only one symptom of diseases such as amyloid neuropathy, certain cancers, or inherited neurologic disorders. Such diseases may affect the **peripheral nervous system** (PNS) and the **central nervous system** (CNS), as well as other body tissues.

To understand peripheral neuropathy and its underlying causes, it may be helpful to review the structures and arrangement of the PNS.

Nerve cells and nerves

Nerve cells are the basic building block of the nervous system. In the PNS, nerve cells can be threadlike (i.e., their width is microscopic, but their length can be measured in feet). The long, spidery extensions of nerve cells are called axons. When a nerve cell is stimulated, by touch or pain, for example, the message is carried along the axon, and neurotransmitters are released within the cell. Neurotransmitters are chemicals within the nervous system that direct nerve cell communication.

Certain nerve cell axons, such as the ones in the PNS, are covered with a substance called myelin. The myelin sheath may be compared to the plastic coating on electrical wires—it is there both to protect the cells and to prevent interference with the signals being transmitted. Protection is also given by Schwann cells, special cells within the nervous system that wrap around both myelinated and unmyelinated axons. The effect is similar to beads threaded on a necklace.

Nerve cell axons leading to the same areas of the body may be bundled together into nerves. Continuing the comparison to electrical wires, nerves may be compared to an electrical cord—the individual components are coated in their own sheaths and then encased together inside a larger protective covering.

Peripheral nervous system

The nervous system is classified into two parts: the CNS and the PNS. The CNS is made up of the brain and the spinal cord, and the PNS is composed of the nerves that lead to or branch off from the CNS.

The peripheral nerves handle a diverse array of functions in the body. This diversity is reflected in the major divisions of the PNS: the afferent and the efferent divisions. The afferent division is in charge of sending sensory information from the body to the CNS. When afferent nerve cell endings, called receptors, are stimulated, they release neurotransmitters. These neurotransmitters relay a signal to the brain, which interprets it and reacts by releasing other neurotransmitters.

Some of the neurotransmitters released by the brain are directed at the efferent division of the PNS. The efferent nerves control voluntary movements, such as moving the arms and legs, and involuntary movements, such as making the heart pump blood. The nerves controlling voluntary movements are called motor nerves, and the nerves controlling involuntary actions are referred to as autonomic nerves. The afferent and efferent divisions continually interact with each other. For example, if a person were to touch a hot stove, the receptors in the skin would transmit a message of heat and pain through the sensory nerves to the brain. The message would be processed in the brain and a reaction, such as pulling back the hand, would be transmitted via a motor nerve.

Neuropathy

NERVE DAMAGE. When an individual has a peripheral neuropathy, nerves of the PNS have been damaged. Nerve damage can arise from a number of causes, including disease, physical injury, poisoning, or malnutrition. These agents may affect either afferent or efferent nerves. Depending on the cause of damage, the nerve cell axon, its protective myelin sheath, or both may be injured or destroyed.

CLASSIFICATION. There are hundreds of peripheral neuropathies. Reflecting the scope of PNS activity, symptoms may involve sensory, motor, or autonomic functions. To aid in diagnosis and treatment, the symptoms are classified into principal neuropathic syndromes based on the type of affected nerves and how long symptoms have been developing. Acute development refers to symptoms that have appeared within days, and subacute refers to those that have evolved over a number of weeks. Early chronic symptoms are those that take months to a few years to develop, and late chronic symptoms have been present for several years.

The classification system is composed of six principal neuropathic syndromes, which are subdivided into more specific categories. By narrowing down the possible diagnoses in this way, specific medical tests can be used more efficiently and effectively. The six syndromes and a few associated causes are listed below:

- Acute motor paralysis, accompanied by variable problems with sensory and autonomic functions. Neuropathies associated with this syndrome are mainly accompanied by motor nerve problems, but the sensory and autonomic nerves may also be involved. Associated disorders include Guillain-Barré syndrome, diphtheritic polyneuropathy, and porphyritic neuropathy.

- Subacute sensorimotor paralysis. The term sensorimotor refers to neuropathies that are mainly characterized by sensory symptoms but also have a minor component of motor nerve problems. Poisoning with heavy metals (e.g., lead, mercury, and arsenic), chemicals, or drugs are linked to this syndrome. Diabetes, Lyme disease, and malnutrition are also possible causes.

- Chronic sensorimotor paralysis. Physical symptoms may resemble those in the above syndrome, but the time scale of symptom development is extended. This syndrome encompasses neuropathies arising from cancers, diabetes, leprosy, inherited neurologic and metabolic disorders, and hypothyroidism.

- Neuropathy associated with mitochondrial diseases. Mitochondria are organelles—structures within cells—responsible for handling a cell's energy requirements. If the mitochondria are damaged or destroyed, the cell's energy requirements are not met and the cell can die.

- Recurrent or relapsing polyneuropathy. This syndrome covers neuropathies that affect several nerves and may come and go, such as Guillain-Barré syndrome, porphyria, and chronic inflammatory demyelinating polyneuropathy.

- Mononeuropathy or plexopathy. Nerve damage associated with this syndrome is limited to a single nerve or a few closely associated nerves. Neuropathies related to physical injury to the nerve, such as carpal tunnel syndrome and sciatica, are included in this syndrome.

Causes and symptoms

Typical symptoms of neuropathy are related to the type of affected nerve. If a sensory nerve is damaged, common symptoms include numbness, tingling in the area, a prickling sensation, or pain. Pain associated with neuropathy can be quite intense and may be described as cutting, stabbing, crushing, or burning. In some cases, a nonpainful stimulus may be perceived as excruciating or pain may be felt even in the absence of a stimulus. Damage to a motor nerve is usually indicated by **weakness** in the affected area. If the problem with the motor nerve has continued over a length of time, muscle shrinkage (atrophy) or lack of muscle tone may be noticeable. Autonomic nerve damage is most noticeable when an individual stands upright and experiences problems such as light-headedness or changes in blood pressure. Other indicators of autonomic nerve damage are lack of sweat, tears, and saliva; constipation; urinary retention; and impotence. In some cases, heart beat irregularities and respiratory problems can develop.

Symptoms may appear over days, weeks, months, or years. Duration of symptoms and the ultimate outcome of the neuropathy are linked to the cause of the nerve damage. Potential causes include diseases, physical injuries, poisoning, malnutrition, or alcohol abuse. In some cases, neuropathy is not the primary disorder, but a symptom of an underlying disease.

Disease

Diseases that cause peripheral neuropathies may either be acquired or inherited; in some cases, it is difficult to make that distinction. The diabetes-peripheral neuropathy link has been well established. A typical pattern of diabetes-associated neuropathic symptoms includes sensory effects that first begin in the feet. The associated pain or pins-and-needles, burning, crawling, or prickling sensations form a typical "stocking" distribution in the feet and lower legs. Other diabetic neuropathies affect the autonomic nerves and have potentially fatal cardiovascular complications.

Several other metabolic diseases have a strong association with peripheral neuropathy. Uremia, or chronic kidney failure, carries a 10–90% risk of eventually developing neuropathy, and there may be an association between liver failure and peripheral neuropathy. Accumulation of lipids inside blood vessels (atherosclerosis) can choke-off blood supply to certain peripheral nerves. Without oxygen and nutrients, the

nerves slowly die. Mild polyneuropathy may develop in persons with low thyroid hormone levels. Individuals with abnormally enlarged skeletal extremities (acromegaly), caused by an overabundance of growth hormone, may also develop mild polyneuropathy.

Neuropathy can also result from severe vasculitides, a group of disorders in which blood vessels are inflamed. When the blood vessels are inflamed or damaged, blood supply to the nerve can be affected, injuring the nerve.

Both viral and bacterial infections have been implicated in peripheral neuropathy. Leprosy is caused by the bacteria *M. leprae*, which directly attack sensory nerves. Other bacterial illness may set the stage for an immune-mediated attack on the nerves. For example, one theory about Guillain-Barré syndrome involves complications following infection with *Campylobacter jejuni*, a bacterium commonly associated with food poisoning. This bacterium carries a protein that closely resembles components of myelin. The immune system launches an attack against the bacteria, but, according to the theory, the immune system confuses the myelin with the bacteria in some cases and attacks the myelin sheath as well. The underlying cause of neuropathy associated with Lyme disease is unknown; the bacteria may either promote an immune-mediated attack on the nerve or inflict damage directly.

Infection with certain viruses is associated with extremely painful sensory neuropathies. A primary example of such a neuropathy is caused by **shingles**. After a case of chickenpox, the causative virus, varicella-zoster virus, becomes inactive in sensory nerves. Years later, the virus may be reactivated. Once reactivated, it attacks and destroys axons. Infection with HIV is also associated with peripheral neuropathy, but the type of neuropathy that develops can vary. Some HIV-linked neuropathies are noted for myelin destruction rather than axonal degradation. Also, HIV infection is frequently accompanied by other infections, both bacterial and viral, that are associated with neuropathy.

Several types of peripheral neuropathies are associated with inherited disorders. These inherited disorders may primarily involve the nervous system, or the effects on the nervous system may be secondary to an inherited metabolic disorder. Inherited neuropathies can fall into several of the principal syndromes, because symptoms may be sensory, motor, or autonomic. The inheritance patterns also vary, depending on the specific disorder. The development of inherited disorders is typically drawn out over several years and may herald a degenerative condition, a condition that becomes progressively worse over time. Even among specific disorders there may be a degree of variability in inheritance patterns and symptoms. For example, Charcot-Marie-Tooth disease is usually inherited as an autosomal dominant disorder, but it can be autosomal recessive or, in rare cases, linked to the X chromosome. Its estimated frequency is approximately one in 2,500 people. Age of onset and sensory nerve involvement can vary. The main symptom is a degeneration of the motor nerves in legs and arms, and resultant muscle atrophy. Other inherited neuropathies have a distinctly metabolic component. For example, in familial amyloid polyneuropathies, protein components that make up the myelin are constructed and deposited incorrectly.

Physical injury

Accidental **falls** and mishaps during sports and recreational activities are common causes of physical injuries that can result in peripheral neuropathy. The common types of injuries in these situations occur from placing too much pressure on the nerve, exceeding the nerve's capacity to stretch, blocking adequate blood supply of oxygen and nutrients to the nerve, and tearing the nerve. Pain may not always be immediately noticeable, and obvious signs of damage may take a while to develop.

These injuries usually affect one nerve or a group of closely associated nerves. For example, a common injury encountered in contact sports such as football is the "burner," or "stinger," syndrome. Typically, a stinger is caused by overstretching the main nerves that span from the neck into the arm. Immediate symptoms are numbness, tingling, and pain that travels down the arm, lasting only a minute or two. A single incident of a stinger is not dangerous, but recurrences can eventually cause permanent motor and sensory loss.

Poisoning

The poisons, or toxins, that cause peripheral neuropathy include drugs, industrial chemicals, and environmental toxins. Neuropathy that is caused by drugs usually involves sensory nerves on both sides of the body, particularly in the hands and feet, and pain is a common symptom. Neuropathy is an unusual side effect of medications; therefore, most people can use these drugs safely. Drugs that have been linked with peripheral neuropathy include metronidazole, an antibiotic; phenytoin, an anticonvulsant; and simvastatin, a cholesterol-lowering medication.

Certain industrial chemicals have been shown to be poisonous to nerves (neurotoxic) following work-related exposures. Chemicals such as acrylamide, allyl chloride, and carbon disulfide have all been strongly linked to development of peripheral neuropathy. Organic compounds, such as N-hexane and toluene, are also encountered in work-related settings, as well as in glue-sniffing and solvent abuse. Either route of exposure can produce severe sensorimotor neuropathy that develops rapidly.

Heavy metals are the third group of toxins that cause peripheral neuropathy. Lead, arsenic, thallium, and mercury usually are not toxic in their elemental form but rather as components in organic or inorganic compounds. The types of metal-induced neuropathies vary widely. Arsenic poisoning may mimic Guillain-Barré syndrome; lead affects motor nerves more than sensory nerves; thallium produces painful sensorimotor neuropathy; and the effects of mercury are seen in both the CNS and PNS.

Malnutrition and alcohol abuse

Burning, stabbing pains, and numbness in the feet and sometimes in the hands are distinguishing features of alcoholic neuropathy. The level of alcohol consumption associated with this variety of peripheral neuropathy has been estimated as approximately 3 L of beer or 300 mL of liquor daily for three years. It is unclear whether alcohol alone is responsible for the neuropathic symptoms because chronic alcoholism is strongly associated with malnutrition.

Malnutrition refers to an extreme lack of nutrients in the diet. It is unknown precisely which nutrient deficiencies cause peripheral neuropathies in alcoholics and famine and starvation patients, but it is suspected that the B vitamins have a significant role. For example, thiamine (vitamin B_1) deficiency is the cause of **beriberi**, a neuropathic disease characterized by heart failure and painful polyneuropathy of sensory nerves. Vitamin E deficiency seems to have a role in both CNS and PNS neuropathy.

Diagnosis

Clinical symptoms can indicate peripheral neuropathy, but an exact diagnosis requires a combination of medical history, medical tests, and possibly a process of exclusion. Certain symptoms can suggest a diagnosis, but more information is commonly needed. For example, painful, burning feet may be a symptom of alcohol abuse, diabetes, HIV infection, or an underlying malignant tumor, among other causes. Without further details, effective treatment would be difficult.

During a physical examination, an individual is asked to describe the symptoms very carefully.

KEY TERMS

Afferent—Refers to peripheral nerves that transmit signals to the spinal cord and the brain. These nerves carry out sensory function.

Autonomic—Refers to peripheral nerves that carry signals from the brain and that control involuntary actions in the body, such as the beating of the heart.

Autosomal dominant or autosomal recessive—Refers to the inheritance pattern of a gene on a chromosome other than X or Y. Genes are inherited in pairs, one gene from each parent; however, the inheritance may not be equal, and one gene may overshadow the other in determining the final form of the encoded characteristic. The gene that overshadows the other is called the dominant gene; the overshadowed gene is the recessive one.

Axon—A long, threadlike projection that is part of a nerve cell.

Central nervous system (CNS)—The part of the nervous system that includes the brain and the spinal cord.

Efferent—Refers to peripheral nerves that carry signals away from the brain and spinal cord. These nerves carry out motor and autonomic functions.

Electromyography—A medical test that assesses nerve signals and muscle reactions. It can determine if there is a disorder with the nerve or if the muscle is not capable of responding.

Inheritance pattern—Refers to dominant or recessive inheritance.

Motor—Refers to peripheral nerves that control voluntary movements, such as moving the arms and legs.

Myelin—The protective coating on axons.

Nerve biopsy—A medical test in which a small portion of a damaged nerve is surgically removed and examined under a microscope.

Nerve conduction—The speed and strength of a signal being transmitted by nerve cells. Testing these factors can reveal the nature of nerve injury, such as damage to nerve cells or to the protective myelin sheath.

Neurotransmitter—Chemicals within the nervous system that transmit information from or between nerve cells.

Peripheral nervous system (PNS)—Nerves that are outside of the brain and spinal cord.

Sensory—Refers to peripheral nerves that transmit information from the senses to the brain.

Detailed information about the location, nature, and duration of symptoms can help exclude some causes or even pinpoint the actual problem. The person's medical history may also provide clues as to the cause, because certain diseases and medications are linked to specific peripheral neuropathies. A medical history should also include information about diseases that run in the family, because some peripheral neuropathies are genetically linked. Information about hobbies, recreational activities, alcohol consumption, and workplace activities can uncover possible injuries or exposures to poisonous substances.

The physical examination also includes blood tests, such as those that check levels of glucose and creatinine to detect diabetes and kidney problems, respectively. A blood count is also done to determine levels of different blood cell types. Iron, vitamin B_{12}, and other factors may be measured as well, to rule out malnutrition. More specific tests, such as an assay for heavy metals or poisonous substances, or tests to detect **vasculitis**, are not typically done unless there is reason to suspect a particular cause.

An individual with neuropathy may be sent to a doctor who specializes in nervous system disorders (**neurologist**). By considering the results of the physical examination and observations of the referring doctor, the neurologist may be able to narrow down the possible diagnoses. Additional tests, such as nerve conduction studies and **electromyography**, which tests muscle reactions, can confirm that nerve damage has occurred and may also be able to indicate the nature of the damage. For example, some neuropathies are characterized by destruction of the myelin. This type of damage is shown by slowed nerve conduction. If the axon itself has suffered damage, the nerve conduction may be slowed, but it will also be diminished in strength. Electromyography adds further information by measuring nerve conduction and muscle response, which determines whether the symptoms are due to a neuropathy or to a muscle disorder.

In approximately 10% of peripheral neuropathy cases, a nerve **biopsy** may be helpful. In this test, a small part of the nerve is surgically removed and examined under a microscope. This procedure is usually the most helpful in confirming a suspected diagnosis, rather than as a diagnostic procedure by itself.

Treatment

Treat the cause

Attacking the underlying cause of the neuropathy can prevent further nerve damage and may allow for a better recovery. For example, in cases of bacterial infection such as leprosy or Lyme disease, antibiotics may be given to destroy the infectious bacteria. Viral infections are more difficult to treat, because antibiotics are not effective against them. Neuropathies associated with drugs, chemicals, and toxins are treated in part by stopping exposure to the damaging agent. Chemicals such as ethylenediaminetetraacetic acid (EDTA) are used to help the body concentrate and excrete some toxins. Diabetic neuropathies may be treated by gaining better control of blood sugar levels, but chronic kidney failure may require dialysis or even kidney transplant to prevent or reduce nerve damage. In some cases, such as compression injury or tumors, surgery may be considered to relieve pressure on a nerve.

In a crisis situation, as in the onset of Guillain-Barré syndrome, plasma exchange, intravenous immunoglobulin, and steroids may be given. Intubation, in which a tube is inserted into the trachea to maintain an open airway, and ventilation may be required to support the respiratory system. Treatment may focus more on symptom management than on combating the underlying cause, at least until a definitive diagnosis has been made.

Pain management

Because pain is associated with many of the neuropathies, a pain management plan may need to be mapped out, especially if the pain becomes chronic. Mild symptoms may be relieved by over-the-counter pain medications and as in any chronic disease, narcotics are best avoided due to the potential for dependence and side effects such as sedation.

The choice of proven drug therapies has broadened during the past decade. Four main classes of drugs are available for nerve pain management, alone or in combination. These include:

- anticonvulsants such as gabapentin (Neurontin), topiramate (Topamax), pregabalin (Lyrica), carbamazepine (Tegretol), and phenytoin (Dilantin)
- antidepressants such as duloxetine hydrochloride (Cymbalta), and Tricyclic antidepressants such as amitriptyline (Elavil), nortriptyline (Pamelor), and imipramine (Tofranil)
- narcotic analgesics such as codeine and morphine
- antiarrhythmics

In addition, topical medications administered via a skin patch (transdermal patch), may be effective for pain relief. The topical anesthetic, Lidocaine, may be administered via patch to the affected area. Capsaicin cream rubbed over the area may be beneficial, as well.

Supportive care and long-term therapy

Some peripheral neuropathies cannot be resolved or require time for resolution. In these cases, long-term monitoring and supportive care is necessary. Medical tests may be repeated to chart the progress of the neuropathy. If autonomic nerve involvement is a concern, regular monitoring of the cardiovascular system may be carried out.

Transcutaneous electrical nerve stimulation (TENS) may be administered via a TENS unit. This therapy utilizes electrodes that adhere to the skin and deliver varying frequencies of electric current. Some patients find minimal to moderate pain relief when this therapy is done on a frequent and ongoing basis.

Physical therapy and physician-directed exercises can help maintain or improve function. In cases in which motor nerves are affected, braces and other supportive equipment can aid an individual's ability to move about.

Prognosis

The outcome for peripheral neuropathy depends heavily on the cause. Peripheral neuropathy ranges from a reversible problem to a potentially fatal complication. In the best cases, a damaged nerve regenerates. Nerve cells cannot be replaced if they are killed, but they are capable of recovering from damage. The extent of recovery is tied to the extent of the damage and a person's age and general health status. Recovery can take weeks to years, because neurons grow very slowly. Full recovery may not be possible and it may also not be possible to determine the prognosis at the outset.

If the neuropathy is a degenerative condition, such as Charcot-Marie-Tooth disease, an individual's condition will become worse. There may be periods of time when the disease seems to reach a plateau, but cures have not yet been discovered for many of these degenerative diseases. Therefore, continued symptoms, potentially worsening to disabilities are to be expected.

A few peripheral neuropathies are eventually fatal. Fatalities have been associated with some cases of diphtheria, botulism, and others. Some diseases associated with neuropathy may also be fatal, but the ultimate cause of death is not necessarily related to the neuropathy, such as with cancer.

Prevention

Peripheral neuropathies are preventable only to the extent that the underlying causes are preventable. Steps that a person can take to prevent potential problems include vaccines against diseases that cause neuropathy, such as polio and diphtheria. Treatment for

QUESTIONS TO ASK YOUR DOCTOR

- What are the indications that I may have peripheral neuropathy?
- What diagnostic tests are needed for a thorough assessment?
- What treatment options do you recommend for me?
- What kind of changes can I expect to see with the medications you have prescribed for me?
- What are the side effects associated with the medications you have prescribed for me?
- Will medications for peripheral neuropathy interact with my current medications?
- Should I see a specialist? If so, what kind of specialist should I contact?
- If surgery is needed, what kind of surgical specialist should I contact?
- What tests or evaluation techniques will you perform to see if treatment has been beneficial for me?
- What changes in my health can I expect to see as my condition progresses?
- What physical limitations do you foresee?
- Does having peripheral neuropathy put me at risk for other health conditions?
- What measures can be taken to prevent peripheral neuropathy?
- How can my quality of life be improved?
- What symptoms or adverse effects are important enough that I should seek immediate treatment?
- Can you recommend an organization that will provide me with additional information about peripheral neuropathy?

physical injuries in a timely manner can help prevent permanent or worsening damage to nerves. Precautions when using certain chemicals and drugs are well advised in order to prevent exposure to neurotoxic agents. Control of chronic diseases such as diabetes may also reduce the chances of developing peripheral neuropathy.

Although not a preventive measure, genetic screening can serve as an early warning for potential problems. Genetic screening is available for some inherited conditions, but not all. In some cases, presence of a particular gene may not mean that a person will necessarily develop the disease, because there may be environmental and other components involved.

Resources

BOOKS

Ali, Naheed. *Diabetes and You: A Comprehensive, Holistic Approach.* Lanham, MD: Rowman & Littlefield, 2011.

Aminoff, Michael J., ed. *Neurology and General Medicine.* 4th ed. New York: Churchill Livingstone, 2007.

Birch, Rolfe. *Surgical Disorders of the Peripheral Nerves.* 2nd ed. New York: Springer, 2011.

Tesfaye, Solomin, and Andrew Boulton. *Diabetic Neuropathy.* New York: Oxford University Press, 2009.

ORGANIZATIONS

American Academy of Neurology (AAN), 1080 Montreal Avenue, Saint Paul, MN 55116, (651) 695-2717, (800) 879-1960, Fax: (651) 695-2791, memberservices@aan.com, http://www.aan.com.

American Academy of Physical Medicine and Rehabilitation, 9700 West Bryn Mawr Avenue, Suite 200, Rosemont, IL 60018-5701, (847) 737-6000, Fax: (847) 737-6001, info@aapmr.org, http://www. aapmr.org.

American Diabetes Association, 1701 North Beauregard Street, Alexandria, VA 22311, (800) DIABETES, askADA@diabetes.org, http://www. diabetes.org.

American Neurological Association, 5841 Cedar Lake Road, Suite 204, Minneapolis, MN 55416, (952) 545-6284, http://www.aneuroa.org.

Juvenile Diabetes Foundation, 26 Broadway, 14th Floor, New York, NY 10004, (800) 533-CURE, info@jdrf.org, http://www.jdf.org.

Myelin Project Headquarters, P.O. Box 39, Pacific Palisades, CA 90272-0039, (310) 459-1071, (800) 8-MYELIN, Fax: (310) 230-4298, http://www. myelin.org.

National Institute of Neurological Disorders and Stroke (NINDS), P.O. Box 5801, Bethesda, MD 20824, (301) 496-5751, (800) 352-9424, http://www.ninds.nih.gov.

National Institutes of Health (NIH), 9000 Rockville Pike, Bethesda, MD 20892, (301) 496-4000, NIHinfo@od.nih.gov, http://www.nih.gov/index.html.

Neuropathy Association, 60 East 42nd Street, Suite 942, New York, NY 10165, (212) 692-0662, Fax: (212) 692-0668, info@neuropathy.org, http://www. neuropathy.org.

U.S. National Library of Medicine, 8600 Rockville Pike, Bethesda, MD 20894, (301) 594-5983, (888) 346-3656, Fax: (301) 402-1384, custserv@nlm. nih.gov, http://www.nlm.nih.gov.

Julia Barrett
Laura Jean Cataldo, RN, EdD

Periventricular leukomalacia

Definition

Periventricular leukomalacia is a brain condition affecting fetuses and newborns in which there is softening, dysfunction, and death of the white matter of the brain.

Description

The brain is composed of outer gray matter and inner white matter. The gray matter is responsible for processing information involved in muscle control, sensory perception, emotion, and memory. The white matter is responsible for transmitting information throughout the brain, to the spinal cord, and outside of the brain to the muscles. The ventricles are four cavities within the brain, all of which are interconnected with each other and with the central spinal canal, and through which the cerebrospinal fluid circulates. "Periventricular" refers to the white matter that surrounds the ventricles. "Leukomalacia" means softening of the white tissue. When the white matter softens, the brain tissue begins to die.

Demographics

Periventricular leukomalacia strikes fetuses and newborns, particularly those who have undergone some kind of oxygen deprivation, such as may occur due to complications of prematurity. Some 4–26% of all premature infants in neonatal intensive care units have evidence of periventricular leukomalacia. As many as 76% of premature infants who die of complications of prematurity have evidence of periventricular leukomalacia on autopsy.

The risk of a baby developing periventricular leukomalacia is higher in those babies with smaller birth weights, who are twins, who are born at less than 32 weeks and require mechanical ventilation, and/or who are born of mothers who have abused cocaine. The following conditions also increase a baby's likelihood of developing periventricular leukomalacia:

- low blood pressure
- increased acidity of the blood
- high blood pressure
- low blood carbon dioxide
- abnormalities of the placenta

Causes and symptoms

Premature babies are at high risk of a variety of complications, including low blood oxygen (hypoxemia), decreased delivery of oxygen to the body's tissues (hypoxia), and/or decreased flow of oxygen-rich blood to the body's tissues (ischemia). All of these complications can result in oxygen deprivation of the susceptible newborn brain tissue, and potentially in subsequent brain damage. Without a constant flow of enough oxygen and nutrients, the oxygen-starved brain tissue will begin to soften and die. Additionally, premature infants have a very high risk of bleeding into the brain (intraventricular hemorrhage). When this occurs, the area around the brain hemorrhage is particularly susceptible to periventricular leukomalacia.

Other risk factors for periventricular leukomalacia include early rupture of the amniotic membranes (the birth sac) prior to delivery of the baby and infections within the mother's uterus during pregnancy and/or labor and delivery of the baby.

Symptoms of periventricular leukomalacia include tight, contracted, spastic leg muscles, delayed motor development, delayed intellectual development, problems with coordination, impaired vision and hearing, and seizures. More than 60% of all babies who have periventricular leukomalacia will actually develop **cerebral palsy**, particularly if the periventricular leukomalacia has been accompanied by intraventricular hemorrhage. Cerebral palsy is a constellation of symptoms that occur due to significant oxygen deprivation of the brain tissue, resulting in lifelong difficulties with coordination between the brain and muscles and sometimes accompanied by **mental retardation**.

Diagnosis

Periventricular leukomalacia can be diagnosed through cranial ultrasound, which allows the brain to be examined using ultrasound techniques through the soft spots, or fontanelles, in the baby's skull. When a baby has periventricular leukomalacia, the ultrasound exam will reveal cysts (fluid-filled compartments) or empty cavities within the brain tissue. Magnetic resonance imaging (MRI) scans of the brain may also reveal the characteristic abnormalities of periventricular leukomalacia.

Treatment team

Most premature babies are treated by a perinatologist (a specialist in the care of premature infants). A pediatric neurologist may be consulted if a baby is suspected of having periventricular leukomalacia or intraventricular bleeding.

Treatment

There is no cure for periventricular leukomalacia. Efforts, instead, are made to help affected children reach their full potential through a variety of modalities throughout childhood.

Recovery and rehabilitation

The rehabilitation team will depend on the extent of a child's physical and intellectual challenges. Physical therapy, occupational therapy, speech and language therapy, and a specialized educational setting may all be necessary.

Prognosis

The prognosis for babies with periventricular leukomalacia is quite variable and is dependent on the other complications of prematurity that a baby may face. Deficits may range from mild to devastating disability or even death.

Special concerns

Some studies have suggested that the risk of periventricular leukomalacia is decreased by the administration of steroids to women in premature labor. Other preventive measures include any steps that may decrease the likelihood of intraventricular hemorrhage, such as careful labor management and monitoring, and care in an experienced neonatal intensive care unit.

Resources

BOOKS

DeGirolami, Umberto, Douglas C. Anthony, and Matthew P. Frosch. "The Central Nervous System." In *Robbins Pathologic Basis of Disease*, edited by Richard E. Behrman, et al. Philadelphia: W.B. Saunders, 1999.

Stoll, Barbara J., and Robert M. Kliegman. "Nervous System Disorders." In *Nelson Textbook of Pediatrics*, edited by Richard E. Behrman, et al. Philadelphia: W.B. Saunders, 2004.

PERIODICALS

Okumara, A. "Abnormal Sharp Transients on Electroencephalograms in Preterm Infants with Periventricular Leukomalacia." *Journal of Pediatrics* 143, no. 1 (July 2003): 26–30.

Sofue, A. "Sharp Wave in Preterm Infants with Periventricular Leukomalacia." *Pediatric Neurology* 29, no. 3 (September 2003): 214–17.

WEBSITES

National Institute of Neurological Disorders and Stroke (NINDS). *Periventricular Leukomalacia Fact Sheet.* (May 23, 2004.) http://www.ninds.nih.gov/health_and_ medical/disorders/periventricular_leukomalacia.htm.

Rosalyn Carson-DeWitt, MD

PET scan *see* **Positron emission tomography (PET)**

Phantom limb

Definition

Phantom limb is the term for abnormal sensations perceived from a previously amputated limb. The abnormal sensations may be painful or nonpainful. It is presumed to be due to central and **peripheral nervous system** reorganization as a response to injury. Phantom limb pain is often considered to be a form of neuropathic pain, a group of pain syndromes associated with damage to nerves.

Demographics

The incidence of phantom limb pain is estimated in 50–80% of all amputees. It is more prevalent in upper limb amputees (82%) than lower limb amputees (54%). There is no known association with age, gender, or which limb is amputated. Studies have shown a decreased incidence of phantom limb syndrome in those born without limbs versus actual amputees.

Description

Silas Weir Mitchell, an American neurologist, coined the term "phantom limb" in 1871. Phantom limb syndrome was first described by Ambroise Pare in 1552. Pare, a French surgeon, noticed this phenomenon in soldiers who felt pain in their amputated limbs. Phantom limb syndrome can be subdivided into phantom limb sensation and phantom limb pain. Stump or residual limb pain refers to pain that may persist at the residual site of amputation and may be grouped under phantom limb syndrome as well.

The onset of pain after amputation usually occurs within days to weeks, although it may be delayed months or years. Pain may last for years and tends to be intermittent rather than constant. Pain may last up to 10–14 hours a day and can vary in severity from mild to debilitating. The abnormal "phantom" sensations and pain are usually located in the distal parts of the missing limb. Pain and tingling may be felt in the fingers and hand and in the lower limbs, in the toes and the feet.

Causes and symptoms

Causes

The exact etiology of phantom limb pain is unknown. Phantom limb is thought to be secondary to the brain plasticity and reorganization. The human brain has an enormous capacity to alter its connections and function in response to everyday learning or to the setting of injury. These processes of reorganization may occur in retained nerves in the amputated limbs, the spinal cord, or various parts of the brain, including the thalamus and the cerebral cortex.

Although phantom pain is presumably a result of a response to amputation injury, phantom limb pain may occur in non-amputees with spinal cord damage causing loss of sensation. This suggests that the phantom limb phenomenon may be a result of damage to pathways responsible for painful sensation in general. Research studies in primates and patients with limb amputation have shown that after amputation, the area of the brain that is responsible for processing

the sensations from the missing limb are taken over by areas neighboring the missing limb.

Symptoms

Patients may feel a variety of sensations emanating from the absent limb. The limb may feel completely intact despite its absence. Nonpainful sensations may include changes in temperature, itching, tingling, shock-like sensations, or perceived motion of the phantom limb. The limb may feel as if it is retracting into the stump, a phenomenon called telescoping. Painful sensations include burning, throbbing, or stabbing in nature. Touching the remaining stump may elicit sensations from the phantom. The quality of the pain may change over time and may not remain constant. Patients may also feel pain from the retained stump itself. Stump pain is often associated with phantom limb sensations and may be related in etiology.

Diagnosis

The diagnosis of phantom limb is a clinical one. A history of previous limb amputation and the subsequent symptoms of abnormal sensations from the missing limb are key to the diagnosis. Spinal cord damage affecting pathways mediating sensation may also be associated with phantom limb. There are no imaging or clinical tests useful in diagnosing phantom limb.

Treatment team

The treatment team for phantom limb pain may involve the participation of neurologists, pain specialists, physical therapists, neurosurgeons, or rehabilitation specialists. Neurologists and pain specialists may help in prescribing medications to treat the phantom limb pain. Physical therapists may help to facilitate and maintain mobility. Neurosurgeons may perform surgery to place electrical nerve stimulators in the spinal cord or lesion procedures to help treat the pain.

Treatment

There are few controlled clinical studies on phantom limb treatment, and therefore no consensus on the best treatment. Treatment is directed toward the management of painful symptoms. Nonpainful symptoms rarely require treatment. Treatment for phantom limb pain involves the use of medications, as well as nonmedical, electrical, and surgical therapy.

Medical treatment of phantom limb pain involves agents typically used for neuropathic pain. Medications such as anticonvulsants, muscle relaxants, and antidepressants may be tried. Opiate medications have also been used. Ketamine, an anesthetic agent, or calcitonin has been shown to be effective in some clinical studies.

Various electrical and nonmedical treatments may be tried. Transcutaneous electrical nerve stimulation (TENS), vibration therapy, and biofeedback may be used. Massage, ultrasound, hypnosis, and **acupuncture** modalities may be tried as well. Training patients to discriminate sensory signals in the stump appears to be helpful in reducing pain. In research studies, allowing individuals to see a reflection of the normal, intact limb moving in the position of the amputated limb helped alleviate symptoms of phantom limb pain.

Mirror box therapy is another treatment modality for phantom limb pain. This therapy, developed in 1995 by Vilayanur Ramachandran, involves artificial visual feedback using two mirrors to train individuals to sense movement and guiding of the phantom limb into a position of comfort. Repeated training is necessary and has led to improvement of pain for some individuals.

Immersive virtual reality is a relatively new treatment modality being developed by a team of researchers at the University of Manchester in England. After attaching their real limb to a specially designed interface, computer simulation allows the individual to view two limbs moving, creating an illusion to "trick" sensory areas in the brain to help decrease discomfort in the phantom limb. Research is ongoing to further develop this therapy.

Surgical treatments for phantom limb pain are limited in benefit. Lesions of various pain centers in the spinal cord and brain can be performed and may provide short-term relief on most occasions.

QUESTIONS TO ASK YOUR DOCTOR

- What diagnostic tests are needed for a thorough assessment?
- What treatment options do you recommend for me?
- Should I see a specialist? If so, what kind of specialist should I contact?
- If surgery is needed, what kind of surgical specialist should I contact?
- Will physical therapy benefit me?
- How can my quality of life be improved?
- What research is being done to learn more about phantom limb syndrome?
- Can you recommend an organization that will provide me with additional information about phantom limb syndrome?
- Can you refer me to a qualified person who can make an assessment of my home and recommend changes to make it safer and easier for me to get around?
- Can you recommend any support groups for me and my family?

Recovery and rehabilitation

Prospective studies of phantom pain show that, in two years, many amputees will experience a reduction of symptoms. Physical and occupational therapists may help in the treatment of phantom limb pain by maintaining range of motion and mobility.

Clinical trials

There are ongoing clinical trials conducted by the National Institute of Neurological Disorders and Stroke (NINDS) studying touch perception in patients with upper limb amputation. Individuals who wish to participate can find a list of clinical trials currently enrolling volunteers at http://clinicaltrials.gov. There is no cost to the patient to participate in a clinical trial.

Prognosis

The prognosis for phantom limb varies from individual to individual. Medical treatment shows the most benefit in treating symptoms. Some studies show that in a two-year period, many amputees will experience a reduction or disappearance of their phantom limb pain. The results of the studies are somewhat limited due to the heterogeneity of the populations studied.

Special concerns

Social needs

Phantom limb may have a chronic course and may lead to feelings of **depression** or anxiety. These feelings may require treatment by a psychiatrist. Patients with phantom limb should continue to be active and participate in community and social activities. There are various support groups for amputees.

Resources

BOOKS

Aminoff, Michael J., editor. *Neurology and General Medicine.* 4th ed. New York: Churchill Livingstone, 2007.

Gallagher, Pamela, Deirdre Desmond, and Malcolm Maclachlan, eds. *Psychoprosthetics.* New York: Springer, 2010.

Moore, Rhonda J., ed. *Biobehavioral Approaches to Pain.* New York: Springer, 2009.

Rosenquist, Richard W. *A Practical Approach to Pain Management.* New York: Lippincott Williams & Wilkins, 2012.

Schaefer, Michael. *Body in Mind: A New Look at the Somatosensory Cortices.* New York: Nova Science, 2010.

Sherman, Richard A. *Phantom Pain.* New York: Springer, 2010.

PERIODICALS

Chapman, Suzanne. "Pain management in patients following limb amputation." *Nursing Standard* 25.19 (2011): 35.

Chernev, Ivan, Delia G. Wilcher, and Kun Yan. "Combined mirror visual and auditory feedback therapy for upper limb phantom pain: a case report." *Journal of Medical Case Reports* 5 (2011): 41.

Jacobs, Michael Bradley, and Richard C. Niemtzow. "Treatment of phantom limb pain with laser and needle auricular acupuncture: a case report." *Medical Acupuncture* 23.1 (2011): 57.

Murray, Craig D. "A review of the use of virtual reality in the treatment of phantom limb pain." *Journal of CyberTherapy and Rehabilitation* 2.2 (2009): 105.

ORGANIZATIONS

American Academy of Neurology (AAN), 1080 Montreal Avenue, Saint Paul, MN 55116, (651) 695-2717, (800) 879-1960, Fax: (651) 695-2791, memberservices@ aan.com, http://www.aan.com.

American Academy of Physical Medicine and Rehabilitation, 9700 West Bryn Mawr Avenue, Suite 200, Rosemont, IL 60018-5701, (847) 737-6000, Fax: (847) 737-6001, info@aapmr.org, http://www.aapmr.org.

American Chronic Pain Association (ACPA), P.O. Box 850, Rocklin, CA 95677, (916) 632-0922, (800) 533-3231, Fax: (916) 632-3208, ACPA@pacbell. net, http:// www.theacpa.org.

American Neurological Association, 5841 Cedar Lake Road, Suite 204, Minneapolis, MN 55416, (952) 545-6284, http://www.aneuroa.org.

American Pain Foundation, 201 North Charles Street, Suite 710, Baltimore, MD 21201, (888) 615-PAIN, info@ painfoundation.org, http://www.pain foundation.org.

National Institute of Neurological Disorders and Stroke (NINDS), P.O. Box 5801, Bethesda, MD 20824, (301) 496-5751, (800) 352-9424, http://www.ninds.nih.gov.

National Institutes of Health (NIH), 9000 Rockville Pike, Bethesda, MD 20892, (301) 496-4000, NIHinfo@ od.nih.gov, http://www.nih.gov/index.html.

The Pain Relief Foundation, Clinical Sciences Centre, University Hospital Aintree, Lower Lane, Liverpool, United Kingdom, L9 7AL, (0151) 529-5820, Fax: (0151) 529-5821, secretary@painrelieffoundation.org.uk, http://www.painrelieffoundation.org.uk.

U.S. National Library of Medicine, 8600 Rockville Pike, Bethesda, MD 20894, (301) 594-5983, (888) 346-3656, Fax: (301) 402-1384, custserv@nlm. nih.gov, http:// www.nlm.nih.gov.

Peter T. Lin, MD
Laura Jean Cataldo, RN, EdD

Pharmacotherapy

Definition

Pharmacotherapy is the use of medicine in the treatment of diseases, conditions, and symptoms.

Description

History of pharmacotherapy

Pharmacotherapy is not a contemporary science. The use of drugs to treat illness is a practice that has been accepted for thousands of years. A famous example is Hippocrates (460–377 BCE), who is generally credited with revolutionizing medicine in ancient Greece by using beneficial drugs to heal illness. Traditionally, plants have been the source of medicinal drugs, but modern day medicine in the United States mostly utilizes synthesized or purified bioactive compounds, rather than an entire sample of plant matter. The advantage to this method of pharmacotherapy is that the dose of medicine rendered is standardized and pure, rather than an unknown drug dosage administered in addition to a wide variety of other chemicals present in the plant. Modern pharmacotherapy is the most common course of treatment for illness in the United States.

Pharmacokinetics and pharmacodynamics

Pharmacokinetics is the study of the concentration of a drug and its metabolites in the body over time. A drug that remains in the body for a longer time period will require lower subsequent doses to maintain a specific concentration. How quickly a drug clears from the body is a function of its absorption, bioavailability, distribution, metabolism, and excretion properties.

The absorption of a drug is the rate at which it leaves its site of administration. The bioavailability of a drug describes the extent to which it is available at the site of action in a bioactive metabolic form. A drug absorbed from the stomach and intestine passes through the liver before reaching the systemic circulation. If the liver biotransforms the drug extensively into an inactive form, its availability in bioactive form would be greatly reduced before it reaches its site of action. This is known as the first pass effect. Sometimes the liver biotransforms an inactive drug into an active form.

Which parts of the body drugs distribute to affects the length of time the drugs remain in the body. Fat-soluble drugs may deposit in fat reservoirs and remain in the body longer than drugs that are not fat-soluble. Drugs are metabolized within cells, often into inactive forms. The rate at which a drug is excreted from the body also affects its pharmacokinetics. Pharmacokinetic information about a drug allows the determination of an optimal dosage regimen and form of administration that will produce a specified drug concentration in the body for a desired period of time.

While pharmacokinetics is the study of drug concentration versus time, pharmacodynamics is the study of drug effect versus concentration, or what effect a drug has on the body. Pharmacodynamics measures a quantifiable drug-induced change in a biochemical or physiological parameter. Pharmacodynamics is the study of the mechanism of action of a drug. Medicinal drugs have targets to reach at the site of action. These targets are usually a specific type of drug receptor. Drug and drug receptor interactions can be measured. Complex pharmacodynamic equations combine with measurable pharmacokinetic values to determine the overall effect of a drug on the body over time.

Pharmacogenetics and pharmacogenomics

Pharmacogenetics is the study of the extent to which genetic differences influence the response of an individual to a medication. This science is still at an early stage in its development, but its importance is well understood. While drug treatment remains the cornerstone of modern medicine, in some cases it has adverse side effects or no effect at all. Adverse drug reactions are a leading cause of disease and death. It has been known for some time that genetic variation often causes these unanticipated situations.

While pharmacogenetics is the term used to describe the relationship between a genetically determined variability and the metabolism of drugs, pharmacogenomics is a separate and much more recent term that expands the concept. Pharmacogenomics includes the identification of all genetic variations that influence the efficacy and toxicity of drugs, describing the junction of pharmaceutical science with knowledge of genes. Pharmacogenomics is the application of the concept of genetic variation to the whole genome. Pharmacogenomics takes the concept of pharmacogenetics to the level of tailoring drug prescriptions to individual genotypes. There is an emerging trend towards defining both terms as pharmacogenomics.

There are many worrisome issues associated with modern pharmacotherapy that necessitate the study of pharmacogenomics. The optimal dose for many drugs is known to vary among individuals. The daily dose for the drug propranolol varies 40-fold, and the dose for warfarin can vary by 20-fold between individuals. Also, the same drug does not always work in every patient. Thirty percent of schizophrenics do not respond to antipsychotic treatment. A major concern is adverse drug reactions. In the United States, adverse effects are a significant cause of death. Research has demonstrated that gene polymorphisms influence drug effectiveness and toxicity, leading to these inconsistencies in patient response, affecting all fields of pharmacotherapy. Some drugs are known to produce potentially fatal side reactions at therapeutically effective doses. The current accepted method of addressing this situation involves determining the correct concentration of the drug for the patient so that therapy can be ceased before potentially irreversible damage. At best this is complicated, time-consuming, and expensive. It is also potentially dangerous for the patient.

The goal of pharmacogenomics is to maximize beneficial drug responses while minimizing adverse effects for individuals. In the future, pharmacogenomics may hold the promise of personalized drugs; however, genetic variation is not solely responsible for variable drug response. Other factors such as health, diet, and drug combinations are all very relevant.

Pharmacotherapy for neurological disorders falls into specific categories, based on the disease category treated. Categories include:

• brain dysfunction

• thrombotic/embolic brain disease

• hypoxic brain disease

- spinal cord disease
- peripheral nervous system disorders
- cranial nerve disorders
- autonomic nervous system disorders
- seizure disorders
- movement disorders
- sleep disorders
- headache
- delirium and dementia
- dizziness and vertigo
- stupor and coma
- traumatic brain injury
- tumors, both malignant and benign
- demyelinating diseases
- infections (including by prions)

Pharmacoepidemiology and pharmacoeconomics

Epidemiology is the study of the distribution and determinants of disease in large populations. Epidemiology has a precise and strict methodology for the study of disease. Pharmacoepidemiology is the application of epidemiology to the study of the effects of drugs in large numbers of people. The discipline of pharmacoepidemiology maintains a close watch on the therapeutic drugs commonly used in society. If the drug monitoring and reviewing process is not implemented, potential adverse effects of drugs and their misuse could have deleterious effects on the population.

Pharmacoepidemiological studies performed on a population seek to address many different issues. Studies are performed to identify and quantify adverse drug effects, including delayed adverse effects, where most research in pharmacoepidemiology has focused. Analyses evaluate the efficiency and toxicity of drugs in specific patient groups such as pregnant and lactating women. Studies are performed on unanticipated side effects of drugs, along with anticipated side effects to monitor their severity. Research is done on the expected beneficial effects of drugs to verify their efficacy. Also, unanticipated beneficial effects of some drugs are examined. Factors that may affect drug therapy are studied to draw correlations between them and effects on pharmacotherapy. Such factors include sudden changes in drug regimen, age, sex, diet, patient compliance, other diseases, concurrent recreational drug usage, and genetics.

Pharmacoepidemiology can be used in conjunction with pharmacogenomics to examine how genetic patterns present in a population may affect a society's use of a specific therapeutic, or the need for

gene-specific pharmacogenomic studies in a population. Studies are performed to examine a few candidate genes where genetic variability has been shown to have biological consequences. Subsequent research attempts to correlate phenotypic markers with genetic characteristics by association studies, involving the analysis of either a specific drug response as a continuous trait or of separate groups (drug responders versus drug non-responders). These genetic association studies are complex and depend on the frequency of the trait, frequency of the genetic variation within the population, the number of contributing genes, and the relative risk associated with the genetic variation. Reviews of drug utilization are generally done on overuse of drugs or use of costly drugs. Expensive drugs may be reviewed in a cost-benefit analysis involving pharmacoeconomics.

Pharmacoeconomics is closely related to the discipline of pharmacoepidemiology. Analysis of cost effectiveness, cost benefit, and cost utility are incorporated in pharmacoepidemiological research. A related topic of controversy is the validity of using economic analysis of pharmaceuticals as a proxy for prescribing medication, or a reason for prescribing one medication over another. The influence of pharmacoeconomic data on the choice of medication prescribed may be considerable. A general concern is whether a physician has the best interest of the patient in mind or of economics when choosing a medication. While the two concerns are not necessarily in contradiction, they sometimes may be. These topics are also being explored in prescribing research.

Resources

BOOKS

Brunton, Laurence, Bruce Chabner, and Bjorn Knollman, eds. *Goodman & Gilman's The Pharmacological Basis of Therapeutics.* 12th ed. New York: McGraw-Hill Professional, 2010.

Venes, Donald, ed. *Taber's Cyclopedic Medical Dictionary*. 21st ed. Philadelphia: F.A. Davis, 2009.

PERIODICALS

Liepert, J. " Pharmacotherapy in restorative neurology." *Current Opinions in Neurology* 21 (December 1, 2008): 639–43.

WEBSITES

Pharmacogenomics Knowledge Base. http://pharmgkb.org/index.jsp (accessed August 27, 2011).

Maria Basile, PhD
Rosalyn Carson-DeWitt, MD

KEY TERMS

Anticonvulsant drugs—Drugs used to prevent convulsions or seizures. They often are prescribed in the treatment of epilepsy.

Hypnotics—A class of drugs that are used as a sedatives and sleep aids.

Sedative—A medication that has a calming effect and may be used to treat nervousness or restlessness. Sometimes used as a synonym for hypnotic.

Phenobarbital

Definition

Phenobarbital is a barbiturate, a drug that has sedative and hypnotic effects. The drug is classed as a **central nervous system** agent and subclassed as an anticonvulsant (antiseizure).

Purpose

Phenobarbital is used to control the seizures that occur in epilepsy and can relieve anxiety. For short-term use, phenobarbital can help those with insomnia fall asleep.

Description

Phenobarbital is available in tablet or capsule form and as a liquid. All three forms are taken orally one to three times each day with or without food. When taken once a day, the drug is typically taken near bedtime.

Recommended dosage

The dosage is prescribed by a physician. Typically, the total daily dose ranges 30–120 mg. For treatment of seizures, the dosage can be 60–200 mg daily. The daily dosage for children is typically 3–6 mg per 2.2 lb (1 kg) of body weight.

Dosages should not be exceeded. It is also important to adhere to the proper timetable for use of the medication. Use of the drug should not be discontinued without consulting a physician.

Precautions

Phenobarbital is potentially habit forming if taken over an extended period of time. When being prescribed to overcome insomnia, the drug should not be used for a period longer than two weeks. Furthermore, phenobarbital should not be taken in a dose that exceeds the prescribed amount. Ingestion of more than the recommended dosage can result in unsteadiness, slurred speech, and confusion. More serious results of overdose include unconsciousness and breathing difficulty.

Long-term use can lead to tolerance, making it necessary to take increased amounts of the drug to achieve the desired effect. This poses a risk of habitual use; however, it should be noted that people with seizure disorders seldom have problems with phenobarbital dependence. Nevertheless, with chemical dependency, symptoms of withdrawal from phenobarbital begin 8–12 hours after the last dose, and progress in severity. Initial symptoms may include anxiousness, insomnia, and irritability. Twitching and tremors in the hands and fingers precludes increasing **weakness**, **dizziness**, nausea, and vomiting. Symptoms can sometimes become severe or life-threatening, with seizures, **delirium**, or **coma**.

While there is evidence of risk to a fetus, the benefits of phenobarbital for a pregnant woman can sometimes warrant its use. This must be determined by a physician.

Side effects

Common side effects include drowsiness, headache, dizziness, **depression**, stomachache, and vomiting. More severe side effects include nightmares, constipation, and pain in muscles and joints. Side effects that require immediate medical attention occur rarely, and include seizures, profuse nosebleeds, fever, breathing or swallowing difficulties, and a severe skin rash.

Interactions

Phenobarbital can interact with a number of prescription and nonprescription medications including **acetaminophen**, anticoagulants such as warfarin, chloramphenicol, monoamine oxidase inhibitors (MAOIs), antidepressants, asthma medicine, cold medicine, antiallergy medicine, sedatives, steroids, tranquilizers, and vitamins. Interactions with these medications can increase the drowsiness caused by phenobarbital. Decreased efficiency of anticoagulants can increase the risk of bleeding. Phenobarbital can also react with oral contraceptives, which can decrease the effectiveness of the birth control medication.

Resources

PERIODICALS

Beghi, E. "Overview of Studies to Prevent Posttraumatic Epilepsy." *Epilepsia* (2003; Suppl): 21–26.

Galindo, P.A., et al. "Anticonvulsant Drug Hypersensitivity." *Journal of Investigative Allergological and Clinical Immunology* (December 2002): 299–304.

Kokwaro, G.O., et al. "Pharmacokinetics and Clinical Effect of Phenobarbital in Children with Severe Falciparum Malaria and Convulsions." *British Journal of Clinical Pharmacology* (October 2003): 453–57.

Pennell, P. B. "Antiepileptic Drug Pharmacokinetics during Pregnancy and Lactation." *Neurology* (September 2003): S35–42.

OTHER

U.S. National Library of Medicine. *Drug Information: Phenobarbital.* MEDLINEplus Health Information. December 28, 2003 (May 23, 2004). http://www.nlm.nih.gov/medlineplus/print/druginfo/medmaster/a682007.html.

ORGANIZATIONS

Epilepsy Foundation. 4351 Garden City Drive, Landover, MD 20785-7223. Tollfree phone: (800) 332-1000. http://www.epilepsyfoundation.org/.

Brian Douglas Hoyle

Phytanic acid storage disease *see* **Refsum disease**

Pick's disease

Definition

Frontotemporal **dementia** (FTD), originally known as Pick's disease, is a rare form of dementia that is associated with shrinking of the frontal and temporal anterior lobes of the brain. The name and classification of FTD has been a topic of discussion for over a century. The current designation of the syndrome groups together Pick's disease, primary progressive **aphasia**, and semantic dementia as FTD. As it is defined today, the symptoms of FTD fall into two clinical patterns that involve either (1) changes in behavior, or (2) problems with language. The first type features behavior that can be either impulsive (disinhibited) or bored and listless (apathetic) and includes inappropriate social behavior; lack of social tact; lack of empathy; distractability; loss of insight into the behaviors of oneself and others; an increased interest in sex; changes in food preferences; agitation or, conversely, blunted emotions; neglect of personal hygiene; repetitive or compulsive behavior; and decreased energy and motivation. The second type primarily features symptoms of language disturbance, including difficulty making or understanding speech, often in conjunction with the behavioral type's symptoms. Spatial skills and memory remain intact. Although the exact etiology of Pick's diseases is not known, there is a strong genetic component to the disease; FTD often runs in families.

Description

Pick's disease was first described by Arnold Pick, a Czechoslovakian physician who was trained in clinical neurology, psychiatry, and neuropathology. In 1892, Pick reported on a 71-year-old man with progressive loss of language and mental deterioration. After the man died, autopsy revealed asymmetrical atrophy of the frontal cortex of the brain. In 1911, Alois Alzheimer confirmed the pattern of atrophy found in brains of patients with Pick's disease. The term Pick's disease was coined by A. Gans in 1922.

The cortical atrophy seen in Pick's disease is different from Alzheimer's disease, although there are major overlaps with Alzheimer's presenile dementia. In Pick's disease, shrinkage is greatest in the frontal and temporal lobes. One of the characteristics of Pick's disease is microtubule-associated tau proteins, which are the main cytoskeletal components modified during the neurodegenerative changes associated with this disease. In Alzheimer's disease, on the other hand, any area of the brain may be affected. Abnormalities called Pick bodies and Pick cells, abnormally swollen nerve cells, are also found in the brains of individuals with Pick's disease. Pick bodies are found inside nerve cells and contain the abnormal form of tau protein that is associated with Pick's disease.

Researchers continue to debate how to classify Pick's disease. Today, few researchers use the term Pick's disease, although it is still used by patients, caregivers, and some health practitioners. Currently,

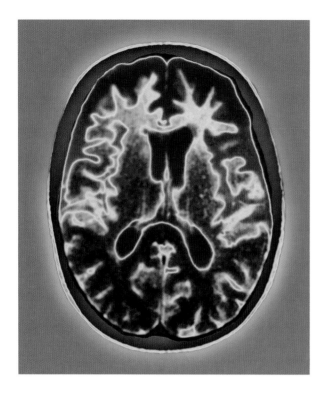

This colored MRI scan shows the progression of Pick's disease as it has caused atrophy in both halves of the brain. *(© Zephyr/Photo Researchers, Inc.)*

Pick's disease is considered to be part of a syndrome that includes not only Pick's disease but also primary progressive aphasia and semantic dementia, which are two related disorders. The syndrome is known as FTD. Some researchers have suggested that some cases of frontotemporal dementia in which Pick bodies or Pick cells are absent may also represent a form of Pick's disease.

Demographics

Pick's disease is rare, affecting less than 1% of the U.S. population. It accounts for about 2–5% of all cases of dementia. Although it sometimes appears in younger or older people, it typically begins in middle age, between the ages of 50 and 60 years. The average age of onset is 54 years, and it tends to occur more often in women than in men.

Causes and symptoms

The symptoms of Pick's disease vary among individuals, but changes in behavior, emotions, and language are frequently associated with neurological problems related to movement and memory. Behavioral changes include disinhibition, inappropriate behavior, compulsions such as a tendency to overeat or eat a particular kind of food, repetitive behavior, social withdrawal, inability to keep a job, difficulty initiating tasks and following through, difficulty maintaining personal hygiene, and a short attention span. Emotional changes include mood swings, inappropriate mood, lack of concern for the feelings of others, apathy, and indifference to behavioral changes. Language changes include decreased ability to read, write, speak, and understand language. Speech difficulties may range from difficulty finding words and diminished vocabulary to a complete inability to speak. Patients also sometimes display echolalia, or a tendency to repeat the words of others. Patients may also experience difficulty with movement and coordination, muscle **weakness** or rigidity, and progressively worsening memory loss. Urinary incontinence may also occur.

In the early stages of Pick's disease, patients frequently demonstrate personality changes that are manifested as inappropriate behavior. This is in contrast to Alzheimer's disease, which, in its early stages, is characterized mainly by memory loss. As Pick's disease progresses, patients become aphonic and apathetic. They eventually lapse into a **vegetative state** and become completely disabled. Death occurs because of malnutrition, infections, or general failure of body systems.

Diagnosis

Diagnosing Pick's disease is difficult, because symptoms overlap with those of other disorders, such as Alzheimer's disease and other dementias that affect the frontal lobes of the brain. According to the National Institutes of Health, at the present time, a definitive diagnosis can only be made with a brain **biopsy**, which is an invasive procedure in which a small sample of brain tissue is surgically removed for examination. Other diagnostic methods are more commonly used, which allow a diagnosis to be made by ruling out other causes of dementia.

Diagnostic procedures include a detailed clinical evaluation to assess personal and family health history, other medical conditions, overall health status, use of prescription or non-prescription drugs, current symptoms, and changes in daily functioning. Blood tests may be done to detect problems in organ function, hormone levels, and vitamin deficiencies. Neurologic exams may be performed to determine which areas of the brain are affected, which can include electroencephalography (EEG), computerized tomography (CT) scans, and magnetic resonance imaging (MRI) scans. A psychiatric evaluation may be carried out to determine whether the patient suffers from disorders such as **depression**, which can mimic or worsen the symptoms of Pick's disease.

Treatments

There is no cure for Pick's disease, and currently, there are no known medications that slow the progression of the disease. Medications that are used to treat Alzheimer's disease should not be used to treat Pick's disease, because they may increase aggression in patients.

Treatments for Pick's disease are designed to manage its symptoms. Behavior modification strategies, which involve rewarding appropriate behavior, may help to decrease unacceptable or dangerous behaviors. Speech therapy may be helpful for increasing language use. Occupational therapy may be used to help patients improve performance of daily living tasks. Encouraging new hobbies may help to relieve boredom in patients and decrease behavior problems.

Disorders that exacerbate confusion, such as heart failure, hypoxia, thyroid disorders, anemia, nutritional deficiencies, infections, and depression, should be treated. Medications that increase confusion, such as **anticholinergics**, analgesics, cimetidine, **central nervous system** depressants, and lidocaine, should be stopped if they are not clearly needed. In some cases, medications may be prescribed to treat aggression, agitation, or dangerous behavior.

In the early stages of Pick's disease, legal advice may help families make ethical decisions about caring for a patient.

As the disease progresses, patients may require constant monitoring and care, either at home or in an institutionalized setting. Help from visiting nurses and aides, volunteer workers, and adult protective services may be needed. Families may benefit from counseling to help them deal with the difficulties of caring for patients. Support groups can also be a helpful resource for families.

Prognosis

The prognosis for Pick's disease is poor. It is a rapidly progressing disease. Death commonly occurs between 2 to 10 years after the onset of the disease.

Prevention

There are currently no known ways of preventing Pick's disease.

Resources

BOOKS

American Psychiatric Association. *Diagnostic and Statistical Manual of Mental Disorders.* 4th ed., Text rev. Washington, D.C.: Author, 2000.

Brookshire, Robert H. *Introduction to Neurogenic Communication Disorders.* 6th ed. St. Louis: Mosby, 2003.

PERIODICALS

Amano, Nanji. "Editorial: Neuropsychiatric Symptoms and Depression in Neurodegenerative Diseases." *Psychogeriatrics* 4 (2004): 1–3.

Hardin, Sonya, and Brenda Schooley. "A Story of Pick's Disease: A Rare Form of Dementia." *Journal of Neuroscience Nursing* 34.3 (2002): 117–23.

Odawara, T., et al. "Short Report: Alterations of Muscarinic Acetylcholine Receptors in Atypical Pick's Disease without Pick Bodies." *Journal of Neurology, Neurosurgery and Psychiatry* 74.7 (2003): 965–68.

Pearce, J. M. S. "Historical Note: Pick's Disease." *Journal of Neurology, Neurosurgery and Psychiatry* 74.2 (2003): 169.

WEBSITES

"Cimetidine." *Medline Plus.* 2003. http://www.nlm.nih.gov/medlineplus/druginfo/medmaster/a682256.html.

"Medical Encyclopedia: Pick's Disease." *Medline Plus.* 2005 http://www.nlm.nih.gov/medlineplus/print/ency/article/000744.htm.

"NINDS Frontotemporal Dementia Information Page." *National Institute of Neurological Disorders and Stroke.* 2006 http://www.ninds.nih.gov/disorders/picks/picks.htm.

ORGANIZATIONS

Association for Frontotemporal Dementias (AFTD),100 North 17th Street, Suite 600, Philadelphia, PA 19103. Telephone: (267) 514-7221, (866) 507-7222.http://www.FTD-Picks.org.

National Aphasia Association, 350 Seventh Ave., Suite 902, New York, NY 10007. Telephone: (800) 922-4622. http://aphasia.org.

NIH Neurological Institute, P.O. Box 5801, Bethesda, MD 20824. Telephone: (800) 352-9424, (301) 496-5751.TTY (for people using adaptive equipment): (301) 468-5981

Pick's Disease Support Group, E-mail: info@pdsg.org.uk. http://www.pdsg.org.uk/index.php.

Ruvanee Pietersz Vilhauer, PhD

Piriformis syndrome

Definition

Piriformis syndrome is a neuromuscular disorder caused by the compression or irritation of the sciatic nerve by the piriformis muscle. It is usually the result of a traumatic injury to the buttocks or hips. The piriformis muscle is a long, narrow, pyramid-shaped muscle located deep in the buttocks that runs from the base of the spine to the top of the femur. Sciatic irritation causes nagging aches, pain, tingling, and numbness in the area extending from the buttocks to the tibia.

Description

Piriformis syndrome is a frequent cause of low **back pain**. Yoeman first described it in 1928, although the term itself was not introduced until 1947, when Robinson correctly identified sciatica as a symptom, not a disease. Diagnosis of the condition remains controversial among physicians.

The condition is caused by the irritation or compression of the proximal sciatic nerve by the piriformis muscle, which at the sacral vertebrae runs through the sciatic notch and inserts at the greater trochanter of the femur. The piriformis muscle is used to help rotate the leg outwards.

Piriformis syndrome is particularly common among skiers, tennis players, long-distance bikers, and truck drivers. In addition, in as much as 20% of the population, the sciatic nerve passes through the piriformis muscle, contributing to the development of the condition.

Demographics

Due to discrepancies in diagnosis, the incidence of piriformis syndrome ranges from very rare to being responsible for approximately 6% of sciatica cases. Women may be affected more frequently than men, with some reports suggesting a six-fold incidence among females. Some reports find that it is most commonly diagnosed in patients between 30 and 40 years old.

Causes and Symptoms

Causes

There is little consensus over the cause of piriformis syndrome. The syndrome is attributed to mechanical or chemical irritation of the sciatic nerve. Approximately 50% of patients have a history of buttocks, lower back, or hip injury, although it is frequently diagnosed in people who sit for long periods of time, presumably because the position leads to compression of the sciatic nerve.

The release of chemical mediators, such as serotonin, prostaglandin E, bradykinin, and histamine, into the region surrounding the sciatic nerve during inflammation contributes to irritation.

Symptoms

Piriformis syndrome is characterized by chronic nagging pain, tingling, or numbness starting at the buttocks and extending along the length of the thigh, sometime descending to the calf. It may worsen with sitting or with lower limb movement.

Diagnosis

Piriformis syndrome is primarily a diagnosis of exclusion, aimed at identifying the piriformis muscle as the primary cause of the pain. Diagnoses should be made through a physical examination and a complete neurologic examination.

Several maneuvers that contract or stretch the piriformis muscle can be performed. Freiberg's maneuver—an inward rotation of the thigh—stretches the piriformis muscle. In sitting patients, Pace's maneuver will elicit pain with the abduction of the affected leg. In Beatty's maneuver, the patient lies on a table on his nonaffected leg, and the knee of the affected leg is bent and placed on the table. Raising the knee several inches off the table causes pain in the buttocks and indicates piriformis syndrome.

Imaging studies of the lower spine can exclude disc protrusion or degeneration, or osteoarthritis, hip and joint disease, and other spinal causes. Nerve conduction studies show delayed F waves and H reflexes.

Treatment Team

The structure of the treatment team will vary on the severity of the condition and on the success of initial interventions. Generally the treatment team is composed of a physiotherapist and a massage therapist. In advanced cases that do not respond to mechanical or pharmacological therapy, surgery may be recommended.

Treatment

Treatment for piriformis syndrome includes avoiding activities that aggravate the condition, such as running and bicycling. Patients who experience pain while sitting for long periods of time, should stand frequently or raise the painful area from the seat.

Physiotherapy aimed at relaxing tight piriformis muscles, hip external rotators, and adductors; that strengthens hip abductors; or that increases the mobility of the sacroiliac joint can be beneficial. Home stretching routines can also be designed for the patient. Ultrasound has been effective for some patients.

Pharmacotherapy, including nonsteroidal anti-inflammatory drugs, analgesics, and muscle relaxants may help. An injection of corticosteroid into the piriformis muscle, close to the sciatic nerve, can also ease pain and reduce swelling. In severe cases, surgical resection of the piriformis muscle can be performed.

KEY TERMS

Corticosteroids—A group of hormones produced naturally by the adrenal gland or manufactured synthetically. They are often used to treat inflammation. Examples include cortisone and prednisone.

Histamine—A substance released by immune system cells in response to the presence of an allergen. It stimulates widening of blood vessels and increased porousness of blood vessel walls so that fluid and protein leak out from the blood into the surrounding tissue, causing localised inflammation of the tissue.

Prostaglandins—A group of hormonelike molecules that exert local effects on a variety of processes including fluid balance, blood flow, and gastrointestinal function. They may be responsible for the production of some types of pain and inflammation.

Sacroiliac joint—The joint between the triangular bone below the spine (sacrum) and the hip bone (ilium).

Serotonin—A widely distributed neurotransmitter that is found in blood platelets, the lining of the digestive tract, and the brain, and that works in combination with norepinephrine. It causes very powerful contractions of smooth muscle and is associated with mood, attention, emotions, and sleep. Low levels of serotonin are associated with depression.

Prognosis

When piriformis syndrome is diagnosed and treated early, prognosis is good.

Special Concerns

Other causes of sciatica must be ruled out. A rapid and accurate diagnosis of piriformis syndrome can localize the cause of the pain and can prevent long-term chronic pain.

Resources

BOOKS

DeLee, J. C., and D. Drez, Jr. *DeLee & Drez's Orthopaedic Sports Medicine, Principles and Practice*, 2nd ed. Philadelphia: Saunders, 2003.

PERIODICALS

Papadopoulos, E. C. and Khan, S. N. "Piriformis syndrome and low back pain: a new classification and review of the literature." *Orthopedic Clinics of North America* 35 (January 2004).

OTHER

"Piriformis Syndrome," Section 5, Chapter 62. In *The Merck Manual of Diagnosis and Therapy*. http://www.merck.com.

ORGANIZATIONS

National Organization of Rare Disorders (NORD). P.O. Box 1968 (55 Kenosia Avenue), Danbury, CT 06813-1968. Phone: (203) 744-0100. Fax: (203) 789-2291. Tollfree phone: (800) 999-NORD (6673). Email: orphan@rarediseases.org. http://www.rarediseases.org.

National Rehabilitation Information Center (NARIC). 4200 Forbes Boulevard, Suite 202, Lanham, MD 20706-4829. Phone: (301) 562-2400. Fax: (301) 562-2401. Tollfree phone: (800) 346-2472. Email: naricinfo@heitechservices.com. http://www.naric.com.

Hannah M. Hoag, MSc

Plexopathies

Definition

Plexopathies are a form of **peripheral neuropathy** (i.e., a form of damage to peripheral nerves).

Common plexopathies include brachial plexopathy affecting the upper thorax (chest and upper back), arm, and shoulder region, cervical plexopathy affecting the neck and head, and lumbosacral plexopathy affecting the lower back and legs.

Description

A branching network of nerves in which individual nerve fibers can pass from one peripheral nerve to another is termed a nerve plexus. Within the **peripheral nervous system**, there are several such plexi (e.g., the cervical plexus, brachial plexus, lumbar plexus, sacral plexus, etc.) that are often associated with neuropathy and pain. These neuropathies are termed plexopathies.

Neural plexi

Neural plexi are branching and interwoven connections among peripheral nerves that allow a redistribution of nerve fibers among the peripheral nerves. As nerves are traced through the peripheral nervous system, they divide into branches that then communicate with branches of nearby nerves. Because peripheral nerves are composed of aggregates or collections of individual nerve fibers, individual fibers are able to pass through the branching connections (e.g., the individual nerve fiber that controls a specific muscle in a distant appendage) to then continue their course within a new peripheral nerve. Although the branching between nerves can be complex, in most cases the nerve fibers pass intact without branching and individual fibers remain separate and distinct.

For example, the brachial plexus is a neural plexus (a grouping and branching of nerves) located deep in the neck, shoulder, and maxilla region that is responsible for the proper innervation and control of the muscles of the shoulder, upper chest, and arms (upper limbs). Because of the complexities of branching nerve roots, trunks, and cords of the brachial plexus, injuries to the brachial plexus region often cause loss or impairments of function at distant muscle groups.

Injury to the median nerve of the brachial plexus can cause a loss of flexion of the fingers. This loss of flexion results in a loss of the critical ability to oppose the thumb with individual fingers. Median nerve impairment can also result in a loss of range of motion of the arm. Individuals who sustain median nerve injury causing loss of index finger flexion may develop an index finger that "points" or remains extended. Because the median nerve ultimately passes through the carpal tunnel of the wrist, injuries or inflammation of the wrist (e.g., **carpal tunnel syndrome**) can result in pain and loss of feeling far away from the wrist itself.

Diverse symptoms

Pain, numbness, tingling, and **weakness** in the area of the affected neural plexus (including the lumbar, sacral, which is also known as the combined lumbsacral pelxi, cervical, brachial, etc.), or in the distal appendage or area of the service by nerve fibers traversing through a particular plexus are symptoms of a potential plexopathy. Trauma, disease, or disorder can result in a plexopathy.

Depending on the source of the damage, treatment for plexopathies can include direct surgical correction, medication to relieve pain, and/or physical therapy.

Plexopathies are often initially diagnosed by a careful evaluation of the patient's history and symptoms, but electromyographic examination and nerve conduction studies are often the most accurate means to localize and determine the exact nature and site of the plexopathy.

Symptoms related to plexpathies can be mild or severe, from diffuse irritation to intense and intractable pain as sometime experienced by cancer patients. In cancer patients, the source of pain may be direct damage to the nerves caused by tumor invasion or by

damage to adjacent tissue (such as by radiation therapy, called a radiation plexopathy).

Damage to the cervical plexus caused by trauma or head and neck tumors often results in pain or a complaint of "aching discomfort" in the neck and head. Cervical plexopathy may be caused by trauma or by head and neck tumors. Brachial plexopathy is commonly related to breast cancer, lung cancer, lymphoma, or metastatic tumor. Similarly, tumors in the pelvis and abdomen may result in plexopathies and pain in the lumar, sacral (lumbosacral) plexi with pain experienced in the abdomen and upper regions of the leg. Specific plexopathy in the sacral region may result in pain in the perineal and perirectal regions.

In many plexopathies, diagnosis can be delayed or made complex by the fact that initial complaints of pain or discomfort may precede (sometimes by weeks, months, or years) the onset of other symptoms of disorder.

Resources

BOOKS

Goetz, C. G., et al. *Textbook of Clinical Neurology*. Philadelphia: W. B. Saunders, 1999.
Goldman, Cecil. *Textbook of Medicine*, 21st ed. New York: W. B. Saunders, 2000.

WEBSITES

"Physical Medicine and Rehabilitation—Plexopathy Articles." *eMedicine.com*. May 9, 2004 (May 27, 2004). http://www.emedicine.com/pmr/PLEXOPATHY.htm.

Paul Arthur

Poliomyelitis

Definition

Poliomyelitis is an infectious disease that is caused by a subgroup of viruses in the Picornavirus family. The hallmark of the disease is the rapid development of paralysis. Poliomyelitis is also commonly called polio and sometimes infantile paralysis. Once a cause of widespread public health measures to control its

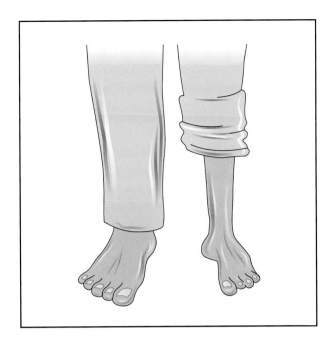

Diagram showing the difference between a healthy leg and foot and one affected by polio. *(Illustration by Electronic Illustrators Group. Reproduced by permission of Gale, a part of Cengage Learning.)*

spread during epidemics, polio is now on the brink of eradication.

Description

The term poliomyelitis comes from the Greek words *polio*, meaning gray, and *myelon*, referring to the spinal cord. The term is accurate, as an important consequence of the disease is the involvement of the spinal cord with resulting paralysis.

Poliomyelitis was first described in 1789, although it likely dates back many centuries prior to that time. Studies of an Egyptian mummy dating from about 3700 B.C. suggest that this individual had polio. Outbreaks occurred in Europe and the United States beginning in the early nineteenth century. For the next hundred years, outbreaks became a regular summer and fall event in northern regions. As time passed, the number of people crippled by the infection rose. By 1952, more than 21,000 people in the United States were paralyzed after surviving a bout of poliomyelitis.

The manufacture and widespread use of several vaccines beginning in the 1950s drastically reduced the number of cases of poliomyelitis. By 1958 an effective oral vaccine was in widespread use in the United States. In the United States, the last reported case of polio acquired from a wild-type (original form of a naturally occurring) virus was in 1979.

Demographics

Humans are the only known carriers of the poliovirus, although polio has been transmitted to monkeys in the laboratory. Poliomyelitis most commonly affects children under the age of five. Several generations ago the disease was much more common than it is now. Even in the 1950s, poliomyelitis was global in its occurrence. Many children in underdeveloped and developed countries, including the United States, were susceptible. With the successful development of vaccines and the implementation of global vaccination and eradication campaigns, the infection has been drastically reduced. Males and females are equally susceptible to polio. Irreversible paralysis, usually in the legs, occurs in about one of every 200 polio infections.

Causes and symptoms

Causes

Poliomyelitis originates with a viral infection. Poliovirus is a member of a group of viruses called enteroviruses. These viruses contain ribonucleic acid (RNA) as their genetic material.

There are three types of poliovirus that are related to each other based on their recognition by the body's immune system. This sort of a relationship is called a serotype. The three poliovirus serotypes are P1, P2, and P3. Even though they are closely related immunologically, developing immunity to one serotype does not provide protection from infection from the other two serotypes. Thus, vaccines are geared towards producing an immune response that will be protective against all three serotypes.

Enteroviruses can be found in the gastrointestinal tract and are not often dissolved by the acidic conditions. Thus, poliovirus can be swallowed and remain intact, capable of causing an infection. As the virus particles lodge at the back of the throat in the pharynx or are swallowed and end up in the intestinal tract, the viruses can begin to multiply. Like all viruses, the multiplication requires a host cell, in this case, cells lining the throat and intestines.

Shortly after the virus enters a person, viral particles can be recovered from the throat and from feces. About one week later, the virus is not usually detectable in the throat, but the virus can continue to be excreted in the feces for several more weeks. During this time, symptoms of the disease do not develop. Thus, the virus can be unknowingly passed to others via the oral or fecal-to-oral route, usually through contaminated food or water. This transmission is a common method of transfer for a variety of viral and bacterial infections in settings such as daycare centers.

Subsequently, the poliovirus invades lymph tissue. From there, the virus can enter the bloodstream and infect cells of the **central nervous system**. This typically takes from 6–20 days after infection. Multiplication of the virus inside motor neurons in the brain destroys the host cells and causes paralysis. The appearance of paralysis is rapid.

Symptoms

Up to 95% of polio infections do not produce any symptoms or damage; however, these individuals will still excrete the virus in their feces and so are capable of infecting others. For every 200 people who are infected with poliovirus, about one person becomes paralyzed.

Approximately 4–8% of polio infections are minor and consist of fairly nonspecific symptoms, including sore throat, fever, nausea, vomiting, abdominal pain, or constipation. Recovery is complete in about a week. Indeed, a person may not know the difference between this polio infection and influenza or some other viral disease. This condition is known as abortive poliomyelitis. There is no involvement of the central nervous system.

In 1–2% of infections, a condition called nonparalytic aseptic **meningitis** occurs. Nonspecific symptoms characterize this condition, followed several days later by stiffness in the neck, back, and/or legs. The symptoms last from 2–10 days. Recovery is complete.

Less than 1% of those who are infected with the poliovirus develop what is termed flaccid paralysis. Paralysis appears anywhere from 1–10 days after symptoms that include loss of reflexes, severe muscle aches, and muscle spasms in the arms, legs, or back. In children, the initial symptoms can begin to fade before paralysis appears. Then over the next few days, the paralysis becomes worse. For many people, muscle strength eventually returns; however, for those who still have weak muscles and/or paralysis a year later, the changes are likely permanent.

Types of paralytic poliomyelitis

Three types of paralysis can develop in poliomyelitis. The first is called spinal polio. This is the most common form of polio-related paralysis, and accounted for nearly 80% of all polio-related paralysis from 1969–1979. This type produces the classical image of a person whose legs have been paralyzed. The second type is known as bulbar polio. This type

accounts for about 2% of known cases. Stiffness and paralysis typically occurs in the neck and head. The third type of polio-related paralysis is called bulbospinal polio. A combination of the previous two conditions, it accounts for nearly 20% of those paralyzed by polio.

Post-polio syndrome

Somewhere between one-fourth and one-half of those who contract polio in childhood will experience muscle pain and **weakness** three or four decades later. This condition is called post-polio syndrome (PPS). PPS is not caused by a recurrence of the viral infection, as no virus can be detected in the feces. Rather, it may result from motor neurons damaged in the initial bout of polio that fail to operate properly decades later. The reason for the failure is not clear, but it appears that the more severe the muscle weakness and disability after initial recovery from polio, the more severe the symptoms of PPS when they appear.

Diagnosis

The diagnosis of poliomyelitis is based on the recovery of the virus from the throat or feces of a person. It is possible to isolate the virus from the cerebrospinal fluid, but this is uncommon. When the virus is recovered, specialized testing can be done to determine if the virus is wild type (that is, it has been acquired from the environment), or whether it is a vaccine type (polio vaccines are made of live, but weakened, polioviruses).

Another means of diagnosis relies on the detection of antibodies that have been produced in response to infection by the virus. Since antibodies are produced as a part of the immunization process, physicians focus on the increasing levels of antibodies over a short time as evidence that the body is battling an active viral infection.

Still another diagnostic test detects increased number of white blood cells and protein in the cerebrospinal fluid. This is a more general response to infections. Other conditions can present similar symptoms, and need to be ruled out when diagnosing poliomyelitis. These include **Guillain-Barré syndrome**, meningitis, and **encephalitis**.

Treatment team

The treatment team ideally consists of the family physician, neurologist, infectious disease specialist, physical therapists, occupational therapists, specialty nurses, and family members. In field conditions in developing countries, the treatment team may consist of a physician and direct caregivers only. World health agencies rapidly mobilize to provide care and vaccinations in order to contain isolated outbreaks in developing countries.

Treatment

Prevention is the watchword for poliomyelitis, and prevention consists of vaccination. There are two polio vaccines available: inactivated (Salk) poliovirus vaccine and oral poliovirus vaccine.

The inactivated vaccine was devised by American physician Jonas Salk (1914–1995) in the 1950s. The vaccine contains all three serotypes of the poliovirus. The viruses, which are inactivated and incapable of causing an infection, are grown in a type of monkey kidney cell. When injected, the viruses stimulate an immune response in humans that is protective. Initially, vaccine impurity caused illness and death in some people who received the Salk vaccine. Refinement of the vaccine preparation eliminated these deleterious effects. Still, in the 1990s, a controversy arose regarding the vaccine as a suggested source of acquired immunodeficiency syndrome (**AIDS**), based on the known presence of the AIDS virus in monkey tissue cells; however, scrupulously conducted examinations ruled out this suggestion.

The oral vaccine was developed by Polish-born American physician Albert Sabin (1906–1993) in the late 1950s and was in widespread use by 1963. This vaccine has largely replaced the injected Salk vaccine. The vaccine contains live but weakened (attenuated) poliovirus.

A series of vaccinations given at 2, 4, and 6–18 months and at 4–6 years produces a lifelong immunity to the three poliovirus serotypes. In regions where poliomyelitis is actively occurring, even a single dose of vaccine can provide improved protection from infection during the outbreak.

As of 2011, in the United States various new formulations of polio vaccine have been approved for use. These include inactivated (dead) polio virus (IPV) alone or in combination vaccines that include IPV plus diphtheria, tetanus, and pertussis (DaTP) vaccine; IPV plus DaTP plus hepatitis B (HepB) vaccine; and IPV plus DaTP plus *Haemophilus influenzae* type b (Hib) vaccine.

Recovery and rehabilitation

There is no cure for poliomyelitis. Some people can partially recover from paralysis, while the condition is irreversible in others. Physical and occupational

KEY TERMS

Disease eradication—A status whereby no further cases of a diseases occur anywhere, and continued control measures are unnecessary.

Flaccid paralysis—Loss of muscle tone resulting from injury or disease of the nerves that innervate the muscles.

Wild-type virus—A virus occurring naturally in the environment or a population in its original form.

therapies can be helpful in providing strengthening exercises and assistive devices for walking, but these are seldom available in remote areas of developing countries where polio outbreaks still occur.

Prognosis

For every 100 people who become paralyzed by the viral infection, 2–5 children and 15–30% of adults will die from polio. Among those who are paralyzed by the viral infection, 5–10% die due to the paralysis of muscles used for breathing.

Special concerns

As of 2010, according to the World Health Organization (WHO), despite extensive vaccination programs, polio has not been eradicated in Afghanistan, India, Nigeria, and Pakistan. Angola, Chad, Democratic Republic of the Congo, and Sudan had at one time eradicated polio, but the disease has re-established itself. In 2010, 13 other countries—Congo, Kazakhstan, Liberia, Mali, Mauritania, Nepal, Niger, Russian Federation, Senegal, Sierra Leone, Tajikistan, Turkmenistan, and Uganda—had outbreaks of polio after the disease was introduced into these country by travelers from infected regions.

Resources

BOOKS

Closser, Svea. *Chasing Polio in Pakistan: Why the World's Largest Public Health Initiative May Fail.* Nashville, TN: Vanderbilt University Press, 2010.

Silver, Julie K. and Daniel Wilson. *Polio Voices: An Oral History from the American Polio Epidemics and Worldwide Eradication Efforts.* Westport, CT: Praeger, 2007

WEBSITES

"Polio and Post-polio Syndrome." MedlinePlus. http://www.nlm.nih.gov/medlineplus/polioandpostpoliosyndrome.html (accessed July 18, 2011).

"Post-polio Information Fact Sheet." National Institute of Neurological Diseases and Stroke. http://www.ninds.nih.gov/disorders/post_polio/detail_post_polio.htm (accessed July 18, 2011).

Vidyadhara, S. "Poliomyelitis." Medscape Reference. http://emedicine.medscape.com/article/1259213-overview (accessed July 18, 2011).

ORGANIZATIONS

National Institute of Neurological Disorders and Stroke (NINDS), P.O. Box 5801, Bethesda, MD 20824, (301) 496-5751, (800) 352-9424, http://www.ninds.nih.gov.

World Health Organization (WHO), Avenue Appia 20, 1211 Geneva 27, Switzerland, 0041 22 791 21 11, Fax: 0041 22 791 31 11, info@who.int, http://www.who.int.

Brian Douglas Hoyle, PhD
Tish Davidson, AM

Polymyositis

Definition

Polymyositis is an inflammatory muscle disease causing **weakness** and pain. **Dermatomyositis** is identical to polymyositis with the addition of a characteristic skin rash.

Description

Polymyositis (PM) is an inflammatory disorder in which muscle tissue becomes inflamed and deteriorates, causing weakness and pain. It is one of several types of inflammatory muscle disease, or **myopathy**. Others include dermatomyositis (DM) and **inclusion body myositis**. All three types are progressive conditions, usually beginning in adulthood. A fourth type, juvenile dermatomyositis, occurs in children. Although PM and DM can occur at any age, 60% of cases appear between the ages of 30 and 60. Females are affected twice as often as males.

Causes and symptoms

Causes

The cause of PM and DM is not known, but it is suspected that a variety of factors may play a role in the development of these diseases. PM and DM may be **autoimmune diseases**, caused by the immune system's attack on the body's own tissue. The reason for this attack is unknown, although some researchers believe that a combination of immune system susceptibility and an environmental trigger may explain at least some cases. Known environmental agents associated with PM and DM include infectious agents such as *Toxoplasma*, *Borrella* (**Lyme disease** bacterium), and coxsackievirus. Most cases, however, have no obvious triggers (direct causative agents). There may also be a genetic component in the development of PM and DM.

Symptoms

The early symptoms of PM and DM are slowly progressing muscle weakness, usually symmetrical between the two sides of the body. PM and DM affect primarily the muscles of the trunk and those closest to the trunk, while the hands, feet, and face usually are not involved. Weakness may cause difficulty walking, standing, and lifting objects. Rarely, the muscles of breathing may be affected. Weakness of the muscles used for swallowing can cause difficulty with swallowing (dysphagia). Joint pain and/or swelling also may be present. Later in the course of these diseases, muscle wasting or shortening (contracture) may develop in the arms or legs. Heart abnormalities, including electrocardiogram (ECG) changes and arrhythmias, develop at some time during the coursed of these diseases in about 30% of patients.

Dermatomyositis is marked by a skin rash. The rash is dusky, reddish, or lilac in color and is most often seen on the eyelids, cheeks, bridge of the nose, and knuckles, as well as on the back, upper chest, knees, and elbows. The rash often appears before the muscle weakness.

Diagnosis

PM and DM are often difficult diseases to diagnose, because they are rare, because symptoms come on slowly, and because they can be mistaken for other diseases that cause muscle weakness, especially limb girdle muscular dystrophy.

Accurate diagnosis involves:

• A neurological exam.

• Blood tests to determine the level of the muscle enzyme creatine kinase, whose presence in the circulation indicates muscle damage.

• Electromyography, an electrical test of muscle function.

• Muscle biopsy, in which a small sample of affected muscle is surgically removed for microscopic analysis. A biopsy revealing muscle cells surrounded by immune system cells is a strong indicator of myositis.

Treatment

PM and DM respond to high doses of immuno-suppressant drugs in most cases. The most common medication used is the corticosteroid prednisone. Prednisone therapy usually leads to improvement within two or three months, at which point the dose can be tapered to a lower level to avoid the significant side effects associated with high doses of prednisone. Unresponsive patients are often given a replacement or supplementary immunosuppressant, such as azathioprine, cyclosporine, or methotrexate. Intravenous immunoglobulin treatments may help some people who are unresponsive to other immunosuppressants.

Pain can usually be controlled with an over-the-counter analgesic, such as aspirin, ibuprofen, or naproxen. A speech-language therapist can help suggest exercises and tips to improve difficulty in swallowing. Avoiding weight gain helps prevent overtaxing weakened muscles.

Alternative treatment

As with all autoimmune conditions, food allergies/intolerances and environmental triggers may be contributing factors. For food allergies and intolerances, an elimination challenge diet can be used under the supervision of a trained practitioner, naturopath, or nutritionist, to identify trigger foods. These foods can then be eliminated from the person's diet. For environmental triggers, it is helpful to identify the source so that it can be avoided or eliminated. A thorough detoxification program can help alleviate symptoms and change the course of the disease. Dietary changes from processed foods to whole foods that do not include allergen triggers can have significant results. Nutrient supplements, especially the antioxidants zinc, selenium, and vitamins A, C, and E, can be beneficial. Constitutional homeopathic treatment can work at a deep level to rebalance the whole person. **Acupuncture** and Chinese herbs can be effective in symptom alleviation and deep healing. Visualization, guided imagery, and hypnosis for pain management are also useful.

Prognosis

The progression of PM and DM varies considerably from person to person. Immunosuppressants can improve strength, although not all patients respond, and relapses may occur. PM and DM can lead to increasing weakness and disability, although the life span usually is not significantly affected. About half of the patients recover and can discontinue treatment within five years of the onset of their symptoms.

About 20% still have active disease requiring ongoing treatment after five years, and about 30% have inactive disease but some remaining muscle weakness.

Prevention

There is no known way to prevent myositis, except to avoid exposure to those environmental agents that may be associated with some cases.

Resources

ORGANIZATIONS

Dermatomyositis and Polymyositis Support Group. 146 Newtown Road, Southampton, SO2 9HR, U.K.

Muscular Dystrophy Association. 3300 East Sunrise Drive, Tucson, AZ 85718. (800) 572-1717. http://www.mdausa.org.

Myositis Association of America. 600-D University Boulevard, Harrisonburg, VA 22801. (540) 433-7686. http://www.myositis.org.

National Institutes of Health. National Institute of Arthritis and Musculoskeletal and Skin Diseases. 900 Rockville Pike, Bethesda, MD 20892. (301) 496-8188. http://www.hih.gov.niams.

Richard Robinson

Pompe disease

Definition

Pompe disease, also called acid maltase deficiency, is a non-sex linked recessive genetic disorder that is the most serious of the glycogen storage diseases affecting muscle tissue. It is one of several known congenital (present at birth) muscular diseases (myopathies), as distinct from a muscular dystrophy, which is a family of muscle disorders arising from faulty nutrition. The Dutch pathologist J. C. Pompe first described this genetic disorder in 1932.

Description

Pompe disease is also known as glycogen storage disease type II (GSD II) because it is characterized by a buildup of glycogen in the muscle cells. Glycogen is the chemical substance muscles use to store sugars and starches for later use. Some of the sugars and starches from the diet that are not immediately put to use are converted into glycogen and then stored in the muscle cells. These stores of glycogen are then broken down into sugars, as the muscles require them. Acid maltase is the chemical substance that regulates the amount of glycogen stored in muscle cells. When too much glycogen begins to accumulate in a muscle cell, acid maltase is released to break down this excess glycogen into products that will be either reabsorbed for later use in other cells or passed out of the body via the digestive system. Individuals affected with Pompe disease have either a complete inability or a severely limited ability to produce acid maltase. Since these individuals cannot produce the amounts of acid maltase required to process excess glycogen in the muscle cells, the muscle cells become overrun with glycogen. This excess glycogen in the muscle cells causes a progressive degeneration of the muscle tissues.

Acid maltase is an enzyme. An enzyme is a chemical that facilitates (catalyzes) the chemical reaction of another chemical or of other chemicals; it is neither a reactant nor a product in the chemical reaction that it catalyzes. As a result, enzymes are not used up in chemical reactions, but rather recycled. One molecule of an enzyme may be used to catalyze the same chemical reaction over and over again several hundreds of thousands of times. All the enzymes necessary for catalyzing the various reactions of human life are produced within the body by genes. Genetic enzyme deficiency disorders, such as Pompe disease, result from only one cause: the affected individual cannot produce enough of the necessary enzyme because the gene designed to make the enzyme is faulty. Enzymes are not used up in chemical reactions, but they do eventually wear out, or accidentally get expelled. Also, as an individual grows, they may require greater quantities of an enzyme. Therefore, most enzyme deficiency disorders will have a time component to them. Individuals with no ability to produce a particular enzyme may show effects of this deficiency at birth or shortly thereafter. Individuals with only a partial ability to produce a particular enzyme may not show the effects of this deficiency until their need for the enzyme, because of growth or maturation, has outpaced their ability to produce it.

The level of ability of individuals with Pompe disease to produce acid maltase, or thier ability to sustain existing levels of acid maltase, are the sole determinants of the severity of the observed symptoms in individuals and the age of onset of these symptoms.

Pompe disease is categorized into three separate types based on the age of onset of symptoms in the affected individual. Type a, or infantile, Pompe disease usually begins to produce observable symptoms in affected individuals between the ages of two and five months. Type b, or childhood, Pompe disease usually begins to produce observable symptoms in affected individuals in early childhood. This type generally progresses much more slowly than infantile Pompe disease. Type c, or adult, Pompe disease generally begins to produce observable symptoms in affected individuals in the third or fourth decades of life. This type progresses even more slowly than childhood Pompe disease.

Genetic profile

The locus of the gene responsible for Pompe disease has been localized to 17q23. The severity of the associated symptoms and the age of onset in affected individuals have been closely tied to the particular mutation at this locus. Three specific mutations and one additional mutation type have been demonstrated to occur along the gene responsible for Pompe disease. Each of these is associated with varying symptoms.

A gene is a particular segment of a particular chromosome. However, within the segment containing a particular gene there are two types of areas: introns and exons. Introns are sections of the segment that do not actively participate in the functioning of the gene. Exons are those sections that do actively participate in gene function. A typical gene consists of several areas that are exons divided by several areas of introns.

One mutation on the gene responsible for the production of acid maltase is a deletion of exon 18. A second mutation on the gene responsible for the production of acid maltase is the deletion of a single base pair of exon 2. Both these mutations are associated with a complete inability of the affected individual to produce acid maltase. Individuals with these mutations will invariably be affected with infantile (type a) Pompe disease.

The third mutation on the gene responsible for the production of acid maltase is a complicated mutation within intron 1 that causes the cutting out of exon 2. This mutation is generally not complete in every copy of the gene within a given individual so it is associated with a partial ability of the affected individual to produce acid maltase. Individuals with this mutation will be affected with either childhood (type b) or, more commonly, adult (type c) Pompe disease. In fact, greater than 70% of all individuals affected with adult Pompe disease possess this particular mutation.

The final mutation class known to occur on the gene responsible for the production of acid maltase is missense at various locations along the various exons. Missense is the alteration of a single coding sequence (codon) that codes for a single amino acid that will be used to build the protein that is the precursor to the acid maltase molecule. These missense mutations generally prevent the production of acid maltase and lead to infantile (type a) Pompe disease.

The exact mutations responsible for the other 30% of the adult (type c) and the remainder of the childhood (type b) Pompe disease cases have not yet been determined.

Demographics

Pompe disease is observed in approximately one in every 100,000 live births. In 2000, it was estimated that between 5,000 and 10,000 people were living somewhere in the developed world with a diagnosed case of Pompe disease. It is observed in equal numbers of males and females and across all ethnic subpopulations.

Since Pompe disease is a recessive disorder, both parents must be carriers of the disorder for it to be passed to their children. In the case of carrier parents with one child affected by Pompe disease, there is a 25% likelihood that their next child will also be affected with the disorder. However, because type c (adult) Pompe disease generally does not show symptoms in the affected individual until that individual is past 30, it is possible for an affected individual to parent children. In this case, the probability of a second child being affected with Pompe disease is 50%. Should two affected individuals bear offspring, the probability of their child being affected with Pompe disease is 100%.

In families with more than one affected child, the symptoms of the siblings will closely correspond. That is, if one child develops infantile Pompe disease, a second child, if affected with the disorder, will also develop the infantile form.

Signs and symptoms

The symptoms of Pompe disease vary depending on the severity of the deficiency of acid maltase in the affected individual. The most acid maltase deficient individuals will develop infantile Pompe disease and will exhibit the most severe symptoms. Likewise, the least acid maltase deficient individuals will develop adult Pompe disease and have less severe symptoms.

Infantile (type a) Pompe disease is characterized by the so-called "floppy baby" syndrome. This condition is caused by extreme **weakness** and lack of tone of the skeletal muscles. This observed weakness in the skeletal muscles is accompanied by the much more serious problems of overall weakness of the heart muscle (cardiomyopathy) and the muscles of the respiratory system, primarily the diaphragm. Enlargement of the heart (cardiomegaly), tongue and liver are also observed. Glycogen accumulation is observed in most tissues of the body.

Childhood (type b) Pompe disease is characterized by weakness of the muscles of the trunk and large muscle mass with little muscle tone. This is due to a buildup of glycogen in the muscle cells. The heart and liver of those affected with childhood maltase deficiency are generally normal. However, there is a progressive weakening of the skeletal and respiratory muscles. The observed muscle weakness in childhood Pompe disease affected individuals gradually progresses from the muscles of the trunk to the muscles of the arms and the legs. Glycogen accumulation is observed primarily in the muscle tissues.

Adult (type c) Pompe disease is characterized by **fatigue** in younger affected individuals and by weakness of the muscles of the trunk in older affected individuals. The observed muscle weakness in adult Pompe disease affected individuals gradually progresses from the muscles of the trunk to the muscles of the arms and the legs. High blood pressure in the artery that delivers blood to the lungs (pulmonary hypertension) is also generally observed in affected adults. Glycogen accumulation is observed primarily in the muscle tissues.

Diagnosis

Infantile Pompe disease is generally diagnosed between the ages of two and five months when symptoms begin to appear. The first indicator of infantile Pompe disease is general weakness and lack of tone (**hypotonia**) of the skeletal muscles, particularly those of the trunk.

A blood test called a serum CK test is the most commonly used test to determine whether muscular degeneration is causing an observed muscular weakness. It is used to rule out other possible causes of muscle weakness, such as nerve problems. To determine the CK serum level, blood is drawn and separated into the part containing the cells and the liquid remaining (the serum). The serum is then tested for the amount of creatine kinase (CK) present. Creatine kinase is an enzyme found almost exclusively in the muscle cells and not typically in high amounts in the bloodstream. Higher than normal amounts of CK in the blood serum indicate that muscular degeneration is occurring: that the muscle cells are breaking open and spilling their contents, including the enzyme creatine kinase (CK) into the bloodstream. Individuals affected with Pompe disease have extremely high serum CK levels. Those affected with infantile Pompe disease have much higher serum CK levels than those affected with the childhood or adult forms. The actual serum CK level, once observed to be higher than normal, can also be used to differentiate between various types of muscular degeneration.

Serum CK levels cannot be used to distinguish Pompe disease from other glycogen storage diseases. Pompe disease (type II glycogen storage disease) is differentially diagnosed from type I glycogen storage disease by blood tests for abnormally low levels of glucose (hypoglycemia) and a low pH, or high acidity, (acidosis). Hypoglycemia and acidosis are both characteristic of type I glycogen storage disease, but neither is characteristic of Pompe disease.

It is sometimes possible to determine the abnormally low levels of the acid maltase enzyme in the white blood cells (leukocytes) removed during the above blood serum tests. If these levels can be determined and they are abnormally low, a definitive diagnosis of Pompe disease can be made. When the results of this leukocyte test are not clear, Pompe disease types a and b may be positively diagnosed by testing muscles cells removed from the affected individual (muscle **biopsy**) for the actual absence or lack of sufficient acid maltase. This test is 100% accurate for type a and type b Pompe disease, but it may give improper results for type c Pompe disease. In these hard-to-identify cases of type c Pompe disease, an identical test to that performed on the leukocytes may be performed on cultured fibroblasts grown from a sample from the affected individual. This test is 100% accurate for type c Pompe disease.

Treatment and management

There is no treatment or cure for Pompe disease. The only potential treatment for this deficiency is enzyme replacement therapy.

Prognosis

Pompe disease of all three types is 100% fatal. Individuals affected with infantile Pompe disease generally die from heart or respiratory failure prior to age one. Individuals affected with childhood

KEY TERMS

Acid maltase—The enzyme that regulates the amount of glycogen stored in muscle cells. When too much glycogen is present, acid maltase is released to break it down into waste products.

Acidosis—A condition of decreased alkalinity resulting from abnormally high acid levels (low pH) in the blood and tissues. Usually indicated by sickly sweet breath, headaches, nausea, vomiting, and visual impairments.

Catalyze—Facilitate. A catalyst lowers the amount of energy required for a specific chemical reaction to occur. Catalysts are not used up in the chemical reactions they facilitate.

Enzyme—A protein that catalyzes a biochemical reaction or change without changing its own structure or function.

Exon—The expressed portion of a gene. The exons of genes are those portions that actually chemically code for the protein or polypeptide that the gene is responsible for producing.

Fibroblast—Cells that form connective tissue fibers like skin.

Glycogen—The chemical substance used by muscles to store sugars and starches for later use. It is composed of repeating units of glucose.

Hypoglycemia—An abnormally low glucose (blood sugar) concentration in the blood.

Intron—That portion of the DNA sequence of a gene that is not directly involved in the formation of the chemical that the gene codes for.

Myopathy—Any abnormal condition or disease of the muscle.

Serum CK test—A blood test that determines the amount of the enzyme creatine kinase (CK) in the blood serum. An elevated level of CK in the blood indicates that muscular degeneration has occurred and/or is occurring.

Pompe disease generally die from respiratory failure between the ages of three and 24. Individuals affected with adult Pompe disease generally die from respiratory failure within 10 to 20 years of the onset of symptoms.

Information about current relevant clinical trials can be found at ClinicalTrials.gov.

Resources

PERIODICALS

Chen, Y., and A. Amalfitano. "Towards a molecular therapy for glycogen storage disease type II (Pompe disease)." *Molecular Medicine Today* (June 2000): 245–51.

Poenaru, L. "Approach to gene therapy of glycogenosis type II (Pompe disease)." *Molecular Genetics and Metabolism* (July 2000): 162-9.

ORGANIZATIONS

Acid Maltase Deficiency Association (AMDA). PO Box 700248, San Antonio, TX 78270-0248. (210) 494-6144 or (210) 490-7161. Fax: (210) 490-7161 or 210-497-3810. *http://www.amda-pompe.org.*

Association for Glycogen Storage Disease (United Kingdom). 0131 554 2791. Fax: 0131 244 8926. *http://www.agsd.org.uk.*

WEBSITES

*Neuromuscular Disease Center*http://www.neuro.wustl.edu/neuromuscular/msys/glycogen.html (February 12, 2001).

*OMIM—Online Mendelian Inheritance in Man.*http://www.ncbi.nlm.nih.gov/htbin-post/Omim/dispmim?232300 (February 12, 2001).

*The Pompe's Disease Page.*http://www.cix.co.uk/~embra/pompe/Welcome.html (February 12, 2001).

OTHER

"Genzyme General and Pharming Group Reports Results From First Two Clinical Trials for Pompe Disease." *Genzyme Corporation Press Release* (October 5, 2000).

Paul A. Johnson

Porencephaly

Definition

Porencephaly is a rare condition in which fluid-filled hollows or cavities develop on the surface of the brain. These cavities usually form at sites where damage has been caused by infection, loss of blood flow, or stroke during brain development, but may also be genetic in origin. Equivalent terms are cerebral porosis, perencephaly, porencephalia, and (no longer in favor) polyporencephaly. The prefix "por" comes from the Latin *porus,* for hole or cavity.

Description

In porencephaly, large dimples, craters, or clefts develop on the surface of the brain. These cavities or cysts are filled with fluid and lined with smooth tissue. They are usually caused by injuries to the fetal or newborn brain before full development of the convolutions or gyri (singular gyrus) on the surface of the cerebrum, especially by infection, ischemia (reduction of blood flow through a vessel), infarction (blockage of blood flow through a vessel), or stroke (bleeding in the brain). The cerebral gyri develop abnormally around a porencephaly cavity, both anatomically and microscopically, and may take on a radiating pattern. Areas of abnormally small gyri (polymicrogyria) may develop on areas of the cerebrum not directly adjacent to a porencephalic cavity.

Porencephaly cavities sometimes develop symmetrically, that is, with a cavity on one side of the brain being matched by a similar cavity on the other side. When a pair of symmetric cavities are very large, they may leave only a thin arch of cerebral cortex running front to back over the top of the brain like a basket handle, a condition termed basket brain. In the most extreme cases, virtually the entire cerebrum may be replaced by fluid, a condition termed **hydranencephaly**.

Demographics

Porencephaly is rare, and its exact incidence is unknown.

Causes and symptoms

Any agent or event that causes localized tissue death in the brain during development can cause porencephaly. The body walls off the injured area with a barrier of smooth tissue (encysts it), and eventually the dead tissue is cleared away and replaced with cerebrospinal fluid. One infectious agent that can cause porencephaly is cytomegalovirus, which can also cause **microcephaly** (small brain). Ischemic brain necrosis, the death of a portion of the brain due to restriction of blood flow through a specific vessel, most often the middle cerebral artery, can also cause porencephaly. Rarely, porencephaly can be caused by a mechanical injury such as accidental penetration of the skull by an amniocentesis needle.

Because porencephaly usually follows from a disruption during development rather than from a genetic defect, it falls into a class of cerebral defects in between primary malformations, those occurring without any specific injury or trigger, and usually genetic in origin, and secondary malformations, those resulting from injury, infection, or some other external cause. The question of whether a given case of porencephaly is primary (genetic) or secondary is important because geneticists wish to provide accurate counseling to prospective parents with family histories of porencephaly. If a familial case of porencephaly is due to infection or injury, there is probably no increased genetic risk for

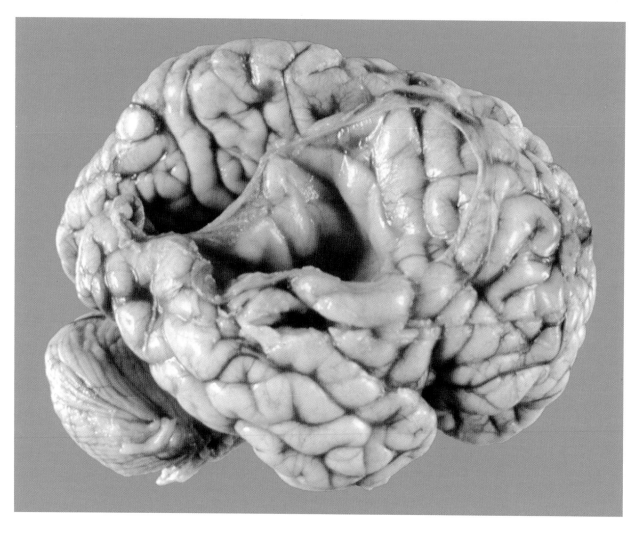

Cavities in a hemisphere of a brain affected with porencephaly. *(© Custom Medical Stock Photo, Inc. Reproduced by permission.)*

future generations. If, on the other hand, a familial case of porencephaly is due to heritable genetic abnormalities affecting clotting factors, for instance, there may be increased risk for a fetus in future pregnancies. Research by the National Institute of Neurological Disorders and Stroke, an arm of the U.S. National Institutes of Health, commenced in 2000 to determine if acquired and/or genetic abnormal coagulation factors in the blood are associated with porencephaly, stroke, and **cerebral palsy**.

The symptoms of porencephaly are varied and depend on the severity of the defects in each individual case. Persons with porencephaly may suffer early death, epilepsy, moderate or severe **mental retardation**, blindness, epilepsy, rigidity, and paralysis.

Diagnosis

Imaging technologies such as ultrasound, x-ray computerized tomography, and magnetic resonance imaging can diagnose porencephaly before or after birth. Ultrasound is preferred for fetal imaging both because it is cheaper than and in most cases just as informative as magnetic resonance imaging or computerized tomography, and because of lingering concerns that magnetic resonance imaging might, by some unknown mechanism, be capable of disrupting the normal formation of organs. (X rays are not used because fetuses are known to be extremely vulnerable to ionizing radiation.) An initial diagnosis can sometimes be made by shining a light through the newborn's skull.

KEY TERMS

Amniocentesis—Surgical withdrawal of a sample of amniotic fluid from a pregnant female for the use in the determination of sex or genetic disorder in the fetus.

Cerebellum—Lower back part of the brain responsible for functions such as maintaining balance, and coordinating and controlling voluntary muscle movement.

Cerebrospinal fluid—Clear fluid that circulates through the brain and spinal cord.

Cerebrum—The main portion of the brain (and the largest part of the central nervous system), occupying the upper portion of the cranial cavity.

Treatment team

As with other severe congenital defects of the brain, the membership of a porencephaly patient's treatment team will depend on the severity and exact nature of the damage. A pediatric neurologist and physical therapist will probably be involved, at minimum.

Treatment

Treatment is addressed to alleviating symptoms, not to curing the underlying problem, as there is no treatment to induce the brain to grow missing sections of the cerebrum. Treatment includes physical therapy for rigidity, **spasticity**, or movement difficulties; medication to prevent seizures; and, if necessary, the installation of a shunt or drain to remove excess cerebrospinal fluid from the inside of the skull.

Clinical trials

Information about current relevant clinical trials can be found at ClinicalTrials.gov.

Prognosis

Most persons with porencephaly die before reaching adulthood. Each individual's prognosis will depend on the location and severity of the lesions on their cerebrum.

Resources

BOOKS

Graham, David I., and Peter L. Lantos. *Greenfield's Neuropathology,* 6th ed. Bath, UK: Arnold, 1997.

OTHER

National Institute of Neurological Disorders and Stroke. *NINDS Porencephaly Information Page.*http://www.ninds.nih.gov/health_and_medical/disorders/porencephaly.htm (April 7, 2004).

ORGANIZATIONS

March of Dimes Birth Defects Foundation. 1275 Mamaroneck Avenue, White Plains, NY 10605. Phone: (914) 428-7100. Fax: (914) 428-8203. Tollfree phone: 888-MODIMES (663-4637). Email: askus@marchofdimes.com. http://www.marchofdimes.com.

National Organization for Rare Disorders. 55 Kenosia Avenue, Danbury, CT 06813-1968. Phone: (203) 744-0100. Fax: (203) 798-2291. Tollfree phone: (800) 999-6673. Email: orphan@rarediseases.org. http://www.rarediseases.org.

Larry Gilman, PhD

Positron emission tomography (PET)

Definition

Positron emission tomography (PET) is a non-invasive scanning technique that utilizes small amounts of radioactive positrons (positively charged particles) to visualize body function and metabolism.

Purpose

PET is the fastest growing nuclear medicine tool in terms of increasing acceptance and applications. It is useful in the diagnosis, staging, and treatment of cancer because it provides information that cannot be obtained by other techniques such as computed tomography (CT) and magnetic resonance imaging (MRI).

PET scans are performed at medical centers equipped with a small cyclotron. Smaller cyclotrons and increasing availability of certain radiopharmaceuticals are making PET a more widely used imaging modality.

Physicians first used PET to obtain information about brain function and to study brain activity in various neurological diseases and disorders including stroke, epilepsy, **Alzheimer's disease**, **Parkinson's disease**, and Huntington's disease; and in psychiatric disorders such as **schizophrenia**, **depression**, obsessive-compulsive disorder, attention-deficit/hyperactivity disorder (**ADHD**), and **Tourette syndrome**. PET is now used to evaluate patients for these cancers: head and neck, lymphoma, melanoma, lung, colorectal, breast, and esophageal. PET also is used to evaluate

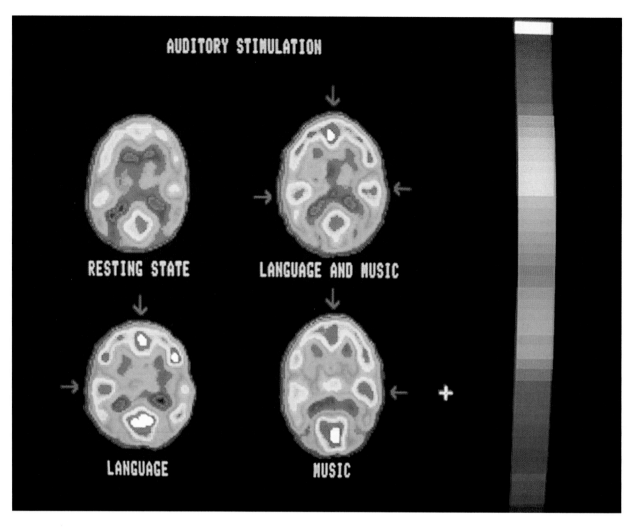

Results of a brain simulation test made with positron emission tomography. *(© Roger Ressmeyer/Corbis)*

heart muscle function in patients with coronary artery disease or cardiomyopathy.

Description

PET involves injecting a patient with a radiopharmaceutical similar to glucose. An hour after injection of this tracer, a PET scanner images a specific metabolic function by measuring the concentration and distribution of the tracer throughout the body.

When it enters the body, the tracer courses through the bloodstream to the target organ, where it emits positrons. The positively charged positrons collide with negatively charged electrons, producing gamma rays. The gamma rays are detected by photomultiplier-scintillator combinations positioned on opposite sides of the patient. These signals are processed by the computer and images are generated.

PET provides an advantage over CT and MRI because it can determine if a lesion is malignant. The two other modalities provide images of anatomical structures, but often cannot provide a determination of malignancy. CT and MRI show structure, while PET shows function. PET has been used in combination with CT and MRI to identify abnormalities with more precision and indicate areas of most active metabolism. This additional information allows for more accurate evaluation of cancer treatment and management.

Resources

BOOKS

Eisenberg, Ronald, and Alexander Margulis. *A Patient's Guide to Medical Imaging.* New York: Oxford University Press, 2011.

KEY TERMS

Electron—One of the small particles that make up an atom. An electron has the same mass and amount of charge as a positron, but the electron has a negative charge.

Gamma ray—A high-energy photon emitted by radioactive substances.

Half-life—The time required for half of the atoms in a radioactive substance to disintegrate.

Photon—A light particle.

Positron—One of the small particles that make up an atom. A positron has the same mass and amount of charge as an electron, but the positron has a positive charge.

QUESTIONS TO ASK YOUR DOCTOR

- What are the indications that I should have a positron emission tomography (PET) scan performed?

- What kind of diagnostic results can be determined with the use of positron emission tomography?

- Should I have other diagnostics tests in addition to a positron emission tomography (PET) scan? If so, what other tests should I have done?

Elgazzar, Abdelhamid E. *A Concise Guide to Nuclear Medicine*. New York: Springer, 2011.

Juweid, Malik E., and Otto S. Hoekstra, eds. *Positron Emission Tomography*. Totowa, NJ: Humana, 2011.

Lin, Eugene, and Abass Alavi. *PET and PET/CT: A Clinical Guide*. New York: Thieme, 2009.

Lynch, T.B., J. Clarke, and G. Cook. *PET/CT in Clinical Practice*. London: Springer-Verlag, 2007.

ORGANIZATIONS

American College of Physicians, 190 North Independence Mall West, Philadelphia, PA 19106-1572, (215) 351-2600, (800) 523-1546, http://www. acponline.org.

American Heart Association, 7272 Greenville Avenue, Dallas, TX 75231, (800) 242-8721, http://www. heart.org.

American Medical Association, 515 N. State Street, Chicago, IL 60654, (800) 621-8335, http://www. ama-assn.org.

National Cancer Institute, 6116 Executive Boulevard, Suite 300, Bethesda, MD, 20892-8322, (800) 422-6237, http:// www.cancer.gov.

Dan Harvey
Lee A. Shratter, MD
Laura Jean Cataldo, RN, EdD

Postinfectious encephalomyelitis *see* **Acute disseminated encephalomyelitis**

Postpolio syndrome

Definition

Postpolio syndrome (PPS) is a condition that strikes survivors of the disease polio. PPS occurs about 20–30 years after the original bout with polio and causes slow but progressive weakening of muscles.

Description

Polio is a disease caused by the poliovirus. It most commonly infects younger children, although it can also infect older children and adults. About 90% of people infected by poliovirus develop only a mild case or no illness at all. However, infected people can continue to spread the virus to others. In its most severe form polio causes paralysis of the muscles of the legs, arms, and respiratory system.

About 1% of all people infected with poliovirus develop the actual disease known as polio. In these cases, the virus (which enters the person's body through the mouth) multiplies rapidly within the intestine. The viruses then invade the nearby lymphatic system. Eventually, poliovirus enters the bloodstream, which allows it to gain access to the **central nervous system** or CNS (the brain and spinal cord). The virus may actually infect a nerve elsewhere in the body, and then spread along that nerve to enter the brain.

The major illness associated with poliovirus often follows a mild illness, which has symptoms of fever, nausea, and vomiting. However, after a symptom-free interval of several days, the patient who is on the way to a major illness develops new symptoms such as headache and back and neck pain. These symptoms are due to invasion of the nervous system. The motor nerves (those nerves responsible for movement of the muscles) become inflamed, injured, and destroyed. The muscles, therefore, no longer receive any messages from the brain or spinal cord. The muscles become weak, floppy, and then totally paralyzed (unable to move). All muscle tone is lost in the affected limb, and the muscle begins to decrease in size (atrophy). The affected muscles are often only on one side (asymmetric paralysis) of the body. Sensation (the person's ability to feel) is not affected in these paralyzed limbs.

The maximum state of paralysis is usually reached within just a few days. The remaining, unaffected nerves then begin the process of attempting to grow branches to compensate (make up for) the destroyed nerves. This process continues for about six months. Whatever function has not been regained in this amount of time will usually be permanently lost.

Causes and symptoms

PPS occurs in about 25% of patients, several decades after their original infection with polio. However, long-term follow-up indicates that two-thirds of polio survivors may experience new **weakness**. Several theories exist as to the cause of this syndrome.

One such theory has looked at the way function is regained by polio survivors. Three mechanisms seem to be at work:

• injured nerves recuperate and begin functioning again
• muscles that still have working nerve connections grow in size and strength, in order to take over for other paralyzed muscles
• working nerves begin to send small branches out to muscles whose original nerves were destroyed by polio

As a person ages, injured nerves that were able to regain function may fail again, as may muscles that have been overworked for years in order to compensate for other paralyzed muscles. Even the uninjured nerves that provided new nerve twigs to the muscles may begin to falter after years of relative over-activity. This theory, then, suggests that the body's ability to compensate for destroyed nerves may eventually begin to fail. The compensating nerves and muscles grow older, and because they've been working so much harder over the years, they wear out relatively sooner than would be expected of normal nerves and muscles. Some researchers look at this situation as a form of premature aging, brought on by overuse.

Other researchers note that normal aging includes the loss of a fair number of motor nerves. When a patient has already lost motor nerves through polio, normal loss of motor nerves through aging may cause the number of remaining working nerves to drop low enough to cause symptoms of weakness.

Other theories of PPS include the possibility that particles of the original polioviruses remain in the body. These particles may exert a negative effect, decades later, or they may cause the body's immune system to produce substances originally intended to fight the invading virus, but which may accidentally set off a variety of reactions within the body that actually serve to interfere with the normal functioning of the nerves and muscles.

Still other researchers are looking at the possibility that polio patients have important spinal cord changes which, over time, affect the nerves responsible for movement.

The symptoms of PPS include generalized **fatigue**, low energy, progressively increasing muscle weakness, shrinking muscle size (atrophy), involuntary twitching of the muscle fibers (fasciculations), painful muscles and joints, difficulties with breathing and swallowing, and sleep problems.

Survivors of polio may also develop arthritis of the spine, shoulders, or arms, related to the long-term use of crutches or overcompensation for weak leg muscles.

Diagnosis

Diagnosis is primarily through history. When a patient who has recovered from polio some decades previously begins to experience muscle weakness, PPS must be strongly suspected.

Treatment

Just as there are no treatments available to reverse the original damage of polio, there are also no treatments available to reverse the damaging effects of post polio syndrome. Attempts can be made to relieve some of the symptoms, however.

Pain and inflammation of the muscles and joints can be treated with anti-inflammatory medications, application of hot packs, stretching exercises, and physical therapy. Exercises to maintain/increase flexibility are particularly important. However, an exercise regimen must be carefully designed, so as not to strain already fatigued muscles and nerves.

Some patients will require new types of braces to provide support for weakening muscles. Others will need to use wheelchairs or motorized scooters to maintain mobility.

Sleep problems and respiratory difficulties may be related to each other. If breathing is labored during sleep, the blood's oxygen content may drop low enough to interfere with the quality of sleep. This

KEY TERMS

Asymmetric—Not occurring equally on both sides of the body.

Atrophy—Shrinking, growing smaller in size.

Flaccid—Weak, soft, floppy.

Paralysis—The inability to voluntarily move.

may require oxygen supplementation or even the use of a machine to aid in breathing.

Prognosis

Prognosis for patients with postpolio syndrome is relatively good. It is a very slow, gradually progressing syndrome. Only about 20% of all patients with PPS will need to rely on new aids for mobility or breathing. It appears that the PPS symptoms reach their most severe about 30–34 years after original diagnosis of polio.

Prevention

There is no way to prevent PPS. However, paying attention to what types of exertion worsen symptoms may slow the progression of the syndrome.

Resources

ORGANIZATIONS

International Polio Network. 4207 Lindell Blvd., Suite 110, St. Louis, MO 63108-2915. (314) 534-0475.

March of Dimes Birth Defects Foundation. 1275 Mamaroneck Ave., White Plains, NY 10605. (914) 428-7100. resourcecenter@modimes.org. http://www.modimes.org.

Polio Survivors Association. 12720 Lareina Ave., Downey, CA 90242. (310) 862-4508.

Rosalyn Carson-DeWitt, MD

Postural hypotension *see* **Orthostatic hypotension**

Prednisone *see* **Glucocorticoids**

Primary lateral sclerosis

Definition

Primary lateral sclerosis (PLS) is a rare disease that causes progressive **weakness** in voluntary muscles such as in the legs, hands, and tongue. PLS is one of the diseases, along with **amyotrophic lateral sclerosis** (or Lou Gehrig's disease) that are grouped together as motor neuron diseases.

Description

Motor neuron diseases like primary lateral sclerosis develop because the nerve cells that normally control the movement of voluntary muscles degenerate and die. The disease is typically detected in middle age, after age 50. The symptoms of the disorder become progressively worse, with muscles typically affected in the following order: legs and feet, main part of the body (the trunk), arms and hands, and face. PLS is not fatal, and people with the disorder can usually maintain mobility with the use of canes or other assistance.

Demographics

Primary lateral sclerosis predominates in those over 50 years of age, although people in their mid-30s can be affected. PLS is rare in younger people, although one case of a 20-year-old has been reported. It is estimated that only about 500 people in the United States have the disease. Due to its historically rare occurrence, it is not yet possible to know if the disease is more prevalent in males or females. The incidence of PLS is uncertain. ALS is known to affect 2–3 people per 100,000. Tentative estimates of the occurrence of PLS are on the order of one person in 10 million, which would make it only about 0.5% as prevalent as the already rare ALS.

Causes and symptoms

The cause of the disease is the progressive degeneration and death of the nerves (neurons) that control the movement of voluntary muscles. There is no evidence of a genetic basis for the disease. Some other process determines the nerve cell death. PLS affects a part of the neuron called the cell body (or soma). Specifically, it is the cell bodies of upper motor neurons that are affected. Upper motor neurons are located in the brain. Their loss affects the transmission of a signal to other neurons that eventually control the muscle activity. This specificity distinguishes PLS from ALS. ALS, the most common motor neuron disease, affects both the upper neurons and also lower motor neurons located in the spinal cord.

PLS is characterized by weakness of voluntary muscles. Typically, the disease is first noticed as a weakening of the legs, hands, or tongue. Other symptoms include difficulty in maintaining balance and clumsiness, sudden muscle spasms, foot dragging, and difficulty in speaking. The neuron death does not affect regions of the brain that control intellect and behavior.

The muscle weakness becomes progressively worse. For some people, this process can stretch over decades. For others, the progression is much faster. While PLS is related to Lou Gehrig's disease, in PLS there is no degeneration of the spinal motor neurons or the wasting away of muscle mass than occurs in ALS.

Diagnosis

Diagnosis is based on the observance of the muscle weakness and the progressive worsening of the weakness. The diagnosis can be delayed because the disease is mistaken for ALS.

Treatment team

Treatment of PLS involves the family physician, a neurologist, and others such as physical therapists. The prolonged nature of the disease means that the energy and commitment of the patient and treatment team must be maintained for a long periods of time, usually decades.

Treatment

The treatment aims to reduce the discomfort and inconvenience of the disease. There is currently no cure for PLS. Medications such as baclofen, **diazepam**, and **gabapentin** have shown effectiveness in reducing muscle spasms in many patients with PLS.

Recovery and rehabilitation

As primary lateral sclerosis is a slowly progressive disorder, emphasis is placed upon maintaining maximum function rather than recovery. Physical therapists can assist with stretching and strengthening exercises to help maintain range of motion and decrease muscle fatigue and spasms. Physical therapists are often involved in assessing gait (manner of walking) and balance and help select the proper type and size of cane or other device to assist with mobility.

Clinical trials

Current information on clinical trials can be found at the National Institutes for Health website on clinical trials at www.clinicaltrials.gov. Aside from clinical trials, research studies seek to develop techniques to diagnose, treat, prevent, and hopefully someday cure motor neuron diseases.

KEY TERMS

Gait—Manner in which a person walks.

Motor neuron disease—A neuromuscular disease, usually progressive, that causes degeneration of motor neuron cells and loss or diminishment of voluntary muscle control.

Prognosis

Because PLS can be a slowly progressing disease, the outlook for a normal life span is good. While life can be greatly changed, a person is still usually able to walk, albeit with the assistance of a cane or other device.

Resources

BOOKS

Parker J. N., and P. M. Parker. *The Official Parent's Sourcebook on Primary Lateral Sclerosis: A Revised and Updated Directory for the Internet Age.* San Diego, Icon Health Publications, 2002.

OTHER

"NINDS Primary Lateral Sclerosis Information Page." *National Institute of Neurological Disorders and Stroke.* http://www.ninds.nih.gov/health_and_medical/disorders/primary_lateral_sclerosis.htm (April 12, 2004).

ORGANIZATIONS

ALS Association (ALSA). 27001 Agoura Road, Suite 150, Calabasas Hills, CA 91301-5104. Phone: (818) 880-9007. Fax: (818) 880-9006. Tollfree phone: (800) 782-4747. Email: info@alsa-national.org. http://www.alsa.org.

National Institute for Neurological Diseases and Stroke (NINDS). 6001 Executive Boulevard, Bethesda, MD 20892. Phone: (301) 496-5751. Tollfree phone: (800) 352-9424. http://www.ninds.nih.gov.

Primary Lateral Sclerosis Newsletter. 101 Pinta Court, Los Gatos, CA 95032. Phone: (408) 356-8227. Fax: (408) 356-8227. Email: 73112.611@compuserve.com.

Brian Douglas Hoyle

Primidone

Definition

Primidone belongs to the class of medications known as anticonvulsants. It is indicated for the control seizures in the treatment of epilepsy and other

---

seizure disorders. Primidome may be prescribed alone or as part of a combination of medications for preventing seizures.

Purpose

Primidone is thought to decrease abnormal activity within the brain that may trigger seizures. While primidone controls some types of seizures associated with epilepsy (grand mal, psychomotor, and focal seizures) there is no known cure for the disorder. Additionally, primidone has shown promise in alleviating some forms of essential tremors but is not approved in the United States for this use.

Description

In the United States, primidone is sold under the names Myidone and Mysoline. Although the precise mechanism by which primidone exerts it therapeutic effects is unknown, it is thought to help slow and control nerve impulses in the brain. The active metabolites of primidone are **phenobarbital** and phenylmethylmalonamide (PEMA), both barbiturate-type compounds with anticonvulsant and sedative properties. Primidone is supplied in chewable tablets (in Canada), tablets to be swallowed whole, and in suspension (syrup) forms for oral administration.

Recommended dosage

Primidone is available in 50 milligram (mg) and 250 mg tablets and is prescribed by physicians in varying dosages. The usual initial dose for adults, teenagers, and children over eight years of age is 100 mg or 125 mg per day. Dosages are gradually increased until arriving at the lowest possible dosage that results in control of seizures. Children under eight year of age typically take an initial daily dose of 50 mg. The maximum daily dose for anyone taking primidone usually is not greater than 2000 mg.

The prescribing physician will schedule a patient's daily dosages, gradually increasing them over the course of several weeks. Primidone may not exert its full therapeutic effect during the initial, dose-increasing period.

Primidone should be taken at approximately the same time every night. If a daily dose is missed, it should be taken as soon as possible. However, if it is almost time for the next dose, the missed dose should be skipped. Double doses of primidone should not be taken.

A patient should consult their physician before they stop taking primidone. Suddenly discontinuing this medicine may cause seizures to return or occur more frequently. When ending treatment including primidone, physicians typically direct patients to taper their daily dosages gradually.

Precautions

A physician should be consulted before taking primidone with nonprescription medications. Patients should avoid alcohol and CNS depressants (medicines that can make one drowsy or less alert, such as antihistimines, sleep medications, and some pain medications) while taking primidone because it can exacerbate their side effects. Primidone may not be suitable for persons with a history of porphyria, asthma or other chronic lung diseases, liver disease, kidney disease, mental illness, high blood presure, angina (chest pain), irregular heartbeats, or other heart problems. Patients should notify their physician if they consume a large amount of alcohol, have a history of drug use, are pregnant, or plan to become pregnant.

Anticonvulsant medications, namely phentoyn and phenobarbital, have been shown to cause birth defects. Physicians usually advise women of childbearing age to use effective birth control while taking this medication. Patients who become pregnant while taking primidone should contact their physician immediately.

Side effects

Patients and their physicians should weigh the risks and benefits of primidone before beginning treatment. Most patients tolerate primidone well but may experience a variety of mild side effects. If any symptoms persist or become too uncomfortable, consult the prescribing physician. The following common side effects usually do not require medical attention and may lessen after taking primidone for several weeks:

- diziness, unsteadiness, or clumsiness
- nausea or vomiting
- decreased sexual desire or ability
- loss of appetite
- mood or mental changes
- tremors

Other, less common side effects of primidone may be serious. Contact a physician immediately if any of the following symptoms occur:

- rash or bluish patches on the skin
- unusual excitement or restlessness (espeically in children, seniors, or patients taking high doasges)

- double vision
- uncontrolled back-and-forth or rolling eye movements
- speech or language problems
- chest pain
- irregular heartbeat
- faintness or loss of consciousness
- persistant, severe headaches
- persistant fever or pain

Interactions

Primidone may have negative interactions with adrenocorticoids (cortisone-like medications), antibiotics, antidepressants, anticoagulants, antihistimines, asthma medications, barbituates, and monoamine oxidase inhibitors (MAOIs). Primidone should be used in conjunction with other seizure prevention medications, especially **valproic acid**, only if advised and closely montiored by a physician. Primidone may decrease the effectiveness of oral contraceptives (birth control pills) that contain estrogen.

Resources

BOOKS

Devinsky, Orrin. *Epilepsy: Patient and Family Guide*, 2nd. ed. Philadelphia: F. A. Davis, 2001.

Weaver, Donald F. *Epilepsy and Seizures: Everything You Need to Know*. Toronto: Firefly Books, 2001.

OTHER

"Primidone (systemic)." *Medline Plus*. National Library of Medicine. http://www.nlm.nih.gov/medlineplus/druginfo/uspdi/202479.html (April 4, 2004).

"Primidone (systemic)." *Thompson Micromedex*. http://health.yahoo.com/health/drug/202479/ (April 4, 2004).

ORGANIZATIONS

American Epilepsy Society. 342 North Main Street, West Hartford, CT 06117-2507. http://www.aesnet.org.

Epilepsy Foundation. 4351 Garden City Drive, Landover, MD 20785-7223. Phone: (800) 332-1000. Tollfree phone: (800) 332-1000. http://www.epilepsyfoundation.org.

Adrienne Wilmoth Lerner

Prion diseases

Definition

Prion diseases are a group of fatal diseases caused by prions, which are infectious agents that consist of protein in a misfolded form. Prion diseases are also called transmissible spongiform encephalopathies (TSEs) because of the sponge-like holes they leave in infected brains. Prions have the ability to transform normal, benign protein molecules into infectious, deadly ones by altering their structure. These deadly proteins initiate a sequence of events in which many benign proteins are transformed into new deadly ones upon contact. Prions are distinct from all other infectious materials in that they do not contain any genetic material. There are multiple prion diseases, including bovine spongiform **encephalopathy** (BSE), or "mad cow disease." Some prion diseases are hereditary, involving a mutation in the gene that encodes for the prion protein. Prion diseases are transmissible within a species and between compatible species.

Description

Research on prion diseases began with Stanley Prusiner (1942—), a neurologist at the University of California, San Francisco. Prusiner spent two decades working on the revolutionary topic of self-reproducing prions. At the time, many other scientists regarded their existence as a preposterous subject. Despite being shunned by the scientific community, Prusiner was able to prove that prions are truly infectious proteins that can cause brain disease in people and animals. The Nobel Prize for Medicine or Physiology was awarded to Prusiner in 1997 for discovering this new genre of disease-causing agents that contain no DNA.

Prion diseases are transmissible between hosts of a single species and different, compatible species. The term "spongiform" in TSE comes from the spongy appearance of the damaged brain tissue. Some examples of infectious prion diseases are scrapie in sheep and goats, **kuru** in cannibalistic humans of Papua New Guinea, and BSE, or mad cow disease, which is

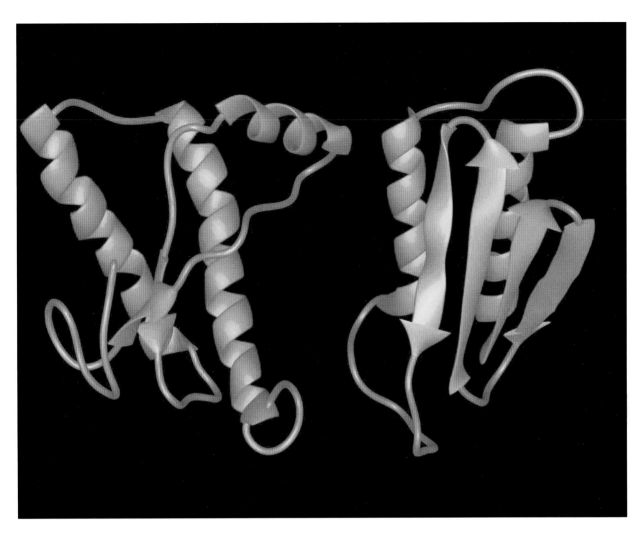

A computer-generated illustration showing, on the left, a human prion protein in its normal shape at the molecular level, and, on the right, a disease-causing, abnormally shaped prion protein. The blue arrow indicates beta strands, the green spiral shapes are alpha helices, and the yellow strands depicts the chain connecting the regions. (© AP Images)

transmitted to humans through infected beef products. Prion diseases can also be transmitted through injections of infected material from a compatible organism. Because of the ability of prions to cross many species barriers, all organisms that carry prion diseases are potential vectors for human infection. These infectious prion diseases are classified as zoonoses. A zoonosis is any disease that can be transmitted from nonhuman animals to humans (or the reverse).

Prion diseases can also be hereditary, as seen in some cases of **Creutzfeldt-Jakob disease** (CJD; pronounced KROYTZ-felt YAH-kob), fatal familial insomnia (FFI), and Gerstmann-Sträussler-Scheinker disease (GSS). Hereditary prion diseases occur when the *PRNP* gene that encodes for the normal human PrP^c

protein, found on the surface of neurons, is mutated so that the prion PrP^{Sc} protein (Sc for scrapie) is formed. The PrP^{Sc} protein has a different conformational structure than the normal protein and is the infectious agent. PrP^{Sc} proteins can convert similar PrP^c proteins upon contact into more infectious agents, thereby reproducing themselves. Prion diseases are inherited when at least one copy of the mutated *PRNP* gene is present. It is the only gene known to be associated with inherited prion diseases as of 2011. Nervous tissue from patients with hereditary prion diseases is also infectious.

A third category of prion disease is sporadic. CJD and FFI sometimes occur in people with no known history of the disease in their family and with no known exposure to infectious materials. The cause of disease in these cases is unknown. Patients with

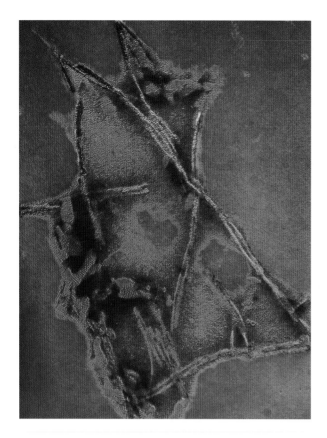

Close-up of prion structure. Amyloid fibrilis form when the protein alters. *(EM Unit, VLA)*

sporadic prion diseases may have a susceptibility polymorphism in their *PRNP* gene and may have spontaneous mutations forming prion proteins.

Demographics

Sporadic CJD, with no recognizable pattern of transmission, has an incidence of about one case per million people per year worldwide. It makes up 85% of total CJD cases and 80% of all prion disease cases. In the United States, there are approximately 200 sporadic CJD cases per year; a recent study indicates that Caucasians are 2.7 times more likely to develop CJD than African Americans. The reason for this difference is not known as of 2011.

Approximately 15% of CJD cases are inherited and associated with a different prion type from that of sporadic CJD. Inherited CJD may show up in geographic clusters. A 60–100-fold increase in CJD is seen in Libya- or Slovakia-born Israelis due to a *PRNP* gene mutation rather than transmission or environmental factors. Other communities genetically at increased risk are located in some areas of Chile. CJD cases caused by

such accidental transmission routes as surgical instruments and transplants are extremely rare and make up less than 1% of total cases. In the United States, CJD cases are almost always diagnosed in patients older than 30 years of age. In the United States, patients under 30 dying of CJD are fewer than one case per 100 million people per year, whereas in the United Kingdom, patients dying of a variant CJD (vCJD) in this age group make up over 50% of the CJD cases.

GSS is rarer than CJD, striking one person in every 10 million people. These figures are likely to be underestimated since prion diseases may be misdiagnosed as other neurological disorders. Kuru occurred in approximately 1% of the indigenous New Guinea population it is associated with. Kuru is found mostly in children older than five years and adult females under 40 years of age.

BSE has been transmitted to humans primarily in the United Kingdom, causing vCJD. An epidemic of mad cow disease began in the United Kingdom in 1985 when cattle feed was contaminated with brain tissue from scrapie-infected sheep. More than 170,000 cattle were infected before the disease was brought under control. Cattle feed containing sheep matter was banned in 1988. In 1989, slaughter techniques that allow nervous tissue to be included in beef intended for human consumption were banned. The mad cow disease epidemic of the United Kingdom reached its peak in 1992 but then declined quickly. More than one million cattle may have been infected with BSE in the United Kingdom. The percentage of BSE cases in cattle reported outside of the United Kingdom is steadily increasing as surveillance increases and disease rates rise. The BSE epidemic in the United Kingdom may have peaked. How much of the population has vCJD in the incubation phase is yet to be determined.

To prevent the spread of BSE to the United States, severe restrictions were placed on the importation of ruminants and ruminant products from Europe. In 1997, the U.S. Department of Agriculture (USDA) also implemented a ban on the use of ruminant tissue in ruminant feed. In 2002, the Centers for Disease Control and Prevention (CDC) reported a case of vCJD in the United States in a 22-year-old patient who was born and grew up in the United Kingdom. Mad cow disease made its first appearance in cattle of the United States in December 2003, when the USDA announced a possible diagnosis in a cow from Washington State. This diagnosis was confirmed within the month at a laboratory in the United Kingdom. The cow was believed to be imported from Canada in 2001 and had been slaughtered for human consumption. The USDA recalled all beef slaughtered at the same slaughter plant on the same date as the infected cow.

Causes and symptoms

Ingested prions are absorbed through Peyer's patches of the small intestine, which are lumps of lymphoid tissue that readily allow the passage of gut antigens. Peyer's patches are a part of the mucosal-associated lymphoid tissue that presents microorganisms to the immune system and would normally facilitate a protective immune response; however, prions do not activate any immune response. Prions passed through Peyer's patches travel to various sites in the lymph system, such as nodes and the spleen. Because many lymph sites are innervated, prions gain access to the nervous system, make their way to the spinal cord, and eventually the brain.

In contrast to bacteria and viruses, prions are not killed by high doses of ultraviolet radiation. Prions are also resistant to high temperatures, strong degradative enzymes, and chemicals. Because of these properties, prions are resistant to many methods of sterilization and to protective, degradative enzymes in the human brain. The plaques formed in the brain by prion proteins are amyloid deposits similar to those seen in **Alzheimer's disease**. Most brain cells contain enzymes that degrade these aggregations. Prions are resistant to these enzymes. The plaques continue to grow and cause damage to the brain, usually along with the formation of large vacuoles that give the brain a spongiform appearance. Brain damage manifests itself in a loss of coordination, paralysis, **dementia**, and wasting, followed by death. Pneumonia also frequently occurs in patients with prion diseases. All prion diseases are inevitably fatal; there are no known cures.

Prion diseases can be inherited in an autosomal dominant matter. This means if one parent carries the mutation on their *PRNP* gene, each offspring has a 50% chance of inheriting the mutation. In this manner, patients with a prion disease have inherited at least one copy of a mutated *PRNP* gene on human chromosome 20. There are a variety of mutations in the gene that cause resultant mutated proteins to be expressed, with each type of mutation resulting in a different prion strain, and a different inherited prion disease. Strains show very different and reproducible patterns of brain degeneration. Extracts of autopsied brain tissue from infected patients have been used for research on prion diseases. It has been demonstrated that only animals whose *PRNP* gene is similar enough

to humans can be infected with human prions. Similarly humans can only be infected by prions from animals whose *PRNP* gene ultimately encodes for a prion protein that is similar to that of humans. Prions transform their normal cellular counterparts into other prions only between prion-compatible species. Infectious prion diseases are transmitted through consumption of infected materials or through injection of ground-up infected tissues. Prion diseases are not contagious in the traditional sense. Individuals who live with patients with prion diseases are at no increased risk. While casual contact does not transmit the disease, brain tissue and cerebrospinal fluid from patients with prion diseases should be avoided.

Inherited prion diseases

GERSTMANN-STRÄUSSLER-SCHEINKER DISEASE. Caused by the GSS prion, this disease was first described in 1928. GSS is associated with variations in at least one *PRNP* gene sequence at positions 102 and 117. It is also highly associated with a polymorphism on both gene copies at position 129 on the human *PRNP* gene. GSS typically occurs between the ages of 35 and 55. It is characterized by progressive cerebellar **ataxia** and associated motor complications, following a time course of 2–10 years before death. Dementia with GSS is less common than with CJD, except in very late stages of disease following a long course. GSS is almost always inherited but has been known to occur sporadically as well.

CREUTZFELDT-JAKOB DISEASE. Caused by the CJD prion, this disease is associated with variations in the *PRNP* gene at positions 178 and 200, along with an insertion of extra DNA in the familial form. CJD was first described in the 1920s as a progressive dementia, following a course of one year, ending in death. CJD presents with a variety of motor disturbances, including twitching. CJD typically occurs between the ages of 50 and 75. While CJD is an inherited disease, the majority of CJD occurs sporadically. Other CJD cases are due to accidental exposure to infected material. The United States has reported fewer than 300 cases of CJD a year in recent years.

FATAL FAMILIAL INSOMNIA. Caused by the FFI prion, FFI is a rare disorder first described in 1986. It is caused by inherited mutations in the *PRNP* gene at position 178 and a polymorphism at position 129. FFI typically occurs between the ages of 40 and 60, and is characterized by progressive sleep disturbance classified as untreatable insomnia, ataxia (motor dysfunction), and dysautonomia (sensory dysfunction). The disease course is 7–18 months, followed by death. Postmortem studies associate this prion disease with severe selective atrophy of the thalamus, a brain region controlling sleep and wakefulness. Sporadic FFI has been reported without the characteristic gene mutation.

ALPERS SYNDROME. Alpers syndrome or Alpers disease is the term used to describe a rare disorder in infants and small children caused by a mutation in the *POLG* gene. It is named for Bernard Jacob Alpers (1900–1981), an American neurosurgeon. Alpers disease is sometimes misdiagnosed as a prion disease in small children; however, it is not an inherited prion disease but is better understood as a genetically determined progressive degeneration of the grey matter of the brain resulting from depletion of mitochondrial DNA.

Infectious prion diseases

SCRAPIE. Caused by the scrapie prion, scrapie is the first prion disease ever studied. Scrapie was first described in sheep and goats more than 200 years ago. It is transmitted through feed contaminated with nervous tissue. It can also be transmitted through pasture infected with placental tissue from infected sheep. The term "scrapie" comes from the behavior of infected sheep that rub up against the fences of their pens to remain upright despite severe ataxia, a loss of muscular coordination due to brain damage. Autopsies of infected animals reveal spongiform encephalopathy. In 1943, scrapie was demonstrated as transmissible when a contaminated vaccine infected healthy sheep.

KURU. Decades after scrapie was first discovered, a similar disorder was described in humans called kuru. Kuru was characterized in 1950 as a progressive cerebellar ataxia associated with a shivering **tremor**, with a disease course of 3–9 months, followed by death. The word *kuru* comes from the Fore (pronounced FOR-ay) language and means "tremor." Caused by the kuru prion, kuru primarily occurred in the Fore highland people of southern New Guinea, whose cultural practice used to involve ritualistic ingestion of the brain tissue of recently deceased family members. The brain tissue was ground into a pale gray soup, heated, and consumed. Statistically, women of the Fore tribe were more likely than men to develop kuru, due to their greater involvement in the preparation of the brain tissue. Infection in the female population was probably via both ingestion and through minor skin abrasions. Clinically, kuru resembles CJD. Since this practice has stopped, the disease has ceased to occur.

BOVINE SPONGIFORM ENCEPHALOPATHY. Humans consuming infected beef are susceptible to the BSE prion strain. Strain typing shows one major strain.

BSE is especially insidious in that it is compatible with and transmissible to a wide variety of species. While food items containing blood or nervous tissue are potential vectors for human infection, milk and milk products from cows are not believed to pose any risk for transmitting the BSE prion to humans (see also vCJD).

On February 18, 2011, the Canadian Food Inspection Agency (CFIA) reported a case of BSE in a dairy cow born in Alberta in 2004. The agency determined that no part of the affected animal's carcass entered the human food chain or animal feed systems. One Canadian epidemiologist noted in 2010 that the risk of BSE in Canada has declined noticeably in recent years. A European team reached the same conclusion about the countries of Western Europe.

ACQUIRED CREUTZFELDT-JAKOB DISEASE. While CJD is an inherited disease it can also be acquired through iatrogenic transmission, which is accidental exposure to CJD prion-contaminated material through a medical procedure using tainted human matter or surgical instruments. Recipients of corneal transplants and of grafts of dura mater (brain-associated connective tissue) have been infected with CJD. The CDC has continued surveillance of reports from Japan concerning this form of transmission up through 2008. Because prions are resistant to many sterilization procedures and to degradation, surgical instruments used in brain surgery have infected new patients two years after being sterilized. More than 100 people have been infected with CJD through injections of human growth hormones prepared from pools of pituitary glands that included materials from humans with CJD. At present, growth hormones are prepared through recombinant DNA technology and surgical instruments used on potentially infected patients have new sterilization guidelines, so the transmission of CJD via these routes has ceased to occur. The National Center for Infectious Diseases has not found any iatrogenic CJD cases linked to contact with pathogens from such surfaces as floors or countertops.

VARIANT CREUTZFELDT-JAKOB DISEASE (VCJD). Variant CJD appeared in 1996 during the mad cow disease epidemic in the United Kingdom. The specific strain found in these patients indicates that they have been infected with prions from contaminated beef, the BSE prion; however, victims of vCJD are homozygous for a polymorphism on the *PRNP* gene at codon 129. Patients with vCJD may develop the disease at an unusually early age with the current median age of 29 years at death, but the incubation time period before the onset of symptoms may be as long as 40 years. The vCJD affects people between 15 and 60 years of age. The clinical symptoms associated with vCJD differ from those seen with CJD, including psychiatric or sensory symptoms early in the course of the disease, delayed onset of neurological abnormalities that follow a pattern identifiable as but different from CJD, and a duration of illness of at least six months, followed by death.

As of May 2011, evidence indicates there has never been a case of vCJD transmitted through direct contact of one person to another. In June 2008 the CDC ruled that the death of a Virginia woman was *not* caused by vCJD. As of March 2010, 215 cases of variant CJD have been reported worldwide: 169 in the United Kingdom, 25 in France, 5 in Spain, 4 in Ireland, 3 in the United States and the Netherlands, 2 in Italy and Portugal, and one each in Canada, Japan, Portugal, and Saudi Arabia.

MISCELLANEOUS INFECTIOUS PRION DISEASES. Cats and mink are susceptible to species-specific forms of TSE known as feline spongiform encephalopathy (FSE) and transmissible mink encephalopathy (TME) respectively. Ostriches have also been found to suffer from a form of spongiform encephalopathy. In many Midwestern states of the United States, elk and mule deer can carry a form of TSE called chronic wasting disease (CWD). CWD prions may possibly be transmissible to humans consuming venison the same way as mad cow disease can be transmitted through contaminated beef; however, there is no evidence as of 2011 that transmission to humans has occurred.

Diagnosis

There is currently no single diagnostic test for any prion disease. Physicians initially rule out such treatable forms of dementia as classical **encephalitis**. Standard diagnostic tests include a spinal tap to exclude other diseases and an electroencephalogram (EEG) to record the patient's brain wave pattern. Computed tomography (CT) scans and magnetic resonance imaging (MRI) can rule out the possibility of stroke and reveal characteristic patterns of brain degeneration associated with various types of prion diseases.

Diagnosis classically relied on clinical symptoms, transmissibility, and postmortem neuropathology. With these diagnostic criteria, many cases of prion diseases may have been misdiagnosed as other neurodegenerative disorders. Modern diagnosis is also dependent on detection of prion proteins and identification of mutations in the *PRNP* gene: A genetic sequence analysis can be performed for a number of different mutations associated with familial CJD. The types of mutations present determine which symptoms will be most prominent, although the presence of these mutations on the *PRNP* gene does not necessarily result in CJD. Most CJD patients contain a specific protein known as the 14-3-3

protein in their cerebrospinal fluid and an abnormal EEG brain wave pattern that is diagnostic for CJD. Confirmation requires neuropathological testing of brain tissue obtained through brain **biopsy** or autopsy. Brain biopsies are usually performed only when required to exclude another condition that may be treatable.

A diagnosis of prion disease is confirmed through examination of the brain tissue. Visible postmortem characteristics of the brain include noninflammatory lesions, vacuoles, amyloid protein deposits forming plaques that follow prion type-specific patterns, and measurable biochemical changes. While dramatic alterations in the brain's appearance are primarily the case, more subtle and non-characteristic changes have also been reported. Some forms of prion disease with shorter durations create plaques in only a small percentage of patients.

Clinical signs of prion disease in sheep and cattle include cerebellar ataxia (loss of muscle coordination), polydipsia (excessive drinking), and an itching syndrome that, along with the lack of coordination, causes the animals to rub up against fences. Animals are not diagnosed with prion disease until brain autopsy reveals neuropathology similar to that seen in humans.

Treatment team

Primary care physicians may notice symptoms of a neurological disorder in a patient and refer them to a neurologist—a specialist in brain disorders. Both doctors, along with nurses and other health care specialists, will act as the treatment team for patients with prion diseases.

Oversight of the BSE Action Plan in the United States is carried out by the Department of Health and Human Services (DHHS). Under this plan, surveillance for human disease is the responsibility of the CDC. Protection against this disease is the responsibility of the Food and Drug Administration (FDA). Research is primarily the responsibility of the National Institutes of Health (NIH).

Treatment

There is no known effective treatment to arrest or cure prion diseases. Treatment focuses on alleviating the patient's symptoms, increasing the patient's comfort, and palliative care at the end of life. Treatment may include medications to control pain and motor disorders, catheters to collect urine, intravenous fluids to maintain hydration, and frequently repositioning the patient to avoid bedsores. Antidepressants have been found helpful in relieving the psychiatric symptoms of prion diseases, and counseling for the patient's family is also beneficial.

Possible future treatments developed may include chemicals that bind to and stabilize PrP^c, agents destabilizing the PrP^{Sc} protein, or agents that interfere with the intereaction between PrP^c and PrP^{Sc}.

Although a vaccine against prion diseases would be highly desirable, researchers in the field report that the development of such a vaccine faces significant obstacles as of 2011 because of the risk to the recipient's immune system. An anti-prion vaccine would have to stimulate the immune system to respond to the presence of a disease agent that has become part of the person's own protein production.

Recovery and rehabilitation

There is no recovery or rehabilitation program as of 2011 for patients diagnosed with a prion disease.

Clinical trials

There were four clinical trials in progress as of early 2011; two are clinical trials of quinacrine, an antimalarial drug sold under the trade name Atabrine, as a treatment for prion diseases. One drawback of quinacrine therapy is its severe side effects, which include anxiety, **depression**, and hallucinations. The remaining two studies involve research for biomarkers to detect prion diseases in their early stages. Information about current relevant clinical trials can be found at ClinicalTrials.gov.

Prognosis

Prions bring about slow degeneration of the **central nervous system**, inevitably leading to death. A very long time period passes between a patient's infection and the initial appearance of clinical symptoms, an incubation process that may take up to 40 years in humans. Once the symptoms appear, the patient generally dies within a few months with rapid, progressive symptoms. As of 2011, prion diseases are fatal.

Special concerns

Highly effective public health control procedures have been implemented in Europe to prevent potential BSE-infected tissue from entering the human food chain. The current risk of becoming infected with vCJD from eating beef and beef products in the United Kingdom is very small, at a rate of one case per 10 billion servings. Other countries have equal or lesser rates of risk. To reduce the risk of being infected with vCJD from food while traveling to geographical

---

KEY TERMS

Ataxia—Lack of movement coordination resulting from loss of function in the parts of the nervous system that control movement.

Autosomal dominant inheritance—A pattern of inheritance in which a trait will be expressed if the gene governing that trait is inherited from either parent.

Electroencephalogram—A recording of the electrical signals produced by the brain.

Encephalopathy—The medical term for a disease or disorder of the brain.

Kuru—A prion disease associated with the cannibalism formerly practiced by the Fore people of Papua New Guinea. Its name comes from a word in the Fore language that means "to shake" or "to tremble."

Polymorphism—A difference in DNA sequence among individuals; genetic variation.

Prion—An infectious agent consisting of protein in a misfolded form. Its name is a combination of "protein" and "infection."

Quinacrine—An antimalarial drug that is being tested as a possible treatment for prion diseases.

Sporadic—Occurring at random in persons with no known risk factors or genetic mutations.

Zoonosis (plural, zoonoses)—Any disease that can be transmitted from nonhuman animals to humans or from humans to nonhuman animals. Some prion diseases are zoonoses.

---

areas associated with risk, travelers who do not wish to avoid eating beef entirely may reduce their risk by selecting beef products in solid pieces, as opposed to ground beef tissue.

Variant CJD (vCJD) is more likely to be transmitted through blood than classical CJD. As of May 2011, there have been two cases reported worldwide of patients developing vCJD following blood transfusions. To reduce the risk of transmission from blood products to humans, those individuals who have lived cumulatively for five or more years in Europe since the year 1980 to the present have been deferred by the FDA from donating blood or blood products. Individuals living specifically in the United Kingdom for three months or more from 1980 to 1996 are also deferred.

The CDC has established a National Prion Disease Pathology Surveillance Center (NPDPSC) that provides high-tech diagnostic services to physicians

QUESTIONS TO ASK YOUR DOCTOR

- What are my risks of acquiring a prion disease from the food supply or a blood transfusion?
- What is my risk of developing an inherited prion disease?
- Would you recommend genetic testing for a defective *PRNP* gene?

in the United States. Relatives of CJD patients who wish to assist research have their physician send brain tissue, blood, cerebrospinal fluid, and urine samples to the center. As of May 1, 2011, the Center charges a fee for diagnostic testing of CJD.

Prion research has been done in yeast, a convenient organism easily used in scientific study. Yeast can be infected with prions, begin forming their own prion proteins, and pass the infection on to further generations of yeast. It has been noted that yeast can be "cured" of their prion disease by increasing the activity of chaperone proteins, which help maintain the normal conformational structure of the PrP^c protein and keep it from being converted to prion conformation.

Resources

BOOKS

Hill, Andrew F., ed. *Prion Protein Protocols*. Totowa, NJ: Humana, 2008.

Lashley, Felissa R., and Jerry D. Durham, eds. *Emerging Infectious Diseases: Trends and Issues*. 2nd ed. New York: Springer, 2007.

Rowland, Lewis P., and Timothy A. Pedley, eds. *Merritt's Neurology*. 12th ed. Philadelphia: Lippincott Williams & Wilkins, 2010.

PERIODICALS

Akritidis, N. "Parasitic, Fungal and Prion Zoonoses: An Expanding Universe of Candidates for Human Disease." *Clinical Microbiology and Infection* 17 (March 2011): 331–35.

Brown, C. "Mad Cow Disease: Risk Now Limited." *Canadian Medical Association Journal* 182 (November 9, 2010): E729–30.

Centers for Disease Control and Prevention. "Update: Creutzfeldt-Jakob Disease Associated with Cadaveric Dura Mater Grafts—Japan, 1978–2008." *Morbidity and Mortality Weekly Report* 57 (October 24, 2008): 1152–54.

Ducrot, C., et al. "Modelling BSE Trend over Time in Europe, a Risk Assessment Perspective." *European Journal of Epidemiology* 25 (June 2010): 411–19.

Holman, R.C., et al. "Human Prion Diseases in the United States." *PLoS One* 5 (January 1, 2010): e8521.

Li, L., et al. "Immunotherapy for Prion Diseases: Opportunities and Obstacles." *Immunotherapy* 2 (March 2010): 269–82.

WEBSITES

"About Human Prion Diseases." National Prion Disease Pathology Surveillance Center (NPDPSC). http://www.cjdsurveillance.com/abouthpd.html (accessed July 18, 2011).

"Bovine Spongiform Encephalopathy (BSE) in North America." Canadian Food Inspection Agency (CFIA). http://www.inspection.gc.ca/english/anima/disemala/bseesb/bseesbe.shtml (accessed July 18, 2011).

"Creutzfeldt-Jakob Disease." Mayo Clinic. http://www.mayoclinic.com/health/creutzfeldt-jakob-disease/DS00531 (accessed July 18, 2011).

Khan, Zartash Zafar. "Kuru." Medscape Reference. http://emedicine.medscape.com/article/220043-overview (accessed July 18, 2011).

Mastrianni, James A. "Genetic Prion Diseases." *GeneReviews*, edited by Roberta A. Pagon, et al. Seattle: University of Washington, 1993–2011. http://www.ncbi.nlm.nih.gov/books/NBK1229/ (accessed July 18, 2011).

"NINDS Alpers' Disease Information Page." National Institute of Neurological Disorders and Stroke (NINDS). http://www.ninds.nih.gov/disorders/alpers disease/alpersdisease.htm (accessed July 18, 2011).

"NINDS Creutzfeldt-Jakob Disease Information Page." National Institute of Neurological Disorders and Stroke (NINDS). http://www.ninds.nih.gov/disorders/cjd/cjd.htm (accessed July 18, 2011).

"Prion Diseases." Centers for Disease Control and Prevention (CDC). http://www.cdc.gov/ncidod/dvrd/prions/ (accessed July 18, 2011).

"Prion Diseases." National Institute of Allergy and Infectious Diseases (NIAID). http://www.niaid.nih.gov/topics/prion/Pages/default.aspx (accessed July 18, 2011).

Thomas, Florian P. "Variant Creutzfeldt-Jakob Disease and Bovine Spongiform Encephalopathy." Medscape Reference. http://emedicine.medscape.com/article/1169688-overview (accessed July 18, 2011).

ORGANIZATIONS

Canadian Food Inspection Agency (CFIA), 1400 Merivale Road, Ottawa ON, Canada, K1A 0Y9, (613) 225-2342, (800) 442-2342, Fax: (613) 228-6601, http://www.inspection.gc.ca.

Centers of Disease Control and Prevention (CDC), 1600 Clifton Road, Atlanta, GA 30333, (800) CDC-INFO, cdcinfo@cdc.gov, http://www.cdc.gov.

Creutzfeldt-Jakob Disease (CJD) Foundation, P.O. Box 5312, Akron, OH 44334, (330) 665-5590, (800) 659-1991, help@cjdfoundation.org, http://www.cjdfoundation.org.

National Institute of Allergy and Infectious Diseases (NIAID), 6610 Rockledge Drive, MSC 6612, Bethesda, MD 20892-6612, (301) 496-5717, (866) 284-4107, Fax: (301) 402-3573, ocpostofficer@niaid.nih.gov, http://www.niaid.nih.gov.

National Institute of Neurological Disorders and Stroke (NINDS), P.O. Box 5801, Bethesda, MD 20824, (301) 496-5751, (800) 352-9424, http://www.ninds.nih.gov.

National Prion Disease Pathology Surveillance Center (NPDPSC), Case Western Reserve University, 2085 Adelbert Road, Room 418, Cleveland, OH 44106-4907, (216) 368-0587, cjdsurv@case.edu, http://www.cjdsurveillance.com.

Maria Basile, PhD
Rebecca J. Frey, PhD

Progressive locomotor ataxia *see* **Tabes dorsalis**

Progressive multifocal leukoencephalopathy

Definition

Progressive multifocal leukoencephalopathy is a rare, fatal disease of the white matter of the brain that almost solely strikes individuals who already have weakened immune systems.

Description

In progressive multifocal leukoencephalopathy, myelin (the substance that wraps around nerve fibers, providing insulation and speeding nerve transmission) is progressively destroyed. Although the disease is caused by a very prevalent virus (called JC virus), it only develops in individuals who are immunocompromised (have weakened immune systems).

Multiple areas of the brain are affected by the demyelination associated with progressive multifocal leukoencephalopathy. Additionally, other abnormalities and bizarre cells take up residence within the brain, causing destruction of normal brain tissue and impairing normal function.

Demographics

The causative virus in progressive multifocal leukoencephalopathy, JC virus, is extremely common. It is thought to be present in upwards of 85% of all children before the age of nine and probably is present in an even greater percentage of adults; however, the JC virus does not cause any symptoms or disease, except in individuals who have severely compromised immune systems. About 62.2% of all progressive multifocal leukoencephalopathy cases occur in individuals with lymphatic cancers (lymphoproliferative disease, such as Hodgkin's disease and

other lymphomas); 6.5% occur in individuals with cancer of bone marrow cells (myeloproliferative disease or leukemias); 2.2% occur in individuals with carcinomatous disease (cancers that affect the lining of tissues or organs of the body); and 10% occur in individuals with any of a number of acquired immunodeficiency states (such as systemic lupus erythematosis, sarcoidosis, and organ transplant survivors). Among patients with acquired immunodeficiency syndrome (AIDS), about 10% of patients develop progressive multifocal leukoencephalopathy. Only 5.6% of all cases of progressive multifocal leukoencephalopathy occur in individuals with no other underlying source of immunocompromise.

Causes and symptoms

Although much is left to be defined about the mechanism whereby progressive multifocal leukoencephalopathy affects an individual, researchers believe that the JC virus resides in the kidneys of most individuals. In normal, nonimmunocompromised individuals, the virus stays within the kidneys, doing no harm. In immunocompromised individuals, the virus is reactivated, travels through the circulatory system to the brain, and selectively destroys myelinated nerve cells.

Patients with progressive multifocal leukoencephalopathy experience a range of symptoms that grow gradually worse over time, including headache and difficulties with speech, thinking, walking, weakness, vision problems (even blindness), memory problems, confusion, slowness of movement, paralysis of half of the body, and seizures. Eventually, patients lapse into a coma and die, usually within just months of the onset of their initial symptoms.

Diagnosis

Diagnosis is usually suggested by a patient's characteristic symptoms of progressive multifocal leukoencephalopathy, in combination with evidence of white matter destruction visualized on CT scan or MRI of the brain. Specialized tests on cerebrospinal fluid (called polymerase chain reactions) may demonstrate the presence of JC virus DNA; however, only brain biopsy can result in an absolutely definitive diagnosis.

Treatment team

Patients with progressive multifocal leukoencephalopathy are usually seen by neurologists, as well as by hematologist/oncologists for patients with lymphoma or leukemia, infectious disease specialists for patients with AIDS, and a rheumatologist for individuals with specific autoimmune disease.

KEY TERMS

Immunocompromise—A condition in which the immune system is weak and ineffective.

Myelin—An insulating layer of fats around nerve fibers that allows nerve impulses to travel more quickly.

Treatment

There are no treatments available to cure progressive multifocal leukoencephalopathy. Some degree of slowing of the relentless progression of the disease has been noted in certain patients treated with the AIDS drug AZT. Other trials are underway to see if the condition responds to the multiple sclerosis drug, natalizumab; the antimalarial drug, mefloquine; antiviral agents such as cidofovir and interleukin-2; or the chemotherapeutic agent, cytarabine.

Prognosis

Progressive multifocal leukoencephalopathy is uniformly fatal, usually within one to four months of the initial symptoms. A few patients have had brief remissions in the disease progression and have lived for several years beyond diagnosis.

Resources

BOOKS

Bradley, W., et al. *Neurology in Clinical Practice*. 5th ed. Philadelphia: Butterworth-Heinemann, 2008.

Goetz, C.G., *Goetz's Textbook of Clinical Neurology*. 3rd ed. Philadelphia: Saunders, 2007.

PERIODICALS

Cei, M. " Progressive multifocal leukoencephalopathy." *Southern Medical Journal* 103, no. 10 (October 1, 2010): 1074–75

Marzocchetti, A. " Determinants of survival in progressive multifocal leukoencephalopathy." *Neurology* 73, no. 19 (November 10, 2009): 1551–58

WEBSITES

"NINDS Progressive Multifocal Leukoencephalopathy Information Page." National Institute of Neurological Disorders and Stroke (NINDS). http://www.ninds.nih. gov/disorders/pml/pml.htm (accessed August 27, 2011).

Rosalyn Carson-DeWitt, MD

Progressive sclerosing poliodystrophy *see* **Alpers' disease**

Progressive supranuclear palsy

Definition

Progressive supranuclear palsy (PSP; also known as Steele-Richardson-Olszewski syndrome) is a rare disease that gradually destroys nerve cells in the parts of the brain that control eye movements, breathing, and muscle coordination. The loss of nerve cells causes palsy, or paralysis, that slowly gets worse as the disease progresses. The palsy affects ability to move the eyes, relax the muscles, and control balance.

Description

Progressive supranuclear palsy is a disease of middle age. Symptoms usually begin in the 60s, rarely before age 45 or after age 75. Men develop PSP more often than women do. It affects 3–4 people per million each year.

Causes and symptoms

PSP affects the brainstem, the basal ganglia, and the **cerebellum**. The brainstem is located at the top of the spinal cord. It controls the most basic functions needed for survival–the involuntary (unwilled) movements such as breathing, blood pressure, and heart rate. The brainstem has three parts: the medulla oblongata, the pons, and the midbrain. The parts affected by PSP are the pons, which controls facial nerves and the muscles that turn the eye outward, and the midbrain, the visual center. The basal ganglia are islands of nerve cells located deep within the brain. They are involved in the initiation of voluntary (willed) movement and control of emotion. Damage to the basal ganglia causes muscle stiffness (**spasticity**) and tremors. The cerebellum is located at the base of the skull. It controls balance and muscle coordination.

Vision is controlled by groups of cells called *nuclei* in the brainstem. In PSP, the nuclei continue to function, but the mechanisms that control the nuclei are destroyed. The term *supranuclear* means that the damage is done above (*supra*) the nuclei. Patients with PSP have difficulty with voluntary (willed) eye movement. At first, the difficulty only occurs in trying to look down. As the disease progresses, ability to move the eyes right and left is also affected. However, reflex or unwilled eye movements remain normal. Thus, when the patient's head is tilted upwards, the eyes move to look down. These reflex movements remain normal until late in the course of the disease. The upper eyelids may be pulled back, the eyebrows raised, and the brow wrinkled, causing a typical wide-eyed stare. Rate of blinking may decrease from the normal 20–30 per minute to 3–5 per minute. It becomes difficult to walk downstairs, to maintain eye contact during conversation, or to move the eyes up and down to read.

The earliest symptoms of PSP may be frequent **falls** or stiff, slow movements of the arms and legs. These symptoms may appear as much as five years before the characteristic vision problems. Walking becomes increasingly awkward, and some patients tend to lean and fall backward. Facial muscles may be weak, causing slurred speech and difficulty swallowing. Sleep may be disturbed and thought processes slowed. Although memory remains intact, the slowed speech and thought patterns and the rigid facial expression may be mistaken for senile **dementia** or **Alzheimer's disease**. Emotional responses may become exaggerated and inappropriate, and the patient may experience anxiety, **depression**, and agitation.

The cause of PSP is not known. Most people who develop PSP come from families with no history of the disease, so it does not seem to be inherited, except in certain rare instances. People who have PSP seem to lack the neurotransmitters dopamine and homovanillic acid in the basal ganglia. Neurotransmitters are chemicals that help carry electrical impulses along the nervous system. Transmitting structures in brain cells called neurofibrils become disorganized (neurofibrillary tangles). Neurofibrillary tangles are also found in Alzheimer's disease, but the pattern is somewhat different.

Diagnosis

PSP is sometimes mistaken for **Parkinson's disease**, which is also associated with stiffness, frequent falls, slurred speech, difficulty swallowing, and decreased spontaneous movement. The facial expression in Parkinson's, however, is blank or mask-like, whereas in PSP it is a grimace and wide-eyed stare. PSP does not cause the uncontrolled shaking (**tremor**) in muscles at rest that is associated with Parkinson's disease. Posture is stooped in Parkinson's disease but erect in PSP. Speech is of low volume in both diseases but is more slurred and irregular in rhythm in PSP.

Multiple strokes or abnormal accumulations of fluid within the skull (hydrocephalus) can also cause balance problems similar to PSP. Magnetic resonance imaging (MRI) scans of the brain may be needed to rule out these conditions. In advanced cases, MRI shows characteristic abnormalities in the brainstem described as "mouse ears."

KEY TERMS

Basal ganglia—Brain structure at the base of the cerebral hemispheres, involved in controlling movement.

Brainstem—Brain structure closest to the spinal cord, involved in controlling vital functions, movement, sensation, and nerves supplying the head and neck.

Cerebellum—The part of the brain involved in coordination of movement, walking, and balance.

Magnetic resonance imaging (MRI)—An imaging technique that uses a large circular magnet and radio waves to generate signals from atoms in the body. These signals are used to construct images of internal structures.

Parkinson's disease—A slowly progressive disease that destroys nerve cells. Parkinson's is characterized by shaking in resting muscles, a stooping posture, slurred speech, muscular stiffness, and weakness.

Treatment

PSP cannot be cured. Drugs are sometimes given to relieve symptoms, but drug treatment is usually disappointing. Dopaminergic medications used in Parkinson's disease, such as levodopa (Sinemet), sometimes decrease stiffness and ease spontaneous movement. Anticholinergic medications, such as trihexyphenidyl (Artane), which restore function to neurotransmitters, or tricyclic drugs, such as amitriptyline (Elavil) may improve speech, walking, and inappropriate emotional responses.

Speech therapy may help manage the swallowing and speech difficulty in PSP. As the disease progresses, the difficulty in swallowing may cause the patient to choke and get small amounts of food in the lungs. This condition can cause aspiration pneumonia. The patient may also lose too much weight. In these cases, a feeding tube may be needed. The home environment should be modified to decrease potential injury from falls. Walkers can be weighted in front to prevent backward falls, and handrails can be installed in the bathroom. Because the patient cannot look down, low objects like throw rugs and coffee tables should be removed. Dry eyes from infrequent blinking can be treated with drops or ointments.

Prognosis

The patient's condition gradually deteriorates. After about seven years, balance problems and stiffness make it nearly impossible for the patient to walk. Persons with PSP become more and more immobile and unable to care for themselves. Death is not caused by the PSP itself. It is usually caused by pneumonia related to choking on secretions or by starvation related to swallowing difficulty. It usually occurs within 10 years, but if good general health and nutrition are maintained, the patient may survive longer.

Prevention

PSP cannot be prevented.

Resources

ORGANIZATIONS

American Academy of Neurology. 1080 Montreal Ave., St. Paul, MN 55116. (612) 695-1940. http://www.aan.com.

Society for Progressive Supranuclear Palsy, Inc. Suite #5065 Johns Hopkins Outpatient Center, 601 N. Caroline St., Baltimore, MD 21287. (800) 457-4777. http://www.psp.org.

Laurie Barclay, MD

Pseudobulbar palsy

Definition

Pseudobulbar palsy refers to a group of symptoms—including difficulty with chewing, swallowing, and speech, as well as inappropriate emotional outbursts—that accompany a variety of nervous system disorders.

Description

Pseudobulbar palsy refers to a cluster of symptoms that can affect individuals suffering from a number of nervous system conditions, such as amyotrophic lateral sclerosis, Parkinson's disease, stroke, multiple sclerosis, or brain damage due to overly rapid correction of low blood sodium levels.

Causes and symptoms

Pseudobulbar palsy occurs when nervous system conditions cause degeneration of certain motor nuclei (nerve clusters responsible for movement) that exit the brainstem.

Patients with pseudobulbar palsy have progressive difficulty with activities that require the use of muscles in the head and neck that are controlled by particular cranial nerves. The first noticeable symptom is often slurred speech. Over time, speech, chewing, and swallowing become more difficult, eventually becoming impossible. Sudden emotional outbursts, in which the patient spontaneously and without cause begins to laugh or cry, are also a characteristic of pseudobulbar palsy.

Diagnosis

Diagnosis is usually made by noting the symptom cluster characteristic of pseudobulbar palsy. Diagnostic tests will be run to determine what underlying neurological disorder has led to the development of pseudobulbar palsy. In particular, neuroimaging (CT scans and MRI) can be used to diagnose many of the conditions that prompt the development of pseudobulbar palsy.

Treatment team

Neurologists usually care for patients with the kinds of conditions that include the symptoms of pseudobulbar palsy.

Treatment

There are no cures for pseudobulbar palsy; the symptoms usually progress over the course of several years, leading to complete disability. Some medications may improve the emotional symptoms associated with pseudobulbar palsy; these include levodopa, amantadine, amitriptyline, and fluoxetine.

Prognosis

The prognosis for pseudobulbar palsy is quite poor. When the symptoms progress to disability, there is a high risk of choking and aspiration (breathing food or liquids into the lungs), which can lead to severe pneumonia and death. The conditions with which pseudobulbar palsy is associated also have a high risk of progression to death.

Resources

BOOKS

Bradley, W., et al. *Neurology in Clinical Practice*. 5th ed. Philadelphia: Butterworth-Heinemann, 2008.

Goetz, C.G., *Goetz's Textbook of Clinical Neurology*. 3rd ed. Philadelphia: Saunders, 2007.

PERIODICALS

Strow, R.E. " Pseudobulbar affect: prevalence and quality of life impact in movement disorders." *Journal of Neurology* 257 (August 1, 2010): 1382–87.

Rosalyn Carson-DeWitt, MD

Pseudotumor cerebri

Definition

Pseudotumor cerebri is a chronic elevation of intracranial pressure that causes papilloedema and possibly blindness, which occurs in the absence of a mass lesion in the brain.

Description

Psuedotumor cerebri primarily affects obese women of childbearing age, and its cause is not known. The disorder is possibly the result of an abnormality in venous blood outflow from the brain, or from an abnormality in cerebrospinal fluid (CSF) flow. The increase in intracranial pressure can result in headache, visual impairment, pain, and hearing problems.

Demographics

Three significant studies concerning pseudotumor cerebri have been conducted in Iowa and Louisiana, the Mayo Clinic in Rochester, Minnesota, and Benghazi, Libya. The incidence of pseudotumor cerebri increases in women between 14 and 44 years of age, who are obese. In the Iowa and Louisiana study, the incidence was 19.3 per 100,000 in women who were 20% over ideal weight. In the Mayo Clinic study, the annual incidence number of new cases between 1976 and 1990 was found to be approximately 8 per 100,000 for obese women 15–44 years old. In the Benghazi study (from 1982–1989), the annual incidence was 21 per 100,000 obese women 15–44 years old. No evidence of any racial or ethnic predilection exists.

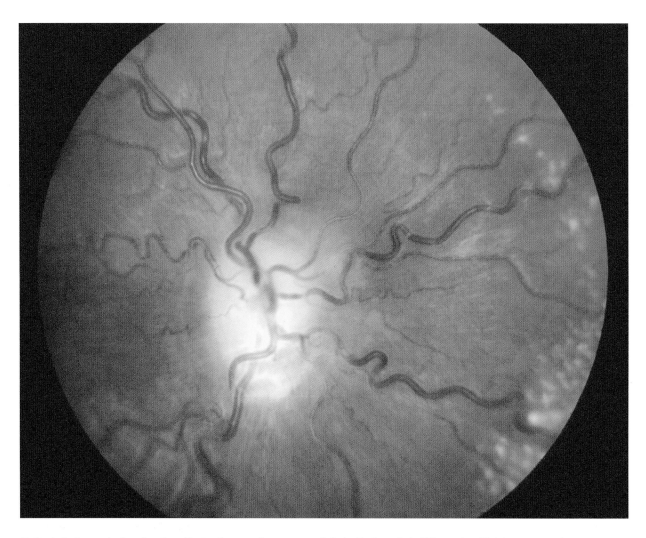

Retinal photograph showing the effects of a pseudotumor cerebri. *(© Barbara Galati/Phototake. All rights reserved.)*

Causes and symptoms

The cause of pseudotumor cerebri is unknown, but it is thought to result from a faulty mechanism in CSF or venous flow from the brain. Certain risk factors have been associated with the disorder that include female gender, menstrual irregularity, obesity, recent weight gain, endocrine (hormone) disorders such as hypothyroidism (underactive thyroid disorder), or medication taken such as cimetidine (anti-ulcer), corticosteroids, lithium (used to treat bipolar disorder), tetracycline, sulfa antibiotics, recombinant human growth hormone, oral contraceptives, and vitamin A intake in infants.

Patients can have symptoms such as headache, ringing sounds in the ears, double vision (diplopia), or pain in the arms. Additionally, patients may have **back pain**, neck pain, or stiffness and arthralgias in the shoulder, knee, and wrist. Patients usually develop papilloedema, which can causes visual obscurations (dimming), progressive loss of peripheral vision, blurring, and sudden visual loss (resulting from intraocular hemorrhage).

Diagnosis

Neuroimaging studies are the best diagnostic tools, especially brain magnetic resonance imaging (MRI) scans. MRI scans provide good images that can reveal other possible disease states that cause increased intracranial pressure. General and special blood tests are typically ordered. CSF studies are also indicated and are usually done by inserting a needle into the lumbar region of the spine to withdraw a fluid sample. CSF studies are done to detect an infection within the **central nervous system**; the sample is used for tumor tests.

Treatment team

Management of pseudotumor cerebri requires a **lumbar puncture** that is performed by a neurologist or internist. Visual problems may be monitored by a neuro-ophthalmologist. Neurosurgical consultations are necessary if treatment does not arrest or reverse the condition quickly, within hours to days.

Treatment

Patients who do not develop visual loss are often treated with a drug called **acetazolamide** (a carbonic anhydrase inhibitor) that lowers intracranial pressure. In persons who present with more severe symptoms such as early loss of vision, a short treatment course with high-dose corticosteroids (prednisone) is recommended. Tapering down from the initial corticosteroid

---

> ## KEY TERMS
>
> **Cerebrospinal fluid**—A colorless and clear fluid that contains glucose and proteins that bath and nourish the brain and spinal cord.
>
> **Recombinant human growth hormone**—A synthetic form of growth hormone that can be given to a patient to help skeletal growth.
>
> **Papilloedema**—Edema or swelling in the optic disk (a portion of the optic nerve that collects nerves from the light sensitive layer of the eye, also called the retina).
>
> **Intraocular**—Inside the eye.

---

dose is individualized and based on the improvement of symptoms. If new visual loss is noted despite treatment, emergency surgical intervention may be indicated. A procedure called a lumboperitoneal shunt is the method of choice utilized for prompt reduction of intracranial hypertension; this is a surgical redirection of fluid flow in the brain, which creates an outflow of fluid from the brain that decreases intracranial pressure.

Recovery and rehabilitation

A formal weight loss and exercise program is required once the diagnosis is established. Admission to the hospital is uncommon, but some patients may be admitted for a short stay for intravenous fluid hydration and pain management in cases of intractable headache. Admission to the hospital is indicated if the patient is a surgical candidate due to severe visual loss. Patients require education concerning blindness and weight reduction. Programs designed to lose weight should include an exercise program and psychological consultations. Many patients do not successfully lose enough weight and may require drastic treatment approaches such as gastric resection or stapling.

Clinical trials

The National Institute of Health has conducted clinical trials concerning the role of thrombosis inside blood vessels and the development of pseudotumor cerebri. Information about current relevant clinical trials can be found at ClinicalTrials.gov.

Prognosis

Typically, persons affected with pseudotumor cerebri can develop blindness, which is the only severe and permanent complication of this disorder. The blindness, which progressively worsens, is due to papilloedema.

Special concerns

Diligent treatment is required since eye deficits in one or both eyes can have a very quick onset and can be disabling. The disorder is not statistically correlated with weight gain during pregnancy; however, both pregnancy and pseudotumor cerebri are linked to weight gain and female gender (within childbearing age).

Resources

BOOKS

Marx, John A., et al, eds. *Rosen's Emergency Medicine: Concepts and Clinical Practice*, 5th ed. St. Louis: Mosby, 2002.

Noble, John, et al., eds. *Textbook of Primary Care Medicine*, 3rd ed. St. Louis: Mosby, 2001.

WEBSITES

Health Topics A-Z. (May 23, 2004.) http://www.medhelp.org.

ORGANIZATIONS

Pseudotumor Cerebri Support Network. 8247 Riverside Drive, Powell, OH 43065. Phone: (614) 895-8814. http://www.pseudotumorcerebri.com.

Laith Farid Gulli, MD
Robert Ramirez, DO
Nicole Mallory, MS,PA-C

Psychogenic neurological disorders

Definition

Psychogenic neurological disorders are conditions with neurological symptoms for which no physiological cause can be identified. The symptoms usually mimic those of known organic disorders but are presumed to be caused by psychological or emotional problems or conflicts.

Description

A condition may be diagnosed as a psychogenic neurological disorder if no organic or physiological basis for neurological symptoms can be identified. Such disorders are sometimes referred to as nonorganic, functional, idiopathic, somatoform, or hysterical disorders. Some may be considered dissociative or conversion psychoneurotic disorders. Dissociative disorders are caused by trauma and are characterized by an abnormal sense of identity or reality. Conversion disorders are characterized by physical symptoms, such as limb paralysis, that have no physiological basis.

Increasingly experts suspect that at least some neurological conversion disorders, such as psychogenic dystonia, represent an underlying disturbance in brain function.

Psychogenic neurological disorders are subconscious and unintentional. The patient's symptoms are real. Patients who report symptoms that they know to be false or who purposely affect symptoms are referred to as malingering, and their disorders are considered factitious rather than psychogenic.

Pain

Psychogenic neurological disorders often manifest as pain. Psychogenic pain is associated with psychological factors, rather than with past injury or disease or any sign of damage to the nervous system or other parts of the body. Among the most common types of psychogenic pain are headaches, muscle pain, **back pain**, and stomach pain. Other examples include idiopathic facial pain, idiopathic toothache, and burning mouth syndrome or oral dysesthesia.

Movement disorders

Movement disorders are relatively common psychogenic disorders. They include psychogenic dystonia, psychogenic or hysterical **tremor**, psychogenic gait abnormalities, and psychogenic paralysis. Dystonia includes a variety of syndromes involving abnormal postures or sustained muscle contractions, which often cause twisting or repetitive movements. Dystonias can be generalized (affecting large portions of the body) or focal (affecting only one part of the body).

In the past, many patients were told that they had psychogenic dystonia and were treated with psychotherapy. By the mid-twentieth century, recognition of hereditary dystonias, the results of surgical treatments and lesion studies, and the limited effectiveness of psychotherapy had revealed an organic basis for many dystonias. Thus, the distinction between organic and psychogenic dystonia is often unclear.

Seizures

Psychogenic seizures mimic epilepsy but have underlying psychological rather than physiological causes. Psychogenic seizures may be called psychogenic non-epileptic seizures (PNES), pseudoseizures, non-epileptic events, non-epileptic paroxysmal events, psychogenic nonepileptic attacks (PNEA), or psychogenic non-epileptic status epilepticus (PNESE). PNES are not true seizures: There is no seizure activity in the brain during PNES, although between 5% and 40% of patients with PNES also have epileptic seizures.

Interestingly, many people with PNES have seizure-response dogs, perhaps because they are more likely than others to have service animals for emotional support. Unfortunately, because many patients with PNES are misdiagnosed as epileptic, they may undergo unnecessary, risky, and expensive epilepsy treatments, while delaying treatment of their psychogenic disorders.

Panic attacks

Panic attacks can also resemble epileptic seizures, especially complex partial epileptic seizures. They may be accompanied by syncope (**fainting**) brought on by hyperventilation. Psychogenic syncope or fainting spells can also be brought on by anxiety or major **depression**.

Dizziness

Psychogenic **dizziness**, also called chronic subjective dizziness, is associated with anxiety and extreme sensitivity to motion stimuli. Situations such as heavy traffic, driving in the rain, or crowded stores or events can exacerbate psychogenic dizziness.

Speech disturbances

Acquired psychogenic speech disturbances take different forms. Psychogenic disfluency is a disfluent speech pattern that arises in the absence of medical factors or a history of developmental **stuttering**. Rarely, spasmodic dysphonia—occasional defective voice use—is psychogenic, although it is usually due to muscle spasms caused by brain abnormalities.

Other psychogenic neurological disorders

Other types of psychogenic neurological disorders include:

• psychogenic visual-field loss or loss of peripheral vision
• psychogenic memory loss or, in extreme cases, psychogenic or dissociative amnesia
• psychogenic erectile dysfunction (ED), which can be either acquired (PAED) or lifelong (PLED), although ED usually has both physiological and psychological components

Demographics

Psychogenic neurological disorders appear to be relatively common. Approximately 30% of all referrals to outpatient neurology clinics have medically unexplainable symptoms, including 5% with conversion disorders that are clearly associated with psychological stress. Although psychogenic dystonia probably accounts for

less than 3% of all dystonia cases, it may be underdiagnosed. In contrast, an estimated 5–10% of outpatients diagnosed with epilepsy and 20–40% of those diagnosed in hospitals or specialized epilepsy centers suffer from PNES rather than epilepsy. Psychogenic neurological disorders are less common in children than in adolescents and adults, although tremor in children is sometimes a psychogenic movement disorder.

Causes and symptoms

Psychogenic neurological disorders can be caused by a variety of factors—including mental and emotional problems, stress, or trauma—that manifest in a variety of symptoms. For example, psychogenic pain disorder may cause, increase, or prolong pain.

Movement disorders

Almost any type of movement disorder can be psychogenic. Many patients with psychogenic dystonia suffer from more than one underlying psychiatric problem, including anxiety, depression, or a personality disorder. Symptoms of psychogenic dystonia are very similar to those of organic dystonias and can be just as disabling, affecting every aspect of daily life. Psychogenic dystonia is sometimes chronic, lasting for many years.

Episodes of psychogenic tremor usually come on suddenly, while the patient is at rest, in a posture, or moving. The frequency of episodes increases with stress, but individual episodes can differ in the type of tremor and the affected body part. Psychogenic tremor decreases significantly or disappears when the patient is distracted. Many patients with psychogenic tremor also have another conversion or mental disorder.

Seizures

Causes of PNES range from an underlying psychiatric disorder to dependence, a need for attention, or avoidance of stressful situations. Older patients sometimes develop late-onset PNES as a result of other severe, frightening, or traumatic medical diagnoses. PNES is characterized by sudden attacks of motor, sensory, or behavioral episodes that are associated with such symptoms as crying, vocalization, or other forms of emotional expression. The seizures can mimic any type of epileptic seizure, but there is no loss of consciousness or abnormal electrical activity in the brain.

Amnesia

Psychogenic amnesia usually results from emotional shock or trauma, such as being victimized by violent crime. Patients with psychogenic amnesia may wander around lost, unable to recall their names, other basic information, or personal memories. Their ability to learn and remember new information is unaffected. Psychogenic amnesia is usually very short-lived and resolves on its own.

Erectile dysfunction

Many men with psychogenic ED also have characteristics of alexithymia—a spectrum of personality traits that involve problems with identifying, differentiating, and communicating emotions. Alexithymia may contribute to the development of psychogenic PAED and the level of alexithymia has been found to correlate with the severity of PAED.

Diagnosis

Because symptoms of psychogenic neurological disorders closely resemble those of organic disorders, diagnosis often involves the elimination of underlying physical conditions. For example, a diagnosis of psychogenic pain may be made after possible causes for the pain have been ruled out or when the pain is not associated with other physical symptoms. Psychogenic visual-field loss is diagnosed by the ability of patients to smoothly and accurately move their eyes to a target that is in their supposed blind spot. Diagnosis of psychogenic neurological disorders often requires the expertise of both medical and mental-health professionals and patients may spend months or years vacillating between neurological and psychiatric diagnoses.

Dystonia

Psychogenic dystonia often resembles other dystonias—especially secondary dystonias—so closely that only an expert in movement disorders may be able to discern subtle differences. Diagnosis usually requires in-depth examinations over time by both a physician experienced in dystonia and other movement disorders and a psychiatrist experienced in conversion disorders. Diagnosis is complicated by the fact that, until fairly recently, organic dystonia was often misdiagnosed as a psychiatric disorder.

Diagnostic criteria for psychogenic dystonia can include symptom inconsistency or distractibility, as well as false neurological signs and potential psychological factors and triggers. Diagnosis usually requires a temporal association between psychological triggers and the onset of neurological symptoms. It also requires ruling out conscious or willful production of symptoms. The presence of another mental disorder is not sufficient for a diagnosis of psychogenic dystonia, since disability caused by dystonia can result in depression or other mental health problems.

Psychogenic seizures

Prompt diagnosis of PNES is important for avoiding potentially risky epilepsy treatments. A distinguishing feature of PNES is that most patients keep their eyes closed throughout the entire episode, whereas most epileptics have their eyes wide open at the outset of a seizure. Other possible distinguishing clinical features of PNES include:

- gradual onset, no loss of consciousness, and variable symptoms
- long event duration and relatively fast recovery
- seizures triggered by suggestion
- motor activity that differs from the usual sequences of various types of epileptic seizures
- bizarre movements of the entire body
- bilateral motor activity
- pelvic movements, especially pelvic thrusting
- side-to-side head movements
- a posture in which the head and lower limbs bend backward and the trunk pushes forward
- complaining and crying during an episode
- avoidance behavior during an episode
- rare tongue biting and, if present, biting of the tip rather than the side of the tongue
- resistance to treatment, especially eye opening, during the event
- whispering or partial motor responses to commands during recovery from the seizure
- post-event serum creatine kinase levels that are lower than those that accompany epileptic seizures

Patients with PNES often have recurrent seizures that lead to emergency department visits or hospitalizations and treatment with high doses of **benzodiazepines**. An implanted port system for emergency intravenous drugs is sometimes a clue that the patient suffers from PNES. Other clues that may suggest PNES include:

- personal, family, or professional experience with epilepsy
- history of sexual or physical abuse
- apathy or excessive emotional responsiveness
- the presence of other psychiatric disorders
- multiple unexplained physical symptoms
- episodes triggered by emotional factors or situations
- episodes that occur only when alone or only in the company of others
- very frequent seizures with no injuries

Alexithymia—An inability to identify and express feelings or emotions.

Amnesia—Partial or complete loss of memory or gaps in memory.

Antiepileptic drug (AED)—Anticonvulsant drug; a medication to prevent epileptic seizures.

Benzodiazepines—A class of tranquilizers or antianxiety drugs, used to treat a variety of conditions including epileptic seizures.

Cognitive-behavioral therapy (CBT)—A treatment that identifies negative thoughts and behaviors and helps develop more positive approaches.

Conversion disorder—A psychoneurotic condition with symptoms, such as paralysis, that are without a physical basis.

Disfluency—An inability to speak fluently.

Dissociative disorder—A reaction in which the mind splits off aspects of a traumatic event from conscious awareness and which can affect memory, sense of reality, and sense of identity.

Dysphonia—Defective use of the voice.

Dystonia—A range of conditions that cause abnormal muscular contractions and movements.

Electroencephalography (EEG)—Monitoring of electrical activity in the brain.

Epilepsy—A brain disorder with symptoms that include seizures.

Erectile dysfunction (ED)—The consistent inability to achieve or maintain a penile erection; psychogenic ED may be acquired (PAED) or lifelong (PLED).

Functional disorder—A condition that affects psychological or physical function without affecting organic structure.

Idiopathic—Occurring spontaneously or from an unknown cause.

Psychogenic non-epileptic seizures (PNES)—Pseudoseizures, non-epileptic events, non-epileptic paroxysmal events, psychogenic non-epileptic status epilepticus (PNESE), or psychogenic non-epileptic attacks (PNEA); seizures, episodes, or events that resemble epilepsy but which are caused by psychological factors rather than by brain abnormalities.

Seizure—A sudden attack, spasm, or convulsion.

Somatoform disorders—A group of psychological disorders characterized by physical complaints for which no physiological explanation can be found and which probably involve psychological factors.

Syncope—Faint; loss of consciousness due to insufficient blood flow to the brain.

Tremor—Trembling or shaking.

One study found that 85% of patients who had at least two seizure events weekly for which at least two **antiepileptic drugs** (AEDs) had proved ineffective, and who had at least two electroencephalograms (EEGs) showing no epileptic-type abnormalities, had PNES. A definitive diagnosis of PNES is made by video-recording typical episodes with simultaneous EEG monitoring that shows the absence of epileptic abnormalities in brain signals. To facilitate video-EEG, seizures are sometimes induced using suggestive techniques, although such inductions are controversial. Nevertheless, it takes an average of seven to nine years from the onset of seizures to arrive at a diagnosis of PNES.

Treatment

Treatment for a psychogenic neurological disorder is usually provided by a psychiatrist or other mental-health professional. It often involves a combination of psychotherapy and medications such as antidepressants.

- Psychogenic pain treatment may include non-narcotic painkillers.
- Treatment of psychogenic movement disorders may require a team that includes a movement-disorder specialist, psychiatrist, and cognitive-behavioral therapist.
- Psychogenic tremor sometimes disappears with treatment of the underlying psychological problem. Physical therapy may be helpful.
- PNES is often treated with cognitive-behavioral therapy.
- Voice therapy can effectively treat psychogenic speech disorders.

Special concerns

In the past, many neurological disorders were considered psychogenic simply because their physiological bases had not yet been identified. For example, Tourette syndrome was long considered to be a rare psychogenic disorder but is now known to be relatively common and to have a genetic basis. Likewise, many types of dystonia were long thought to be psychogenic and are now known to have physiological bases. Other disorders, such as ED, are often caused by multiple factors, which may include psychological components. It is possible that in the future an organic basis will be identified for some disorders that are currently considered to be psychogenic. Misdiagnosis of an organic disorder as psychogenic can delay delay effective treatment and cause undue hardship and suffering. Conversely, misdiagnosis of a psychogenic disorder as organic can expose a patient to risky and aggressive treatments while delaying treatment of an underlying psychological problem.

Resources

BOOKS

Evans, Hilary, and Robert E. Bartholomew. *Outbreak! The Encyclopedia of Extraordinary Social Behavior*. San Antonio, TX: Anomalist Books, 2009.

Henry, Gregory L. *Neurologic Emergencies*. 3rd ed. New York: McGraw-Hill Medical, 2010.

Schachter, Steven C., W. Curt LaFrance, and John R. Gates. *Gates and Rowan's Nonepileptic Seizures*. 3rd ed. New York: Cambridge University Press, 2010.

PERIODICALS

Plug, L., B. Sharrack, and M. Reuber. "Seizure Metaphors Differ in Patients' Accounts of Epileptic and Psychogenic Nonepileptic Seizures." *Epilepsia* 50, no. 5 (2009): 994–1000.

Reuber, M. "The Etiology of Psychogenic Non-Epileptic Seizures: Toward a Biopsychosocial Model." *Neurologic Clinics* 27, no. 4 (November 2009): 909–24.

Syed, T.U., et al. "A Self-Administered Screening Instrument for Psychogenic Nonepileptic Seizures." *Neurology* 72, no. 19 (May 2009): 1646–52.

WEBSITES

Bodde, N.M.G., et al. "Psychogenic Non-Epileptic Seizures—Definition, Etiology, Treatment and Prognostic Issues: A Critical Review." *Seizure* 18, no. 8 (October 2009): 543–53. http://www.seizure-journal.com/article/S1059-1311(09)00128-9/fulltext (accessed July 19, 2011).

Munts, Alexander G., and Peter J. Koehler. "How Psychogenic is Dystonia? Views from Past to Present." *Brain* 133, no. 5 (2010): 1552–64. http://www.medscape.com/viewarticle/722007 (accessed July 19, 2011).

"Psychogenic Dystonia." Dystonia Medical Research Foundation. http://www.dystonia-foundation.org/pages/more_info/86.php (accessed July 19, 2011).

Rowe, James B. "Conversion Disorder: Understanding the Pathogenic Links Between Emotion and Motor Systems in the Brain." *Brain* 133, no. 5 (2010): 1295–97. http://www.medscape.com/viewarticle/722165 (accessed July 19, 2011).

ORGANIZATIONS

Dystonia Medical Research Foundation, One East Wacker Drive, Suite 2810, Chicago, IL, United States, 60601-1905, (312) 755-0198, (800) 377-DYST (3978), Fax: (312) 803-0138, dystonia@dystonia-foundation.org, http://www.dystonia-foundation.org.

National Institute of Neurological Disorders and Stroke (NINDS), P.O. Box 5801, Bethesda, MD, United States, 20824, (301) 496-5751, (800) 352-9424, http://www.ninds.nih.gov.

Margaret Alic, PhD

Pyridostigmine *see* **Cholinergic stimulants**

R

Radiation

Definition

Radiation and radioisotopes allow physicians to image internal structures and processes *in vivo* (in the living body) with a minimum of invasion to the patient. Higher doses of radiation are also used to kill cancerous cells.

Radiation is actually a term that includes a variety of physical phenomena. In essence, all these phenomena can be divided in two classes: phenomena connected with nuclear radioactive processes, the so-called radioactive radiation (RR); and electromagnetic radiation (EMR).

Both classes of radiation are used in diagnoses and treatment of neurological disorders.

Description

Three kinds of radiation are useful to medical personnel: alpha, beta, and gamma radiation. Alpha radiation is a flow of alpha particles, beta radiation is a flow of electrons, and gamma radiation is electromagnetic radiation.

Radioisotopes, containing unstable combinations of protons and neutrons, are created by neutron activation. This involves the capture of a neutron by the nucleus of an atom, resulting in an excess of neutrons (neutron rich). Proton-rich radioisotopes are manufactured in cyclotrons. During radioactive decay, the nucleus of a radioisotope seeks energetic stability by emitting particles (alpha, beta, or positron) and photons (including gamma rays).

Radiation—produced by radioisotopes—allows accurate imaging of internal organs and structures. Radioactive tracers are formed from the bonding of short-lived radioisotopes with chemical compounds that, when in the body, allow the targeting of specific body regions or physiologic processes. Emitted gamma rays (photons) can be detected by gamma cameras and computer enhancement of the resulting images and allows quick and relatively noninvasive (compared to surgery) assessments of trauma or physiological impairments.

Because the density of tissues is unequal, x rays (a high frequency and energetic form of electromagnetic radiation) pass through tissues in an unequal manner. The beam passed through the body layer is recorded on special film to produce an image of internal structures; however, conventional x rays produce only a two-dimensional picture of the body structure under investigation.

Tomography (from the Greek *tomos*, meaning "to slice") is a method developed to allow the detailed construction of images of the target object. Initially using the x rays to scan layers of the area in question, with computer assisted tomography, a computer then analyzes data of all layers to construct a 3D image of the object.

Computed tomography (CT) and computerized axial tomography (CAT) scans use x rays to produce images of anatomical structures.

Single proton (or photon) emission computed tomography (SPECT) produces three-dimensional images of an organ or body system. SPECT detects the presence and course of a radioactive substance that is injected, ingested, or inhaled. In neurology, a SPECT scan can allow physicians to examine and observe the cerebral circulation. SPECT produces images of the target region by detecting the presence and location of a radioactive isotope. The photon emissions of the radioactive compound containing the isotope can be detected in a manner that is similar to the detection of x rays in computed tomography (CT). At the end of the SPECT scan, the stored information can be integrated to produce a computer-generated composite image.

Positron emission tomography (PET) scans utilize isotopes produced in a cyclotron. Positron-emitting radionuclides are injected and allowed to accumulate in the target tissue or organ. As the radionuclide decays, it emits a positron that collides with nearby electrons to result in the emission of two identifiable gamma photons. PET scans use rings of detectors that surround the patient to track the movements and concentrations of radioactive tracers. PET scans have attracted the interest of physicians because of their potential use in research into metabolic changes associated with mental diseases such as schizophrenia and depression. PET scans are used in the diagnosis and characterizations of certain cancers and heart disease, as well as clinical studies of the brain. PET uses radio-labeled tracers, including deoxyglucose, which is chemically similar to glucose and is used to assess metabolic rate in tissues and to image tumors and dopa within the brain.

Electromagnetic radiation

In contrast to imaging produced through the emission and collection of nuclear radiation (e.g., x rays, **CT scans**), **magnetic resonance imaging** (MRI) scanners rely on the emission and detection of electromagnetic radiation.

Electromagnetic radiation are oscillations of components of electric and magnetic fields. In the simplest cases, these oscillations occur with definite frequencies (the unit of frequency measurement is 1 Hertz (Hz), which is one oscillation per second). Electromagnetic radiation at all frequencies travels at the speed of light. Another characteristic of electromagnetic radiation is wavelength, which can be thought of as the distance between the crests of two successive waves. Because the product of the wavelength and frequency must equal the velocity of light, the greater the frequency, the smaller the wavelength (and vice versa).

MRI scanners rely on the principles of atomic nuclear-spin resonance. Using strong magnetic fields and radio waves, MRIs collect and correlate deflections caused by atoms into images. MRIs allow physicians to see internal structures with great detail and also allow earlier and more accurate diagnosis of disorders.

MRI technology was developed from nuclear magnetic resonance (NMR) technology. Groups of nuclei brought into resonance, that is, nuclei absorbing and emitting photons of similar electromagnetic radiation such as radio waves, make subtle yet distinguishable changes when the resonance is forced to change by altering the energy of impacting photons. The speed and extent of the resonance changes permit a non-destructive (because of the use of low-energy photons) determination of anatomical structures.

MRI images do not utilize potentially harmful ionizing radiation generated by three-dimensional x-ray CT scans but rely on the atomic properties (nuclear resonance) of protons in tissues when they are scanned with radio frequency radiation. The protons in the tissues, which resonate at slightly different frequencies, produce a signal that a computer uses to tell one tissue from another. MRI provides detailed three-dimensional soft tissue images.

These methods are used successfully for brain investigations.

Radiation therapy (radiotherapy)

Radiotherapy requires the use of radioisotopes and higher doses of radiation that are used diagnostically to treat some cancers (including brain cancer) and other medical conditions that require destruction of harmful cells.

Radiation therapy is delivered via external radiation or via internal radiation therapy (the implantation/injection of radioactive substances).

Cancer, tumors, and other rapidly dividing cells are usually sensitive to damage by radiation. The goal of radiation therapy is to deliver the minimally sufficient dosage to kill cancerous cells or to keep them from dividing. Cancer cells divide and grow at rates more rapid than normal cells and so are particularly susceptible to radiation. Accordingly, some cancerous growths can be restricted or eliminated by radioisotope irradiation. The most common forms of external radiation therapy use gamma and x rays. During the last half of the twentieth century, the radioisotope cobalt-60 was the frequently used source of radiation used in such treatments. Subsequent methods of irradiation include the production of x rays from linear accelerators.

Iodine-131, phosphorus-32 are commonly used in radiotherapy. More radical uses of radioisotopes include the use of boron-10 to specifically attack tumor cells. Boron-10 concentrates in tumor cells and is then subjected to neutron beams that result in highly energetic alpha particles that are lethal to the tumor tissue.

Precautions

Radiation therapy is not without risk to healthy tissue and to persons on the health care team, and precautions (shielding and limiting exposure) are taken to minimize exposure to other areas of the patient's body and to personnel on the treatment team.

Therapeutic radiologists, radiation oncologists, and a number of technical specialists use radiation and other methods to treat patients who have cancer or other tumors.

Care is taken in the selection of the appropriate radioactive isotope. Ideally, the radioactive compound used loses its radioactive potency rapidly (this is expressed as the half-life of a compound). For example, gamma-emitting compounds used in SPECT scans can have a half-life of just a few hours. This is beneficial for the patients, as it limits the contact time with the potentially damaging radioisotope.

The selection of radioisotopes for medical use is governed by several important considerations involving dosage and half-life. Radioisotopes must be administered in sufficient dosages so that emitted radiation is present in sufficient quantity to be measured. Ideally the radioisotope has a short enough half-life that, at the delivered dosage, there is insignificant residual radiation following the desired length of exposure.

New areas of radiation therapy that may prove more effective in treating brain tumors (and other forms of cancers) include three-dimensional conformal radiation therapy (a process where multiple beans are shaped to match the contour of the tumor) and stereotactic radiosurgery (used to irradiate certain brain tumors and obstructions of the cerebral circulation). Gamma knives use focused beams (with the patient often wearing a special helmet to help focus the beams), while cyberknifes use hundreds of precise pinpoint beams emanating from a source of irradiation that moves around the patient's head.

Resources

BOOKS

Bradley, W., et al. *Neurology in Clinical Practice*. 5th ed. Philadelphia: Butterworth-Heinemann, 2008.

Goetz, C.G., *Goetz's Textbook of Clinical Neurology*.3rd ed. Philadelphia: Saunders, 2007.

Grainger R.G., et al. *Grainger & Allison's Diagnostic Radiology: A Textbook of Medical Imaging*. 5th ed. Philadelphia: Saunders, 2008.

Mettler, F.A., *Essentials of Radiology*. 2nd ed. Philadelphia: Saunders, 2005.

PERIODICALS

Bick, A.S. "From research to clinical practice: Implementation of functional magnetic imaging and white matter tractography in the clinical environment." *J Neurol Sci* (August 22, 2011): epub.

Plummer, C. "Ischemic Stroke and Transient Ischemic Attack After Head and Neck Radiotherapy: A Review." *Stroke* (August 4, 2011).

WEBSITES

"What Is Nuclear Medicine?" Society of Nuclear Medicine. http://www.snm.org/index.cfm?PageID=3106&RPID (accessed August 27, 2011).

Alexander Ioffe
Rosalyn Carson-DeWitt, MD

Radiculopathy

Definition

Radiculopathy refers to disease of the spinal nerve roots (from the Latin *radix* for root). Radiculopathy produces pain, numbness, or **weakness** radiating from the spine.

Description

At the joints between the vertebrae, sensory nerves (nerves conducting sensory information toward the **central nervous system**) and motor nerves (nerves conducting commands to muscles away from the central nervous system) connect to the spinal cord. Each spinal nerve divides or fans out just before merging with the spinal cord. These smaller, separate nerve bundles are termed the roots of the nerve because they are reminiscent of the way the roots of a plant divide in the ground.

Damage to the spinal nerve roots can lead to pain, numbness, weakness, and paresthesia (abnormal sensations in the absence of stimuli) in the limbs or trunk. Pain may be felt in a region corresponding to a dermatome, an area of skin innervated by the sensory fibers of a given spinal nerve or a dynatome, an area in which pain is felt when a given spinal nerve is irritated. Dynatomes and dermatomes may overlap but do not necessarily coincide.

Radiculopathies are categorized according to which part of the spinal cord is affected. Thus, there are cervical (neck), thoracic (middle back), and lumbar (lower back) radiculopathies. Lumbar radiculopathy is also known a sciatica. Radiculopathies may be further categorized by what vertebrae they are associated with. For example, radiculopathy of the nerve roots at the level of the

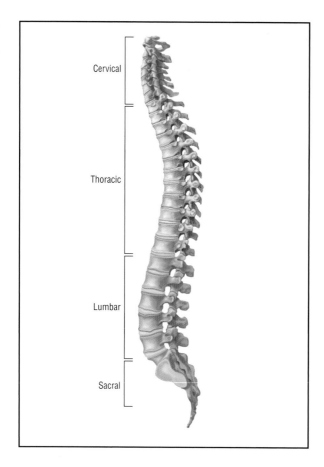

Radiculopathies are categorized according to which part of the spinal cord is affected and by which vertebrae they are associated with. *(Illustration by PreMediaGlobal. © 2012 Cengage Learning.)*

seventh cervical vertebra is termed C7 radiculopathy; at the level of the fifth cervical vertebra, C5 radiculopathy; at the level of the first thoracic vertebra, T1 radiculopathy; and so on.

Radiculopathy is to be distinguished from myelopathy, which involves pathological changes in or functional problems with the spinal cord itself rather than the nerve roots. Sometimes, radiculopathy is also distinguished from radiculitis, the latter being defined as irritation (hence the "itis" suffix) of a nerve root that causes pain in the dermatome or dynatome corresponding to that nerve. Radiculopathy, by contrast, denotes spinal nerve dysfunction (not just irritation) presenting with pain, altered reflex, weakness, and nerve-conduction abnormalities. Pain may not be present with radiculopathy but is always present with radiculitis.

Demographics

Millions of persons experience some form of radiculopathy at some point in their lives. Because many of

the causes of radiculopathy are long-term diseases (e.g., ankylosing spondylosis, diabetes) or diseases that tend to affect the elderly (e.g., arthritis), radiculopathy occurs more often in the middle-aged and elderly than in the young. However, injuries due to sports, heavy lifting, or bad posture affect the young as well. Cervical **disc herniation** with radiculopathy (mostly involving the C4 to C5 levels) affects 5.5 per 100,000 adults every year, with the highest risk being among adults 35 to 55 years old.

Causes and symptoms

Radiculopathy can be caused by any disease or injury process that compresses or otherwise injures the spinal nerve roots. Violent blows or **falls**, cancer, some infections such as flu and **Lyme disease**, diseases that lead to degeneration of the vertebrae and/or intervertebral discs (osteoarthritis), slipped or herniated discs, scoliosis, and other factors can cause radiculopathy. For example, extreme backward bending of the neck can trigger cervical radiculopathy. This has given rise to a recently recognized category of radiculopathy termed "salon sink radiculopathy," so-called because salon patrons are asked to tip their heads sharply backward into sinks for shampooing. Spondylosis (immobilization and growing-together of one or more vertebral joints, often due to osteoarthritis) can deform the structures of bone, cartilage, and ligament through which spinal nerves must pass, leading to cervical and lumbar radiculopathy. Thoracic and lumbar radiculopathies are a common result of diabetes, which can impair blood flow to the spinal nerve roots.

Diagnosis

Radiculopathy is a possible diagnosis when numbness, pain, weakness, or paresthesia of the extremities or torso are reported by a patient, especially in a dermatomal pattern. However, these symptoms can also be caused by **nerve compression** remote from the spine, and the physician must rule out this possibility before ruling in favor of radiculopathy. Electrodiagnostic studies can help distinguish radiculopathy from other diagnoses. These techniques include current perception threshold testing, which tests patient ability to sense alternating electric currents at several frequencies; electromyographic nerve conduction tests; and testing of sensory evoked potentials (changes in brain waves in response to sensory stimuli).

When radiculopathy is diagnosed, the location of the affected nerve roots and, ultimately, the cause of their dysfunction must be determined. Diagnosticians look at the precise features of radicular symptoms in order to determine the spinal level of the affected root or roots. For example, radiculopathy at the C7 level (the nerve root most often affected by herniated cervical disc) is characterized by weak triceps and wrist extensor muscles and a numb middle finger. Radiculopathy at the L3 (third lumbar disc) level is characterized by decreased patellar (kneecap) reflex, loss of sensation and/or pain in the anterior (forward) part of the thigh, and weakness in quadriceps muscle; and so on.

X ray or MRI may be used to confirm the diagnosis. A herniated disc, for example, will be revealed by imaging. A herniated disc is one that has partly popped or bulged out from between the vertebra above and below it. This may place pressure on the nerve roots and on the spinal cord itself.

In persons with spinal cancer or other progressive disorders, the appearance of radiculopathy may be an important sign that pressure is beginning to be exerted by the tumor or some other changing structure. This may signal that it is time for surgical intervention.

Treatment team

Diagnosis of radiculopathy will usually involve a neurologist. An orthopedist will usually be involved as well. Other specialists will be required depending on the cause of the radiculopathy (e.g., oncologist, if cancer is present). Treatment will usually call for a physical therapist. An orthopedic surgeon would perform any necessary surgery.

Treatment

Treatment for radiculopathy varies with the nature and severity of the disease process or injury that has caused the disorder. Conservative (non-surgical) treatment is often attempted first. This consists primarily of rest, exercise, and medication. Patient-specific exercises are prescribed by a physical therapist for the targeted strengthening of muscles and other supporting tissues to relieve pressure on affected spinal nerve roots. Weight loss may be advised to decrease stress on the spine. Medications may include oral opioids (e.g., morphine) or other analgesic (anti-pain) medications. In severe cases, injection of an opioid by an external or implanted pump directly into the affected area may be prescribed. Epidural corticosteroid injections, selective nerve root block, and epidural lysis (destruction) of adhesions are also used to treat radiculopathy. A soft neck collar may be prescribed for persons with cervical radiculopathy.

When conservative treatment fails, surgery may be necessary. The primary purpose of surgery is to take pressure off the affected nerve roots or the blood vessels

KEY TERMS

Dermatome—An area of skin that receive sensations through a single nerve root.

Dynatome—An area in which pain is felt when a given spinal nerve is irritated.

Motor nerves—Nerves conducting commands to muscles away from the central nervous system.

Sensory nerves—Nerves conducting sensory information toward the central nervous system.

that serve them and to stabilize spinal structure, but surgery may also sever nerves in order to relieve severe pain. Fusion of vertebrae (i.e., removal of the flexible intervertebral disc and joining of the adjacent vertebrae so that they grow into a single bone) was for many decades a common treatment for intractable radiculopathy, but later the Bryan disc was developed. The Bryan disc is a flexible disc or ring of titanium and Teflon that is used to replace the intervertebral disc in patients with degenerative disc disease: one cervical (for the neck) and the other lumbar (for the lower back).

Recovery and rehabilitation

Exercise is key to the treatment of both conservative and surgical treatment of radiculopathy. It may even be curative in some cases. It is also an important aspect of recovery from surgery. Exercise is done as directed by a physical therapist.

Clinical trials

Information about current relevant clinical trials can be found at ClinicalTrials.gov.

Prognosis

Prognosis varies with the underlying process causing the radiculopathy. For sports injuries, at one extreme, the prognosis is excellent; for degenerative disc disorders, even surgery may not completely or permanently resolve the problem. However, new surgical techniques are improving outcomes.

Resources

PERIODICALS

Kilcline, Bradford A. "Acute Low Back Pain: Guidelines for Treating Common and Uncommon Syndromes." *Consultant* (October 1, 2002).

Lenrow, David A. "Chronic Neck Pain: Mapping Out Diagnosis and Management; Part 1: Step-by-step Algorithms Can Show the Way to Effective Treatment." *Journal of Musculoskeletal Medicine* (June 1, 2002).

OTHER

"Cervical Radiculopathy." *Neuroland.* http://neuroland.com/spine/c_radi.htm (April 29, 2004).

Skelton, Alta. "Lumbar radiculopathy." http://www.spineuniverse.com/displayarticle.php/article1469.html (April 29, 2004).

ORGANIZATIONS

National Institute for Neurological Diseases and Stroke (NINDS). 6001 Executive Boulevard, Bethesda, MD 20892. Phone: (301) 496-5751. Tollfree phone: (800) 352-9424. http://www.ninds.nih.gov.

Larry Gilman

Ramsay-Hunt syndrome type II

Definition

Ramsay-Hunt syndrome type II is a very rare, progressive neurological disorder that causes epilepsy, **tremor**, mental impairment, and eventually death.

Description

Ramsay-Hunt syndrome type II begins in adulthood. It is a relentlessly progressive degenerative disease that culminates in death, characterized by Parkinson-like tremors and muscle jerks (**myoclonus**).

Demographics

The average age of onset is about 30 years.

Causes and symptoms

Some cases seem to be caused by abnormalities of the mitochondria within the cell. Mitochondria are the cells' power stations. They are organelles within each cell that are responsible for producing energy.

Some cases of Ramsay-Hunt syndrome type II appear to be inherited in an autosomal dominant fashion, meaning that a child who has one parent with the abnormal gene has a 50:50 chance of inheriting the disorder. Other cases appear to be inherited in an autosomal recessive fashion, meaning that individuals who develop the disease have inherited defective genes from both parents.

Ramsay-Hunt syndrome type II begins as an intention tremor in the limbs, particularly the arms.

An intention tremor is an involuntary shaking or trembling that occurs when an individual is attempting a purposeful movement; the tremor is not manifested when the individual is at rest. The intention tremor generally occurs in just one limb. Over time, the entire muscular system is affected. In addition to the tremor, individuals with Ramsay-Hunt syndrome type II experience sudden twitching or contraction of muscle groups, called myoclonus. Some individuals experience progressive hearing impairment. As the disease progresses, the individual experiences decreased muscle tone, increasing **weakness**, disturbances of fine motor control, difficulty walking, epilepsy, and (in some cases) mental deterioration. The disease usually progresses over the course of about 10 years, ultimately resulting in the death of the patient.

Diagnosis

An electroencephalogram (EEG) may reveal certain abnormalities of the electrical patterns in the brain. Muscle **biopsy** may or may not reveal mitochondrial abnormalities.

Treatment team

Ramsay-Hunt syndrome type II is usually diagnosed and treated by a neurologist. In an effort to maintain functioning as long as possible, other treatment members may include physical therapists, occupational therapists, and speech and language therapists.

Treatment

There is no cure for Ramsay-Hunt syndrome type II. Seizures may respond to antiseizure medications such as **phenobarbital**, clonazepam, or **valproic acid**. The involuntary muscle jerking (myoclonus) may decrease with such medication as valproic acid; **benzodiazepines** such as clonazepam; L-tryptophan; 5-hydroxytryptophan with carbidopa; or piracetam.

Prognosis

Ramsay-Hunt syndrome type II generally progresses to death within about 10 years of the onset of symptoms.

Resources

BOOKS

Foldvary-Schaefer, Nancy, and Elaine Wyllie. "Epilepsy." In *Textbook of Clinical Neurology*, edited by Christopher G. Goetz. Philadelphia: W.B. Saunders 2003.

WEBSITES

National Institute of Neurological Disorders and Stroke (NINDS). *Ramsay-Hunt Syndrome Type II Fact Sheet.* (May 23, 2004.) http://www.ninds.nih.gov/health_and_medical/disorders/ramsey2.htm.

ORGANIZATIONS

National ataxia Foundation. 2600 Fernbrook Lane, Suite 119, Minneapolis, MN 55447-4752. Phone: (763) 553-0020. Fax: (763) 553-0167. Email: naf@ataxia.org. http://www.ataxia.org.

WE MOVE. 204 West 84th Street, New York, NY 10024. Fax: (212) 875-8389. Tollfree phone: (800) 437-MOV2. Email: wemove@wemove.org. http://www.wemove.org.

Rosalyn Carson-DeWitt, MD

Rasmussen's encephalitis

Definition

Rasmussen's **encephalitis**, also termed Rasmussen's syndrome, is a rare degenerative brain disease that initially affects only one side of the brain. It first manifests in childhood with the onset of epileptic seizures. Later, it progresses to paralysis of one side of the body (hemiparesis), blindness in one eye (**hemianopsia**), and loss of mental function. The seizures in Rasmussen's encephalitis usually resist therapy with anticonvulsant drugs but respond well to hemispherectomy, the surgical removal of the entire affected side of the brain.

Description

Rasmussen's encephalitis usually appears in children but may also strike in adulthood. It initially affects only one side (hemisphere) of the brain. The disease causes uncontrollable seizures and other symptoms that become progressively worse. The affected hemisphere shows changes characteristic of chronic inflammation, including long-term atrophy or shrinkage, hence, the term encephalitis (inflammation of the brain). Unless the affected hemisphere is removed, the disorder eventually spreads to the brain's other hemisphere.

Demographics

Rasmussen's encephalitis is very rare; between 1958, when the syndrome was first identified, and 2000, barely 100 cases were identified. The medical literature does not describe a higher incidence of this disease in either gender or in any particular racial group or geographical area.

Causes and symptoms

For many years, the cause of Rasmussen's encephalitis was a mystery. It seemed to resemble a viral infection, but despite much research, no organism could be consistently found in the brains of those who had suffered from the disorder. Finally, in the early 1990s, it was discovered that Rasmussen's encephalitis is an autoimmune disease, that is, a disorder in which the body is attacked by its own immune system.

Specifically, the body responds to one of the glutamate receptors, GluR3, as if it were an invading organism. Glutamate is a neurotransmitter, or one of the chemicals that neurons use to signal to each other. A receptor is a complex molecule embedded in the cell membrane of a neuron that detects the presence of a specific neurotransmitter and responds by causing some change in the neuron itself, such as admitting a flow of sodium, potassium, or calcium ions into the cell. There are at least 20 distinct receptors for glutamate in the brain, one of which is denoted GluR3. In Rasmussen's encephalitis, the body (for reasons still unknown) produces anti-GluR3 antibodies. Attracted by these antibodies, groupings of special immune system proteins, termed complement, gather on neurons in the affected parts of the brain, eventually forming "membrane attack complexes" that damage the neurons. It is still not known why this autoimmune response attacks only one side of the brain at first, but it has been hypothesized that a breach in the blood-brain barrier in one part of the brain might allow initial access of antibodies to neurons. The arrival of lymphocytes in the affected area, with consequent swelling of tissues, may then cause further damage to the blood-brain barrier and allow more anti-GluR3 antibodies access to the neurons. Finally, it remains possible that infection by cytomegalovirus may play a role in triggering the autoimmune processes of Rasmussen's encephalitis. Cytomegalovirus DNA has been detected in the brains of some patients.

The first symptom of Rasmussen's encephalitis is seizures, usually beginning suddenly before the age

KEY TERMS

Aphasia—Total or partial loss of the ability to use or understand language; usually caused by stroke, brain disease, or injury.

Autoimmune disorder—Disorders in which the body mounts a destructive immune response against its own tissues.

Blood-brain barrier—The protective membrane that separates circulating blood from brain cells, allowing some substances to enter while others, such as certain drugs, are prevented from entering brain tissue.

Cytomegalovirus—A herpes type of virus that may be transmitted through blood or body fluids and can be fatal in people with weakened immune systems.

Encephalitis—Inflammation of the brain.

Hemiparesis—Muscle weakness on one side of the body.

Neurotransmitter—A chemical that is released during a nerve impulse that transmits information from one nerve cell to another.

of 10. Loss of control over voluntary movements, loss of speech ability (**aphasia**), hemiparesis (**weakness** on one side of the body), **dementia**, **mental retardation**, and eventually, death, will follow if untreated.

Diagnosis

Rasmussen's encephalitis is diagnosed by the sudden onset of epileptic seizures in childhood, gradual worsening of seizures, gradual intellectual deterioration, the onset of hemiparesis and other one-sided symptoms, and the elimination of other possible causes for these symptoms.

Treatment

Early in the progress of Rasmussen's encephalitis, anticonvulsant drugs may help control seizures. Use of the anti-cytomegalovirus drug ganciclovir early in the syndrome produces improvement in some patients. Also, some patients have shown dramatic positive response to removal of anti-GluR3 antibodies from the blood by a process known as plasmapheresis. Researchers have explored the hypothesis that drugs to prevent the formation of membrane-attack complexes might slow or halt the progression of Rasmussen's encephalitis as well as of other neurodegenerative diseases. However, the treatment of choice remained

hemispherectomy, surgical removal of the affected half of the brain.

Remarkably, children may show little or no change in personality and no loss of intelligence or memory after having half their brain removed. Some children are irritable, withdrawn, or depressed immediately after surgery, but these symptoms are not permanent. So flexible is brain development that a child with a hemispherectomy may become fluent in one or more languages even if the left side of the brain, where the speech centers are usually located, is removed. Blindness or vision loss in one eye usually results from hemispherectomy, but normal hearing in both ears may be recovered. The older patients are when the surgery is performed, however, the more likely they are to suffer permanent sensory, speech, and motor losses.

Recovery and rehabilitation

Rehabilitation begins immediately after hemispherectomy with passive range-of-motion exercises. Physical, occupational, and speech therapists are required. For children of school age, neuropsychological testing can help determine what academic setting or grade level is best. Children with hemispherectomies are often able to participate in school at the level appropriate for their age.

Prognosis

The prognosis for children below the age of 10 who are treated early in the course of the syndrome is good. This group can often achieve normal psychosocial and intellectual functioning. Without hemispherectomy, however, persons with Rasmussen's encephalitis eventually suffer near-continuous seizures, mental retardation, and death.

Resources

BOOKS

Graham, David I., and Peter L. Lantos. *Greenfield's Neuropathology*, 6th ed. Bath, UK: Arnold, 1997.

PERIODICALS

Cleaver, Hannah. "Girl Left with Half a Brain Is Fluent in Two Languages." *Daily Telegraph* (London, England), May 23, 2002.

Duke University. "Mild Injury May Render Brain Cells Vulnerable to Immune System Attack." *Ascribe Higher Education News Service* October 23, 2002.

Lilly, Donna J. "Functional Hemispherectomy: Radical Treatment for Rasmussen's Encephalitis." *Journal of Neuroscience Nursing* April 1, 2000.

Mercadante, Marcos T. "Genetics of Childhood Disorders: XXX. Autoimmune Disorders, Part 3: Myasthenia Gravis and Rasmussen's Encephalitis." *Journal of the*

American Academy of Child and Adolescent Psychiatry (September 1, 2001).

Zuckerberg, Aaron. "Why Would You Remove Half a Brain? The Outcome of 58 Children after Hemispherectomy— The Johns Hopkins Experience: 1968–1996." *Pediatrics* (August 1, 1997).

OTHER

"NINDS Rasmussen's Encephalitis Information Page." *National Institute of Neurological Disorders and Stroke.* March 30, 2004 (June 2, 2004). http://www.ninds.nih. gov/health_and_medical/disorders/rasmussn_doc.htm.

ORGANIZATIONS

National Organization for Rare Disorders (NORD). P.O. Box 1968 (55 Kenosia Avenue), Danbury, CT 06813-1968. Phone: (203) 744-0100. Fax: (203) 798-2291. Tollfree phone: (800) 999-NORD. Email: orphan@ rarediseases.org. http://www.rarediseases.org.

Larry Gilman, PhD

Reflex sympathetic dystrophy

Definition

Reflex sympathetic dystrophy is the feeling of pain associated with evidence of minor nerve injury. Reflex sympathetic dystrophy may also referred to as complex regional pain syndrome (CRPS).

Demographics

Reflex sympathetic dystrophy affects between 200,000 and 1.2 million Americans and is two to three times more frequent in females than males. It occurs across all age groups, with a mean age at diagnosis of 42 years.

Description

Historically, reflex sympathetic dystrophy (RSD) was noticed during the American Civil War in patients who suffered pain following gunshot wounds that affected the median nerve (a major nerve in the arm). In 1867 the condition was called causalgia from the Greek term meaning "burning pain." Causalgia refers to pain associated with major nerve injury. The exact causes of RSD are still unclear.

There are two types of RSD. Type 1 is defined as one in which the nerve injury cannot be immediately identified. Type 2 is defined as one in which a distinct nerve injury has occurred.

> **KEY TERMS**
>
> **Atrophy**—Abnormal changes in a cell that lead to loss of cell structure and function.
>
> **Osteoporosis**—Reduction in the quantity of bone.

Patients usually develop a triad of phases. In the first phase, pain and sympathetic activity is increased. Patients will typically present with swelling (edema), stiffness, pain, increased vascularity (resulting in increasing warmth), hyperhydrosis (abnormally increased perspiration), and x-ray changes demonstrating loss of minerals in bone (demineralization). The second phase develops 3–9 months later and is characterized by increased stiffness and changes in the extremity that include a decrease in warmth and atrophy of the skin and muscles. The late phase commencing several months to years later, presents with a pale, cold, painful, and atrophic extremity. Patients at this stage will also have osteoporosis.

It has been thought that each phase relates to a specific nerve defect that involves nerve tracts from the periphery spinal cord to the brain. Both sexes are affected, but the number of new cases is higher in women, adolescents, and young adults. Reflex sympathetic dystrophy has been associated with other terms such as Sudeck's atrophy, post-traumatic osteoporosis, causalgia, shoulder-hand syndrome, and reflex neuromuscular dystrophy.

Causes and symptoms

The exact causes of RSD are not clearly understood as of 2011. There are several theories such as sympathetic overflow (over activity), abnormal circuitry in nerve impulses through the sympathetic system, and as a post-operative complication for both elective and traumatic surgical procedures. Patients typically develop pain, swelling, temperature, color changes, and skin and muscle wasting.

Diagnosis

The diagnosis is confirmed by a local anesthetic block along sympathetic nerve paths in the hand or foot, depending on whether an arm or leg is affected. A test called the erythrocyte sedimentation rate (ESR) can be performed to rule out diseases with similar presentation and arising from other causes.

QUESTIONS TO ASK YOUR DOCTOR

- What are the indications that I may have reflex sympathetic dystrophy?
- What diagnostic tests are needed for a thorough assessment?
- What treatment options do you recommend for me?
- Should I see a specialist? If so, what kind of specialist should I contact?
- If surgery is needed, what kind of surgical specialist should I contact?
- What kind of changes can I expect to see with the medications you have prescribed for me?
- What are the side effects associated with the medications you have prescribed for me?
- What physical limitations do you foresee?
- What tests or evaluation techniques will you perform to see if treatment has been beneficial for me?
- What symptoms are important enough that I should seek immediate treatment?

Treatment

The preferred method to treat RSD includes sympathetic block and physical therapy. Pain is reduced as motion of the affected limb improves. Patients may also require tranquilizers and mild analgesics. Although RSD is not a psychological syndrome, when faced with family and friends who may not believe their recurring complaint of pain, many individuals may benefit from psychological support. Patients who received repeated blocks should consider surgical symathectomy (removal of the nerves causing pain).

Prognosis

The prognosis for treatment during phase one is favorable. As the disease progresses undetected into phase two or three the prognosis for recovery is poor.

Prevention

There is no known prevention since the cause is not clearly understood.

Resources

BOOKS

Aminoff, Michael J., ed. *Neurology and General Medicine.* 4th ed. New York: Churchill Livingstone, 2007.

Hayek, Salim, and Nagy Mekhail. *Complex Regional Pain Syndrome: Redefining Reflex Sympathetic Dystrophy and Causalgia.* 5th ed. Berwyn, PA: JTE Multimedia, 2010.

Icon Group International. *Reflex Sympathetic Dystrophy— A Medical Dictionary, Bibliography, and Annotated Research Guide to Internet References,* 2nd ed. San Diego, CA: Author, 2010.

WEBSITES

"NINDS Complex Regional Pain Syndrome Information Page." National Institute of Neurological Disorders and Stroke. http://www.ninds.nih.gov/disorders/ reflex_sympathetic_dystrophy/reflex_sympathetic_ dystrophy.htm (accessed July 19, 2011).

ORGANIZATIONS

American Academy of Neurology (AAN), 1080 Montreal Avenue, Saint Paul, MN 55116, (651) 695-2717, (800) 879-1960, Fax: (651) 695-2791, memberservices@aan. com, http://www.aan.com.

American Neurological Association, 5841 Cedar Lake Road, Suite 204, Minneapolis, MN 55416, (952) 545-6284, http://www.aneuroa.org.

National Institutes of Health (NIH), 9000 Rockville Pike, Bethesda, MD, United States, 20892, (301) 496-4000, NIHinfo@od.nih.gov, http://www.nih.gov/index.html.

Reflex Sympathetic Dystrophy Syndrome Association of America, P.O. Box 502, Milford, CT 06460, (203) 877-3790, (877) 662-7737, Fax: (203) 882-8362, info@rsds.org, http://www.rsds.org.

Laith Farid Gulli, MD
Robert Ramirez, BS
Laura Jean Cataldo, RN, EdD

Refsum disease

Definition

Refsum disease is an inherited disorder in which the enzyme responsible for processing phytanic acid is defective. Accumulation of phytanic acid in the tissues and the blood leads to damage of the brain, nerves, eyes, skin, and bones.

Description

Refsum disease was first characterized by the Norwegian physician, Sigvald Refsum, in the 1940s and is known by other names, such as classical Refsum disease, adult Refsum disease, phytanic acid alpha-hydroxylase deficiency, phytanic acid storage disease, hypertrophic neuropathy of Refsum, heredopathia atactica polyneuritiformis, and hereditary motor and sensory neuropathy IV. Refsum disease should not be confused with infantile Refsum disease, which was once thought to be a variant of the disorder but is now known to be a genetically and biochemically distinct entity. Sometimes infantile Refsum disease is simply referred to as "Refsum disease," furthering the confusion.

Living bodies are made up of millions of individual cells that are specifically adapted to carry out particular functions. Within cells are even smaller structures, called organelles, that perform jobs and enable the cell to serve its ultimate purpose. One type of organelle is the peroxisome, whose main function is to break down waste materials or to process materials that, if allowed to accumulate, would prove toxic to the cells.

Phytanic acid is a substance found in foods, such as dairy products, beef, lamb, and some fish. Normally, phytanic acid is processed by a set of enzymes within the cell to convert it to another form. In the past, scientists were unsure where in the cell this process took place, hypothesizing that it may occur in the peroxisome or another organelle, called the mitochondrion. However, recent research has definitively determined that the enzymes responsible for processing phytanic acid are located in the peroxisome.

Refsum disease is an inherited disorder in which one of the peroxisomal enzymes, phytanic acid hydroxylase (also called phytanic acid oxidase, or phytanyl CoA hydroxylase), is defective, resulting in unprocessed phytanic acid. Consequently, phytanic acid builds up in the tissues of the body and the bloodstream, causing damage to different organ systems.

Genetic profile

Refsum disease is a genetic condition and can be inherited or passed on in a family. The genetic defect for the disorder is inherited as an autosomal recessive trait, meaning that two abnormal genes are needed to display the disease. A person who carries one abnormal gene does not display the disease and is called a carrier. A carrier has a 50% chance of transmitting the gene to his or her children. A child must inherit the same abnormal gene from each parent to display the disease.

Refsum disease is caused by a deficiency in an enzyme, phytanic acid hydroxylase. The gene encoding for this enzyme, called PAHX or PHYH, was identified in 1997 and mapped to human chromosome 10 (locus: 10pter-p11.2). Several common mutations have been identified in the gene that result in Refsum disease.

Demographics

Refsum disease is rare, but the exact incidence and prevalence of the disorder in the general population is not known. Refsum disease may not be distributed equally among geographical areas or different ethnic groups, as most of the diagnosed cases have been found in children and young adults of Scandinavian heritage.

Signs and symptoms

Patients with Refsum disease generally do not show obvious defects at birth, and growth and development initially appears normal. The onset of clinical symptoms varies from early childhood to age 50, but symptoms usually appear before 20 years of age. The manifestations of Refsum disease primarily involve the nervous system, the eye, the skin, the bones, and, in rare cases, the heart and kidneys.

Phytanic acid deposits in the fatty sheaths surrounding nerves, causing damage and resulting in **peripheral**

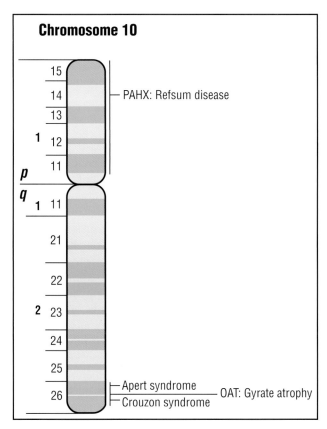

Refsum disease, on chromosome 10. *(Illustration by Argosy, Inc. Reproduced by permission of Gale, a part of Cengage Learning.)*

neuropathy in 90% of patients with Refsum disease. Peripheral neuropathy is the term for dysfunction of the nerves outside of the spinal cord, causing loss of sensation, muscle **weakness**, pain, and loss of reflexes. Nerves leading to the nose and ears can also be affected, resulting in **anosmia** (loss of the sense of smell) in 35% of patients and **hearing loss** or deafness in 50% of patients. Finally, Refsum disease results in cerebellar **ataxia** in 75% of patients. Cerebellar ataxia is a defect in a specific part of the brain (the **cerebellum**), resulting in loss of coordination and unsteadiness. In contrast to infantile Refsum disease, people with Refsum disease do not show **mental retardation** and generally have normal intelligence.

Accumulation of phytanic acid also results in disorders of the eye. The most common finding is retinitis pigmentosa, a degeneration of the retina resulting in poor nighttime vision and sometimes blindness. Disorders of pupil movement and nystagmus (uncontrollable movements of the eye) may also be present due to related nervous system damage. Other eye manifestations of Refsum disease may include glaucoma (abnormally high pressure in the eye, leading to vision loss) and cataracts (clouding of the lens of the eye).

People with Refsum disease often develop dry, rough, scaly skin. These skin changes, called ichthyosis, can occur over the entire body but sometimes will appear only on the palms and soles of the feet. In addition to these skin abnormalities, 60% of affected people may experience abnormal bone growth, manifesting as shortened limbs or fingers, or abnormal curvatures of the spine.

Patients with Refsum disease usually first present to a physician complaining of weakness in the arms and legs, physical unsteadiness and/or nightblindness or failing vision. The symptoms associated with Refsum disease are progressive and, if untreated, will become more numerous and severe as the patient ages. For reasons that are not completely understood, clinical deterioration can sometimes be interrupted by periods of good health without symptoms.

Diagnosis

Refsum disease is diagnosed though a combination of consistent medical history, physical exam findings, and laboratory and genetic testing. When patients with Refsum disease present to their physicians complaining of visual problems or muscle weakness, physical signs of retinitis pigmentosa, peripheral neuropathy, cerebellar ataxia, or skin and bone changes (as discussed above) are often noted. These findings raise suspicion

for a genetic syndrome or metabolic disorder, and further tests are conducted.

Laboratory tests reveal several abnormalities. Normally, phytanic acid levels are essentially undetectable in the plasma. Thus, the presence of high levels of phytanic acid in the bloodstream is highly indicative of Refsum disease. If necessary, a small portion of the patient's connective tissue can be sampled and grown in a laboratory and tested to demonstrate a failure to process phytanic acid appropriately. Other associated laboratory abnormalities include the presence of high amounts of protein in the fluid that bathes the spinal cord, or abnormal electrical responses recorded from the brain, muscles, heart, ears, retina, and various nerves as a result of nervous system damage.

Genetic testing can also be performed. When a diagnosis of Refsum disease is made in a child, genetic testing of the PAHX/PHYH gene can be offered to determine if a specific gene change can be identified. If a specific change is identified, carrier testing can be offered to relatives. In families where the parents have been identified to be carriers of the abnormal gene, diagnosis of Refsum disease before birth is possible. Prenatal diagnosis is performed on cells obtained by amniocentesis (withdrawal of the fluid surrounding a fetus in the womb using a needle) at about 16–18 weeks of pregnancy or from the chorionic villi (a part of the placenta) at 10–12 weeks of pregnancy.

Treatment and management

There is no cure for Refsum disease, thus treatment focuses on reducing levels of phytanic acid in the bloodstream to prevent the progression of tissue damage. Phytanic acid is not made in the human body and comes exclusively from the diet. Restriction of phytanic acid-containing foods can slow progress of the disease or reverse some of the symptoms. Patients are advised to maintain consumption of phytanic acid below 10 mg/day (the normal intake is approximately 100 mg/day). Sources of high levels of phytanic acid to be avoided include meats (beef, lamb, goat), dairy products (cream, milk, butter, cheese), and some fish (tuna, cod, haddock). Plasma levels of phytanic acid can be monitored periodically by a physician to investigate the effectiveness of the restricted diet and determine if changes are required. As a result of dietary restriction, nutritional deficiencies may result. Consultation with a nutritionist is recommended to assure proper amounts of calories, protein, and vitamins are obtained through the diet, and nutritional supplements may be required.

KEY TERMS

Autosomal recessive—A pattern of genetic inheritance where two abnormal genes are needed to display the trait or disease.

Carrier—A person who possesses a gene for an abnormal trait without showing signs of the disorder. The person may pass the abnormal gene on to offspring.

Cerebellar ataxia—Unsteadiness and lack of coordination caused by a progressive degeneration of the part of the brain known as the cerebellum.

Enzyme—A protein that catalyzes a biochemical reaction or change without changing its own structure or function.

Ichthyosis—Rough, dry, scaly skin that forms as a result of a defect in skin formation.

Mutant—A change in the genetic material that may alter a trait or characteristic of an individual or manifest as disease.

Organelle—Small, sub-cellular structures that carry out different functions necessary for cellular survival and proper cellular functioning.

Peripheral neuropathy—Any disease of the nerves outside of the spinal cord, usually resulting in weakness and/or numbness.

Peroxisome—A cellular organelle containing different enzymes responsible for the breakdown of waste or other products.

Phytanic acid—A substance found in various foods that, if allowed to accumulate, is toxic to various tissues. It is metabolized in the peroxisome by phytanic acid hydroxylase.

Phytanic acid hydroxylase—A peroxisomal enzyme responsible for processing phytanic acid. It is defective in Refsum disease.

Plasmapheresis—A procedure in which the fluid component of blood is removed from the bloodstream and sometimes replaced with other fluids or plasma.

Retinitis pigmentosa—Progressive deterioration of the retina, often leading to vision loss and blindness.

Because phytanic acid is stored in fat deposits within the body, it is important for patients with Refsum disease to have regular eating patterns; with even brief periods of fasting, fat stores are converted to energy, resulting in the release of stored phytanic acid into the blood stream. Thus, unless a patient assumes a regular eating pattern, repeated and periodic liberation of phytanic acid stores results in greater tissue damage and symptom development. For these same reasons, intentional weight loss through calorie-restricted diets or vigorous exercise is discouraged.

Another useful adjunct to dietary treatment is plasmapheresis. Plasmapheresis is a procedure by which a determined amount of plasma (the fluid component of blood that contains phytanic acid) is removed from the blood and replaced with fluids or plasma that do not contain phytanic acid. Regular utilization of this technique allows people who fail to follow a restricted diet to maintain lower phytanic acid levels and experience less tissue damage and symptoms.

Patients with Refsum disease should be seen regularly by a multidisciplinary team of health care providers, including a pediatrician, neurologist, ophthalmologist, cardiologist, medical geneticist specializing in metabolic disease, nutritionist, and physical/occupational therapist. People with Refsum disease, or those who are carriers of the abnormal gene or who have an relative with the disorder, can be referred for genetic counseling to assist in making reproductive decisions.

Prognosis

The prognosis of Refsum disease varies dramatically. The disorder is slowly progressive and, if left untreated, severe symptoms will develop with considerably shortened life expectancy. However, if diagnosed early, strict adherence to a phytanic acid-free dietary regimen can prevent progression of the disease and reverse skin disease and some of the symptoms of peripheral neuropathy. Unfortunately, treatment cannot undo existing damage to vision and hearing.

Resources

BOOKS

"Peroxisomal Disorders." In *Nelson Textbook of Pediatrics.* Edited by R. E. Behrman. Philadelphia: W.B. Saunders, 2000. 318–84.

WEBSITES

"Entry 266500: Refsum Disease." *OMIM—Online Mendelian Inheritance in Man.* http://www.ncbi.nlm.nih.gov/htbin-post/Omim/dispmim?266500.

Oren Traub, MD, PhD

Repetitive motion disorders

Definition

Repetitive motion disorders are a group of syndromes caused by injuries to muscles, tendons, nerves, or blood vessels from repeated or sustained exertions of different body parts. Most of these disorders involve the hands, arms, or neck and shoulder area. Other names for repetitive motion disorders include repetitive trauma disorders, repetitive strain injuries (RSIs), overuse syndrome, work-related disorders, and regional musculoskeletal disorders.

Description

Repetitive motion disorders are characterized by pain, loss of strength and coordination, numbness or tingling, and sometimes redness or swelling in the affected area. The symptoms come on gradually and are usually relieved temporarily by resting or avoiding the use of the affected body part. Repetitive motion disorders are commonly thought of as work related, but they can occur as a result of academic, leisure-time, or household activities as well.

Demographics

The demographics of repetitive motion disorders vary according to the specific syndrome. About 50% of all industrial injuries in the United States and Canada are attributed to overuse disorders. Professional athletes, dancers, and musicians experience one of these disorders at a much higher percentage at some point in their careers.

Race is not known to be a factor in repetitive motion disorders. Gender has a significant effect on the demographics of some disorders, but it is not clear whether the higher incidence of some disorders in women reflects different occupational choices for men and women, or whether it reflects biological differences. For example, de Quervain's syndrome is a common overuse disorder in women involved with childcare, because repeated lifting and carrying of small children places severe strains on the wrist joint. However, some researchers think that the greater frequency of this disorder in women is related to the effects of female sex hormones on connective tissue, as women's ligaments are slightly looser during pregnancy and at certain points in the menstrual cycle.

Some repetitive motion disorders appear to be age related. **Carpal tunnel syndrome** is more common in middle-aged than in younger women and trigger finger is most common in people aged 55–60. It is not yet known whether the widespread use of computers in the workplace will change the age distribution of repetitive motion disorders as present workers grow older.

Causes and symptoms

Causes

SOFT TISSUE DAMAGE. Repetitive motion disorders are the end result of a combination of factors. One basic cause of repetitive motion disorders, however, is microtraumas, which are tiny damages to or tears in soft tissue that occur from routine stresses on the body or repeated use of specific muscles and joints. When microtraumas are not healed during sleep or daily rest periods, they accumulate over time, causing tissue damage, inflammation, and the activation of pain receptors in peripheral nerves.

NERVE COMPRESSION. Some repetitive motion disorders are associated with entrapment neuropathies, which are functional disorders of the **peripheral nervous system**. In an entrapment neuropathy, a nerve is damaged by compression as it passes through a bony or fibrous tunnel. Carpal tunnel syndrome, de Quervain's syndrome, ulnar nerve syndrome, and **thoracic outlet syndrome** are examples of entrapment neuropathies.

Compression damages peripheral nerves by limiting their blood supply. Even slight pressures on a nerve can limit the flow of blood through the smaller blood vessels surrounding the nerve. As the pressure increases, transmission of nerve impulses is affected and the patient's sensation and coordination are affected, with further increases in **nerve compression** producing greater distortion of sensation and range of motion.

TECHNOLOGICAL AND SOCIAL FACTORS. Economic and social factors that have affected people's occupations and leisure-time activities over the past two centuries have contributed to the increase in repetitive motion disorders. The Industrial Revolution led to increased job specialization, which meant that more and more workers were employed doing one task repeatedly rather than many different tasks. In addition, industrialization brought about the invention of complex tools and machinery that affect the tissues and organs of the human body in many ways. The high levels of psychological and emotional tension in modern life also contribute to repetitive stress injuries by increasing the physical stresses on muscles and joints.

INDIVIDUAL RISK FACTORS. Risk factors that are associated with repetitive stress injuries include the following:

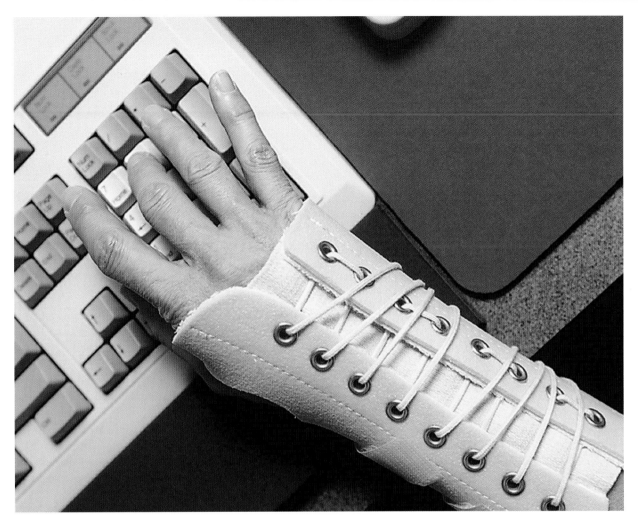

The Industrial Revolution led to increased job specialization, which meant that more and more workers were employed doing one task repeatedly rather than many different tasks. Office work is a case in point. *(© Photo Researchers, Inc.)*

- Awkward or incorrect body postures. Each joint in the body has a position within its range of motion in which it is least likely to become injured. This position is called the neutral position. Any deviation from the neutral position puts increased strain on body tissues. Inadequate work space, using athletic or job-related equipment that is not proportioned to one's height, or improper technique are common reasons for RSIs related to body posture.

- Use of excessive force to perform a task. Pounding on piano keys or hammering harder than is necessary to drive nails are examples of this risk factor.

- Extended periods of static work. This type of work requires muscular effort, but no movement takes place. Instead, the muscles contract, preventing blood from reaching tissues to nourish the cells and carry away waste products. Over time, the muscle tissue

loses its ability to repair microtraumas. Examples of static work include sitting at a desk for hours on end or holding the arms over the head while painting a ceiling.

- Activities that require repetitive movements. Assembly-line work and word processing are examples of job-related repetitive motion. In addition, such leisure-time activities as knitting, embroidery, gardening, model construction, and golf or tennis can have the same long-term effects on the body as work-related activities.

- Mechanical injury. Tools with poorly designed handles that cut into the skin or concentrate pressure on a small area of the hand often contribute to overuse disorders.

- Vibration. There are two types of vibration that can cause damage to the body. One type is segmental vibration, which occurs when the source of the vibration affects only the part of the body in direct contact with it. An example of segmental vibration is a dentist's use of a high-speed drill. Overexposure of the hands to segmental vibration can eventually damage the fingers, leading to Raynaud's phenomenon. The second type is whole-body vibration, which occurs when the vibrations are transmitted throughout the body. Long-distance truckers and jackhammer operators often develop back injuries as the result of long-term whole-body vibration.

- Temperature extremes. Cold temperatures decrease blood flow in the extremities, while high temperatures lead to dehydration and rapid fatigue. In both cases, blood circulation is either decreased or redirected, thus slowing down the process of normal tissue recovery.

- Psychological stress. People who are worried, afraid, or angry often carry their tension in their neck, back, or shoulder muscles. This tension reduces blood circulation in the affected tissues, thus interfering with tissue recovery. In addition, emotional stress has been shown to influence people's perception of physical pain; workers who are unhappy in their jobs, for example, are more likely to seek treatment for work-related disorders.

- Structural abnormalities. These abnormalities include congenital deformities in bones and muscles, changes in the shape of a bone from healed breaks or fractures, bone spurs, and tumors. Overdevelopment of certain muscle groups from athletic workouts may result in entrapment neuropathies in the shoulder area.

- Other systemic conditions or diseases. People with such disorders as rheumatoid arthritis (RA), joint infections, hypothyroidism, or diabetes are at increased risk of developing repetitive motion disorders. Pregnancy is a risk factor for overuse disorders affecting the hands because of the increased amount of fluid in the joints of the wrists and fingers.

Symptoms

The symptoms of repetitive motion disorders include the following:

- Pain. The pain of an RSI is typically felt as an aching sensation that gets worse if the affected joint(s) or limb is moved or used. The pain may be severe enough to wake the patient at night.

- Paresthesias. Paresthesia refers to an abnormal sensation of pricking, tingling, burning, or "insects crawling beneath the skin" in the absence of an external stimulus.

- Numbness, coldness, or loss of sensation in the affected area.
- Clumsiness, weakness, or loss of coordination.
- Impaired range of motion or locking of a joint.
- Popping, clicking, or crackling sounds in a joint.
- Swelling or redness in the affected area.

Diagnosis

History and physical examination

The diagnosis of a repetitive motion disorder begins with taking the patient's history, including occupational history. The doctor will ask about the specific symptoms in the affected part, particularly if the patient suffers from rheumatoid arthritis, diabetes, or other general conditions as well as overuse of the joint or limb.

The next step is physical examination of the affected area. The doctor will typically palpate (feel) or press on the sore area to determine whether there is swelling as well as pain. He or she will then perform a series of maneuvers to evaluate the range of motion in the affected joint(s), listen for crackles or other sounds when the joint is moved, and test for **weakness** or instability in the limb or joint. There are simple physical tests for specific repetitive motion disorders. For example, the Finkelstein test is used to evaluate a patient for de Quervain's syndrome. The patient is asked to fold the thumb across the palm of the affected hand and then bend the fingers over the thumb. A person with de Quervain's will experience sharp pain when the doctor moves the hand sideways in the direction of the elbow. Tinel's test is used to diagnose carpal tunnel syndrome. The doctor gently taps with a rubber hammer along the inside of the wrist above the median nerve to see whether the patient experiences paresthesias.

Laboratory tests

Laboratory tests of blood or tissue fluid are not ordinarily ordered unless the doctor suspects an infection or wishes to rule out diabetes, anemia, or thyroid imbalance.

Imaging studies

Imaging studies may be ordered to rule out other conditions that may be causing the patient's symptoms or to identify areas of nerve compression. When surgery is being planned, x rays may be helpful in identifying stress fractures, damage to cartilage, or other abnormalities in bones and joints. Magnetic resonance imaging (MRI) can be used to identify injuries to tendons, ligaments, and muscles as well as areas of nerve entrapment.

Electrodiagnostic studies

The most common electrodiagnostic tests used to evaluate repetitive motion disorders are **electromyography** (EMG) and nerve conduction studies (NCS). In EMG, the doctor inserts thin needles in specific muscles and observes the electrical signals that are displayed on a screen. This test helps to identify which muscles and nerves are affected by pain. Nerve conduction studies are done to determine whether specific nerves have been damaged. The doctor positions two sets of electrodes on the patient's skin over the muscles in the affected area. One set of electrodes stimulates the nerves supplying that muscle by delivering a mild electrical shock; the other set records the nerve's electrical signals on a machine.

Treatment team

A mild repetitive motion disorder may be treated by a primary care physician. If conservative treatment is ineffective, the patient may be referred to an orthopedic surgeon or neurosurgeon for further evaluation and surgical treatment. Patients whose disorders are related to job dissatisfaction or who have had to give up their occupation or favorite activity because of their disorder may benefit from psychotherapy.

Physical therapists and occupational therapists are an important part of the treatment team, advising patients about proper use of the injured body part and developing a home exercise program. Some patients benefit from having their workplace and equipment evaluated by the occupational therapist or an ergonomics expert. Professional athletes, dancers, or musicians usually consult an expert in their specific field for evaluation of faulty posture or technique.

Treatment

Conservative treatment

Conservative treatment for overuse injuries typically includes:

- Resting the affected part. Complete rest should last no longer than 2–3 days, however. What is known as "relative rest" is better for the patient because it maintains range of motion in the affected part, prevents loss of muscle strength, and lowers the risk of "sick behavior." Sick behavior refers to using an injury or illness to gain attention or care and concern from others.
- Applying ice packs or gentle heat.

- Oral medications. These may include mild pain relievers (usually NSAIDs); amitriptyline or another tricyclic antidepressant; or vitamin B_6.
- Injections. Corticosteroids may be injected into joints to lower inflammation and swelling. In some cases, local anesthetics may also be given by injection.
- Splinting. Splints are most commonly used to treat overuse injuries of the hand or wrist; they can be custom-molded by an occupational therapist.
- Ergonomic corrections in the home or workplace. These may include changing the height of chairs or computer keyboards; scheduling frequent breaks from computer work or musical practice; correcting one's posture; and similar measures.
- Transcutaneous electrical nerve stimulation (TENS). TENS involves the use of a patient-controlled portable device that sends mild electrical impulses through injured tissues via electrodes placed over the skin. It is reported to relieve pain in 75–80% of patients treated for repetitive motion disorders.

Surgery

Repetitive motion disorders are treated with surgery only when conservative measures fail to relieve the patient's pain after a trial of 6–12 weeks. The most common surgical procedures performed for these disorders are nerve decompression, tendon release, and repair of loose or torn ligaments.

Complementary and alternative (CAM) treatments

Complementary and alternative treatments that have been shown to be effective in treating repetitive motion disorders include:

- Acupuncture. Studies funded by the National Center for Complementary and Alternative Medicine (NCCAM) since 1998 have found that acupuncture is an effective treatment for pain related to repetitive motion disorders.
- Sports massage, Swedish massage, and shiatsu.
- Yoga and tai chi. The gentle stretching in these forms of exercise helps to improve blood circulation and maintain range of motion without tissue damage.
- Alexander technique. The Alexander technique is an approach to body movement that emphasizes correct posture, particularly the proper position of the head with respect to the spine. It is often recommended for dancers, musicians, and computer users.

KEY TERMS

Alexander technique—A form of movement therapy that emphasizes correct posture and the proper positioning of the head with regard to the spine.

de Quervain's syndrome—Inflammation of the tendons contained within the wrist, associated with aching pain in the wrist and thumb. Named for the Swiss surgeon who first described it in 1895, the syndrome is sometimes called washerwoman's sprain because it is commonly caused by overuse of the wrist.

Entrapment neuropathy—A disorder of the peripheral nervous system in which a nerve is damaged by compression as it passes through a bony or fibrous passage or canal. Many repetitive motion disorders are associated with entrapment neuropathies.

Ergonomics—The branch of science that deals with human work and the efficient use of energy, including anatomical, physiological, biomechanical, and psychosocial factors.

Median nerve—The nerve that supplies the forearm, wrist area, and many of the joints of the hand.

Neuropathy—Any diseased condition of the nervous system.

Paresthesia—The medical term for an abnormal touch sensation, usually tingling, burning, or prickling, that develops in the absence of an external stimulus. Paresthesias are a common symptom of repetitive motion disorders.

Peripheral nervous system—The part of the human nervous system outside the brain and spinal cord.

Raynaud's phenomenon—A disorder characterized by episodic attacks of loss of circulation in the fingers or toes. Most cases of Raynaud's are not work-related; however, the disorder occasionally develops in workers who operate vibrating tools as part of their job, and is sometimes called vibration-induced white finger.

Transcutaneous electrical nerve stimulation (TENS)—A form of treatment for chronic pain that involves the use of a patient-controlled device for transmitting mild electrical impulses through the skin over the injured area.

Trigger finger—An overuse disorder of the hand in which one or more fingers tend to lock or "trigger" when the patient tries to extend the finger.

Ulnar nerve—The nerve that supplies some of the forearm muscles, the elbow joint, and many of the short muscles of the hand.

• Hydrotherapy. Warm whirlpool baths improve circulation and relieve pain in injured joints and soft tissue.

Recovery and rehabilitation

Recovery from a repeated motion disorder may take only a few days of rest or modified activity, or it may take several months when surgery is required.

Rehabilitation is tailored to the individual patient and the specific disorder involved. Rehabilitation programs for repetitive motion disorders focus on recovering strength in the injured body part, maintaining or improving range of motion, and learning ways to lower the risk of reinjuring the affected part. Professional musicians, dancers, and athletes require highly specialized rehabilitation programs.

Clinical trials

Information about current relevant clinical trials can be found at ClinicalTrials.gov.

Prognosis

The prognosis for recovery from repetitive motion disorders depends on the specific disorder, the degree of damage to the nerves and other structures involved, and the patient's compliance with exercise or rehabilitation programs. Most patients experience adequate pain relief from either conservative measures or surgery. Some, however, will not recover full use of the affected body part and must change occupations or give up the activity that produced the disorder.

Resources

BOOKS

National Research Council and Institute of Medicine (IOM). *Musculoskeletal Disorders and the Workplace: Low Back and Upper Extremities.* Washington, DC: National Academy Press, 2001.

"Neurovascular Syndromes: Carpal Tunnel Syndrome." Section 5, Chapter 61 in *The Merck Manual of Diagnosis and Therapy,* edited by Mark H. Beers and Robert Berkow. Whitehouse Station, NJ: Merck Research Laboratories, 2002.

Pelletier, Kenneth R., *The Best Alternative Medicine,* Part II, "CAM Therapies for Specific Conditions: Carpal

Tunnel Syndrome." New York: Simon & Schuster, 2002.

"Tendon Problems: Digital Tendinitis and Tenosynovitis." Section 5, Chapter 61 in *The Merck Manual of Diagnosis and Therapy*, edited by Mark H. Beers and Robert Berkow. Whitehouse Station, NJ: Merck Research Laboratories, 2002.

PERIODICALS

Andersen, J. H., J. F. Thomsen, E. Overgaard, et al. "Computer Use and Carpal Tunnel Syndrome: A 1-Year Follow-Up Study." *Journal of the American Medical Association* 289 (June 11, 2003): 2963–69.

Hogan, K. A., and R. H. Gross. "Overuse Injuries in Pediatric Athletes." *Orthopedic Clinics of North America* 34 (July 2003): 405–15.

Kern, R. Z. "The Electrodiagnosis of Ulnar Nerve Entrapment at the Elbow." *Canadian Journal of Neurological Sciences/ Journal canadien des sciences neurologiques* 30 (November 2003): 314–19.

Kryger, A. I., J. H. Andersen, C. F. Lassen, et al. "Does Computer Use Pose An Occupational Hazard for Forearm Pain; from the NUDATA Study." *Occupational and Environmental Medicine* 60 (November 2003): e14.

Leclerc, A., J. F. Chastang, I. Niedhammer, et al. "Incidence of Shoulder Pain in Repetitive Work." *Occupational and Environmental Medicine* 61 (January 2004): 39–44.

Nourissat, G., P. Chamagne, and C. Dumontier. "Reasons Why Musicians Consult Hand Surgeons." [in French] *Revue de chirurgie orthopédique et réparatrice de l'appareil moteur* 89 (October 2003): 524–31.

Tallia, A. F., and D. A. Cardone. "Diagnostic and Therapeutic Injection of the Wrist and Hand Region." *American Family Physician* 67 (February 15, 2003): 745–50.

Valachi, B., and K. Valachi. "Mechanisms Leading to Musculoskeletal Disorders in Dentistry." *Journal of the American Dental Association* 134 (October 2003): 1344–50.

WEBSITES

Fuller, David A., MD. "Carpal Tunnel Syndrome." eMedicine 15 October 2003 (March 23, 2004). http://www. emedicine. com/orthoped/topic455.htm.

Kale, Satischandra, MD. "Trigger Finger." eMedicine 25 February 2002 (March 23, 2004). http://www.emedicine. com/orthoped/topic570.htm.

Kaye, Vladimir, and Murray E. Brandstater. "Transcutaneous Electrical Nerve Stimulation." eMedicine 29 January, 2002 (March 23, 2004). http://www.emedicine. com/pmr/topic206.htm.

Meals, Roy A., MD. "De Quervain Tenosynovitis." eMedicine 15 April 2002 (March 23, 2004). http://www.emedicine.com/ orthoped/topic482.htm

National Institute of Neurological Disorders and Stroke (NINDS). *NINDS Thoracic Outlet Syndrome Information Page*. (March 23, 2004.) http://www.ninds.nih.gov/ health_and_medical/disorders/thoracic_doc.htm.

Stern, Mark, and Scott P. Steinmann, "Ulnar Nerve Entrapment." eMedicine 8 January 2004 (March 23, 2004). http://www.emedicine.com/orthoped/ topic574.htm.

Strober, Jonathan B., MD. "Writer's Cramp." eMedicine 18 January 2002 (March 23, 2004). http://www.emedicine. com/neuro/topic614.htm.

Strum, Scott, MD. "Overuse Injury." eMedicine 14 September 2001 (March 23, 2004). http://www.emedicine.com/pmr/ topic97.htm.

ORGANIZATIONS

American Academy of Orthopaedic Surgeons (AAOS). 6300 North River Road, Rosemont, IL 60018-4262. Phone: (847) 823-7186. Fax: (847) 823-8125. Tollfree phone: (800) 346-AAOS. http://www.aaos.org.

American Society for Surgery of the Hand (ASSH). 6300 North River Road, Suite 800, Rosemont, IL 60018. Phone: (847) 384-8300. Fax: (847) 384-1435. Email: info@hand-surg.org. http://www.hand-surg.org.

National Institute for Occupational Safety and Health (NIOSH). Centers for Disease Control and Prevention, 1600 Clifton Road, Atlanta, GA 30333. Phone: (404) 639-3534. Tollfree phone: (800) 311-3435. http:// www.cdc.gov/niosh/homepage.html.

National Institute of Arthritis and Musculoskeletal and Skin Diseases (NIAMS) Information Clearinghouse, National Institutes of Health. 1 AMS Circle, Bethesda, MD 20892-3675. Phone: (301) 495-4844. Fax: (301) 718-6366. Tollfree phone: (877) 22-NIAMS. Email: NIAMSinfo@mail.nih.gov. http:// www.niams.nih.gov.

National Institute of Neurological Disorders and Stroke (NINDS). 9000 Rockville Pike, Bethesda, MD 20892. Phone: (301) 496-5751. Tollfree phone: (800) 352-9424. http://www.ninds.nih.gov.

Rebecca J. Frey, PhD

Repetitive stress injuries *see* **Repetitive motion disorders**

Respite

Definition

Respite literally means a period of rest or relief. Respite care provides a caregiver temporary relief from the responsibilities of caring for individuals with chronic physical or mental disabilities. Respite care is often referred to as a gift of time.

Purpose

Respite was developed in response to the deinstitutionalization movement of the 1960s and 1970s. Maintaining individuals in their natural homes rather than placing them in long-term care facilities was viewed as beneficial to the individual, the involved family, and society (in terms of lowered health care costs). The primary purpose of respite care is to relieve caregiver stress, thereby enabling the caregiver to continue caring for the individual with a disability.

Respite care is typically provided for individuals with disorders related to aging (**dementia**, frail health), terminal illnesses, chronic health issues, or developmental disabilities. More recently, children with behavior disorders have also been eligible for respite care. Respite care is usually recreational and does not include therapy or treatment for the individual with the disability.

Caregivers frequently experience stress in the forms of physical **fatigue**, psychological distress (resentment, frustration, anxiety, guilt, **depression**), and disruption in relations with other family members. The emotional aspects of caring for a family member are often more taxing than the physical demands. Increased caregiver stress may result in health problems such as ulcers, high blood pressure, difficulty sleeping, weight loss or gain, or breathing difficulties.

Types of respite

Length of respite care can be anywhere from a few hours to several weeks. Services may be used frequently or infrequently, such as for emergencies, vacations, one day per week or month, weekends, or everyday.

A variety of facilities provide respite care services. The type of service available is often closely related to the characteristics of the facility, including:

- In-home respite services consist of a worker who comes to the family home while the caregiver is away. These services are usually provided by agencies that recruit, screen, and train workers. This type of respite is usually less disruptive to the individual with the disability, provided there is a good match between the worker and the individual. However, issues of reliability and trustworthiness of the worker can be an additional source of stress for the caregiver.

- Respite centers are residential facilities specifically designed for respite care. Adult day care programs and respite camps also fall into this category. This type of respite offers more peace of mind to the caregiver and may provide a stimulating environment for the individual with the disability. However, centers

usually restrict length of stay and may exclude individuals based on severity of disability.

- Institutional settings sometimes reserve spaces to be used for respite purposes. These include skilled nursing facilities, intermediate care facilities, group homes, senior housing, regular day care or after-school programs for children, and hospitals. Some of these facilities provide higher levels of care but are less homelike. The individual with the disability may oppose staying in an institutional setting or may fear abandonment.

- Licensed foster care providers can also provide respite services in their homes.

Funding

Costs of respite care present a financial burden to many families. Community mental health centers often fund respite services if the individual meets certain criteria, including eligibility for Medicaid. Wraparound programs (also accessed through community mental health centers) for children with emotional or behavioral disorders also pay for respite services. Veteran's Administration hospitals provide respite care at little or no charge if the individual receiving the care is a veteran (but not if the caregiver is a veteran). Private insurance companies rarely pay for respite, and many respite providers do not accept this form of payment. Some respite facilities have sliding-scale fees. Other facilities operate as a co-op, where caregivers work at the facility in exchange for respite services.

In addition, respite agencies may have difficulty recruiting and retaining qualified employees, because limited funding prevents agencies from offering desirable salaries. The high turnover and unavailability of employees may result in delays in service delivery or family dissatisfaction with services. Advocacy for policy changes regarding funding is needed.

Barriers to using respite services

Recent research suggests that families who use respite tend to have higher levels of perceived stress, lower levels of support from others, and fewer resources. In many of these families, the individuals in need of care have more severe disabilities, problem behaviors such as aggression or self-injury, and communication difficulties; are school-aged; and are more dependent for basic needs such as eating, toileting, and dressing.

It has been well documented that many families eligible for respite care never utilize these services. Research regarding the use, availability, and effectiveness of respite care is still in the preliminary stages. Various reasons for non-utilization of respite include:

- Unfamiliarity: Some families are unaware that such services exist or may be uncertain about how to access services. This implies a need for improved referral services.

- Funding: Limited funding may prevent some families from receiving services.

- Caregiver qualities: Some caregivers experience guilt or anxiety over allowing someone else to care for their loved one. Being able to maintain one's family independently may be tied to gender roles or cultural customs. Relatives and friends may assist in caregiving, making formal respite unnecessary.

- Care recipient qualities: Occasionally individuals with the disability are opposed to respite care. They may not trust strangers or may refuse to leave home. In other instances, individuals may have behaviors, or require physical care, that are too challenging for the respite provider.

- Program qualities: Many researchers believe that respite programs are not adequately meeting the needs of families. In some cases, times that services are offered are inconvenient. Individuals with severe disabilities who pose the most need for services are sometimes excluded.

Many caregivers obtain respite in informal ways not offered by respite services. Some researchers have suggested that respite care should be just one form of service available to caregivers. Other services that may alleviate caregiver stress could include home-delivered meals, transportation assistance, recreational resources, or care skills training.

Resources

BOOKS

Ownby, Lisa L. *Partners Plus: Families and Caregivers in Partnerships: A Family-Centered Guide to Respite Care.* Washington, DC: Child Development Resources, U.S. Department of Education, Office of Educational Research and Improvement, Educational Resources Information Center, 1999.

Tepper, Lynn M., and John A. Toner, eds. *Respite Care: Programs, Problems, and Solutions.* Philadelphia: Charles Press, 1993.

PERIODICALS

Chan, Jeffrey B., and Jeff Sigafoos. "A Review of Child and Family Characteristics Related to the Use of Respite Care in Developmental Disability Services." *Child and Youth Care Forum* 29, no. 1 (2000): 27–37.

Chappell, Neena L., R. Colin Reid, and Elizabeth Dow. "Respite Reconsidered: A Typology of Meanings Based on the Caregiver's Point of View." *Journal of Aging Studies* 15, no. 2 (2001): 201–16.

ORGANIZATIONS

The Arc National Headquarters, P.O. Box 1047, Arlington, TX 76004. (817) 261-6003; (817) 277-0553 TDD. the-arc@metronet.com. http://www.thearc.org.

ARCH National Respite Network and Resource Center. Chapel Hill Training-Outreach Project, 800 Eastowne Drive, Suite 105, Chapel Hill, NC 27514. (888) 671-2594; (919) 490-5577. http://www.chtop.com.

National Aging Information Center. Administration on Aging, 330 Independence Avenue, SW, Room 4656, Washington, DC 20201. (202) 619-7501. http://www.aoa.gov/naic.

National Information Center for Children and Youth with Disabilities. P.O. Box 1492, Washington, DC 20013. (800)-695-0285. http://www.nichcy.org.

OTHER

Senior Care Web. http://www2.seniorcareweb.com.

Sandra L. Friedrich, MA

Restless legs syndrome

Definition

Restless legs syndrome (RLS) is a neurological disorder characterized by uncomfortable sensations in the legs and, less commonly, the arms. These sensations are exacerbated (heightened) when the person with RLS is at rest. The sensations are described as crawly, tingly, prickly, and occasionally painful. They result in a nearly insuppressible urge to move around. Symptoms are often associated with sleep disturbances.

Demographics

Studies have found that between 5% and 10% of the population of the United States and Europe experience from some degree of RLS symptoms. Almost twice as many women are affected as men, and Caucasians are more often affected than African Americans. The age of onset varies greatly. People with more severe disturbances tend to have an earlier onset, often in childhood or adolescence. Many other people report that symptoms severe enough to disturb sleep do not develop until they are in their fifties. People with familial (inherited) RLS on average report symptoms at age 45.

Description

Restless legs syndrome is a sensory-motor disorder that causes uncomfortable feelings in the legs, especially during periods of inactivity. Some people also report sensations in the arms, but this occurs much less frequently. The sensations occur deep in the legs and are usually described with terms that imply movement such as prickly or creepy-crawly and result in an irrepressible urge to move the leg. Symptoms are temporarily relieved when the person voluntarily moves. RLS symptoms tend to be worse in the night or during periods of inactivity (e.g., sitting on an airplane).

Restless legs syndrome is associated with another disorder called periodic limb movements in sleep (PLMS). It is estimated that four out of five patients with RLS also suffer from PLMS. PLMS is characterized by jerking leg movements while sleeping that may occur as frequently as every 20 seconds. These jerks disrupt sleep by causing continual arousals throughout the night.

People with both RLS and PLMS are prone to abnormal levels of exhaustion during the day because they are unable to sleep properly at night. They may have trouble concentrating at work, at school or during social activities. They may also have mood swings and difficulty with interpersonal relationships. **Depression** and anxiety may also result from the lack of sleep. RLS affects people who want to travel or attend events that require sitting for long periods of time.

Causes and symptoms

Restless legs syndrome is categorized in two ways. Primary RLS occurs in the absence of other medical symptoms, while secondary RLS usually is associated with some other medical disorder. Although the cause of primary RLS is currently unknown, a large amount of research suggests that there may be multiple causes. These include:

• a disruption in iron balance in the brain
• a deficiency of specific dopamine receptors (D2 receptors) in the brain
• a defect in serotonin transmission in the brain

Dopamine and serotonin are both neurotransmitters, chemicals critical to regulating nerve impulse transmission. In addition, genetic changes (mutations) have been found on various chromosomes in people with RLS. Some of these mutations are inherited in an autosomal dominant pattern, meaning that the presence of a mutated gene inherited from one parent will cause symptoms. Others are inherited in an autosomal recessive pattern, meaning that two copies of the mutated gene, one from each parent, must be present for symptoms of the disease to appear in the offspring. Multiple interacting causes may explain the variability of age of onset and type and severity of symptoms among individuals with

RLS. RLS is three to five times more common in an immediate family member of someone who has RLS than in the general population.

In many people, other medical conditions play a role in the development of RLS. When this is true, the disorder is classified as secondary RLS. People with peripheral neuropathies (injury to nerves in the arms and legs) may experience RLS. Such neuropathies can result from diabetes or alcoholism. Other chronic diseases such as kidney disorders and rheumatoid arthritis may result in RLS. Iron deficiencies and blood anemias are associated with RLS. Symptoms of RLS often decrease once blood iron levels have been corrected. According to the Restless Legs Syndrome Foundation, attention-deficit/hyperactivity disorder (**ADHD**) is common in both children and adults with RLS, and up to one-fourth of pregnant women develop RLS symptoms. These symptoms normally disappear after the pregnancy has ended. Some people find that high levels of caffeine intake may result in RLS.

All symptoms of RLS are associated with unpleasant feelings in the limbs. The words used to describe these feelings are various, but include such adjectives as deep-seated crawling, jittery, tingling, burning, aching, pulling, painful, itchy, or prickly. The sensations are usually not described as a muscle cramp or numbness. Most often the sensations occur during periods of inactivity. They are characterized by an urge to get up and move. Such movements include stretching, walking, jogging, or simply jiggling the legs. The feelings worsen in the evening.

A variety of symptoms are associated with RLS, but may not be characteristic of every case. Some people with RLS report involuntary arm and leg movements during the night. Eighty-five percent of RLS patients either have difficulty falling asleep or wake several times during the night, and almost half experience daytime **fatigue** or sleepiness. It is common for the symptoms to be intermittent. They may disappear for several months and then return for no apparent reason. Two-thirds of patients report that their symptoms become worse with time. Some older patients claim to have had symptoms since they were in their early 20s but were not diagnosed until their 50s. Suspected underdiagnosis of RLS may be attributed to the difficulty experienced by patients in describing their symptoms.

Diagnosis

A careful history enables the physician to distinguish RLS from similar types of disorders that cause night time discomfort in the limbs, such as muscle cramps, burning

KEY TERMS

Anemia—A condition that affects the size and number of red blood cells. It often results from lack of iron or certain B vitamins and may be treated with iron or vitamin supplements.

Dopamine—A neurochemical made in the brain that is involved in many brain activities, including movement and emotion.

Neurotransmitter—One of a group of chemicals secreted by a nerve cell (neuron) to carry a chemical message to another nerve cell, often as a way of transmitting a nerve impulse. Examples of neurotransmitters are acetylcholine, dopamine, serotonin, and norepinephrine.

Periodic limb movements in sleep (PLMS)—Random movements of the arms or legs that occur at regular intervals of time during sleep.

Serotonin—5-Hydroxytryptamine; a substance that occurs throughout the body with numerous effects including neurotransmission. Low serotonin levels are associated with mood disorders, particularly depression and obsessive-compulsive disorder.

feet syndrome, and damage to nerves that detect sensations or cause movement (polyneuropathy).

The most important tool the doctor has in diagnosis is the history obtained from the patient. Several common medical conditions are known to either cause or to be closely associated with RLS. The doctor may link the patient's symptoms to one of these conditions, which include anemia, diabetes, disease of the spinal nerve roots (lumbosacral **radiculopathy**), **Parkinson's disease**, late-stage pregnancy, kidney failure (uremia), and complications of stomach surgery. In order to identify or eliminate such a primary cause, blood tests may be performed to determine the presence of serum iron, ferritin, folate, vitamin B $_{12}$, creatinine, and thyroid-stimulating hormones. The physician may also ask if symptoms are present in any close family members since it is common for RLS to run in families and the inherited type is sometimes more difficult to treat.

In some cases, sleep studies such as polysomnography are undertaken to identify the presence of PLMS that are reported to affect 70–80% of people who suffer from RLS. The patient is often unaware of these movements, since they may not cause him to wake; however, the presence of PLMS with RLS can leave the person more tired because it interferes with

deep sleep. A patient who also displays evidence of some neurologic disease may undergo **electromyography** (EMG). During EMG, a very small, thin needle is inserted into the muscle and electrical activity of the muscle is recorded. A doctor or technician usually performs this test at a hospital outpatient department.

Treatment

The first step in treatment is to treat existing conditions that are known to be associated with RLS and that will be identified by blood tests. If the patient is anemic, iron (iron sulfate) or vitamin supplements (folate or vitamin B$_{12}$) will be prescribed. If kidney disease is identified as a cause, treatment of the kidney problem will take priority.

After treating underlying disorders, treatment for restless legs syndrome is generally two-pronged. Although there are no drugs to cure RLS, drug therapy may be used to control symptoms. Lifestyle changes also can help reduce symptoms.

Drugs

Dopaminergic agents are the first type of drug prescribed in the treatment of RLS. Commonly prescribed dopaminenergic drugs include pramipexole (Mirapex), pergolide (Permax), ropinirole (Requip), Ropinirole (Requip), and Bromocriptine mesylate (Parlodel). Carbidopa/levodopa (Sinemet) is prescribed frequently than other drugs in treating RLS because a problem known as augmentation has been associated with its use. When augmentation develops, symptoms of RLS will return earlier in the day and increasing the dose will not improve the symptoms.

Benzodiazepines are drugs that sedate and are typically taken before bedtime so that a patient with RLS can sleep more soundly. They include clonazepam (Klonopin), temazepam (Restoril), and alprazolam (Xanax)

Opioids are synthetic narcotics that relieve pain and cause drowsiness. They are usually taken in the evening. Because of their potential for addiction, opiods normally are prescribed in low doses only in severe cases where other treatment does not provide relief. Opioids that may be prescribed for RLS include codeine, oxycodone hydrochloride (Roxicodone), methadone hydrochloride (Dolophine), and levorphanol tartrate (Levo-Dromoran)

Antiepileptic drugs are those used for people with seizures. These are also useful in the treatment of moderate to severe RLS, and include **gabapentin** (Horizant, Neurontin) and pregabalin (Lyrica).

A few drugs have been found to worsen symptoms of RLS, and patients exhibiting RLS symptoms should avoid them. These include antihistamines, such as Benadryl, that are found in many over-the-counter cold and allergy drugs; anti-nausea drugs such as Antivert, Atarax, Compazine, and Phenergan; certain antidepressants; and certain drugs used to treat bipolar disorder and **schizophrenia**.

Lifestyle changes

Simple changes to diet have proven effective for some people suffering from RLS. Healthy diet, regular exercise, and practicing good sleep hygiene help some people. Vitamin supplements, based on the result of blood tests and taken as directed by a physician, maybe helpful. Reducing or eliminating caffeine and alcohol consumption has been effective in other patients. Patients should check with their doctor or pharmacist to make sure that other drugs (including herbal supplements) will not worsen symptoms.

Alternative treatment

Complementary therapy that includes alternative treatments and conventional approaches may help reduce RLS symptoms. Alternative therapies may include:

- Acupuncture. Patients who also have rheumatoid arthritis may especially benefit from acupuncture to relieve RLS symptoms. Acupuncture may stimulate those parts of the brain that are involved in RLS.

- Homeopathy. Homeopaths believe that disorders of the nervous system are especially important because the brain controls so many other bodily functions. Homeopathic remedies are tailored to the individual patient and are based on individual symptoms as well as the general symptoms of RLS.

- Reflexology. Reflexologists claim that the brain, head, and spine all respond to indirect massage of specific parts of the feet.

- Nutritional supplements. Supplementation of the diet with iron, vitamin E, calcium, magnesium, and folic acid may be helpful for people with RLS. The most effective supplementation is based on results of blood tests.

Some alternative methods may treat the associated condition that is suspected to cause restless legs. These include:

- Anemia or low ferritin levels. Chinese medicine emphasizes stimulation of the spleen as a means of improving blood circulation and vitamin absorption. Other treatments may include acupuncture

QUESTIONS TO ASK YOUR DOCTOR

- What kinds of tests will be required to verify that I have RLS and not some other condition?
- What types of treatments are available?
- What types of side effects from treatments can I expect? What are your recommendations to help me deal with those side effects?
- Are there any lifestyle changes that I should make?

and herbal therapies, such as ginseng (*Panax ginseng*) for anemia-related fatigue.

- Late-stage pregnancy. Few conventional therapies are available to pregnant women because most of the drugs prescribed are not recommended for use during pregnancy. Pregnant women may benefit from alternative techniques that focus on body work, including yoga, reflexology, and acupuncture.

Prognosis

RLS usually does not indicate the onset of other neurological disease. It may remain static, although two-thirds of patients get worse with time. The symptoms usually progress gradually and intermittently. Drug therapy may be effective in moderate to severe cases that include significant PLMS, but many of the drugs use in treatment produce significant side effects, and continued successful treatment may depend on carefully monitored use of combination drug therapy. The prognosis is usually best if RLS symptoms are recent and can be traced to another treatable condition (secondary RLS). Some associated conditions are not treatable. In these cases, such as for rheumatoid arthritis, complementary treatment that includes alternative therapies such as **acupuncture** may be helpful.

Prevention

Diet may help to prevent RLS. A preventive diet will include an adequate intake of iron and the B vitamins, especially B_{12} and folic acid. Strict vegetarians should take vitamin supplements to obtain sufficient vitamin B_{12}. Ferrous gluconate may be easier on the digestive system than ferrous sulfate if iron supplements are prescribed. Some drugs may cause or worsen symptoms of RLS. Patients should check with their doctor about these possible side effects, especially if symptoms first occur after starting a new medication. Caffeine, alcohol, and nicotine use should be minimized or eliminated. Even a hot bath before bed has been shown to help prevent symptoms for some individuals.

Resources

BOOKS

Chokroverty, Sudhansu. *100 Questions & Answers About Restless Legs Syndrome*. Sudbury, MA: Jones & Bartlett Learning, 2011.

Ferri, Fred, ed. *Ferri's Clinical Advisor 2010*. Philadelphia: Mosby Elsevier, 2009.

WEBSITES

Bozorg, Ali M. "Restless Legs Syndrome." Medscape Reference April 19, 2011. http://emedicine.medscape. com/article/1188327-overview (accessed June 17, 2011).

"Restless Legs." MedlinePlus. http://www.nlm.nih.gov/ medlineplus/restlesslegs.html (accessed July 19, 2011).

"Restless Legs Syndrome Fact Sheet." National Institute of Neurological Disorders and Stroke. http://www.ninds. nih.gov/disorders/restless_legs/detail_restless_legs.htm (accessed July 19, 2011).

"What Is Restless Legs Syndrome?" National Heart, Lung, and Blood Institute. http://www.nhlbi.nih.gov/health/ dci/Diseases/rls/rls_WhatIs.html (accessed July 19, 2011).

ORGANIZATIONS

National Institute of Neurological Disorders and Stroke (NINDS), P.O. Box 5801, Bethesda, MD, 20824, (301) 496-5751, (800) 352-9424, http://www.ninds.nih.gov.

National Sleep Foundation, 1010 N. Glebe Road, Suite 310, Arlington, VA, 22210, (703) 243-1697, nsf@ sleepfoundation.org, http://www.sleepfoundation.org.

Restless Legs Syndrome Foundation, 1610 14th St NW, Suite 300, Rochester, MN, 55901, (507) 287-6465, Fax: (507) 287-6312, rlsfoundation@rls.org, http:// www.rls.org.

Ann M. Haren
Tish Davidson, AM

Retrovirus-associated myelopathy *see* **Tropical spastic paraparesis**

Rett syndrome

Definition

Rett syndrome is a progressive neurological disorder seen almost exclusively in females. The most common symptoms include decreased speech, cognitive disabilities, severe lack of muscle control, small head size, and unusual hand movements.

Demographics

Rett syndrome affects almost only females. Males who carry the same gene mutation gene typically are miscarried before birth or die as infants. Rett syndrome usually is fatal in males because they have a single X chromosome, and the Y chromosome they carry cannot compensate for this mutation on their X chromosome. Females with a mutation in the gene that causes Rett Syndrome are able to survive because the presence of the second normal X chromosome partially compensates for the mutation on the other X chromosome. Rett syndrome is believed to affect all ethnic groups and nationalities with an equal frequency of about 1 case for every 10,000 to 15,000 live female births.

Description

Rett syndrome is an X-linked dominant condition. This means that the mutation (genetic change) responsible for Rett syndrome affects a gene located on the X chromosome. Females have two X chromosomes, one from each parent. Males have one X chromosome from their mother and one Y chromosome from their father.

Dr. Andreas Rett first reported females with the symptoms of Rett syndrome in 1966. Females with this X-linked dominant genetic condition are healthy and of average size at birth. During infancy, head growth is abnormally slow and **microcephaly** (small head size) develops. Babies with Rett syndrome initially have normal development. At approximately one year of age, development slows and eventually stops. Children with Rett syndrome develop autistic features. Involuntary hand movements are a classic feature of Rett syndrome.

Females with Rett syndrome also may develop seizures, curvature of the spine (scoliosis), irregular breathing patterns, swallowing problems (dysphagia), motor control problems, and difficulties walking. Some females with Rett syndrome are completely unable to walk unassisted. There is currently no cure for Rett syndrome. Most girls with Rett syndrome live into adulthood.

If a woman has a mutation in her MECP2 gene, she has a 50% risk with any pregnancy to pass on her X chromosome with the mutation. However, it is uncommon for women with Rett syndrome to have children due to the severity of the disorder. The gene responsible for Rett syndrome has been identified with genetic testing.

Causes and symptoms

The mutated gene on the X chromosome that is responsible for causing Rett syndrome is the methyl

CpG-binding protein 2 (MECP2) gene. This gene makes a protein that regulates other genes. When a mutation occurs in MECP2, the protein it makes does not work properly. This is thought to prevent normal neuron (nerve cell) development. The severity of the syndrome in females is related to the type of mutation in the MECP2 gene and the percentage of cells that carry a normal copy of the MECP2 gene.

Infants with Rett syndrome typically have normal size at birth. They develop normally until approximately 6–18 months of age. Development then slows, eventually stops, and soon regresses so that affected individuals are unable to do things they were once able to do. Girls with Rett syndrome lose the ability to speak, become uninterested in interacting with others, and lose many motor functions they had previously mastered. The loss of language and eye contact causes girls with Rett syndrome to display some symptoms similar to those seen in **autism**. Between one and three years of age, girls with Rett syndrome typically develop the unusual hand movements that are associated with the disease. These include wringing or clapping their hands and putting their hands in their mouth involuntarily. Some individuals with Rett syndrome also lose the ability to walk. If the ability to walk is maintained, the gait is often ataxic (uncoordinated, clumsy).

By preschool age the developmental deterioration of girls with Rett syndrome stops, but they continue to lack coherent speech, are unable to understand language at a normal level, show poor eye contact, and have a range of cognitive disabilities. Other common symptoms associated with Rett syndrome include seizures, constipation, irregular breathing, scoliosis, swallowing problems, teeth grinding, sleep disturbances, and poor circulation. As individuals with Rett syndrome get older the deterioration usually stops and some symptoms, such as repetitive hand movements and lack of eye contact can improve.

Diagnosis

The diagnosis of Rett syndrome is made when the majority of the symptoms associated with the disease are present. If a physician suspects an individual has Rett syndrome, DNA testing is recommended. DNA testing can be performed on a blood sample or other tissue from the body. If a mutation is found in the MECP2 gene, the diagnosis of Rett syndrome is confirmed.

Treatment

There is no cure for Rett syndrome. Treatment of patients with Rett syndrome focuses on improving the symptoms present. Treatment may include medications that inhibit seizures, reduce **spasticity**, and prevent sleep disturbances. Nutrition is monitored in females with Rett syndrome due to their small stature and the constipation associated with the disorder.

Most treatment for Rett syndrome focuses on helping individuals with the syndrome have the happiest, most productive lives possible. This can involve the use of assistive equipment to help the individual walk and move more independently or the use of adaptive tools to help the individual participate more fully in the tasks of daily living. For some individuals with Rett syndrome, special educational or vocational training can help them take a more full role in managing their own lives.

Prognosis

In the absence of severe medical problems, most females with Rett syndrome live into adulthood. Because research on this syndrome did not start in any significant way until the 1980s, there is not a wide body of research documenting outcomes. It is believed that an average life expectancy for women with Rett syndrome is around age 40.

Prevention

There is no known way to prevent Rett syndrome. Women who may be carriers for the MECP2 gene can have their fetus tested for the presence of the mutation.

It is believed that most cases of Rett syndrome are due to a spontaneous mutation of the MECP2 gene, meaning that the parents are not carries of the mutation. Because Rett syndrome is rare, genetic testing of the fetus is not usually recommended unless another child in the family has the syndrome.

Resources

BOOKS

Hunter, Kathy. *The Rett Syndrome Handbook*, 2nd ed. Clinton, MD: International Rett Syndrome Association, 2007.

Judd, Sandra J., ed. *Autism and Pervasive Developmental Disorders Sourcebook*. Detroit: Omnigraphics, 2007.

Lindberg, Barbro. *Understanding Rett Syndrome: A Practical Guide for Parents, Teachers, and Therapists*, 2nd rev. ed. Cambridge, MA : Hogrefe & Huber, 2006.

OTHER

Rett Syndrome. Medline Plus. December 22 2009. http://www.nlm.nih. gov/medlineplus/rettsyndrome.html

ORGANIZATIONS

Alliance of Genetic Support Groups, 4301 Connecticut Ave. NW, Suite 404, Washington, DC, 20008-2369, (202) 966-5557, Fax: (202) 966-8553, info@geneticalliance. org, http://www.geneticalliance.org.

International Rett Syndrome Association, 4600 Devitt Drive, Cincinnati , OH, 45246, (800) 818-7388, Fax: 513-874-2520 , http://www.rettsyndrome.org.

National Organization for Rare Disorders (NORD), PO Box 1968, Danbury, CT, 06813-1968, (203) 744-0100, (800) 999-6673, Fax: (203)798-2291, orphan@rarediseases. org, http://www.rarediseases.org.

Holly A. Ishmael, MS, CGC
Tish Davidson, A.M.

Reye's syndrome

Definition

Reye's syndrome is a disorder principally affecting the liver and brain, marked by rapid development of life-threatening neurological symptoms.

Description

Reye's syndrome is an emergency illness chiefly affecting children and teenagers. It almost always follows a viral illness such as a cold, the flu, or chicken pox. Reye's syndrome may affect all the organs of the body, but most seriously affects the brain and liver. Rapid development of severe neurological symptoms, including lethargy, confusion, seizures, and **coma**, make Reye's syndrome a life-threatening emergency.

Reye's syndrome is a rare illness, even rarer now than when first described in the early 1970s. The incidence of the disorder peaked in 1980, with 555 cases reported. The number of cases declined rapidly thereafter due to decreased use of aspirin compounds for childhood fever, an important risk factor for Reye's syndrome development. Because of its rarity, it is often misdiagnosed as **encephalitis**, **meningitis**, diabetes, or poisoning, and the true incidence may be higher than the number of reported cases indicates.

Causes and symptoms

Reye's syndrome causes fatty accumulation in the organs of the body, especially the liver. In the brain, it causes fluid accumulation (edema), which leads to a rise in intracranial pressure. This pressure squeezes blood vessels, preventing blood from entering the brain. Untreated, this pressure increase leads to brain damage and death.

Although the cause remains unknown, Reye's syndrome appears to be linked to an abnormality in the energy-converting structures (mitochondria) within the body's cells.

Reye's syndrome usually occurs after a viral, fever-causing illness, most often an upper respiratory tract infection. Its cause is unknown. It is most often associated with use of aspirin during the fever, and for this reason aspirin and aspirin-containing products are not recommended for people under the age of 19 during fever. Reye's syndrome may occur without aspirin use, and in adults, although very rarely.

After the beginning of recovery from the viral illness, the affected person suddenly becomes worse, with the development of persistent vomiting. This may

KEY TERMS

Acetylsalicylic acid—Aspirin; an analgesic, antipyretic, and antirheumatic drug prescribed to reduce fever and for relief of pain and inflammation.

Edema—The abnormal accumulation of fluid in interstitial spaces of tissue.

Mitochondria—Small rodlike, threadlike, or granular organelle witin the cytoplasm that function in metabolism and respiration.

be followed rapidly by quietness, lethargy, agitation or combativeness, seizures, and coma. In infants, diarrhea may be more common than vomiting. Fever is usually absent at this point.

Diagnosis

Reye's syndrome may be suspected in a child who begins vomiting three to six days after a viral illness, followed by an alteration in consciousness. Diagnosis involves blood tests to determine the levels of certain liver enzymes, which are highly elevated in Reye's syndrome. Other blood changes may occur as well, including an increase in the level of ammonia and amino acids, a drop in blood sugar, and an increase in clotting time. A liver **biopsy** may also be done after clotting abnormalities are corrected with vitamin K or blood products. A **lumbar puncture** (spinal tap) may be needed to rule out other possible causes, including meningitis or encephalitis.

Treatment

Reye's syndrome is a life-threatening emergency that requires intensive management. The likelihood of recovery is greatest if it is recognized early and treated promptly. Children with Reye's syndrome should be managed in an intensive-care unit.

Treatment in the early stages includes intravenous sugar to return levels to normal and plasma transfusion to restore normal clotting time. Intracranial pressure is monitored and, if elevated, is treated with intravenous mannitol and hyperventilation to constrict the blood vessels in the brain. If the pressure remains high, barbiturates may be used.

Prognosis

The mortality rate for Reye's syndrome is between 30–50%. The likelihood of recovery is increased to 90% by early diagnosis and treatment. Almost all children who survive Reye's syndrome recover fully, although recovery may be slow. In some patients, permanent neurologic damage may remain, requiring physical or educational special services and equipment.

Prevention

Because Reye's syndrome is so highly correlated with use of aspirin for fever in young people, avoidance of aspirin use by children is strongly recommended. Aspirin is in many over-the-counter and prescription drugs, including drugs for headache, fever, menstrual cramps, muscle pain, nausea, upset stomach, and arthritis. It may be used in drugs taken orally or by suppository.

Any of the following ingredients indicates that aspirin is present:

- aspirin
- acetylsalicylate
- acetylsalicylic acid
- salicylic acid
- salicylate

Teenagers who take their own medications without parental consultation should be warned not to take aspirin-containing drugs.

Resources

ORGANIZATIONS

National Reye's Syndrome Foundation. P.O. Box 829, Bryan, OH 43506-0829. (800) 233-7393. http:// www.bright.net/~reyessyn.

Richard Robinson

Rivastigmine *see* **Cholinesterase inhibitors**

S

Sacral nerve root cysts *see* **Perineural cysts**

Sacral radiculopathy *see* **Radiculopathy**

Saint Vitus Dance *see* **Sydenham's chorea**

Salivary gland disease *see* **Cytomegalic inclusion body disease**

Sandhoff disease

Definition

Sandhoff disease is a relatively rare, genetically inherited disease that results in the progressive deterioration of the **central nervous system**. In Sandhoff disease, abnormal lipid (fat) accumulation due to a storage defect causes damage to the brain as well as other organs of the body.

Description

Sandhoff disease is an autosomal recessive disorder, meaning that having an affected offspring requires both unaffected parents to be carriers. Parents who carry the disorder will have a 25% risk of having an affected offspring in subsequent pregnancies. This disease is similar to a related disorder known as **Tay-Sachs disease**, although Sandhoff disease is more severe.

Demographics

As Sandhoff disease is a recessive disorder, males and females are affected with equal frequency. This disorder is more common in people with non-Jewish descent, unlike Tay-Sachs disease, which is prevalent mainly in individuals with Jewish ancestry.

Causes and symptoms

Sandhoff disease is caused by mutations in two different genes that encodes a subunits that makeup a protein called hexosaminidase. Hexosaminidase is an enzyme that breaks down certain fats in the brain. This enzyme is either composed of an alpha and a beta subunit (HexA) or two beta subunits (HexB). Sandhoff disease is caused by a mutation in a gene that is distinct from the gene that causes Tay-Sachs disease. In Tay-Sachs disease, a mutation that affects the alpha subunit of the enzyme causes a deficiency in HexA. Sandhoff disease is caused by mutations that affect the beta subunit, rendering both the HEXA and HEXB enzymes deficient. A deficiency of this enzyme leads to the accumulation of GM2 ganglioside, a fatty material found in the brain.

The beta subunit is encoded by a gene localized to chromosome 5, while the alpha subunit is encoded by a gene on chromosome 13. There is also another gene on chromosome 5 that encodes an activator that is required for either enzyme to be functional. Similar symptoms are observed in diseases arising from mutations that affect any of these three genes. Only biochemical genetic analysis of enzyme activity can pinpoint the cause and specify the disorder. However, Sandhoff disease can be distinguished from Tay-Sachs disease clinically by virtue of skeletal system or abdominal organ involvement (if present) in the later disease.

At birth, infants tend to be without symptoms and usually do not develop them until approximately six months of age. The symptoms begin with motor deficits (lack of normal movement) and a characteristic startle reaction to various sounds. Babies with Sandhoff disease progressively deteriorate in terms of motor function, and they often have seizures and **myoclonus**. Myoclonus is abnormal, exaggerated muscle contractions. Blindness can also be part of the symptoms. The loss of motor function includes the ability to swallow, and the affected

KEY TERMS

Autosomal recessive mutation—A pattern of genetic inheritance where two abnormal genes are needed to display the trait or disease.

Lipids—Organic compounds not soluble in water, but soluble in fat solvents such as alcohol. Lipids are stored in the body as energy reserves and are also important components of cell membranes. Commonly known as fats.

Myoclonus—Involuntary contractions of a muscle or an interrelated group of muscles. Also known as myoclonic seizures.

infant has an increased risk for inhaling feedings into the lungs, frequently leading to pneumonia.

A typical physical feature of Sandhoff disease is the presence of cherry-red spots in the back of the eyes. Additionally, affected children have an abnormally enlarged head and appear to have a doll-like appearance.

Diagnosis

Because Sandhoff disease and Tay-Sachs disease have similar clinical symptoms, distinguishing them requires biochemical analysis. This involves a test to measure enzyme activity of the two hexosaminidase enzymes. If the enzyme activity results indicate that there is no hexosaminidase activity, it means that the patient has Sandhoff disease. If, however, there is still B subunit activity, then this indicates that the patient might have Tay-Sachs disease.

Treatment

There is no cure for Sandhoff disease, and treatment is based on lessening the symptoms once they begin. Medication is usually given to reduce seizures, for example, and a feeding tube may be inserted to prevent aspiration of feedings into the lungs.

Recovery and rehabilitation

Emphasis is placed on comfort rather than recovery, due to the progressive nature of Sandhoff disease. Because of the nature of the disorder, rehabilitation is not usually applicable to help with improving the motor deficits that develop. Physical therapy may be helpful to maintain muscle tone and skeletal alignment for as long as possible, while positional strategies and devices

provided by an occupational therapist may increase comfort as symptoms progress.

Clinical trials

Information about current relevant clinical trials can be found at ClinicalTrials.gov.

Prognosis

The prognosis for Sandhoff disease is poor. Affected babies usually do not survive past the age of three and typically, death occurs due to complications associated with respiratory infections.

Special concerns

Children that are affected with Sandhoff disease will require full time supervision and caretaking responsibilities. Psychological counseling for family members is often helpful. Genetic counseling for reproductive risks is recommended. There are also several support groups operated and composed of other families nationwide with Sandhoff disease.

Resources

BOOKS

Icon Health Publications. *The Official Parent's Sourcebook on Sandhoff Disease: A Revised and Updated Directory for the Internet Age.* New York: Icon Group International, 2002.

Nussbaum, Robert L., Roderick R. McInnes, and Huntington F. Willard. *Genetics in Medicine.* Philadelphia : Saunders, 2001.

PERIODICALS

Gilbert, F., et al. "Tay-Sachs' and Sandhoff's diseases: the assignment of genes for hexosaminidase A and B to individual human chromosomes." *Proc. Nat. Acad. Sci.* 72 (1975): 263–67.

Neufeld, E. F. "Natural history and inherited disorders of a lysosomal enzyme, beta-hexosaminidase." *J. Biol. Chem.* 264 (1989): 10927–30.

OTHER

"NINDS Sandhoff Disease Information Page." National Institute of Neurological Disorders and Stroke. http://www.ninds.nih.gov/health_and_medical/disorders/sandhoff.htm (February 1, 2004).

"What every family should know: Sandhoff disease." *The National Tay-Sachs & Allied Diseases Association.* http://www.ntsad.org/pages/sandhoff.htm (February 1, 2004).

ORGANIZATIONS

National Organization for Rare Disorders (NORD). P.O. Box 1968 (55 Kenosia Avenue), Danbury, CT 06813-1968. Phone: (203) 744-0100. Fax: (203) 798-2291.

Tollfree phone: (800) 999-NORD (6673). Email: orphan@rare diseases.org. http://www.rarediseases.org.

National Tay-Sachs and Allied Diseases Association. 2001 Beacon Street Suite 204, Brighton, MA 02135. Phone: (617) 277-4463. Fax: (617) 277-0134. Tollfree phone: (800) 90-NTSAD (906-8723). Email: info@ntsad.org. http://www.ntsad.org.

Bryan Richard Cobb, PhD

Schilder's disease

Definition

Schilder's disease is a form of **multiple sclerosis** that strikes in childhood.

Description

Schilder's disease is a very rare progressive degenerative disease that affects children. It resembles multiple sclerosis both in its symptoms (difficulties with movement and speech) and its pathology (widespread demyelination of the brain). Demyelination refers to the destruction of the myelin that normally encases nerve fibers. Myelin is the fatty white substance that wraps around nerve fibers, providing insulation and allowing nerve signals to move quickly. Without myelin, nervous transmission is significantly slowed. As the disease progresses, larger and larger patches of demyelination occur, interfering with motor movement, speech, personality, hearing and vision. Ultimately, the vital functions (respiration, heart rate, blood pressure) are affected, leading to the individual's death.

Demographics

Schilder's disease is exceedingly rare. Because there are no specific criteria for the diagnosis, there continues to be debate among researchers and clinicians regarding the most appropriate way to definitively diagnose the disease and collect data on its frequency and incidence. Some sources suggest that there have only been nine cases of definitively diagnosed Schilder's disease since it was originally described in the German medical literature in 1912.

Most patients with Schilder's disease are diagnosed between seven and twelve years of age.

Causes and symptoms

The underlying cause of Schilder's disease is unknown. Symptoms of the disease are caused by widespread patches of demyelination throughout the brain and spinal cord, resulting in slowed, faulty nervous transmission.

Symptoms of Schilder's disease include **weakness** of one side of the body (hemiparesis), slowness of movement (psychomotor retardation), paralysis of all four extremities (quadraparesis), seizures, difficulty with speech (**dysarthria**), visual and hearing impairment, irritability, memory problems, personality changes, gradual loss of awareness and responsiveness. Over time, patients become unable to maintain their nutritional status and become increasingly thin and malnourished. Bowel and bladder function are often lost as the disease progresses.

Some children have a relentlessly progressive course of the disease, culminating in death. Other children have remissions and exacerbations, with each subsequent exacerbation more severe and each remission less complete, until death supervenes.

Diagnosis

Because researchers and clinicians have not been able to delineate a clear-cut list of criteria for the diagnosis of Schilder's disease, definitive diagnosis is difficult. EEG studies may show some abnormalities. MRI studies will certainly reveal demyelination. Other lab studies (blood tests, test on cerebrospinal fluid obtain via **lumbar puncture**, brain **biopsy**) are usually performed in an effort to rule out some other cause for the patients symptoms, such as an infectious, malignant, or metabolic condition; in Schilder's disease, these will all come back normal.

Treatment team

The treatment team for a child with Schilder's disease usually consists of neurologists, specialists in multiple sclerosis, and rheumatologists. Support from physical therapists, occupational therapists, and speech and language therapists can help a child maintain as much functioning as possible.

Treatment

There is no cure for Schilder's disease. Treatments are aimed at slowing the inexorable course of the disease and are similar to treatments used for multiple sclerosis, such as high dose steroids, beta interferon, and immunosuppressants.

KEY TERMS

Demyelination—Destruction of the myelin that should normally wrap around nerve fibers.

Dysarthria—Disturbances of speech and communication.

Hemiparesis—Weakness of one side of the body.

Myelin—The fatty white substance that wraps around nerve fibers, providing insulation and allowing for speedier nervous transmission.

Psychomotor retardation—Slowing of movement and speech.

Quadriparesis—Weakness of all four limbs.

Prognosis

Schilder's disease is uniformly fatal.

Resources

BOOKS

Ferri, Fred F., ed. *Ferri's Clinical Advisor: Instant Diagnosis and Treatment.* St. Louis: Mosby, 2004.

Goetz, Christopher G., ed. *Textbook of Clinical Neurology.* Philadelphia: W. B. Saunders, 2003.

PERIODICALS

Fernández-Jaén, A. "Schilder's diffuse myelinoclastic sclerosis." *Review of Neurology* 33, no. 1 (1 July 2001): 16–21.

Kotil, K. "Human Prion Diseases." *British Journal of Neurosurgery* 16, no. 5 (1 October 2002): 516–19.

WEBSITES

National Institute of Neurological Disorders and Stroke (NINDS). *NINDS Schilder's Disease Information Page.* July 24, 2001. http://www.ninds.nih.gov/health_and_medical/disorders/schilder's.htm.

ORGANIZATIONS

National Multiple Sclerosis Society. 733 Third Avenue, 6th Floor, New York, NY 10017-3288. Phone: 212-986-3240. Fax: 212-986-7981. Tollfree phone: 800-344-4867 (FIGHTMS). Email: nat@nmss.org. http://www.nationalmssociety.org.

Multiple Sclerosis Association of American. 706 Haddonfield Road, Cherry Hill, NJ 08002. Phone: 856-488-4500. Fax: 856-661-9797. Tollfree phone: 800-532-7667. Email: msaa@msaa.com. http://www.msaa.com.

Multiple Sclerosis Foundation. 6350 North Andrews Avenue, Ft. Lauderdale, FL 33309-2130. Phone: 954-776-6805. Fax: 954-351-0630. Tollfree phone: 888-MSFocus (673-6287).

Rosalyn Carson-DeWitt, MD

Schizencephaly

Definition

Schizencephaly, or "split brain," is a neurological disease caused by abnormal development of the brain, leading to the characteristic appearance of abnormal clefts in either one or both cerebral hemispheres. The exact etiology is unknown, although it is classified as a type of neuronal migration disorder and thought to be due to a defect in development that occurs during the period of one to seven months of fetal gestation.

Description

Schizencephaly may have different forms. The appearance of the abnormal schizencephalic brain varies depending on the size and extent of the clefts. Clefts may be unilateral or bilateral and usually extend from the surface of the brain to the fluid-filled ventricles. Clefts are usually located next to the Sylvian fissure, but may be located in any part of the hemispheres. Separation of the walls of the cleft is referred to as open-lip schizencephaly, whereas apposed walls are referred to as closed-lip schizencephaly.

Schizencephaly differs from **porencephaly**, another developmental disorder that is due to early injuries to the developing fetal brain. Porencephaly results from injured brain tissue that subsequently dissolves and leaves a fluid-filled area known as a porencephalic cyst. This cyst can resemble the cleft seen in schizencephaly. Whereas schizencephaly is thought to be a primary disorder of development or neuronal migration, porencephaly is thought to be due to secondary brain damage, although the distinction is not entirely clear. Some theories of schizencephaly also propose early brain injury as contributory, but at an earlier stage of development than in porencephaly. Differentiation between the two often requires brain imaging such as magnetic resonance imaging (MRI) to identify the nature of the brain tissue lining the cleft. In porencephaly, scar tissue and white matter is often present, whereas in schizencephaly, gray matter lines the cleft.

Demographics

Schizencephaly is a rare disorder and the incidence is unknown. It usually is noticed in infancy or childhood, although it may be diagnosed in adulthood with the onset of seizures.

Causes and symptoms

Causes

The cause of schizencephaly is unknown, although environmental and genetic factors have been proposed.

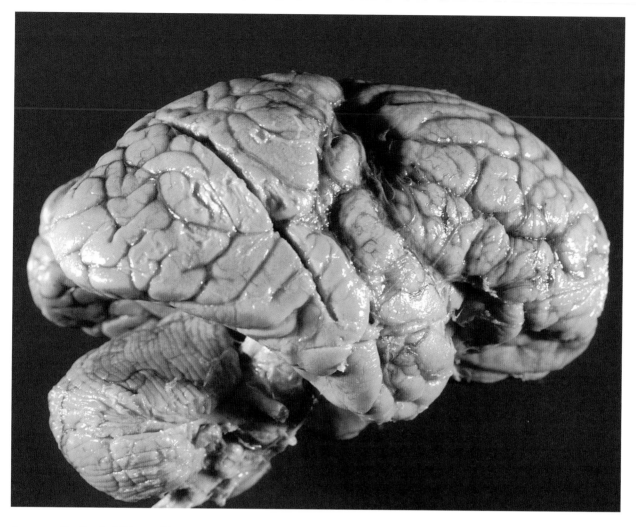

A gray-matter lined cleft in a schizencephalic brain. *(© Custom Medical Stock Photo, Inc. Reproduced by permission.)*

Various theories exist as to the timing and nature of the defect in development. Early injury to the brain during the second trimester of pregnancy has been proposed to cause the characteristic clefts. These insults may be due to infection, poor blood flow causing stroke, or genetic abnormalities. The earlier onset of injury leading to absence of scar tissue around the defect presumably differentiates schizencephaly from porencephaly. A mutation in the EMX2 gene has been associated with schizencephaly in some familial cases, providing evidence for genetic causes. EMX2 is a transcription factor on human chromosome 10 that is important in early brain formation in mice and flies. The clefts in schizencephaly are often lined by normal brain tissue, but may often be surrounded by abnormal brain tissue that has an unusually high density of folding (polymicrogyria). Schizencephaly may also be associated with abnormal nerve clusters called heterotopias in different parts of the brain. Polymicrogyria and heterotopias are thought to be due to defective neuronal migration, and their association with schizencephaly suggests a common underlying mechanism.

Symptoms

Symptoms can vary widely depending on the extent and the size of the cleft. Patients may show developmental delay that can range from mild to severe. Bilateral and open-lip clefts are associated with more severe delay. Affected individuals may have small heads (**microcephaly**) or increased pressure due to fluid accumulation inside the brain, known as hydrocephalus. Paralysis of the limbs may be present. The paralysis may be on one or both sides of the body depending on the location of the clefts. Abnormal muscle tone, including decreased tone (**hypotonia**) and increased tone (**spasticity**), can be seen. Some patients may have only seizures. Seizures usually present before three years of age, but patients may present with seizures in later life as their only symptom and then be diagnosed with schizencephaly by brain imaging.

Diagnosis

Diagnosis is made by imaging of the brain. A computed tomography scan (CT) or MRI demonstrates the abnormal clefts, which may be bilateral or unilateral, open or closed lip. The clefts may appear symmetric or asymmetric. MRI may show evidence of polymicrogyria lining the clefts. There is no genetic testing available at this time for schizencephaly.

Treatment team

Treatment for patients with schizencephaly differs among patients due to the wide variety of clinical manifestations and symptoms. The team responsible for medical care may include a pediatrician and pediatric neurologist. A pediatric neurosurgeon may be involved in performing a shunt procedure for hydrocephalus. An orthopedic surgeon may perform surgeries to improve the mobility of spastic limbs. Physical and occupational therapists can help with improving mobility. A case manager may help in coordinating care and treatments.

Treatment

There is no cure for schizencephaly at this time. The treatment of schizencephaly is directed towards the symptoms caused by the abnormally formed brain. Seizures may require anticonvulsant drug therapy. Seizures that cannot be controlled with medications may be treated by surgical removal of the abnormal tissue surrounding the cleft. With complications of hydrocephalus, a surgical shunt procedure may be necessary to relieve fluid accumulation and pressure.

Recovery and rehabilitation

Due to the congenital nature of schizencephaly, symptoms tend to be unchanging and there is little recovery. Physical therapy may be useful in relieving symptoms of spasticity or paralysis and in improving mobility and ambulation. Occupational therapists may help maintain hand function in those with impaired ability.

Clinical trials

Information about current relevant clinical trials can be found at ClinicalTrials.gov.

KEY TERMS

Neuronal migration—A step of early brain development in which nerve cells travel over large distances to different parts of the brain.

Sylvian fissure—The lateral fold separating the brain hemisphere into the frontal and temporal lobes.

Transcription factor—A protein that acts to regulate the expression of genes.

Ventricle—The spaces in the cerebral hemispheres containing cerebrospinal fluid, a nutrient-rich fluid that bathes the brain.

Prognosis

The prognosis for individuals with schizencephaly depends on the amount of neurologic deficiency associated with the malformation. Some patients with unilateral clefts may only have seizures and no other cognitive or motor abnormalities. Seizures may respond to medications or require surgery if unmanageable. Patients with severe **mental retardation** and paralysis will often require lifelong dependent care and may have a shortened lifespan as a result of infections such as pneumonias. Bilateral clefts are associated with earlier onset of seizures and seizures that are more difficult to treat.

Special Concerns

Educational and Social Needs

Due to developmental disability, individuals with schizencephaly may benefit from special education programs. Various state and federal programs are available to help individuals and their families with meeting these needs.

Resources

BOOKS

Menkes, John H., and Harvey Sarnat, eds. *Childhood Neurology*, 6th edition. Philadelphia: Lippincott Williams & Wilkins, 2000.

"Congenital Anomalies of the Nervous System," Section 7, Chapter 585. In *Nelson Textbook of Pediatrics*, 17th edition, edited by Richard E. Behrman, Robert M. Kliegman, and Hal B. Jenson. Philadelphia: Saunders 2004.

PERIODICALS

Guerrini, R., and R. Carrozzo. "Epilepsy and Genetic Malformations of the Cerebral Cortex." *American Journal of Medical Genetics* 106 (2001): 160–73.

Ross, M. E., and C. A. Walsh. "Human Brain Malformations and Their Lessons for Neuronal Migration." *Annual Review of Neuroscience* 24 (2001): 1041–70.

WEBSITES

National Institutes of Neurological Disorders and Stroke (NINDS). Cephalic Disorders Information Page. (February 26, 2004.) http://www.ninds.nih.gov/ health_and_medical/pubs/cephalic_disorders.htm.

National Institutes of Neurological Disorders and Stroke (NINDS). *Schizencephaly Information Page.* (February 26, 2004.) http://www.ninds.nih.gov/health_and_ medical/disorders/schizencephaly.htm.

ORGANIZATIONS

March of Dimes Birth Defects Foundation. 1275 Mamaroneck Avenue, White Plains, NY 10605. Phone: (914) 428-7100. Fax: (914) 428-8203. Tollfree phone: (888) MODIMES. Email: askus@marchofdimes.com. http://www. marchofdimes.com.

National Information Center for Children and Youth with Disabilities. P.O. Box 1492, Washington, DC 20013-1492. Phone: (202) 884-8200. Fax: (202) 884-8441. Tollfree phone: (800) 695-0285. Email: nichcy@aed.org. http:// www.nichcy.org.

National Institute of Child Health and Human Development (NICHD). Bldg. 31, Rm. 2A32, Bethesda, MD 20892-2425. Phone: (301) 496-5133. Tollfree phone: (800) 370-2943. Email: NICHDClearinghouse@mail. nih.gov. http://www.nichd.nih.gov.

Walsh Lab. 4 Blackfan Circle, Boston, MA 02115. Phone: (617) 667-0813. Fax: (617) 667-0815. Email: cwalsh@- bidmc.harvard.edu. http://walshlab.bidmc. harvard.edu.

Peter T. Lin, MD

Schizophrenia

Schizophrenia is a psychotic disorder or group of disorders marked by severely impaired thinking, emotions, and behaviors. It is sometimes called a psychotic disorder or a psychosis. Schizophrenic patients are typically unable to filter sensory stimuli and may have enhanced perceptions of sounds, colors, and other features of their environment. Most schizophrenics, if untreated, gradually withdraw from interactions with other people and lose their ability to take care of personal needs and grooming.

The term *schizophrenia* was coined by the Swiss psychiatrist Eugen Bleuler (1857–1939) around 1910. It comes from two Greek words that mean "split" and "mind" and refers to the splitting apart or separation of mental functions that Bleuler considered the essential characteristic of the disorder. Prior to Bleuler, schizophrenia was called **dementia** praecox, or precocious dementia, because it occurred in young people in contrast to the senile dementia of the elderly. Schizophrenia is often mislabeled in popular usage; it does *not* mean "split personality." It should also not be confused with the personality fragments, or alters, found in patients with dissociative identity disorder (DID). Schizophrenia is the end result of a combination of genetic, biochemical, and environmental factors, whereas DID is almost always caused by severe abuse in childhood.

As of 2011 there is ongoing debate among mental health professionals as to whether schizophrenia is a single disorder or a collection of separate syndromes, because of the many combinations of symptoms that patients may have. The successor to the present fourth edition of the *Diagnostic and Statistical Manual of Mental Disorders* (*DSM-IV*), *DSM-5*, due for publication in 2013, is proposing to replace the current category "Schizophrenia and Other Psychotic Disorders" with "Schizophrenia Spectrum and Other Psychotic Disorders."

Demographics

According to the World Health Organization (WHO), schizophrenia is estimated to afflict about 0.3–0.7% of the population worldwide, mostly in the 15–35 year age group. Though the incidence is low (3 in 10,000), the prevalence is high due to chronicity. It is also estimated that more than 50% of persons with schizophrenia are not receiving appropriate care and that 90% of people with untreated schizophrenia live in developing countries. Schizophrenia affects about 3 million people in the United States, according to the National Institute of Mental Health (NIMH); some 280,000 in Canada, 285,000 in Australia, and 250,000 in the United Kingdom. It ranks among the top ten causes of disability in developed countries worldwide.

The disease typically begins in early adulthood between the ages of 15 and 25. Men tend to develop schizophrenia slightly earlier than women: Most men become ill between 16 and 25 years old, while most women develop symptoms several years later. The average age of onset is 18 in men and 25 in women. The onset of the disorder is quite rare in children under the age of 10, and in people over 40 years of age.

As far as is known, schizophrenia is equally common in all racial and ethnic groups worldwide.

Description

The course of schizophrenia in adults can be divided into three phases or stages. In the acute phase, the

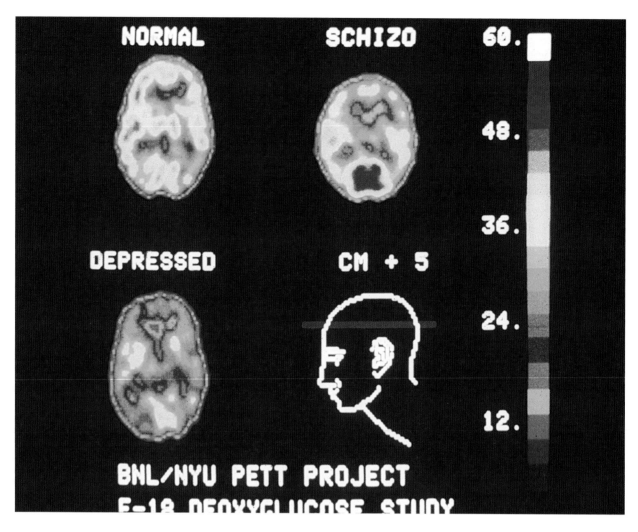

PET scans of normal, schizophrenic, and depressed human brains. *(© NIH/Science Source/Photo Researchers, Inc.)*

patient has an overt loss of contact with reality (psychotic episode) that requires intervention and treatment. In the second or stabilization phase, the initial psychotic symptoms have been brought under control but the patient is at risk for relapse if treatment is interrupted. In the third or maintenance phase, the patient is relatively stable and can be kept indefinitely on antipsychotic medications. Even in the maintenance phase, relapses are not unusual, and patients do not always return to full functioning.

DSM-IV specifies five subtypes of schizophrenia; however, the working group for *DSM-5* is recommending that these subtypes be dropped in the forthcoming edition.

Paranoid

The key feature of this subtype of schizophrenia is the combination of false beliefs (delusions) and hearing voices (auditory hallucinations), with more nearly normal emotions and cognitive functioning (cognitive functions include reasoning, judgment, and memory). The delusions of paranoid schizophrenics usually involve thoughts of being persecuted or harmed by others or exaggerated opinions of their own importance but may also reflect feelings of jealousy or excessive religiosity. The delusions are typically organized into a coherent framework. Paranoid schizophrenics function at a higher level than other subtypes but are at risk for suicidal or violent behavior under the influence of their delusions.

Disorganized

Disorganized schizophrenia (formerly called hebephrenic schizophrenia) is marked by disorganized speech, thinking, and behavior on the patient's part, coupled with flat or inappropriate emotional responses to a situation (affect). The patient may act silly or withdraw socially to an extreme extent. Most patients in this category have weak personality structures prior to their initial acute psychotic episode.

Catatonic

Catatonic schizophrenia is characterized by disturbances of movement that may include rigidity, stupor, agitation, bizarre posturing, and repetitive imitations of the movements or speech of other people. These patients are at risk for malnutrition, exhaustion, or self-injury. This subtype is uncommon in Europe and the United States. Catatonia as a symptom is most commonly associated with mood disorders.

Undifferentiated

Patients in this category have the characteristic positive and negative symptoms of schizophrenia but do not meet the specific criteria for the paranoid, disorganized, or catatonic subtypes.

Residual

This category is used for patients who have had at least one acute schizophrenic episode but do not presently have strong positive psychotic symptoms, such as delusions and hallucinations. They may have negative symptoms, such as withdrawal from others, or mild forms of positive symptoms, which indicate that the disorder has not completely resolved.

Risk factors

In sum, the risk factors for schizophrenia include:

- Age. Schizophrenia is largely a disorder of adolescents and young adults. It is rare in children, although cases have been reported in children as young as 5. It is also rare for schizophrenia to develop in adults over 45.
- Sex. Males are more likely to develop schizophrenia in the late teens and early 20s and to have more severe symptoms. Females are more likely to develop symptoms in their late 20s or early 30s.
- A family history of schizophrenia. A child of a schizophrenic parent has a 10% chance of developing the disorder; if both parents have schizophrenia, the child's risk increases to 40%. The risk is highest for the identical twin of a person with schizophrenia; he or she has a 40–65% chance of developing the disorder.
- Exposure to viruses or malnutrition prior to birth or surviving a difficult childbirth
- Experimentation with recreational drugs during the early teens

- Having a father who was over 40 at the time of one's birth
- Living in a large city

Causes and symptoms

Causes

One of the reasons for the ongoing difficulty in classifying schizophrenic disorders is incomplete understanding of their causes. As of 2011, it is thought that these disorders are the end result of a combination of genetic, neurobiological, and environmental causes. A leading neurobiological hypothesis looks at the connection between the disease and excessive levels of dopamine, a chemical that transmits signals in the brain (neurotransmitter). The genetic factor in schizophrenia has been underscored by recent findings that first-degree biological relatives of schizophrenics are ten times as likely to develop the disorder as are members of the general population.

Prior to recent findings of abnormalities in the brain structure of schizophrenic patients, several generations of psychotherapists advanced a number of psychoanalytic and sociological theories about the origins of schizophrenia. These theories ranged from hypotheses about the patient's problems with anxiety or aggression to theories about stress reactions or interactions with disturbed parents. Psychosocial factors are now thought to influence the expression or severity of schizophrenia rather than cause it directly.

Another hypothesis suggests that schizophrenia may be caused by a virus that attacks the hippocampus, a part of the brain that processes sense perceptions. Damage to the hippocampus would account for schizophrenic patients' vulnerability to sensory overload.

Symptoms

Patients with a possible diagnosis of schizophrenia are evaluated on the basis of a set or constellation of symptoms; there is no single symptom that is unique to schizophrenia. Doctors classify the symptoms of schizophrenia into three groups: positive, negative, and cognitive. Positive symptoms refer to behaviors that indicate a loss of contact with reality:

- Hallucinations, or seeing or hearing things that are not really there. People with schizophrenia commonly have auditory (hearing-related) hallucinations, often voices telling them to do something, including harming other people.
- Delusions. Delusions are false ideas that a person continues to hold even after they are shown to be false.

- Disorganized thought and speech. This symptom may include making up words that have no meaning or stringing words together in nonsensical ways. Disorganized thought processes are marked by such characteristics as looseness of associations, in which the patient rambles from topic to topic in a disconnected way; tangential, which means that the patient gives unrelated answers to questions; and "word salad," in which the patient's speech is so incoherent that it makes no grammatical or linguistic sense.
- Disorganized behavior. Disorganized behavior means that the patient has difficulty with any type of purposeful or goal-oriented behavior, including personal self-care or preparing meals. Other forms of disorganized behavior may include dressing in odd or inappropriate ways, sexual self-stimulation in public, or agitated shouting or cursing.
- Movement disorders. The patient may be clumsy and uncoordinated or may sit motionless for hours, a condition called catatonia.

Negative symptoms refer to losses or deficiencies in relating to others or in general functioning:

- Lack of emotion in the voice or facial expressions. This symptom is sometimes referred to as affective flattening.
- Social isolation
- Neglecting personal cleanliness and grooming
- Inability to take pleasure in things that most people enjoy
- Problems in starting and organizing tasks or activities
- Refusing to speak even when spoken to

In general, the negative symptoms of schizophrenia are more difficult for doctors to evaluate than the positive symptoms.

Cognitive symptoms refer to problems with thinking, memory, and the ability to pay attention. These are the symptoms that interfere most severely with the patient's education and employment in adult life.

Diagnosis

People with schizophrenia are usually unaware that they are suffering from a mental illness; it is often necessary for family or friends to get help for them. If the person is threatening suicide or appears to be a danger to others, family or friends (or even bystanders) should call 911; first responders can take the affected person to a hospital for evaluation and (when needed) emergency hospitalization. The diagnosis of schizophrenia itself may be made by a psychiatrist during a lengthy office examination or in a hospital emergency department.

Examination

A doctor must make a diagnosis of schizophrenia on the basis of a standardized list of outwardly observable symptoms, not on the basis of internal psychological processes. There are no specific laboratory or imaging tests as of 2011 that can be used to diagnose schizophrenia; however, researchers have discovered that patients with schizophrenia have certain abnormalities in the structure and functioning of the brain compared to normal test subjects. These discoveries have been made with the help of imaging techniques such as computed tomography (CT) scans.

When a psychiatrist assesses a patient for schizophrenia, he or she will begin by excluding physical conditions that can cause abnormal thinking and some other behaviors associated with schizophrenia. These conditions include organic brain disorders (including traumatic injuries of the brain), temporal lobe epilepsy, Wilson's disease, Huntington's **chorea**, thyroid disorders, late-stage syphilis, AIDS-related dementia, and **encephalitis**. The doctor will also need to rule out substance abuse disorders, especially amphetamine use.

The role of drug and alcohol abuse in schizophrenia is complicated. On the one hand, the disorder itself is not caused by alcoholism or drug abuse. On the other, schizophrenics are more likely than others to abuse drugs and alcohol, often as a way of coping with their symptoms. One problem with drug and alcohol abuse is that it makes schizophrenia harder to treat. Drugs such as PCP ("angel dust"), marijuana, or cocaine can make the symptoms of schizophrenia worse; they also make patients less likely to follow their treatment plan. The drug that is most commonly abused by schizophrenics, however, is nicotine: 75–90% of people with schizophrenia are heavy smokers, compared with 25–30% in the general population.

After ruling out organic disorders, the clinician will consider other psychiatric conditions that may include psychotic symptoms or symptoms resembling psychosis. These disorders include mood disorders with psychotic features; delusional disorder; dissociative disorder not otherwise specified (DDNOS) or multiple personality disorder; schizotypal, schizoid, or paranoid personality disorders; and atypical reactive disorders. In the past, many individuals were incorrectly diagnosed as schizophrenic. Some patients who were diagnosed prior to the changes in categorization introduced by *DSM-IV* should have their diagnoses and treatment reevaluated. In children, the doctor must distinguish between psychotic symptoms and a vivid fantasy life and also identify learning

KEY TERMS

Affective flattening—A loss or lack of emotional expressiveness. It is sometimes called blunted or restricted affect.

Akathisia—Agitated or restless movement, usually affecting the legs and accompanied by a sense of discomfort. It is a common side effect of neuroleptic medications.

Antipsychotics—A group of drugs used to treat schizophrenia. The older antipsychotic drugs are also called neuroleptics.

Auditory—Pertaining to the sense of hearing.

Catatonia—A condition in which a person sits motionless for long periods of time and does not respond to others.

Delusion—In medicine, a false belief that a person holds to despite evidence or proof that it is false.

Depot dosage—A form of medication that can be stored in the patient's body tissues for several days or weeks, thus minimizing the risk of the patient forgetting daily doses. Haloperidol and fluphenazine can be given in depot form.

Dopamine receptor antagonists (DAs)—The older class of antipsychotic medications, also called neuroleptics. These primarily block the site on nerve cells that normally receive the brain chemical dopamine.

Dystonia—Painful involuntary muscle cramps or spasms.

Extrapyramidal symptoms (EPS)—A group of side effects associated with antipsychotic medications. EPS include parkinsonism, akathisia, dystonia, and tardive dyskinesia.

Hallucination—Perceiving something that is not really there. Hallucinations can affect any of the five senses.

Huntington's chorea—A hereditary disease that typically appears in midlife, marked by gradual loss of brain function and voluntary movement. Some of its symptoms resemble those of schizophrenia.

Negative symptoms—Symptoms of schizophrenia characterized by the absence or elimination of certain behaviors. *DSM-IV* specifies three negative symptoms: affective flattening, poverty of speech, and loss of will or initiative.

Neuroleptic—Another name for the older type of antipsychotic medications given to schizophrenic patients.

Parkinsonism—A set of symptoms originally associated with Parkinson's disease that can occur as side effects of neuroleptic medications. The symptoms include trembling of the fingers or hands, a shuffling gait, and tight or rigid muscles.

Positive symptoms—Symptoms of schizophrenia that are characterized by the production or presence of behaviors that are grossly abnormal or excessive, including hallucinations and thought-process disorder.

Poverty of speech—A negative symptom of schizophrenia, characterized by brief and empty replies to questions. It should not be confused with shyness or reluctance to talk.

Psychosis—Severe mental illness marked by hallucinations and loss of contact with the real world.

Relapse—Recurrence of an illness after a period of improvement.

Serotonin dopamine antagonists (SDA)—The newer second-generation antipsychotic drugs, also called atypical antipsychotics. SDAs include clozapine (Clozaril), risperidone (Risperdal), aripiprazole (Abilify), and olanzapine (Zyprexa).

Tardive dyskinesia—A movement disorder that may result from long-term treatment with the older antipsychotic drugs. Its symptoms include uncontrollable tongue thrusting, lip smacking, and facial grimacing.

Wilson's disease—A rare hereditary disease marked by high levels of copper deposits in the brain and liver. It can cause psychiatric symptoms resembling those of schizophrenia.

Word salad—Speech that is so disorganized that it makes no linguistic or grammatical sense.

problems or disorders. After other conditions have been ruled out, the patient must meet a set of criteria specified by *DSM-IV*:

• Characteristic symptoms. The patient must have two (or more) of the following symptoms during a one-month period: delusions; hallucinations; disorganized speech; disorganized or catatonic behavior; negative symptoms

• Decline in social, interpersonal, or occupational functioning, including self-care

• Duration. The disturbed behavior must last for at least six months.

• Diagnostic exclusions. Mood disorders, substance abuse disorders, medical conditions, and developmental disorders have been ruled out.

Treatment

Traditional

The treatment of schizophrenia depends in part on the patient's stage or phase. Patients in the acute phase are hospitalized in most cases, to prevent harm to the patient or others and to begin treatment with antipsychotic medications. A patient having a first psychotic episode may be given a CT or MRI (**magnetic resonance imaging**) scan to rule out structural brain disease.

Most schizophrenics can benefit from psychotherapy once their acute symptoms have been brought under control by antipsychotic medication. Psychoanalytic approaches are not recommended; however, behavior therapy is often helpful in assisting patients to acquire skills for daily living and social interaction. It can be combined with occupational therapy to prepare the patient for eventual employment.

Family therapy is often recommended for the families of schizophrenic patients to relieve the feelings of guilt that they often have as well as to help them understand the patient's disorder. The family's attitude and behaviors toward the patient are key factors in minimizing relapses (for example, by reducing stress in the patient's life), and family therapy can often strengthen the family's ability to cope with the stresses caused by the illness. Family therapy focused on communication skills and problem-solving strategies is particularly helpful. In addition to formal treatment, many families benefit from support groups and similar mutual help organizations for relatives of schizophrenics.

Drugs

The primary form of treatment of schizophrenia is antipsychotic medication. Antipsychotic drugs help to control almost all the positive symptoms of the disorder. They have minimal effects on disorganized behavior and negative symptoms. Between 60% and 70% of schizophrenics respond to antipsychotics. In the acute phase of the illness, patients are usually given medications by mouth or by intramuscular injection. After the patient has been stabilized, the antipsychotic drug may be given in a long-acting form called a depot dose. Depot medications last two to four weeks; they have the advantage of protecting the patient against the consequences of forgetting or skipping daily doses. In addition, some patients who do not respond to oral neuroleptics have better results with depot form. Patients whose long-term treatment includes depot medications are introduced to the depot form gradually during their stabilization period. Most people with schizophrenia are kept on antipsychotic medications indefinitely during the maintenance phase of their disorder to minimize the possibility of relapse.

The most frequently used antipsychotics fall into two classes: the older dopamine receptor antagonists, or DAs, and the newer serotonin dopamine antagonists, or SDAs. (Antagonists block the action of some other substance; for example, dopamine antagonists counteract the action of dopamine.) The exact mechanisms of action of these medications are not known, but it is thought that they lower the patient's sensitivity to sensory stimuli and so indirectly improve the patient's ability to interact with others.

DOPAMINE RECEPTOR ANTAGONISTS. The dopamine antagonists include the older antipsychotic (also called neuroleptic) drugs, such as haloperidol (Haldol), chlorpromazine (Thorazine), and fluphenazine (Prolixin). These drugs have two major drawbacks: It is often difficult to find the best dosage level for the individual patient, and a dosage level high enough to control psychotic symptoms frequently produces extrapyramidal side effects, or EPS. EPS includes parkinsonism, in which the patient cannot walk normally and usually develops a **tremor**; dystonia, or painful muscle spasms of the head, tongue, or neck; and akathisia, or restlessness. A type of long-term EPS is called tardive dyskinesia, which features slow, rhythmic, automatic movements. Schizophrenics with **AIDS** are especially vulnerable to developing EPS.

SEROTONIN DOPANINE ANTAGONISTS. The serotonin dopamine antagonists, also called atypical antipsychotics, are newer medications that include clozapine (Clozaril), risperidone (Risperdal), aripiprazole (Abilify), and olanzapine (Zyprexa). In October 2010 the Food and Drug Administration approved a new drug, lurasidone (Latuda), which appears to have fewer side effects than other atypical antipsychotics. As a group, the SDAs have a better effect on the negative symptoms of schizophrenia than do the older drugs and are less likely to produce EPS than the older compounds. The newer drugs are significantly more expensive in the short term, although the SDAs may reduce long-term costs by reducing the need for hospitalization. They are also presently unavailable in injectable forms. The SDAs are commonly used to treat patients who respond poorly to the DAs. Many psychotherapists now regard the use of these atypical antipsychotics as the treatment of first choice. There are side effects of atypical antipsychotic medications, however, which include weight gain, increased risk of diabetes, and high blood cholesterol levels. Lurasidone appears to be less likely to cause these side effects that the other SDAs.

ANTIDEPRESSANTS. Patients with schizophrenia have a lifetime prevalence of 80% for major **depression**; others suffer from phobias or other anxiety disorders. These patients may be prescribed antidepressants or a short course of **benzodiazepines** along with their antipsychotic medications.

Alternative

Alternative and complementary therapies that are being investigated for the treatment of schizophrenia include gingko biloba, an Asian shrub, and vitamin therapy. One Chinese study reported that a group of patients who had not responded to conventional antipsychotic medications benefited from a 13-week trial of gingko extract, with significantly fewer side effects. Vitamin therapy is recommended by naturopathic practitioners on the grounds that many hospitalized patients with schizophrenia suffer from nutritional deficiencies. The supplements recommended include folic acid, niacin, vitamin B_6, and vitamin C.

Clinical trials

There were 1,556 clinical trials of various treatments and interventions for schizophrenia under way as of mid-2011. The trials include approaches to smoking cessation and weight reduction in schizophrenia patients; various therapies to improve cognitive function; trials of several investigational drugs, including memantine, cariprazine, dipyridamole, and unnamed compounds identified as AQW051 and MK8998; family therapy and genetic counseling; the effectiveness of vitamin supplementation; and various anti-inflammatory agents.

Prognosis

One important prognostic sign is the patient's age at onset of psychotic symptoms. Patients with early onset of schizophrenia are more often male, have a lower level of functioning prior to onset, a higher rate of brain abnormalities, more noticeable negative symptoms, and worse outcomes. Patients with later onset are more likely to be female, with fewer brain abnormalities and thought impairment, and more hopeful prognoses.

The average course and outcome for schizophrenics are less favorable than those for most other mental disorders, although a few patients do recover completely. Most have periodic relapses and need group homes or long-term structured programs in order to function in the community. In addition to problems with drug abuse and dependence, patients with schizophrenia also have a very high rate of suicide, around 10%. The average life expectancy for patients diagnosed with schizophrenia is 12 to 15 years shorter than that of people who do not have the disorder; this difference is largely the result of health problems due to lack of proper self-care, heavy smoking, and the increased risk of substance abuse and suicide.

Two factors that influence outcomes are stressful life events and a hostile or emotionally intense family environment. Schizophrenics with a high number of stressful changes in their lives, or who have frequent contact with critical or emotionally over-involved family members, are more likely to relapse. Overall, the most important component of long-term care of schizophrenic patients is complying with their regimen of antipsychotic medications.

Prevention

There is no proven way as of 2011 to prevent the onset of schizophrenia. Researchers have investigated the possibility of treating schizophrenia before symptoms start (such as when the likelihood of hereditary transmission is high). Other areas of research include the links between schizophrenia and family stress, drug use, and exposure to certain infectious agents.

Resources

BOOKS

American Psychiatric Association. *Diagnostic and Statistical Manual*. 4th ed. Washington, DC: Author, 2000.

Beck, Aaron T., et al. *Schizophrenia: Cognitive Theory, Research, and Therapy*. New York: Guilford, 2008.

Brown, Alan S., and Paul H. Patterson, eds. *The Origins of Schizophrenia*. New York: Columbia University Press, 2012.

DeLisi, Lynn. *100 Questions and Answers about Schizophrenia: Painful Minds*. 2nd ed. Sudbury, MA: Jones and Bartlett, 2011.

Kaye, Randye. *Ben Behind His Voices: One Family's Journey from the Chaos of Schizophrenia to Hope*. Lanham, MD: Rowman and Littlefield, 2011.

Lieberman, Jeffrey A., T. Scott Stroup, and Diana O. Perkins, eds. *Essentials of Schizophrenia*. Washington, DC: American Psychiatric Publishing, 2012.

North, Carol S., and Sean H. Yutzy. *Goodwin and Guze's Psychiatric Diagnosis*. 6th ed. New York: Oxford University Press, 2010.

Snyder, Kurt, et al. *Me, Myself, and Them: A Firsthand Account of One Young Person's Experience with Schizophrenia*. New York: Oxford University Press, 2007.

PERIODICALS

Carlisle, L.L., and J. McClellan. "Psychopharmacology of Schizophrenia in Children and Adolescents." *Psychiatric Clinics of North America* 58 (February 2011): 205–18.

Citrome, L. "Lurasidone for Schizophrenia: A Brief Review of a New Second-generation Antipsychotic." *Clinical Schizophrenia and Related Psychoses* 4 (January 2011): 239–50.

Felmet, K., et al. "Elderly Patients with Schizophrenia and Depression: Diagnosis and Treatment." *Clinical Schizophrenia and Related Psychoses* 4 (January 2011): 251–57.

Gershon, E.S., et al. "After Genome-Wide Association Studies: Searching for Genetic Risk for Schizophrenia and Bipolar Disorder." *American Journal of Psychiatry* 168 (March 2011): 253–56.

Gur, R.E. "Neuropsychiatric Aspects of Schizophrenia." *CNS Neuroscience and Therapeutics* 17 (February 2011): 45–51.

Kleinman, J.E., et al. "Genetic Neuropathology of Schizophrenia: New Approaches to an Old Question and New Uses for Postmortem Human Brains." *Biological Psychiatry* 69 (January 15, 2011): 140–45.

Large, M.M., et al. "The Predictive Value of Risk Categorization in Schizophrenia." *Harvard Review of Psychiatry* 19 (January–February 2011): 25–33.

Lawrence, D., et al. "The Epidemiology of Excess Mortality in People with Mental Illness." *Canadian Journal of Psychiatry* 55 (December 2010): 752–60.

Moore, T.A. "Schizophrenia Treatment Guidelines in the United States." *Clinical Schizophrenia and Related Psychoses* 5 (April 2011): 40–49.

Van Sant, S.P., and P.F. Buckley. "Pharmacotherapy for Treatment-refractory Schizophrenia." *Expert Opinion on Pharmacotherapy* 12 (February 2011): 411–34.

Vyas, N.S., et al. "Neurobiology and Phenotypic Expression in Early Onset Schizophrenia." *Early Intervention in Psychiatry* 5 (February 2011): 3–14.

WEBSITES

Frankenburg, Frances R. "Schizophrenia." Medscape Reference. http://emedicine.medscape.com/article/288259-overview (accessed July 19, 2011).

Gerstein, Paul S. "Emergent Treatment of Schizophrenia." Medscape Reference. http://emedicine.medscape.com/article/805988-overview (accessed July 19, 2011).

"Schizophrenia." Mayo Clinic. http://www.mayoclinic.com/health/schizophrenia/DS00196 (accessed July 19, 2011).

"Schizophrenia." National Institute of Mental Health. http://www.nimh.nih.gov/health/topics/schizophrenia/index.shtml (accessed July 19, 2011).

"Schizophrenia Spectrum and Other Psychotic Disorders." American Psychiatric Association. DSM-5 Development. http://www.dsm5.org/proposedrevision/Pages/SchizophreniaSpectrumandOtherPsychoticDisorders.aspx (accessed July 19, 2011).

"What Is Schizophrenia?" National Alliance on Mental Illness (NAMI). http://www.nami.org/Template.cfm?Section = Schizophrenia9&Template = /ContentManagement/ContentDisplay.cfm&ContentID = 117961 (accessed July 19, 2011).

ORGANIZATIONS

American Psychiatric Association (APA), 1000 Wilson Boulevard, Suite 1825, Arlington, VA 22209-3901, (703) 907-7300, (888) 35-PSYCH, apa@ psych.org, http://www.psych.org/.

National Alliance on Mental Illness (NAMI), 3803 N. Fairfax Dr., Suite 100, Arlington, VA 22203, (703) 524-7600, (800) 950-NAMI, Fax: (703) 524-9094, http://www.nami.org.

National Institute of Mental Health (NIMH), 6001 Executive Boulevard, Room 8184, MSC 9663, Bethesda, MD 20892-9663, (301) 443-4513, (866) 615-6464, Fax: (301) 443-4279, nimhinfo@nih.gov, http://www.nimh.nih.gov/index.shtml.

U.S. Food and Drug Administration, 10903 New Hampshire Avenue, Silver Spring, MD 20993-0002, (888) 463-6332, http://www.fda.gov.

Laith Farid Gulli, MD
Rebecca J. Frey, PhD

Sciatic neuropathy

Definition

Sciatica is a term given to any painful condition of the leg that originates in the lower back and descends down the leg. Because it tends to involve a single nerve tract it is designated as mononeuropathy (localized nerve disorder).

The cause of this pain is the neuropathy defined by the inflammation and swelling of the large sciatic nerve that originates from the exit of an intervertebral nerve plexus between one of the large lumbar vertebral discs. A portion of the sciatic nerve also originates from the sacrum. The name for the region from which this nerve emanates is the sacral plexus. It encompasses the lumbar vertebra L 4–5 through the sacral vertebra S 1–3. The intervertebral nerves join to form one of the larger nerve tracts in the body, the sciatic nerve. This nerve tract winds over the pelvic bones and down the proximal posterior side of the femurs (either right or left). From there it branches into the tibial and common peroneal nerve. Further branching produces the deep peroneal nerve.

An inflammation or irritation of this nerve can produce pain that ranges anywhere from mild discomfort to extreme distress. Many sufferers describe a constant pain that does not ease with change in body position or conventional medications. The pain can extend from a small area of the lower back to along the hip and down the leg past the ankle to the foot.

Additional symptoms of sciatic neuropathy that distinguish it from peripheral neuropathy include sensation changes. These occur on the soles of the foot and up the leg. They may include numbness and tingling and even a burning sensation. Difficulty in walking is common, and, in serious conditions, there may be an inability to move the foot or knee.

Description

The most common source of inflammation of the sciatic nerve and its branches is injury to an intervertebral disc. This neuritis (nerve inflammation) may occur when pressure on the disc forces it to rupture, squeezing some of the softer, more gelatinous interior against the nerve. In turn, this constant pressure begins to irritate the sciatic nerve until eventual swelling from inflammation occurs. The irritation is transmitted to the brain and the patient experiences constant or intermittent pain of varying degrees.

Depending on the degree of herniation to the disc, the pain may eventually go away or the patient may consider lower back surgery. Surgery is the most extreme form of treatment for this condition, as most cases will be relieved with exercise and anti-inflammatory medications. Healing may be slow and take up to six weeks.

A common source of sciatic neuropathy is wounding of the sciatic nerve. This condition presents itself when a person has been forced to lie down for extended lengths of time. The resulting pressure on the nerve and lack of movement produces neuropathy. This condition is often confused with tibial nerve dysfunction or common nerve dysfunction.

Wounds to the sciatic nerve may result from fractures of the pelvis, wounds from gunshots or blunt objects such as a bat or stick. Car injuries may often produce damage to the sciatic nerve. Physiological damage can also result from diabetes. In some patients, long-lasting sciatica has been found to be caused by infection, which may have started after the spine suffered a minor injury.

Another possible cause of pressure on the sciatic nerve is that imposed by a tumor. Again, surgery may be considered to treat this form of sciatica. The physician may offer alternative therapies to treat the tumor, but therapies are case dependent and vary widely. In cases where tumors are present, the primary cause of the sciatica usually requires treatment that is are not aimed specifically at resolving the sciatica.

The sciatic nerve is closely associated with the piriformis muscle, and in some patients the nerve may actually pass through this muscle. If the muscle is injured or inflamed, pressure on the nerve, and thus sciatica, can result. This condition is known as piriformis syndrome, pseudosciatica, wallet sciatica, or hip socket neuropathy.

Direct trauma to the sciatic nerve may also produce inflammation. A fall or a puncture from an injection can produce insult to the nerve tissues and result in sciatica. In these cases, the treatment is simple and effective. Movement and anti-inflammatory medications usually improve the situation until it eventually resolves.

Demographics

While there are varying demographics regarding sciatica, there are conditions that may alert a physician to look for underlying cause of the condition. People under 20 or over 55 are often examined for additional symptoms of other disorders. Associated pain in the back of the chest is a concern along with recent major injury as the type sustained from a traffic injury.

Included in the groups of patients who receive additional examination when they complain of sciatica are those who have lost weight recently, have had cancer, are on steroids, have worsening pain, and those who have developed other nervous system disorders in the past.

A study conducted in Finland found that women who had been overweight as teenagers showed an increased risk for sciatica severe enough to require hospitalization. For men, the same study found a connection between sciatica that required hospital treatment with two factors: the men's weight as teenagers and smoking.

Causes and symptoms

As previously noted, the most common cause of sciatica is a slipped or herniated disk, also called a prolapsed intervertebral disk (PID) or a herniated nucleus pulposus. Any trauma or injury to the nerve will result in swelling and inflammation. While this healing condition persists, the nerve will respond with pain, which in turn will often reduce normal movement.

Rarely, sciatic neuropathy has been reported after surgical procedures that required the patient to be immobilized in the operating room for long periods of time or in positions that may have irritated the sciatic nerve.

Diagnosis

Sciatica is in itself a symptom of some other condition which must be diagnosed by a physician. The root causes of the disorder may vary. Only a professional who is trained in recognizing the information provided by the patient and laboratory results can determine if or whether the condition is an isolated symptom or a symptom of a more general or serious disorder of the patient.

Although the diagnosis is based primarily upon symptoms of pain, the physician will usually test for muscle strength, reflexes, and flexibility while considering a diagnosis of sciatic neuropathy. Areas of spinal problems that may cause sciatic nerve irritation or compression are usually visible on MRI or CT scan. Occasionally, further nerve function tests may be necessary.

Treatment team

Physicians are the first contact to be made in a treatment team. It is the physician who must first make the diagnosis. A radiologist or laboratory technician may take x rays of the area to look for bone spurs or disk protrusions. Once the diagnosis is made, the pharmacist may be called to provide appropriate medication for treatment. In more severe cases, a physical therapist may be used to keep the patient active and performing physical tasks that help reduce the pain. With intractable pain, a neurosurgeon may be consulted for surgery.

Among the non-surgical health care professionals who work with sciatica patients are physical therapists, pain medicine specialists, chiropractors, osteopaths, and physiatrists.

Treatment

The immediate treatment of most cases of sciatica is to recommend medications specific to the inflammation. Staying active is also highly recommended, while avoiding activities that put pressure on the back. Studies have

found that a simple combination of anti-inflammatory medication such as ibuprofen and mild exercise, such as walking, are effective treatment for most cases of common sciatica. Sometimes an epidural injection (an injection to the epidural space of the spine) may provide pain relief. Surgery for a herniated disk is an aggressive alternative, and includes more risk.

Recovery and rehabilitation

Approximately half the patients suffering with sciatica recover within six weeks, and 90% are better within 12 weeks. While the pain may be intense for some sufferers, it is usually temporary. With treatment, person has an excellent chance for reduction or resolution of the neuropathy pain of sciatica.

Clinical trials

A variety of clinical trials have examined the effectiveness of various treatments for sciatica, including the administration of topiramate, adalimumab, epidurals, and predisone, as well as **exercise**. Information on additional clinical trials can be found at the U.S. National Institutes of Health Web site for clinical trials: http://clinicaltrials.gov.

Prognosis

The prognosis for the pain relief of most cases of sciatica is excellent. With a combined use of anti-inflammatory drugs and mild exercise, such as walking, sciatica can be reduced and even eliminated. If the underlying cause is more serious, the prognosis varies with the degree of severity and type of condition.

Special concerns

One of the myths associated with sciatica is the need to rest in bed. In fact, mild exercise is one of the best treatments for the pain. Prolonged sitting is a primary cause of many cases of sciatica. If a job requires extended periods of sitting, it is wise to take short walks or perform mild stretches to keep compression of the lower lumbar vertebrae from occurring.

Resources

BOOKS

Dagenais, Simon, and Scott Haldeman. *Evidence-Based Management of Low Back Pain.* New York: Mosby, 2011.

Fonseca, David, and Joanne L. Martins, eds. *The Sciatic Nerve: Blocks, Injuries and Regeneration.* Hauppauge, NY: Nova Science, 2011.

PERIODICALS

Rivinoja, A.E., et al. "Sports, smoking, and overweight during adolescence as predictors of sciatica in adulthood: a 28-year follow-up study of a birth cohort." *American Journal of Epidemiology* 173, no. 8 (April 2011): 890–97.

WEBSITES

Hochschuler, S.H. "What You Need to Know about Sciatica." Spine-health. www.spine-health.com/conditions/sciatica/what-you-need-know-about-sciatica (accessed August 28, 2011).

"Sciatica." Medline Plus. http://www.nlm.nih.gov/medlineplus/sciatica.html (accessed August 28, 2011).

ORGANIZATIONS

American Chronic Pain Association (ACPA), P.O. Box 850, Rocklin, CA 95677, (916) 632-0922, (800) 533-3231, Fax: (916) 632-3208, ACPA@pacbell. net, http://www.theacpa.org.

National Institute of Arthritis and Musculoskeletal and Skin Diseases (NIAMS), 1 AMS Circle, Bethesda, MD 20892-3675, (301) 495-4484, (877) 226-4267, NIAMSinfo@mail.nih.gov, http://www.niams.nih.gov.

Brook Ellen Hall, PhD
Fran Hodgkins

Seizure disorder *see* **Epilepsy**

Seizures

Definition

A seizure is a sudden change in behavior characterized by changes in sensory perception (sense of feeling) or motor activity (movement) due to an abnormal firing of nerve cells in the brain. **Epilepsy** is a condition characterized by recurrent seizures that may include repetitive muscle jerking called convulsions.

Description

Seizure disorders and their classification date back to the earliest medical literature accounts in history. In 1964, the Commission on Classification and Terminology of the International League Against Epilepsy (ILAE) devised the first official classification of seizures, which was revised in 1981 and again in 1989. They then proposed to use a diagnostic scheme of five diagnostic levels or axes, rather than a classification scheme, for characterizing seizures. These axes are (1) the events that occur during the seizure; (2) the type of seizure, chosen from a list that can include where the seizure localizes in the brain and what stimulates it; (3) the type of epileptic syndrome most closely associated with the seizure; (4) the underlying medical or other causes of the syndrome; and (5) the level of impairment the seizure causes. These are proposed recommendations that are still under discussion.

The ILAE classification, meanwhile, is accepted worldwide and is based on electroencephalographic (EEG) studies. Based on this system, seizures can be classified as either focal or generalized. Each of these categories can also be further subdivided.

Focal seizures

A focal (partial) seizure develops when a limited, confined population of nerve cells fire their impulses abnormally on one hemisphere of the brain. (The brain has two portions or cerebral hemispheres—the right and left hemispheres.) Focal seizures are identified as simple or complex based on the level of consciousness (wakefulness) during an attack. Simple partial seizures occur in patients who are conscious, whereas complex partial seizures demonstrate impaired levels of consciousness.

Generalized seizures

A generalized seizure results from initial abnormal firing of brain nerve cells throughout both the left and right hemispheres. Generalized seizures can be classified as follows:

- tonic-clonic seizures: This is the most common type among all age groups and is categorized into several phases beginning with vague symptoms that appear hours or days before an attack. These seizures are sometimes called grand mal seizures.

- tonic seizures: These are typically characterized by a sustained nonvibratory contraction of muscles in the legs and arms. Consciousness is also impaired during these episodes.

- atonic seizures (also called "drop attacks"): These are characterized by sudden, limp posture and a brief period of unconsciousness, and last for one to two seconds.

- clonic seizures: These are characterized by a rapid loss of consciousness with loss of muscle tone, tonic spasm, and jerks. The muscles become rigid for about 30 seconds during the tonic phase of the seizure and alternately contract and relax during the clonic phase, which lasts 30–60 seconds.

- absence seizures: These are subdivided into typical and atypical forms based on duration of attack and level of consciousness. Absence (petit mal) seizures generally begin at about the age of four and stop by the time the child becomes an adolescent. They usually begin with a brief loss of consciousness and last 1–10 seconds. People having petit mal seizures become very quiet and may blink, stare blankly, roll their eyes, or move their lips. A petit mal seizure lasts 15–20 seconds. When it ends, individuals resume whatever they were doing before the seizure began, will not remember the seizure, and may not realize that anything unusual happened. Untreated, petit mal seizures can recur as many as 100 times a day and may progress to grand mal seizures.
- myoclonic seizures: These are characterized by rapid muscular contractions accompanied with jerks in facial and pelvic muscles.

Subcategories are commonly diagnosed based on electroencephalographic (EEG) results. Terminology for classification in infants and newborns is still controversial.

Causes and symptoms

Causes

Simple partial seizures can be caused by congenital abnormalities (abnormalities present at birth), tumor growths, head trauma, stroke, and infections in the brain or nearby structures. Generalized tonic-clonic seizures are associated with drug and alcohol abuse, and low levels of blood glucose (blood sugar) and sodium. Certain psychiatric medications, antihistamines, and even antibiotics can precipitate tonic-clonic seizures. Absence seizures are implicated with an abnormal imbalance of certain chemicals in the brain that modulate nerve cell activity (one of these neurotransmitters is called gamma-aminobutyric acid or GABA, which functions as an inhibitor). Myoclonic seizures are commonly diagnosed in newborns and children.

Symptoms

Symptoms for the different types of seizures are specific.

Partial seizures

SIMPLE PARTIAL SEIZURES. Multiple signs and symptoms may be present during a single simple partial seizure. These symptoms include specific muscles tensing and then alternately contracting and relaxing, speech arrest, vocalizations, and involuntary turning of the eyes or head. There could be changes in vision, hearing, balance, taste, and smell. Additionally, patients with simple partial seizures may have a sensation in the abdomen, sweating, paleness, flushing, hair follicles standing up (piloerection), and dilated pupils (the dark center in the eye enlarges). Seizures with psychological symptoms include thinking disturbances and hallucinations, or illusions of memory, sound, sight, time, and self-image.

COMPLEX PARTIAL SEIZURES. Complex partial seizures often begin with a motionless stare or arrest of activity; this is followed by a series of involuntary movements, speech disturbances, and eye movements.

Generalized seizures

Generalized seizures have a more complex set of signs and symptoms.

TONIC-CLONIC SEIZURES. Tonic-clonic seizures usually have vague prodromal (pre-attack) symptoms that can start hours or days before a seizure. These symptoms include anxiety, mood changes, irritability, weakness, dizziness, lightheadedness, and changes in appetite. The tonic phases may be preceded with brief (lasting only a few seconds in duration) muscle contractions on both sides of affected muscle groups. The tonic phase typically begins with a brief flexing of trunk muscles, upward movement of the eyes, and pupil dilation. Patients usually emit a characteristic vocalization. This sound is caused by contraction of trunk muscles that forces air from the lungs across spasmodic (abnormally tensed) throat muscles. This is followed by a very short period (10–15 seconds) of general muscle relaxation. The clonic phase consists of muscular contractions with alternating periods of no movements (muscle atonia) that gradually increase duration until abnormal muscular contractions stop. Tonic-clonic seizures end in a final generalized spasm. The affected person can lose consciousness during tonic and clonic phases of seizure.

Tonic-clonic seizures can also produce chemical changes in the body. Patients commonly experience lowered carbon dioxide (hypocarbia) due to breathing alterations, increased blood glucose (blood sugar), and an elevated level of the hormone prolactin. Once affected people regain consciousness, they are usually weak and have a headache and muscle pain. Tonic-clonic seizures can cause serious medical problems such as trauma to the head and mouth, fractures in the spinal column, pulmonary edema (water in the lungs), aspiration pneumonia (a pneumonia caused by a foreign body being lodged in the lungs), and sudden death. Attacks are generally one minute in duration.

TONIC SEIZURES. Tonic and atonic seizures have distinct differences but are often present in the same patient. Tonic seizures are characterized by nonvibratory muscle contractions, usually involving flexing of arms and relaxing or flexing of legs. The seizure usually lasts less than ten seconds but may be as long as one minute. Tonic seizures are usually abrupt and patients lose consciousness. Tonic seizures commonly occur during non-rapid eye movement (non-REM) sleep and drowsiness. Tonic seizures that occur during wakeful states commonly produce physical injuries due to abrupt, unexpected falls.

ATONIC SEIZURES. Atonic seizures, also called "drop attacks," are abrupt, with loss of muscle tone lasting one to two seconds, but with rapid recovery. Consciousness is usually impaired. The rapid loss of muscular tone could be limited to head and neck muscles, resulting in head drop, or it may be more extensive involving muscles for balance, causing unexpected falls with physical injury.

CLONIC SEIZURES. Generalized clonic seizures are rare and seen typically in children with elevated fever. These seizures are characterized by a rapid loss of consciousness, decreased muscle tone, and a generalized spasm that is followed by jerky movements.

ABSENCE SEIZURES. Absence seizures are classified as either typical or atypical. The typical absence seizure is characterized by unresponsiveness and behavioral arrest, abnormal muscular movements of the face and eyelids, and lasts less than ten seconds. In atypical absence seizures, the affected person is generally more conscious, the seizures begin and end more gradually and do not exceed ten seconds in duration.

MYOCLONIC SEIZURES. People with myoclonic seizures commonly exhibit rapid muscular contractions. Myoclonic seizures are seen in newborns and children who have either symptomatic or idiopathic (cause is unknown) epilepsy.

Demographics

Epilepsy and seizures affect a reported 3 million—or 1%—of Americans of all ages, although up to 10% of the population may experience at least one seizure during their lives; some of these events are febrile convulsions associated with high fevers in childhood. Every year, about 200,000 new cases are diagnosed and about 300,000 people have their first convulsion. The annual costs of treatment for seizure and epilepsy, in direct and indirect costs, is about $12.5 billion. Men are slightly more likely than women to develop epilepsy, and its prevalence is higher among minority populations in the United States.

Seizures caused by fever have a recurrence rate of 51% if the attack occurred in the first year of life, whereas recurrence rate is decreased to 25% if the seizure took place during the second year. Approximately 88% of children who experience seizures caused by fever in the first two years experience recurrence.

About 45 million people worldwide are affected by epilepsy. The incidence is highest among young children (under age 2) and the elderly (over age 65). High-risk groups include people with a previous history of brain injury or lesions; children with mental retardation, cerebral palsy, or both; patients with Alzheimer's disease or stroke; and children with at least one parent who has epilepsy.

Diagnosis

Patients seeking help for seizures should first undergo an EEG that records brain-wave patterns emitted between nerve cells. Electrodes are placed on the head, sometimes for 24 hours, to monitor brain-wave activity and detect both normal and abnormal impulses. Imaging studies such as **magnetic resonance imaging** (MRI) and computerized axial tomography (CAT)—that take still "pictures"—are useful in detecting abnormalities in the temporal lobes (parts of the brain associated with hearing) or for helping diagnose tonic-clonic seizures. A complete blood count (CBC) can be helpful in determining whether a seizure is caused by a neurological infection, which is typically accompanied by high fever. If drugs or toxins in the blood are suspected to be the cause of the seizure(s), blood and urine screening tests for these compounds may be necessary.

Antiseizure medication can be altered by many commonly used medications such as sulfa drugs, erythromycin, warfarin, and cimetidine. Pregnancy may also decrease serum concentration of antiseizure medications; therefore, frequent monitoring and dose adjustments are vital to maintain appropriate blood concentrations of the antiseizure medication—known as the therapeutic blood concentration. Some medications taken during pregnancy could affect the fetus, and women must discuss with their doctors the costs and benefits of any medication taken during pregnancy.

Diagnosis requires a detailed and accurate history, and a physical examination is important because this may help identify neurological or systemic causes. In cases in which a central nervous system (CNS) infection (e.g., meningitis or encephalitis) is suspected, a lumbar puncture (or spinal tap) can help detect an increase in immune cells (white blood cells) that develop to fight the specific infection. (A lumbar puncture involves removing a small amount of cerebrospinal fluid—the fluid that bathes and nourishes the brain and spinal cord—from the spinal chord by syringe.)

Treatments

Treatment is targeted primarily to do the following:

- assist the patient in adjusting psychologically to the diagnosis and in maintaining as normal a lifestyle as possible
- reduce or eliminate seizure occurrence
- avoid side effects of long-term drug treatment

Simple and complex partial seizures respond to drugs such as carbamazepine, valproic acid (valproate), phenytoin, gabapentin, tiagabine, lamotrigine, and topiramate. Tonic-clonic seizures tend to respond to valproate, carbamazepine, phenytoin, and lamotrigine. Absence seizures seem to be sensitive to ethosuximide, valproate, and lamotrigine. Myoclonic seizures can be treated with valproate and clonazepam. Tonic seizures seem to respond favorably to valproate, felbamate, and clonazepam.

People treated with a class of medications called barbiturates (Mysoline, Mebral, phenobarbital) have adverse cognitive (thinking) effects. These cognitive effects can include decreased general intelligence, attention, memory, problem solving, motor speed, and visual motor functions. The drug phenytoin (Dilantin) can adversely affect speed of response, memory, and attention. Other medications used for treatment of seizures do not have substantial cognitive impairment.

Surgical treatment may be considered when medications fail. Advances in medical sciences and techniques have improved methods of identifying the parts of the brain that generate abnormal discharge of nerve impulses. The most common type of surgery is the extra-temporal cortical resection. In this procedure, a small part of the brain responsible for causing the seizures is removed. An option of last resort for people with extreme, uncontrollable seizures is functional hemispherectomy, in which communication between the two hemispheres of the brain is severed. Surgical intervention may be considered a feasible treatment option in any of the following cases:

- the site of seizures is identifiable and localized
- surgery can remove the seizure-generating (epileptogenic) area
- surgical procedure will not cause damage to nearby areas

Vagus nerve stimulation involves the implantation of a stimulator under the skin of the chest. Wires run from the stimulator to the vagus nerve and deliver short bursts of electrical energy. The electricity runs up to the brain through the vagus nerve, and serves to interrupt the seizure-causing electrical activity in the brain.

Another treatment approach that has been found to reduce seizures in some children is the ketogenic diet. This diet reduces available glucose in the body, forcing the child's body to turn to fat stores for energy. It is a high-fat diet that results in the person getting about 80% of their calories from fat. No one is exactly sure why this diet, which mimics starvation in the body, works to prevent seizures. It also does not work for every child, and the reasons for that are unclear.

Prognosis

About 30% of patients with severe seizures (starting in early childhood), continue to have attacks and usually never achieve a remission state. In the United States, the prevalence of treatment-resistant seizures is about one to two per 1,000 people. About 60–70% of people achieve a five-year remission within ten years of initial diagnosis. Approximately half of these patients become seizure-free. Usually the prognosis is better if seizures can be controlled by one medication, the frequency of seizures decreases, and there is a normal EEG and neurological examination prior to medication cessation.

People affected by seizures have increased death rates compared with the general population. Patients who have seizures of unknown cause have an increased chance of dying due to accidents (primarily drowning). Other causes of seizure-associated death include abnormal heart rhythms, water in the lungs, or heart attack.

Prevention

There are no gold-standard recommendations for prevention because seizures can be caused by genetic factors, blood abnormalities, many medications, illicit drugs, infection, neurologic conditions, and other systemic diseases. If a person has had a previous attack or has a genetic propensity, care is advised when receiving medical treatment or if diagnosed with an illness correlated with possible seizure development.

Resources

BOOKS

Goetz, Christopher G. *Textbook of Clinical Neurology*. 3rd ed. Philadelphia: W. B. Saunders, 2007.
Goldman, Lee, et al. *Cecil Textbook of Medicine*. 24th ed. Philadelphia: W. B. Saunders, 2011.
Goroll, Allan H. *Primary Care Medicine*. 6th ed. Philadelphia: Lippincott Williams and Wilkins, 2009.

PERIODICALS

Benbadis, S. "The differential diagnosis of epilepsy: a critical review." *Epilepsy and Behavior* 15 (May 1, 2009): 15–21.

Kellinghaus, C." Frequency of seizures and epilepsy in neurological HIV-infected patients."*Seizure* 47.9 (January 1, 2008): 27–33.

WEBSITES

"Seizures." Medline Plus. http://www.nlm.nih.gov/medline plus/seizures.html (accessed August 28, 2011).

ORGANIZATIONS

The Epilepsy Foundation, 8301 Professional Place, Landover, MD 20785-7223, (800) 332-1000, http://www.epilepsyfoundation.org.

International League Against Epilepsy, 342 North Main Street, West Hartford, CT 06117-2507, (860) 586-7547, Fax: (860) 586-7550, http://www.ilae-epilepsy.org/.

Laith Farid Gulli, MD
Alfredo Mori, MD, FACEM
Emily Jane Willingham, PhD
Rosalyn Carson-DeWitt, MD

Septo-optic dysplasia

Definition

Septo-optic dysplasia (SOD) is a rare, congenital disorder. Findings include optic nerve hypoplasia with a thin or absent septum pellucidum and/or corpus callosum and pituitary dysfunction. Optic nerve hypoplasia is mandatory for the diagnosis of SOD.

Description

SOD, also known as DeMorsier's syndrome, is a combination of optic nerve underdevelopment (hypoplasia) with abnormalities of a part of the brain called the septum pellucidum and/or corpus callosum. Endocrine disorders such as dwarfism, decreased thyroid gland function (hypothyroidism), dehydration, delayed or precocious puberty, and reduced blood sugar may occur from dysfunction of the pituitary gland of the brain. SOD has also been associated with congenital architectural brain anomalies.

Demographics

There is no sex predilection in patients with SOD.

Causes and symptoms

The cause of SOD is thought to be related to intrauterine viral infections or diabetes during pregnancy. Antiseizure medications, alcohol, and illicit drugs have also been linked to SOD. In addition, vascular abnormalities and, less commonly, genetics are thought to play a role.

Patients afflicted with SOD can present at any age depending on the severity of the symptoms. Signs and symptoms such as failure to thrive, prolonged jaundice, body temperature dysregulation, decreased blood sugar, small genitalia, or muscular flaccidity can herald the diagnosis of SOD in newborns.

Older children may complain of visual difficulties and be found to have strabismus (crossed eyes), nystagmus (involuntary, jerky eye movements), or inability to fixate on an object. In addition pupillary and color vision abnormalities may be noted. The optic nerves will appear small and grey or pale in color and can be surrounded by a yellowed halo signifying hypoplasia or atrophy.

A large percentage of SOD patients will have endocrine disorders. By far growth hormone deficiencies are the most common in patients with optic nerve hypoplasia. Growth hormone deficiency can lead to reduced blood sugar, while abnormal levels of reproductive hormones can result in unusual pubertal development. Reduced levels of thyroid-stimulating hormone will cause suboptimal thyroid gland functioning (hypothyroidism). Other endocrine problems include increased urination, dehydration, and death.

In some instances patients will have behavioral and cognitive problems resulting from brain maldevelopment or endocrinologic disorders.

Diagnosis

Suspicion for the diagnosis of SOD is based on clinical findings described above. In addition magnetic resonance imaging (MRI) of the brain focusing on the visual pathways, hypothalamus-pituitary region and other midline structures, and septum pellucidum is invaluable for solidifying the diagnosis.

Treatment team

Pediatricians, endocrinologists, optometrists, ophthalmologists, neuro-ophthalmologists, and neurologists can all contribute to patient care.

Treatment

SOD is treated symptomatically. Hormone deficiencies are managed with hormone replacement therapy, while the best possible visual acuity is achieved with corrective spectacle lenses.

Recovery and rehabilitation

Patients with extremely poor vision may benefit from a low vision specialist who may be able to

KEY TERMS

Corpus callosum—The largest commissure connecting the right and left hemispheres of the brain.

Septum pellucidum—Two-layered thin wall separating the right and the left anterior horn of lateral ventricle.

prescribe a visual apparatus to maximally improve visual function.

Clinical trials

Information about current relevant clinical trials can be found at ClinicalTrials.gov.

Special concerns

Patients with severe visual depression may have difficulty obtaining a driver's license or gainful employment.

Resources

BOOKS

Liu, Grant T., Nicholas J. Volpe, and Steven L. Galetta. *Neuro-Ophthalmology Diagnosis and Management*, 1st ed. Philadelphia: W. B. Saunders, 2001.

PERIODICALS

Campbell, Carrie. "Septo-optic dysplasia: a literature review." *Optometry* 72, no. 7 (July 2003): 417–26.

ORGANIZATIONS

National Eye Institute. Bldg. 31, Rm. 6A32, Bethesda, MD 20892-2510. Phone: 301-496-5248. Email: 2020@b31.nei.nih.gov. http://www.nei.nih.gov.

National Organization for Rare Disorders. PO Box 1968, Danbury, CT 06813-1968. Phone: 202-744-1000. Fax: 203-798-2291. Tollfree phone: 800-999-NORD. Email: orphan@rarediseases.org. http://www.rarediseases.org.

Adam J. Cohen, MD

Shaken baby syndrome

Definition

Shaken baby syndrome is a severe form of head injury caused by the forcible shaking of a child. The force is sufficient to cause the brain to bounce against the baby's skull, causing injury or damage to the brain.

Description

Shaking an infant forcibly transfers a great deal of energy to the infant. When the shaking occurs as the infant is being held, much of the force is transferred to the neck and head. The force can be so great that the brain can move within the skull, rebounding from one side of the skull to the other. The bashing can be very destructive to the brain, causing bruising, swelling, or bleeding. Bleeding of the brain is also called intracerebral hemorrhage. The force of shaking can also damage the neck.

As its name implies, shaken baby syndrome is often the result of deliberate abuse. The brain damage can also be the result of an accident. The force and length of the force necessary to cause shaken baby syndrome is debatable. What is clear is that not much time is needed, since most shaking events likely tend to last only 20 seconds or less. It is the explosive violence of the shaking that exacts the damage.

Demographics

Reliable statistics on the prevalence of shaken baby syndrome do not exist. Estimates in the United States approach 50,000 cases each year. Nearly 25% of infants with shaken baby syndrome die from the brain injuries sustained. The victims of this syndrome range in age from just a few days to five years, with an average age of 6–8 months. Statistics point to men as the usual perpetrators, typically young men (i.e., early 20s). Females who shake babies tend to be caregivers. As reliable statistics emerge, it would not be unexpected to find the actual number of cases greatly exceeds these estimates. Abuse of children is a hidden event, so many cases of abuse, including shaken baby syndrome, are not reported or are presented in some other form (such as a fall or an accident).

Causes and symptoms

The cause of the brain, neck, and spine damage that can result from shaken baby syndrome is brute force. The violent shaking of a baby by a much stronger adult conveys a tremendous amount of energy to the infant. Partly the damage is explained by the fact that an infant's head is much larger than the rest of the body, in relation to an older child or an adult. This, combined with neck muscles that are still developing and are incapable of adequately supporting the head, can make shaking an explosively destructive event. The amount of brain damage depends on how hard the shaking is and how long an infant is shaken. If accidental, the force and length of the head trauma similarly determines the extent of injury.

The damage to the brain can have dire consequences that include permanent and severe brain damage or death. Other symptoms that can develop include behavioral changes, lack of energy or motivation, irritable behavior, loss of consciousness, paling of the skin color or development of a bluish tinge to the skin, vomiting, and convulsions. These symptoms are the result of the destruction of brain cells that occurs directly due to the trauma of the blow against the skull and secondarily as a result of oxygen deprivation and swelling of the brain. The banging of the brain against the sides of the skull causes inflammation and swelling as well as internal bleeding. Increased intracranial pressure can be damaging to the structure and function of the brain.

Additionally, because the neck and head can absorb a tremendous amount of energy due to the shaking force of the adult, bones in the neck and spine can be broken and muscles can be torn or pulled. The eyes can also be damaged by the explosive energy of shaking. Retinal damage occur in 50–80% of cases. The damage can be so severe as to permanently blind an infant.

Shaken baby syndrome is also known as abusive head trauma, shaken brain trauma, pediatric **traumatic brain injury**, **whiplash** shaken infant syndrome, and shaken impact syndrome.

Diagnosis

Diagnosis depends on the detection of a blood clot below the inner layer of the dura (a membrane that surrounds the brain) but external to the brain. The clot is also known as a **subdural hematoma**. Two other critical features of shaken baby syndrome used in diagnosis are brain swelling and hemorrhaging in the eyes.

An infant may also have external bruising on parts of the body that were used to grip him or her during shaking. Bone or rib fractures can also be apparent. However, these external features may not always be present. Diagnosis can also involve the nondestructive imaging of the brain using the techniques of computed tomography (CT), skull x ray, or **magnetic resonance imaging** (MRI). Typically, these procedures are done after an infant has been stabilized and survival is assured.

KEY TERMS

Increased intracranial pressure—Increased overall pressure inside the skull.

Subdural hematoma—A collection of blood or a clot trapped under the dura matter, the outermost membrane surrounding the brain and spinal cord, often causing neurological damage due to pressure on the brain.

Treatment team

Treatment in an emergency setting typically involves nurses and emergency room physicians. A neurosurgeon is usually consulted when shaken baby syndrome is suspected. Depending on the extent of injury, neurosurgeons can become involved if surgery for brain repair is needed.

Police officers and **social workers** also become involved in cases of shaken baby syndrome, who work to ensure that the child is placed in a safe environment.

Treatment

Initially, treatment is provided on an emergency basis. Life-saving measures can include stopping internal bleeding in the brain and relieving pressure that can build up in the brain because of bleeding and swelling of the brain.

Recovery and rehabilitation

If the infant survives the initial injury from shaken baby syndrome, rehabilitation focuses on recovering as much function as possible. Physical and occupational therapies can offer exercises for caregivers to provide the child, as well as any supportive or positional devices required. The full effects of the brain injury sustained in infants who survive shaken baby syndrome may not become apparent until delays in developmental milestones such as sitting alone, walking, or acquiring speech are noticed.

Clinical trials

No clinical trials on shaken baby syndrome are underway in the United States. However, agencies such as the National Institute of Neurological Disorders and Stroke fund studies that seek to better understand the basis of the damage. Other agencies attempt to lessen the occurrence of the syndrome through counseling, anger management, and interventions in abusive situations.

Prognosis

The prognosis for children with shaken baby syndrome is usually poor. Twenty percent of cases result in death within the first few days. If infants survive, they are most often left with intellectual and developmental disabilities such as **mental retardation** or **cerebral palsy**. Damage to the eyes can cause partial or total loss of vision. Survivors are likely to require specialized care for the remainder of their lives.

Resources

BOOKS

Lazoritz, Stephen, and Vincent J. Palusci, eds. *Shaken Baby Syndrome: A Multidisciplinary Approach.* Binghamton, NY: Haworth Press, 2002.

PERIODICALS

Geddes, J. F., and J. Plunkett. "The Evidence Base for Shaken Baby Syndrome." *British Medical Journal* (March 2004): 719–20.

Harding, B., R. A. Risdon, and H. F. Krous. "Shaken Baby Syndrome." *British Medical Journal* (March 2004): 720–21.

OTHER

"NINDS Shaken Baby Syndrome Information Page." *National Institute of Neurological Disorders and Stroke.* May 13, 2004 (May 27, 2004). http://www.ninds.nih. gov/health_and_medical/disorders/shakenbaby.htm.

ORGANIZATIONS

The Arc of the United States. 1010 Wayne Avenue, Suite 650, Silver Spring, MD 20910. Phone: (301) 565-3842. Fax: (301) 565-3843. Email: info@thearc.org. http://www.thearc.org.

National Center on Shaken Baby Syndrome. 2955 Harrison Blvd., #102, Ogden, UT 84403. Phone: (801) 627-3399. Fax: (801) 627-3321. Tollfree phone: (888) 273-0071. Email: dontshake@mindspring.com. http://www.dontshake.com.

National Institute of Child Health and Human Development. 31 Center Drive, Rm. 2A32 MSC 2425, Bethesda, MD 20892-2425. Phone: (301) 496-5133. Fax: (301) 496-7101. http://www.nichd.nih.gov.

Think First Foundation [National Injury Prevention Program]. 5550 Meadowbrook Drive, Suite110, Rolling Meadows, IL 60008. Phone: (847) 290-8600. Fax: (847) 290-9005. Tollfree phone: (800) 844-6556. Email: thinkfirst@thinkfirst.org. http://www.thinkfirst.org.

Brian Douglas Hoyle, PhD

Shingles

Definition

Shingles, or herpes zoster, is a condition caused by the reactivation of the varicella zoster virus (VZV) that causes chickenpox (varicella). After a bout of chickenpox, the virus remains dormant in the sensory nerve ganglia that are adjacent to the spinal cord and brain. Years later the virus reemerges, traveling along the nerves to the skin where it causes red rashes that develop into blisters. In the process the virus can damage nerves, leading to a very painful inflammation called post-herpetic neuralgia (PHN), which can persist long after the rash disappears.

Demographics

Anyone who has had chickenpox or been vaccinated against varicella can develop shingles. Virtually all American adults have had chickenpox, even if the disease was so mild as to pass unnoticed. Nearly one in three Americans eventually develops shingles and there are at least one million cases in the United States each year.

Although shingles can occur at any age, even in children, the incidence increases steadily with age. About half of all cases occur in people aged 60 or older. About 20% of people with shingles develop PHN. It is more common in women than in men. In the United States between 120,000 and 200,000 people suffer from PHN each year. It occurs more frequently among the elderly and is one of the most

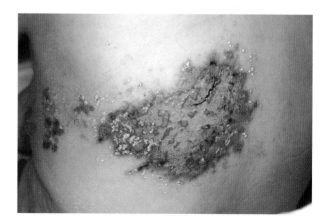

Following primary infection of the varicella-zoster virus (VZV), shingles develops as an infection of the dorsal root ganglia of the spine, which migrates through the sensory nerves to the skin. This leads to fluid-filled vesicles or bumps that erupt on the skin. *(© Dr. M.A, Ansary/Photo Researchers, Inc.)*

common causes of pain-related suicide in older adults. The incidence of PHN increases with age and tends to last longer in older patients:

• PHN is rare in those under age 30.

• By age 40 the risk of PHN lasting longer than one month is 33%.

• By age 70 the risk increases to 74%.

Some scientists believe that the incidence of shingles is likely to increase over the next 40–50 years, due to the introduction of a childhood vaccine against chickenpox in 1995. With far fewer children contracting chickenpox, adults have far less exposure to the virus, which would otherwise boost the immunity they acquired during childhood and help prevent reactivation of latent virus in their bodies.

Description

Varicella zoster virus is a member of the herpesvirus family. It causes chickenpox or varicella, which is highly contagious and spreads through the air. Following this initial or primary VZV infection, which usually occurs in childhood, the virus remains in an inactive or latent state in nerve tissue. Years later—usually after age 50—VZV can be reactivated to cause herpes zoster or shingles. The name "varicella" is derived from "variola," the Latin name for smallpox, a now-eradicated deadly disease, which can resemble chickenpox. "Zoster" is the Greek word for girdle and "shingles" derives from "cingulum," the Latin word for belt or girdle, which refer to the shingles lesions or blisters that form on one side of the waist. Scientists suspected as early as 1909 that chickenpox and shingles were caused by the same virus. This was confirmed in 1958.

Shingles is an infection of the **central nervous system**, particularly the dorsal root ganglia of the spine. From there the virus migrates through sensory nerve fibers to the skin, usually on the trunk, where it causes painful, fluid-filled eruptions or vesicles. Because the sensory nerves serve sharply bounded, non-overlapping areas of the skin called dermatomes, the shingles lesions appear within these dermatomes and do not cross the midline of the body.

Unlike chickenpox, shingles is not contagious because the virus is not usually in the lungs from which it could spread through the air. However, the fluid-filled eruptions on the skin contain large amounts of virus, which can be transmitted through direct contact and infect a person, usually a child, who has not previously been exposed to VZV. The infected person will develop a case of primary chickenpox. A vaccine that prevents or ameliorates the symptoms of shingles became available in 2006. Immunization against chickenpox does not prevent shingles, although it may reduce its incidence.

Risk factors

Anyone who has ever had chickenpox or been vaccinated against it is at risk for shingles. Overall approximately 20% of those who had chickenpox as children eventually develop shingles. Susceptibility to shingles appears to be genetically determined and the condition runs in families. The risk of shingles increases with age and with any condition that weakens the immune system. Those at particular risk for shingles include:

• children who had chickenpox in infancy or whose mothers had chickenpox late in pregnancy

• bone marrow and other transplant recipients

• those with compromised immune systems from diseases such as HIV/AIDS

• those with suppressed immune systems from chemotherapy drugs or other medications

Causes and symptoms

It is not clear why VZV reactivates to cause shingles, but it appears to be related to a decreased immune response due to advancing age, emotional or physical stress, **fatigue**, certain medications, chemotherapy, or diseases such as cancer or HIV/AIDS. Shingles is sometimes an early sign of immunodeficiency in people infected with HIV. In some cases the virus appears to be reactivated by mechanical irritation or minor surgical procedures.

Mild cases of shingles often go unnoticed. The earliest signs may be vague and can easily be mistaken for other illnesses. The condition may begin with fever, chills, gastrointestinal discomfort, and malaise (a vague feeling of **weakness** or discomfort). Lymph nodes may swell. Within two to four days localized areas of intense pain, itching, and numbness/tingling (paresthesia) or extreme sensitivity to touch (hyperesthesia) can develop, usually on the trunk. The second most common place is on one side of the face around the eye (ophthalmic shingles) or on the forehead. However, shingles can occur on the arms, legs, or elsewhere on the body. The pain may be continuous or intermittent, usually lasting from one to four weeks. The pain may accompany skin eruptions or precede the eruptions by days.

KEY TERMS

Acyclovir—An antiviral drug that is available in oral, intravenous, and topical forms and that blocks replication of the varicella zoster virus.

Antibody—A specific protein produced by the immune system in response to a specific foreign protein or particle called an antigen.

Capsaicin—An active ingredient from hot chili peppers that is used in topical ointments to relieve pain. It appears to work by reducing the levels of a chemical substance involved in transmitting pain signals from nerve endings to the brain.

Corticosteroids—A group of hormones produced by the adrenal glands or manufactured synthetically. They are often used to treat inflammation. Examples include cortisone and prednisone.

Famciclovir—An oral antiviral drug that blocks the replication of the varicella zoster virus.

Ganglion—A mass of nerve tissue outside of the central nervous system.

Immunocompromised—A weakened or poorly functioning immune system due to disease.

Immunosuppressed—Suppression of the immune system by medications during the treatment of diseases such as cancer or following an organ transplantation.

Post-herpetic neuralgia (PHN)—Long-lasting nerve pain caused by herpes zoster.

Tzanck preparation—A procedure in which skin cells from a blister are stained and examined under the microscope.

Valacyclovir—An oral antiviral drug that blocks the replication of the varicella zoster virus.

Vesicle—A small, raised lesion filled with clear fluid.

The red rash or oozing blisters appear along the course of the affected nerve. There is usually a vague streak or band from the spine along the path of the nerve on one side of the body. About five days after they appear, the vesicles begin to crust or scab and the disease resolves within the next 2–3 weeks. There may be no visible aftereffects or a slight scarring from the vesicles.

Shingles can be more debilitating in the elderly or those in poor health. The eruptions may be more extensive and inflammatory and may include bleeding blisters, areas of skin death, secondary bacterial infection, or extensive and permanent scarring. Ophthalmic shingles can cause painful eye infections and vision loss. Shingles infections within or near the ear can cause hearing or balance problems. Sometimes shingles can cause temporary or permanent tremors or paralysis. Rarely shingles can spread to the brain or spinal cord and cause stroke or **meningitis**.

Shingles pain usually subsides when the rash disappears, but it may last much longer, especially in the elderly. PHN can persist for months or years. It is caused by damage to the dorsal root ganglia, with the nerves becoming either spontaneously active—which is perceived as chronic pain—or hypersensitive to slight stimuli such as light touch. In the most severe cases, PHN can cause insomnia, weight loss, **depression**, and disability.

Diagnosis

Examination

Diagnosis of shingles is based on a medical history and physical examination. A definite diagnosis is difficult before eruption of the characteristic vesicles or bumps on the skin. The vesicles have a clear dermatome-bounded distribution, usually on the midsection of the body.

Tests

Tests for shingles are rarely necessary but may include:

- polymerase chain reaction (PCR) testing for viral DNA

- viral culture of skin lesions

- a Tzanck preparation—stained cells from a blister, which will appear under the microscope to have many very large dark nuclei if infected with VZV

- a complete blood count (CBC) to test for elevated white blood cells that are indicative of infection

- blood serum levels of antibodies against VZV

Treatment

Traditional

Shingles almost always resolves spontaneously within a few weeks. Unless complicated by conditions such as HIV/AIDS or cancer, a primary care physician can provide treatment for easing painful symptoms. Rarely, transcutaneous electrical nerve stimulation (TENS) or a permanent nerve block is used to relieve the pain of PHN.

Drugs

The **antiviral drugs** acyclovir, valacyclovir, and famciclovir are used to treat shingles. These drugs can shorten the course of the illness. If started within 72 hours of the onset of the rash, antiviral therapy can heal the blisters more rapidly and sometimes even halt the disease. If taken after the disease has progressed, these drugs are less effective but may still lessen the pain. Antiviral drug treatment reduces the incidence of PHN by about one half and may also shorten its duration. Severely immunocompromised individuals, such as those with HIV/AIDS, may require intravenous administration of antiviral drugs or taking the drugs on an ongoing basis.

Various other drugs may be prescribed for shingles and PHN:

- corticosteroids, such as prednisone, to reduce inflammation from shingles, especially if the eye or other facial nerves are involved, and to reduce severe pain
- anticonvulsants such as pregabalin (Lyrica) or gabapentin to relieve pain
- the tricylcic antidepressants (TCAs) desipramine and nortriptyline
- opioid painkillers such as oxycodone, morphine, tramadol, or methadone
- tranquilizers or sedatives
- topical local anesthetics for application to the painful skin area and for post-herpetic itch; especially lidocaine, available as a cream, gel, spray, or patch
- capsaicin cream, which is available without a prescription, but which usually causes burning pain during application

Alternative

Alternative remedies and therapies will not cure shingles, but they may relieve pain, reduce inflammation, and speed recovery:

- The amino acid lysine has also been reported to ease the symptoms of shingles and other herpes infections. Foods that are high in lysine include soybeans, black bean sprouts, lentils, parsley, and peas.
- Vitamin B12 supplementation during the first two days of the illness and ongoing vitamin B complex, vitamin C with bioflavonoids, and calcium supplements may boost the immune system.
- Echinacea can boost the immune system and help fight viral infections.
- Red pepper (capsicum or cayenne) is an ingredient in commercial ointments, including Zostrix and Capzasin-P. It should be applied only to healed blisters and

is useful for treating painful PHN. Seasoning food with red pepper may also provide relief.
- Calendula or licorice (*Glycyrrhiza glabra*) ointment or lotion may help treat shingles.
- Topical applications of lemon balm (*Melissa officinalis*), licorice, or peppermint (*Mentha piperita*) may reduce pain and blistering. These can also be consumed as teas.
- Sedative herbs such as passionflower can be brewed for a tea to treat PHN.
- Vervain helps relieve pain and inflammation.
- St. John's wort, lavender, chamomile, and marjoram help relieve inflammation.
- Homeopathic remedies include *Rhus toxicodendron* for blisters, *Mezereum* and *Arsenicum album* for pain, and *Ranunculus* for itching.
- Several drops of "Rescue Remedy" placed under the tongue or taken in water throughout the day are prescribed for relieving stress.
- Ayurvedic treatments for shingles include the application of turmeric paste.
- Acupuncture and acupressure can alleviate pain and PHN.
- Biofeedback or spinal cord stimulators may help relieve PHN.
- Relaxation techniques such as hypnotherapy and yoga may help relieve pain.
- Reflexology may help balance the body.

Practitioners of traditional Chinese medicine (TCM) may recommend herbal remedies:

- Chinese gentian root is used to treat the liver.
- Skullcap root in water is a Chinese folk remedy for shingles.
- Long Dan Xie Gan Tang is used to quell the accumulation of damp, toxic heat in the liver.
- For damp, infected, painful eruptions on the torso, Huang Qin Gao can be applied to the surrounding area.

Home remedies

Home remedies for shingles include plenty of rest, a healthy diet, regular exercise, and minimizing stress. The skin should be kept clean and contaminated items should not be reused. Cool, wet compresses may help reduce pain from blisters. Blisters or crusting can be treated with compresses made with one-quarter cup (60 ml) of white vinegar in two quarts (1.9 l) of lukewarm water and applied twice daily for 10 minutes. The compresses should be discontinued when the blisters have dried up. Soothing baths and lotions with

QUESTIONS TO ASK YOUR DOCTOR

- Why do you think I have shingles?
- Will you perform diagnostic tests?
- Will you prescribe an antiviral drug? Which one?
- How long will the shingles last?
- Am I likely to suffer from post-herpetic neuralgia?
- Can I get shingles again?

colloidal oatmeal, starch, or calamine may help to relieve itching and discomfort. If the skin become dry, tight, and cracked as the crusts and scabs separate, a small amount of plain petroleum jelly can be applied three or four times daily. The pain of PHN may be relieved with hot and cold compresses.

Prognosis

Shingles is almost never life-threatening in otherwise healthy patients and usually resolves without treatment in a few weeks. Because shingles boosts the immune response to VZV, repeat episodes are rare, occurring in less than 4% of patients. Although PHN usually diminishes over time, it can be disabling and difficult to treat.

Shingles can be much more severe in immunocompromised patients. The condition can last for months, recur frequently, and spread to the lungs, liver, gastrointestinal tract, brain, or other vital organs. Complications of shingles in immunocompromised or immunosuppressed patients may resemble those of primary varicella infection in adults, including viral pneumonia, male sterility, acute liver failure, and birth defects in children born to infected mothers. Depletion of CD4+ T lymphocytes in HIV/AIDS patients is associated with severe and chronic or recurrent VZV infection.

Prevention

A lifestyle that promotes immune system function and overall health may help prevent shingles. Factors include a well-balanced diet rich in essential vitamins and minerals, adequate sleep, regular exercise, and reduced stress. Patients with shingles should avoid contact with anyone who has not had chickenpox or been vaccinated against the disease, particularly pregnant women, newborns, and those with weakened immune systems.

In the United States it is now recommended that all children between 18 months and adolescence be immunized against chickenpox. Because a weakened (attenuated) form of the virus is used in this vaccine, it is thought that vaccination will reduce the likelihood of shingles later on in life. A single-dose vaccine against shingles (Zostavax) became available in 2006 and is recommended for most people aged 60 and older who have previously had chickenpox. It appears to prevent shingles in about 50% of vaccinated people and reduces the pain associated with shingles in others. It also can help prevent post-herpetic neuralgia.

Resources

BOOKS

Kirschmann, John D. *Nutrition Almanac,* 6th ed. New York: McGraw-Hill, 2007.

Shannon, Joyce Brennfleck. *Pain Sourcebook,* 3rd ed. Detroit: Omnigraphics, 2008.

Siegel, Mary-Ellen, and Gray Williams. *Shingles: New Hope for an Old Disease,* updated ed. Lanham, MD: M. Evans, 2008.

PERIODICALS

Froelich, Janis D. "How Did a Gal Like Me Come Down with Shingles?" *Tampa Tribune* (June 21, 2008): 16.

Gutpa, Sanjay. "Rash Redux." *Time* 172, no. 4 (July 28, 2008): 53.

OTHER

"Herpes Zoster." *American Academy of Dermatology.*http://www.aad.org/public/publications/pamphlets/viral_herpes_zoster.htm

Office of Communications and Public Liaison, National Institute of Neurological Disorders and Stroke. "Shingles: Hope Through Research." *NIH Publication No. 06-307.*http://www.ninds.nih.gov/disorders/shingles/detail_shingles.htm

"Shingles." *National Institute of Allergy and Infectious Diseases.*http://www3.niaid.nih.gov/topics/shingles/

"Shingles & After-Shingles Pain." *AfterShingles.com.*http://www.aftershingles.com/after-shingles-pain.aspx

"Shingles (Herpes Zoster) Vaccination." *Vaccines & Immunizations.*http://www.cdc.gov/vaccines/vpd-vac/shingles/default.htm

ORGANIZATIONS

American Academy of Dermatology, PO Box 4014, Schaumburg, IL 60168, (847) 240-1280, (866) 503-SKIN (7546), Fax: (847) 240-1859, http://www.aad.org.

American Botanical Council, 6200 Manor Rd., Austin, TX 78723, (512) 926-4900, Fax: (512) 926-2345, abc@herbalgram.org, http://cms.herbalgram.org.

National Institute of Allergy and Infectious Diseases (NIAID), Office of Communications and Public Liaison, 6610 Rockledge Drive, Bethesda, MD 20892-66123, (866) 284-4107, http://www3.niaid.nih.gov.

National Institute of Neurological Disorders and Stroke (NINDS), NIH Neurological Institute, PO Box 5801,

Bethesda, MD 20824, (301) 496-5751, (800) 352-9424, http://www.ninds.nih.gov.

National Shingles Foundation, 590 Madison Ave., 21st Floor, New York, NY 10022, (212) 222-3390, Fax: (212) 222-8627, http://www.vzvfoundation.org.

U.S. Centers for Disease Control and Prevention (CDC), 1600 Clifton Road, Atlanta, GA 30333, 800-CDC-INFO (232-4636), cdcinfo@cdc.gov, http://www.cdc.gov.

Rebecca J. Frey, PhD
Larry Gilman, PhD
Margaret Alic, PhD

Shy-Drager syndrome *see* **Multiple system atrophy**

Single proton emission computed tomography

Definition

Single proton (or photon) emission computed tomography (SPECT) allows a physician to see three-dimensional images of a person's particular organ or body system. SPECT detects the course of a radioactive substance that is injected, ingested, or inhaled. In neurology, a SPECT scan is often used to visualize the brain's cerebral blood flow and thereby indicate metabolic activity patterns in the brain.

Purpose

SPECT can locate the site of origin of a seizure, can confirm the type of seizure that has occurred, and can provide information that is useful in the determination of therapy. Other uses for SPECT include locating tumors, monitoring the metabolism of oxygen and glucose, and determining the concentration of neurologically relevant compounds such as dopamine.

Research in the United States has focused on brain receptors for the neurotransmitter acetylcholine. The aim of this study was to determine the usefulness of the technique in charting the progress of the brain deterioration associated with **Parkinson's disease**.

Precautions

The exposure to radiation, particularly to the thyroid gland, is minimized as described below in the sections on preparation and aftercare.

Description

Since its development in the 1970s, single proton emission computed tomography has become a critical and routine facet of a clinician's diagnostic routine. A SPECT scan is now a typical part of the diagnosis of coronary artery disease, cancer, stroke, liver disease, bone and spinal abnormalities, and lung maladies.

SPECT produces two-dimensional and three-dimensional images of a target region in the body by detecting the presence and location of a radioactive compound given prior to the test. The photon emissions of the radioactive compound can be detected in a manner that is similar to the detection of x rays in computed tomography (CT). The image produced is a compilation of data collected over time following introduction of the tracer.

The radioactive compound that is introduced typically loses its radioactive potency rapidly (this is expressed as the half-life of a compound). For example, gamma-emitting compounds can have a half-life of just a few hours. This is beneficial for the patients, as it limits the contact time with the potentially damaging radioisotope.

The emitted radiation is collected by a gamma-camera through thousands of round or hexagonal channels that are arranged in parallel in a part of the machine called the collimator. Only gamma rays can pass through the channels. At the other end of the channel, the radiation contacts a crystal of sodium iodide. The interaction produces a photon of light (hence, the name of the technique). The light is subsequently detected and the time and body location of the light-producing radiation is stored computationally. At the end of the SPECT scan, the stored information can be integrated to produce a composite image.

Typically, a patient is stationary. The SPECT scanner can move completely around the patient. Usually patients lie on a bed with their head restrained in a holder. Scans are taken for periods up to six hours following the injection of the tracer.

Monitoring of the heartbeat (electrocardiogram), respiration, and blood pressure are accomplished just prior to the start of the scan, five minutes after the introduction of the tracer, and 30–60 minutes after injection. Blood and urine samples are often collected towards the end of the scan.

Preparation

On the night before a scan, patients take an oral dose of potassium iodide. This protects the thyroid gland from the radioactive tracer. If a patient is allergic to potassium iodide, potassium perchlorate can be taken instead. Just prior to a scan, small radioisotope markers that contain the element 99Tc are attached with adhesive to the patient's head. Two intravenous catheters are usually placed in veins, through which the radioactive tracer is injected, and so that blood samples can be withdrawn during the scan.

Aftercare

Oral doses of potassium iodide or potassium perchlorate are taken daily for four days following a scan. Patients are asked to urinate every two hours for the first 12 hours following the scan to eliminate the tracer from their body as quickly as possible.

Risks

The use of radiation poses a risk of cellular or tissue damage. However, the injection of the radioactive tracer results in the swift movement of the tracer through the body and its rapid elimination.

Normal results

The image of the target region of the body is compared to an image of the healthy target region. Analysis of the images by a qualified physician determines the result.

Resources

BOOKS

Brant, Thomas. *Neurological Disorders: Course and Treatment*, 2nd. ed. Philadelphia: Academic Press, 2002.

OTHER

"Psychopharmacology–The Fourth Generation of Progress." *Positron and Single Photon Emission Tomography. Principles and Applications in Psychopharmacology*. American College of Neuropsychopharmacology. http://www.acnp.org/g4/GN401000088/CH087.html (January 27 2004).

Brian Douglas Hoyle, PhD

Sixth nerve palsy

Definition

Cranial nerve six supplies the lateral rectus muscle allowing for outward (abduction) eye movement. A sixth nerve palsy, also known as abducens nerve palsy, is a neurological defect resulting from an impaired sixth nerve or the nucleus that controls it. This may result in horizontal double vision (diplopia) with in turning of the eye and decreased lateral movement.

Description

Isolated sixth nerve palsies usually manifest as a horizontal diplopia worse when looking toward the affected eye, with a decreased ability to abduct. Since the sixth nerve only innervates the lateral rectus muscle, isolated palsies will only manifest in this fashion.

Demographics

Sixth nerve palsies have no predilection for males or females and can occur at any age.

Causes and symptoms

For all intensive purposes causes of abducens nerve palsy can be classified as congenital or acquired. Isolated congenital sixth nerve palsy is quite uncommon. If congenital the usual presentation is accompanied by other cranial nerve deficits as seen with Duane's retraction or Mobius syndromes. Strabismus, commonly known as "lazy eye," may mimic the appearance of abducens nerve palsy and may go undetected until adulthood because of compensatory mechanisms allowing for alignment of the eyes when focusing. Abduction deficits may also result from **myasthenia gravis**, thyroid eye disease, inflammation and orbital fractures which imitate sixth nerve palsies.

A myriad of causes resulting in abducens nerve palsies have been reported. In order to better differentiate these one must take into account the patient's age and underlying illnesses. In children, trauma and tumors were reported as the most common causes. Therefore, if no trauma has occurred one must consider a tumor of the **central nervous system** in the pediatric population. Other causes include idiopathic intracranial hypertension, inflammation following viral illness or immunization, **multiple sclerosis**, fulminant ear infections, Arnold-Chiari malformations, and **meningitis**.

New onset palsies in adults can stem from myasthenia gravis, diabetes, meningitis, microvascular disease (atherosclerotic vascular disease) or giant cell arteritis (arterial inflammation. Other causes include **Lyme disease**, syphilis, cancers, autoimmune disorders, central nervous system tumors, and vitamin deficiencies.

Children may be found to have head tilt or in turning of the affected eye, with reduction of outward gaze. They will very rarely complain of double vision while adults may describe two images, side by side (horizontal diplopia), which are furthest apart when looking towards the affected eye. Covering of one eye, no matter which one is covered, and gazing away from the affected eye will resolve their diplopia. Patients may also note muscle **weakness** possibly heralding myasthenia gravis or headache and jaw pain raising the possibility of giant cell arteritis.

Optic nerve swelling or jumpy eye movements (nystagmus) may occur at any age and warrants immediate work-up for a central nervous system tumor.

Diagnosis

Diagnosis of sixth nerve palsy is based on history and clinical findings. Once the diagnosis has been established the work-up should be tailored based on the patient's age and medical history.

Pediatric patients with no apparent trauma should undergo magnetic resonance imaging of the brain with contrast enhancement to rule out a central nervous system structural lesion (tumor or aneurysm). If the imaging is without abnormal findings a **lumbar puncture** (spinal tap) should be done to exclude increased intracranial pressure or infection. If this is normal, consideration of a post-viral or post-immunization palsy may be safely entertained.

Isolated abducens palsies in the adult population should be approached in a more conservative manner. If a patient is known to have diabetes, high blood pressure, or atherosclerotic vascular disease, a small stroke is likely. If diplopia worsens or no improvement occurs at eight weeks time, a more extensive work-up, including **magnetic resonance imaging** of the brain with contrast and blood work to exclude infections, autoimmune disorders, vitamin deficiencies, or inflammation, is warranted. A potentially devastating, blinding disorder known as cranial arteritis may occur in patients usually over 50 years of age. Headache, jaw pain worsened with chewing, night sweats, fevers, weight loss, or muscle aches necessitates blood work to rule out this inflammatory disorder.

Treatment team

Ophthalmologists, neuro-ophthalmologists, optometrists, neurologists, and pediatricians are medical specialists who can evaluate and diagnose a patient with a sixth nerve palsy. Usually an optometrist or ophthalmologist will initially see a patient complaining of diplopia or displaying findings of sixth nerve palsy. A referral will then likely be made to a neurologist or neuro-ophthalmologist for evaluation and work-up.

Treatment

Treatment of sixth nerve palsies is dictated by the underlying causes. Older patients who are thought to have had a mini-stroke are observed for several months because of likely spontaneous resolution. Causes related to masses of the central nervous system or systemic disease should be managed and treated promptly by the appropriate specialist.

Children who are at risk for amblyopia can be treated with patching to reduce the risk of permanent visual loss. Older patients may elect to use a prism incorporated into a spectacle to reduce or eliminate their double vision. Prisms or fogging of one eye are excellent options for the older patient being observed for spontaneous resolution of their palsy.

If diplopia persists for more than six months and prisms cannot realign the images surgical intervention is an option. Depending on the amount of lateral rectus muscle function one or two surgical options are used. If muscle function remains, weakening of the medial rectus muscle and tightening of the affected lateral rectus muscle may resolve the patient's complaint. If no function exists, then a muscle transposition surgery can help restore some abduction ability.

Botulinum toxin may also be used to weaken the medial rectus muscle of the affected eye. This weakening effect is short-lived and repeat injections are necessary.

Clinical trials

Information about current relevant clinical trials can be found at ClinicalTrials.gov.

Prognosis

Isolated abducens nerve palsies in the older population are usually related to a small stroke and resolve within a several months. Palsies related to trauma or brain masses have a guarded prognosis, and recovery, if any, may take up to one year. Treatment of systemic disorders, such as myasthenia gravis, have an excellent

KEY TERMS

Multiple sclerosis—A slowly progressive CNS disease characterized by disseminated patches of demyelination in the brain and spinal cord, resulting in multiple and varied neurologic symptoms and signs, usually with remissions and exacerbations.

Myasthenia gravis—A disease characterized by episodic muscle weakness caused by loss or dysfunction of acetylcholine receptors.

Strabismus—Deviation of one eye from parallelism with the other.

prognosis, while inflammation related to multiple sclerosis are likely to improve as well. Unfortunately there is no hard and fast rules regarding recovery of any sixth nerve palsy.

Special concerns

Patients afflicted with a sixth nerve palsy should refrain from driving unless an eye patch is used. In addition, certain types of employment may warrant a medical leave or temporary change of duties.

Resources

BOOKS

Beers, Mark H., and Robert Berkow, eds. *The Merck Manual of Diagnosis and Therapy.* Whitehouse Station, NJ: Merck Research Laboratories, 1999.

Burde, Ronald M., Peter J. Savino, and Jonathan D. Trobe. *Clinical Decisions in Neuro-Ophthalmology,* 3rd ed. St. Louis: Mosby, 2002.

Liu, Grant T., Nicholas J. Volpe, and Steven L. Galetta. *Neuro-Ophthalmology Diagnosis and Management,* 1st ed. Philadelphia: W. B. Saunders, 2001.

Adam J. Cohen, MD

Sjögren-Larsson syndrome

Definition

Sjögren-Larsson syndrome is an inherited disorder characterized by ichthyosis (scaly skin), speech abnormalities, **mental retardation**, and **spasticity** (a state of increased muscle tone with heightened reflexes). Severity is variable.

Description

Sjögren-Larsson syndrome is a rare genetic disorder inherited in an autosomal recessive fashion, which was characterized by Swedish psychiatrist Torsten Sjögren in 1956 and by Sjögren and Tage Larsson in 1957. Sjögren and Tage Larsson suggested that all Swedes with the syndrome are descended from one ancestor in whom a mutation (a genetic change) occurred about 600 years ago. The highest incidence of the disease occurs in northern Sweden.

In infancy, development of various degrees of scaling and reddened skin occurs, often accompanied by hyperkeratosis (thickening of the skin) on the outer skin layer. After infancy, skin on the arms, legs, and abdomen often is dark, scaly, and lacking redness. Seizures and speech abnormalities may accompany skin symptoms. About half of children affected with the syndrome experience degeneration of the pigment in the retina of the eye.

Sjögren-Larsson syndrome is also sometimes known as SLS; congenital ichthyosis-mental retardation-spasticity syndrome; ichthyosis-spastic neurologic disorder-oligophrenia syndrome; fatty aldehyde dehydrogenase deficiency (FALDH deficiency); fatty aldehyde dehydrogenase 10 deficiency (FALDH10 deficiency); or disorder of cornification 10 (Sjögren-Larsson Type). Sjögren-Larsson syndrome is not to be confused with Sjögren syndrome; it is sometimes called the T. Sjögren syndrome to distinguish it from Sjögren syndrome (characterized by dry eyes and mouth), which was described by Swedish ophthalmologist Henrick Sjögren.

Genetic profile

Inheritance of Sjögren-Larsson syndrome is autosomal recessive. In autosomal recessive inheritance, a single abnormal gene on one of the autosomal chromosomes (one of the first 22 "non-sex" chromosomes) from both parents can cause the disease. Both of the parents must be carriers in order for the child to inherit the disease since recessive genes are expressed only when both copies in the pair have the same recessive instruction. Neither of the parents has the disease (since it is recessive).

A child with both parents who carry the disease has a 25% chance having the disease; a 50% chance of being a carrier of the disease (but not affected by the disease, having both one normal gene and one gene with the mutation for the disorder); and a 25% chance of receiving both normal genes, one from each parent, and being genetically normal for that particular trait.

The gene for the Sjögren-Larsson syndrome, FALDH, is located on chromosome number 17 in band 17p11.2. The gene mutation that is responsible for the disorder is located near the center of the chromosome and is strongly associated the gene markers D17S805 and ALDH10.

Demographics

Sjögren-Larsson syndrome is a rare disorder. The highest incidence occurs in northern Sweden. The mutation responsible for the disease is present in approximately 1% of the population in northern Sweden. All Swedes with the syndrome are believed to be descendents of one ancestor in whom a genetic change occurred about 600 years ago. (The phenomenon wherein everyone is descended from one person within what was once a tiny group of people is called founder effect.) The disease also occurs in members of families of other European, Arabic, and Native American descent, but is less prevalent. Sjögren-Larsson syndrome affects both males and females.

Signs and symptoms

There are several signs and symptoms of Sjögren-Larsson syndrome. The major features of the disorder are the following:

• Skin: In infancy, development of various degrees of scaling and reddened skin occurs (ichthyosis), often accompanied by hyperkeratosis (thickening of the skin) on the outer skin layer. After infancy, skin on the arms, legs, and abdomen is often dark and scaly and lacking redness. Bruises are present at birth or soon after.

• Hair: Hair may be brittle.

• Extremities: Joint contracture and hypertonia cause resistance of joints to movement and of muscles to stretching. Most individuals with the syndrome never walk.

• Eyes: About half of the individuals with this syndrome have retinitis pigmentosa (pigmentary degeneration of the retina). Glistening white or yellow-white dots on the retina (ocular fundus) are characteristic. They may be an early sign of the disease, presenting at age 1–2 and may increase with age.

• Nervous system: Spastic diplegia or tetraplegia (paralysis) affecting arms and/or legs. About half of the individuals with this disorder have seizures.

• Urogenital system: Kidney diseases may be associated with this syndrome.

• Growth and development: Individuals with the disorder tend to be unusually short in stature. Mental retardation is characteristic. Speech disorders may be present.

Speech abnormalities, mental retardation, and seizures usually occur during the first two or three years of life.

Diagnosis

The clinical features of Sjögren-Larsson syndrome are often distinctive, and a pattern of anomalies may suggest the diagnosis. In addition to ichthyosis and spasticity at birth, glistening white or yellow-white dots on the retina may be an early sign of the disease, presenting in the first or second year of life. If they occur, speech abnormalities, mental retardation, and seizures are also present during the first two or three years of life.

Laboratory findings are important in diagnosing Sjögren-Larsson syndrome. A laboratory test for deficiency of an enzyme (a protein that catalyzes chemical reactions in the human body) called fatty aldehyde dehydrogenase 10 (FALDH10) will determine presence of the disease. Sjögren-Larsson is due to a deficiency of FALDH10, and the gene for the Sjögren-Larsson syndrome is the same as the FALDH10 gene.

Positive laboratory results for Sjögren-Larsson will include the following findings:

• Hexadeconal elevated in fibroblasts

• Fatty alcohol NAD+ deficient in Sjögren-Larsson syndrome fibroblasts

• Fatty aldehyde dehydrogenase (FALDH) deficiency

Genetic counseling

Individuals with a family history of Sjögren-Larsson syndrome may benefit from genetic counseling to learn about the condition, including treatments, inheritance, testing, and options available to them, so that they can make informed decisions appropriate to their families. A child with both parents who carry the Sjögren-Larsson gene mutation has a 25% chance having the disorder. Couples who have had one affected child have a 25% risk of having another child with the disorder in each pregnancy.

Prenatal testing

Families at risk for having a child with Sjögren-Larsson syndrome may have the option of prenatal diagnosis. DNA can be extracted from fetal cells obtained by either chorionic villus sampling (usually done until 12 weeks gestation) or amniocentesis (usually done at 16–18 weeks gestation) and tested to determine if the altered gene in the family is present. These techniques usually require that the alteration in

KEY TERMS

Contracture—A tightening of muscles that prevents normal movement of the associated limb or other body part.

Diplegia—Paralysis affecting like parts on both sides of the body, such as both arms or both legs.

Hypertonia—Excessive muscle tone or tension, causing resistance of muscle to being stretched.

Ichthyosis—Rough, dry, scaly skin that forms as a result of a defect in skin formation.

Retinitis pigmentosa—Progressive deterioration of the retina, often leading to vision loss and blindness.

Spasticity—Increased muscle tone, or stiffness, which leads to uncontrolled, awkward movements.

Tetraplegia—Paralysis of all four limbs. Also called quadriplegia.

the gene has been identified previously in an affected family member.

Chorionic villus sampling is a procedure to obtain chorionic villi tissue for testing. Chorionic villi are microscopic, finger-like projections that emerge from the chorionic membrane and eventually form the placenta. The cells of the chorionic villi are of fetal origin so laboratory analysis can identify a number of genetic abnormalities of the fetus. Because the villi are attached to the uterus, however, there is a chance that maternal tissue may be analyzed rather than the fetal cells. If the sample is too small, it may be necessary to repeat the procedure. In addition, the quality of the chromosome analysis is usually not as good with chorionic villus sampling as with amniocentesis. The chromosomes may not be as long, and so it may not be possible to identify some of the smaller bands on the chromosomes.

Amniocentesis is a procedure that involves inserting a thin needle into the uterus, into the amniotic sac, and withdrawing a small amount of amniotic fluid (a liquid produced by the fetal membranes and the fetus that surrounds the fetus throughout pregnancy). DNA can be extracted from the fetal cells contained in the amniotic fluid and tested for the specific mutation known to cause Sjögren-Larsson syndrome.

Treatment and management

Individuals with Sjögren-Larsson syndrome should be under routine health supervision by a physician who is familiar with the disorder, its complications, and its treatment. Supportive resources for individuals with

Sjögren-Larsson syndrome and their families should be provided. Some clinical improvement has been reported to occur with fat restriction in the diet and supplementation with medium-chain triglycerides.

Other treatment of the disorder is generally symptomatic.

• For dermatologic symptoms, various skin softening ointments are useful in reducing symptoms. Plain petroleum jelly may be effective, especially when applied while the skin is still moist, such as after bathing. Salicylic acid gel may also be effective. When using the ointment, skin is covered at night with an airtight, waterproof dressing. Lactate lotion is another effective treatment for the dermatologic symptoms.

• For ocular symptoms, regular care from a qualified ophthalmologist is important.

• To control seizures, anti-convulsant medications may be helpful.

• Speech therapy and special education services may be helpful.

Prognosis

Prognosis is variable depending upon the severity of the disease. Sjögren-Larsson does not generally lead to shortened life span.

Resources

BOOKS

Jorde, Lynn B., et al. *Medical Genetics*, 2nd ed. St. Louis: Mosby, 1999.

PERIODICALS

Willemsen, M.A., et al. "Sjögren-Larsson Syndrome." *Journal of Pediatrics* 136 (February 2000): 261.

ORGANIZATIONS

Arc (a National Organization on Mental Retardation). 1010 Wayne Ave., Suite 650, Silver Spring, MD 20910. (800) 433-5255. http://www.thearclink.org.

Foundation for Ichthyosis and Related Skin Types. 650 N. Cannon Ave., Suite 17, Landsdale, PA 19446. (215) 631-1411 or (800) 545-3286. Fax: (215) 631-1413. http://www.scalyskin.org.

National Institute of Arthritis and Musculoskeletal and Skin Diseases. National Institutes of Health, One AMS Circle, Bethesda, MD 20892. http://www.nih.gov/niams.

WEBSITES

Online Mendelian Inheritance in Man.http://www.ncbi.nlm. nih.gov:80/entrez/query.fcgi?db=OMIM.

Jennifer F. Wilson, MS

Sleep apnea

Definition

Sleep apnea is a condition in which breathing stops for more than ten seconds during sleep. Sleep apnea is a major, though often unrecognized, cause of daytime sleepiness. It can have serious negative effects on a person's quality of life and is thought to be considerably underdiagnosed in the United States, as it is a common disorder that can become more serious.

Demographics

Approximately 6–7% of the U.S. population, or 18 million Americans, are thought to have sleep apnea, but only 10 million have symptoms, and only 0.6 million have yet been diagnosed. In Americans aged 30–60 years, obstructive sleep apnea affects nearly one in four men and one in ten women; men are twice as likely as women to have sleep apnea. As sleep apnea seldom occurs in premenopausal females, it is suggested that hormones may play some role in the disorder.

Other predisposing factors include age, as nearly 20–60% of the elderly may be affected; overweight status or obesity; or use of alcohol or sedatives. Some studies have demonstrated that elderly African Americans are more than twice as likely as elderly whites to suffer from sleep apnea. Up to 50% of people with sleep apnea also suffer from high blood pressure. Losing as little as 10% of body weight can also reduce the number of times with sleep apnea that breathing stops during sleep. Some families appear to have increased incidence of sleep apnea. Children can also have sleep apnea, and it is often linked to attention deficit hyperactivity disorder (ADHD).

Description

A sleeping person normally breathes continuously and uninterruptedly throughout the night. Individuals with sleep apnea have frequent episodes (up to 400–500 per night) in which they stop breathing. This interruption of breathing is called apnea. Breathing stops for about 30 seconds, then the person usually startles awake with a loud snort and begins to breathe again, gradually falling back to slep.

There are two forms of sleep apnea. In obstructive sleep apnea (OSA), breathing stops because tissue in the throat closes off the airway. In central sleep apnea (CSA), the brain centers responsible for breathing fail to send messages to the breathing muscles. OSA is much more common than CSA. It is thought that about 1–10% of adults are affected by OSA; only about one-tenth of that number have CSA. OSA can affect people of any age and of either sex, but it is most common in middle-aged, somewhat overweight men, especially those who use alcohol.

Causes and symptoms

Obstructive sleep apnea

Obstructive sleep apnea occurs when part of the airway is closed off (usually at the back of the throat) while a person is trying to inhale during sleep. People whose airways are slightly narrower than average are more likely to be affected by OSA. Obesity, especially obesity in the neck, can increase the risk of developing OSA, because the fat tissue tends to narrow the airway. In some people, the airway is blocked by enlarged tonsils, an enlarged tongue, jaw deformities, or growths in the neck that compress the airway. Blocked nasal passages may also play a part in some people.

When a person begins to inhale, the expansion of the lungs lowers the air pressure inside the airway. If the muscles that keep the airway open are not working hard enough, the airway narrows and may collapse, shutting off the supply of air to the lungs. OSA occurs during sleep because the neck muscles that keep the airway open are not as active then. Congestion in the nose can make collapse more likely, since the extra effort needed to inhale will lower the pressure in the airway even more. Drinking alcohol or taking tranquilizers in the evening worsens this situation, because these cause the neck muscles to relax. (These drugs also lower the respiratory drive in the nervous system, reducing breathing rate and strength.)

People with OSA almost always snore heavily, because the same narrowing of the airway that causes snoring can also cause OSA. Snoring may actually help cause OSA as well, because the vibration of the throat tissues can cause them to swell; however, most people who snore do not go on to develop OSA.

Other risk factors for developing OSA include being male, being pregnant, having a family history of the disorder, and smoking. With regard to gender, it has been found that male sex hormones sometimes cause changes in the size or structure of the upper airway. The weight gain that accompanies pregnancy can affect a woman's breathing patterns during sleep, particularly during the third trimester. With regard to family history, OSA is known to run in families even though no gene or genes associated with the disorder have been identified as of 2011. Smoking increases the risk of developing OSA because it causes inflammation, swelling, and narrowing of the upper airway.

Some patients being treated for head and neck cancer develop OSA as a result of physical changes in the muscles and other tissues of the neck and throat. Doctors recommend prompt treatment of the OSA to improve the patient's quality of life.

Central sleep apnea

In central sleep apnea, the airway remains open, but the nerve signals controlling the respiratory muscles are not regulated properly. This can cause wide fluctuations in the level of carbon dioxide (CO_2) in the blood. Normal activity in the body produces CO_2, which is brought by the blood to the lungs for exhalation. When the blood level of CO_2 rises, brain centers respond by increasing the rate of respiration, clearing the CO_2. As blood levels fall again, respiration slows down. Normally, this interaction of CO_2 and breathing rate maintains the CO_2 level within very narrow limits. CSA can occur when the regulation system becomes insensitive to CO_2 levels, allowing wide fluctuations in both CO_2 levels and breathing rates. High CO_2 levels cause very rapid breathing (hyperventilation), which then lowers CO_2 so much that breathing becomes very slow or even stops. CSA occurs during sleep because when a person is awake, breathing is usually stimulated by other signals, including conscious awareness of breathing rate.

A combination of the two forms is also possible and is called mixed sleep apnea. Mixed sleep apnea episodes usually begin with a reduced central respiratory drive, followed by obstruction.

OSA and CSA cause similar symptoms. The most common symptoms are:

• daytime sleepiness
• morning headaches
• a feeling that sleep is not restful
• disorientation upon waking
• poor judgment
• personality changes

Sleepiness is caused not only by the frequent interruption of sleep but by the inability to enter long periods of deep sleep, during which the body performs numerous restorative functions. OSA is one of the leading causes of daytime sleepiness and is a major risk factor for motor vehicle accidents. Headaches and disorientation are caused by low oxygen levels during sleep, from the lack of regular breathing.

Other symptoms of sleep apnea may include sexual dysfunction, loss of concentration, memory loss, intellectual impairment, and behavioral changes such as anxiety and depression.

Sleep apnea is also associated with night sweats and nocturia, or increased frequency of urination at night. Bedwetting in children is also linked to sleep apnea.

Sleep apnea can cause serious changes in the cardiovascular system. Daytime hypertension (high blood pressure) is common. An increase in the number of red blood cells (polycythemia) is possible, as is an enlarged left ventricle of the heart (cor pulmonale), and left ventricular failure. In some people, sleep apnea causes life-threatening changes in the rhythm of the heart, including heartbeat slowing (bradycardia), racing (tachycardia), and other types of arrhythmias. Sudden death may occur from such arrhythmias. Patients with Pickwickian syndrome (named after a character in the Charles Dickens novel *The Pickwick Papers,* who seems to have this disease) are obese (obesity is the primary cause of the syndrome) with excessive daytime sleepiness, shortness of breath due to elevated blood carbon dioxide pressure, disturbed sleep at night, and flushed face. The skin can also have a bluish tint, and the patient may have high blood pressure, an enlarged liver, and an abnormally high red blood cell count.

Diagnosis

Excessive daytime sleepiness is the complaint that usually brings a person to see the doctor. A careful medical history includes questions about alcohol or tranquilizer use, snoring (often reported by the person's partner), and morning headaches or disorientation. A physical exam includes examination of the throat to look for narrowing or obstruction. Blood pressure is also measured. Measuring heart rate or blood levels of oxygen and CO_2 during the daytime will not usually be done, since these are abnormal only at night in most patients.

In some cases the person's dentist may suggest the diagnosis of OSA on the basis of a dental checkup or evaluation of the patient for oral surgery.

Confirmation of the diagnosis usually requires making measurements while the person sleeps. These tests are called a polysomnography study and are conducted during an overnight stay in a specialized sleep laboratory. During a sleep study, surface electrodes are put on the face and scalp and send recorded electrical signals to the measuring equipment. These signals, which are generated by brain and muscle activity, are then recorded digitally. Belts are placed around the

KEY TERMS

Continuous positive airway pressure (CPAP)—A ventilation system that blows a gentle stream of air into the nose to keep the airway open.

Genioplasty—An operation performed to reshape the chin. Genioplasties are often done to treat OSA because the procedure changes the structure of the patient's upper airway.

Mandible—The medical term for the lower jaw. One type of oral appliance used to treat OSA pushes the mandible forward in order to ease breathing during sleep.

Nocturia—Excessive need to urinate at night. Nocturia is a symptom of OSA and often increases the patient's daytime sleepiness.

Polysomnography—A group of tests administered to analyze heart, blood, and breathing patterns during sleep.

Tracheotomy—A surgical procedure in which a small hole is cut into the trachea, or windpipe, below the level of the vocal cords.

Uvulopalatopharyngoplasty (UPPP)—An operation to remove excess tissue at the back of the throat to prevent it from closing off the airway during sleep.

chest and abdomen to measure breathing. A bandage-like oximeter probe is put on the patient's finger to measure the amount of oxygen in the blood. Important parts of the polysomnography study include measurements of the following:

- heart rate
- airflow at the mouth and nose
- respiratory effort
- sleep stage (light sleep, deep sleep, dream sleep, etc.)
- oxygen level in the blood, using a noninvasive probe (ear oximetry)

Simplified studies done overnight at home are also possible and may be appropriate for people whose profile strongly suggests the presence of obstructive sleep apnea; that is, middle-aged, somewhat overweight men, who snore and have high blood pressure. The home-based study usually includes ear oximetry and cardiac measurements. If these measurements support the diagnosis of OSA, initial treatment is usually suggested without polysomnography. Home-based measurements are not used to rule out OSA, and if the measurements do not support the OSA

diagnosis, polysomnography may be needed to define the problem further.

Other sleep tests may include an EEG (electroencephalogram) to measure and record brain wave activity; an EMG (electromyogram) to record muscle activity such as face twitches, teeth grinding, and leg movements, and to determine the presence of REM stage sleep. During REM sleep, intense dreams often occur as the brain undergoes heightened activity; an EOG (electro-oculogram) records eye movements. These movements are important in determining the different sleep stages, particularly REM stage sleep; an ECG (electrocardiogram) records heart rate and rhythm. Oftentimes a nasal airflow sensor is used to record airflow or a snore microphone to record snoring activity.

Treatment

Behavioral changes

Treatment of obstructive sleep apnea begins with reducing the use of alcohol or tranquilizers in the evening, if these have been contributing to the problem. Weight loss is also effective, but if the weight returns, as it often does, so does the apnea. Changing sleeping position may be effective; snoring and sleep apnea are both most common when a person sleeps on his back. Turning to sleep on the side may be enough to clear up the symptoms. Raising the head of the bed may also help. Opening of the nasal passages can provide some relief. There are a variety of nasal devices such as clips, tapes, or holders that may help, though discomfort may limit their use. Nasal decongestants may be useful but should not be taken for sleep apnea without the consent of the treating physician.

Oxygen and drug therapy

Supplemental nighttime oxygen can be useful for some people with either central and obstructive sleep apnea. Tricyclic antidepressant drugs such as protriptyline (Vivactil) may help by increasing the muscle tone of the upper airway muscles, but their side effects may severely limit their usefulness.

Mechanical ventilation

For moderate to severe sleep apnea, the most successful treatment is nighttime use of a ventilator, called a CPAP machine. CPAP (continuous positive airway pressure) blows air into the airway continuously, preventing its collapse. CPAP requires the use of a nasal mask. The appropriate pressure setting for the CPAP machine is determined by polysomnography in the sleep lab. Its effects are dramatic; daytime sleepiness usually disappears within one to two days after treatment begins. CPAP is used to treat both obstructive and central sleep apnea.

CPAP is tolerated well by about two-thirds of patients who try it. Bilevel positive airway pressure (BiPAP) is an alternative form of ventilation. With BiPAP, the ventilator reduces the air pressure when the person exhales. This is more comfortable for some. CPAP is the most common, noninvasive treatment for moderate to severe sleep apnea.

Surgery

Surgery can be used to correct obstructions in the airways. The most common surgery is called UPPP, for uvulopalatopharngyoplasty. This surgery removes tissue from the rear of the mouth and top of the throat. The tissues removed include parts of the uvula (the flap of tissue that hangs down at the back of the mouth), the soft palate, and the pharynx. Tonsils and adenoids are usually removed in this operation. This operation significantly improves sleep apnea in slightly more than half of all cases.

Reconstructive surgery is possible for those whose OSA is due to constriction of the airway by lower jaw deformities. Genioplasty, which is a procedure that plastic surgeons usually perform to reshape a patient's chin to improve his or her appearance, is now being done to reshape the upper airway in patients with OSA.

When other forms of treatment are not successful, obstructive sleep apnea may be treated by a tracheostomy. In this procedure, an opening is made into the trachea (windpipe) below the obstruction, and a tube inserted to maintain an air passage. A tracheostomy requires a great deal of care to prevent infection of the tracheostomy site. In addition, since air is no longer being filtered and moistened by the nasal passages before entering the lungs, the lower airways can become dry and susceptible to infection as well. Tracheostomy is usually reserved for those whose apnea has led to life-threatening heart arrhythmias and who have not been treated successfully with other treatments.

Tonsillectomy and/or adenoidectomy removes the tonsils and/or the adenoids. It is an option for individuals who have enlarged tonsils and adenoids that are blocking their airway during sleep. This is often the first treatment option for children because enlarged tonsils and adenoids are usually the cause of their sleep apnea. If none of these options is used, some people opt for bariatric surgery, which is done for weight loss for extremely overweight persons.

Oral appliances

Another approach to treating OSA involves the use of oral appliances intended to improve breathing either by holding the tongue in place or by pushing the lower jaw forward during sleep to increase the air volume in the upper airway. The first type of oral appliance is known as a tongue retaining device or TRD. The second type is variously called an oral protrusive device (OPD) or mandibular advancement splint (MAS), because it holds the mandible, or lower jaw, forward during sleep. These oral devices appear to work best for patients with mild-to-moderate OSA and in some cases can postpone or prevent the need for surgery. Their rate of patient compliance is about 50%; most patients who stop using oral appliances do so because their teeth are in poor condition. TRDs and OPDs can be fitted by dentists; however, most dentists work together with the patient's physician following a polysomnogram rather than prescribing the device by themselves.

Clinical Trials

As of 2011, there were several active clinical trials for sleep apnea. For information on clinical trials, go to http://clinicaltrials.gov.

Prognosis

The combination of behavioral changes, ventilation assistance, drug therapy, and surgery allow most people with sleep apnea to be treated successfully, although it may take some time to determine the most effective and least intrusive treatment. Polysomnography testing is usually required after beginning a treatment to determine how effective it has been.

Prevention

For people who snore frequently, weight control, avoidance of evening alcohol or tranquilizers, and adjustment of sleeping position may help reduce the risk of developing obstructive sleep apnea.

Resources

BOOKS

Libby, P. et al. *Braunwald's Heart Disease*. 8th ed. Philadelphia: Saunders, 2007.

Cummings, C.W., et al. *Otolayrngology: Head and Neck Surgery*. 4th ed. St. Louis: Mosby, 2005.

Goetz, C.G. *Goetz's Textbook of Clinical Neurology*. 3rd ed. Philadelphia: Saunders, 2007.

Goldman L., and D. Ausiello, eds. *Cecil Textbook of Internal Medicine*. 23rd ed. Philadelphia: Saunders, 2008.

PERIODICALS

Chasens, E.R., and M.G. Umlauf. "Nocturia: A Problem That Disrupts Sleep and Predicts Obstructive Sleep Apnea." *Geriatric Nursing* 24 (March-April 2003): 76–81, 105.

Chung, S.A., et al. "How, What, and Why of Sleep Apnea. Perspectives for Primary Care Physicians." *Canadian Family Physician* 48 (June 2002): 1073–80.

Edwards, N., et al. "Sleep Disordered Breathing and Pregnancy." *Thorax* 57 (June 2002): 555–58.

Freire A.O., et al. "Treatment of moderate obstructive sleep apnea syndrome with acupuncture: A randomised, placebo-controlled pilot trial." *Sleep Medicine* 8, no. 1 (January 2007): 43–50.

Hirshkowitz M., et al. "Adjunct armodafinil improves wakefulness and memory in obstructive sleep apnea/hypopnea syndrome." *Respiratory Medicine* 101, no. 3 (March 2007): 616–27.

Hisanaga, A., et al. "A Case of Sleep Choking Syndrome Improved by the Kampo Extract of Hange-Koboku-To." *Psychiatry and Clinical Neuroscience* 56 (June 2002): 325–27.

Kapur, V., et al. "Underdiagnosis of Sleep Apnea Syndrome in U.S. Communities." *Sleep and Breathing* 6 (June 2002): 49–54.

Koliha, C.A. "Obstructive Sleep Apnea in Head and Neck Cancer Patients Post Treatment ... Something to Consider?" *ORL—Head and Neck Nursing* 21 (Winter 2003): 10–14.

Neill, A., et al. "Mandibular Advancement Splint Improves Indices of Obstructive Sleep Apnoea and Snoring but Side Effects Are Common." *New Zealand Medical Journal* 115 (June 21, 2002): 289–92.

Redolfi S., et al. "Relationship between overnight rostral fluid shift and obstructive sleep apnea in nonobese men." *American Journal of Respiratory and Critical Care Medicine* 179, no. 3 (February 2009): 241–46.

Shiomi, T., et al. "Falling Asleep While Driving and Automobile Accidents Among Patients with Obstructive Sleep Apnea-Hypopnea Syndrome." *Psychiatry and Clinical Neuroscience* 56 (June 2002): 333–34.

Stanton, D.C. "Genioplasty." *Facial Plastic Surgery* 19 (February 2003): 75–86.

Umlauf, M.G., and E.R. Chasens. "Bedwetting—Not Always What It Seems: A Sign of Sleep-Disordered Breathing in Children." *Journal for Specialists in Pediatric Nursing* 8 (January-March 2003): 22–30.

Veale, D., et al. "Identification of Quality of Life Concerns of Patients with Obstructive Sleep Apnoea at the Time of Initiation of Continuous Positive Airway Pressure: A Discourse Analysis." *Quality of Life Research* 11 (June 2002): 389–99.

Viera, A.J., M.M. Bond, and S.J. Yates. "Diagnosing Night Sweats." *American Family Physician* 67 (March 1, 2003): 1019–24.

WEBSITES

"What Is Sleep Apnea?" National Heart, Lung, and Blood Institute (NHLBI). http://www.nhlbi.nih.gov/health/dci/Diseases/SleepApnea/SleepApnea_WhatIs.html (accessed August 28, 2011).

ORGANIZATIONS

American Academy of Otolaryngology—Head and Neck Surgery, 1650 Diagonal Road, Alexandria, VA 22314-2857, (703) 836-4444, http://www. entnet.org.

American Dental Association, 211 East Chicago Avenue, Chicago, IL 60611-2678, (312) 440-2500, http://www.ada.org.

American Sleep Apnea Association, 6856 Eastern Avenue, NW, Suite 203, Washington, DC United States, 20012, (202) 293-3650, (888) 293-3650, Fax: (202) 293-3656, http://www.sleepapnea.org.

National Sleep Foundation, 1010 N. Glebe Road, Suite 310, Arlington, VA 22210, (703) 243-1697, nsf@sleepfoundation.org, http://www.sleep foundation.org.

Richard Robinson
Rebecca J. Frey, PhD
Karl Finley

Sleep disorders or parasomnias

Definition

Sleep disorders are common conditions ranging from difficulty falling asleep or staying asleep to sleeping for extended periods or falling asleep inappropriately. Parasomnias are undesirable sleep experiences.

Description

Sleep is essential for bodily function, including nervous system function. The brain has various mechanisms for controlling the sleep-wake cycle, including circadian rhythms controlled by a biological clock and chemical messengers in the brain called neurotransmitters. A variety of physical, psychological, and emotional factors can disrupt these mechanisms, resulting in sleep disorders.

Of more than 80 recognized sleep disorders, most fall into one of five categories:

- insomnia
- sleep apnea or sleep-related breathing problems
- restless legs syndrome (RLS), often accompanied by periodic limb movement disorder (PLMD)

- narcolepsy
- parasomnias

Insomnia

Insomnia includes difficulty falling asleep, staying asleep, or obtaining restful sleep, leading to daytime impairment. Insomnia can be short-term or chronic—occurring at least three nights per week for more than a month—and ranges from mild to severe. Many other sleep disorders involve at least some degree of insomnia.

Sleep apnea

Sleep apnea is a major cause of daytime sleepiness. Apnea interrupts sleep by momentarily suspending breathing. These interruptions may occur 5–30 times per hour. Obstructive sleep apnea—the most common type—usually results from blockage or collapse of the airway. Central sleep apnea, which is less common, is a neurological disorder in which the brain fails to send correct signals to the breathing muscles, leading to brief periods when no effort is made to breathe. It is not uncommon to have both types of sleep apnea simultaneously.

Restless legs syndrome

RLS is one of the most common sleep disorders, especially in older adults. It involves a strong urge to move one's legs, along with unpleasant sensations in the legs, making it difficult to fall asleep and remain asleep. RLS that begins before age 45—and can be as early as childhood—tends to run in families and is usually a lifelong syndrome, with symptoms slowly worsening and becoming more frequent. RLS that begins later in life usually starts abruptly and does not worsen over time.

Narcolepsy

Narcolepsy causes severe daytime sleepiness and repeated "sleep attacks,"—falling asleep suddenly, even while talking, eating, or engaged in another activity. Most people with narcolepsy have nighttime insomnia. They typically fall into rapid eye moment (REM) sleep quickly, wake up directly from REM sleep, and have vivid dreams or hallucinations while falling asleep or waking up.

Parasomnias

Parasomnias are abnormal activities occurring during sleep. Examples include:

- hallucinations
- sleep paralysis
- sleepwalking (somnambulism)
- nightmares or sleep terrors
- sleep-related eating disorder
- confusional arousals
- sleep talking (somniloquy)
- REM sleep behavior disorder (RBD)—the vigorous acting out of dreams
- groaning
- head banging
- bedwetting
- teeth grinding
- sleep aggression
- sexsomnia or "sleep sex"—sexual activity while asleep

Parasomnias can occur at any point in the sleep cycle. Hallucinations and sleep paralysis usually happen while falling asleep or awakening. Somnambulism usually occurs in early deep sleep or during arousals from slow-wave sleep. Sleep terrors—in which the sleeper sits up in fright, screaming or crying—usually occur during arousal from slow-wave sleep. Sleepwalking, sleep terrors, sleep-related eating disorder, and confusional arousals may be accompanied by abrupt, partial awakenings. Sleepwalking is usually a random event that does not indicate a problem or require treatment, unless it involves unusual or dangerous behaviors.

Somniloquy can occur on its own or as a symptom of another sleep disorder. It may or may not be intelligible speech. Although the talk is usually harmless, it may sometimes be vulgar or harsh, emotional, and loud, especially if it is associated with sleep terrors or RBD.

RBD is a brain disorder that usually affects men over age 50 and patients with neurological disorders such as **Parkinson's disease**, narcolepsy, or stroke. It also can be caused by medications such as antidepressants.

Other sleep disorders

Other sleep disorders include:

- circadian rhythm sleeping disorder (CRSD)
- hypersomnia, characterized by frequent daytime naps and prolonged nighttime sleep
- Kleine-Levin syndrome

CRSD is a persistent or recurring pattern of sleep disruption caused by an altered circadian rhythm. Circadian rhythms regulate sleep-wake cycles through the production and release of the hormone melatonin, which is derived from the neurotransmitter serotonin. Types of CRSDs include:

- delayed sleep phase
- advanced sleep phase

- irregular sleep-wake rhythm
- jet lag
- shift-work-induced
- free-running (non-entrained) or non-24-hour sleep-wake cycle
- medical-condition-induced
- drug- or substance-induced

Demographics

An estimated 40 million Americans suffer from chronic sleep disorders.

- One in three adults has occasional insomnia and one in ten suffers from chronic insomnia. The incidence of insomnia increases with age, with women somewhat more affected than men.
- An estimated 18 million Americans have sleep apnea, although most cases go undiagnosed.
- RLS affects up to 12 million Americans.
- Narcolepsy, which usually develops in adolescence or young adulthood, affects an estimated 250,000 Americans.
- About 10% of Americans have parasomnias, which are especially common in children. Sleepwalking is most common in children between the ages of 8 and 12. About 50% of young children and 5% of adults sleep talk.
- Delayed-sleep-phase CRSD affects up to 7% of teens and 4% of adults. As many as 60% of night-shift workers have CRSD. Non-24-hour sleep-wake syndrome most often affects people who are totally blind.
- Kleine-Levin syndrome is rare, primarily affecting teenage males.

Causes and symptoms

Sleep disorders have a variety of causes. Some sleep disorders run in families and have a genetic basis. Most people with mental disorders—including **depression**, anxiety, posttraumatic stress disorder (PTSD), and schizophrenia—have sleep disturbances. Sleep disorders are early symptoms of some neurodegenerative diseases such Alzheimer's and Parkinson's. Underlying medical conditions, medications, drugs and alcohol, stress, and sleeping habits can cause or contribute to sleep disorders.

General symptoms of a sleep disorder may include:

- consistently taking more than 30 minutes to fall asleep
- waking up several times each night
- awakening too early in the morning
- waking up feeling tired
- excessive daytime sleepiness
- frequent naps
- hyperactivity or poor concentration in children

Insomnia

Primary insomnia may be caused by long-term stress or emotional upset; however, about 80% of insomnias are secondary to another medical condition or neurological, emotional, or sleep disorder. Insomnias can also be caused by medications or substances such as caffeine or other stimulants, tobacco or other nicotine products, alcohol, or sedatives. Symptoms of insomnia may include **fatigue**, poor concentration, irritability, anxiety, or depression.

Sleep apnea

Obstructive sleep apnea is caused by blockage or collapse of the windpipe. In overweight people, the windpipe wall may thicken with fat and narrow the opening. A buildup of fat or loss of muscle tone with age can also cause the throat and tongue muscles to relax during sleep, blocking the opening or collapsing the windpipe. In small children, enlarged tonsils can block the opening. When oxygen levels drop significantly, the brain triggers a sleep disturbance that tightens the upper airway muscles and opens the windpipe to restore normal breathing. This is usually accompanied by a snort or choking sound. Obstructive sleep apnea is frequently associated with parasomnias and loud snoring caused by the air squeezing through.

Central sleep apnea may be caused by a malfunction in neurons that control breathing during sleep and is usually associated with another medical condition or a medication. Sleep apnea has been linked to high blood pressure, an increased risk of heart attack and stroke, and even sudden death from respiratory failure.

Restless legs syndrome

The primary cause of RLS appears to be iron insufficiency or poor utilization of iron in the brain. The brain requires iron to produce the neurotransmitter dopamine, which helps control movement. Iron deficiency or poor utilization can be inherited. It is also linked to a variety of conditions, including pregnancy, anemia, diabetes, kidney failure, Parkinson's disease, and rheumatoid arthritis. Nerve damage from diabetes or other conditions can also cause or contribute to RLS, as can certain medications.

The following symptoms constitute a diagnosis of RLS:

- a strong urge to move one's legs, often accompanied by tingling, prickling, crawling, itching, burning, or creeping sensations, and aches in the legs
- onset or worsening of symptoms at night or during inactivity
- relief of symptoms by moving, especially walking

Narcolepsy

Narcolepsy is usually caused by an inherited defect in a gene that affects hypocretin, a brain chemical that promotes wakefulness. Narcolepsy also requires a second causative factor such as one of the following:

- infection
- another neurological disorder or brain injury
- an autoimmune disorder such as rheumatoid arthritis
- low levels of histamine, a chemical in the blood that promotes wakefulness
- possibly an environment toxin, such as a heavy metal, pesticide, herbicide, or secondhand smoke

Narcolepsy can cause cataplexy, a sudden muscle **weakness** lasting seconds to minutes, or sleep paralysis, an inability to move or speak while falling asleep or waking up. Sleep paralysis usually goes away after a few minutes.

Parasomnias

Sleepwalking, sleep talking, and some other parasomnias appear to run in families, suggesting that they have a genetic component. Children are particularly likely to sleepwalk if both of their parents sleepwalk. Parasomnias can be triggered by obstructive sleep apnea and other sleep disorders, various medical conditions, mental disorders, medications, or substance abuse. Pediatric parasomnias often disappear by late childhood or adolescence.

Other sleep disorders

There are many causes of CRSD. Frequent flying across multiple time zones and shift work are common causes. CRSD can also be caused by stress, medications, herbs, nutritional supplements, caffeine, liver disease, and substance abuse. CRSD is common in **dementia** patients.

Hypersomnia usually first appears during childhood or adolescence and may involve a genetic predisposition. Known causes of hypersomnia are:

- another sleep disorder, such as sleep apnea or narcolepsy
- an autonomic nervous system dysfunction
- a central nervous system injury, such as a tumor or head trauma
- certain medications or withdrawal from medications
- drug or alcohol abuse

Symptoms of hypersomnia include difficulty awakening and feeling disoriented upon awakening. Other symptoms may include slow thinking and speech, appetite loss, anxiety, irritation, low energy, restlessness, hallucinations, and memory difficulties.

Kleine-Levin syndrome may be related to malfunction of the thalamus and hypothalamus, which control sleep and appetite. It is characterized by recurring periods of sleeping as much as 20 hours per day. Episodes often begin abruptly, sometimes with flu-like symptoms, and may last a few days to a few weeks. Episodes may include excessive eating, irritability, disorientation, hallucinations, childlike behaviors, uninhibited sex drive, and depression. Individuals are normal between episodes. Intensity and frequency of episodes decrease over a period of 8 to 12 years.

Diagnosis

Sleep disorders may be diagnosed by a primary-care physician, neurologist, or sleep specialist. Diagnosis begins with a medical and family history and lifestyle questions. A physical examination, including a neurological exam, may uncover an underlying cause. Sleep history, habits, and symptoms are analyzed. Patients often keep sleep diaries, detailing when they sleep, awaken, nap, and feel sleepy, and the timing of any medications or other substances. The Epworth Sleepiness Scale may be used to rate sleep. Sometimes patients wear an actigraph on their wrists for one to two weeks, to record active and inactive periods throughout the day and night.

Other diagnostic tests and procedures may include:

- blood tests to measure melatonin or iron levels or detect thyroid problems or other conditions
- computed tomography (CT) scans or magnetic resonance imaging (MRI) to detect underlying conditions
- an overnight sleep study, called a polysomnogram (PSG), which records electrical activity in the brain, eye movements, heart rate, blood pressure, blood oxygen levels, breathing, muscle activity, and arm and leg movements throughout the night

Apnea—A transient cessation of breathing.

Cataplexy—A sudden loss of muscle control that is a characteristic symptom of narcolepsy.

Chronotherapy—A sleep disorder treatment that involves adjusting sleep and wake times to reset one's biological clock.

Circadian rhythm—An approximately 24-hour cycle of physiological and behavioral activity.

Circadian rhythm sleep disorder (CRSD)—A disruption of the circadian rhythm sleep-wake cycle.

Cognitive-behavioral therapy (CBT)—A treatment that identifies negative thoughts and behaviors and helps develop more positive approaches.

Dopamine—A neurotransmitter in the brain; low levels are associated with restless legs syndrome.

Hypersomnia—Episodes of sleeping excessively, followed by periods of normal sleep.

Hypocretin—A brain chemical that promotes wakefulness; low levels are associated with narcolepsy.

Insomnia—Prolonged or abnormal inability to obtain adequate sleep.

Melatonin—A hormone involved in regulation of the sleep-wake cycle and other circadian rhythms.

Multiple sleep latency test (MSLT)—A measurement of brain activity during daytime naps.

Narcolepsy—A condition characterized by brief attacks of deep sleep.

Neurotransmitters—Chemicals that transmit nerve impulses from one nerve cell to another.

Over-the-counter (OTC)—A drug that can be purchased without a doctor's prescription.

Periodic limb movement disorder (PLMD)—A neurological disorder that often accompanies restless legs syndrome.

Polysomnogram (PSG)—A recording of various physiological measures during overnight sleep.

Rapid eye movement (REM)—A stage of the normal sleep cycle characterized by rapid eye movements, increased forebrain and midbrain activity, and dreaming.

REM sleep behavior disorder (RBD)—The acting out of wild or violent dreams and hallucinations during REM sleep; an early symptom of Parkinson's disease.

Restless legs syndrome (RLS)—A neurological disorder characterized by aching, burning, or creeping sensations in the legs and an urge to move the legs, often resulting in insomnia.

Serotonin—A neurotransmitter found primarily in the brain and blood.

Slow-wave sleep—Deep, usually dreamless sleep, that occurs regularly between intervals of REM sleep.

Somnambulism—Motor actions, such as walking, during sleep.

Somniloquy—Sleep talking.

• a multiple sleep latency test (MSLT) to measure daytime sleepiness via brain activity—often performed throughout the day following a PSG

• use of a simple device for detecting sleep apnea

• muscle or nerve tests for RLS

• hypocretin levels in cerebrospinal fluid obtained through a lumbar puncture (spinal tap) to diagnose narcolepsy

Treatment

Most sleep disorders can be effectively treated or managed. Sometimes lifestyle changes or adjustment of sleep habits is all that is required:

• avoiding caffeine, tobacco, stimulants, chocolate, and alcohol in the hours before bed

• avoiding large meals and beverages before bed

• avoiding over-the-counter (OTC) and prescription medications, such as some cold and allergy medicines, that can disrupt sleep

• daily exercise, but not within three hours of bed

• avoiding bright lights before bed

• relaxing before bed

• creating a sleep-friendly bedroom that is cool, dark, and quiet

• sleeping and waking around the same time every day, even on weekends

• allowing about 20 minutes to fall asleep or fall back asleep and then getting up and engaging in a relaxing activity until sleepy

• weight loss or not sleeping on one's back for sleep apnea

• regular daytime naps to help prevent falling asleep inappropriately due to narcolepsy

Treatments for sleep disorders may include:

- cognitive-behavioral therapy (CBT) to identify thoughts and behaviors that contribute to sleep problems and replace them with good sleep habits
- relaxation training, such as meditation, hypnosis, or muscle relaxation
- biofeedback techniques
- for sleep apnea—mouthpieces, breathing devices, or surgery to correct an airway obstruction
- for CRSD—sunlight, light therapy, or chronotherapy (changing sleeping and waking times) to reset one's biological clock

Drugs

There are many prescription sleep medications for short-term use. Certain sedatives/hypnotics may be prescribed long term. Some drugs help only with falling asleep; others also help with staying asleep. Some drugs treat both insomnia and depression. Sleep apnea cannot be treated with sedatives or sleeping medications because these may prevent awakening to breathe. RLS and PLMD can be effectively treated with Parkinson's disease medications that increase dopamine levels or mimic its activities. Narcolepsy may be treated with stimulants to reduce daytime sleepiness, nighttime sleep aids, a drug that helps compensate for low hypocretin levels, and/or antidepressants to help prevent cataplexy, hallucinations, and sleep paralysis.

Over-the-counter sleep aids usually contain antihistamines, which can have side effects and quickly lose their effectiveness. Other products promoted as insomnia treatments include melatonin and L-tryptophan, an amino-acid precursor of serotonin. Herbal remedies for insomnia include valerian, lemon balm, chamomile, kava kava, passionflower, lavender, and St. John's wort. It is not clear whether any of these products is safe or effective.

Clinical trials

Sleep disorders are a very active area of research. There are a large number of ongoing clinical trials for determining the effectiveness of lifestyle changes, drug therapies, and other treatments. Information about current relevant clinical trials can be found at ClinicalTrials.gov.

Resources

BOOKS

Colligan, L.H. *Sleep Disorders.* New York: Marshall Cavendish Benchmark, 2009.

Foldvary-Schaefer, Nancy. *The Cleveland Clinic Guide to Sleep Disorders.* New York: Kaplan, 2009.

Judd, Sandra J. *Sleep Disorders Sourcebook.* 3rd ed. Detroit: Omnigraphics, 2010.

Kotler, Ronald, and Maryann Karinch. *365 Ways to Get a Good Night's Sleep.* Avon, MA: Adams Media, 2009.

Marcovitz, Hal. *Sleep Disorders.* San Diego, CA: Reference-Point, 2010.

Marcus, Mary Brophy. *Sleep Disorders.* New York: Chelsea House, 2009.

Pollak, Charles, Michael J. Thorpy, and Jan Yager. *The Encyclopedia of Sleep and Sleep Disorders.* 3rd ed. New York: Facts on File, 2010.

Ramlakhan, Nerina. *Tired but Wired: The Essential Sleep Toolkit: How to Overcome Sleep Problems.* London: Souvenir, 2010.

Stores, Gregory. *Insomnia and Other Adult Sleep Problems.* New York: Oxford University Press, 2009.

PERIODICALS

Babson, Kimberly A., et al. "Cognitive Behavioral Therapy for Sleep Disorders." *Psychiatric Clinics of North America* 33, no. 3 (September 2010): 629–40.

Hauw, J.J., et al. "Neuropathology of Sleep Disorders: A Review." *Journal of Neuropathology and Experimental Neurology* 70, no. 4 (April 2011): 243–52.

Mascarelli, Amanda Leigh. "Dread of Night; Sleep Apnea is on the Rise in the U.S., and Despite Treatments to Maintain Air Flow, There is No Cure-All." *Los Angeles Times* (February 28, 2011): E1.

Pigeon, Wilfred R. "Treatment of Adult Insomnia with Cognitive-Behavioral Therapy." Journal of Clinical Psychology 66, no. 11 (November 2010): 1148–60. http://onlinelibrary.wiley.com/doi/10.1002/jclp.20737/full (accessed July 19, 2011).

WEBSITES

"Insomnia: Prescription Sleeping Pills: What's Right for You?" Mayo Clinic. http://www.mayoclinic.com/print/sleeping-pills/SL00010/ (accessed July 19, 2011).

"Insomnia Treatment: Cognitive Behavioral Therapy Instead of Sleeping Pills." Mayo Clinic. http://www.mayoclinic.com/print/insomnia-treatment/SL00013/ (accessed July 19, 2011).

"Polysomnography (Sleep Study)." Mayo Clinic. http://www.mayoclinic.com/health/polysomnography/MY00970/ (accessed July 19, 2011).

Schenck, Carlos H. "Sleep and Parasomnias." National Sleep Foundation. http://www.sleepfoundation.org/article/ask-the-expert/sleep-and-parasomnias (accessed July 19, 2011).

"Sleep Disorders." MedlinePlus. http://www.nlm.nih.gov/medlineplus/sleepdisorders.html (accessed July 19, 2011).

"Sleep Disorders." National Heart, Lung, and Blood Institute. http://www.nhlbi.nih.gov/health/dci/Browse/Sleep.html (accessed July 19, 2011).

"Sleep Disorders and CAM: At a Glance." National Center for Complementary and Alternative Medicine. http://nccam.nih.gov/health/sleep/ataglance.htm (accessed July 19, 2011).

ORGANIZATIONS

American Academy of Sleep Medicine, 2510 North Frontage Road, Darien, IL 60561, (630) 737-9700, Fax: (630) 737-9790, inquiries@aasmnet.org, http://www.aasmnet.org.

National Heart, Lung, and Blood Institute Health Information Center, P.O. Box 30105, Bethesda, MD, 20824-0105, (301) 592-8573, Fax: (240) 629-3246, nhlbiinfo@nhlbi.nih.gov, http://www.nhlbi.nih.gov.

National Institute of Neurological Disorders and Stroke (NINDS), P.O. Box 5801, Bethesda, MD 20824, (301) 496-5751, (800) 352-9424, http://www.ninds.nih.gov.

National Sleep Foundation, 1010 N. Glebe Road, Suite 310, Arlington, VA 22210, (703) 243-1697, nsf@sleepfoundation.org, http://www.sleepfoundation.org.

Margaret Alic, PhD

Sleeping sickness *see* **Encephalitis lethargica**

Social workers

Definition

A social worker is a helping professional who is distinguished from other human service professionals by a focus on both the individual and his or her environment. Generally, social workers have at least a bachelor's degree from an accredited education program, and in most states they must be licensed, certified, or registered. A master's in social work is required for those who provide psychotherapy or work in specific settings such as hospitals or nursing homes.

Description

Social workers comprise a profession that had its beginnings in 1889 when Jane Addams founded Hull House and the American settlement house movement in Chicago's West Side. The ethics and values that informed her work became the basis for the social work profession. They include respect for human beings, especially those who are vulnerable, an understanding that people are influenced by their environment, and a desire to work for social change that rectifies gross or unjust differences.

The social work profession is broader than most disciplines with regard to the range and types of problems addressed, the settings in which the work takes place, the levels of practice, interventions used, and populations served. It has been observed that social work is defined in its own place in the larger social environment, continuously evolving to respond to and address a changing world. Although several definitions of social work have been provided throughout its history, common to all definitions is the focus on both the individual and the environment, distinguishing it from other helping professions.

Social workers may be engaged in a variety of occupations ranging from hospitals, schools, clinics, police departments, public agencies, court systems to private practices or businesses. They provide the majority of mental health care to persons of all ages in the United States, and in rural areas they are often the sole providers of services. In general, they assist people to obtain tangible services; help communities or groups provide or improve social and health services; provide counseling and psychotherapy with individuals, families, and groups; and participate in policy change through legislative processes. The practice of social work requires knowledge of human development and behavior; of social, economic and cultural institutions; and of the interaction of all these factors.

Resources

ORGANIZATIONS

National Association of Social Workers. 750 First St. NE, Washington, D.C. 20002-4241. http://www.naswdc.org.

OTHER

National Association of Social Workers. *Choices: Careers in Social Work.* (2002). http://www.naswdc.org/pubs/choices/choices.htm..

National Association of Social Workers. *Professional Social Work Centennial: 1898–1998, Addams' Work Laid the Foundation.* 1998 (2002). http://www.naswdc.org/nasw/centennial/addams.htm.

Judy Leaver, M.A.

Sodium oxybate

Definition

Sodium oxybate is primarily used to treat cataplexy attacks (episodes of weak or paralyzed muscles) in patients with **narcolepsy**, a condition that causes excessive sleepiness.

Purpose

There is no known cure for narcolepsy. Sodium oxybate is specifically indicated only for the treatment of cataplexy; it does not promote wakefulness or relieve excessive sleepiness, the main symptom of narcolepsy.

Description

Sodium oxybate is also sold in the United States under the name Xyrem. It is a Schedule III, federally controlled substance. Sodium oxybate has a high potential for abuse and is commonly known by its nonmedical name, GHB. Patients who are prescribed soduim oxybate should use care when storing and disposing of the medication and its containers.

Recommended dosage

Sodium oxybate is taken as an oral solution, mixed with water. Physicians prescribe it in varying dosages. Sodium oxybate is usually taken in two divided doses, the first administered at bedtime and the second 2.5–4 hours later. As the medication induces sleep quickly, an alarm clock is sometimes needed to wake the person for the second dose. Typical adult daily dosages range .17–.31 oz/ (5–9 g). If the first half of a daily divided dose is missed, it should be taken as soon as possible. If the second half of a daily divided dose is missed, that dose should be skipped and no more sodium oxybate should be taken until the following day. Two doses of sodium oxybate should never be taken at the same time.

Sodium oxybate works quickly, relaxing muscles and inducing sleep. As food will decrease the amount of sodium oxybate absorbed into the body, patients should not take the medication with meals.

Precautions

Sodium oxybate may be habit forming and has a high potential for nonmedical abuse. When taking the medication, it is important to follow physician instructions precisely.

Sodium oxybate is sleep inducing and takes effect quickly. It should, therefore, be taken only at bedtime and while in bed. It may also cause clumsiness and impair thinking. It can exacerbate the side effects of alcohol and other medications. A physician should be consulted before taking sodium oxybate with certain nonprescription medications. Patients should avoid alcohol and **central nervous system** (CNS) depressants (medications that can make one drowsy or less alert, such as antihistimines, sleep medications, and some pain medications) while taking sodium oxybate because they can exacerbate the side effects.

Sodium oxybate may not be suitable for persons with a history of hypopnea (abnormally slow breathing), sleep apnea, liver or kidney disease, **depression**, metabolic disorders, high blood pressure, angina (chest pain), or irregular heartbeats and other heart problems.

Before beginning treatment with sodium oxybate, patients should notify their physician if they have a history of consuming a large amount of alcohol or a history of drug use. In these cases, dependence on sodium oxybate may be more likely to develop.

Patients who become pregnant while taking sodium oxybate should contact their physician immediately. Taking sodium oxybate while pregnant may cause fetal harm.

Side effects

Research indicates that sodium oxybate, when used under a physician's direction, is generally well tolerated. However, sodium oxybate may cause a variety of usually mild side effects. These side effects usually do not require medical attention, and may diminish with continued use of the medication. They include:

- flu-like feeling
- abdominal pain
- difficulty sleeping
- nightmares
- nervousness or anxiety
- depression
- diarrhea
- dry mouth
- runny nose
- neck pain or stiffness
- back pain
- nausea or vomiting
- headache

Other, uncommon side effects of sodium oxybate can be potentially serious. Individuals taking soduim oxybate who experience any of the following symptoms should immediately contact their physician:

- sleepwalking
- change in vision
- ringing or pounding in the ears
- problems with memory
- numbness or tingling feelings on the skin
- disorientation, fainting, or loss of consciousness
- irregular heartbeat
- shortness of breath
- hives, rashes, or bluish patches on the lips and skin
- chest pain
- severe headache

Interactions

Sodium oxybate may have negative interactions with some anticoagulants (blood thinners), antidepressants, antifungals, antibiotics, asthma medications, barbiturates, and monoamine oxidase inhibitors (MAOIs). Seizure prevention medications, **diazepam** (Valium), **phenobarbital** (Luminal, Solfoton), phenytoin (Dilantin), and propranolol (Inderal); rifampin (Rifadin, Rimactane) may also adversely react with sodium oxybate.

Resources

BOOKS

Parker, James N., and Philip N. Parker. *The Official Patient's Sourcebook on Narcolepsy.* San Diego: ICON Health, 2002.

OTHER

"Sodium Oxybate (Systemic)." *Medline Plus.* National Library of Medicine. May 13, 2004 (May 27, 2004). http://www.nlm.nih.gov/medlineplus/druginfo/uspdi/500407.html.

"Xyrem (Sodium Oxybate) Oral Solution Medication Guide." *U.S. Food and Drug Administration Center for Drug Evaluation and Research.* May 13, 2004 (May 27, 2004). http://www.fda.gov/cder/drug/infopage/xyrem/medicationguide.htm.

ORGANIZATIONS

Center for Narcolepsy. 701B Welch Road; Room 146, Palo Alto, CA 94304-5742. Phone: (650) 725-6517. Fax: (650) 725-4913. http://www-med.stanford.edu/school/Psychiatry/narcolepsy/.

Adrienne Wilmoth Lerner

Sotos syndrome

Definition

Sotos syndrome is a genetic condition causing excessive growth and a distinctive head and facial appearance. It has in the past been known as cerebral gigantism. It is often accompanied by delayed development, low muscle tone, and impaired speech.

Description

Sotos syndrome was first described in 1964 and is primarily classified as an overgrowth syndrome, which means that the individual affected with it experiences rapid growth. A number of different symptoms occur in Sotos syndrome, however, it primarily results in rapid growth beginning in the prenatal period and continuing through the infancy and toddler years and into the elementary school years. It is also strongly associated with the bones developing and maturing more quickly (advanced bone age), in a distinctive appearing face, and in developmental delay.

The excessive prenatal growth often results in the newborn being large with respect to length and head circumference; weight is usually average. The rapid growth continues through infancy and into the youth years with the child's length/height and head circumference often being above the 97th percentile, meaning that out of 100 children of the same age, the child is longer/taller and has a larger head than 97 of the children. The rate of growth appears to decrease in later childhood and adolescence and final heights tend to be within the normal ranges.

The facial features of individuals with Sotos syndrome change over time. In infants and toddlers, the face is round with the forehead being prominent and the chin small. As the child grows older and becomes an adolescent, the face becomes long with the chin being more prominent, usually with a pointed or square shape. In adults, faces are usually long and thin. The head remains large from birth through adulthood.

Hypotonia is present at birth in nearly every child with Sotos syndrome. Hypotonia means that there is significantly less tone in the muscles. Bodies with hypotonia are sometimes referred to as "floppy." Muscle tone improves as the child grows older but even in adults, it is still present to some degree. Hypotonia affects many aspects of the baby's development. It can cause difficulty in sucking and swallowing and many babies are diagnosed with failure to thrive in the newborn period. This, however, usually lasts for about three to four months and then goes away. Hypotonia makes attaining fine motor skills (grasping, playing with toys, babbling) and gross motor skills (rolling, crawling, walking) difficult and these developmental milestones are usually delayed. Speech is also affected by hypotonia but as the child grows older and the hypotonia resolves or goes away, speech improves. Although the child may have delayed development, intellect typically is borderline to normal. Special attention may be needed in certain subjects, such as reading comprehension and arithmetic. Severe **mental retardation** is rarely seen.

There are a number of other features that have been associated with Sotos syndrome including jaundice in the newborn period, coordination problems and a tendency for clumsiness. Behavioral problems and emotional immaturity are commonly reported. About half of the children with Sotos syndrome experience a seizure associated with fever. Dental problems such as early eruption of teeth, excessive wear, discoloration, and gingivitis are common. Teeth may also be aligned incorrectly due to changes in the facial structure.

Infections tend to develop in the ear, upper respiratory tract and urinary tract. In some children, hearing may be disrupted due to recurrent ear infections, and in these situations, a referral to an otolaryngologist (a doctor specializing in the ear, nose and throat) may be necessary for assessment of hearing. Urinary tract infections occur in about one out of five children with Sotos syndrome. These have been associated with structural problems of the bladder and ureters; consequently, if urinary tract infections occur, the child should undergo further evaluations.

Congenital heart problems and development of tumors have been reported in individuals with Sotos syndrome. However, information regarding the actual risks of these problems is not definitive and medical screening for these conditions is not routinely recommended.

Genetic profile

Sotos syndrome is for the most part a sporadic condition, meaning that a child affected by it did not inherit it from a parent. In a very few families, autosomal dominant inheritance has been documented, which means that both a parent and his/her child is affected by Sotos syndrome. The cause of Sotos syndrome is not known, and the gene(s) that are involved in it have not been identified.

Demographics

Sotos syndrome is described by different groups as being both "fairly common" and "rare." Incidence numbers have not been determined. Sotos syndrome occurs in both males and females and has been reported in several races and countries.

Signs and symptoms

A variety of clinical features are associated with Sotos syndrome.

- Newborns are large with respect to length and head circumference; weight is usually average. The rapid growth continues through infancy and into childhood with the child's length/height and head circumference often being above the 97th percentile. The rate of growth appears to decrease in later childhood and adolescence.
- Respiratory and feeding problems (due to hyoptonia) may develop in the neonatal period.
- Infants have a round face with prominent forehead and small chin. As the child grows into adolescence and then adulthood the face becomes long and thin, and the chin becomes more prominent.
- Hypotonia is present at birth. This affects the development of fine and gross motor skills, and developmental milestones are usually delayed. Speech is also affected by hypotonia but as the child grows older and the hypotonia resolves or goes away, speech improves.
- Intellect typically is borderline to normal.
- Behavioral problems and emotional immaturity are commonly reported.
- Dental problems such as early eruption of teeth, excessive wear, discoloration, and gingivitis are common.

Diagnosis

Diagnosis of Sotos syndrome is based upon clinical examination, medical history and x ray data. There are no laboratory tests that can provide a diagnosis. The clinical criteria that are considered to be diagnostic for Sotos syndrome are excessive growth during the prenatal and postnatal period, advanced bone age, developmental delay, and a characteristic facial appearance. It should be noted that although features suggestive of Sotos syndrome may be present at birth or within 6-12 months after birth, making a diagnosis in infancy is not clear cut and may take multiple evaluations over several years.

There are many conditions and genetic syndromes that cause excessive growth, consequently, a baby and/or child who has accelerated growth needs to be thoroughly examined by a physician knowledgeable in overgrowth and genetic syndromes. The evaluation includes asking about health problems in the family as well as asking about the growth patterns of the parents and their final height. In some families, growth patterns are different and thus may account for the child's excessive growth. The child will also undergo a complete physical examination. Additional examination of facial appearance, with special attention paid to the shape of the head, width of the face at the level of the eyes, and the appearance of the chin and forehead is necessary as well. Measurement of the head circumference, arm length, leg length, and wing span should be taken. Laboratory testing such as chromosome analysis (karyotype) may be done along with testing for another genetic syndrome called fragile-X. A bone age will also be ordered. Bone age is determined by x rays of the hand. If the child begins to lose developmental milestones or appears to stop developing, metabolic testing may be done to evaluate for a metabolic condition.

Treatment and management

There is no cure or method for preventing Sotos syndrome. However, the symptoms can be treated and managed. In the majority of cases, the symptoms developed by individuals with Sotos syndrome are treated and managed the same as in individuals in the general population. For example, physical and occupational therapy may help with muscle tone, speech therapy may improve speech, and behavioral assessments may assist with behavioral problems.

Managing the health of a child with Sotos syndrome includes regular measurements of the growth parameters, i.e. height, head circumference and weight, although excessive growth is not treated. Regular eye and dental examinations are also recommended. Medical screening for congenital heart defects and tumors is not routinely recommended, although it has been noted that symptoms should be evaluated sooner rather than later.

Prognosis

With appropriate treatment, management and encouragement, children with Sotos syndrome can

---

KEY TERMS

Advanced bone age—The bones, on x ray, appear to be those of an older individual.

Congenital—Refers to a disorder which is present at birth.

Failure to thrive—Significantly reduced or delayed physical growth.

Jaundice—Yellowing of the skin or eyes due to excess of bilirubin in the blood.

Karyotype—A standard arrangement of photographic or computer-generated images of chromosome pairs from a cell in ascending numerical order, from largest to smallest.

Tumor—An abnormal growth of cells. Tumors may be benign (noncancerous) or malignant (cancerous).

---

do well. Adults with Sotos syndrome are likely to be within the normal range for height and intellect. Sotos syndrome is not associated with a shortened life span.

Resources

BOOKS

Anderson, Rebecca Rae, and Bruce A. Buehler. *Sotos Syndrome: A Handbook for Families*. Omaha, NB: Meyer Rehabilitation Institute, 1992.

Cole, Trevor R.P. "Sotos Syndrome." In *Management of Genetic Syndromes,* edited by Suzanne B. Cassidy and Judith E. Allanson. New York: Wiley-Liss, 2001. 389–404.

WEBSITES

Family Village. http://www.familyvillage.wisc.edu/index.htmlx.

Genetic and Rare Conditions Site. http://www.kumc.edu/gec/support/.

ORGANIZATIONS

Sotos Syndrome Support Group. Three Danda Square East #235, Wheaton, IL 60187. (888) 246-SSSA or (708) 682-8815. http://www.well.com/user/sssa/.

Cindy L Hunter, CGC

Spasticity

Definition

Spasticity is a form of muscle overactivity. A spastic muscle is one in which a muscle resists being stretched out, and the resistance to stretch is increased the faster

---

the muscle is moved. Spasticity is often used as an umbrella term for other forms of muscle overactivity that often occur at the same time in the same patient.

Description

Spasticity occurs following damage to the neurons, or nerve cells, that send signals from the brain to the muscles to cause movement. These neurons, which run from the brain through the spinal cord, are called upper motor neurons, and damage to them produces an upper motor neuron syndrome. The upper motor neuron syndrome may be caused by stroke, **traumatic brain injury**, spinal cord injury, **multiple sclerosis**, or numerous other less common causes of damage to the motor neurons. Damage to the brain occurring prior to or shortly after birth is called **cerebral palsy** (CP), which is the most common cause of an upper motor neuron syndrome in children.

The other forms of muscle overactivity common in the upper motor neuron syndrome are:

• Clonus, a relatively slow rhythmic contraction and relaxation of a muscle, typically occurring after a stimulus such as movement or while attempting to hold the muscle still. Clonus can be mild or severe in intensity.

• Spasms, strong and sustained contractions of muscles, which are often painful

• Increased reflexes, in which the normal reflexes (such as knee extension in response to tapping) is greatly exaggerated.

Together, all these forms of muscle overactivity can cause significant disability in a patient, interfering with dressing, bathing, feeding, mobility, and other activities of daily living. The upper motor neuron syndrome also involves **weakness** and loss of dexterity, which may be even more disabling to the patient, and may be much less amenable to treatment.

Clinical patterns and problems

Spasticity may affect any muscle or group of muscles, but common patterns are often seen. Each causes its own set of impairments. For instance, the forearm may be drawn up and in toward the chest, making it difficult to put on or take off a shirt. The thighs may be pulled close together, not only making dressing difficult, but narrowing the base of support for standing and walking. The fingers may be clenched tight, driving the nails into the palm and preventing access for cleaning, resulting in infections and skin breakdown. One of the most common patterns is termed equinus, in which the calf muscles

tighten, preventing the ankle from flexing completely and leading to walking on the toes.

When the muscle that is overactive is also very strong, it can lead to more severe complications, including partial dislocation. Hip dislocation is a common complication of spasticity in cerebral palsy. A constant imbalance in the forces across a joint due to spasticity can cause the bone to form new tissue in response, leading to bony deformities.

Inactivity brought on by disability can lead to a host of other problems, including pressure sores, osteoporosis, respiratory infections, and social isolation.

Contracture

The resistance to stretch that characterizes spasticity may be mild and infrequent, or it may be severe and quite frequent. In the latter case, the patient can rarely attain a fully stretched position for the muscle, and the muscle spends more time than normal in a partially shortened position. When this occurs, a muscle can develop contracture. A contracture is the loss of full range of motion of a joint due to changes in the soft tissues (muscles and tendons) surrounding that joint. In contracture, the muscle fibers remodel themselves to accommodate this shorter length, thus shortening the muscle overall. In addition, the muscle may develop more fibrous tissue that cannot stretch as much, further increasing its resistance to stretch.

A muscle that develops contracture becomes almost impossible to stretch out to its full length, further worsening the clinical problems of the person with spasticity.

Treatments

Spasticity or other forms of muscle overactivity should be treated if they interfere with function, comfort, or care, or have the potential to lead to deformity that will later require treatment. Treatments available include physical therapy, oral medications, chemical denervation, intrathecal baclofen, **neurosurgery**, and orthopedic surgery.

Physical therapy

Physical therapy includes daily stretching exercises to maintain the full range of motion for the affected muscles. In mild spasticity, this may be the only treatment needed, while in severe spasticity, it is a part of the full therapy plan. Physical therapy also includes instructions in how to perform activities that are energy-efficient and do not worsen spasticity, including ways to transfer in and out of bed, sitting positions, and hygiene activities.

Bracing may be used to support a weak muscle or to prevent excess contraction of a spastic muscle. A knee-ankle-foot brace is common to help correct equinus, for instance. Serial casting may be used to stretch out a contracted muscle, with a series of casts at increasing joint angles applied over time. The physical therapist also provides advice on assistive equipment such as wheelchairs and walkers.

Oral medications

Four main medications are used to treat spasticity and other forms of muscle overactivity. Each causes sedation, and thus their uses are limited in patients for whom excess sedation is a significant problem. Oral medications are typically most useful in patients with mild, widespread spasticity, or those for whom sedation is not a problem. They may also be useful at night, to improve comfort during sleep.

Benzodiazepines include **diazepam** and clonazepam. They are most commonly used in spinal cord injury and multiple sclerosis and may be especially effective against painful spasms. They also reduce anxiety, which may be useful in some patients. Typical side effects include weakness, sedation, and confusion.

Oral baclofen is primarily used for patients with spinal cord injury or multiple sclerosis (MS). A special caution with baclofen is that sudden withdrawal may cause seizures and hallucinations. Tizanidine is also used widely in those with spinal cord injury or MS, and is also used in other patients. It is less likely to cause weakness than some other oral medications.

Dantrolene sodium is used for patients with stroke, cerebral palsy, MS, and spinal cord injury. It is somewhat less likely to cause confusion and sedation than other medications, and may be more effective against clonus than some of the other medications. Diarrhea is a side effect in some patients, and monitoring for liver damage is required.

In rare cases, a pump may be inserted into the spinal fluid to directly deliver medicine to the nervous system.

Chemodenervation

Chemodenervation refers to use of a chemical to prevent a nerve from stimulating its target muscle. This reduces spasticity. Chemodenervation is performed with phenol, ethyl alcohol, or **botulinum toxin**. Chemodenervation is most appropriate in patients with localized spasticity in one or two large muscles or several small muscles.

Phenol and ethyl alcohol are injected directly onto the nerve, causing the nerve fiber to degenerate so that it cannot send messages to the muscle. Benefits may last from one month to six months or more, when the nerve regrows. Advantages of the procedure are that the chemicals are inexpensive and can be used repeatedly. Disadvantages are that the injection requires a high degree of skill, may cause pain due to damage to nerves carrying sensory information, and has a somewhat unpredictable duration of action.

Botulinum toxin is injected into the overactive muscle. It prevents the nerve endings from releasing the chemical they use to stimulate the muscle. The effect lasts approximately three months. Benefits include a simpler and easier injection procedure, with more predictable and reproducible results, with no risk of pain. Disadvantages include high cost and the potential to develop antibodies against the toxin after repeat injections, rendering it ineffective.

Intrathecal baclofen

Intrathecal baclofen (ITB) delivers baclofen directly to the spinal cord, via a tube from an implanted pump. It is most commonly used in patients with widespread spasticity, especially children with cerebral palsy. The pump is implanted in the wall of the abdomen, and the tube is inserted between the vertebrae in the lower or mid-back, releasing the drug into the space surrounding the spinal cord. This allows a much smaller amount of baclofen to be used than if delivered orally, reducing side effects. The baclofen is contained in a reservoir within the pump, and is refilled approximately every three months. The dose can be adjusted to match activities, for instance, increasing at night to aid sleep and decreasing in the morning to increase stiffness slightly to aid getting out of bed. Risks include pump failure and sudden withdrawal from baclofen, which can be dangerous or even fatal, as well as surgery and anesthesia risks. Benefits include reduced spasticity without excess sedation.

Neurosurgery

Selective dorsal rhizotomy (SDR) is used to treat spasticity in cerebral palsy. During SDR, certain overactive nerves entering the spinal cord are cut, reducing the activity that leads to spasticity. Children receiving SDR tend to be able to walk more normally, assuming they have good underlying strength before the operation. SDR is a major surgery requiring general anesthesia. Long-term results indicate children receiving SDR require slightly fewer orthopedic surgeries later in life.

Griggs, R., R. Jozefowicz, and M. Aminoff. "Chapter 418: Approach to the Patient with Neurologic Disease." In *Cecil Medicine*, 23rd ed., edited by L. Goldman and D. Ausiello. Philadelphia: Saunders Elsevier, 2007.

Hammerstad J. "Strength and Reflexes." In *Chapter 15: Textbook of Clinical Neurology*, 3rd ed., edited by C.G. Goetz. Philadelphia: Saunders Elsevier, 2007.

KEY TERMS

Equinus—Excess contraction of the calf, causing toe walking.

PERIODICALS

Ada, Louise, et al. "Muscle strengthening in children and adolescents with spastic cerebral palsy: considerations for future resistance training protocols." *Physical Therapy* (July 2011): 1130.

Anderson, Lisa C., et al. "Clinical measurement of limb spasticity in adults: state of the science." *Journal of Neuroscience Nursing* (April 2011): 104.

Hugos, Cinda. "MS Spasticity: Take Control!" *Paraplegia News* 64.12 (2010): 40.

Logan, Lynne Romeiser. "Rehabilitation techniques to maximize spasticity management." *Topics in Stroke Rehabilitation* 18.3 (2011): 203.

ORGANIZATIONS

Worldwide Education and Awareness for Movement Disorders (WE MOVE), 5731 Mosholu Avenue, Bronx, NY 10471, (347) 843-6132, Fax: (718) 601-5112, wemove@wemove.org, http://www.wemove.org.

Orthopedic surgery

This type of surgery is performed on muscle or bone, in order to correct deformity, including contracture. The most common surgery is tendon lengthening to treat equinus. In this procedure, the Achilles tendon is cut and the leg is placed in a cast in a more normal position. The tendon regrows to a longer length, reducing the equinus. Other tendon lengthening procedures are performed at the hips and knees. An osteotomy may also be performed to remove abnormal bone growth.

Spasticity and Botox

Botox injections may help relieve spasticity symptoms in some patients. Botox was first approved by the Food and Drug Administration (FDA) over 20 years ago. Botox is a prescription-only medical product that contains tiny amounts of highly purified botulinum toxin protein from the bacterium, *Clostridium botulinum*. Botox has a unique, protected molecular structure that stabilizes the core toxin in Botox from degradation. When injected into muscles, it diffuses locally and produces temporary reduction in the overacting muscle or gland, usually lasting up to approximately 3 to 6.7 months depending on the individual patient and indication.

In 2010, the FDA approved the use of Botox (onabotulinumtoxinA) for the treatment of increased muscle stiffness in the elbow, wrist, and fingers in adults with upper limb spasticity. Spasticity impacts approximately 1 million Americans, many of whom suffer from spasticity in the upper limbs following a stroke.

Allergan, the manufacturer of Botox, has conducted multiple studies evaluating the use of Botox to treat upper limb spasticity, including three double-blind, placebo-controlled studies, two of which were published in the *New England Journal of Medicine* and *Archives of Physical and Medical Rehabilitation*.

Resources

BOOKS

Brashear, Allison, and Elie Elovic. *Spasticity: Diagnosis and Management*. New York: Demos Medical, 2010.

Espay, Alberto J. and José Biller. *Concise Neurology*. Philadelphia: Lippincott Williams & Wilkins, 2011.

Richard Robinson
Karl Finley

SPECT scan *see* **Single proton emission computed tomography**

Speech synthesizer

Definition

A speech synthesizer is a computerized device that accepts input, interprets data, and produces audible language.

It is capable of translating any text, predefined input, or controlled nonverbal body movement into audible speech. Such inputs may include text from a computer document, coordinated action such as keystrokes on a computer keyboard, simple action such as directional interpretation of a joystick, or basic functions such as eye, head, or foot movement.

Purpose

According to a study by the American Speech and Hearing Association, approximately 1.5 million people in the United States are unable to communicate through vocal language; this number does not include hearing impaired. A speech synthesizer can provide an electronic means of verbal communication for individuals who are unable to speak or have visual impairments. Since spoken language is the primary means of communication in most societies, it is often essential for people who are unable to speak on their own to capture that ability.

Individuals with motor neuron disease (MND) often lose their ability to speak due to weakened vocal cords. MND is a classification for disorders that cause muscle **weakness** and wasting such as **amyotrophic lateral sclerosis** (ALS), progressive bulbar palsy (PBP), **primary lateral sclerosis** (PLS), and progressive muscular atrophy (PMA). In patients with **cerebral palsy**, the area of the brain controlling vocal muscles is damaged resulting in speech loss.

Speech synthesizers can also be useful for people who are visually impaired. Although they may be able to produce oral speech, they are unable to read or produce written text in a non-Braille format. In the example of a student who is visually impaired, the ability to take notes during a lecture and to then review those notes later is not possible. However, with a speech synthesizer, the student can type lecture notes into a laptop and have a text-to-speech software program read them back for review and revision. Without this technology, the more time-consuming method of transcribing audio-recorded lectures into Braille is used.

Precautions

There are many considerations involved in selecting a method for speech synthesis. Key factors are the type of technology used, costs, and equipment. Technology can be overpriced or can quickly become obsolete. When considering the purchase of a speech synthesizer, it is important to determine the reliability of the manufacturer as well as policies regarding maintenance and upgrades of equipment or software. The most cost-effective tools are a laptop computer equipped with appropriate software and hardware. Unfortunately, many insurance companies will not cover the purchase of speech synthesizers or related assistive communication devices.

Description

There are many technologies involved in the production of speech with speech synthesizers. The two most definitive segments are how the user inputs information to be spoken and how the sounds for the words are actually interpreted and produced.

The first step to produce the speech is the composition of text to be spoken. In some cases, it is as simple as loading a computer text file into a software program. In other cases, a more complicated input system is required.

There are many different input devices, but the most prevalent is a keyboard or other similar typing board (such as a touchscreen). Patients with severe mobility restrictions may instead use a joystick device. Special input devices are created that act as switches. These switches are programmed to accept and decipher the motions of the user, even blinking of the eyes. Essentially any muscular movement can be interpreted as a switch and programmed to produce language.

The second step is deciphering the input and producing the desired audio speech. Data are gathered or assembled through the input device until the user indicates that the information is complete. The computer then interprets and speaks the words, phrases, or sentences. Complicated logic is involved when translating written text into spoken language. For example, there are many words that are spelled the same, but pronounced differently in different contexts. The software must make that determination.

Depending on the device, multiple shortcuts may be available to the user. Examples include:

- storing phrases or sentences to reuse at a later time
- translation of abbreviations such as ASAP, which can also be programmed to speak the full phrase, i.e., "as soon as possible"
- software programs that "guess" what the user wants to say and predicts the output as input is gathered; if correct, the user can acknowledge the completion, thereby speeding up the entry of data

Preparation

Even with the advanced technology available for speech synthesizers, a bottleneck of information often occurs with the input. A typical spoken conversation takes place at a rate of 150–200 words per minute. While some individuals can become proficient at touch-typing, allowing for greater success with interactive conversations, many individuals are challenged to produce even 15 words per minute with communication devices.

The typical setup for individuals who use a computer or touchscreen includes a computer, keyboard, monitor, and speakers. In many cases, this equipment can be attached to a wheelchair or bed frame, allowing the user access to "speech" at any time. Other users may simply carry a laptop, batteries, and the necessary connection cables.

For those users unable to manipulate a computer or keyboard-style input device, there is a period of learning and acclamation required to become accustom to the switch-style inputs. The user must learn how to complete the step-by-step process of composing thoughts into text for output.

A major challenge for individuals who are visually impaired is the presence of graphics in text. Because graphics typically lack a textual equivalent, they are not recognized and spoken by the synthesizer. This may cause the user to miss some information on the screen.

Aftercare

Once an individual has selected a speech synthesis device, there is little follow-up necessary. Hardware and software updates frequently evolve and so there is potential to upgrade devices periodically. Depending on the underlying cause of speech loss, some patients may need to change devices as they lose or regain the ability to speak or move.

Normal results

Through a speech synthesizer, nonvocal users can communicate with spoken words and people who are visually impaired can hear written text. The challenge of becoming proficient with these devices may be greater for some individuals based on physical restrictions.

Resources

BOOKS

Holmes, John, and Wendy Holmes. *Speech Synthesis and Recognition*, 2nd ed. New York: Taylor & Francis, 2002.

PERIODICALS

Sasso, Len. "Voices from the Machine." *Electronic Musician* February 1, 2004.

WEBSITES

Maxey, H. David. "Smithsonian Speech Synthesis History Project." *National Museum of Natural History, Smithsonian Institute*. July 1, 2002 (cited March 23, 2003 [June 3, 2004]). http://www.mindspring.com/~sshp/ssshp_cd/dk_779.htm#V.
Olshan, Michael. "Voice Lessons: Speaking with ALS." *American Speech-Language-Hearing Association*. 2004 (cited March 23,2004 [June 3, 2004]). http://www.asha.org/public/speech/disorders/als-voice-lessons-speaking-with-als.htm.

"What is MND?" *Motor Neuron Diesease Association*. March 26, 2004 (cited March 26, 2004 [June 3, 2004]). http://www.mndassociation.org/full-site/what/index.htm.

ORGANIZATIONS

American Speech-Language-Hearing Association. 10801 Rockville Pike, Bethesda, MD 20852. Tollfree phone: (800) 638-8255. Email: actioncenter@asha.org. http://www.asha.org.
Motor Neuron Disease Association. P.O. Box 246, Northampton, United Kingdom NN1 2PR. Phone: 01604 250505. Fax: 01604 638289/624726. Email: enquiries@mndassociation.org. http://www.mndassociation.org.

Stacey L. Chamberlin

Spina bifida

Definition

Spina bifida belongs to a group of disorders known as neural tube defects (NTDs). It is a serious birth abnormality characterized by the incomplete development of the brain, spinal cord, and/or **meninges**.

Demographics

According to the National Institute of Neurological Disorders and Stroke (NINDS), spina bifida is the most common neural tube defect (NTD) in the United States, affecting 1,500 to 2,000 of the more than 4 million babies born each year. The Centers for Disease Control and Prevention (CDC) reports that NTDs are more common among white women than black women and more common among Hispanic women than non–Hispanic women.

Spina bifida occurs worldwide, but there has been a steady downward trend in occurrence rates over the past 50–70 years, particularly in regions of high prevalence. The highest prevalence rates, about one in 200 pregnancies, have been reported in certain northern provinces in China. Intermediate prevalence rates, about one in 1,000 pregnancies, have been found in Central and South America. The lowest prevalence rates, less than one in 2,000 pregnancies, have been found in European countries.

Description

Spina bifida is also known by the name spinal dysraphism. Spina bifida may appear in the body midline anywhere from the neck to the buttocks. In its most severe form, termed spinal rachischisis, the entire spinal canal is open, exposing the spinal cord and nerves. More commonly, the abnormality appears as a localized mass on the back that is covered by skin or by the meninges, the three–layered membrane that surrounds the spinal cord. Spina bifida is usually readily apparent at birth because of the malformation of the back and paralysis below the level of the abnormality.

Names of various forms of spina bifida are meningomyelocele, myelomeningocele, spina bifida aperta, open spina bifida, myelodysplasia, spinal dysraphism, spinal rachischisis, myelocele, and meningocele. The term meningocele is used when the spine malformation contains only the protective covering (meninges) of the spinal cord. The other terms indicate involvement of the spinal cord and nerves in the malformation. A related term, spina bifida occulta, indicates that one or more of the bony bodies in the spine are incompletely hardened but that there is no abnormality of the spinal cord itself.

Risk factors

In the United States, 95% of neural tube defects (NTDs) occur in women with no family history of these conditions. The CDC outlines some of the risk factors associated with NTDs and by extension, with spina bifida. They include the occurrence of a previous NTD–affected pregnancy or of maternal insulin–dependent diabetes as well as the use of certain anticonvulsant medications (such as Valproic acid/Depakene, and Carbamazapine/Tegretol). Medically diagnosed obesity is also considered a risk factor. The recurrence risk after the birth of an infant with isolated spina bifida is 3–5%. Recurrence may be for spina bifida or another type of spinal abnormality.

Causes and symptoms

Spina bifida occurs because the neural tube, around the area of the spine, fails to close during fetal development. Spina bifida may occur as an isolated abnormality or in the company of other malformations. As an isolated abnormality, spina bifida is caused by the combination of genetic factors and environmental influences that bring about malformation of the spine and spinal column. The specific genes and environmental influences that contribute to the many–factored causes of spina bifida are not precisely known. An insufficiency of folic acid is known to be one influential nutritional factor. Changes (mutations) in genes involving the metabolism of folic acid are believed to be significant genetic risk factors.

Spina bifida may arise because of chromosome abnormalities, single gene mutations, or specific environmental insults such as maternal diabetes mellitus or prenatal exposure to certain anticonvulsant drugs. The recurrence risk varies with each of these specific causes.

In most cases, spina bifida is obvious at birth because of malformation of the spine. The spine may be completely open, exposing the spinal cord and nerves. More commonly, the spine abnormality appears as a mass on the back covered by membrane (meninges) or skin. Spina bifida may occur anywhere from the base of the skull to the buttocks. About 75% of abnormalities occur in the lower back (lumbar) region. In rare instances, the spinal cord malformation may occur internally, sometimes with a connection to the gastrointestinal tract.

In spina bifida, many complications arise, dependent in part on the level and severity of the spine malformation. As a rule, the nerves below the level of the abnormality develop in a faulty manner and fail to function, resulting in paralysis and loss of sensation below the level of the spine malformation. Since most abnormalities occur in the lumbar region, the lower limbs are paralyzed and lack sensation. Furthermore, the bowel and bladder have inadequate nerve connections, causing an inability to control bowel and bladder function. Most infants also develop hydrocephaly, an accumulation of excess fluid in the four cavities of the brain. At least one of every seven cases develop findings of Chiari II malformation, a condition in which the lower part of the brain is crowded and may be forced into the upper part of the spinal cavity.

There are a number of mild variant forms of spina bifida, including multiple vertebral abnormalities, skin dimples, tufts of hair, and localized areas of skin deficiency over the spine. Two variants, lipomeningocele and lipomyelomeningocele, typically occur in the lower back area (lumbar or sacral) of the spine. In these conditions, a tumor of fatty tissue becomes isolated among the nerves below the spinal cord, which may result in tethering of the spinal cord and complications similar to those with open spina bifida.

Diagnosis

Examination

Few disorders are to be confused with open spina bifida. The diagnosis is usually obvious based on the external findings at birth. Paralysis below the level of the abnormality and fluid on the brain (hydrocephaly) may contribute to the diagnosis. Other spine abnormalities such as congenital scoliosis and kyphosis, or soft tissue tumors overlying the spine, are not likely to have these accompanying findings. In cases in which there are no external findings, the diagnosis is more difficult and may not become evident until neurological abnormalities or hydrocephaly develop weeks, months, or years following birth.

Tests

Prenatal diagnosis may be made in most cases with ultrasound examination after 12–14 weeks of pregnancy. Ultrasounds cannot identify every structural problem in a developing baby, so some cases of spina bifida (especially mild forms) may be missed. However, it is a risk–free method to use that gives immediate results.

Prenatal blood screening is often offered to women between 15 and 21 weeks in a pregnancy. This screening measures the levels of various chemicals naturally found in a mother's blood, including alpha-fetoprotein (AFP). For this reason, the screening is often called AFP screening. AFP is a protein normally made by a developing fetus, so it is naturally present in maternal serum and called MS-AFP. When a fetus has spina bifida, the levels of MS-AFP may be higher than usual because it leaks out of the hole in the spine. If a woman's AFP screen comes back abnormal with a high MS–AFP value, she often is at a higher risk for having a baby with spina bifida. This may prompt her physician to offer her a detailed ultrasound, as well as other medical options that might give her more information about the baby.

Once spina bifida is seen outwardly, imaging scans like x rays, ultrasound, magnetic resonance imaging (MRI), or computed tomography (CT) can be helpful to see the extent of it. It is also a good way to identify whether someone has associated neurological complications like hydrocephalus.

Some genetic testing, like chromosome studies, may identify a diagnosis or cause for the spina bifida. Abnormal genetic test results cannot be changed or reversed, but may provide answers about why the spina bifida occurred.

Procedures

One option to find spina bifida is a procedure called amniocentesis. Amniocentesis involves removing a small amount of fluid from around the baby, using a fine needle. This fluid naturally contains AFP, which may also be elevated if the baby has spina bifida. There is a small risk of miscarriage, about 1 in 200, with this procedure. As such, every women usually receives proper counseling through their doctor or a genetic counselor before having the test done.

Treatment

There is no known cure for spina bifida. Treatment primarily focuses on dealing with symptoms as they arise, since they vary so greatly from person to person.

Traditional

Aggressive surgical and medical management have improved the survival and function of infants with spina bifida. Initial surgery may be carried out during the first days of life, providing protection against injury and infection. Subsequent surgery is often necessary to protect against excessive curvature of the spine, and in the presence of hydrocephaly, to place a mechanical shunt to decrease the pressure and amount of cerebrospinal fluid in the cavities of the brain. Because of **weakness** or paralysis below the level of the spine abnormality, most children require physical therapy, bracing, and other orthopedic assistance to enable them to walk. A variety of approaches including periodic bladder

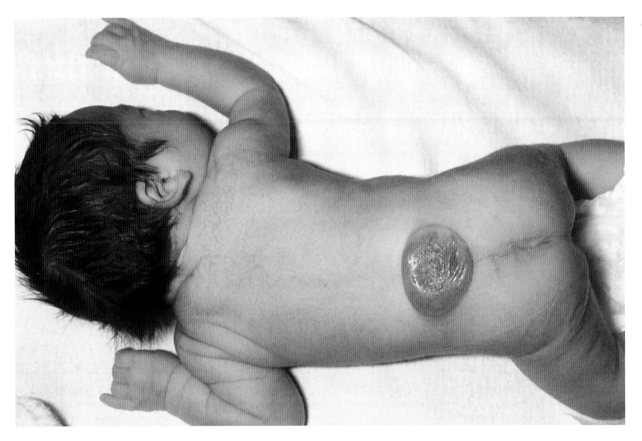

An infant with spina bifida. (© *Custom Medical Stock Photo, Inc. Reproduced by permission.*)

catheterization, surgical diversion of urine, and antibiotics are used to protect urinary function.

Although most individuals with spina bifida have normal intellectual function, learning disabilities or mental impairment does occur. This may result, in part, from hydrocephaly and/or infections of the nervous system. Children so affected may benefit from early educational intervention, physical therapy, and occupational therapy. Counseling to improve self-image and lessen barriers to socialization becomes important in late childhood and adolescence.

Drugs

Medications are widely available to treat those who develop seizures, and these may need periodic adjustments. Those who have problems with bowel or bladder control may also require medications.

Alternative

Open fetal surgery has been performed for spina bifida during the last half of pregnancy. After direct closure of the spine malformation, the fetus is returned to the womb. By preventing chronic intrauterine exposure to mechanical and chemical trauma, prenatal surgery improves neurological function and leads to fewer complications after birth. Fetal surgery is considered experimental, and results have been mixed.

Prognosis

Prognosis in spina bifida is extremely varied and unpredictable. Years ago with far less intervention and fewer treatments available, someone with severe spina bifida had a high chance of dying from complications. Today, more than 80% of infants born with spina bifida survive with surgical and medical management. Although complications from paralysis, hydrocephaly, Chiari II malformation, and urinary tract deterioration threaten the well-being of the survivors, the outlook for normal intellectual function is good.

Prevention

Prevention of isolated spina bifida and other spinal abnormalities has become possible during recent decades. The major prevention is through the use of the

B vitamin folic acid for several months prior to and following conception. The CDC recommends the intake of 400 micrograms of synthetic folic acid every day for all women of childbearing years.

Resources

BOOKS

Appelmann, Larry E. *Living with Spina Bifida: Speaking Out About My Disability*. Victoria, BC: Trafford, 2006.

Lutkenhoff, Marlene, editor. *Children with Spina Bifida: A Parents' Guide*, 2nd ed. Bethesda, MD: Woodbine House, 2007.

The Official Parent's Sourcebook on Spina Bifida: A Revised and Updated Directory for the Internet Age. San Diego, CA: ICON Health Publications, 2003.

Sandler, Adrian. *Living with Spina Bifida: A Guide for Families and Professionals*. Chapel Hill University of North Carolina Press, 20039.

Watson, Stephanie. *Spina Bifida*. New York: Rosen, 2008.

PERIODICALS

Dennis, M., et al. "Upper limb motor function in young adults with spina bifida and hydrocephalus." *Child's Nervous System* 25, no. 11 (November 2009): 1447–1453.

Dicianno, B. E., et al. "Mobility, assistive technology use, and social integration among adults with spina bifida." *American Journal of Physical Medicine & Rehabilitation* 88, no. 7 (July 2009): 533–41.

Holmbeck, G. N., et al. "Family functioning in children and adolescents with spina bifida: an evidence–based review of research and interventions." *Journal of Developmental and Behavioral Pediatrics* 27, no. 3 (June 2006): 249–77.

Jandasek, B., et al. "Trajectories of family processes across the adolescent transition in youth with spina bifida" *Journal of Family Psychology* 23, no. 5 (October 2009): 726–38.

Van Der Vossen, S. et al. "Role of prenatal ultrasound in predicting survival and mental and motor functioning in children with spina bifida." *Ultrasound in Obstetrics & Gynecology* 34, no. 3 (September 2009): 253–58.

OTHER

"FAQ About Spina Bifida." *Spina Bifida Association*. Information Page. http://www.spinabifidaassociation. org/site/c.liKWL7PLLrF/b.2642327/k.5899/FAQ_About_Spina_Bifida.htm (accessed October 25, 2009)

"Spina Bifida." *NICHCY*. Information Page. http://www.nichcy.org/Disabilities/Specific/Pages/SpinaBifida.aspx (accessed October 27, 2009)

"Spina Bifida." *Medline Plus*. Health Topic. http://www.nlm.nih.gov/medlineplus/spinabifida.html (accessed October 27, 2009)

"Spina Bifida Fact Sheet." *NINDS*. Information Page. http://www.ninds.nih.gov/disorders/spina_bifida/detail_spina_bifida.htm (accessed October 27, 2009)

ORGANIZATIONS

Disabled Sports USA, 451 Hungerford Drive, Suite 100, Rockville, MD, 20850, (301) 217-0960, Fax: (301) 217-0968, dsusa@dsusa.org, http://www.dsusa.org.

March of Dimes Foundation, 1275 Mamaroneck Avenue, White Plains, NY, 10605, (914) 428-7100, (888) MODIMES, Fax: (914) 428-8203, askus@marchofdimes.com, http://www.marchofdimes.com.

National Dissemination Center for Children with Disabilities (NICHCY), PO Box 1492, Washington, DC, 20013-1492, (800) 695-0285, Fax: (202) 884-8441, nichcy@aed.org, http://www.nichcy.org.

National Institute of Neurological Disorders and Stroke (NINDS), PO Box 5801, Bethesda, MD, 20824, (301) 496-5751, (800) 352-9424, http://www.ninds.nih.gov.

Spina Bifida Association of America, 4590 MacArthur Blvd. NW, Suite 250, Washington, DC, 20007-4266, (202) 944-3285, (800) 621-3141, Fax: (202) 944-3295, sbaa@ sbaa.org, http://www.spinabifida association.org.

Deepti Babu, MS, CGC
Roger E. Stevenson, MD
Monique Laberge, PhD

Spinal cord infarction

Definition

Spinal cord infarction (sometimes called spinal stroke) refers to injury to the spinal cord due to oxygen deprivation.

Description

Spinal cord infarction occurs when one of the three major arteries that supply blood (and therefore oxygen) to the spinal cord is blocked. As a result of such an occlusion, the spinal cord is deprived of oxygen, resulting in injury and destruction of the very vulnerable nerve fibers. The resulting disability will depend on what level of the spinal cord suffers the injury; everything below the area of the occlusion will be affected.

Demographics

Spinal cord infarction is a relatively rare condition, affecting about 12 in 100,000 people in the population.

Causes and symptoms

A variety of conditions can result in occlusion of the spinal arteries and spinal cord infarction:

• atherosclerosis of the aorta
• a dissecting aortic aneurysm (as well as surgical accidents that occur when clipping aortic aneurysms)
• a tumor or abscess impinging on an artery
• blockages in smaller blood vessels due to diabetes, polyarteritis nodosa, systemic lupus erythematosus, neurosyphilis, tuberculous meningitis, pneumococcal meningitis
• severe low blood pressure
• blood clots
• vasculitis

Rare cases of spinal cord infarction have resulted from conditions that exert pressure on the spine (pregnancy, back injury, exercise), resulting in the core of a spinal disc (nucleus pulposus) extruding out of the disc and entering into a spinal artery, resulting in a blockage of blood flow.

Depending on the mechanism underlying spinal cord infarction, the symptoms may begin abruptly and acutely or slowly and gradually. Specific symptoms depend on where in the spinal cord the infarction occurs. Symptoms can include pain; **paraplegia**; quadriplegia; initially limp, floppy muscles that become tightly contracted (spastic) over the next several days; initial loss of reflexes, which become overactive (hyperreflexia) over the next several days; loss of the sense of pain and temperature; loss of bladder and bowel control.

Diagnosis

Diagnosis is often made by excluding other conditions that might account for the patient's symptoms. Although many tests will not actually reveal spinal cord infarction as the reason for a patient's loss of function, it is important that a variety of tests are performed in order to search for potentially reversible causes of disability. MRI scanning may be helpful in this effort; it may not actually reveal images indicative of spinal cord infarction, however.

Treatment team

Individuals with spinal cord infarction are usually cared for by neurologists, physiatrists, physical therapists, and occupational therapists. Complications of spinal cord infarction may require consultation with urologists and pulmonologists.

Treatment

Once an individual has suffered a spinal cord infarction, there are no treatments that will reverse the damage. Some degree of functioning may return as the acute inflammation decreases. Underlying conditions that may have predisposed the individual to spinal cord infarction should certainly be addressed and treated.

Recovery and rehabilitation

Rehabilitation will involve teaching the individual new ways of being as independent as possible, based on the new limitations rendered by the disabilities of spinal cord infarction. The efforts of physical and occupational therapists are crucial in this endeavor.

Prognosis

The prognosis of spinal cord infarction tends to be very poor. There is a high risk of death, either during the acute phase of infarction or over the long term, particularly due to blood clots in the lungs (pulmonary emboli) or infection of bladder, lungs, or skin ulcerations secondary to inactivity and debilitation. Disability is significant, with a risk of paraplegia or quadriplegia.

Special concerns

The sudden loss of normal functioning and independence that can occur due to spinal cord infarction can prompt severe **depression**. Supportive psychotherapy can be an important adjunctive aid to optimal recovery.

Resources

BOOKS

Hauser, Stephen L. "Diseases of the Spinal Cord." In *Harrison's Principles of Internal Medicine*, edited by Eugene Braunwald, et al. New York: McGraw-Hill Professional, 2001.
Perron, Andrew D., and J. Stephen Huff. "Spinal Cord Disorders." In *Rosen's Emergency Medicine: Concepts and Clinical Practice*, 5th ed., edited by Lee Goldman, et al. St. Louis: Mosby, 2002.

KEY TERMS

Aneurysm—A weakness and ballooning of the wall of an artery, which can burst with potentially catastrophic ramifications.

Aorta—The major artery that carries oxygenated blood from the heart to be delivered by arteries throughout the body.

Atherosclerosis—A disease in which fatty deposits line the blood vessel walls, eventually threatening to block blood flow.

Infarction—Tissue injury and death due to blocked blood flow and oxygen delivery.

Occlusion—Blockage.

Vasculitis—A condition in which inflammation of the blood vessels sometimes interferes with normal blood flow to various organs and tissues.

Pryse-Phillips, William, and T. Jock Murray. "Infectious diseases of the nervous system." In *Noble: Textbook of Primary Care Medicine*, edited by John Noble, et al. St. Louis: W. B. Saunders, 2001.

WEBSITES

National Institute of Neurological Disorders and Stroke (NINDS). *NINDS Spinal Cord Infarction Information Page.* January 28, 2003. http://www.ninds.nih.gov/health_and_medical/disorders/spinal_infarction.htm (June 3, 2004).

ORGANIZATIONS

Christopher Reeve Paralysis Foundation / Paralysis Resource Center. 500 Morris Avenue , Springfield, NJ 07081 . Phone: 973-379-2690 . Fax: 973-912-9433 . Tollfree phone: 800-225-0292 . Email: info@crpf.org; research@crpf.org. http://www.christopherreeve.org.

National Spinal Cord Injury Association. 6701 Democracy Blvd. #300-9, Bethesda, MD 20817. Phone: 301-214-4006. Fax: 301-881-9817. Tollfree phone: 800-962-9629. Email: info@spinalcord.org. http://www.spinalcord.org.

Rosalyn Carson-DeWitt, MD

▌Spinal cord injury

Definition

Spinal cord injury is damage to the spinal cord that causes loss of sensation and motor control.

Description

Approximately 10,000 new spinal cord injuries (SCIs) occur each year in the United States. About 250,000 people are currently affected. Spinal cord injuries can happen to anyone at any time of life; however, the typical patient is a man between the ages of 19 and 26, injured in a motor vehicle accident (about 50% of all SCIs), a fall (20%), an act of violence (15%), or a sporting accident (14%). Alcohol or other drug abuse plays an important role in a large percentage of all spinal cord injuries. Six percent of people who receive injuries to the lower spine die within a year, and 40% of people who receive the more frequent higher spine injuries die within a year.

Short-term costs for hospitalization, equipment, and home modifications are approximately $140,000 for an SCI patient capable of independent living. Lifetime costs may exceed one million dollars. Costs may be three to four times higher for the SCI patient who needs long-term institutional care. Overall costs to the American economy in direct payments and lost productivity are more than $10 billion per year.

Causes and symptoms

Causes

The spinal cord is about as big around as the index finger. It descends from the brain down the back through hollow channels of the backbone. The spinal cord is made of nerve cells (neurons). The nerve cells carry sensory data from the areas outside the spinal cord (periphery) to the brain, and they carry motor commands from brain to periphery. Peripheral neurons are bundled together to make up the 31 pairs of peripheral nerve roots. The peripheral nerve roots enter and exit the spinal cord by passing through the spaces between the stacked vertebrae. Each pair of nerves is named for the vertebra from which it exits. These are named as follows:

- C1–8: these nerves enter from the eight cervical or neck vertebrae.
- T1–12: these nerves enter from the thoracic or chest vertebrae.
- L1–5: these nerves enter from the lumbar vertebrae of the lower back.
- S1–5: these nerves enter through the sacral or pelvic vertebrae.
- Coccygeal: these nerves enter through the coccyx or tailbone.

Peripheral nerves carry motor commands to the muscles and internal organs, and they carry sensations from these areas and from the body's surface. (Sensory data from the head, including sight, sound, smell, and taste, do not pass through the spinal cord and are not affected by most SCIs.) Damage to the spinal cord interrupts these signals. The interruption damages motor functions that allow the muscles to move, sensory functions such as feeling heat and cold, and autonomic functions such as urination, sexual function, sweating, and blood pressure.

Spinal cord injuries most often occur where the spine is most flexible, in the regions of C5–C7 of the neck, and T10–L2 at the base of the rib cage. Several physically distinct types of damage are recognized. Sudden and violent jolts to nearby tissues can jar the cord. This jarring causes a temporary spinal concussion. Concussion symptoms usually disappear completely within several hours. A spinal contusion or bruise is bleeding within the spinal column. The pressure from the excess fluid may kill spinal cord neurons. Spinal compression is caused by some object, such as a tumor, pressing on the cord. Lacerations or tears cause direct damage to cord neurons. Lacerations can be caused by bone fragments or missiles such as bullets. Spinal transection describes the complete severing of the cord. Most spinal cord injuries involve two or more of these types of damage.

Symptoms

PARALYSIS AND LOSS OF SENSATION. The extent to which movement and sensation are damaged depends on the level of the spinal cord injury. Nerves leaving the spinal cord at different levels control sensation and movement in different parts of the body. The distribution is roughly as follows:

- C1–C4: head and neck
- C3–C5: diaphragm (chest and breathing)
- C5–T1: shoulders, arms, and hands
- T2–T12: chest and abdomen (excluding internal organs)
- L1–L4: abdomen (excluding internal organs), buttocks, genitals, and upper legs
- L4–S1: legs
- S2–S4: genitals and muscles of the perineum

Damage below T1, which lies at the base of the rib cage, causes paralysis and loss of sensation in the legs and trunk below the injury. Injury at this level usually does no damage to the arms and hands. Paralysis of the legs is called paraplegia. Damage above T1 involves the arms as well as the legs. Paralysis of all four limbs is called quadriplegia or tetraplegia. Cervical or neck injuries not only cause quadriplegia but also may cause difficulty in breathing. Damage in the lower part of the neck may leave enough diaphragm control to allow unassisted breathing. Patients with damage at C3 or above, just below the base of the skull, require mechanical assistance to breathe.

Symptoms also depend on the extent of spinal cord injury. A completely severed cord causes paralysis and loss of sensation below the wound. If the cord is only partially severed, some function will remain below the injury. Damage limited to the front portion of the cord causes paralysis and loss of sensations of pain and temperature. Other sensation may be preserved. Damage to the center of the cord may spare the legs but paralyze the arms. Damage to the right or left half causes loss of position sense, paralysis on the side of the injury, and loss of pain and temperature sensation on the opposite side.

DEEP VENOUS THROMBOSIS. Blood does not flow normally to a paralyzed limb that is inactive for long periods. The blood pools in the deep veins and forms clots, a condition known as deep vein thrombosis. A clot or thrombus can break free and lodge in smaller arteries in the brain, causing a stroke, or in the lungs, causing pulmonary embolism.

PRESSURE ULCERS. Inability to move also leads to pressure ulcers or bed sores. Pressure ulcers form where skin remains in contact with a bed or chair for a long time. The most common sites of pressure ulcers are the buttocks, hips, and heels.

SPASTICITY AND CONTRACTURE. A paralyzed limb is incapable of active movement, but the muscle still has tone, a constant low level of contraction. Normal muscle tone requires communication between the muscle and the brain. Spinal cord injury prevents the brain from telling the muscle to relax. The result is prolonged muscle contraction or spasticity. Because the muscles that extend and those that bend a joint are not usually equal in strength, the involved joint is bent, often severely. This constant pressure causes deformity. As the muscle remains in the shortened position over several weeks or months, the tendons remodel and cause permanent muscle shortening or contracture. When muscles have permanently shortened, the inner surfaces of joints, such as armpits or palms, cannot be cleaned and the skin breaks down in that area.

HETEROTOPIC OSSIFICATION. Heterotopic ossification is an abnormal deposit of bone in muscles and tendons that may occur after injury. It is most common in the hips and knees. Initially heterotopic ossification causes localized swelling, warmth, redness, and stiffness of the muscle. It usually begins one to four months after the injury and is rare after one year.

AUTONOMIC DYSREFLEXIA. Body organs that regulate themselves, such as the heart, gastrointestinal tract, and glands, are controlled by groups of nerves called autonomic nerves. Autonomic nerves emerge from three different places: above the spinal column, in the lower back from vertebrae T1–L4, and from the lowest regions of the sacrum at the base of the spine. In general, these three groups of autonomic nerves operate in balance. Spinal cord injury can disrupt this balance, a condition called autonomic dysreflexia or autonomic hyperreflexia. Patients with injuries at T6 or above are at greatest risk.

In autonomic dysreflexia, irritation of the skin, bowel, or bladder causes a highly exaggerated response from autonomic nerves. This response is caused by the uncontrolled release of norepinephrine, a hormone similar to adrenaline. Uncontrolled release of norepinephrine causes a rapid rise in blood pressure and a slowing of the heart rate. These symptoms are accompanied by throbbing headache, nausea, anxiety, sweating, and goose bumps below the level of the injury. The elevated blood pressure can rapidly cause loss of consciousness, seizures, cerebral hemorrhage, and death. Autonomic dysreflexia is most often caused by an over-full bladder or bladder infection; impaction or hard impassable fecal mass in the bowel; or skin irritation from tight clothing, sunburn, or other irritant. Inability to sense these irritants before the autonomic reaction begins is a major cause of dysreflexia.

LOSS OF BLADDER AND BOWEL CONTROL. Bladder and bowel control require both motor nerves and the autonomic nervous system. Both of these systems may be damaged by SCI. When the autonomic nervous system triggers an urge to urinate or defecate, continence is maintained by contracting the anal or urethral sphincters. A sphincter is a ring of muscle that contracts to close off a passage or opening in the body. When the neural connections to these muscles are severed, conscious control is lost. In addition, loss of feeling may prevent sensations of fullness from reaching the brain. To compensate, the patient may help empty the bowel or bladder by using physical maneuvers that stimulate autonomic contractions before they would otherwise begin; however, the patient may not be able to relax the sphincters. If the sphincters cannot be relaxed, the patient will retain urine or feces.

Retention of urine may cause muscular changes in the bladder and urethral sphincter that make the problem worse. Urinary tract infection is common. Retention of feces can cause impaction. Symptoms of impaction include loss of appetite and nausea. Untreated impaction may cause perforation of the large intestine and rapid overwhelming infection.

SEXUAL DYSFUNCTION. Men who have sustained SCI may be unable to achieve an erection or ejaculate. Sperm formation may be abnormal too, reducing fertility. Fertility and the ability to achieve orgasm are less impaired for women. Women may still be able to become pregnant and deliver vaginally with proper medical care.

Diagnosis

The location and extent of spinal cord injury is determined with computed tomography (CT) scans, **magnetic resonance imaging** (MRI), and x rays. X rays may be enhanced with an injected contrast dye.

Treatment

A person who may have a spinal cord injury should not be moved. Treatment of SCI begins with immobilization. This strategy prevents partial injuries of the cord from severing it completely. Use of splints to completely immobilize suspected SCI at the scene of the injury has helped reduce the severity of spinal cord injuries since the late twentieth century. Intravenous methylprednisone, a steroidal anti-inflammatory drug, is given during the first 24 hours to reduce inflammation and tissue destruction.

Rehabilitation after spinal cord injury seeks to prevent complications, promote recovery, and make the most of remaining function. Rehabilitation is a complex and long-term process. It requires a team of professionals, including a neurologist, physiatrist or rehabilitation specialist, physical therapist, and occupational therapist. Other specialists who may be needed include a respiratory therapist, vocational rehabilitation counselor, social worker, speech-language pathologist, nutritionist, special education teacher, recreation therapist, and clinical psychologist. Support groups provide a critical source of information, advice, and support for SCI patients.

Scientists continue to experiment with stem cells to treat spinal cord injuries. Research in rats that used embryonic stem cells may lead to new therapies in humans. Stem cells have the potential to become any cell type in the body depending on what chemical signals they get when they mature. Researchers hope that by triggering stem cells to become nerve cell precursors and then transplanting these precursor cells into the injured area they can promote healing of the spinal cord. Stem cell research is relatively new and controversial; however, it offers the hope of treating these kinds of injuries more successfully in the future.

Paralysis and loss of sensation

Some limited mobility and sensation may be recovered, but the extent and speed of this recovery cannot be predicted. Experimental electrical stimulation has been shown to allow some control of muscle contraction in paraplegia. This experimental technique offers the possibility of unaided walking. Further development of current control systems will be needed before useful movement is possible outside the laboratory.

The physical therapist focuses on mobility to maintain range of motion of affected limbs and reduce contracture and deformity. Physical therapy helps compensate for lost skills by using those muscles that are still functional. It also helps to increase any residual strength and control in affected muscles. A physical therapist suggests adaptive equipment such as braces, canes, or wheelchairs.

An occupational therapist works to restore ability to perform the activities of daily living, such as eating and grooming, with tools and new techniques. The occupational therapist also designs modifications of the home and workplace to match the individual impairment.

A pulmonologist or respiratory therapist promotes airway hygiene through instruction in assisted coughing techniques and postural drainage. The respiratory professional also prescribes and provides instruction in the use of ventilators, facial or nasal masks, and tracheostomy equipment where necessary.

Pressure ulcers

Pressure ulcers are prevented by turning in bed at least every two hours. The patient should be turned more frequently when redness begins to develop in sensitive areas. Special mattresses and chair cushions can distribute weight more evenly to reduce pressure. Electrical stimulation is sometimes used to promote muscle movement to prevent pressure ulcers.

Spasticity and contracture

Range of motion (ROM) exercises help to prevent contracture. Chemicals can be used to prevent contractures from becoming fixed when ROM exercise is inadequate. Phenol or alcohol can be injected onto the nerve or botulinum toxin directly into the muscle. Botulinum toxin is associated with fewer complications, but it is more expensive than phenol and alcohol. Contractures can be released by cutting the shortened tendon or transferring it surgically to a different site on the bone where its pull will not cause as much deformity. Such tendon transfers may also be used to increase strength in partially functional extremities.

Heterotopic ossification

Etidronate disodium (Didronel), a drug that regulates the body's use of calcium, is used to prevent heterotopic ossification. Treatment begins three weeks after the injury and continues for 12 weeks. Surgical removal of ossified tissue is possible.

Autonomic dysreflexia

Autonomic dysreflexia is prevented by bowel and bladder care and attention to potential irritants. It is treated by prompt removal of the irritant. Drugs to lower blood pressure are used when necessary. People with SCI should educate friends and family members about the symptoms and treatment of dysreflexia, because immediate attention is necessary.

Loss of bladder and bowel control

Normal bowel function is promoted through adequate fluid intake and a diet rich in fiber. Evacuation is stimulated by deliberately increasing the abdominal pressure, either voluntarily or by using an abdominal binder.

Bladder care involves continual or intermittent catheterization. The full bladder may be detected by feeling its bulge against the abdominal wall. Urinary tract infection is a significant complication of catheterization and requires frequent monitoring.

Sexual dysfunction

Counseling can help in adjusting to changes in sexual function after spinal cord injury. Erection may be enhanced through the same means used to treat erectile dysfunction in the general population.

Prognosis

The prognosis of SCI depends on the location and extent of injury. Injuries of the neck above C4 with significant involvement of the diaphragm hold the gravest prognosis. Respiratory infection is one of the leading causes of death in long-term SCI. Overall, 85% of SCI patients who survive the first 24 hours are alive ten years after their injuries. Recovery of function is impossible to predict. Partial recovery is more likely after an incomplete wound than after the spinal cord has been completely severed.

Prevention

Risk of spinal cord injury can be reduced through prevention of the accidents that lead to it. Chances of injury from automobile accidents, the major cause of

SCIs, can be significantly reduced by driving at safe speeds, avoiding alcohol while driving, and using seat belts.

Resources

BOOKS

Bradley, W., et al. *Neurology in Clinical Practice.* 5th ed. Philadelphia: Butterworth-Heinemann, 2008.

Goetz, C.G. *Goetz's Textbook of Clinical Neurology.* 3rd ed. Philadelphia: Saunders, 2007.

Palmer, Sara, et al. *Spinal Cord Injury: A Guide for Living.* Baltimore: Johns Hopkins University Press, 2008.

PERIODICALS

Adoni, Tarso, et al. "Complete motor recovery after acute paraparesis caused by spontaneous spinal epidural hematoma: case report." *BMC Emergency Medicine* 11 (2011): 10.

Al-Habib, Amro F., et al. "Clinical predictors of recovery after blunt spinal cord trauma: systematic review." *Journal of Neurotrauma* 28.8 (2011): 1431.

Barchi, Soraya, et al. "The impact of specialized centers of care for spinal cord injury on length of stay, complications, and mortality: a systematic review of the literature." *Journal of Neurotrauma* 28.8 (2011): 1363.

McCallister, Patrick. "Breakthrough therapy for SCI?" *Paraplegia News* 65.8 (2011): 47.

ORGANIZATIONS

Canadian Paraplegic Association, 1101 Prince of Wales Drive, 230, Ottawa, ONT, Canada, K2C 3W7, (613) 723-1913, Fax: (613) 723-1060, info@canparaplegic. org, http://www.canparaplegic.org.

National Spinal Cord Injury Association, 75-20 Astoria Boulevard, Suite 120, Jackson Heights, NY 11370, (718) 512-0010, (800) 962-9629, Fax: (866) 387-2196, info@spinalcord.org, http://www.spinalcord.org.

Spinal Cord Injuries Australia, 1 Jennifer Street, Little Bay, NSW, Australia, 2036, (02) 9661 8855, Fax: (02) 9661 9598, office@scia.org.au, http://scia.org.au.

Richard Robinson
Ken R. Wells
Rosalyn Carson-DeWitt, MD

Spinal cord tumors *see* **Brain and spinal tumors**

Spinal muscular atrophy

Definition

Spinal muscular atrophy (SMA) is a disease characterized by degradation of the anterior horn cells of the spinal cord and has similar characteristics to Spinobulbar muscular atrophy (SBMA). SBMA differs from SMA in its mode of inheritance, the disease-determining gene, the mutational events that trigger disease and the cellular specificity of the disease pathology.

Description

The anterior horn cells control the voluntary muscle contractions from large muscle groups such as the arms and legs. For example, if an individual

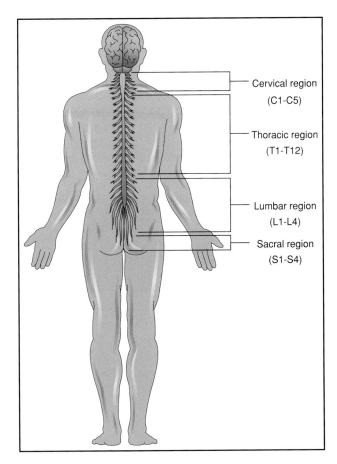

The extent of sensory and motor loss resulting from a spinal cord injury depends on the level of the injury because nerves at different levels control sensation and movement in different parts of the body. The distribution is as follows: C1-C4: head and neck; C3-C5: diaphragm; C5-T1: shoulders, arms, and hands; T2-T12: chest and abdomen (excluding internal organs); L1-L4: abdomen (excluding internal organs), buttocks, genitals, upper legs; L4-S3: legs; S2-S4: genitals, muscles of the perineum. *(Illustration by Electronic Illustrators Group. Reproduced by permission of Gale, a part of Cengage Learning.)*

wants to move his/her arm, electrical impulses are sent from the brain down the anterior horn cells to the muscles of the arm, which then stimulates the arm muscles to contract allowing the arm to move. Degradation is a rapid loss of functional motor neurons. Loss of motor neurons results in progressive symmetrical atrophy of the voluntary muscles. Progressive symmetrical atrophy refers to the loss of function of muscle groups from both sides of the body. For example, both arms and both legs are equally effected to similar degrees of muscle loss and the inability to be controlled and used properly. Progressive loss indicates that muscle loss is not instantaneous, rather, muscle loss occurs over a period of time. These

muscle groups include those skeletal muscles that control large muscle groups such as the arms, legs and torso. The **weakness** in the legs is generally greater than the weakness in the arms.

Spinal muscular atrophy (SMA) arises primarily from degradation of the anterior horn cells of the spinal cord, resulting in proximal weakness and atrophy of voluntary skeletal muscle. Proximal weakness effects the limbs positioned closer to the body, such as arms and legs, rather than more distant body parts such as hands, feet, fingers, or toes.

Spinal muscular atrophy only affects the motor neurons of the spinal cord and voluntary muscles of the limb and trunk. Patients do not display sensory loss, heart problems, or **mental retardation**. There are numerous secondary complications seen in SMA, including bending of the legs and arms and pneumonia. SMA development involves an initial substantial loss of motor units, followed by a stabilization of the surviving motor units. Motor units refer to an entire motor neuron and the connections within a muscle required for neuronal function.

Clinical subgroups

The childhood form of SMA is subdivided into three main clinical subgroups, Type I, II, and III, depending upon the age of onset and severity. A fourth subgroup, Type O, was recently discovered in London.

Type I

Type I SMA, or Werdnig-Hoffmann disease, is the acute or severe form, characterized by severe muscle atrophy. Guido-Werdig, an Austrian doctor, first identified the disease in 1891. He described two brothers displaying progressive muscle weakness from the age of 10 months, starting in the legs and progressing to the back and arms. The first brother died at the age three years with respiratory problems. The second brother survived to the age of six years.

Symptoms emerge in the first three months of life with the affected children never gaining the ability to sit, stand, or walk. Swallowing and feeding may be difficult, and the child may show difficulties with their own secretions. There is general weakness in the intercostals and accessory respiratory muscles (the muscles situated between the ribs). The chest may appear concave (sunken in) due to the diaphragmatic (tummy) breathing.

Type II

Type II SMA was first described in 1964. It is less severe than type I, with clinical symptoms emerging between three and 15 months of age. Most patients can sit but are unable to stand or walk unaided. Feeding and swallowing problems are uncommon in patients with Type II SMA. Again, as with patients diagnosed with type I SMA, the intercostal muscles are affected, with diaphragmatic breathing a main characteristic of children with type II. Most patients will survive beyond the age of four years and, depending upon how their respiratory system is affected, may live through adolescence.

Type III

The chronic form of SMA, Type III (Kugelberg-Welander disease) was first described in 1956. The clinical symptoms manifest after the age of four. It produces proximal muscle weakness, predominantly in the lower body. Affected individuals can walk unaided and have a normal life span depending upon the extent of respiratory muscles loss.

Type O

Clinicians in London identified a fourth form of the childhood disease, Type 0 SMA. This form appears to have a fetal-onset in that affected individuals display reduced movement within the uterus and are born with severe muscular atrophy with massive motor neuronal cell death. Therefore, these patients have very few functional motor neurons and motor units.

Diagnosis

One of the main diagnostic tools is **electromyography** (EMG). Contraction of voluntary muscle is controlled by electrical impulses originating from the brain. These impulses pass down the motor neurons of the spinal cord to the connecting muscles, where it triggers the contraction. The EMG records this electrical impulse and determines whether the electric current is the same as in normal individuals. Metal needles are inserted into the arms and thigh and the electrical impulse is recorded.

In addition, the speed at which the electric impulse passes down the motor neuron can also be used as a diagnostic test. In SMA patients, both the nerve conduction velocity (NVC) and the EMG readings are reduced.

The third test is an invasive procedure called a muscle **biopsy**. This involves a surgeon removing a small section of muscle. This is then tested for signs of degradation.

Genetic profile

All forms of childhood SMA are autosomal recessive, with both parents needing to be carriers to pass

the disease on. If both parents are carriers, there is a 25% chance of their child being affected.

All three forms are caused by a decrease in the production of a protein, termed Survival of Motor Neuron (SMN). The SMN protein is encoded by two nearly identical genes located on chromosome 5; SMN-1 and SMN-2 (previously referred to as telomeric and centomeric SMN, respectively). Remarkably, only mutations or deletions of SMN-1 result in disease development.

In most individuals who do not have SMA, each chromosome (maternal and paternal) contains one copy of SMN-1 and one copy of SMN-2. Therefore, in most unaffected individuals, there are two SMN-1 and two SMN-2 genes. Importantly, a subset of SMA-causing mutations are intragenic SMN-1 single amino acid substitutions. Intragenic indicates that mutations are within an otherwise intact SMN gene, but that there is a small and very subtle mutation that is only found within the SMN gene. This is in contrast to large genomic deletions that can delete the SMN gene and also neighboring genes. The intragenic or small mutations thereby confirms SMN-1 as the SMA-determining gene.

Signs and symptoms

Research shows that, in SMA, the reduced SMN protein levels result in motor neuronal cell degradation. How and why this occurs is still not known.

Demographics

Approximately one in 10,000 live births are affected with SMA, which is slightly lower than expected since the carrier frequency is between one in 40 and one in 50. Since this is a recessive disease, meaning two copies of the abnormal gene must be present for the disease to occur, carriers are unaffected because only one copy of the abnormal gene is present.

The genomic SMN region is remarkably unstable, and *de novo* mutations (mutations that are new and not inherited from the parents) are quite frequent, accounting for nearly 2% of all SMA cases. In 90% of patients, death occurs before the age of two due to respiratory failure. In North America and Europe, type I SMA accounts for one in every 25,000 infant mortalities. SMA is the leading genetic cause of infantile death and is the second most common autosomal recessive disorder behind cystic fibrosis. Carrier frequencies and disease frequencies are similar throughout the world, although slight variations can exist. Asian populations have a slightly reduced carrier frequency although it is not known why this discrepancy has occurred.

KEY TERMS

Anterior horn cells—Subset of motor neurons within the spinal cord.

Atrophy—Wasting away of normal tissue or an organ due to degeneration of the cells.

Degradation—Loss or diminishing.

Dorsal root ganglia—The subset of neuronal cells controlling impulses in and out of the brain.

Intragenic—Occuring within a single gene.

Motor neurons—Class of neurons that specifically control and stimulate voluntary muscles.

Motor units—Functional connection with a single motor neuron and muscle.

Sensory neurons—Class of neurons that specifically regulate and control external stimuli (senses: sight, sound).

Transcription—The process by which genetic information on a strand of DNA is used to synthesize a strand of complementary RNA.

Voluntary muscle—A muscle under conscious control, such as arm and leg muscles.

Treatment and management

To date, there is no treatment for childhood SMA. However, there are possible mechanisms through which treatment could be developed. Gene therapy could be used for SMA to replace the abnormal SMN-1 gene. Such treatment is not yet available or possible.

Prognosis

In Type I SMA, eating and swallowing can become difficult as the muscles of the face are affected. Due to the degradation of the respiratory muscles breathing can also be labored. It is therefore essential for patients to undergo chest physiotherapy (CPT). CPT is a standard set of procedures designed to trigger and aid coughing in patients. Coughing is important as it clears the patients lungs and throat of moisture and prevents secondary problems, such as pneumonia.

As symptoms progress, patients may require a ventilator to aid breathing. There are two main forms of ventilation systems. Negative Pressure Ventilation can be achieved by placing the patient in a Port-A-Lung. This machine ensures that the air pressure around the patient is lower than the air pressure within the patient's lungs, enabling easier breathing. The pressure can be raised or lowered if the patients ventilation rate increases or decreases.

The second method is called Bi-Pap (Biphasic Positive Airway Pressure). This procedure involves the insertion of a small tube down the nose into the patient's lungs, through which oxygen is pumped into the lungs and waste carbon dioxide is removed. This system allows maximum inspiration and expiration levels to be reached.

Of all the forms of childhood SMA, Type II is the most diverse. It is therefore hard to tell when muscle weakness will occur and how severe the disease will be. With the aid of leg braces and walking devices, some children may gain the ability to stand. Unlike Type I SMA, not all children with Type II are affected by respiratory weakness. The main cause of death in patients with Type II is respiratory failure resulting from a respiratory infection. It is therefore important to ensure that mucus does not build up in patients' respiratory tracts as this could aid viral and bacterial infections.

Resources

PERIODICALS

Crawford, T. O., and C. A. Pardo. "The neurobiology of childhood spinal muscular atrophy." *Neurobiology of Disease* 3 (1996): 97-110.

WEBSITES

Families of Spinal Muscular Atrophy. http://www.fsma.org.
The Andrew's Buddies web site. *FightSMA.com* http://www.andrewsbuddies.com/news.html.

ORGANIZATIONS

Muscular Dystrophy Association. 3300 East Sunrise Dr., Tucson, AZ 85718. (520) 529-2000 or (800) 572–1717. http://www.mdausa.org.

Philip J. Young
Christian L. Lorson, PhD

Spinal surgery *see* **Laminectomy**

Spinocerebellar ataxia

Definition

The spinocerebellar ataxias (SCAs) are a group of inherited conditions that affect the brain and spinal cord, causing progressive difficulty with coordination. Some types of SCA also involve impairment of speech and eye movement.

Description

The SCAs are named for the parts of the nervous system that are affected in this condition. *Spino* refers to the spinal cord and *cerebellar* refers to the **cerebellum**, or back part of the brain. The cerebellum is the area of the brain that controls coordination. In people with SCA, the cerebellum often becomes atrophied or smaller. Symptoms of SCA usually begin in the 30s or 40s, but onset can be at any age. Onset from childhood through the 70s has been reported.

At least 25 different types of SCA have been described. This group is numbered 1–26, and each is caused by mutations, or changes, in a different gene. Although the category of SCA9 has been reserved, there is no described condition for SCA9 and no gene has been found. Spinocerebellar **ataxia** has also been called **olivopontocerebellar atrophy**, Marie's ataxia, and cerebellar degeneration. SCA3 is sometimes called **Machado-Joseph disease**, named after two of the first families described with this condition. All affected people in a family have the same type of SCA.

Genetic profile

Although each of the SCAs is caused by mutations in different genes, the types of mutations are the same in all of the genes that have been found. Most genes come in pairs; one member of a pair comes from a person's mother and the other one comes from the person's father. The genes are made up of deoxyribonucleic acid (DNA), which is made up of chemical bases that are represented by the letters C, T, G, and A. This is the DNA alphabet. The letters are usually put together in three-letter words.

In each of the genes that cause SCA, there is a section of the gene where a three-letter DNA word is repeated a certain number of times. In most of the types of SCA, the DNA word that is repeated is CAG. So there is a part of the gene that reads CAGCAGCAG-CAGCAG and so on. In people who have SCA, this DNA segment is repeated too many times, making this section of the gene too big. This is called a trinucleotide repeat expansion. In SCA8, the DNA word that is repeated is CTG. In SCA10, the repeated DNA word is five DNA letters long and is ATTCT. This is called a pentanucleotide expansion. The actual number of DNA repeats that is normal or that causes SCA is different in each type of SCA.

In each type of SCA, there are a certain range or number of repeats that still fall within the normal range. People who have repeat numbers in the normal range will not develop SCA and cannot pass it to their children. There are also a certain number of repeats that

cause SCA (the affected range). People who have repeat numbers in the affected range will go on to develop SCA sometime in their lifetime, if they live long enough. People with repeat numbers in the affected range can pass SCA onto their children. Between the normal and affected ranges, there is a gray range. People who have repeat numbers in the gray range may or may not develop SCA in their lifetime. Why some people with numbers in the gray zone develop SCA and others do not is not known. People with repeat numbers in the gray range can also pass SCA onto their children.

In general, the more repeats in the affected range that someone has, the earlier the age of onset of symptoms and the more severe the symptoms. However, this is only a general rule. It is not possible to look at a person's repeat number and predict at what age that person will begin to have symptoms or how their condition will progress.

Sometimes when a person who has repeat numbers in the affected or gray range has children, the DNA expansion grows larger during the passing on of genes. This is called anticipation. Anticipation can result in an even earlier age of onset in children than in their affected parent. Anticipation does not occur in SCA6. However, significant anticipation can occur in SCA7. It is not unusual for a child with SCA7 to be affected before their parent or even grandparent begins to show symptoms. In most types of SCA, anticipation happens more often when a father passes SCA on to his children then when a mother passes it. However, in SCA8, the opposite is true; anticipation happens more often when a mother passes SCA8 to her children. Occasionally, repeat sizes stay the same or even get smaller when they are passed to a person's children.

The SCAs are passed on by autosomal dominant inheritance. This means that males and females are equally likely to be affected. It also means that only one gene in the pair needs to have the mutation in order for a person to become affected. Since a person only passes one copy of each gene on to their children, there is a 50%, or one in two, chance that a person who has SCA will pass it on to each of their children. A person who has repeat numbers in the gray range also has a 50%, or one in two, chance of passing the gene onto each of their children. However, whether their children will develop SCA depends on the number of their repeats. A person who has repeat numbers in the normal range cannot pass SCA onto their children.

Usually a person with SCA has a long family history of the condition. However, sometimes a person with SCA appears to be the only one affected in the family. This can be due to a couple reasons. First, it is possible that one of their parents is or was affected, but died before they began to show symptoms. It is also possible that their parent had a mutation in the gray range and was not affected, but the mutation expanded into the affected range when it was passed on. Other family members may also have SCA but have been misdiagnosed with another condition or are having symptoms, but have no definitive diagnosis. It is also possible that a person has a new mutation for SCA. New mutations are changes in the gene that happen for the first time in an affected person. Although a person with a new mutation may not have other affected family members, they still have a 50%, or one in two, chance of passing it on to their children.

Demographics

SCA has been found in people from all over the world. However, some of the types of SCA are more common in certain areas and ethnic groups. SCA types 1, 2, 3, 6, 7, and 8 are the most commonly documented autosomal dominant SCA. SCA1 accounts for at least 25% of SCA cases in South Africa and Italy. SCA2 accounts for 25% of SCA cases in Singapore, India, and Italy. SCA3 appears to be the most common type and was first described in families from Portugal. SCA3 accounts for almost 100% of SCA cases in Brazil. SCA3 also accounts for the majority of SCA cases in Portugal, the Netherlands, Germany, China, and Singapore, and a significant proportion in Japan. SCA6 accounts for a significant proportion of SCA cases in the Netherlands, Germany, and Japan. In the United States, SCA2, SCA3, and SCA6 account for the majority of documented cases; these three types also account for 51% of cases worldwide. SCA1, SCA7, and SCA8 each account for less than 10% of SCA cases worldwide.

SCA types 4, 5, and 10 through 26 are rare and have each only been described in a few families. The first family described with SCA5 may have been distantly related to President Abraham Lincoln and was first called Lincoln ataxia. SCA10 has only been described in Mexican families, SCA13 and 25 have each only been described in single French families, SCA14 and 16 have each only been described in single families from Japan, and SCA19 and 23 have each only been described in single Dutch families.

Signs and symptoms

Although different genes cause each of the SCAs, they all have similar symptoms. All people with SCA have ataxia or a lack of muscle coordination. Walking is affected, and eventually the coordination of the arms and hands and of the speech and swallowing is also affected. One of first symptoms of SCA is often problems with walking and difficulties with balance. The muscles that control speech and swallowing usually become affected. This results in **dysarthria**, or slurred speech, and difficulties with eating. Choking while eating can become a significant problem and can lead to a decrease in the number of calories a person can take in. The age of the onset of symptoms can vary greatly—anywhere from childhood through the seventh decade have been reported. The age of onset and severity of symptoms can also vary between people in the same family.

As the condition progresses, walking becomes more difficult, and it is necessary to use a cane, walker, and often a wheelchair. Because of the uncoordinated walking that develops, it is not uncommon for people with SCA to be mistaken for being intoxicated. Carrying around a note from their doctor explaining their medical condition is helpful.

Some of the SCA types can also have other symptoms, although not all of these are seen in every person with that particular type. SCA2 may have slower eye movements; this does not usually interfere with a person's sight. People with SCA1 and 3 may develop problems with the peripheral nerves, which carry information to and from the spinal cord. This can lead to decreased sensation and **weakness** in the hands and feet. In SCA3, people may also have twitching in the face and tongue, and bulging eyes. SCA4 may cause a loss of sensation, but affected individuals often have a normal lifespan. SCA5 often has an adult onset, and is slowly progressive, not affecting the lifespan. SCA6 often has a later onset, progresses very slowly, and does not shorten the lifespan. SCA7 involves progressive visual loss that eventually leads to blindness. SCA8 may cause sensory loss, but people have a normal lifespan. SCA10 may cause affected individuals to develop seizures. SCA11 is a relatively mild type, resulting in a normal lifespan for the affected person. SCA12 cases often develop a **tremor** as the first noticeable symptom, and the people may eventually develop **dementia**. SCA13 may cause individuals to be shorter than average and have mild **mental retardation**. SCA14 may have an early onset, between 12 and 42 years of age, with an average of 28 years of age. SCA15 and 22 may be slow to progress, with SCA22 sometimes being early onset. SCA16 may involve tremors, SCA17 may involve mental deterioration, and SCA19 may involve both. SCA20 may result in calcification of some brain areas that shows up on brain imaging tests. SCA21 can be early onset, but involve only mild cognitive impairment. SCA23 is late onset and may involve sensory loss. SCA25 may also cause sensory loss. SCA26 may involve irregular eye movements.

Diagnosis

Genetic forms of ataxia must be distinguished from nongenetic types that may have their own treatment. Nongenetic causes of ataxia are not types of SCA, and include alcoholism, vitamin deficiencies, **multiple sclerosis**, vascular disease, and some cancers. The genetic forms of ataxia, such as SCA, are diagnosed by family history, physical examination, and brain imaging.

An initial workup of people who are having symptoms of ataxia will involve a medical history and a physical examination. Magnetic resonance imaging (MRI) of the brain in people with SCA will usually show degeneration, or atrophy, of the cerebellum and may be helpful in suggesting a diagnosis of SCA. A thorough family history should be taken to determine if others in the family have similar symptoms and the inheritance pattern in the family.

Since there is so much overlap between symptoms in the different types of SCA, it is not usually possible to tell the different types apart based on clinical symptoms. The only way to definitively diagnose SCA and determine a specific subtype is by genetic testing, which involves drawing a small amount of blood. The DNA in the blood cells is then examined, and the number of CAG repeats in each of the SCA genes is counted. Clinical testing is available to detect the mutations that cause SCA1, 2, 3, 6, 7, 8, 10, 12, 14, and 17. These tests may be offered as two sequential groups based on population frequency. Testing is often first performed for the more common ataxias, SCA1 through SCA7. Testing for the less common hereditary ataxias are often individualized as appropriate. Factors that may indicate testing for less common SCA types may include factors, such as ethnic background (SCA10 in the Mexican population), or specific symptoms, such as the presence of a tremor (SCA12). In these cases, testing can be performed for a single disease. If genetic testing is negative for the available testing, it does not mean that a person does not have SCA. It could mean that the person has a type of SCA for which genetic testing is not yet available.

It is possible to test individuals who are at risk for developing SCA before they are showing symptoms to see whether they inherited an expanded trinucleotide repeat. This is called predictive testing. Predictive testing cannot determine the age of onset or the course of the disease. The decision to undergo this testing is personal. Some people choose to have testing so that they can make decisions about having children or about their future education, career, or finances. Protocols for predictive testing have been developed, and only certain centers perform this testing. Most centers require that the diagnosis of SCA has been confirmed by genetic testing in another family member.

Individuals who are interested in testing will be seen by a team of specialists over the course of a few visits. Often they will meet a neurologist who will perform a neurological examination to see if they may be showing early signs of the condition. If individuals have symptoms, testing may be performed to confirm the diagnosis. They will also meet with a genetic counselor to talk about SCA, how it is inherited, and what testing can and cannot tell someone. They will also explore reasons for testing and what impact the results may have on their life, their family, their job, and their insurance. Most centers also require individuals going through predictive testing to meet a few times with a psychologist. The purpose of these visits is to make sure that they have thought through the decision to be tested and are prepared to deal with whatever the results may be.

If children are having symptoms, it is appropriate to perform testing to confirm the cause of their symptoms. However, testing will not be performed on children who are at risk for developing SCA, but are not having symptoms. Children can make their own choice when they are old enough. Testing a child who does not have symptoms could lead to possible problems with their future relationships, education, career, and insurance.

Testing a pregnant woman to determine whether an unborn child is affected is possible if genetic testing in a family has identified a certain type of SCA. This can be done between 10 and 12 weeks gestation by a procedure called chorionic villus sampling (CVS) that involves removing a tiny piece of the placenta and examining the cells. It can also be done by amniocentesis after 16 weeks gestation by removing a small amount of the amniotic fluid surrounding the fetus and analyzing the cells in the fluid. Each of these procedures has a small risk of miscarriage associated with it. Continuing a pregnancy that is found to be affected is like performing predictive testing on a child. Therefore, couples interested in these options should have genetic counseling to carefully explore all of the benefits and limitations of these procedures.

There is also another procedure, called preimplantation diagnosis, that allows a couple to have a child that is unaffected with the genetic condition in their family. This procedure is experimental and not widely available.

Treatment and management

Although there is a lot of ongoing research, no cure currently exists for the SCAs. Although vitamin

KEY TERMS

Anticipation—Increasing severity in disease with earlier ages of onset, in successive generations; a condition that begins at a younger age and is more severe with each generation

Ataxia—A deficiency of muscular coordination, especially when voluntary movements are attempted, such as grasping or walking.

Calcification—The addition of calcium deposits.

Trinucleotide repeat expansion—A sequence of three nucleotides that is repeated too many times in a section of a gene.

supplements are not a cure or treatment for SCA, they may be recommended if a person is taking in fewer calories because of feeding difficulties. Different types of therapy might be useful to help people maintain as independent a lifestyle as possible. An occupational therapist may be able to suggest adaptive devices to make the activities of daily living easier. Canes, walkers, and wheelchairs are often useful. A speech therapist may recommend devices that may make communication easier as speech progressively becomes affected. As swallowing becomes more difficult, a special swallow evaluation may lead to better strategies for eating and to help lessen the risk of choking.

Genetic counseling helps people and their families make decisions about their medical care, genetic testing, and having children. It can also help people to deal with the medical and emotional issues that arise when there is a genetic condition diagnosed in the family.

Prognosis

Most people with the SCAs do have progression of their symptoms that leads to fulltime use of a wheelchair. The duration of the disease after the onset of symptoms is about 10–30 years, but can vary depending in part to the number of trinucleotide repeats and age of onset. In general, people with a larger number of repeats have an earlier age of onset and more severe symptoms. Choking can be a major hazard because, if food gets into the lungs, a life-threatening pneumonia can result. As the condition progresses, it can become difficult for people to cough and clear secretions. Most people die from respiratory failure or pulmonary complications.

Resources

PERIODICALS

Evidente, V. G. H., et al. "Hereditary Ataxias." *Mayo Clinic Proceedings* (2000): 475–90.

Zohgbi, H. Y., and H. T. Orr. "Glutamine Repeats and Neurodegeneration." *Mayo Clinic Proceedings* (2000): 217–47.

ORGANIZATIONS

National Ataxia Foundation. 2600 Fernbrook Lane, Suite 119, Minneapolis, MN 55447. (763) 553-0020. Fax: (763) 553-0167. E-mail: naf@ataxia.org. (April 23, 2005.) http://www.ataxia.org.

WE MOVE (Worldwide Education and Awareness for Movement Disorders). 204 E. 84th St., New York, NY 10024. (212) 875-8312 or (800) 437-MOV2. Fax: (212) 875-8389. E-mail: wemove@wemove.org. (April 23, 2005.) http://www.wemove.org.

WEB SITES

Hereditary Ataxia Overview. (April 23, 2005.) http://www.geneclinics.org/profiles/ataxias/details.html.

International Network of Ataxia Friends (INTERNAF). (April 23, 2005.) http://www.internaf.org.

Online Mendelian Inheritance in Man. (April 23, 2005.) http://www.ncbi.nlm.nih.gov/entrez/query.fcgi?db=OMIM.

Maria Basile, PhD

Status epilepticus

Definition

Status epilepticus is a term describing a state of continuous seizure activity. In the past, 30 minutes of continuing seizure or frequent attacks that prevent recovery was required for the definition of status to be met; however, since most seizures last less than 4–5 minutes, it is now understood that any seizure that continues five minutes or longer should be considered as status epilepticus and managed accordingly.

Description

Nearly all types of seizures have the potential of occurring in a continuous or repeated fashion. There are two general categories: generalized status and focal status, depending on the clinical features of the situation. Generalized status can preferentially manifest with tonic, clonic, absence, and/or myoclonic seizures. Hence, status can be merely a prolongation of commonly observed individual seizure types. Nonconvulsive status epilepticus can manifest with sustained or repeating complex partial seizures with a change in mental status, or simply as a focal seizure with limited physical signs but without alteration of consciousness. Status can occur in individuals who have epilepsy already, but in some cases, the first seizure that a person experiences can be status epilepticus.

Demographics

The epidemiology of status epilepticus varies depending on the study. In the United States the incidence is approximately up to 40 per 100,000 individuals. Therefore more than 100,000 cases of status occur annually. Up to 10% of all first-time seizures are situations of status epilepticus. The mortality of status epilepticus is roughly 20%. Those most at risk are the very young or the elderly. The causes of death vary depending on the age of the patient, presence of medical complications, duration of the uncontrollable seizures, and the underlying cause of the status epilepticus.

Causes and symptoms

Causes

The exact pathophysiology of why a seizure evolves into status is complex and not fully understood. Status epilepticus has many causes, some of which are the same as causes of seizures in general. In infants, status can occur in the setting of perinatal hypoxia or anoxia (low oxygen or lack of oxygen) that injures the brain. Also, illness such as meningitis that can cause seizures can also be severe enough to cause status epilepticus. Metabolic disorders of infancy and childhood that can be causes of epilepsy can also produce status epilepticus. In adults, infections of the brain, strokes, brain tumors, and severe head trauma can cause seizures and, hence, status epilepticus.

Symptoms

Clinically, status epilepticus is basically a prolonged seizure situation. Individual seizures occurring frequently enough to impair full recovery to baseline function can be a manifestation of status epilepticus as well. A limited seizure such as an arm jerking without alteration of consciousness is called a simple or focal seizure. If it occurs continuously, the term epilepsy partialis continua is used. This is the least serious of the different types of status epilepticus. The more dangerous type is, of course, generalized tonic/clonic status. This is because cardiac arrhythmias or blood pressure changes can be life threatening. Also, breathing and oxygenation can be compromised, and patients may require ventilator assistance. Complex partial seizures and absence seizures are manifested with an alteration of consciousness. When these particular seizures become status, patients may simply appear confused or agitated. Since they are not having convulsions, they may be misdiagnosed as having a psychiatric symptom. Nevertheless, prompt and accurate diagnosis is important for proper management.

Diagnosis

When convulsions are occurring, status is typically easily recognized, but subtle status, as in complex partial or absence status, may necessitate an electroencephalogram (EEG) for diagnosis. The EEG is not only used for initial diagnosis, but is often left running for longer periods to monitor response to treatment. The recognition of seizure activity is only one of the urgent tasks in the care of the patient. The other major issue is to rapidly identify the cause of seizures and the status epilepticus. This involves testing blood for at least glucose, electrolytes, liver function, and illicit substances. Very low blood glucose or extreme changes in sodium, for example, can cause seizures. Infections such as meningitis can cause status. Rapidly assessed levels of older, commonly used seizure medications such as phenytoin, phenobarbital, carbamazepine, and valproic acid are sometimes sought in cases where there is no available history from the patient. Indeed, one of the most frequent causes of status is low anticonvulsant levels in a patient with a history of epilepsy.

Treatment team

Patients in status epilepticus will often necessitate a neurologist to guide the management from the emergency department through the rest of the hospital stay. Social workers are important for discharge plans because many patients who survive status epilepticus need skilled nursing or rehabilitation to fully recover prior to being discharged home.

Treatment

The treatment of status depends on identifying quickly the underlying cause, if any. In cases of hypoglycemia, thiamine must be administered just prior to glucose supplementation. This is because some individuals, alcoholics for example, may be deficient in thiamine and a correction of glucose levels without thiamine supplementation can cause a condition known as Wernicke's encephalopathy. Sodium must be corrected slowly or a condition called central pontine myelinolysis can occur. A computed tomography (CT) scan of the brain is often ordered to evaluate for any brain trauma. A lumbar puncture may be performed to determine if there is meningitis so appropriate antibiotics can be used. Overall, in cases that an identifiable cause of status can be found, the key to successful treatment is the management of the underlying cause itself. There are published guidelines for the treatment of seizures themselves.

Initially, a sedative such as lorazepam or diazepam or buccal midazolam is given, which can stop many seizures, at least temporarily, while a longer-acting anticonvulsant such as phenytoin takes effect. If seizures persist, then phenobarbital, valproate, levetiracetam, and/or lacosamide is typically added. Since some of these particular medications, when fully loaded, can cause respiratory depression, an anesthesiologist is consulted to manage ventilator assistance. Status epilepticus is managed and treated in an intensive care unit with EEG monitoring to continually assess the response to seizure medications. When phenobarbital fails to stop the ongoing seizures, a number of other medications are considered, such as a midazolam drip or propofol. Anesthetic dosages of these particular medications are usually effective in suppressing seizure activity. Approximately every 24 hours, the dosage is reduced to determine if seizures recur or not.

The severity of status can vary widely. Sometimes it is effectively treated within 1–2 hours and other times the status is severe and extremely resistant to treatment and lasts for weeks. In such cases, the mortality rate is increased because of risk of medical complications such as pneumonia and blood clots. Immunological therapy may also be instituted to treat particularly refractory status epilepticus.

Recovery and rehabilitation

The recovery from status epilepticus will depend on its duration. If status can be effectively stopped in a relatively short period of time, complete neurological recovery is possible. The longer the seizures persist, the greater the chance of cerebral injury. Also, the longer the status epilepticus, the more difficult it is to stop. A complication of status epilepticus can actually be the development of epilepsy in some cases.

Clinical trials

As of August 2011, there were seven clinical trials examining various aspects of status. See the ClinicalTrials.gov site for the latest information.

Prognosis

The prognosis with status epilepticus will depend on the duration of status and coexisting medical problems. The prognosis is good for recovery if status can be stopped in a relatively short period of time (hours) and there are no complications such as infection, active cardiac problems, or other medical issues. Prognosis for complete recovery is less favorable as status persists for long periods of time. Coexisting medical problems will complicate management and chance for a negative outcome.

Special concerns

It is important to be on the lookout for subtle status situations that may go unrecognized. An EEG is a relatively easy way to determine the presence of active seizures. It is crucial to respond urgently to status epilepticus because the longer seizures continue the more difficult they are to stop.

Resources

BOOKS

Bradley, W., et al. *Neurology in Clinical Practice.* 5th ed. Philadelphia: Butterworth-Heinemann, 2008.

Goetz, C.G. *Goetz's Textbook of Clinical Neurology.* 3rd ed. Philadelphia: Saunders, 2007.

PERIODICALS

Abend, N. "Treatment of refractory status epilepticus: literature review and a proposed protocol." *Pediatric Neurology* 38 (June 1, 2008): 377–90.

Shearer P. "Generalized convulsive status epilepticus in adults and children: treatment guidelines and protocols." *Emergency Medical Clinics of North America* 29 (February 1, 2011): 51–64.

ORGANIZATIONS

American Epilepsy Society, 342 North Main Street, West Hartford, CT 06117-2507, (860) 586-7505, http://www.aesnet.org.

Epilepsy Foundation, 8301 Professional Place, Landover, MD 20785-7223, (800) 332-1000, http://www.epilepsyfoundation.org.

International League Against Epilepsy, 342 North Main Street, West Hartford, CT 06117-2507, (860) 586-7547, Fax: (860) 586-7550, http://www.ilae-epilepsy.org/.

Roy Sucholeiki, MD
Rosalyn Carson-DeWitt, MD

Steele-Richardson-Olszewski syndrome *see* **Progressive supranuclear palsy**

Stem cell therapy

Definition

Stem cell therapy is the utilization of stem cells to repair or replace damaged cells or tissues. Stem cells are unspecialized (undifferentiated) cells that can reproduce themselves indefinitely or differentiate into specialized cell types.

Purpose

Blood-forming (hematopoietic) stem cells have been used for decades in bone marrow stem cell transplants to treat blood and immune system disorders, including leukemia and lymphoma. They are also used to treat loss of bone marrow function from cancer treatments. Tissue grafts for treating certain diseases of the skin, bone, and cornea may depend on stem cells present in the grafted tissue.

Most types of stem cell therapy, other than bone marrow transplants, are considered experimental. For example, umbilical cord blood stem cells have been used to treat heart problems and other conditions in children with rare metabolic disorders and certain types of anemia. Stem cell therapy holds great promise for treating a wide range of conditions and disorders, including **multiple sclerosis** (MS), **Parkinson's disease**, and spinal cord injuries. Stem cell therapy for such conditions may be available in the United States as part of a clinical trial. In other countries, stem cell therapies are available to treat various disorders, including MS.

Precautions

In the United States, bone marrow stem cell transplants to treat leukemia, sickle-cell disease, and certain other conditions are the only approved uses of stem cell therapy; however, in a phenomenon called "medical tourism," many patients travel to other countries for stem cell therapy, sometimes at great expense. These therapies have not been shown to be safe and effective, and unregulated clinics in other countries vary considerably in the quality of care. Some may be outright scams.

Embryonic stem cells (ESCs) have the potential to differentiate into any cell type in the body and may someday be used to treat a wide range of human disorders. These cells are available only from human embryos and cannot yet be used directly for stem cell therapy, since they are unlikely to form the required cell type and may cause tumors.

There are many other types of stem cells that derive from various bodily tissues. Tissue-specific or adult stem cells primarily form only the cell types found in the tissues from which they are derived. For example, hematopoietic or blood-forming stem cells in the bone marrow can differentiate into various types of blood cells. Neural stem cells in the brain differentiate into different types of brain cells. Some clinics use adult, tissue-specific stem cells for treating a wide range of disorders, but these cells are unlikely to be effective for treating disorders in tissues other than those from which they were derived. For example, it is unlikely that a single type of stem cell therapy could effectively treat both diabetes and Parkinson's disease, since very different cell types are required. Stem cell therapy for neurological disorders can be particularly challenging, because it may require that the stem cells develop into specific types of neurons and form appropriate connections with other neurons.

The United States and many other countries require that treatments such as stem cell therapy undergo controlled clinical trials before being declared safe and effective. Many stem cell clinics use patient testimonials to advertise their services; however, patients may improve for a variety of reasons other than stem cell therapy. Placebo effects are particularly important: a patient's strong desire for positive results, as well as beneficial effects of medical attention in any form, can lead to an improvement in symptoms. Furthermore, the symptoms of many disorders wax and wane over time. For example, MS cycles through periods of remission, so it can take years to determine whether a specific treatment is effective. Many stem cell clinics also prescribe diet, medication, physical therapy, and relaxation and other alternative techniques, making it difficult to identify the source of any improvement. Undergoing an unproven stem cell treatment may make a patient ineligible for participating in a recognized clinical trial.

Description

Stem cell types

Stem cells divide continually, replacing themselves or "self-renewing" indefinitely. They do not age and die out after a finite number of cell divisions like most other cells. Under appropriate conditions, stem cells give rise to daughter progenitor cells that mature or differentiate into a specific cell type.

Human embryonic stem cells (hESCs) are totipotent or pluripotent and can develop into every type of cell in the human body. hESCs exist only during early stages of development. They are isolated from blastocysts—the balls of cells that have developed by about five days after fertilization. Most hESCs are derived from excess blastocysts that were created by *in vitro* fertilization (IVF).

Adult or tissue-specific stem cells, also called somatic stem cells, are multipotent. They can give rise to the different cell types present in a specific tissue or organ. Although they originate during fetal development, adult stem cells remain in the body throughout life to replace dying cells. The most easily isolated multipotent stem cells are hematopoietic cells in the bone marrow, which can differentiate into different types of blood cells. Adult multipotent stem cells can also be isolated from circulating blood, from the umbilical cord blood of newborns, and from skin.

Scientists have engineered cells that are similar to ESCs and can differentiate into various cell types. These induced pluripotent stem (iPS) cells are obtained by reprogramming specialized adult cells, such as skin cells.

Stem cell therapy can be autologous—utilizing the patient's own stem cells—or allogeneic—using donor stem cells from another person or embryonic stem cells. For autologous stem cell therapy, the patient's stem cells are removed, grown in the laboratory or treated in some way, and returned to the patient's body. These cells are recognized as "self" by the patient's immune system and are not rejected. Allogeneic stem cells are used when a patient's own stem cells are unavailable or defective. Unless the donor cells are a close match to the patient's cells, the patient's immune system may reject them as "foreign," as sometimes happens with organ transplants from an unrelated donor.

Neurological disorders

Clinical trials of stem cell therapies for neurological conditions include neural stem cell treatments for ischemic stroke and hESC treatments for acute spinal cord injury. One such trial involves the injection of several million oligodendrocyte progenitor cells, derived from hESCs, directly into the site of a recent spinal cord lesion. Stem cell therapy trials for neural tube defects—the failure of the neural tube to close properly during fetal development—are also underway. Researchers are working to develop stem cell therapies for other common neurological disorders, including Parkinson's disease and **Alzheimer's disease**.

There are two major approaches to stem cell therapy for MS. One approach is to reboot the patient's immune system in hopes of overcoming the autoimmunity that causes demyelination of nerve cells with MS. In this approach, stem cells are obtained from patients' own blood and their immune systems are then destroyed with chemotherapy. The stem cells are injected back into the patients, in the hope that their immune systems will reset and no longer attack the myelin covering of nerve cells. The other approach is to try to repair damage already caused by MS. In this therapy, stem cells from a patient's bone marrow are injected into the patient's blood and spinal cord, in the hope that the cells will migrate to the sites of nerve damage and promote healing. These therapies are undergoing early clinical trials in the United States and are available at some foreign university centers. However stem cell clinics in Mexico, Costa Rica, China, and elsewhere sometimes use donor umbilical cord blood or placental cells that are not necessarily safe or effective. Furthermore, stem cell therapy is known to be ineffective for later-stage MS.

Other stem cell therapies

Clinical trials of stem cell therapy for various heart problems are ongoing. For example, heart attack patients have been treated with autologous bone marrow from their hip bones. Either whole bone marrow or stem cells removed from bone marrow and grown in the laboratory are injected directly into the patient's damaged heart chamber. In one early trial, this treatment significantly reduced heart size and scar tissue and greatly improved heart function, even when the damage occurred years previously.

Other trials are using hESC-derived retinal cells to treat eye diseases, including age-related macular degeneration and Stargardt's macular dystrophy. These cells are injected directly into the damaged eyes. Stem cell therapy is also being investigated as a treatment for burned corneas, in cases where the stem cells that normally renew and repair the cornea have also been destroyed.

Risks

Even bone marrow stem cell transplants that have been in use for decades carry significant risks. Allogeneic stem cell therapies carry the risk of rejection by the patient's immune system: as with organ transplants, the closer the match of donor tissue to that of the recipient, the lower the risk of rejection; however, allogeneic stem cell therapy may require lifelong use of immunosuppressants to prevent rejection.

Although autologous stem cell therapy is unlikely to trigger an immune response, there are still risks involved in the procedures for acquiring, growing, and reintroducing the stem cells. Stem cells removed from a patient's body are manipulated in ways that can change their characteristics. During growth in laboratory culture—a process called expansion—stem cells may lose their

KEY TERMS

Allogeneic—Donor cells or tissues that are genetically distinct from those of the recipient.

Autoimmunity—An immune response to one's own bodily constituents.

Autologous—Donor cells or tissues that are derived from the recipient.

Blastocyst—A very early embryo, consisting of a ball of 150–200 cells with an inner cell mass from which embryonic stem cells are derived.

Demyelination—Loss or destruction of the myelin sheath surrounding nerve fibers.

Differentiation—The process by which a cell increases in complexity and specialization of function.

Embryo—The stage of development between a fertilized egg and a fetus.

Embryonic stem cell (ESC)—Cells from the inner cell mass of a blastocyst that can reproduce themselves indefinitely and differentiate into any cell type in the body; also called human embryonic stem cell (hESC).

Expansion—Growing cells in laboratory culture to increase their numbers.

Hematopoietic stem cells—Cells in the blood and bone marrow that can become various types of blood cells.

Immunosuppressant—A drug that suppresses the immune response.

In vitro fertilization (IVF)—A procedure in which an egg cell is fertilized with sperm in a laboratory and allowed to form an embryo, which can be implanted in a woman's uterus to initiate pregnancy.

Induced pluripotent stem cell (iPS cell)—A specialized cell, such as a skin cell, that has been induced or reprogrammed to return to a pluripotent or nonspecialized state similar to an embryonic stem cell.

Medical tourism—Traveling to a foreign country for a medical treatment that is not available in one's home country.

Multiple sclerosis (MS)—A demyelinating, autoimmune, progressive degenerative disease.

Multipotent stem cell—A stem cell that has the potential to differentiate into several types of cells found in a specific organ or tissue, but not into all cell types. For example, blood stem cells can differentiate into various types of blood cells, but not into cells of other tissues or organs.

Myelin—The white, fatty substance that covers and protects nerves.

Pluripotent stem cell—A stem cell that can differentiate into any of the cell types found in an organism.

Progenitor—A cell that has differentiated from a stem cell and is committed to developing into a specific cell type.

Self-renewal—The process by which stem cells divide and replace themselves indefinitely.

Tissue-specific stem cell—Adult or somatic stem cell; a multipotent stem cell that can differentiate into the specialized cell types of the tissue from which it was derived.

---

ability to mature into the required cell type or may lose mechanisms for controlling their growth. There is also potential for contamination with viruses, bacteria, or other pathogens. Injection of stem cells back into a patient carries the risk of introducing infection or damaging tissues.

Each type of stem cell therapy has its own particular risks. For example, stem cell therapies that involve first destroying the immune system leave patients nearly defenseless against infection for weeks.

Special concerns

Stem cell therapy holds great promise for curing or preventing the progression of many debilitating and fatal conditions, including many neurological disorders. Some researchers, physicians, and patients believe that the United States is moving too slowly toward making stem cell therapy available to the millions of patients who could potentially benefit, but many physicians also worry about patients flocking to unregulated treatment centers, both domestic and foreign, for therapies that have been proven neither safe nor effective. Stem cell therapy is very expensive and most treatments are not covered by insurance. Participation in a registered clinical trial is usually free of cost.

The U.S. Food and Drug Administration (FDA) allows a patient's stem cells to be removed and replaced, as long as they are not significantly altered in the process. If these autologous stem cells are treated with growth factors or other compounds, the FDA

QUESTIONS TO ASK YOUR DOCTOR

- What are the treatment options for my condition?
- Is there a stem cell therapy available?
- Might I be eligible for a clinical trial?
- What is the evidence that the stem cell therapy for my condition is safe and effective?
- If I pursue stem cell therapy, will it affect my ability to enter a future clinical trial or obtain other treatment?

regulates them as drugs. Some U.S.-based clinics collect stem cells from patients' blood, bone marrow, or fatty tissues and re-infuse them into damaged or diseased sites in the body. Most of these procedures have not been subjected to scientific scrutiny and some patients have been harmed.

The destruction of human embryos to obtain hESCs has been a major source of controversy in the United States and elsewhere, even though the embryos would otherwise be discarded. Restrictions on the use of hESCs have, at times, significantly interfered with stem cell therapy research. Although some of the barriers to hESC research were removed in 2009, court cases and temporary injunctions have continued to frustrate researchers.

Even some proponents of stem cell therapy have expressed concern over clinical trials that they believe to be premature. They are particularly concerned that failures or patient harm will further impede progress in stem cell therapy, as has happened in the past. Some critics are also concerned that patients who have been recently diagnosed with a life-altering disease or suffered a traumatic spinal cord injury may not be capable of fully comprehending the risks of undergoing an unproven therapy.

Resources

BOOKS

Capps, Benjamin J., and Alastair V. Campbell, eds. *Contested Cells: Global Perspectives on the Stem Cell Debate.* London: Imperial College Press, 2010.

Koka, Prasad S. *Stem Cell Therapy and Uses in Medical Treatment.* Hauppauge, NY: Nova Science, 2011.

Smith, Robin. *Stem Cell Medicine: The New Adult Stem Cell Regenerative Therapy for Cancer, Spinal Injuries, Multiple Sclerosis, Parkinson's and Other Conditions.* Long Island City, NY: Hatherleigh, 2009.

PERIODICALS

Ackerman, Todd. "A New Hope: MS Patients Going Abroad to Find Help: Promising Stem-Cell Therapies Remain Hard to Obtain in U.S." *Houston Chronicle* (February 21, 2011): 1.

Banerjee, Soma, et al. "Human Stem Cell Therapy in Ischaemic Stroke: A Review." *Age and Aging* 40, no. 1 (January 2011): 7–13.

Caplan, Arthur, and Bruce Levine. "Hope, Hype and Help: Ethically Assessing the Growing Market in Stem Cell Therapies." *Current* no. 524 (July/August 2010): 33.

Dhaulakhandi, Dhara B., Seema Rohilla, and Kamal Nain Rattan. "Neural Tube Defects: Review of Experimental Evidence on Stem Cell Therapy and Newer Treatment Options." *Fetal Diagnosis and Therapy* 28, no. 2 (August 2010): 72–78.

Hyun, Insoo. "Allowing Innovative Stem Cell-Based Therapies Outside of Clinical Trials: Ethical and Policy Challenges." *Journal of Law, Medicine & Ethics* 38, no. 2 (Summer 2010): 277–85.

Johnson, Carolyn Y. "ACT Wins FDA's Approval to Test Stem Cell Therapy." *Boston Globe* (November 22, 2010): B7.

Parker, Graham C. "Stem Cell Therapy for Stroke." *Journal of Pediatric Neurology* 8, no. 3 (2010): 333–41.

Pownall, Mark. "Experts Warn Against 'Tourist Trap' Stem Cell Therapies." *British Medical Journal* 341, no. 7771 (September 4, 2010): 477.

Stein, Rob. "First Patient to Have Experimental Stem Cell Therapy Comes Forward." *Washington Post* (April 7, 2011): A13.

Svodboda, Elizabeth. "Offshore Operations." *Popular Science* 277, no. 1 (July 2010): 64–72.

WEBSITES

International Society for Stem Cell Research. "Top Ten Things to Know About Stem Cell Treatments." A Closer Look at Stem Cell Treatments. http://www.closerlookatstemcells.org/Top_10_Stem_Cell_Treatment_Facts.htm (accessed July 19, 2011).

National Institutes of Health. "Stem Cells and Diseases." Stem Cell Information. http://stemcells.nih.gov/info/health.asp (accessed July 19, 2011).

"Stem Cell Statement and Fact Sheet." Pulmonary Hypertension Association. http://www.phassociation.org/page.aspx?pid=918 (accessed July 19, 2011).

ORGANIZATIONS

International Society for Stem Cell Research, 111 Deer Lake Road, Suite 100, Deerfield, IL 60015, (847) 509-1944, Fax: (847) 480-9282, isscr@isscr.org, http://www.isscr.org.

U.S. Food and Drug Administration, 10903 New Hampshire Avenue, Silver Spring, MD 20993-0002, (888) 463-6332, http://www.fda.gov.

Margaret Alic, PhD

Stem cell transplant

Definition

A stem cell transplant (SCT) is the infusion into a vein of healthy stem cells to replace blood-cell-forming (hematopoietic) bone marrow cells that have been removed or destroyed. A stem cell transplant is also called a bone marrow transplant (BMT), a hematopoietic stem cell transplant (HSCT), a peripheral blood stem cell (PBSC), or umbilical cord blood transplant, depending on the source of the stem cells.

Purpose

An estimated 45,000–50,000 SCTs are performed worldwide every year to treat life-threatening diseases and conditions. SCTs primarily treat diseases of the blood and immune system or restore blood-forming cells that have been destroyed by cancer treatments. SCTs can enable the bone marrow to make healthy new red blood cells, immune-system white blood cells, and platelets. Conditions that are often treated with SCTs include:

- myelodysplastic syndromes—disorders of blood-forming cells in the bone marrow
- leukemias and lymphomas, including acute lymphoblastic leukemia that involves the central nervous system (CNS)
- multiple myeloma and other disorders of plasma cells
- anemias
- inherited immune system disorders
- inherited metabolic disorders, including leukodystrophies—progressive diseases that destroy (demyelinate) the myelin sheaths surrounding nerve cells in the brain, spinal cord, and peripheral nerves

Technological advances, increasing long-term experience with SCTs, and the results of clinical trials are rapidly expanding the pool of eligible patients, as well as the conditions for which SCT may become a standard treatment option. These include neurological disorders such as the following:

- certain CNS tumors in children, especially neuroblastomas—malignant nerve cell tumors that are the most common cancers in infants
- recurrent or treatment-resistant CNS cancers
- globoid-cell leukodystrophy (GLD) or Krabbe disease, a rare, inherited, and often fatal CNS disorder
- aggressive multiple sclerosis (MS) that has not responded to other treatments
- epilepsy
- Parkinson's disease
- Tay-Sachs and Sandhoff diseases—inherited disorders of lipid metabolism that result in lipid accumulation in nervous tissue
- severe, treatment-resistant myasthenia gravis—an autoimmune disorder that interferes with the transfer of nerve impulses to muscles

Precautions

The decision to undergo SCT requires in-depth consultations and careful consideration. Although they are often successful, SCTs are painful procedures that may involve lengthy preparation and convalescence and that carry the risk of serious complications. Furthermore, it can be weeks or months before the results of a transplant are known. SCTs are best tolerated by younger patients, those in the early stages of disease, and those who have not already undergone extensive treatments.

SCTs for many conditions are either unavailable in the United States or available only as part of a clinical trial with strict eligibility requirements. Although these procedures may be available in other countries, many foreign stem cell clinics are unregulated and may offer very expensive procedures that have not been shown to be either safe or effective.

Description

Stem cells are cells that are not yet committed to developing into a single cell type—they have the potential to differentiate into some or all cell types. Stem cells divide and multiply indefinitely, unlike most other cells that divide only a finite number of times before dying. Hematopoietic stem cells are multipotent, meaning that they can develop into any type of blood cell—red blood cells, various kinds of immune system white blood cells, and platelets, which are involved in blood clotting. Hematopoietic stem cells continue to form new blood cells in the bone marrow throughout life. They are also found in the peripheral or circulating blood. Umbilical cord blood obtained from newborns is rich in hematopoietic stem cells and is supplied in cord blood units.

SCTs can be autologous or allogeneic. Autologous transplants utilize the patient's own stem cells. Allogeneic transplants utilize stem cells from a family member, an unrelated donor, or a cord blood unit. The donor or cord blood must match the recipient's HLA (human leukocyte antigen) tissue type. This reduces the risk that the new immune system formed from the transplanted stem cells will react to the recipient's tissues as foreign, resulting in graft-versus-host disease (GVHD). A syneneic transplant is an unusual type of allogeneic transplant in which the donor and recipient are identical twins or triplets and therefore have identical tissue types. The proportion of allogeneic SCTs using unrelated donors or cord blood units is increasing. When family members are not suitable donors and a transplant must be performed quickly, it is often easier to find suitably matched cord blood than an unrelated adult donor.

SCTs can be performed with whole bone marrow, hematopoietic stem cells isolated from bone marrow or peripheral blood, or cord blood. When peripheral blood is used, the donor is first treated to increase the number of circulating stem cells. For an autologous SCT, the harvested cells may be treated to destroy cancer cells or to remove other disease-causing cells. Bone marrow for an allogeneic transplant is harvested in an operating room, processed in a laboratory, and immediately transplanted or frozen for later use.

SCTs are performed in hospitals or outpatient clinics. About two million stem cells are infused through an intravenous catheter. If the bone marrow or stem cells were frozen, they are thawed in warm water immediately before infusion. The patient may be given medication that reduces the risk of side effects from preservatives added to the frozen cells. The infusion process usually takes between one and five hours. The stem cells migrate to the bone cavities, where they form new bone marrow and stem cells and begin to produce normal-functioning blood cells and a new immune system. With an allogeneic SCT, the new immune system may help destroy any remaining cancer cells.

Preparation

Eligibility

The first step in preparing for SCT is determining eligibility. Although SCTs can cure some diseases, they are physically and emotionally draining and complications can be fatal. Some SCT centers set age limits for patients, such as 50 for allogeneic transplants and 60–65 for autologous transplants. Coexisting major medical problems, such as heart, lung, liver, or kidney disease, may disqualify a patient. Transplants are usually most successful in patients who are otherwise in good health. For many diseases, transplants performed early in the disease progression carry lower risks for transplant-related mortality and disease recurrence. SCTs are usually most successful for cancers that are sensitive to chemotherapy and performed when the patient is in remission or has only a small number of tumors. Sometimes comprehensive cancer treatment plans include accommodation for a possible future SCT, since multiple cycles of chemotherapy or previous radiation increase the risk of post-transplant complications.

Autologous transplant patients should not have active disease in their bone marrow and must have adequate hematopoietic cells to collect from their peripheral blood. For allogeneic transplants, a close HLA match must be located and other donor factors may also be relevant.

Previous infections can be reactivated by SCT and patients with active infections at the time of transplant have a very high mortality rate. Most clinics will not accept HIV/AIDS patients, although some centers have special autologous protocols for them.

Tests and procedures

Preparation may include:

- complete medical history and physical examination
- neurological exam
- blood tests
- chest x ray or pulmonary function tests
- tests of heart, liver, and kidney function
- computed tomography (CT) scans or magnetic resonance imaging (MRI)
- bone marrow biopsy
- treatment of any dental problems
- Karnofsky Performance Score to evaluate the patient's ability to perform normal activities
- psychological and emotional evaluations
- identification of a primary caregiver
- HLA tissue typing of patient and siblings or search for an unrelated donor or cord blood unit
- consultations with the transplant team

A catheter may be inserted into a large vein in the upper chest for apheresis to harvest stem cells for an autologous transplant, as well as for infusing the transplanted cells. It is also used to administer chemotherapy or other medications, collect blood samples, and provide blood transfusions or nutrition if required.

Conditioning

Prior to SCT—and after harvesting stem cells for an autologous transplant—the patient's bone marrow may be destroyed with high-dose chemotherapy and/or total body irradiation (TBI). This process is called conditioning, immunosuppressive therapy, bone marrow preparation, or myeloablation. Conditioning may be required for the following purposes:

- make space in the bone cavities for transplanted stem cells to develop
- suppress the patient's immune system to lessen the risk of rejection of the transplanted cells

KEY TERMS

Allogeneic—A transplant in which the donor and recipient are genetically distinct individuals.

Anemia—A deficiency in red blood cells, in the hemoglobin component of red blood cells, or in total blood volume.

Apheresis—The process of withdrawing blood, removing one or more blood components, and transfusing the remaining blood back into the donor.

Autoimmune disorder—A disorder in which the immune system reacts to the body's own molecules, cells, or tissues.

Autologous—A transplant in which the patient is both the donor and recipient.

Bone marrow transplant (BMT)—The infusion of blood-forming stem cells for incorporation into the recipient's bone marrow or bone cavities.

Central nervous system (CNS)—The brain and spinal cord.

Conditioning—Bone marrow preparation; also known as myeloablation or immunosuppressive therapy; the destruction of bone marrow by chemotherapy and/or radiation in preparation for a stem cell transplant.

Demyelinate—The loss or destruction of the myelin sheaths surrounding nerve fibers.

Epilepsy—Chronic disorders marked by abnormal electrical discharges in the brain.

Globoid-cell leukodystrophy (GLD)—Krabbe disease; a rare, inherited, and usually fatal disorder that causes demyelination of nerves in the central nervous system.

Graft-versus-host disease (GVHD)—A condition in which immune system cells from a stem cell transplant react against recipient cells and tissues.

Hematopoietic stem cell transplant (HSCT)—Infusion of blood-forming stem cells from donor bone marrow, circulating blood, or umbilical cord blood.

Human leukocyte antigen (HLA)—The major tissue compatibility complex, which determines whether transplanted donor cells will be compatible with those of the recipient.

Immunosuppressive therapy—Destruction of the immune system with chemotherapy and/or radiation treatment to prevent rejection of transplanted cells; drug treatment to suppress the donor immune system following a stem cell transplant, to prevent graft-versus-host disease.

Leukodystrophy—Any of several inherited diseases characterized by the degeneration of myelin in the brain, spinal cord, and peripheral nerves.

Multiple sclerosis (MS)—A demyelinating autoimmune disease that affects the brain or spinal cord.

Myelin—The white, fatty substance that covers and protects nerves.

Peripheral blood stem cells (PBSC)—Blood-cell-forming stem cells in circulating blood.

Platelet—A blood component that assists clotting.

Synegeneic—A transplant in which the donor and recipient are identical twins or triplets.

Total body irradiation (TBI)—Whole-body irradiation therapy; used for conditioning to destroy bone marrow prior to a stem cell transplant.

• eliminate abnormal or dysfunctional bone marrow cells

• destroy cancer cells

A mini stem cell transplant, also called a reduced-intensity conditioning transplant or a nonmyeloablative transplant, is a less aggressive conditioning process that relies on the transplanted cells to fight the cancer. It is typically used for patients in poorer health or with a slowly progressing disease.

Aftercare

Immunodeficient post-transplant patients must restrict their activities to reduce the risk of infection, and sometimes long hospital stays are required. Patients

generally stay at the transplant center until the following are achieved:

• They have 48 hours without a fever.

• Medication can be swallowed and kept down for 48 hours.

• Nausea, vomiting, and diarrhea are controlled with medication.

• Red blood cell, neutrophil (a white blood cell), and platelet counts have reached certain levels.

• There is a caregiver at home.

It usually takes two to six weeks for transplanted cells to begin multiplying and producing blood cells. It takes about a year for blood cells and the immune system to return to normal levels. Patients may take antibiotics, and possibly antifungal and **antiviral drugs**, until their white blood cell counts reach safe levels. Many patients require intravenous antibiotics and transfusions of red blood cells and platelets. Supplemental nutrition may be required because of vomiting and diarrhea. Patients also may require treatment for toxicity related to the conditioning or transplant, graft failure or transplant rejection, drug reactions, or recurrence of the underlying disease. GVHD must be treated with immunosuppressive drugs. Replacement hormones may be required because of hypothyroidism resulting from radiation treatments. Children undergoing SCTs often suffer from growth retardation and may require synthetic growth hormone.

Risks

SCTs can cause serious side effects and complications up to a year or more post-transplant. Although most medical problems are related to conditioning, specific risks associated with SCT include:

- transplant failure
- infections
- lung, kidney, liver, or heart problems from organ damage
- poor thyroid function
- cataracts
- secondary cancers
- infertility or early menopause
- sexual problems
- fatigue
- activity limitations
- memory loss
- poor concentration
- depression, anxiety, emotional distress, or body-image disorders
- social isolation or relationship changes
- job or insurance discrimination

Between 30% and 70% of allogeneic transplant patients develop GVHD. It can occur immediately after an SCT or develop months or even years later. Although chronic GVHD is a serious and potentially life-threatening complication, most cases resolve within five years.

About 45% of pediatric SCT patients experience retarded growth and development for two years post-transplant. This is especially true for children receiving TBI. Radiation can also interfere with dental and facial development, especially in children under seven. Therefore pediatric SCT patients receive chemotherapy-only conditioning if possible.

QUESTIONS TO ASK YOUR DOCTOR

- Am I a candidate for a stem cell transplant?
- Can my own stem cells be used or do I require donor stem cells?
- How will you obtain the donor stem cells?
- Is it likely that my stem cell transplant will be successful?
- What are the risks involved in a stem cell transplant?

Results

The success of SCT depends on many factors, including the type and severity of the disorder, the type of SCT, and the age and overall health of the patient. SCTs can cure some diseases and put others into remission. Many SCT patients go on to live normal lives. Recovery from an autologous transplant is usually faster than from an allogeneic transplant.

Resources

BOOKS

Treleaven, Jennifer, and A.J. Barrett. *Hematopoietic Stem Cell Transplantation*. New York: Churchill Livingstone/Elsevier, 2009.

PERIODICALS

Duffner, Patricia K., et al. "The Long-Term Outcomes of Presymptomatic Infants Transplanted for Krabbe Disease." *Genetics in Medicine* 11, no. 6 (June 2009): 450–54.

WEBSITES

"Curing Epilepsy: The Promise of Research." National Institute of Neurological Disorders and Stroke. http://www.ninds.nih.gov/disorders/epilepsy/epilepsy_research.htm (accessed July 20, 2011).

"Globoid-Cell Leukodystrophy (Krabbe Disease) and Transplant." National Marrow Donor Program. http://www.marrow.org/PATIENT/Undrstnd_Disease_Treat/Lrn_about_Disease/Metabolic_Storage/GLD_and_Tx/index.html (accessed July 20, 2011).

"Recommended Post-Transplant Care—Part I: Long-Term Screening." National Marrow Donor Program. http://www.marrow.org/PHYSICIAN/Patient_Care_Post_Tx/PDF/QuickRefGuidelines_Long-term_screening_Part%20I.pdf (accessed July 20, 2011).

"Recommended Post-Transplant Care—Part II: Screening for Chronic GVHD." National Marrow Donor Program. http://www.marrow.org/PHYSICIAN/Patient_Care_Post_Tx/PDF/QuickRefGuidelines_cGVHD_screening_Part%20II.pdf (accessed July 20, 2011).

"Stem Cell Transplant." Mayo Clinic. http://www.mayoclinic.com/print/stem-cell-transplant/MY00089/ (accessed July 20, 2011).

"Stem Cell Transplant Marks New 'Birthday' for Woman with MS." *MS Connection* (Winter/Spring 2010): 4. http://www.nationalmssociety.org/download.aspx?id=18499 (accessed July 20, 2011).

"Stem Cell Transplant (Peripheral Blood, Bone Marrow, and Cord Blood Transplants)." American Cancer Society. http://www.cancer.org/Treatment/Treatments andSideEffects/TreatmentTypes/BoneMarrowand PeripheralBloodStemCellTransplant/stem-cell-transplant-transplant-process (accessed July 20, 2011).

"Transplant Indications, Timing & Referral." National Marrow Donor Program. http://www.marrow.org/PHYSICIAN/Tx_Indications_Timing_Referral/index.html (accessed July 20, 2011).

"Understanding Bone Marrow Transplantation as a Treatment Option." Health Resources and Services Administration. http://bloodcell.transplant.hrsa.gov/TRANSPLANT/Understanding_Tx/index.html (accessed July 20, 2011).

ORGANIZATIONS

National Institute of Neurological Disorders and Stroke (NINDS), P.O. Box 5801, Bethesda, MD 20824, (301) 496-5751, (800) 352-9424, http://www.ninds.nih.gov.

National Marrow Donor Program, 3001 Broadway Street NE, Suite 100, Minneapolis, MN 55413-1753, (612) 627-5800, (800) MARROW2 (627-7692), http://www.marrow.org.

National Multiple Sclerosis Society, 733 Third Avenue, New York, NY 10017, (800) 344-4867, http://www.nmss.org.

Margaret Alic, PhD

Stiff person syndrome

Definition

Stiff person syndrome (SPS) is an extremely rare progressive neurological disorder characterized by persistent rigidity and spasms of certain voluntary muscles, especially those of legs and feet. In some cases, muscles of the neck, trunk, and shoulders may also be involved. SPS may begin as recurring (intermittent) episodes of stiffness and spasms, often precipitated by surprise or minor physical contact.

Description

SPS is a rare progressive neurological disorder characterized by constant painful contractions and spasms of voluntary muscles, particularly the muscles of the back and upper legs. In 1956, scientists at the Mayo Clinic also coined the term "stiff man syndrome," and clearly described the stiff person syndrome as a neurological disorder. The rigidity, which is characterized by tightness and stiffness, begins slowly over several months at the axial muscles, especially the thoracic and lumbar spine, and spreads to the legs. The stiffness may worsen when the affected individual is anxious or exposed to sudden motion or noise. Affected muscles may become twisted and contracted, resulting in bone fractures in the most severe cases.

Another abnormality in SPS is called co-contraction: when the person attempts to contract a muscle to move in one direction, muscles that pull in the opposite direction are involuntarily activated. Individuals with SPS may have difficulty making sudden movements and may have a stiff-legged unsteady gait (manner of walking). The muscle contractions are usually reduced with extra rest.

Eventually, persons with stiff person syndrome may develop a hunched posture (kyphosis) or a swayback (lordosis).

Demographics

The frequency of SPS worldwide or in the United States is unknown, but the syndrome is rare. Unlike many **autoimmune diseases**, which have a higher incidence in women, SPS is found more frequently in men, occurring in men in approximately 70% of all cases. The syndrome also occurs in children younger than three years, most commonly in infants. Onset in adults is most frequent in the third to fifth decades of life.

Causes and symptoms

Causes

The cause of stiff person syndrome is unknown; however, researchers theorize that SPS may be an autoimmune disorder. An autoimmune disorder involves a malfunction of the immune system, where the body produces antibodies against its own tissues. Antibodies are proteins produced by the body as part of its defense against foreign bacteria, viruses, or other harmful substances. Other autoimmune disorders such as diabetes, pernicious anemia (a chronic, progressive blood disorder), and thyroiditis (inflammation of the thyroid gland) may occur more frequently in patients with SPS.

Often SPS, antibodies are produced against glutamic acid decarboxylase (GAD), an enzyme largely found in the **central nervous system**. However, GAD antibodies alone appear to be insufficient to cause SPS, as some persons with stiff person disease do not have the GAD antibodies, and GAD antibodies are associated with a number of diseases.

Symptoms

Symptoms may occur gradually, spreading from the back and legs to involve the arms and neck. Initially, the patient has an exaggerated upright posture and may experience back discomfort, stiffness, or pain in the entire back, which worsens with tension or stress. Some persons with SPS, in the early stages, show brief episodes of rather dramatic severe worsening that resolve spontaneously within hours or days. Later in the disease, upper limb muscles also begin to be involved, particularly when the person is stimulated, surprised, angered, upset, or frightened. This sort of stimulation may evoke painful severe spasms in the upper arm and leg muscles that resolve slowly. The person with SPS begins to move very slowly because rapid movement induces severe spasms. Even the lower extremities may become involved when moved rapidly. In the end stages of the disease, few muscles in the body are spared. However, facial and pharyngeal muscles may be especially affected.

Babies and young children are less rigid between attacks. Involvement of lower arm and leg muscles is often more evident, particularly during muscle spasms.

Diagnosis

During physical examination, the physician who suspects SPS looks for stiffness, rigidity, or increased tone, spasm, or pain. The areas of involvement may include the face, neck, abdomen, or arms, but more typically the legs or lumbar spine are involved. Evaluation may include tests to rule out other causes of stiffness such as **multiple sclerosis**. When overwhelming anxiety and fear overshadow the stiffness, it may be difficult to distinguish SPS from an emotional disorder.

Laboratory procedures assess the presence of specific autoantibodies called anti-GAD, which are found at high levels in the blood of a person with SPS. These examinations include immunocytochemistry, Western blotting, ELISA (enzyme-linked immunosorbent assay), and radioimmunoassay (RIA). The last two procedures have the advantage of quantitatively assessing the amount of anti-GAD antibody a patient produces.

Electromyography (EMG) is an important diagnostic tool to determine an abnormal firing pattern in the muscles sometimes seen in persons with SPS. The EMG findings of SPS may be subtle in patients who are fully treated for symptoms of SPS. Except for global muscle stiffness, results of a neurological examination are usually normal. Results of conventional computed tomography and magnetic resonance imaging of the brain are also normal.

Treatment team

The treatment team for a person with SPS is often composed of physical and occupational therapists, nutritionists, neurosurgeons, and neurologists.

Treatment

SPS is clinically elusive, but potentially treatable. Traditional treatment for SPS starts with medications such as baclofen or a benzodiazepine. Commonly used **benzodiazepines** are **diazepam** (Valium) or lorazepam (Ativan). Both benzodiazepine and baclofen increase the activity of the central inhibitory systems. Although no studies have been performed, tizanidine (Zanaflex) may be a less sedating alternative, and prednisone is also a commonly prescribed drug for treatment of SPS.

In some patients, plasmapheresis, a process of filtering the blood to remove excess antibodies, has been demonstrated to be useful in removing anti-GAD antibodies from the bloodstream. In the hospital setting, intravenous immunoglobulin (IVIG) has also been used in the treatment of SPS.

Recovery and rehabilitation

Physical therapy and occupational therapy are critical to the recovery of patients under treatment. Medical treatment can make the patient feel weak, a feeling that may be alleviated by therapy. The person with SPS may also have problems with voluntary movements and fine motor skills. Occupational and physical therapists devise strategies to compensate for these weaknesses during the common daily activities of living.

Clinical trials

Information about current relevant clinical trials can be found at ClinicalTrials.gov.

Prognosis

There is no cure for SPS and the long-term prognosis is variable. Many patients have a slow course of the disorder that is mostly without symptoms, punctuated by occasional episodes of stiffness. Other patients may have a much more aggressive course, rapidly progressing to the late stages of disease. Other forms of the disease have been described that are accompanied by brain disorders and other central nervous system abnormalities, but whether they are separate diseases or different manifestations of the same disease is unclear. Management of the disorder with drug therapy usually provides significant improvement and relief of symptoms.

Special concerns

Many of the medications prescribed for SPS are not indicated during pregnancy. Elderly persons with SPS may have increased chances of falling and injury because of concurrent disability from other causes. As with all autoimmune disorders, dietary changes sometimes helpful. For best results, dietary changes should be made under the supervision of a physician experienced in nutritional medicine.

Resources

BOOKS

Larsen, Povl K. Egeberg, J. Schousboe, A. *Glutamate and GABA Receptors and Transporters.* New York: Taylor & Francis, 2001.
The Official Patient's Sourcebook on Stiff-Person Syndrome: A Revised and Updated Directory for the Internet Age. San Diego: Icon Group International, 2002.

PERIODICALS

Gerschlager, W. et al. "Quality of life in stiff person syndrome."*Movement Disorders* 17(2002): 1064–67.

OTHER

"NINDS Stiff-Person Syndrome Information Page" *National Institute of Neurological Disorders and Stroke*http://www.ninds.nih.gov/health_and_medical/disorders/stiffperson_doc.htm (March 11, 2004).

ORGANIZATIONS

National Institute of Arthritis and Musculoskeletal and Skin Diseases (NIAMS). Bldg. 31, Rm. 4C05, Bethesda, Maryland 20892-2350. Phone: (301) 496-8188. Tollfree Email: NIAMSInfo@mail.nih.gov. http://www.nih.gov/niams.
National Organization for Rare Disorders (NORD). 55 Kenosia Avenue, Danbury, Connecticut 06813-1968. Phone: (203) 744-0100. Fax: (203) 798-2291. Tollfree Email: orphan@rarediseases.org. http://www.rarediseases.org.
National Rehabilitation Information Center (NARIC). 4200 Forbes Boulevard; Suite 202, Lanham, Maryland 20706-4829. Phone: (301) 562-2400. Fax: (301) 562-2401. Tollfree phone: (800) 346-2742. Email: naricinfo@heitechservices.com. http://www.naric.com.

Bruno Verbeno Azevedo
Iuri Drumond Louro, MD, PhD

Striatonigral degeneration

Definition

Striatonigral degeneration is a neurodegenerative disease caused by disruption of two areas, the striatum and substantia nigra, which work together to enable movement and balance.

Description

Striatonigral degeneration was described by Adam in 1961 and 1964. However, since the disorder has common manifestations seen in multiple diseases (e.g., the Shy-Drager syndrome, where autonomic nervous system failure predominates, and sporadic olivopontocerebellar degeneration, where **cerebellum** deficits predominate), it was necessary to clarify the nomenclature. In 1999, the name striatonigral degeneration was replaced with the accepted new names, multiple system atrophy-Parkinson (MSA-P), if **Parkinson's disease** symptoms predominate, or MSA-cerebellum (MSA-C), if cerebellar **ataxia** is the main feature. Patients who have MSA have characteristic pathological changes in common, but in variable degrees. Affected neurons in the brain have inclusion bodies that cause neuronal loss, by a mechanism of programmed cell death called apoptosis. The presence of inclusion bodies in neurons causes a reaction to self-destruct following a programmed sequence of chemical reactions that promotes cell death.

Demographics

The prevalence of MSA-P is difficult to establish with accuracy since the disorder is frequently misdiagnosed in the United States and internationally. It is estimated to account for 5–22% of cases in patients with Parkinson's or Parkinson-like disorders. Approximately 80% of patients present with MSA-P symptoms and

20% exhibit symptoms of cerebellar ataxia (MSA-C subtype). It is estimated that the prevalence of this disorder is 1.9–4.9 cases per 100,000. The age range of diagnosis is between 33 and 76 years of age. MSA-P has never been identified in a person younger than 30 years. The mean survival time after the onset of symptoms is 7–9 years. There is no racial predilection, and males and females are affected equally. The mean age of diagnosis is 53 years. For the majority of MSA-P affected persons, the full clinical picture evolves within five years after onset of symptoms.

Causes and symptoms

The cause of MSA has not been identified. MSA occurs in the general population in a sporadic manner. The disorder is degenerative and progressively worsens. The natural history of the disorder is chronic, symptoms progressively worsen, and the disorder often results in death, after multiple treatment efforts.

Common symptoms of MSA-P (which may be asymmetric) include bradykinesia (slowness of movement) characterized by an irregular jerky postural **tremor**. It is uncommon for the tremor to occur at rest. Additionally, patients often exhibit rigidity, postural instability, and a characteristic quivering high-pitched **dysarthria**. Many patients with MSA-P also develop orofacial and craniocervical dystonia. Patients with the MSA-C subtype also develop gait and limb ataxia, eye abnormalities, and scanning dysarthria. Other symptoms can include **depression**, emotional lability (fluctuations of emotional state), hyperreflexia, extensor plantar (sole) response, **myoclonus**, or laryngeal stridor. Failure of the autonomic nervous system (ANS) is a characteristic of both subtypes (MSA-P and MSA-C), which primarily consists of urogenital problems and **orthostatic hypotension**. ANS failure causes early male erectile dysfunction, and urinary dysfunction causing problems with frequency, urgency, retention, and incontinence. Additionally, patients frequently develop postprandial (after food) postural hypotension and episodes of syncope (loss of consciousness), due to lack of oxygen to the brain (cerebral hypoperfusion).

Diagnosis

No specific lab tests are indicated. High-resolution neuroimaging studies may demonstrate neuronal abnormalities and/or atrophy in the brain. The diagnosis is based on history, physical examination, and family history (to detect genetic correlations). A definite diagnosis can be obtained by pathological examination of brain neurons. A probable diagnosis is made by the presence of ANS failure, poor response to medications, or cerebellar dysfunction (cerebellar ataxia). Neuroimaging studies using magnetic resonance imaging (MRI) indicate that that there is volume loss (neuronal loss) in associated areas in the brain (the striatum and substantia nigra). Functional neuroimaging techniques (which take images of neuron function) indicate that neuron receptor binding is defective and there is low metabolism (low level of vital chemical reactions).

Treatment team

The treatment team can typically include a neurologist and respiratory care providers, when management of breathing difficulties requires professional intervention. A physical therapist can help with postural and movement difficulties. An audiologist is utilized for speech and eating difficulties.

Treatment

No surgical treatment exists for striatonigral degeneration, and pharmacological treatment is not effective in the long term. Approximately 30% of patients demonstrate initial improvement with the medication levodopa-carbidopa. However, symptomatic improvement is temporary; approximately 90% patients are unresponsive to levodopa in the long term. Dystonia can be treated with **botulinum toxin**, which tends to control involuntary muscular movements. Affected persons who develop failure of the autonomic nervous system may develop orthostatic hypotension. Patients who develop low blood pressure symptoms should avoid activities such as overeating, straining at stool passage, and exposure to extreme heat. Elevating the head of the bed, use of pressure stockings, and increased sodium intake (which causes water retention, which in turn stabilizes blood pressure) are treatments for hypotension. Additionally, medication to correct hypotension can be prescribed, including fludrocortisone, ephedrine, and midodrine. Medication to treat postprandial hypotension (octreotide) or bladder symptoms (oxybutynin) can be given when needed. Overall, however, the results of medical treatment for MSA is poor.

Recovery and rehabilitation

Rehabilitation can include patient, family, and caretaker education concerning the possibilities of respiratory failure, aspiration pneumonia, trauma, and syncope. Patients can develop paresis of the larynx or pharynx, central chronic respiratory failure (a chronic respiratory failure due to destruction of neurons in the brain), or sudden death. Patients require physical therapy to help maintain mobility and prevent permanent

KEY TERMS

Ataxia—Muscular incoordination and irregularity of muscular action.

Autonomic nervous system (ANS)—Consists of neurons that are not under one's conscious control. The ANS is comprised of two subdivisions called the parasympathetic nervous system, which slows heart rate, increases intestinal and gland activity, and relaxes the sphincter muscles; and the sympathetic nervous system, which accelerates heart rate, raises blood pressure, and constricts blood vessels.

Cerebellar ataxia—Disorders of the cerebellum that cause a loss of muscular coordination.

Dysarthria—Nerve damage that causes disturbances in muscular control, resulting in impaired speech articulation.

Dyskinesias—A group of disorders characterized by involuntary movements of muscles.

Dystonia—Abnormal tone in a group of muscles.

Hyperreflexia—An increased reaction to reflexes.

Incontinence—Inability to control excretory functions such as defecation and urination.

Laryngeal stridor—Constriction of the voice box, causing vocal hoarseness.

Myoclonus—Spasm or twitching of a muscle or a group of muscles.

Orthostatic hypotension—A reduction of blood pressure (systolic blood pressure that occurs when the heart contracts or diastolic pressure that occurs when the heart muscle relaxes).

Paresis—A slight paralysis.

Parkinson's disease—A neurodegenerative disorder characterized by slowness of voluntary movements, mask-like facial expression, and a rhythmic tremor of the limbs and stooped posture.

Receptor—A structure located on the outside of a cell's membrane that causes the cell to attach to specific molecules; the molecules are then internalized, taken inside the cell.

Striatum—Area located deep within the brain.

Substantia nigra—An area located in the middle portion of the brain that can become depleted of a specific neurotransmitter called dopamine, causing symptoms of Parkinson's disease.

Syncope—Loss of consciousness.

Tremor—An involuntary movement characterized by quivering and trembling.

muscular contractures. Speech therapy can improve speech impairments and difficulty with swallowing (dysphagia) mechanisms. Dysphagia may necessitate tube placement and feedings. Patients eventually require occupational therapy to limit handicap from disability. A wheelchair is indicated depending on liability to **falls** due to gait (walking) ataxia, and postural instability. Psychological support is necessary for the patient and family member caretakers.

Clinical trials

Clinical trials are being done to find methods to prevent and treat MSA-P. The Mayo Clinic in Rochester, Minnesota, currently has projects and investigations concerning new techniques for diagnosis using **PET** scan technology. This technology is likely to be available in the near future.

Prognosis

The disorder is degenerative and the mean survival time in confirmed cases is seven years. The range of survival for persons with MSA-P is 2–15 years.

Approximately 50% of affected patients who receive levodopa develop side effects that can include dyskinesia of orofacial and neck muscles.

Special concerns

Episodes of syncope can cause severe trauma, usually from falls. Patients are advised to lie or sit down when symptoms of low blood present appear. Family members and caretakers should be aware of the syncope and the dangers associated with falls and trauma.

Resources

PERIODICALS

Wenning, Gregor, and Werner Poewe. "Multiple System Atrophy." *Lancet Neurology* 3:2 (February 2004).

WEBSITES

National Organization for Rare Disorders (NORD). (May 23, 2004.) http://www.rarediseases.org.

Mayo Clinic. *Clinical Information.* (May 23, 2004.) http://www.mayoresearch.mayo.edu.

ORGANIZATIONS

Worldwide Education & Awareness for Movement Disorders (WE MOVE). 204 West 84th Street, New York, NY 10024. Phone: (212) 875-8312. Fax: (212) 875-8389. Tollfree phone: (800) 437-6682. Email: wemove@wemove. org. http://www.wemove.org.

Laith Farid Gulli, MD
Nicole Mallory, MS, PA-C

Stroke

Definition

Stroke is a life-threatening condition that occurs when the blood supply to a part of the brain is suddenly cut off or when brain tissue is damaged by bleeding into the brain. There are two main types of stroke. Ischemic stroke occurs when a clot blocks an artery to the brain; this type accounts for about 80 percent of strokes. The other type, hemorrhagic stroke, occurs when a blood vessel in the brain bursts, allowing blood to spill out

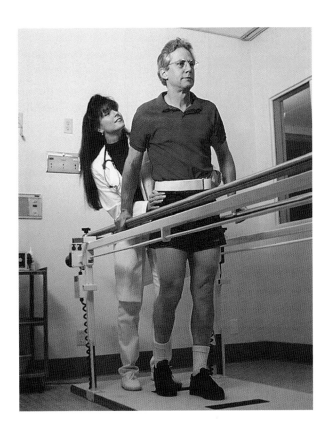

A man who suffered a stroke is helped with rehabilitation by a physical therapist. (© *Custom Medical Stock Photo, Inc. Reproduced by permission.*)

into brain tissue. The blood upsets the chemical balance that the nerve cells in the brain need to function.

Demographics

According to the Centers for Disease Control and Prevention (CDC), stroke is the fourth leading cause of death in the United States as of 2009, being responsible for about 128,000 deaths each year. About 795,000 Americans have strokes each year, 550,000 for the first time and 245,000 having a second or third stroke. Of these cases, approximately 625,000 are ischemic strokes. The total cost of stroke to the U.S. economy per year as of 2009 is approximately $68.9 billion. By the year 2025, the annual number of strokes is expected to reach 1 million. As of 2009, more than 4.4 million people in the United States are stroke survivors. Worldwide, the World Health Organization estimatesáthat 15 million people suffer a stroke each year, resulting in 5 million deaths and 5 million permanently disabled survivors.

About 50,000 Americans have a transient ischemic attack (TIA) in an average year; of this group, 35 percent will have a severe stroke at some point in the future.

Strokes can affect people in any age group; however, the risk increases sharply in people over 55 years of age, doubling every decade over age 55. Seventy-five percent of all strokes in Canada and the United States occur in people over 64. Men are 1.25 times more likely to have strokes than women; however, women are more likely to die of stroke because they are usually older when they have their first stroke.

Strokes in children are rare—about six cases per 100,000 children per year in North America. About one-third of these cases are in newborns.

African Americans have an increased risk of stroke compared to other racial and ethnic groups in the United States, and they are also more likely to suffer a stroke at younger ages. Hispanics are at lesser risk of stroke than African Americans, but they also tend to have strokes at relatively young ages. African Americans between the ages of 45 and 55 die from stroke 4–5 times more often that Caucasians in the same age group.

Description

Stroke is usually a sudden occurrence. A stroke occurs when blood flow is interrupted to part of the brain. Without blood to supply oxygen and nutrients and to remove waste products, brain cells quickly begin to die. Depending on the region of the brain affected, a stroke may cause paralysis, speech impairment, loss of memory and reasoning ability, coma, or death. A stroke also is sometimes called a brain attack or a cerebrovascular accident (CVA).

Some people have a warning event called a transient ischemic attack (TIA) or mini-stroke. A TIA has the same symptoms as a full-blown stroke but goes away in a few minutes or hours, leaving no permanent effects. It is, however, an indication that the person is at risk of a major stroke and should see their doctor right away. A TIA offers the person an opportunity to take preventive action.

Stroke is a medical emergency requiring immediate treatment. Prompt treatment improves the chances of survival and increases the degree of recovery that may be expected. A person who may have suffered a stroke should be seen in a hospital emergency room without delay. Treatment to break up a blood clot, the major cause of stroke, must begin within three hours of the stroke to be effective. Improved medical treatment of all types of stroke has resulted in a dramatic decline in death rates in recent decades. In 1950, nine in ten stroke patients died, compared to slightly less than one in three in the twenty-first century. However, about two-thirds of stroke survivors have disabilities ranging from moderate to severe.

Risk factors

Risk factors for stroke in adults include:

- Hypertension (high blood pressure), the most important single risk factor for stroke
- High blood cholesterol levels
- Age over 55
- A family history of stroke, TIA, or heart attack
- Diabetes
- Smoking, which doubles a person's risk of ischemic stroke
- Personal history of previous stroke or TIA
- Obesity
- Heavy use of cocaine
- Irregular heart rhythm
- High alcohol consumption, which raises a person's blood pressure
- Use of birth control pills or hormone replacement therapy

Risk factors for stroke in children include:

- Congenital (present at birth) malformations of blood vessels and other structures in the brain
- Infections of the brain like encephalitis and meningitis
- Head trauma
- Blood disorders, particularly sickle cell disease

Causes and symptoms

Causes

Stroke is caused by a loss of blood supply to the brain resulting either from a clot blocking an artery or from bleeding into or around the brain. Ischemic stroke can result from two types of clots. The first is an embolus, which is a free-floating clot produced in the heart or somewhere else in the body that travels to a blood vessel in the brain. The second type of clot is called a thrombus. It is formed within an artery in the head or neck and grows there until it is large enough to block the artery. Atherosclerosis, a disease of the blood vessels in which fatty deposits build up along the walls of the vessels, is a common cause of this type of clot.

ISCHEMIC STROKE. A cerebral embolism occurs when a blood clot from elsewhere in the circulatory system breaks free. If it becomes lodged in an artery supplying the brain, either in the brain or in the neck, it can cause a stroke. The most common cause of cerebral embolism is atrial fibrillation, a disorder of the heart beat. In atrial fibrillation, the upper chambers (atria) of the heart beat weakly and rapidly instead of slowly and steadily. Blood within the atria is not completely emptied. This stagnant blood may form clots within the atria, which can then break off and enter the circulation. Atrial fibrillation is a factor in about 15% of all strokes. The risk of a stroke from atrial fibrillation can be dramatically reduced with daily use of anticoagulant medication.

Cerebral thrombosis occurs when a blood clot, or thrombus, forms within the brain itself, blocking the flow of blood through the affected vessel. Clots most often form due to "hardening" (atherosclerosis) of brain arteries. Cerebral thrombosis occurs most often at night or early in the morning. Cerebral thrombosis is often preceded by a transient ischemic attack, or TIA, sometimes called a "mini-stroke." In a TIA, blood flow is temporarily interrupted, causing short-lived stroke-like symptoms. Recognizing the occurrence of a TIA and seeking immediate treatment is an important step in stroke prevention.

HEMORRHAGIC STROKE. Hemorrhagic stroke can occur when an aneurysm—a weak spot in the wall of an artery—suddenly bursts. High blood pressure is the most common cause of this type of hemorrhagic stroke. Hemorrhagic stroke can also occur when the walls of an artery become thin and brittle; they can then break and leak blood into the brain. Hemorrhagic stroke can take one of two forms: The blood can leak directly into brain tissue from an artery in the brain, or it can leak from an artery near the surface of the brain into the space between the skull and the membranes covering the brain.

The vessels most likely to break are those with preexisting defects such as an aneurysm. An aneurysm is a bulge or pouch in a blood vessel caused by weakening of the arterial wall. Brain aneurysms are surprisingly common; according to autopsy studies, about 6% of all Americans have them. Aneurysms rarely cause symptoms until they burst, however. Aneurysms are most likely to burst when blood pressure is highest, and controlling blood pressure is an important preventive strategy.

Intracerebral hemorrhage affects vessels within the brain itself, while subarachnoid hemorrhage affects arteries at the brain's surface, just below the protective arachnoid membrane. Intracerebral hemorrhages represent about 10% of all strokes, while subarachnoid hemorrhages account for about 7%.

In addition to depriving affected tissues of blood supply, the accumulation of fluid within the inflexible skull creates excess pressure on brain tissue, which can quickly lead to death. Nonetheless, recovery may be more complete for a person who survives hemorrhage than for one who survives a clot, because the effects of blood deprivation usually are not as severe.

The death of brain cells triggers a chain reaction in which toxic chemicals created by cell death affect other nearby cells. This is one reason why prompt treatment can have such a dramatic effect on final recovery.

Symptoms

Stroke has five major signs or symptoms:

- Walk: Is the person having trouble with balance or coordination?
- Talk: Is speech difficult or slurred? Is the person's face drooping?
- Reach: Is one side of the body weak or numb?
- See: Is vision partly or entirely lost?
- Feel: Does the person have a sudden severe headache with no obvious cause?

Other symptoms of stroke that some patients experience are drooling, uncontrollable eye movements, personality or mood changes, drowsiness, loss of memory, or loss of consciousness.

A person with stroke can have more than one of these symptoms at the same time. The important feature to keep in mind is that the symptoms of an embolic ischemic stroke come on suddenly, which helps in distinguishing stroke from other causes of dizziness, vision problems, or headache. The symptoms of a thrombotic stroke come on more gradually.

A child having a stroke may lose bladder control, have a seizure, or have nausea and vomiting as well as the symptoms associated with stroke in adults.

Diagnosis

The diagnosis of stroke includes taking the patient's history and obtaining an account of the patient's present symptoms. In younger patients, the doctor will ask about recent drug use, head trauma, use of oral contraceptives, or bleeding disorders. In middle-aged and older patients, the doctor will ask about such risk factors as hypertension, diabetes, tobacco use, high cholesterol, and a history of coronary artery disease, coronary artery bypass surgery, or atrial fibrillation.

An important part of the history-taking is finding out when the symptoms began and when the patient was last seen normal. Information from family, bystanders, or emergency personnel is often critical to prompt diagnosis and treatment, particularly when tissue plasminogen activator (tPA) therapy is an option. If the patient has awakened with the symptoms of stroke, then the time of onset is defined as the time the patient was last seen without symptoms.

Examination

The next step is a complete physical and neurological examination to rule out the possibility that the patient's symptoms are being caused by a brain tumor. The examination has several purposes: checking the patient's airway, breathing, and circulation; identifying any neurological deficits; identifying the potential cause(s) of the stroke; and identifying any comorbid conditions the patient may have. The neurologist may use the National Institutes of Health Stroke Scale (NIHSS), which is a checklist that allows the doctor to record the patient's level of consciousness; visual function; ability to move; ability to feel sensations; ability to move the facial muscles; and ability to talk.

Tests

Other tests used to diagnose stroke are:

- Blood tests. These can reveal the existence of blood disorders that increase a person's risk of stroke.
- Computed tomography (CT) scan. This type of imaging test is one of the first tests given to a patient suspected of having a stroke. It helps the doctor determine the cause of the stroke and the extent of brain injury.

KEY TERMS

Aneurysm—A pouchlike bulging of a blood vessel. Aneurysms can rupture, leading to stroke.

Atrial fibrillation—A disorder of the heart beat associated with a higher risk of stroke. In this disorder, the upper chambers (atria) of the heart do not completely empty when the heart beats, which can allow blood clots to form.

Cerebral embolism—A blockage of blood flow through a vessel in the brain by a blood clot that formed elsewhere in the body and traveled to the brain.

Cerebral thrombosis—A blockage of blood flow through a vessel in the brain by a blood clot that formed in the brain itself.

Comorbid—Referring to the presence of one or more diseases or disorders in addition to the patient's primary disorder.

Deficit—In medicine, the loss or impairment of a function or ability.

Dysphagia—The medical term for difficulty in swallowing.

Embolus—The medical term for a clot that forms in the heart and travels through the circulatory system to another part of the body.

Intracerebral hemorrhage—A cause of some strokes in which vessels within the brain begin bleeding.

Ischemia—Loss of blood supply to a tissue or organ resulting from the blockage of a blood vessel.

Platelets—Small irregularly shaped blood cells involved in the formation of blood clots.

Statins—A group of medications given to lower blood cholesterol levels that work by inhibiting an enzyme involved in cholesterol formation. Statins are also known as HMG-CoA reductase inhibitors.

Subarachnoid hemorrhage—A cause of some strokes in which arteries on the surface of the brain begin bleeding.

Thrombus—A blood clot that forms inside an intact blood vessel and remains there.

Tissue plasminogen activator (tPA)—A substance that is sometimes given to patients within three hours of a stroke to dissolve blood clots within the brain.

Transient ischemic attack (TIA)—A brief stroke lasting from a few minutes to 24 hours. TIAs are sometimes called mini-strokes.

- Magnetic resonance imaging (MRI). This imaging test is useful in pinpointing the location of small or deep brain injuries.
- Electroencephalogram (EEG). This test measures the brain's electrical activity.
- Blood flow tests. These are done to detect the location and size of any blockages in the blood vessels. One type of blood flow test uses ultrasound to produce an image of the arteries in the neck leading into the brain. Another type of blood flow test, called angiography, uses a special dye injected into blood vessels that will show up on an x-ray.
- Echocardiography. This type of test uses ultrasound to produce an image of the heart. It can be useful in determining whether an embolus from the heart caused the patient's stroke.

Treatment

Traditional

Treatment of stroke depends on whether it is ischemic or hemorrhagic. Ischemic stroke is treated first with blood thinners, often aspirin or warfarin. If the patient is seen by a specialized stroke team within 3 hours of the attack, he or she may be treated with a drug called tissue plasminogen activator or tPA, described more fully in the next section. It is critical, however, to be sure that the patient has an ischemic rather than a hemorrhagic stroke, as blood-thinning drugs can make a hemorrhagic stroke worse.

Ischemic stroke can also be treated by surgery. The two procedures most commonly used are endarterectomy, a procedure in which the surgeon removes the fatty deposits caused by atherosclerosis from the inside of one of the main arteries to the brain and places a tube made of metallic mesh called a stent inside the artery to prevent recurrent narrowing of the artery.

Hemorrhagic stroke is treated by removing pooled blood from the brain and repairing damaged blood vessels. To prevent another hemorrhagic stroke, the surgeon may use a procedure called aneurysm clipping. In this procedure, the surgeon clamps the weak spot in the artery away from the rest of the blood vessel, which reduces the chances that it will burst and bleed. Endovascular treatment may be used for aneurysms that are difficult to reach surgically. In this procedure, a catheter is guided from a larger artery up into the brain to reach the aneurysm. Small coils of wire are discharged into the aneurysm, which plug it and block off blood flow from the main artery.

Drugs

Emergency treatment of stroke from a blood clot is aimed at dissolving the clot. This "thrombolytic therapy" currently is performed most often with tissue plasminogen activator, or tPA. This drug must be administered within three hours of the stroke event. Therefore, patients who awaken with stroke symptoms are ineligible for tPA therapy, as the time of onset cannot be accurately determined. tPA therapy has been shown to improve recovery and decrease long-term disability in selected patients. tPA therapy carries a 6.4% risk of inducing a cerebral hemorrhage, however, and is not appropriate for patients with bleeding disorders, very high blood pressure, known aneurysms, any evidence of intracranial hemorrhage, or incidence of stroke, head trauma, or intracranial surgery within the past three months. Patients with clot-related (thrombotic or embolic) stroke who are ineligible for tPA treatment may be treated with heparin or other blood thinners, or with aspirin or other anti-clotting agents in some cases.

Emergency treatment of hemorrhagic stroke is aimed at controlling intracranial pressure. Intravenous urea or mannitol plus hyperventilation is the most common treatment. Corticosteroids also may be used. Patients with reversible bleeding disorders, such as those due to anticoagulant treatment, should have these bleeding disorders reversed, if possible.

Rehabilitation

Rehabilitation refers to a comprehensive program designed to regain function as much as possible and compensate for permanent losses. Approximately 10% of stroke survivors recover without any significant disability and able to function independently. Another 10% are so severely affected that they must remain institutionalized for severe disability. The remaining 80% can return home with appropriate therapy, training, support, and care services.

Rehabilitation is coordinated by a team of medical professionals and may include the services of a neurologist, a physician who specializes in rehabilitation medicine (physiatrist), a physical therapist, an occupational therapist, a speech-language pathologist, a nutritionist, a mental health professional, and a social worker. Rehabilitation services may be provided in an acute care hospital, rehabilitation hospital, long-term care facility, outpatient clinic, or at home.

The rehabilitation program is based on the patient's individual deficits and strengths. Strokes on the left side of the brain primarily affect the right half of the body, and vice versa. In addition, in left-brain dominant people, who constitute a significant majority of the population, left-brain strokes usually lead to speech and language deficits. Right-brain strokes may affect spatial perception. Patients with right brain strokes also may deny their illness, neglect the affected side of their body, and behave impulsively.

Rehabilitation may be complicated by cognitive losses, including diminished ability to understand and follow directions. Poor results are more likely in patients with significant or prolonged cognitive changes, sensory losses, language deficits, or incontinence.

PREVENTION OF COMPLICATIONS. Rehabilitation begins with prevention of stroke recurrence and other medical complications. The risk of stroke recurrence may be reduced with many of the same measures used to prevent stroke, including quitting smoking and controlling blood pressure.

One of the most common medical complications following stroke is deep venous thrombosis, in which a clot forms within a limb immobilized by paralysis. Clots that break free often become lodged in an artery feeding the lungs. This type of pulmonary embolism is a common cause of death in the weeks following a stroke. Resuming activity within a day or two after the stroke is an important preventive measure, along with use of elastic stockings on the lower limbs. Drugs that prevent clotting may be given, including intravenous heparin and oral warfarin.

Weakness and loss of coordination of the swallowing muscles may impair swallowing (dysphagia), and allow food to enter the lower airway. This may lead to aspiration pneumonia, another common cause of death shortly after a stroke. Dysphagia may be treated with retraining exercises and temporary use of pureed foods.

Depression occurs in 30–60% of stroke patients. Antidepressants and psychotherapy may be used in combination. Other medical complications include urinary tract infections, pressure ulcers, falls, and seizures.

TYPES OF REHABILITATIVE THERAPY. Brain tissue that dies in a stroke cannot regenerate. In some cases, other brain regions may "take over" the functions of that tissue after a training period. In other cases, compensatory actions may be developed to replace lost abilities.

Physical therapy is used to maintain and restore range of motion and strength in affected limbs, and to maximize mobility in walking, wheelchair use, and transferring (from wheelchair to toilet or from standing to sitting, for instance). The physical therapist advises on mobility aids such as wheelchairs, braces, and canes. In the recovery period, a stroke patient may develop muscle spasticity and contractures, or abnormal contractions. Contractures may be treated with a combination of stretching and splinting.

Occupational therapy improves such self-care skills as feeding, bathing, and dressing, and helps develop effective compensatory strategies and devices for activities of daily living. A speech-language pathologist focuses on communication and swallowing skills. When dysphagia is a problem, a nutritionist can advise alternative meals that provide adequate nutrition.

Mental health professionals may be involved in the treatment of depression or loss of thinking (cognitive) skills. A social worker may help coordinate services and ease the transition out of the hospital back into the home. Both social workers and mental health professionals may help counsel the patient and family during the difficult rehabilitation period. Caring for a person affected with stroke requires learning a new set of skills and adapting to new demands and limitations. Home caregivers may develop stress, anxiety, and depression. Caring for the caregiver is an important part of the overall stroke treatment program.

Support groups can provide an important source of information, advice, and comfort for stroke patients and for caregivers. Joining a support group can be one of the most important steps in the rehabilitation process.

First aid

It is useful for friends, coworkers, or bystanders to know the basics of first aid for stroke victims. If someone appears to be having a stroke, the most important first step is to call for emergency help *at once*. Stroke is a medical emergency; the sooner the person is evaluated and treated, the better their chances of recovery. The drug presently considered most useful in treating stroke must be given within 3 hours of the attack to be effective.

Additional measures that can be taken to help the affected person while waiting for the emergency response team:

- If the person stops breathing, give them mouth-to-mouth resuscitation.
- If they are vomiting, tilt their head to one side to prevent them from swallowing the material.
- Do *not* give them anything to eat or drink.

Prognosis

The prognosis of stroke depends on the person's age, the type and location of the stroke, and the amount of time elapsed between diagnosis and treatment. In general, patients with ischemic stroke have a better prognosis than those with hemorrhagic stroke. In one study in the Boston area, 19 percent of patients with ischemic stroke died within the first 30 days of the attack compared to 35 percent with hemorrhagic stroke.

Stroke is fatal for about 27% of white males, 52% of black males, 23% of white females, and 40% of black females. Stroke survivors may be left with significant deficits. Emergency treatment and comprehensive rehabilitation can significantly improve both survival and recovery. One recent study found that treating stroke survivors with certain antidepressant medications, even if they were not depressed, could increase their chances of living longer. People who received the treatment were less likely to die from cardiovascular events than those who did not receive antidepressant drugs.

About 10 percent of stroke patients recover enough function to live independently without help; another 50 percent can remain at home with outside assistance. The remaining 40 percent require long-term care in a nursing home.

Stroke in children can be devastating. Between 20% and 35% of newborns who survive a stroke will go on to have a second stroke. More than 66% of older children who suffer strokes will have cognitive deficits, seizures, behavioral problems, changes in personality, or physical disabilities. Unlike adult survivors, children who survive strokes may develop mental retardation, epilepsy, or cerebral palsy.

Prevention

Many strokes are preventable with proper self-care. People cannot change some risk factors for stroke, such as race, age, sex, or family history, but they can control several other risk factors:

- They can quit smoking, drinking heavily, or using cocaine.
- They can keep their weight at a healthy level.

QUESTIONS TO ASK YOUR DOCTOR

- What is my risk of having a stroke?
- How would I or those around me know that I am having a stroke?
- Would you recommend preventive medications to lower my risk of stroke?
- What changes should I make in my lifestyle to lower my risk of stroke?

- They can exercise regularly, eat a healthy diet, and take medications for high blood pressure if they are diagnosed with it.
- They can take steps to lower their risk of diabetes or high blood cholesterol levels.
- They can lower the level of emotional stress in their life or learn to manage stress more effectively.
- They can get regular checkups for abnormal heart rhythms if they have been diagnosed with such problems.
- They can see their doctor at once if they have a TIA.

People with no previous history of stroke may be given certain drugs as preventive measures. These drugs include statins (drugs that lower blood cholesterol levels) and platelet antiaggregants (medications intended to prevent platelets in the blood from forming clumps that may lead to clots). Among the latter medications are aspirin, aspirin with extended release dipyridamole, clopidogrel (Plavix) and ticlopidine (Ticlid).

Damage from stroke may be significantly reduced through emergency treatment. Knowing the symptoms of stroke is as important as knowing those of a heart attack. Patients with stroke symptoms should seek emergency treatment without delay, which may mean dialing 911 rather than their family physician.

Treatment of atrial fibrillation may significantly reduce the risk of stroke. Preventive anticoagulant therapy may benefit those with untreated atrial fibrillation. Warfarin (Coumadin) has proven to be more effective than aspirin for patients at higher risk of stroke. Warfarin is, however, complicated to use because it interacts with a large number of other drugs and requires frequent monitoring by the patient's physician.

A recent innovation is the use of computer technology to allow stroke experts in one hospital to evaluate and diagnose a patient in another hospital that might not have a specialist available. Called Tele-Stroke, the network allows a patient to be evaluated for ischemic stroke within the three-hour time limit for the effective use of tPA. TeleStroke networks are now established in more than 20 states.

Resources

BOOKS

Brainin, Michael, and Hans-Dieter Heiss, eds. *Textbook of Stroke Medicine.* New York: Cambridge University Press, 2010.

Gillen, Glen. *Stroke Rehabilitation.* New York: Mosby, 2010.

Palmer, Sara, and Jeffrey B. Palmer. *When Your Spouse Has a Stroke: Caring for Your Partner, Yourself, and Your Relationship.* Baltimore: Johns Hopkins University Press, 2011.

Williams, Olajide. *Stroke Diaries: A Guide for Survivors and Their Families.* New York: Oxford University Press, 2010.

PERIODICALS

Alvarez-Sabin, J., et al. "Therapeutic Interventions and Success in Risk Factor Control for Secondary Prevention of Stroke." *Journal of Stroke and Cerebrovascular Diseases* 18 (November/December 2009): 460–65.

Birns, Jonathan. "Stroke." *GP* August 6, 2010, 29.

Jellinger, K.A. "Stroke Medicine." *European Journal of Neurology* 17 (8) (August 2010): 66.

Mathews, M.S., et al. "Safety, Effectiveness, and Practicality of Endovascular Therapy within the First 3 Hours of Acute Ischemic Stroke Onset." *Neurosurgery* 65 (November 2009): 860–65.

Reiss, A.B., and E. Wirkowski. "Statins in Neurological Disorders: Mechanisms and Therapeutic Value." *Scientific World Journal* 9 (November 1, 2009): 1242–59.

Zivin, J.A. "Acute Stroke Therapy with Tissue Plasminogen Activator (tPA) Since It Was Approved by the U.S. Food and Drug Administration (FDA)." *Annals of Neurology* 66 (July 2009): 6–10.

OTHER

Brain Aneurysm Foundation. *Act Now: Brain Aneurysm Basics That Can Save Your Life.* http://www.bafound.org/sites/default/files/BAF_Brain_Aneurysm_Basics_0.pdf (accessed August 10, 2011).

Centers for Disease Control and Prevention (CDC). *Stroke Home Page.* http://www.cdc.gov/stroke/index.htm (accessed August 10, 2011).

Jausch, Edward C. "Acute Management of Stroke." *eMedicine*, April 6, 2011. http://emedicine.medscape.com/article/1159752-overview (accessed August 10, 2011).

Mayo Clinic. *Stroke.* http://www.mayoclinic.com/health/stroke/DS00150.

National Heart, Lung, and Blood Institute (NHLBI). *What Is an Aneurysm?* http://www.nhlbi.nih.gov/health/dci/Diseases/arm/arm_what.html (accessed August 10, 2011).

National Institute of Neurological Disorders and Stroke (NINDS). *Cerebral Aneurysm Fact Sheet.* http://www.ninds.nih.gov/disorders/cerebral_aneurysm/detail_cerebral_aneurysm.htm.

National Institute of Neurological Disorders and Stroke (NINDS). *Stroke: Hope through Research.* November 2009. http://www.ninds.nih.gov/disorders/stroke/detail_stroke.htm (accessed August 10, 2011).

National Stroke Association (NSA). *Stroke 101 Fact Sheet.* http://www.stroke.org/site/DocServer/STROKE_101_ Fact_Sheet.pdf?docID=4541 (accessed August 10, 2011).

St. John's Hospital (Springfield, IL). *Children and Stroke.* http://www.st-johns.org/services/stroke_center/Children.aspx (accessed August 10, 2011).

ORGANIZATIONS

American Academy of Neurology (AAN), 1080 Montreal Avenue, Saint Paul, MN 55116, 651-695-2717, 800-879-1960, Fax: 651-695-2791, http://www.aan.com/.

American Stroke Association (ASA), 7272 Greenville Avenue, Dallas, TX 75231, 888-4-STROKE, Fax: 214-706-5231, strokeassociation@heart.org, http://www.strokeassociation.org/presenter.jhtml?identifier=1200037.

Brain Aneurysm Foundation (BAF), 269 Hanover Street, Building 3, Hanover, MA 02339, 781-826-5556, 888-272-4602, office@bafound.org, http://www.bafound.org/.

National Heart, Lung, and Blood Institute (NHLBI), Health Information Center, P.O. Box 30105, Bethesda, MD 20824-0105, 301-592-8573, Fax: 240-629-3246, nhlbiinfo@nhlbi.nih.gov, http://www.nhlbi.nih.gov/.

National Institute of Neurological Disorders and Stroke (NINDS), P.O. Box 5801, Bethesda, MD 20824, (800) 352-9424, (301) 496-5751, http://www.ninds.nih.gov/index.htm.

National Stroke Association (NSA), 9707 E. Easter Lane, Centennial, CO 80112, (800) 787-6537, Fax: (303) 649-1328, info@stroke.org, http://www.stroke.org.

Richard Robinson
Teresa G. Odle
Rebecca J. Frey, PhD
Fran Hodgkins

Sturge-Weber syndrome

Definition

Sturge-Weber syndrome (SRS) is a condition involving specific brain changes that often cause seizures and mental delays. It also includes port-wine colored birthmarks (or "port-wine stains"), usually found on the face.

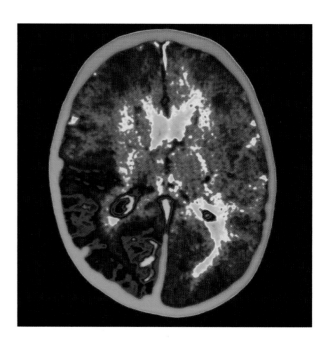

This magnetic resonance image of the brain shows a patient with Sturge-Weber syndrome. The front of the brain is at the top. Green colored areas indicate fluid-filled ventricles. The blue area is where the brain has become calified. (© *Mehau Kulyk/SPL/Photo Researchers, Inc.*)

Description

The brain finding in SRS is leptomeningeal angioma, which is a swelling of the tissue surrounding the brain and spinal cord. These angiomas cause seizures in approximately 90% of people with SWS. A large number of affected individuals are also mentally delayed.

Port-wine stains are present at birth. They can be quite large and are typically found on the face near the eyes or on the eyelids. Vision problems are common, especially if a port-wine stain covers the eyes. These vision problems can include glaucoma and vision loss.

Facial features, such as port-wine stains, can be very challenging for individuals with SWS. These birthmarks can increase in size with time, and this may be particularly emotionally distressing for the individuals, as well as their parents. A state of unhappiness about this is more common during middle childhood and later than it is at younger ages.

Genetic profile

The genetics behind Sturge-Weber syndrome are still unknown. Interestingly, in other genetic conditions involving changes in the skin and brain (such as **neurofibromatosis** and **tuberous sclerosis**) the genetic causes are well described. It is known that most people with SRS are the only ones in their family with the condition; there is usually not a strong family history of the disease. However, a gene known to cause SRS is still not known. For now, SRS is thought to be caused by a random, sporadic event.

Demographics

Sturge-Weber syndrome is a sporadic disease that is found throughout the world, affecting males and females equally. The total number of people with Sturge-Weber syndrome is not known, but estimates range between one in 400,000 to one in 40,000.

Signs and symptoms

People with SWS may have a larger head circumference (measurement around the head) than usual. Leptomeningeal angiomas can progress with time. They usually only occur on one side of the brain, but can exist on both sides in up to 30% of people with SWS. The angiomas can also cause great changes within the brain's white matter. Generalized wasting, or regression, of portions of the brain can result from large angiomas. Calcification of the portions of the brain underlying the angiomas can also occur. The larger and more involved the angiomas are, the greater the expected amount of mental delays in the individual. Seizures are common in SWS, and they can often begin in very early childhood. Occasionally, slight paralysis affecting one side of the body may occur.

Port-wine stains are actually capillaries (blood vessels) that reach the skin's surface and grow larger than usual. As mentioned earlier, the birthmarks mostly occur near the eyes; they often occur only on one side of the face. Though they can increase in size over time, port-wine stains cause no direct health problems for the person with SWS.

Vision loss and other complications are common in SWS. The choroid of the eye can swell, and this may lead to increased pressure within the eye in 33–50% of people with SWS. Glaucoma is another common vision problem in SWS and is more often seen when a person has a port-wine stain that is near or touches the eye.

In a 2000 study about the psychological functioning of children with SRS, it was noted that parents and teachers report a higher incidence of social problems, emotional distress, and problems with compliance in these individuals. Taking the mental delays into account, behaviors associated with attention-deficit hyperactivity disorder (**ADHD**) were noted; as it turns out, about 22% of people with SWS are eventually diagnosed with ADHD.

Diagnosis

Because no genetic testing is available for Sturge-Weber syndrome, all diagnoses are made through a careful physical examination and study of a person's medical history.

Port-wine stains are present at birth, and seizures may occur in early childhood. If an individual has both of these features, SWS should be suspected. A brain MRI or CT scan can often reveal a leptomeningeal angioma, brain calcifications, as well as any other associated white matter changes.

Treatment and management

Treatment of seizures in SWS by anti-epileptic medications is often an effective way to control them. In the rare occasion that an aggressive seizure medication therapy is not effective, surgery may be necessary. The general goal of the surgery is to remove the portion of brain that is causing the seizures, while keeping the normal brain tissue intact. Though most patients with SWS only have brain surgery as a final attempt to treat seizures, some physicians favor earlier surgery because this may prevent some irreversible damage to the brain (caused by the angiomas).

Standard glaucoma treatment, including medications and surgery, is used to treat people with this complication. This can often reduce the amount of vision loss.

There is no specific treatment for port-wine stains. Because they contain blood vessels, it could disrupt blood flow to remove or alter the birthmarks.

Prognosis

The prognosis for people with SWS is directly related to the amount of brain involvement for the leptomeningeal angiomas. For those individuals with smaller angiomas, prognosis is relatively good, especially if they do not have severe seizures or vision problems.

Resources

BOOKS

Charkins, Hope. *Children with Facial Difference: A Parent's Guide*. Bethesda, MD: Woodbine House, 1996.

ORGANIZATIONS

Sturge-Weber Foundation. PO Box 418, Mount Freedom, NJ 07970. (800) 627-5482 or (973) 895-4445. Fax: (973) 895-4846. swfoffice@aol.com. http://www.sturge weber.com/.

WEBSITES

"Sturge-Weber Syndrome." *Family Village*.http://www. familyvillage.wisc.edu/lib_stur.htm.
Sturge-Weber Syndrome Support Group of New Zealand. http://www.geocities.com/HotSprings/Spa/1563/.

Deepti Babu, MS

▌Stuttering

Definition

There is no standard definition of stuttering, but most attempt to define stuttering as the blockages, discoordination, or fragmentations of the forward flow of speech (fluency). These stoppages, referred to as disfluencies, are often excessive and characterized by specific types of disfluency. These types of disfluencies include repetitions of sounds and syllables, prolongation of sounds, and blockages of airflow. Individuals who stutter are often aware of their stuttering and feel a loss of control when they are disfluent. Both young and older stutterers expend an excessive amount of physical

and mental energy when speaking. Older children and adults who stutter show myriad negative reactive behaviors, feelings, and attitudes. These behaviors, referred to as "secondary behaviors," make the disorder more severe and difficult.

Description

Stuttering is a confusing and often misunderstood developmental speech and language disorder. Before discussing stuttering, it is important to understand the concepts of speech fluency and disfluency. Fluency is generally described as the forward flow of speech. For most speakers, fluent speech is easy and effortless. Fluent speech is free of any interruptions, blockages, or fragmentations. Disfluency is defined as a breakdown or blockage in the forward flow of speech, or fluency. For all speakers, some occurrence of disfluency is normal. For example, people may insert short sounds or words, referred to as "interjections," when speaking; examples of such are "um," "like," or "uh." Also, speakers might repeat phrases, revise words or phrases, or sometimes repeat whole words for the purpose of clarification. For young children, disfluency is a part of the normal development of speech and language, especially during the preschool years (between the ages of two and five years).

The occurrence of disfluency is not the same as stuttering, though stuttered speech is characterized by an excessive amount of disfluency. The disfluencies produced by people who stutter will often be similar to those in the speech of individuals who do not stutter; however, certain types of disfluent behavior are likely to appear only in the speech of people who stutter. These disfluencies are sound and syllable repetitions (i.e., ca-ca-ca-cat), sound prolongations ("sssss-salad," "fffff-fish"), and complete blockages of airflow. These behaviors, often referred to as stuttering type disfluencies, distinguish stuttered speech from nonstuttered speech.

Unlike speakers who do not stutter, most people who stutter react negatively to their disfluencies. A person may develop a number of physical reactions, including tension of the muscles involved in speech (tongue, jaw, lips, or chest, for example) and tension in muscles not related to speech (such as shoulders, limbs, and forehead). In addition to these physiological reactions, people who stutter will often have negative emotional reactions to the disorder. Among the emotions that people who stutter report are embarrassment, guilt, and frustration.

Finally, many people who stutter will develop a number of negative attitudes and beliefs regarding themselves and speaking—because of their stuttering. These may be negative attitudes and beliefs in certain speaking situations, with people with whom they interact, and in their own abilities. These physiological, emotional, and attitudinal (cognitive) reactions to stuttering, described as secondary stuttering behaviors, are often very disruptive to the communication process and the person's life.

Stuttering behaviors can develop and vary throughout the life span. Sometimes, children will experience periods when the stuttering appears to "go away," only to return in a more severe pattern. Many children, (estimates range between 50 and 80%) will develop normal fluency after periods of stuttering. For those who continue to stutter during late childhood, adolescence, and into adulthood, stuttering can become a chronic problem. Lifelong efforts will be needed to cope successfully with the behavior.

Due to the effect that stuttering has on communication, the person who stutters may experience certain difficulties in various parts of his/her life. These problems might be secondary to factors inside the person (symptoms of stuttering) and outside the person (society's attitudes toward stuttering and other barriers). For example, many people who stutter report difficulties in social settings. Children who stutter often experience teasing and other social penalties. Adolescents and adults also report a variety of social problems. Academic settings may be difficult for children who stutter because of the emphasis schools place on verbal performance.

Finally, there appears to be some evidence that people who stutter might confront barriers in employment. These barriers might take the form of inability to do certain tasks easily (talking on the phone, for example), limitations in job choices, and discrimination in the hiring and promotion processes.

Causes and symptoms

Though research has not identified a single cause, there appears to be several factors that are viewed as being important to the onset and development of stuttering. Therefore, stuttering is often described as being related to multiple factors and having possibly multiple causes. First, there is a genetic predisposition to stutter, as evidenced by studies of families and twins. A second important factor in stuttering the onset of stuttering is the physiological makeup of people who stutter. Research suggests that the brains of people who stutter may function abnormally during speech production. These differences in functioning may lead to breakdowns in speech production and to the development of disfluent speech.

Third, there is some evidence that speech and language development is an important issue in understanding the development of stuttering. Studies have found some evidence that children who are showing stuttering type behaviors may also have other difficulties with speech-language. Additionally, children with speech-language delays will often show stuttering type behaviors. Finally, environmental issues have a significant impact on the development of stuttering behaviors. An environment that is overly stressful or demanding may cause children to have difficulties developing fluent speech. Though the environment, in particular parental behaviors, does not cause stuttering, it is an important factor that might adversely affect a child who is operating at a reduced capacity for developing fluent speech.

There is no evidence that stuttering is secondary to a psychological disturbance. It is reasonable to assume that stuttering might have some effect on psychological adjustment and a person's ability to cope with speaking situations. People who stutter might experience a lower self-esteem and some might report feeling depressed. These feelings and difficulties with coping are most likely the result and not the cause of stuttering. In addition, several research studies have reported that many people who stutter report high levels of anxiety and stress when they are talking and stuttering. These feelings, psychological states, and difficulties with coping are most likely the result and not the cause of stuttering.

Generally, children begin to stutter between the ages of two and five years. Nevertheless, there are instances when individuals begin to show stuttering type behaviors in late childhood or as adults. These instances are often related to specific causes such as a stroke or a degenerative neurological disease. This type of stuttering, stuttering secondary to a specific neurological process, is referred to as neurogenic stuttering. In other cases, stuttering may be secondary to a psychological conversion disorder due to a psychologically traumatic event. When stuttering has abrupt onset secondary to a psychological trauma, it is described as psychogenic stuttering.

As stated earlier, the primary symptoms of stuttering include excessive disfluency, both stuttering and normal types (core behaviors), as well as physical, emotional, and cognitive reactions to the problem. These behaviors will vary in severity across people who stutter from very mild to very severe. Additionally, the behaviors will vary considerably across different speaking situations. There are specific situations when people tend to experience more stuttering (such as talking on the phone or with an authority figure) or less stuttering (speaking with a pet or to themselves, for example). It is likely that this variability might even extend to people having periods (days and even weeks) when they can maintain normally fluent or nonstuttered speech.

Demographics

Stuttering is a relatively low-prevalence disorder. Across all cultures, roughly 1% of people currently has a stuttering disorder. This differs from incidence, or number of individuals who have been diagnosed with stuttering at some point in their lives. Research suggests that roughly 5% of the population has ever been diagnosed with a stuttering disorder. This difference suggests that a significant number of individuals who stutter will someday develop through or "grow out of" the problem. Research suggests that roughly 50–80% of all children who begin to stutter will stop stuttering. In addition, approximately three times as many men stutter as women. This ratio seems to be lower early in childhood, with a similar number of girls and boys stuttering. The ratio of boys to girls appears to get larger as children become older. This phenomenon suggests that males are more likely to continue to stutter than females.

Diagnosis

Speech-language pathologists are responsible for making the diagnosis and managing the treatment of adults and children who stutter. Preferably, a board-certified speech-language pathologist board should be sought for direct intervention or consulting. Diagnosis of stuttering, or identifying children at risk for stuttering, is difficult because most children will show excessive disfluencies in their speech. With children, diagnostic procedures include the collection and analysis of speech and disfluent behaviors in a variety of situations. In addition, the child's general speech-language abilities will be evaluated.

Finally, the speech-language pathologist will interview parents and teachers regarding the child's general developmental, speech-language development, and their perceptions of the child's stuttering behaviors. For adults and older children, the diagnostic procedures will also include gathering and analyzing speech samples from a variety of settings. In addition, the speech-language pathologist will conduct a lengthy interview with the person about

their stuttering and history of their stuttering problem. Finally, the person who stutters might be asked to report his/her attitudes and feelings related to stuttering, either while being interviewed or by completing a series of questionnaires.

Treatments

General considerations

It is generally accepted that conducting interventions with children and families early in childhood (preschool) is the most effective means of total recovery from stuttering. The chances for a person to fully recover from stuttering by obtaining near-normal fluency are reduced as the person ages. This is why early intervention is critical. For older children and adults for which stuttering has become a chronic disorder, the focus of therapy is on developing positive coping mechanisms for dealing with the problem. This therapy varies in success based on the individual.

Treatment options for young children

Treatment of young children generally follows one of two basic approaches. These approaches may also be combined into a single treatment program. The first type of approach, often referred to as indirect therapy, focuses on altering the environment to allow the child opportunities to develop fluent speech. With this approach, counseling parents regarding the alteration of behaviors that affect fluency is the focus. For example, parents may be taught to reduce the amount of household stress or in the level of speech-language demands being placed on the child. In addition, parents may be advised to change characteristics of their speech, such as their speech rate and turn-taking style; this is done to help their children develop more fluent speech.

The other basic approach in treatment with young children targets the development of fluent speech. This type of approach, often referred to as direct therapy, teaches children to use skills that will help them improve fluency and they are sometimes given verbal rewards for producing fluent speech.

Treatment options for older children and adults

Treatment approaches for older children and adults usually take one of two forms. These approaches target either helping the person to modify his/her stuttering or modify his/her fluency. Approaches that focus on modifying stuttering will usually teach individuals to reduce the severity of their stuttering behaviors by identifying and eliminating all of the secondary or reactive behaviors. Individuals will also work to reduce the amount of emotional reaction toward stuttering.

Finally, the speech-language pathologist will help the individual to learn techniques that allow them to stutter in an easier manner. Therapy does not focus on helping the individual to speak fluently, though most individuals will attain higher levels of fluency if this approach is successful. The other groups of approaches will focus on assisting adults and children who stutter to speak more fluently. This type of therapy, which focuses less on changing secondary and emotional reactions, helps the person to modify their speech movements in a specific manner that allows for fluent sounding speech. These procedures require the individual to focus on developing new speech patterns. This often requires a significant amount of practice and skill. The successful outcome of these approaches is nonstuttered, fluent sounding speech. Many therapists will integrate stuttering modification and fluency shaping approaches into more complete treatment programs. In addition, psychological counseling may be used to supplement traditional speech therapy.

Prognosis

Complete alleviation of recovery from stuttering is most likely possible when children and their families receive treatment close to the time of onset. Thus, early identification and treatment of stuttering is critical. For older children and adults, stuttering becomes a chronic problem that requires a lifetime of formal and self-directed therapy. For individuals who show this more chronic form of the disorder, internal motivation for change and support from significant others is going to be an important part of recovery.

Resources

BOOKS

Bloodstein, O. *A Handbook on Stuttering*. 5th ed., rev. San Diego, CA. Singular, 1995.

Guitar, B. *Stuttering: An Integrated Approach to Its Nature and treatment*. 2nd ed., text rev. Baltimore: Lippincott Williams and Willkins, 1998.

Manning, W. H. *Clinical Decision Making in Fluency Disorders*. 2nd. ed., rev. San Diego, CA. Singular, 2001.

ORGANIZATIONS

National Stuttering Association. 5100 East La Palma, Suite #208, Anaheim Hills, CA 92807. http://www.nsastutter.org.

Stuttering Foundation of America. 3100 Walnut Grove Road, Suite 603, P.O. Box 11749, Memphis, TN 38111-0749. http://www.stuttersfa.org.

Rodney Gabel, PhD

Subacute sclerosing panencephalitis

Definition

Subacute sclerosing panencephalitis is a rare, progressive brain disorder caused by an abnormal immune response to the measles virus.

Description

This fatal condition is a complication of measles and affects children and young adults before the age of 20. It occurs in boys more often than in girls but is extremely rare, appearing in only one out of a million cases of measles.

Causes and symptoms

Experts believe this condition is a form of measles **encephalitis** (swelling of the brain), caused by an improper response by the immune system to the measles virus.

The condition begins with behavioral changes, memory loss, irritability, and problems with school work. As the neurological damage increases, the child experiences seizures, involuntary movements, and further neurological deterioration. Eventually, the child starts suffering from progressive **dementia**. The optic nerve begins to shrink and weaken (atrophy) and subsequently the child becomes blind.

Diagnosis

Blood tests and spinal fluid reveal high levels of antibodies to measles virus, and there is a characteristically abnormal electroencephalogram (EEG), or brain wave test. Typically, there is a history of measles infection two to ten years before symptoms begin.

Treatment

There is no standard treatment, and a number of **antiviral drugs** have been tested with little success. Treatment of symptoms, including the use of anticonvulsant drugs, can be helpful.

Prognosis

While there may be periodic remissions during the course of this disease, it is usually fatal (often from pneumonia) within one to three years after onset.

Resources

ORGANIZATIONS

National Institute of Allergy and Infectious Disease. Building 31, Room 7A-50, 31 Center Drive MSC 2520,

Bethesda, MD 20892-2520. (301) 496-5717. http://www.niaid.nih.gov/default.htm.

National Organization for Rare Disorders. P.O. Box 8923, New Fairfield, CT 06812-8923. (800) 999-6673. http://www.rarediseases.org.

Carol A. Turkington

Subarachnoid hemorrhage *see* **Aneurysm**

Subcortical arteriosclerotic encephalitis *see* **Binswanger disease**

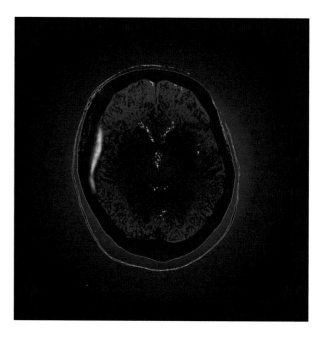

Between the dura and arachnoid is a collection of blood known as a subdural hematoma. *(© Living Art Enterprises/ Photo Researchers, Inc.)*

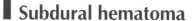

Subdural hematoma

Definition

A subdural hematoma is a collection of blood in the space between the outer layer (dura) and middle layers of the covering of the brain (the **meninges**). It is most often caused by torn, bleeding veins on the inside of the dura as a result of a blow to the head.

Description

Subdural hematomas most often affect people who are prone to falling. Only a slight hit on the head or even a fall to the ground without hitting the head may be enough to tear veins in the brain, often without fracturing the skull. There may be no external evidence of the bruising on the brain's surface.

Small subdural hematomas may not be very serious, and the blood can be slowly absorbed over several weeks. Larger hematomas, however, can gradually enlarge over several weeks, even though the bleeding has stopped. This enlargement can compress the brain itself, possibly leading to death if the blood is not drained.

The time between the injury and the appearance of symptoms can vary from less than 48 hours to several weeks, or more. Symptoms appearing in less than 48 hours are due to an acute subdural hematoma. This type of bleeding is often fatal, and results from tearing of the venous sinus. If more than two weeks have passed before symptoms appear, the condition is called a chronic subdural hematoma, resulting from tearing of the smaller vein. The young and the old are most likely to experience a chronic condition. This chronic form is less risky, as pressure of the veins against the skull lessens the bleeding. Prompt medical care can reduce the probability of permanent brain damage.

Causes and symptoms

A subdural hematoma is caused by an injury to the head that tears blood vessels. In childhood, hematomas are a common complication of **falls**. A subdural hematoma also may be an indication of child abuse, as evidenced by **shaken baby syndrome**.

Symptoms tend to fluctuate, and include:

- headache
- episodes of confusion and drowsiness
- one-sided weakness or paralysis
- lethargy
- enlarged or asymmetric pupils
- convulsions or loss of consciousness after head injury
- coma

Corticosteroids—A group of drugs similar to natural corticosteroid hormones produced by the adrenal glands. The drugs have a wide variety of applications, including use for inflammatory disorders and swelling.

Diuretics—A group of drugs that helps remove excess water from the body by increasing the amount lost by urination.

Fontanelle—One of the two soft areas on a baby's scalp; a membrane-covered gap between the bones of the skull.

A doctor should be contacted immediately if symptoms appear. Because these symptoms mimic the signs of a stroke, the patient should tell the doctor about any head injury within the previous few months.

In an infant, symptoms may include increased pressure within the skull, growing head size, bulging fontanelle (one of two soft spots on a infant's skull), vomiting, irritability, lethargy, and seizures. In cases of child abuse, there may be fractures of the skull or other bones.

Diagnosis

A chronic subdural hematoma can be difficult to diagnose, but a slow loss of consciousness after a head injury is assumed to be a hematoma unless proven otherwise. The hematoma can be confirmed with **magnetic resonance imaging** (MRI), which is the preferred type of scan; a hematoma can be hard to detect on a computed tomography scan (CT scan), depending on how long after the hemorrhage the CT is done.

Treatment

Small hematomas that do not cause symptoms may not need to be treated. Otherwise, the hematoma should be surgically removed. Liquid blood can be drained from burr holes drilled into the skull. The surgeon may have to open a section of skull to remove a large hematoma or to tie off the bleeding vein.

Corticosteroids and diuretics can control brain swelling. After surgery, anticonvulsant drugs (such as phenytoin) may help control or prevent seizures, which can begin as late as two years after the head injury.

Prognosis

If treatment is provided soon enough, recovery is usually complete. Headache, amnesia, attention problems, anxiety, and giddiness may continue for some time after surgery. Most symptoms in adults usually disappear within six months, with further improvement over several years. Children tend to recover much faster.

Prevention

Because a subdural hematoma usually follows a head injury, preventing head injury can prevent a hematoma.

Resources

ORGANIZATIONS

American Academy of Neurology. 1080 Montreal Ave., St. Paul, MN 55116. (612) 695-1940. http://www.aan.com.

Brain Injury Association of America. 105 North Alfred St., Alexandria, VA 22314. (800) 444-6443. http://www.biausa.org.

Head Injury Hotline. P.O. Box 84151, Seattle WA 98124. (206) 621- 8558. http://www.headinjury.com.

Head Trauma Support Project, Inc. 2500 Marconi Ave., Ste. 203, Sacramento, CA 95821. (916) 482-5770.

Carol A. Turkington

Succinamides

Definition

Succinamides are a sub-class of anticonvulsants, indicated for the treatment of seizures associated with epilepsy.

Purpose

Although there is no known cure for epilepsy, succinamides are used to control and prevent absence (petit mal) seizures associated with the disorder. Succinamides are most often used in conjunction with other anticonvulsant medications to control other types of seizures (such as other generalized tonic-clonic or grand mal seizures) as part of a comprehensive course of treatment for epilepsy and other disorders.

Description

Succinamides are sold under several names, including ethosuximide (Zarontin) and celontin. Zarontin is the only succinamide that is regularly used in the United States, as celontin has a higher rate of side effects. Zarontin effectively controls partial seizures, but in some individuals may actually increase the likelihood of generalized seizures. It is often, therefore, prescribed in combination with other anticonvulsants to minimize the chances of generalized seizures.

Recommended dosage

Succinamides are taken orally and are available in tablet or suspension form. For the treatment of epilepsy, succinamides may be taken by both adults and children. Succinamides are prescribed by physicians in varying dosages, but typical total daily dosages range from 250 mg to 1.5 g.

When beginning a course of treatment that includes succinamides, most physicians recommend a gradual dose-increasing regimen. Patients typically take a reduced dose at the beginning of treatment. The prescribing physician will determine the proper initial dosage, and then will periodically raise the patient's daily dosage until seizure control is achieved.

A double dose of any succinamide should not be taken together. If a daily dose is missed, take it as soon as possible. However, if it is within four hours of the next dose, then skip the missed dose. Physicians typically direct patients to gradually taper their daily dosages when ending treatment that includes succinamides. Stopping the medicine suddenly may cause seizures to return, occur more frequently, or become more severe.

Precautions

A physician should be consulted before taking succinamides with certain nonprescription medications. Persons should avoid alcohol and CNS depressants (medicines that can make one drowsy or less alert, such as antihistimines, sleep medications, and some pain medications) while taking succinimides or any other anticonvulsants. They can exacerbate the side effects of alcohol and other medications. Succinamides are not habit-forming.

A course of treatment including succinamides may not be appropriate for persons with gastro-intestional disorders, stroke, anemia, mental illness, diabetes, high blood presure, angina (chest pain), irregular heartbeats, or other heart problems.

Succinamides may not be suitable for persons with a history of liver or kidney disease. In rare cases, succinamides may cause abnormalities in theblood and abnormal liver or kidney function. Periodicblood, kidney, and liver function tests are advised for all patients

using the medicine. To check for rare blood disorders and symptoms of infection, periodic blood tests may be necessary while taking succinamides.

Before beginning treatment with succinamides, patients should notify their physician if they consume a large amount of alcohol, have a history of drug use, are pregnant, nursing, or plan on becoming pregnant. Although succinamides have not been associated with problems during pregnancy, other anticonvulsant medications may cause birth defects. Patients are often advised to use effective birth control while taking succinamides in combination with other anticonvulsants. Women who become pregnant while taking succinamides should contact their physician immediately.

Side effects

Patients should discuss with their physicians the risks and benefits of treatment including succinamides before taking the medication. Succinamides are usually well tolerated, but may case a variety of usually mild side effects. Diziness, nausea and drowsiness are the most frequently reported side effects. Most side effects do not require medical attention, and usually diminish with continued use of the medication. Possible side effects include:

- unusual tiredness or weakness
- clumbsiness
- hiccups
- loss of appetite
- nausea, vomiting, stomach cramps

If any symptoms persist or become too uncomfortable, the prescribing physician should be consulted.

Other, uncommon side effects of succinamides can be serious or could indicate an allergic reaction. Patients who experience any of the following symptoms should immediately contact a physician:

- nightmares and sleeplessness
- rash or blusih patches on skin
- persistent nosebleed
- ulcers or white spots on lips
- extreme mood or mental changes
- shakiness or unsteady walking
- severe unsteadiness or clumsiness
- speech or language problems
- difficulty breathing
- chest pain
- irregular heartbeat
- faintness or loss of consciousness
- severe cramping

KEY TERMS

Absence seizure—A type of generalized seizure where the person may temporarily appear to be staring into space and/or have jerking or twitching muscles. Previously called a petit mal seizure.

Epilepsy—A disorder associated with disturbed electrical discharges in the central nervous system that cause seizures.

Seizure—A convulsion, or uncontrolled discharge of nerve cells that may spread to other cells throughout the brain, resulting in abnormal body movements or behaviors.

Tonic-clonic seizure—A type of seizure involving loss of consciousness, generalized involuntary muscular contractions, and rigidity.

- persistant, severe headaches
- persistant sore throat, fever or pain

Interactions

Succinamides may have negative interactions with some antihistimines, antidepressants, antibiotics, and monoamine oxidase inhibitors (MAOIs). Other medications such as **Diazepam** (Valium), **phenobarbital** (Luminal, Solfoton), nefazodone, metronidazole, and certain anesthetics may react with succinamides.

Resources

BOOKS

Weaver, Donald F. *Epilepsy and Seizures: Everything You Need to Know*. Toronto: Firefly Books, 2001.

OTHER

"Ethosuximide Oral." *Medline Plus*.http://www.nlm.nih.gov/medlineplus/druginfo/medmaster/a682327.html (May 1, 2004).
"Zarontin." *RxMed*.http://www.rxmed.com/b.main/b2.pharmaceutical/b2.1.monographs/CPS-%20Monographs/CPS-%20(General%20Monographs-%20Z)/ZARONTIN.html (May 1, 2004).

ORGANIZATIONS

American Epilepsy Society. 342 NorthMain Street, West Hartford, CT 06117-2507. http://www.aesnet.org.
Epilepsy Foundation. 4351 Garden City Drive, Landover, MD 20785-7223. Phone: (800) 332-1000. Tollfree phone: (800) 332-1000. http://www.epilepsyfoundation.org.

Adrienne Wilmoth Lerner

Sunsetting of eyes *see* **Visual disturbances**

Swallowing disorders

Definition

Swallowing disorders include a number of diseases and conditions that cause difficulty in passing food or liquid from the mouth to the stomach.

Description

Although normally swallowing is automatic, it is a complex process involving several phases and 29 muscles. Saliva helps soften food as it is chewed. The tongue helps move food to the back of the mouth, triggering a swallowing reflex that passes food through the pharynx. The epiglottis helps keep food from mistakenly going down the windpipe and into the esophagus, the canal that carries food to the stomach. Swallowing disorders can occur at any phase in the swallowing process. The medical term for difficult swallowing is dysphagia.

Each year, about 10 million people in the United States require medical evaluation for swallowing problems. Some experts say that about 10% of Americans develop symptoms of swallowing disorders in adulthood. Elderly people are the most likely to have problems with swallowing.

Causes and symptoms

Swallowing disorders often result from other conditions and diseases. For example, **Parkinson's disease**, **cerebral palsy**, stroke, head injury, and other **central nervous system** conditions can damage the muscles and nerves involved in swallowing. Some people are born with abnormalities in the swallowing structures, such as infants with cleft palate.

Some cancers can lead to swallowing disorders. Esophageal cancer can cause narrowing and eventual blockage of the esophagus. Surgery and radiation therapy for head and neck cancer can restrict or weaken tongue motion, paralyze vocal cords, or cause muscle damage that affects swallowing. An inflamed esophagus, often resulting from gastroesophageal reflux disease (GERD), can cause painful or difficult swallowing. Infections of the esophagus also can inflame it and cause it to narrow. Swallowing difficulty may result from aging, though researchers are not certain why.

The most common symptoms people report are choking and the feeling that food is stuck in the throat. Other symptoms include needing to swallow many times to clear food from the mouth and throat, a gurgly, wet sound to the voice after swallowing, having to clear the throat after eating, coughing, pain while swallowing, bringing food back up (regurgitation), food or acid backing up into the throat, unexpected weight loss, and not being able to swallow at all. Children also may gag during meals and may have excessive drooling or leaking of food or liquid from their mouths during meals. They may have difficulty breathing when eating or drinking, spit up frequently and lag behind in weight gain. They also may have recurring pneumonia or respiratory infections.

Diagnosis

A physician should perform a full head and neck examination based on the patient's symptoms. Speech-language pathologists may aid in the diagnosis. Physicians also might order a swallowing test to study how the patient swallows. The patient will be asked to drink a liquid with a contrast agent called barium that will show up on x rays of the throat and upper chest. The exam might be imaged with a technique called video fluoroscopy, which will take motion camera images in addition to still images. For this exam, the patient may be asked to swallow liquid, paste, and solids. A speech pathologist may work with the radiologist to perform this exam.

If the physician thinks the problem originates in the lower esophagus or has concerns about an abnormality in the esophagus, an endoscopy may be ordered. This test involves passing a thin, flexible instrument called an endoscope down the throat. The lighted endoscope helps the physician view the esophagus. Other tests may be used, including ultrasound.

Treatment

Treatment will depend on the cause of the swallowing problem. Special exercises may help strengthen the muscles used for chewing and swallowing. Problems originating in the mouth may be treated with artificial saliva, improved hydration or better dental care. Esophageal problems will be treated depending on the cause. Patients with GERD will receive medications and instructions on how to better manage the disease. Esophageal cancer is a life-threatening disease that will involve coordinating care with an oncologist. Many patients will receive help with their disorders from speech pathologists. Special liquid diets may be ordered for patients who continue to have trouble chewing or swallowing. In severe cases, the patient may need a feeding tube that bypasses the part of the swallowing system that does not work.

KEY TERMS

Cleft palate—An opening or hole in the roof of the mouth that occurs at birth when the roof fails to fully develop in the infant.

Epiglottis—A thin layer of cartilage behind the tongue that helps block food from entering the windpipe.

Pharynx—The muscular cavity that leads from the mouth and nasal passages to the larynx and esophagus.

Alternative treatment

Some herbs that may help improve swallowing are oil of peppermint and licorice. Valerian may be used as a tea. Homeopathic physicians may suggest some remedies aimed at improving bloating, indigestion, or cough. Alternative care should be sought from licensed practitioners and coordinated with physician care.

Prognosis

In many cases, these disorders can be corrected. If not treated, swallowing disorders can lead to serious complications, including dehydration and malnutrition. There also is a risk of food entering the airway (aspiration) as a person attempts to swallow, which can lead to aspiration pneumonia as the food particles enter the lungs.

Prevention

Many causes of swallowing disorders cannot be prevented. Slowly and fully chewing food helps. People with GERD should manage it to lower the risk of developing swallowing difficulties.

Resources

PERIODICALS

"Disorders of Swallowing." *Harvard Men's Health Watch* (Sept. 2003).

"The Evaluation and Management of Swallowing Disorders in the Elderly." *Geriatric Times* (Nov. 1, 2003): 17.

ORGANIZATIONS

American Academy of Otolaryngology-Head and Neck Surgery. One Prince St., Alexandria, VA 22314-3357. 703-836-4444. http://www.entnet.org.

American Speech-Language Association (ASHA). 10801 Rockville Pike, Rockville, MD 20852. 800-638-8255. http://www.asha.org.

National Institute of Dental and Craniofacial Research (NIDCR). 45 Center Dr., Rm 4AS19 MSC 6400, Bethesda, MD 20892-6400. 301-496-4261. http://www.nidr.nih.gov.

OTHER

Dysphagia. National Institute on Deafness and Other Communication Disorders, 2005. http://www. nidcd. nih.gov/health/voice/dysph.asp.

*NINDS Swallowing Disorders Information Page.*Web page. National Institute of Neurological Disorders and Stroke, 2005. http://www.ninds.nih.gov/disorders/ swallowing_disorders/swallowing_disorders.htm.

Teresa G. Odle

Sydenham's chorea

Definition

Sydenham's **chorea** is an acute but self-limited movement disorder that occurs most commonly in children between the ages of 5 and 15, and occasionally in pregnant women. It is closely associated with rheumatic fever following a throat infection. The disorder is named for Thomas Sydenham (1624–1689), an English doctor who first described it in 1686. Other names for Sydenham's chorea include simple chorea, chorea minor, acute chorea, rheumatic chorea, juvenile chorea, and St. Vitus' dance. The English word "chorea" itself comes from the Greek word *choreia*, which means "dance." The disorder takes its name from the rapid involuntary jerking or twitching movements of the patient's face, limbs, and upper body.

Description

Sydenham's chorea is a disorder that occurs in children and is associated with rheumatic fever. Rheumatic fever is an acute infectious disease caused by certain types of streptococci bacteria. It usually starts with strep throat or tonsillitis. These types of streptococci are able to cause disease throughout the body. The most serious damage caused by rheumatic fever is to the valves in the heart. At one time, rheumatic fever was the most common cause of damaged heart valves, and it still is in most developing countries around the world. Rheumatic fever and rheumatic heart disease are still present in the industrialized countries, but the incidence has dropped substantially.

Both acute rheumatic fever and Sydenham's chorea are relatively uncommon disorders in the United States. According to the Centers for Disease Control and Prevention (CDC), only 1%–3% of people with streptococcal throat infections develop acute rheumatic fever (ARF); thus the incidence of ARF in the United States is thought to be about 0.5 per 100,000 patients between 5 and 17 years of age.

With regard to age, the incidence of Sydenham's chorea is higher in childhood and adolescence than in adult life. It occurs more frequently in females than in males; the gender ratio is thought to be about 2 F: 1 M. Since the peak incidence of rheumatic fever in North America occurs in late winter and spring, Sydenham's chorea is more likely to occur in the summer and early fall. There is no evidence that the disorder selectively affects specific racial or ethnic groups.

Rheumatic fever may appear in several different forms. Sydenham's chorea is one of five major criteria for the diagnosis of rheumatic fever. There are also four minor criteria and two types of laboratory tests associated with the disease. The "Jones criteria" define the diagnosis. They require laboratory evidence of a streptococcal infection plus two or more of the criteria. The laboratory evidence may be identification of streptococci from a sore throat or antibodies to streptococcus in the blood. The most common criteria are arthritis and heart disease, occurring in half to three-fourths of the patients. Sydenham's chorea, characteristic nodules under the skin, and a specific type of skin rash occur only 10% of the time.

About 20% of patients diagnosed with Sydenham's chorea experience a recurrence of the disorder, usually within two years of the first episode. Most women who develop Sydenham's during pregnancy have a history of acute rheumatic fever in childhood or of using birth control pills containing estrogen.

Causes and symptoms

Sydenham's is caused by certain types of streptococci called Group A beta-hemolytic streptococci or GAS bacteria. In general, streptococci are spherical-shaped anaerobic bacteria that occur in pairs or chains. GAS bacteria belong to a subcategory known as pyogenic streptococci, which means that the infections they cause produce pus. These particular germs seem to be able to create an immune response that attacks the body's own tissues along with the germs. Those tissues are joints, heart valves, skin, and brain.

The initial throat infection that leads to Sydenham's chorea is typically followed by a symptom-free period of 1–5 weeks. The patient then develops an acute case of rheumatic fever (ARF), an inflammatory disease that affects multiple organ systems and tissues of the body. In most patients, ARF is characterized by fever, arthritis in one or more joints, and carditis, or inflammation of the heart. In about 20% of patients, however, Sydenham's chorea is the only indication of ARF. Sydenham's is considered a delayed complication of rheumatic fever; it may begin as late as 12 months after the initial sore throat, and it may start only after the patient's temperature and other physical signs have returned to normal. The average time interval between the pharyngitis and the first symptoms of Sydenham's, however, is 8–9 weeks.

It is difficult to describe a "typical" case of Sydenham's chorea because the symptoms vary in speed of onset as well as severity. Most patients have an acute onset of the disorder, but in others, the onset is insidious, which means that the symptoms develop slowly and gradually. In some cases, the child's physical symptoms are present for 4–5 weeks before they become severe enough for the parents to consult a doctor. In other cases, emotional or psychiatric symptoms precede the clumsiness and involuntary muscular movements that characterize the disorder. The psychiatric symptoms that may develop in patients with Sydenham's chorea are one reason why it is sometimes categorized as a **PANDAS** disorder. PANDAS stands for Pediatric Autoimmune Neuropsychiatric Disorders Associated with Streptococcal Infections.

Behavioral or emotional disturbances that have been observed with Sydenham's include:

• frequent mood changes

• episodes of uncontrollable crying

• behavioral regression; that is, acting like much younger children

• mental confusion

• general irritability

• difficulty concentrating

• impulsive behavior

Some researchers think that children who have had Sydenham's are at increased risk of developing obsessive-compulsive disorder (OCD). OCD is characterized by obsessions, which are unwanted recurrent thoughts, images, or impulses, and by compulsions, which are repetitive rituals, mental acts, or behaviors. Obsessions in children often take the form of fears of intruders or harm coming to a family member. Compulsions may include such acts as counting silently, washing the hands over and over, insisting on keeping items in a specific order, checking repeatedly to make sure a door is locked, and similar behaviors.

Diagnosis

Because rheumatic fever is such a damaging disease, a complete evaluation should be done whenever it is suspected. This includes cultures for streptococci, blood tests, and usually an electrocardiogram (heartbeat mapping to detect abnormalities).

The diagnosis of Sydenham's is also based on the doctor's observation of the patient's involuntary movements. Unlike **tics**, the movements associated with chorea are not repetitive; and unlike the behavior of hyperactive children, the movements are not intentional. The recent onset of the movements rules out a diagnosis of **cerebral palsy**. If the doctor suspects Sydenham's, he or she may ask the patient to stick out the tongue and keep it in that position, or to squeeze the doctor's hand. Many patients with Sydenham's cannot hold their mouth open and keep the tongue out for more than a second or two. Another characteristic of Sydenham's is an inability to grip with a steady pressure; when the patient squeezes the doctor's hand, the strength of the grip will increase and decrease in an erratic fashion. This characteristic is sometimes called the "milking sign."

Treatment

Suspected streptococcal infections must be treated. All the other manifestations of rheumatic fever, including Sydenham's chorea and excluding heart valve damage, remit with the acute disease and do not require treatment. Sydenham's chorea generally lasts for several months.

Most patients with Sydenham's chorea recover after a period of bed rest and temporary limitation of normal activities. In most cases the symptoms disappear gradually rather than stopping abruptly.

Most doctors recommend ongoing treatment with penicillin to prevent a recurrence of rheumatic fever or Sydenham's chorea, although there is some disagreement as to whether this treatment should continue for 5 years after an acute attack or for the rest of the patient's life. The penicillin may be given orally or by injection. Patients who cannot take penicillin may be given erythromycin or sulfadiazine.

Prognosis

Syndenham's chorea usually clears up without complications when the rheumatic fever is treated. The heart valve damage associated with rheumatic fever may lead to heart trouble and require a surgical valve repair or replacement.

KEY TERMS

Arthralgia—Joint pain.

Chorea—A term that is used to refer to rapid, jerky, involuntary movements of the limbs or face that characterize several different disorders of the nervous system, including chorea of pregnancy and Huntington's chorea as well as Sydenham's chorea.

Electrocardiogram—Mapping the electrical activity of the heart.

Insidious—Developing in a stealthy or gradual manner. Sydenham's chorea may have an insidious onset.

PANDAS disorders—A group of childhood disorders associated with such streptococcal infections as scarlet fever and "strep throat." The acronym stands for Pediatric Autoimmune Neuropsychiatric Disorders Associated with Streptococcal Infections. Sydenham's chorea is considered a PANDAS disorder.

Pharyngitis—Inflammation of the throat, accompanied by dryness and pain. Pharyngitis caused by a streptococcal infection is the usual trigger of Sydenham's chorea.

Rheumatic fever—Chiefly childhood disease marked by fever, inflammation, joint pain, and Syndenham's chorea. It is often recurrent and can lead to heart valve damage.

St. Vitus' dance—Another name for Sydenham's chorea. St. Vitus was a fourth-century martyr who became the patron saint of dancers and actors during the Middle Ages. He was also invoked for protection against nervous disorders, epilepsy, and the disease that bears his name.

Streptococcus (plural, streptococci)—A genus of spherical-shaped anaerobic bacteria occurring in pairs or chains. Sydenham's chorea is considered a complication of a streptococcal throat infection.

Tonsillitis—Inflammation of the tonsils, which are in the back of the throat.

In most cases of Sydenham's, the patient recovers completely, although a recurrence is possible. In a very few cases—about 1.5% of patients diagnosed with Sydenham's— there may be increasing muscle stiffness and loss of muscle tone resulting in disability. This condition is occasionally referred to as paralytic chorea

Prevention

All cases of strep throat in children should be treated with a full 10 days of antibiotics (penicillin or erythromycin). Treatment may best be delayed a day or two to allow the body to build up its own antibodies. In addition, for those who have had an episode of rheumatic fever or have damaged heart valves from any other cause, prophylactic antibiotics should be continued to prevent recurrence.

It is possible to eradicate dangerous GAS bacteria from a community by culturing everyone's throat and treating everyone who tests positive. This is worth doing wherever a case of rheumatic fever appears, but it is expensive and requires many resources.

Resources

BOOKS

Beers, Mark H., and Robert Berkow, eds. "Sydenham's Chorea (Chorea Minor; Rheumatic Fever; St. Vitus' Dance)." In *The Merck Manual of Diagnosis and Therapy*. Whitehouse Station, NJ: Merck Research Laboratories, 2004.

PERIODICALS

Bhidayasiri, R., and D. D. Truong. "Chorea and Related Disorders." *Postgraduate Medical Journal* 80 (September 2004): 527–34.

Bonthius, D. J., and B. Karacay. "Sydenham's Chorea: Not Gone and Not Forgotten." *Seminars in Pediatric Neurology* 10 (March 2003): 11–19.

Dale, R. C., I. Heyman, R. A. Surtees, et al. "Dyskinesias and Associated Psychiatric Disorders following Streptococcal Infections." *Archives of Disease in Childhood* 89 (July 2004): 604–10.

Kim, S. W., et al. "A Possible Association of Recurrent Streptococcal Infections and Acute Onset of Obsessive-Compulsive Disorder." *Journal of Neuropsychiatry and Clinical Neurosciences* 16 (Summer 2004): 252–60.

Korn-Lubetzki, I., A. Brand, and I. Steiner. "Recurrence of Sydenham Chorea: Implications for Pathogenesis." *Archives of Neurology* 61 (August 2004): 1261–64.

Snider, L. A., and S. E. Swedo. "Post-Streptococcal Autoimmune Disorders of the Central Nervous System." *Current Opinion in Neurology* 16 (June 2003): 359–65.

ORGANIZATIONS

American Academy of Child and Adolescent Psychiatry (AACAP). 3615 Wisconsin Avenue, NW, Washington, DC 20016-3007. (202) 966-7300. Fax: (202) 966-2891. http://www.aacap.org.

American Academy of Family Physicians (AAFP). 11400 Tomahawk Creek Parkway, Leawood, KS 66211-2672. (800) 274-2237 or (913) 906-6000. *lt;http://www.aafp.org.

National Institute of Neurological Disorders and Stroke (NINDS). NIH Neurological Institute, P. O. Box 5801, Bethesda, MD 20824. (800) 352-9424 or (301) 496-5751. http://www.ninds.nih.gov.

OTHER

American Academy of Child and Adolescent Psychiatry (AACAP). AACAP Facts for Families, No. 60. *Obsessive-Compulsive Disorder in Children and Adolescents.*http://www.aacap.org/publications/factsfam/ocd.htm.

Herrera, Maria Alejandra, MD, and Nestor Galvez-Jiminez, MD. "Chorea in Adults." eMedicine February 1, 2002. http://www.emedicine.com/neuro/topic62.htm.

National Institute of Neurological Disorders and Stroke (NINDS). *NINDS Sydenham Chorea Information Page.* http://www.ninds.nih.gov/health_and_medical/disorders/sydenham.htm.

J. Ricker Polsdorfer, MD
Rebecca J. Frey, PhD

Syncope *see* **Fainting**

Syphilitic spinal sclerosis *see* **Tabes dorsalis**

Syringohydromyelia *see* **Hydromyelia, Syringomyelia**

Syringomyelia

Definition

The term syringomyelia refers to a collection of differing conditions characterized by damage to the spinal cord that is caused by formation of abnormal fluid-filled cavities (syrinx) within the cord. In 1827, French physician Charles-Prosper Ollivier d'Angers (1796–1845) suggested the term syringomyelia after the Greek *syrinx*, meaning pipe or tube, and *myelos*, meaning marrow. Later, the term hydromyelia was used to indicate a dilatation of the central canal, and syringomyelia referred to cystic cavities separate from the central spinal canal.

Description

The cavities may be a result of spinal cord injury, tumors of the spinal cord, or congenital defects. An idiopathic form of syringomyelia (a form of the disorder without known cause) is also described in medical literature. The fluid-filled cavity, or syrinx, expands slowly and elongates over time, causing progressive damage to the nerve centers of the spinal cord due to

the pressure exerted by the fluid. This damage results in pain, **weakness**, and stiffness in the back, shoulders, arms, or legs. People with syringomyelia experience different combinations of symptoms. In many cases, the disorder is related to abnormal lesions of the foramen magnum, the opening in the occipital bone that houses the lower portion of the medulla oblongata, the structure that links the brain and spinal cord. An additional cause of syringomyelia involves a Chiari malformation, a condition in which excess cerebral matter extends downward toward the medulla oblongata, crowding the outlet to the spinal canal. Some familial cases of syringomyelia have been observed, although this is rare. Types of syringomyelia include:

- syringomyelia with fourth ventricle communication
- syringomyelia due to blockage of cerebrospinal fluid (CSF) circulation (without fourth ventricular communication)
- syringomyelia due to spinal cord injury
- syringomyelia and spinal dysraphism (incomplete closure of the neural tube)
- syringomyelia due to intramedullary tumors
- idiopathic syringomyelia

Demographics

Syringomyelia occurs in approximately 8 in every 100,000 individuals. The onset is most commonly observed between ages 25 to 40. Rarely, syringomyelia may develop in childhood or late adulthood. Males are affected with the condition more often than females. No geographic difference in the prevalence of syringomyelia is known, and the occurrence of syringomyelia in different races is also unknown. Familial cases have been described.

Causes and symptoms

Most people with syringomyelia experience headaches, along with intermittent pain in the arms or legs, usually more severe on one side of the body. The pain may begin as dull or achy and slowly increases, or may occur suddenly, often as a result of coughing or straining. Pain in the extremities frequently becomes chronic. Additionally, numbness and tingling in the arm, chest, or back is often reported. The inability to feel the ground under the foot, or tingling in the legs and feet is also frequently experienced. Weakness of an extremity, leading to clumsiness in grasping objects or difficulty walking may also occur in individuals with syringomyelia. Eventually, functional use of the limb may be lost.

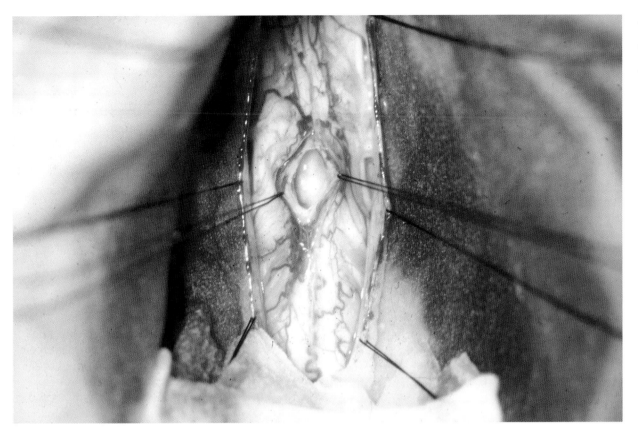

A spinal cord cyst associated with syringomyelia. *(© Custom Medical Stock Photo, Inc. Reproduced by permission.)*

The cause of syringomyelia remains unknown. Not a single clear theory at the present can properly explain the basic mechanisms of cyst formation and enlargement. One theory proposes that syringomyelia results from pulsating CSF pressure between the fourth ventricle of the brain and the central canal of the spinal cord. Another theory suggests that syrinx development, particularly in people with Chiari malformation, occurs after a difference in intracranial pressure and spinal pressure. A third theory contends that syrinx formation is caused by the cerebellar tonsils acting as a piston to produce large pressure waves in the spinal subarachnoid space, and this action forces fluid through the surface of the spinal cord into the central canal. Syringomyelia usually progresses slowly; the course may extend over many years. Infrequently, the condition may have a more acute course, especially when the brainstem is affected.

Diagnosis

Examination by a neurologist may reveal loss of sensation or movement caused by compression of the spinal cord. Diagnosis is usually reached by magnetic resonance imaging (MRI) of the spine, which can confirm syringomyelia and determine the exact location and extent of damage to the spinal cord. The most common place for a syrinx to develop is in the cervical spine (neck), with the second most common in the thoracic spine (chest and rib areas). The least likely place for a syrinx is in the lumbar spine (lower back). MRI of the head can be useful to determine the presence of any additional lesions present, as well as the presence of hydrocephalus (excess CSF in the ventricles of the brain). As the syrinx grows in size, it may cause scoliosis (abnormal curvature of the spine), which is best determined by x ray of the spine.

Treatment team

Diagnosis and treatment of syringomyelia require specialized physicians, including neurologists, radiologists, neurosurgeons, and orthopedists, along with specialized nurses. Physical therapy is often useful to maximize muscular function and assist with gait (walking).

Treatment

Treatment, usually surgery, is aimed at stopping the progression of spinal cord damage and maximizing functioning. Surgical procedures are often performed if there is an identifiable mass compressing the spinal cord. Additional surgical options to minimize the syrinx include correction of spinal deformities and various CSF-shunting procedures. Fetal spinal cord tissue implantation has recently been used in an attempt to obliterate syrinx. Surgery results in stabilization or modest improvement in symptoms for most patients. Many physicians advocate surgical treatment only for patients with progressive neurological deterioration or pain. Delay in treatment when the condition is progressive may result in irreversible spinal cord injury, and post-traumatic syringomyelia remains difficult to manage.

Medications (vasoconstrictors) are often prescribed to help reduce fluid formation around the spinal cord. Avoiding vigorous activity that increases venous pressure is often recommended. Certain exercises such as bending the trunk so the chest rests on the thighs may reduce the risk of syrinx expansion. People with progressive symptoms of syringomyelia, whether or not surgically treated, usually are monitored by their physician and have MRI scans completed every 6–12 months.

Recovery and rehabilitation

Despite reports of neurological recovery following surgery, most people achieve stabilization or only mild improvement in symptoms. Syringomyelia in children has a much lower incidence of sensory disturbance and pain than occurs with adolescents and adults and is associated with a high incidence of scoliosis that is more favorable to surgical treatment. Additionally, all cases of syringomyelia do not progress at the same rate. Some people, usually with milder symptoms, experience stabilization in their symptoms for a period of years. A frequent complication of symptom progression is the person's ongoing need to adjust to evolving functional losses that accompany syringomyelia. These adjustments may result in loss of independence and loss of personal privacy. Rehabilitation may focus on maintaining functionality for as long as practically possible with the use of exercises and adaptive equipment, or, especially in the case of children, may focus on recovery from scoliosis caused by the syringomyelia.

Clinical trials

The National Institute of Neurological Disorders and Stroke (NINDS) does sponsor trials regarding

syringomyelia, and information regarding them can be found online at ClinicalTrials.gov.

Prognosis

The prognosis for persons with syringomyelia depends on the underlying cause of the syrinx and on the type of treatment. Untreated syringomyelia is compatible with long-term survival without progression in 35–50% of cases. In patients treated by shunting for syringomyelia due to spinal cord injury, long-lasting pain relief and improved strength are usually observed. Some studies have revealed an unsatisfactory long-term prognosis due to high rates of syrinx recurrence in other forms of syringomyelia. Surgery (posterior fossa decompression) in syringomyelia associated with a Chiari malformation is described as a surgically safe procedure with a considerable chance of clinical improvement. In pediatric syringomyelia, surgery is effective in improving or stabilizing scoliosis.

Resources

BOOKS

Anson, John A., Edward C. Benzel, and Issam A. Awad. *Syringomyelia & the Chiari Malformation.* Rolling Hills, IL: American Association of Neurological Surgeons, 1997.

Icon Health Publications Staff. *The Official Patient's Sourcebook on Syringomyelia: A Revised and Updated Directory for the Internet Age.* San Diego: Icon Group International, 2002.

Klekamp, Joerg. *Syringomyelia: Diagnosis & Treatment* New York: Springer-Verlag, 2001.

PERIODICALS

Brodbelt, A. R., and M. A. Stoodley. "Post-traumatic Syringomyelia: A Review." *J Clin Neurosci.* 10, no. 4 (July 2003): 401–08.

Todor, D. R., T. M. Harrison, and T. H. Milhorat. "Pain and Syringomyelia: A Review." *Neurosurg Focus* 8, no. 3 (2000): 1–6.

OTHER

"Syringomyelia Fact Sheet." *National Institute of Neurological Disorders and Stroke*. February 10, 2004 (April 4, 2004). http://www.ninds.nih.gov/health_and_medical/pubs/syringomyelia.htm.

ORGANIZATIONS

American Syringomyelia Alliance Project (ASAP). P.O. Box 1586, Longview, TX 75606-1586. Phone: (903) 236-7079. Fax: (903) 757-7456. Tollfree phone: (800) ASAP-282 (272-7282). Email: info@asap.org. http://www.asap.org.

National Institute for Neurological Disorders and Stroke. P.O. Box 5801, Bethesda, MD 20824. Phone: (301) 496-5761. Tollfree phone: (800) 352-9424. http://www.ninds.nih.gov.

Antonio Farina, MD, PhD

Systemic lupus erythematosus *see* **Lupus**

Tabes dorsalis

Definition

Tabes dorsalis is a late manifestation of untreated syphilis and is characterized by a triad of clinical symptoms namely gait unsteadiness, lightning pains, and urinary incontinence. It occurs due to a slow and progressive degeneration of nerve cells and fibers in spinal cord. It is one of the forms of tertiary syphilis or neurosyphilis.

Description

The first description of the disorder was given by the French neurologist Guillame Duchenne in 1858 who called it *L'Ataxie Locomotrice Progressive* (Progressive Locomotor **Ataxia**). But the term tabes dorsalis was coined in 1836 even before the actual cause was discovered. *Tabes* in Latin means "decay" or "shriveling"; *dorsalis* means "of the back." These indicate the location and type of damage occurring in the spinal cord. It is also called as "spinal syphilis" or "syphilitic myelopathy."

Syphilis was widespread in the early part of the twentieth century but there has been a ten-fold decrease in incidence since then due to better screening measures and effective antibiotic therapy. Therefore classic, full blown forms of tabes dorsalis are seldom seen in the twenty-first century.

Demographics

The Centers for Disease Control (CDC) reports the annual incidence of syphilis and from this, an estimate of the number of tabes dorsalis cases can be made. In 2009, there was around 14.7/100,000 population or 44,828 new cases of syphilis reported. Three percent to 7 percent of untreated patients develop neurosyphilis, of whom about 5 % develop tabes dorsalis. Normally, fifteen or twenty years elapse after the initial syphilis infection, but this is shortened in patients with **AIDS**. Tabes dorsalis is more common in middle-aged males, homosexuals, and inner city population in New York, San Francisco, and the southern part of the United States.

Causes and symptoms

Causes

Syphilis is a sexually transmitted disease caused by the bacteria *Treponema pallidum*. During initial infection, the bacteria spread through the blood stream into remote sites like the brain and spinal cord, but remain silent in these areas. If proper treatment is not instituted, neurological disorders arise about a decade later called neurosyphilis. Damage to the spinal cord substance due to syphilis is called tabes dorsalis.

Inflammation occurs in the dorsal columns of the spinal cord. These columns are in the portion of the spinal cord closest to the back and have nerve fibers that carry sensory information like deep pain and position sense (proprioception) from the legs and arms to the brain. As a result of this, the nerve fibers lose their insulation and start atrophying. The pathological process starts in the lowermost portion of the spinal cord that receives information from the legs and spreads upwards. The inflammation can also involve other nerves that control vision, hearing, eye movements, bladder and bowel.

Symptoms

In the twenty-first century, mostly atypical cases of tabes dorsalis are seen due to previous partial antibiotic treatment. Much of the description of the classic disease comes from scientific articles and patient reports more than fifty years ago. The earliest and probably the most troublesome symptom is pain. This is often described as "stabbing" or "lightning-like" and is intense. It appears very suddenly, usually in the legs, spreads rapidly to other parts of the body and then disappears quickly. Unfortunately, this cycle can repeat itself several times a day and for days together, making the patients' life miserable. They also experience uncomfortable abnormal sensations or "paresthesias," like tingling, burning or coldness. Later the feet become progressively numb. "Visceral crisis" develop either spontaneously or after stress in about 15% of patients due to autonomic nerve dysfunction. These episodes are frightening and severe but rarely life threatening. They consist of excruciating abdominal pain and vomiting or vocal cord spasm or burning rectal pain.

A characteristic unsteady gait called "sensory ataxia" develops. Due to degeneration of nerves that carry position sense from the legs, patients are unable to judge the position of their feet in relation to the ground while walking. They become very unsteady especially while walking in a straight line, on uneven surfaces, or while turning suddenly. This becomes dramatically accentuated in the dark or while closing the eyes as visual compensation is removed. A person with tabes dorsalis walks stooped forward with a wide based "high-stepping" gait and eyes glued to the ground in order to prevent falling. With progression of the disease, they become unable to walk although muscle strength is intact.

Visual symptoms are quite common and include double vision, blurred vision, narrowed field of vision and finally blindness. The pupils are characteristically small and non-reactive to light and called "Argyll-Robertson" pupils. Urine overflow incontinence is very common as the bladder loses its muscular tone. Constipation, impotence, deafness, painless foot ulcers, and painless hip and knee arthritis are other features. Decreased memory, disorientation, personality changes and sometimes frank psychiatric illness can also occur.

Diagnosis

Diagnosis is mainly clinical. Syphilis has often been called "the great mimicker" and requires an astute physician to diagnose. There are three steps in diagnosis.

Firstly, the physician has to suspect the diagnosis. The classic signs seen in tabes dorsalis are a triad of 3A's; Argyll Robertson pupil, Areflexia (absent tendon reflexes), and Ataxia. Poor visual acuity, asymmetrical eye movement, deafness, clumsy hand and leg movements are other telltale signs.

Secondly, it has to be differentiated from other disorders that can present similarly. This is done with the help of CAT scans, MRI scans, spinal tap and certain screening blood tests. The most common screening blood test is called Venereal Disease Research Laboratory (VDRL) test. This measures the level of certain antibodies that are elevated in the blood in syphilis. It reflects disease activity and therefore may be falsely negative in very late "burnt out" cases of tabes. However, it may be falsely elevated in a host of other medical conditions. Therefore, it is a sensitive but not a very specific test. It is only a screening test and any positive result has to be confirmed with other blood tests. The cerebrospinal fluid (CSF) circulates around the brain and spinal cord and reflects underlying inflammation. In tabes, the white cell count and protein level in the CSF are elevated. A positive VDRL test in the CSF is a definitive diagnostic test for tabes dorsalis.

Thirdly, confirmatory tests should be done on the spinal fluid and blood. There are two confirmatory tests for syphilis, namely the Fluorescent Treponemal Antibody Absorption (FTA-ABS) and Micro Hemagglutination of Treponema Pallidum (MHA-TP). These detect very specific antibodies in the blood that are present when the person has syphilis and not otherwise. FTA-ABS in the CSF is a very sensitive test and a negative result virtually rules out tabes dorsalis. It is mandatory that all patients with syphilis undergo testing for HIV. Elevated white cells and protein in the CSF with a positive CSF VDRL test in a person with appropriate clinical findings is diagnostic for tabes dorsalis.

Treatment team

The team consists of an adult neurologist, an internist, an infectious disease specialist, psychiatrist and sometimes a pain management specialist. They will closely interact with physical therapists and occupational therapists.

Treatment

Treatment is aimed at curing the infection and hopefully halting the progression of neurologic damage. Treatment is unfortunately limited in reversing the damage already done and the degree of recovery depends on the extent of damage when therapy is started. Appropriate treatment, however, does reduce future nerve damage, reduces symptoms and normalizes the CSF abnormalities.

The CDC of the United States Department of Health and Human Services has extensive guidelines for treatment of tabes. It recommends antibiotic treatment with intravenous aqueous crystalline Penicillin G for two weeks. If the patient has penicillin allergy, he should be desensitized first before treatment. Otherwise, the antibiotic Ceftriaxone can be used as an

KEY TERMS

AIDS—Acquired immune deficiency syndrome is a sexually transmitted disease caused by the human immunodeficiency virus (HIV). It weakens the immune system and makes a person susceptible to many infections and malignancies.

Ataxia—Clumsiness or loss of co-ordination of the arms and legs due a variety of causes. It is a symptom of an underlying disease process of the nervous system.

Cerebrospinal fluid—A colorless fluid that is produced in the brain and circulates around the brain and spinal cord in the subarachnoid space.

Dementia—A chronic condition where there is loss of mental capacity due to an underlying organic cause. It may involve progressive deterioration of thinking, memory, behavior and personality.

Dorsal columns—Nerve fiber tracts that run in the portion of the spinal cord that is closest to the back. They carry sensory information like position sense and deep pain from the legs and arms to the brain.

Locomotor—Means of or pertaining to movement or locomotion.

Myelopathy—Disease of the spinal cord.

Neurosyphilis—Slow, progressive destruction of the brain and spinal cord due to untreated tertiary syphilis. It can be asymptomatic or cause different disorders like tabes dorsalis, general paresis and meningovascular syphilis.

Paresthesia—Abnormal sensation of the body like numbness or prickling.

Proprioception—The ability to sense the location and postion and orientation and movement of the body and its parts.

Spinal cord—The part of the central nervous system that extends from the base of the skull and runs through the vertebral column in the back. It acts as a relay to convey information between the brain and the periphery.

Syphilis—Sexually transmitted disease caused by a corkscrew shaped bacterium called Treponema pallidum. It is characterized by three clinical stages namely primary, secondary and tertiary or late syphilis.

Tendon reflex—A simple circuit that consists of a stimulus like a sharp tap delivered to a tendon and the response is one of the appropriate muscle contraction. It is used to test the integrity of the nervous system.

---

alternative but the adequacy of this has not been fully approved by the CDC. Serum VDRL titers are checked every three months till they start declining. CSF is checked at six and twelve months and if still abnormal, rechecked at two years. Re-treatment is recommended if neurological damage progresses, if CSF white cell count does not normalize in six months, VDRL titers do not decline or show a four-fold increase and if the first course of treatment was suboptimal. Symptomatic analgesic treatment is given for pain. This can range from simple over-the-counter medications such as aspirin or Tylenol or more potent analgesics like narcotics. Certain anti-seizure medications like Phenytoin, **Carbamazepine** and **Valproic acid** are efficacious in treating resistant pain. If patients become demented and have behavioral issues, anti-psychotic medications can be given.

Primary and secondary prevention of syphilis is important to prevent development of tabes dorsalis. Safe sex like using a condom is a way of primary prevention. Screening, detection and treatment of early syphilis are measures of secondary prevention. Sexually active people should consult a physician about any rash or sore in the genital area. Those who have been treated for another sexually transmitted infection, such as gonorrhea, should be tested for syphilis and HIV. Persons who have been exposed sexually to another person who has syphilis of any stage should be clinically evaluated, undergo testing, and even be presumptively treated in certain instances.

Recovery and rehabilitation

Assistance or supervision may be needed for self-care activities such as eating, showering, and dressing. Patients may require assistive devices such as a cane, walker or wheelchair to overcome gait difficulty. Diapers or urinary catheters are used for urinary incontinence. Surgery can help replace joints destroyed by arthritis. Patients need a good bowel regimen to avoid constipation, which can trigger a visceral crisis. Since this is a chronic illness, **respite** care should be provided for the caregivers.

Clinical trials

There is no trial open for tabes dorsalis, but there is an ongoing Phase three multicenter randomized trial. Information about current relevant clinical trials can be found at ClinicalTrials.gov.

Prognosis

Tabes dorsalis is a chronic, annoying, and incapacitating disease but is *per se* seldom fatal. If tabes is diagnosed in its very early stages, fairly good recovery is possible. Pain is quite bothersome and has a serious impact on quality of life. Ataxia, **dementia** and blindness are incapacitating. Death usually occurs due to rupture of enlarged blood vessels and damage to heart valves, which occur as a part of tertiary syphilis. Rarely, a urinary infection will lead to sepsis and death.

Special concerns

Tabes dorsalis can affect thinking and memory and all patients must have neuropsychological testing for dementia. They will need to get legal advice for estate and financial planning and their wishes for future medical care.

Resources

BOOKS

Aminoff, Michael J., ed. *Neurology and General Medicine*, 3rd ed. New York: Churchill Livingstone, 2001.

Rowland, Lewis P., ed. *Merritt's Neurology*, 10th ed. Philadelphia: Lippincott Williams & Wilkins, 2000.

Victor, Maurice, and Allan H. Ropper, eds. *Principles of Neurology*, 7th ed. New York: McGraw-Hill, 2001.

PERIODICALS

Golden, R. M., M. M. Christina, and K. K. Holmes. "Update on Syphilis: Resurgence of an Old Problem." *Journal of American Medical Association* 290 (September 2003): 1510–14.

WEBSITES

Clinical Trials Website. http://www.clinicaltrials.gov.

ORGANIZATIONS

Centers for Disease Control and Prevention. 1600 Clifton Road, Atlanta, GA 30333. Tollfree phone: (800) 232-3228. http://www.cdc.gov.

National Institute of Allergy and Infectious Diseases. 31 Center Drive, MSC 2520, Bethesda, MD 20892-2520. Phone: (301) 496-5717. http://www.niaid.nih.gov.

Chitra Venkatasubramanian, MBBS, MD

Tacrine *see* **Cholinesterase inhibitors**

Tarlov cysts *see* **Perineural cysts**

Tay-Sachs disease

Definition

Tay-Sachs disease is a genetic disorder caused by a missing enzyme that results in the accumulation of a fatty substance in the nervous system. This results in disability and death.

Description

Gangliosides are fatty substances necessary for the proper development of the brain and nerve cells (nervous system). Under normal conditions, gangliosides are continuously broken down, so that an appropriate balance is maintained. In Tay-Sachs disease, the enzyme necessary for removing excess gangliosides is missing. This allows gangliosides to accumulate throughout the brain and is responsible for the disability associated with the disease.

Tay-Sachs disease is particularly common among Jewish people of Eastern European and Russian (Ashkenazi) origin. About one out of every 3,600 babies born to Ashkenazi Jewish couples will have the disease. Tay-Sachs is also more common among certain French-Canadian and Cajun French families.

Causes and symptoms

Tay-Sachs is caused by a defective gene. Genes are located on chromosomes and serve to direct specific development/processes within the body. The genetic defect in Tay-Sachs disease results in the lack of an enzyme hexosaminidase A. Without this enzyme, gangliosides cannot be degraded. They build up within the brain, interfering with nerve functioning. Because Tay-Sachs is a recessive disorder, only people who receive two defective genes (one from the mother and one from the father) will actually have the disease. People who have only one defective gene and one normal gene are called carriers. They carry the defective gene and thus the possibility of passing the gene and/or the disease onto their offspring.

When a carrier and a non-carrier have children, none of their children will actually have Tay-Sachs. It is likely that 50% of their children will be carriers themselves. When two carriers have children, their children have a 25% chance of having normal genes, a 50% chance of being carriers of the defective gene, and a 25% chance of having two defective genes. The two defective genes cause the disease itself.

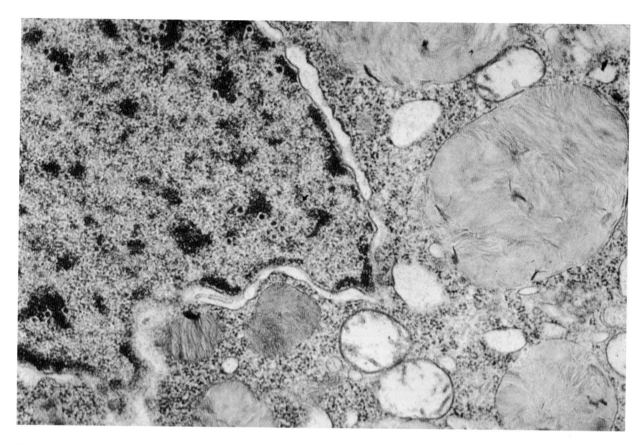

Scanning electron micrograph of cerebromacular degeneration as a result of Tay-Sachs disease. *(© Custom Medical Stock Photo, Inc. Reproduced by permission.)*

Classic Tay-Sachs disease strikes infants around the age of six months. Up until this age, the baby will appear to be developing normally. When Tay-Sachs begins to show itself, the baby will stop interacting with other people and develop a staring gaze. Normal levels of noise will startle the baby to an abnormal degree. By about one year of age, the baby will have very weak, floppy muscles, and may be completely blind. The head will be quite large. Patients also present with loss of peripheral (side) vision, inability to breathe and swallow, and paralysis as the disorder progresses. Seizures become a problem between ages one and two, and the baby usually dies by about age four.

A few variations from this classical progression of Tay-Sachs disease are possible:

• Juvenile hexosaminidase A deficiency. Symptoms appear between ages two and five; the disease progresses more slowly, with death by about 15 years.

• Chronic hexosaminidase A deficiency. Symptoms may begin around age five or may not occur until age 20–30. The disease is milder. Speech becomes slurred. The individual may have difficulty walking due to weakness, muscle cramps, and decreased coordination of movements. Some individuals develop mental illness. Many have changes in intellect, hearing, or vision.

Diagnosis

Examination of the eyes of a child with Tay-Sachs disease will reveal a characteristic cherry-red spot at the back of the eye (in an area called the retina). Tests to determine the presence and quantity of hexosaminidase A can be performed on the blood, specially treated skin cells, or white blood cells. A carrier will have about half of the normal level of hexosaminidase A present, while a patient with the disease will have none.

Treatment

There is no treatment for Tay-Sachs disease.

Prognosis

Sadly, the prognosis for a child with classic Tay-Sachs disease is certain death. Adults with the chronic form of Tay-Sachs experience milder symptoms and life expectancy is not always affected, though the disease is still progressive and may be disabling.

Prevention

Prevention involves identifying carriers of the disease and providing them with appropriate information concerning the chance of their offspring having Tay-Sachs disease. When the levels of hexosaminidase A are half the normal level, a person is a carrier of the defective gene. Blood tests of carriers reveals reduction of hexosaminidase A.

When a woman is already pregnant, tests can be performed on either the cells of the baby (aminocentesis) or the placenta (chorionic villus sampling) to determine whether the baby will have Tay-Sachs disease.

Resources

ORGANIZATIONS

Late Onset Tay-Sachs Foundation. 1303 Paper Mill Road, Erdenheim, PA 19038. (800)672-2022.
March of Dimes Birth Defects Foundation. 1275 Mamaroneck Avenue, White Plains, NY 10605. (888) 663-4637. resourcecenter@modimes.org. http://www.modimes.org.

Laith Farid Gulli, M.D.

Temporal arteritis

Definition

The term temporal arteritis literally means "inflammation of the temporal arteries." As implied by the name, these blood vessels run along the temples after they branch off from the carotid artery in the neck. They provide the blood supply to portions of the scalp, jaw muscles, and salivary glands. Inflammation of these arteries, probably resulting from an abnormal immune reaction, disrupts this blood supply, resulting in a variety of symptoms, ranging from relatively minor jaw pain or headache to major symptoms, including temporary or permanent blindness.

Temporal arteritis is also called giant cell arteritis or cranial arteritis. It is a rheumatic disease that affects large and medium-sized arteries throughout the body and can occur in a variety of patients. Although the temporal arteries are most commonly affected, other arteries throughout the body may be affected. The disease seems to target arteries containing elastic tissue. Veins are rarely affected. Temporal arteritis is a type of **vasculitis**.

Description

Temporal arteritis almost always occurs in people over 50, and it becomes more common as people age. About 20 out of 100,000 people over the age of 50 suffer from temporal arteritis. Women are affected twice as often as men. Some authorities say that temporal arteritis is more common in Caucasians (especially Scandinavians) than in people of other races. Close relatives of patients with temporal arteritis may be more likely than others to get the disease.

Patients with temporal arteritis are diagnosed and overlap with a broader disorder called giant cell arteritis. This can affect parts of the body in addition to the scalp, eyes, and jaw. Sometimes the disease can cause restricted circulation to both arms or both legs, producing pain in the affected limbs. With other blood vessels involved, patients with advanced forms of the disease may experience strokes or transient ischemic attacks (TIA). These result in brief episodes of pain caused by decreased blood flow. Even heart attacks are occasionally caused by giant cell arteritis.

Causes and symptoms

This disease is one of a group of diseases in which the linings of large- or medium-sized blood vessels become inflamed. The elastic layer of these vessels is attacked by "giant" cells and chemicals produced by the immune system. This reaction reduces blood flow through the blood vessels, and the limited blood supply causes the symptoms.

The disease usually begins with "flu-like" symptoms, including a mild fever (100–101°F), general body discomfort, and a persistent, dull headache. The scalp may be tender to the touch over the affected blood vessels. Jaw muscles sometimes become painful when the patient chews.

As the disease progresses, more severe symptoms occur. These include blurred vision or temporary blindness that typically lasts ten minutes or less. Eventually, permanent loss of vision can occur. Transient ischemic attacks, strokes, and heart attacks may occur when the disease is far advanced.

Diagnosis

Doctors from a number of specialties develop experience in diagnosing and treating temporal arteritis. These include internists, who treat a broad range of diseases; rheumatologists, who focus on rheumatic diseases; geriatricians, who treat older people; ophthalmologists, who treat eye and vision disorders; neurologists, who treat headaches and problems of the optic nerve; and vascular surgeons, who treat blood vessel problems.

The doctor will generally take a medical history first. The patient can help the doctor tremendously by reviewing all symptoms—both major and minor—from the last two or three months. If possible, the patient should ask family or close friends for help in recalling his/her ailments from recent months. Then the doctor will conduct a complete physical examination. Often, he or she will detect a tender, swollen artery on the scalp.

The doctor will order blood tests as well. A standard and inexpensive test called the erythrocyte sedimentation rate (ESR or "sed" rate) is particularly helpful. Results from this test, which measures inflammation in the body, will almost always be higher than normal. Tests of the red blood cells may show mild anemia. Sometimes blood tests for liver function will also be abnormal.

The definitive diagnostic test is a temporal artery **biopsy**. A doctor will make one or more tiny incisions under local anesthesia to remove samples of the suspect artery. Under the microscope, a pathologist usually can identify the typical damage caused by temporal arteritis.

Treatment

The mainstay of treatment is a course of corticosteroids (steroid hormones that have an anti-inflammatory effect), usually prednisone. The initial prescription involves a fairly high dose of steroids (40–60 mg/day) which is gradually tapered down to a maintenance dose. Because of the high incidence of blindness in untreated cases, steroid therapy should be started immediately rather than waiting for biopsy results. Patients typically take this maintenance dose for periods of one to three years. Sometimes nonsteroidal anti-inflammatory drugs (NSAIDs) are prescribed for muscle aches or headaches, especially while steroid doses are being reduced.

KEY TERMS

Anemia—Lower than normal level of red blood cells, or of the oxygen-carrying chemical hemoglobin.

Biopsy—Removal and examination of a sample tissue from the body for diagnostic purposes.

Corticosteroids—A group of hormones, produced naturally by the adrenal gland and other organs. They are used to treat a wide variety of disorders, including many rheumatic disorders.

Erythrocyte sedimentation rate—The speed at which red blood cells sink in a tube of freshly drawn blood, which is a rough measure of clotting disorders or inflammation.

Prednisone—A corticosteroid often used to treat inflammation.

Rheumatic disease—A type of disease involving inflammation of muscles, joints, and other tissues.

Transient ischemic attack—A brief experience of stroke-like symptoms (for instance, numbness, paralysis, problems in speaking or understanding speech) that go away within hours, with no permanent damage. Also known as TIA.

Vasculitis—An inflammation of the blood vessels.

Prognosis

The outlook for most patients with temporal arteritis is good, especially if the disorder is diagnosed early. Symptoms often diminish within a month once patients begin to take steroids. Although physicians do not talk about a "cure" for temporal arteritis, symptoms typically do not return after a full course of steroid treatment. Unfortunately, if the diagnosis is made late in the disease, lost vision may not return.

Prevention

There is no medically proven approach to prevention. The best way to prevent severe, permanent damage is to obtain expert medical advice if the patient or the family physician suspects this problem.

Resources

ORGANIZATIONS

National Headache Foundation. 428 W. St. James Place, Chicago, IL 60614. (800) 843-2256. http://www.headaches.org.

Richard H. Lampert

Temporal lobe epilepsy

Definition

Temporal lobe epilepsy (TLE) refers to a condition where seizures are generated in the portion of the brain called the temporal lobe. Either the right or the left temporal lobe can be involved, and in rare cases both temporal lobes can be involved in a particular individual.

Description

Under the broad category of TLE, there are a number of specific types. In mesial TLE (MTLE), there are characteristic abnormalities in the mesial aspect of the temporal lobe. This variably involves sclerosis (scarring), loss of nerve cells in the hippocampus and mossy cell fiber sprouting. Of course, there are other pathologies that can be seen in the temporal lobe including tumors, stroke, multiple sclerosis plaques, and tubers (as seen in tuberous sclerosis). Another type of TLE is lateral TLE. This is where the seizures originate in the lateral portion of the particular temporal lobe. Again, various pathologies can be found such as cortical malformations and stroke; however, imaging studies, such as magnetic resonance imaging (MRI), often may not show any obvious lesions or abnormalities. As more information is gathered regarding the genetics that may be involved in some cases, the classification of TLE will likely change.

Demographics

TLE, as a whole, constitutes a common type of epilepsy. The exact incidence is not clear but it is suspected to make up a significant proportion of medication-resistant epilepsy. Approximately 30% (of the 2.7 million cases of epilepsy in the United States) do not adequately respond to medications. Up to one-half of these may be due to TLE. One of the risk factors that may predispose children to, in particular, mesial TLE is complicated or prolonged febrile convulsions before the age of five years. Mesial TLE can run in some families.

Causes and symptoms

Causes

The abnormalities most associated with mesial TLE are sclerosis (scarring) of the hippocampus, neuronal cell loss in the hippocampal area, and inappropriate sprouting (growth) of mossy cell fibers. The cause of these variable pathological findings is still being studied. There is some evidence that mesial TLE may be a progressive condition where seizures become more resistant to medications over time. Likely, seizures over time play a role in the changes seen in the mesial temporal lobe. Likewise, the mesial temporal abnormalities contribute to the epileptogenicity (seizure potential) of that region. Although these pathologies are the most common findings in cases of mesial TLE, other lesions can be the suspected cause of epilepsy such as stroke, multiple sclerosis plaques, tumors, and cortical malformations. Lateral TLE can also be affected by strokes, cortical malformations, and multiple sclerosis plaques, and be the cause of seizures from this area. In the rare condition of benign familial TLE the cause is genetic and runs in families. Exactly how any of the previously mentioned abnormalities actually cause groups of neurons to generate seizure activity is complex and not fully understood. Because there can be different lesions, there can also be different mechanisms of generating a seizure. The temporal lobe epilepsies should not be considered diseases. Rather, they are syndromes (groups of physical signs and symptoms) with many causes.

Symptoms

The age of onset of TLE is highly variable depending on the cause. In mesial TLE, seizure can begin as early as childhood or even later in adulthood. There is a characteristic remission that can occur during childhood, lasting a few years, but then seizures resume in adulthood.

The seizures that occur in TLE are simple partial seizures or complex partial seizures. Uncommonly, a generalized tonic-clonic seizure may occur. The simple partial seizures can take the form of auras. Although these are viewed as seizure warnings, they are actually minor seizures that do not affect consciousness. The most common aura is a visceral sensation. This can take the form of a rising feeling in stomach. Other kinds of auras can be déjà vu (a sense of familiarity) or *jamais vu* (the opposite of déjà vu, a sense of unfamiliarity or uniqueness); distortion of perceptions of size, or movement (vertigo); or olfactory (odors) distortions and buzzing sounds depending on what portion of the temporal lobe is involved. Emotional auras can also occur; fear, for example. Still other auras are too difficult for patients to describe. All these minor seizures are usually not serious unless they are occurring frequently and are disturbing to the person.

Seizures that affect or alter consciousness are present in the majority of people with TLE. These complex partial seizures variably involve cessation of activity, a certain degree of staring off, and lip smacking or other oral movements. Moreover, the arm contralateral (opposite) the temporal lobe displays a posturing action. The arm ipsilateral (same side) as the affected temporal lobe has automatisms (semi-purposeful motions). During this phase of the seizure, the person has little-to-no awareness of the environment and will virtually be unresponsive to those around him or her. The aura plus the complex partial seizure phase typically lasts less than 2–3 minutes. Then there is a variable period of confusion lasting longer. If the seizure involves primarily the dominant (usually left) hemisphere (where language is processed) then a so-called postictal (after seizure) aphasia (loss of language) can occur and last several minutes. All these behavioral features can help decide which hemisphere, if not temporal lobe, is involved.

Diagnosis

The diagnosis of TLE can be made by a careful history (of an accurate description of the seizures) coupled with abnormalities on high resolution MRI of the brain and electroencephalogram (EEG). MRIs are sensitive, but subtle lesions such as mesial temporal sclerosis can be missed either by routine MRIs or inexperienced radiologists. The routine EEG (usually 30 minutes of testing) can be normal between seizures but may sometimes show occasional characteristic wave patterns in the temporal regions suggesting the location of seizure generation. Long-term monitoring with EEG/closed circuit TV (LTME) is extremely helpful to determining which temporal lobe is abnormal.

Treatment

The treatment goal of any epilepsy is freedom from seizures with no side-effects of medications. Although this is the goal, it is frequently not attained. There may be a highly variable response to medications. There are over 20 seizure medications available. It is important to understand that if a trial of up to three different well-chosen medications, alone or in combination, fails to control seizures, then the likelihood that some other medication will work is slim. Therefore, the general belief is that not all medications and combinations need to be tried to know if an epilepsy will be resistant. A timely referral to a comprehensive epilepsy center should be done to explore other treatment options, such as surgery. In mesial TLE, medications frequently fail to adequately control the seizures. Fortunately, this particular epilepsy is most responsive to surgical treatment. Brain surgery should not be viewed as a last resort when pharmocoresistant epilepsies are considered. With modern screening methods and neurosurgical technique,

complications are rare. The surgery for mesial TLE offers up to an 80% chance of cure. The surgery involves the removal of a portion of the affected temporal lobe. However, seizures that are generated from other areas of the temporal lobe are more complicated.

Vagus nerve stimulation involves the implantation of a stimulator under the skin of the chest. Wires run from the stimulator to the vagus nerve, and deliver short bursts of electrical energy. The electricity runs up to the brain through the vagus nerve, and serves to interrupt the seizure-causing electrical activity in the brain.

Recovery and rehabilitation

Recovery and rehabilitation is a consideration if epilepsy surgery is performed. If a partial temporal lobectomy has been done, the patient remains in the hospital for several days. Postoperatively, there can be headaches and nausea that are managed with medications and resolved in one to three days. Complications of surgery are rare but include infection (managed with antibiotics) and bleeding (which, if severe, may require a transfusion). Neurological deficits are uncommon; when they are present they are usually mild. This includes a limited visual field deficit, contralateral (opposite to surgical side) weakness or speech difficulty. When neurological complications occur, they usually improve with time and are not disabling.

Clinical trials

As of August 2011, there were 15 active clinical trials examining various aspects of temporal lobe epilepsy. The National Institutes of Health clinical trials Web site at http://clinicaltrials.gov has information on other recruiting and ongoing studies of TLE.

Prognosis

The prognosis for TLE varies considerably depending on the type of TLE. Although medications should be tried initially, mesial TLE and many of the lateral TLEs are often resistant. Timely referral to an epilepsy center that can determine the nature of the seizure disorder and offer other kinds of treatment approaches should be undertaken. Epilepsy surgery for mesial TLE offers up to an 80% chance of sustained seizure freedom and the possibility of discontinuing medications.

Special concerns

Long-standing, poorly controlled epilepsy has a number of psychosocial ramifications. These can include (but are not limited to) memory difficulty, reduced self-esteem, depression, reduced ability for gainful employment, and greater difficulty with interpersonal relationships. These issues may be underestimated in the setting of treating the seizure disorder. Recognizing the psychosocial wellbeing of the patient will greatly help in improving quality of life.

Resources

BOOKS

Browne, T.R., and G.L. Holmes. *Handbook of Epilepsy*. 4th ed. Baltimore: Lippincott Williams & Wilkins, 2008.

Engel Jr. J., and T.A. Pedley. *Epilepsy: A Comprehensive Textbook*. 2nd ed. 3 vols. Baltimore: Lippincott Williams & Wilkins, 2007.

Wyllie, E. *The Treatment of Epilepsy: Principles and Practice*. 5th ed. Baltimore: Lippincott Williams & Wilkins, 2010.

PERIODICALS

Micallef, S. "Psychological outcome profiles in childhood-onset temporal lobe epilepsy." *Epilepsia* 51 (October 1, 2010): 2066–73.

Uijl, S. "Prognosis after temporal lobe epilepsy surgery: the value of combining predictors." *Epilepsia* 49 (August 1, 2008): 1317–23.

ORGANIZATIONS

American Epilepsy Society, 342 North Main Street, West Hartford, CT 06117-2507, (860) 586-7505, http://www.aesnet.org.

The Epilepsy Foundation, 8301 Professional Place, Landover, MD 20785-7223, (800) 332-1000, http://www.epilepsyfoundation.org.

International League Against Epilepsy, 342 North Main Street, West Hartford, CT 06117-2507, (860) 586-7547, Fax: (860) 586-7550, http://www.ilae-epilepsy.org.

Roy Sucholeiki, MD
Rosalyn Carson-DeWitt, MD

Tension headache *see* **Headache**

Tethered spinal cord syndrome

Definition

Tethered spinal cord syndrome (TSCS), also known as Occult Spinal Dysraphism Sequence, is a congenital condition that causes the spinal cord, before or after birth, to become attached to the spinal column at some point along its length, most often in the lower (lumbar) portion. TSCS is related to **spina bifida**, since both disorders arise from a failure of the neural tube to close completely during embryonic development. There are differing forms and degrees of severity of tethered spinal cord syndrome, including tight filum terminale, lipomeningomyelocele, split cord malformations, and dermal sinus tracts.

Description

The normal spinal cord, a cable of nerves, extends vertically from the base of the brain to the lumbar region, or lower back, contained within the hollow cylinder formed by the bony vertebrae and soft tissues of the spinal column. The spinal cord hangs freely within the spinal column, cushioned by cerebrospinal fluid, and is attached at its lower end to a strand of elastic tissue, the *filum terminale*, which is in turn attached to the lower end of the spinal column and which secures the lower end of the cord but allows it to be stretched without injury. Beyond the lower end of the cord proper, the major afferent and efferent nerves for the muscles of the legs, lower bowel, and bladder, the *cauda equina*, continue down the spinal canal and branch to those areas.

TSCS is initiated by incomplete closure, during embryonic development, of the *neural tube*, the early embryonic foundation of the spinal cord and column, resulting in malformations of the spinal column and cord. One disorder brought about by the malformation is *spina bifida*, in which the spine is open on its dorsal surface, somewhere along its length. Spina bifida can range in severity from not being visible externally, or *spina bifida occulta*, to a visible, open cavity with major impairment of the spinal cord at and below that spot. Among these extremes, tethered spinal cord may occur in the invisible forms or spina bifida occulta.

In cases of relatively mild spina bifida that result in TSCS, the flaw occurs most often along the lower (lumbar) portion of the spinal column and cord. Cases of tethered cord in the cervical and thoracic regions of the spinal column are known but are extremely rare.

The developmental flaw causes soft tissues of the spinal column to grow into the hollow containing the spinal cord and to attach to the spinal cord, anchoring it at that spot. Since the spinal cord grows more slowly than the spinal column, a tethered spinal cord becomes stretched and stressed over time, causing neurological damage in the cord and the nerves of the cauda equina that results in physical problems that manifest in a range of diagnostic symptoms and signs. Bending or stretching movements of the body put additional tension on the tethered cord.

As the cord is stretched, circulation of blood to the lower portion and cauda equina may be reduced as the blood vessels there are compressed by the tension in the cord. This in turn results in hypoxia, or loss of oxygen, delivered in the blood to that part of the cord, eventually causing damage and loss of function in the neurons.

If left untreated, the stress induced in the tethered cord can cause permanent damage and malfunction to the nerves and muscles that control movements of the legs, feet, bowel and bladder. Severe consequences can be deformed feet and legs, paralysis and incontinence.

Other forms of tethered cord include tight filum terminale syndrome, in which malformations in the embryonic neural tube at its lowermost point result in a defective filum terminale, the normally flexible anchor of the cord's lower end. A defective filum terminale is short and fibrous, with reduced elasticity or none, thus tethering the spinal cord at its lower end.

A lipomeningomyelocele is an abnormal growth of fatty tissue at the base of the developing spinal cord that entangles the lower end of the cord and thus tethers it.

In diastematomyelia, or split cord syndrome, an abnormal growth of bony or fibrous tissue forms a spur within the spinal canal, parting longitudinally (not severing) the nerves of the spinal cord, which rejoin into a single tract below the spur. The spinal cord can become tethered at the location of the split.

A dermal sinus tract is a canal lined with epithelial (skin) tissue, one end of which shows as an opening in the lumbar skin, the other end connecting with the tissues of the spinal cord or canal, or with adjacent tissues. Tumors form in the internal end of the sinus in about half of all cases, the tumors often bringing about spinal cord tethering.

TSCS may also develop following surgery for spina bifida, when scar tissue resulting from surgery grows and snags the spinal cord, thus tethering it.

Demographics

Tethered spinal cord is a relatively rare disorder. Its exact frequency is unknown, mostly because of a general lack of research on the disorder, and because the mildest forms may never be detected. TSCS in all forms affect both sexes and all races and ethnic groups.

Causes and symptoms

Congenital tethered spinal cord syndrome is initiated by incomplete closure of the neural tube during embryonic development. During the eighteenth to twenty-second day of embryonic development, the beginning structure of the neural tube, which will become the spinal column and cord, is formed by ectodermal tissue on the back of the embryo that forms a groove, which deepens and forms into a hollow tube, still open dorsally along its length. The tube begins to close itself, starting in the thoracic region, then moving on toward the head and lumbar regions. During the twenty-eighth to forty-eighth day of development, ectodermal tissue in the tail area of the embryo forms a separate, short length of neural tube, the conus medullaris, whose anterior end meets and fuses with the main neural tube while the posterior forms the filum terminale. The conus medullaris also produces the cauda equinae nerves.

Symptoms of TSCS may be visible at birth or appear later, even in adulthood, but most often in childhood. The symptoms may be visible or behavioral. Various visible signs on the skin of the lower back, along and near the spinal cord, are:

- Lipomas, or fatty tumors below the skin
- Hairy patches
- Spots of increased pigmentation
- Dimples that may indicate dermal sinus tracts
- Skin lesions
- Skin tags or outgrowths
- *Angiomas*, or port-wine stains

Behavioral symptoms manifest as
- Chronic lower back pains
- Progressive scoliosis, or curvature of the spine
- Foot deformities
- Numbness and loss of sensation in the legs or feet
- Awkward gait and stumbling
- Weakness in legs or feet
- Unequal growth in the legs or feet
- Progressive loss of control over bladder and bowel functions (incontinence)
- Urinary tract infections

Diagnosis

The initial indicators of TSCS are the physical and behavioral ones listed above. A newborn that carries any of the symptomatic skin defects should be diagnosed further for possible TSCS. Among the behavioral signs, a child will likely complain to parents of lower back pains, while other behavioral symptoms will become obvious to parents. An adult who shows any of the physical or behavioral symptoms should bring these to the attention of his family physician, who should suspect TSCS as the cause. Symptoms, physical or behavioral, may not appear until many years after birth, including well into adulthood, depending on the time of tethering, degree of stretching of the spinal cord, and severity of damage to the nerves of the cord.

The next steps in diagnosis of TSCS are taking x-ray images of the spine to detect bone abnormalities, followed by the application of diagnostic neuroimaging by means of MRI (magnetic resonance imaging) to produce three-dimensional images of the spinal column and spinal cord. Since a defect in the spinal cord or column makes it likely that there are other defects in the cord, column, or brain, an entire imaging of the brain and spinal column is recommended. **Electromyography** (EMG) can be used to check for or assess damage to nerve conduction in the spinal cord and the nerves of the cauda equinae. Ultrasound imaging can be used to monitor unborn infants for evidence of TSCS, should there be a reason to suspect it.

Since the muscles of the bladder are often affected by TSCS, urodynamics testing is recommended to discover the extent of the damage.

Treatment team

A family doctor is probably the person most likely to first link symptoms in a child or adult to TSCS, when parents bring in a child for a routine health check or because of the physical and behavioral signs and problems. Following the tentative diagnosis, the patient will be sent to neurologists, MRI imaging technicians, EMG technicians, urologists, surgeons and neurophysiologists if surgery is called for, and the personnel monitoring recovery.

Treatment

TSCS is corrected by surgery to detach the cord at its place of tethering. Follow-up examinations are necessary because the freed spinal cord sometimes becomes retethered to growing scar tissue.

In the case of tight filum terminale, the filum terminale is severed, allowing the cord to float freely.

Surgery for TSCS generally takes four to six hours and is conducted according to the form of TSCS in the patient. The spinal column is opened from behind to reach the site of tethering. Neurophysiologists are present to monitor spinal cord and nerve functioning to reduce the risk of damage to nerves and other tissues.

Recovery and rehabilitation

The degree of recovery is based on the amount of damage induced by the TSCS and the success of the surgery. Nearly all patients improve or at least show no worsening of signs. A successful operation leaves two percent or less possibility of the symptoms getting worse, and a fifty percent likelihood of sensation and movement problems becoming normal. **Back pain** usually is reduced or eliminated and strength to the lower part of the body improves. On the other hand, bladder dysfunction usually does not improve.

Ongoing monitoring of a patient following surgery for TSCS is required, in case the spinal cord should retether.

Clinical trials

Information about current relevant clinical trials can be found at ClinicalTrials.gov.

Prognosis

The prognosis for tethered spine syndrome is favorable, since skin symptoms may be visible at birth or later, allowing early detection and treatment, while behavioral symptoms manifest slowly enough for diagnosis and treatment before the condition becomes severe.

Special concerns

Spinal surgery is always risky because of possible damage to the nerves of the spinal cord. The patient may also have to deal with permanent damage caused by TSCS that surgery cannot improve.

Resources

BOOKS

Parker; James N. and Philip M. Parker. *The Official Patient's Sourcebook on Tethered Spinal Cord Syndrome*. Rev. and updated. San Diego, CA: ICON Health Publications, San Diego, CA., 2002.

Weinstein, Stuart L. *Pediatric Spine Surgery*. Philadelphia: Lippincott Williams & Wilkins Publishers, 2001.

PERIODICALS

Baskaya, M. K., J. A. Menendez, and B. K. Willis. "Late presentation of tethered spinal cord in a 73-year-old patient." *Journal of the American Geriatric Society* 49, no. 5 (May 2000): 682–83.

Witkamp, T. D., W. P. Vandertop, F. J. Beek, et al. "Medullary cone movement in subjects with a normal spinal cord and in patients with a tethered spinal cord." *Radiology* 220, no. 1 (July 2001): 208–12.

WEBSITES

NINDS Tethered Spinal Cord Syndrome Information Page. National Institute of Neurological Disorders and Stroke. http://www.ninds.nih.gov/health_and_medical/disorders/tethered_cord.htm.

ORGANIZATIONS

National Organization for Rare Disorders (NORD). P.O. Box 1968 (55 Kenosia Avenue), Danbury, CT 06813-1968. Phone: 203-744-0100. Fax: 203-798-2291. Voice Mail: 800-999-NORD (6673). Email: orphan@rarediseases.org. http://www.rarediseases.org.

Spina Bifida Association of America. 4590 MacArthur Blvd. NW, Suite 250, Washington, DC 20007-4266. Phone: 202-944-3285. Fax: 202-944-3295. Tollfree phone: 800-621-3141. Email: sbaa@sbaa.org. http://www.sbaa.org.

Kevin Fitzgerald

Third nerve palsy

Definition

Third nerve palsy describes a condition involving the third cranial nerve (also called the oculomotor nerve), which is responsible for innervating some of the muscles responsible for eye movement.

Description

Third nerve palsy results in an inability to move the eye normally in all directions. Injury to the third nerve can occur anywhere along its path, from where it originates within the brain to where it innervates the muscles that move the eyeball. Third nerve palsy prevents the proper functioning of the medial, superior, and inferior recti, and inferior oblique muscles. As a result, the eye cannot move up, down, or in. When at rest, the eye tends to look down and to the side, due to an inequality of muscle functioning. The muscle responsible for keeping the upper eyelid open (levator palpebrae superioris) is also affected, resulting in a drooping upper eyelid (ptosis).

Causes and symptoms

A wide variety of conditions can result in third nerve palsy, including pressure and damage from tumors; blocked arteries or **aneurysms** leading to oxygen deprivation of nerves; **meningitis**; vascular complications of diabetes or high blood pressure; complications of migraine headaches; traumatic injury; birth injury; congenital defects; and conditions that strip nerve fibers of their myelin coating, resulting in slowed nervous transmission.

Some patients have severe pain and double vision (diplopia), in addition to problems moving their eyes normally. The affected eye tends to move down and out, due to an inequality in muscle functioning. The eye cannot move up, down, or in. In some cases, the pupil remains fixed in a dilated state. The upper eyelid is droopy (ptosis). The eyeball itself may actually be slightly displaced, pushed more forward than normal (proptosis).

Additionally, after the acute phase of third nerve palsy, as the nerve attempts to regenerate, a phenomenon called oculomotor synkinesis may take place. In this associated condition, nerve sprouts accidentally misdirect nerve transmission, so that efforts to utilize certain muscle groups accidentally prompt the functioning of other muscle groups. Therefore, attempts to accomplish certain muscular tasks actually result in different muscular tasks occurring. For example, as an individual with oculomotor synkinesis attempts to look down, the eyelid may raise up; when attempting to look up, the eye instead moves toward the midline; when attempting to look toward the midline, the pupil constricts.

Diagnosis

Eye muscle dysfunction is usually revealed during the course of a basic physical examination, which should always include testing of eye movements and examination of the pupils. MRI, CT, or **angiography** (a dye test that lights up the arteries throughout the brain, allowing the arteries to be better visualized on CT or MRI) may reveal the underlying cause of third nerve palsy.

Treatment team

Ophthalmologists and neurologists may work together to care for patients with third nerve palsy. In addition, physicians who manage diabetes, high blood pressure, or other underlying causative conditions will be involved in the patients' care.

Treatment

Steroids may treat pain and double vision. Special lenses with prisms may improve diplopia. Surgery on the eye muscles or eyelid may be necessary in some cases, although most clinicians recommend waiting six months from onset so that the patients' condition stabilizes.

Prognosis

In individuals who have no pupil involvement, and whose third nerve palsy is due to complications of diabetes or high blood pressure, symptoms may actually resolve within 3–6 months of onset. Other patients have a variable outcome, depending on the underlying condition responsible for the third nerve palsy.

Resources

BOOKS

Donahue, Sean P. "Nuclear and Fascicular Disorders of Eye Movement." In *Opthalmology*, edited by Myron Yanoff, et al. St. Louis: Mosby, 2003.

Goodwin, James. "Cranial Nerves III, IV, and VI: The Oculomotor System." In *Textbook of Clinical Neurology*, edited by Christopher G. Goetz. Philadelphia: W. B. Saunders, 2003.

Noble, John, et al., eds. *Noble: Textbook of Primary Care Medicine*. St. Louis: W. B. Saunders, 2001.

Rosalyn Carson-DeWitt, MD

Thoracic outlet syndrome

Definition

Thoracic outlet syndrome refers to a group of disorders that cause pain and abnormal nerve sensations in the neck, shoulder, arm, and/or hand.

Description

The thoracic outlet is an area at the top of the rib cage, between the neck and the chest. Several anatomical structures pass through this area, including the esophagus, trachea, and nerves and blood vessels that lead to the arm and neck region. The area contains the first rib; collar bone (clavicle); the arteries beneath the collar bone (subclavian artery), which supply blood to the arms; a network of nerves leading to the arms (brachial plexus); and the top of the lungs.

Pain and other symptoms occur when the nerves or blood vessels in this area are compressed. The likelihood of blood vessels or nerves in the thoracic outlet being compressed increases with increased size of body tissues in this area or with decreased size of the thoracic outlet. The pain of thoracic outlet syndrome is sometimes confused with the pain of angina that indicates heart problems. The two conditions can be distinguished from each other because the pain of thoracic outlet syndrome does not appear or increase when walking, while the pain of angina does. Also, the pain of thoracic outlet syndrome usually increases if the affected arm is raised, which does not happen in cases of angina.

There are three types of thoracic outlet syndrome:

- True neurogenic thoracic outlet syndrome is caused by a compression of the nerves in the brachial plexus. Abnormal muscle or other tissue causes the problem.

- Arterial thoracic outlet syndrome is caused by compression of the major artery leading to the arm, usually by a rib.

- Disputed thoracic outlet syndrome describes conditions in patients who have chronic pain in the shoulders and arms and have no other disease or syndrome, but the underlying cause cannot be accurately determined.

Thoracic outlet syndrome is most common in women who are 35 to 55 years of age.

Causes and symptoms

Compression of blood vessels or nerves in the thoracic outlet causes pain and/or abnormal nerve sensations. Compression usually occurs at the location where the blood vessels and nerves pass out of the thoracic outlet into the arm.

There are several factors that contribute to thoracic outlet syndrome. Poor posture is a major cause and is easy to treat. A person's physical makeup also can cause thoracic outlet syndrome. For example, abnormalities of certain anatomical structures can put pressure on blood vessels or nerves. Typical abnormalities that can cause problems are malformed ribs and too narrow an opening between the collar bone and the first rib.

Normal Anatomy

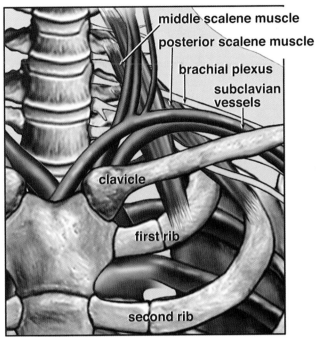

middle scalene muscle

posterior scalene muscle

brachial plexus

subclavian vessels

clavicle

first rib

second rib

Post-Accident Condition

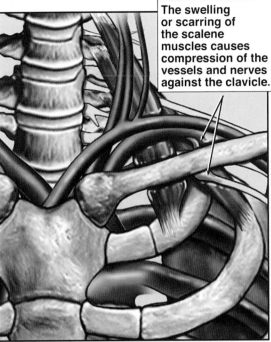

The swelling or scarring of the scalene muscles causes compression of the vessels and nerves against the clavicle.

ANTERIOR VIEW OF LEFT SHOULDER REGION

Post-Operative Condition

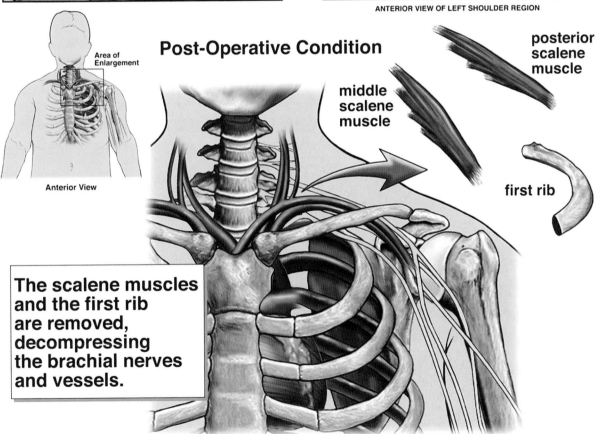

Area of Enlargement

Anterior View

posterior scalene muscle

middle scalene muscle

first rib

The scalene muscles and the first rib are removed, decompressing the brachial nerves and vessels.

(© Nucleus Medical Art, Inc./Alamy)

The main symptom is pain in the affected area. The patient can also develop **weakness** in the arm and hands, tingling nerve sensations, and a condition called Raynaud's syndrome. In Raynaud's syndrome, exposure to cold causes small arteries in the fingers to contract, cutting off blood flow. This causes the fingers to turn pale. In very severe cases of blood vessel compression, gangrene can result. Gangrene is the death of tissue caused by the blood supply being completely cut off.

In the case of arterial thoracic outlet syndrome, the artery beneath the collar bone leading to the arm is compressed, causing the artery to increase in size. Blood clots (thrombi) may form in the blood vessel. When blood vessels are compressed, the hands, arms, and shoulders do not receive proper blood supply. They can swell and turn blue from a lack of blood.

In the case of true neurogenic thoracic outlet syndrome, the nerves most affected are those of the network of nerves supplying the chest, shoulder, arm, forearm, and hand (brachial plexus). When a nerve is affected in thoracic outlet syndrome it produces a tingling sensation (paresthesia). It can also cause weakness in the hand and reduced sensation in the palm and fingers.

Diagnosis

There are no specific diagnostic tests for thoracic outlet syndromes. The diagnosis is made by ruling out other diseases and by observing the patient. Two non-specific tests that can suggest the presence of thoracic outlet syndrome are the Adson test and the Allen test. In the Adson test, the patient takes a deep breath and tilts his or her head back and turns it to one side. The physician tests to see if the strength of the patient's pulse is reduced in the wrist on the arm on the opposite side of the head turn. In the Allen test, the arm in which the patient is experiencing symptoms is raised and rotated while the head is turned to the opposite side. The physician tests to see if the pulse strength at the wrist is reduced. If the strength of the pulse is reduced in either of these two tests it indicates compression of the subclavian artery.

Occasionally, examination with a stethoscope may reveal abnormal sounds in affected blood vessels. X rays can reveal constrictions in blood vessels if a special dye is injected into the blood stream to make the blood vessels visible (**angiography**).

Certain tests are available to help with the diagnosis of **nerve compression**. These include the nerve conduction velocity test and somatosensory evoked potential test. In the nerve conduction velocity test, electrodes are placed at various locations on the skin along a nerve that is being tested. A mild electrical

KEY TERMS

Angina—A severe constricting pain in the chest, usually caused by a lack of oxygen to the heart.

Neurogenic—Caused by nerves; originating in the nerves.

Subclavian—Located beneath the collarbone (clavicle).

impulse is delivered through an electrode at one end of the nerve and the electrical activity is recorded by the other electrodes. The time it takes for the electrical impulse to travel down the nerve from the stimulating electrodes to the recording electrodes is used to calculate the nerve conduction velocity. This can be used to determine if any nerve damage exists.

In a somatosensory evoked potential test, electrodes are placed on the skin at the scalp, neck, shoulder, and wrist. A mild electrical impulse is delivered at the wrist, and a recording is made of the response by the brain and spinal cord. This test also can determine the presence of nerve damage.

Treatment

The main treatment for thoracic outlet syndrome is physical therapy. Exercises aimed at improving the posture of the affected person are also useful. In some cases, surgery can be performed to remove the cervical rib if this is causing the problem and physical therapy has failed to work. However, surgery is generally not used to treat thoracic outlet syndrome.

Prognosis

Treatment of true neurogenic and arterial thoracic outlet syndromes is usually successful. Treatment of disputed thoracic outlet syndrome is often unsuccessful. This may relate to the uncertainty of the underlying cause of the pain.

Resources

BOOKS

Porter, Robert. S., ed. *Merck Manual of Medical Information*. 3rd. ed. Whitehouse Station, NJ: Merck Research Laboratories, 2009.

John T. Lohr, PhD

Thoracic radiculopathy *see* **Radiculopathy**

Thyrotoxic myopathy

Definition

Thyrotoxic **myopathy** is a neuromuscular disorder that occurs due to overproduction of thyroid hormone and is characterized by excessive fatigability, muscle wasting, and **weakness**. It mainly affects muscles of the shoulder, hips, and hands. The adverse effects of thyroid hormone on the structure and function of muscles gives rise to this myopathy. Although diagnosis can be tricky, this disorder is reversible with appropriate treatment.

Description

Thyrotoxic myopathy is known by several other names such as hyperthyroid myopathy, Graves and Basedow's myopathy, and Basedow **paraplegia**. It was first recognized in the early nineteenth century by Graves and Von Basedow as occurring infrequently in severe hyperthyroidism. In the middle of the twentieth century, researchers found that up to 80% of hyperthyroid patients manifested at least some degree of muscle weakness, and this was confirmed on electromyographic studies.

Myopathy or muscle disease is categorized based on the underlying cause, for example, inheritance pattern. One of the broader categories is endocrine myopathies, which occur when there is an abnormal level of endocrine hormones in the body. The thyroid gland produces the hormone thyroxine, which regulates maturation of the nervous system, growth and metabolism. Of all the endocrine myopathies, the myopathy due to dysfunction of the thyroid gland is the commonest.

Demographics

Although some degree of muscle weakness is common in most hyperthyroid patients, it is still a rare disorder overall, and there are no accurate estimates of incidence. In one group of hyperthyroid patients, 67% had symptoms attributable to myopathy. In another group of 100 hyperthyroid patients only 33%–64% of patients complained of weakness but 61%–82% actually had demonstrable weakness on examination. Although hyperthyroidism is more common among women, symptomatic myopathy is more common among middle-aged hyperthyroid men. Unlike the classic myopathy, periodic paralysis, which is an unusual neuromuscular complication of hyperthyroidism, is seen among young Asian males.

Causes and symptoms

Causes

Much research has been done to elucidate how thyroxine affects muscle function. A brief overview of normal muscle structure and function helps to understand this. Muscle is made up of thousands of individual muscle fibers and myofibrils. The latter have myofilaments that are composed of contractile proteins called actin and myosin. In order for a muscle to contract, the command originates from the brain, travels along the spinal cord and then the nerve to terminate on the muscle. This impulse is then transmitted via a complicated process to the myofilaments that contract and relax appropriately. Adenosine triphosphate (ATP) is a chemical that supplies the necessary energy for contraction. Calcium, which is released during contraction, is taken up to cause muscle relaxation. Muscle fibers are of two types, slow and fast twitch. The slow or type 1 fibers are needed for sustained effort like standing and are more responsive to thyroxine. The fast type 2 fibers are needed for short rapid bursts like sprinting.

In hyperthyroidism, there is an accelerated production of ATP and reuptake of calcium. This leads to very rapid contraction and relaxation. When this occurs repetitively, the structure and mechanics of the slow fiber are changed to that of a fast fiber. Hyperthyroidism increases the body's basal metabolic rate, and much of this energy is inefficiently used for muscle contraction. In turn, the muscles lose their endurance, fatigue easily, and become weak and wasted.

Hyperthyroidism can have several causes. Of these, only two are commonly associated with myopathy. One of them is multinodular goiter, when the thyroid gland becomes studded with nodules, enlarges, and overproduces thyroxine. The other is Graves disease, where the body launches an autoimmune attack on the thyroid gland and causes it to produce excess thyroxine.

Symptoms

A hyperthyroid person who has muscle weakness may or may not have other recognizable manifestations of hyperthyroidism. Myopathy can sometimes be the first presentation of the underlying hyperthyroid state. There are several types depending on the rapidity of symptom development and patterns of muscle involvement.

Chronic Thyrotoxic Myopathy: The symptom onset is insidious, so much so that patients very often do not notice the wasting or weakness. An average of six months elapse before the diagnosis is made, as the symptoms are subtle and the progress is gradual. As mentioned earlier, only around 30% of patients complain of neuromuscular symptoms, whereas around 80% show muscle weakness on testing. Patients complain of low exercise tolerance, easy fatigability, difficulty in doing certain tasks, muscle stiffness, muscle twitching, and sometimes muscle wasting. Shoulder, hand, and then pelvic muscles are affected, and tasks like climbing stairs, getting up from a low chair, or lifting arms above the shoulders become strenuous. Due to the weakness, movements become clumsy and effortful. The degree of wasting varies among individuals. It is usually mild to moderate but on occasions can be so severe that the scapulae look "winged." Despite a remarkable degree of wasting and weakness, patients remain ambulatory. If the myopathy progresses untreated, then facial muscles, swallowing, and respiratory muscles are involved with resultant difficulty swallowing and breathing. Muscles that control eye movement can also be affected, leading to double vision and squint.

Acute Thyrotoxic Myopathy: This was first described by Laurent in 1944 and is a much rarer form that the chronic myopathy. It is rapidly progressive with profound muscle weakness developing over a few days. Muscle pain, cramps, and muscle breakdown develop and lead to rhabdomyolysis. Patients are confused, have very weak respiratory muscles, and develop severe respiratory failure necessitating artificial ventilation.

Ocular Myopathy: This is also called dysthyroid opthalmopathy or exopthalmic opthalmoplegia. It is more common in females, can be unilateral, and may or may not be associated with chronic thyrotoxic myopathy. It can occur even after treatment for hyperthyroidism. The eye muscles become swollen and weak due to inflammation from an autoimmune attack. Eyes are bulging, the cornea is inflamed, and eye movements are restricted especially in the horizontal direction. In severe cases, the cornea is ulcerated, and blindness occurs. It progresses over six to eighteen months, and longer delays in treatment result in severe residual deficit.

Thyrotoxic Periodic Paralysis: This is very rare and occurs mostly in young adult males of Asian ancestry around the third decade. It is characterized by sudden episodes of muscle weakness involving the trunk and limb muscles, developing over few minutes to hours and lasting for hours to a couple of days. It is due to altered muscle membrane excitability secondary to low potassium levels. Although it is reversible spontaneously or with administration of potassium, death can occur due to cardiac arrhythmias.

Diagnosis

The diagnosis is clinical and is usually made by a neurologist who has expertise in neuromuscular disorders. There should be a high index of clinical suspicion as the pattern of muscle weakness is nonspecific and often patients do not know that they are hyperthyroid. The combination of symptoms in a severe case of hyperthyroid myopathy, such as muscle wasting, difficulty swallowing, and muscle twitching can lead to a mistaken diagnosis of Lou-Gehrig's disease (ALS). A classic picture is that of a patient, who despite a ravenous appetite has significant muscle wasting, weakness and brisk tendon reflexes. Associated hyperthyroid features such as enlarged thyroid gland, **tremor**, bulging eyes, and a fast heart rate may be seen.

Blood tests show an elevated thyroxine level. In Graves disease, antibodies against the thyroid gland are present. Levels of creatine phosphokinase (CPK), a muscle enzyme, is normal except when there is acute muscle breakdown. **Electromyography** is a technique used to diagnose myopathies by studying the response of muscle contraction to an electrical stimulus. In hyperthyroid myopathy, this measure may be normal or show a "polyphasic" or "myopathic" response. Muscle **biopsy** again may be normal or show some degenerating fibers in a nonspecific pattern. CAT scans or MRI scans can be used to see the swollen eye muscles.

Treatment team

Treatment for hyperthyroid myopathy involves a neuromuscular specialist, an endocrinologist, a surgeon, and an ophthalmologist. Physiatrists and physical and occupational therapists are also part of the team helping in rehabilitation.

Treatment

Hyperthyroid myopathy is fortunately reversible provided the underlying hyperthyroidism is corrected, and a normal thyroid state (euthyroidism) is restored. This can be done with medications, radiation or surgery. Treatment is also aimed at symptomatic relief, prevention, and treatment of complications.

Medications

Beta-blockers are used to block the effects of adrenaline on peripheral tissues, as adrenergic systems are upregulated in hyperthyroidism. This affords symptomatic but temporary relief. Definitive treatment, however, aims at reducing the output of thyroxine from the thyroid gland. Propylthiouracil and methimazole are medications that inhibit production

Amyotrophic Lateral Sclerosis (ALS)—Also called Lou-Gehrig's disease, a progressive neuromuscular condition due to degeneration of the motor nerve cells and fiber tracts in the spinal cord. The cause is not yet well defined. It leads to progressive weakening of the limb muscles and that of swallowing and breathing and leads to death within a couple of years of onset.

Autoimmune—An immune response by the body against its own tissues or cells.

Contracture—Loss of range of motion at a joint due to abnormal shortening of soft tissues around the joint.

Creatine phosphokinase—A muscle enzyme present in various skeletal muscles and the heart which is released due to any type of muscle injury and this can be measured in the blood.

Electromyography—Technique used to measure the function of muscles by studying their contraction response to an electrical stimulus. A needle is inserted into the muscle, an electrical stimulus is given, and the resulting contraction is recorded from which normal and abnormal patterns can be interpreted.

Euthyroid—State of normal function of the thyroid gland.

Goiter—A swelling or enlargement of the thyroid gland.

Hormone—Chemical substance produced by certain endocrine glands, which are released into the bloodstream where they control and regulate functioning of several other tissues.

Hyperthyroid—State of excess thyroid hormone in the body.

Myofilament—Ultrastructural microscopic unit of a muscle, which is made up of proteins that contract.

Myopathy—Disease of muscle.

Opthalmoplegia—Paralysis of the muscles that control eye movements.

Paraplegia—Paralysis of the legs and lower part of the body.

Rhabdomyolysis—Breakdown of muscle fibers resulting in release of muscle contents into the blood.

Thyroxine—Hormone produced by the thyroid gland.

and release of thyroxine and also block tissue effects of thyroxine. Radiation in the form of oral radio-iodine therapy destroys the overactive thyroid gland. Steroids, other anti-inflammatory medications or radiation is used to treat the ocular myopathy. Artificial tears and lubricating ointments are used to prevent corneal ulceration. Potassium chloride given intravenously will reverse the thyrotoxic periodic paralysis.

Surgical treatment

Surgical removal of portions of the enlarged and unsightly thyroid gland can be done to restore euthyroid state. In severe cases of ocular myopathy, surgical widening of the walls of the orbit allows the eyes to decompress. Corneal grafting can be done to treat corneal ulceration.

Recovery and rehabilitation

When proper treatment is given, full recovery of the myopathy is possible, and complications can be avoided. Physical therapists can help in devising muscle strengthening exercises and in preventing muscle contractures.

Protective eye glasses and eye patches are used to prevent corneal exposure and ulceration.

Clinical trials

Information about current relevant clinical trials can be found at ClinicalTrials.gov.

Prognosis

Prognosis is quite good. In two to four months after euthryoid state is achieved, muscle weakness improves. But it may take up to a year for muscle bulk to return. Respiratory failure is very rare. Patients have a normal life expectancy and lead normal lives if properly and promptly treated.

Resources

BOOKS

"Thyroid disorders and the nervous system." Chapter 19. In *Neurology and General Medicine*, edited by Michael J. Aminoff. Philadelphia: Churchill Livingstone, 2001.
"Electrophysiologic Testing and Laboratory aids in the diagnosis of neuromuscular disease." Chapter 45. In

Principles of Neurology, edited by Maurice Victor and Allan H. Ropper. New York: McGraw-Hill, 2001.

"Principles of Clinical Myology: Diagnosis and Classification of Muscle Diseases-General Considerations." Chapter 48. In *Principles of Neurology*, edited by Maurice Victor and Allan H. Ropper. New York: McGraw-Hill, 2001.

"The Metabolic and Toxic Myopathies." Chapter 51. In *Principles of Neurology*, edited by Maurice Victor and Allan H. Ropper. New York: McGraw-Hill, 2001.

PERIODICALS

Alshekhlee, A., H. J. Kaminski, and R. L. Ruff. "Neuromuscular manifestations of endocrine disorders." *Neurologic Clinics* 20 (February 2002): 35–58.

Horak, H., and R. Pourmand. "Endocrine myopathies." *Neurologic Clinics* 18 (February 2000): 203–13.

Klein, I., and K. Ojamaa. "Thyroid (neuro)myopathy." *Lancet* 356 (August 2000): 614.

WEBSITES

National Institutes of Neurological Disorders and Stroke (NINDS). *Thyrotoxic Myopathy Information Page*.http://www.ninds.nih.gov/health_and_medical/disorders/thyrotoxic_myopathy.htm.

ORGANIZATIONS

Muscular Dystrophy Association. 3300 East Sunrise Drive, Tucson, AZ 85718-3208. Phone: (520) 529-2000. Toll-free phone: (800) 572-1717. Fax: (520) 529-5300. Email: mda@mdusa.org. http://www.mdusa.org.

National Institute of Health Neurological Institute. P.O.Box 5801, Bethesda, MD 20824. Phone: (301) 496-5751. Toll-free phone: (800) 352-9424. http://www.ninds.nih.gov/.

Chitra Venkatasubramanian, MBBS, MD

Tiagabine

Definition

Tiagabine is an anticonvulsant medication indicated for the control seizures in the treatment of epilepsy. Epilepsy is a neurological disorder in which excessive surges of electrical energy are emitted in the brain, causing seizures.

Purpose

Tiagabine decreases abnormal electrical activity within the brain that may trigger seizures. Although tiagabine controls some types of seizures associated with epilepsy, especially partial seizures, there is no known cure for the disorder.

Description

In the United States, tiagabine is sold under the brand name Gabitril. While the exact mechanism by which tiagabine reduces seizures is unknown, the drug boosts the levels of GABA, a neurotransmitter, in the brain. Neurotransmitters such as GABA are naturally occurring chemicals that transmit messages from one neuron (nerve cell) to another. When one neuron releases GABA, it normally binds to the next neuron, transmitting information and preventing the transmission of extra electrical activity. When levels of GABA are reduced, there may not be enough GABA to sufficiently bond to the neuron, leading to extra electrical activity in the brain and seizures. Tiagabine works to block GABA from being re-absorbed too quickly into the tissues, thereby increasing the amount available to bind to neurons.

Recommended dosage

Tiagabine is taken by mouth in tablet form and is prescribed by physicians in varying dosages.

Beginning a course of treatment with tiagabine requires a gradual dose-increasing regimen. Adults and teenagers 16 years or older typically take 4 mg a day at the beginning of treatment. The prescribing physician may raise a patient's daily dosage gradually over the course of several weeks. The usual dose is not greater than 56 mg per day. The full benefits of tiagabine may not be realized until after several weeks of therapy.

A person should not take a double dose of tiagabine. If a daily dose is missed, the next dose should be taken as soon as possible. However, if it is almost time for the next dose, the missed dose is skipped.

When discontinuing treatment with tiagabine, physicians typically direct patients to gradually reduce their daily dosages. Stopping the medicine suddenly may cause seizures to return or occur more frequently.

Precautions

A physician should be consulted before taking tiagabine with certain nonprescription medications. Patients should avoid alcohol and CNS depressants (medicines that can make one drowsy or less alert, such as antihistimines, sleep medications, and some pain medications) while taking tiagabine. Tiagabine can exacerbate the side effects of alcohol and other medications.

Tiagabine may not be suitable for persons with a history of liver or kidney disease, mental illness, high blood presure, angina (chest pain), irregular heartbeats, or other heart problems. Before beginning treatment with tiagabine, patients should notify their physician if they consume a large amount of alcohol, have a history of drug use, are pregnant, or plan to become pregnant. Physicians often advise the use of effective birth control while patients take tiagabine. Studies in animals indicate that tiagabine may cause birth defects. Patients who become pregnant while taking tiagabine should contact their physician immediately.

Side effects

Patients and their physicians should weigh the risks and benefits of tiagabine before beginning treatment. Tiagabine is usually well-tolerated but may case a variety of usually mild side effects. Diziness, nausea, and drowsiness are the most frequently reported side effects of tiagabine. Other possible side effects include:

• Trouble sleeping
• Fever
• Headache
• Unusual tiredness or weakness
• Tremors
• Abdominal pain
• Increased appetite
• Vomiting, diarrhea or constipation
• Heartburn or indigestion
• Aching joints and muscles or chills
• Unpleasant taste in mouth or dry mouth
• Tingling or prickly feeling on the skin

Many of these side effects disappear or occur less frequently during treatment as the body adjusts to the medication. However, if any symptoms persist or become too uncomfortable, the perscribing physician should be notified.

Certain uncommon side effects of tiagabine can be serious. Patients taking tiagabine who experience any of the following symptoms should contact their physician:

• Rash or bluish patches on the skin
• Mood or mental changes
• Shakiness or unsteady walking
• Excessive anxiety
• Dificulty with memory
• Double vision
• Numbness in a limb
• Unsteadiness or clumsiness
• Speech or language problems
• Difficulty breathing
• Chest pain

• Irregular heartbeat
• Faintness or loss of consciousness
• Persistant, severe headaches
• Persistant fever or pain

Interactions

Tiagabine may have negative interactions with some antihistimines, antidepressants, antibiotics, and monoamine oxidase inhibitors (MAOIs). Other medications such as **diazepam** (Valium), **phenobarbital** (Luminal, Solfoton), nefazodone, metronidazole, **acetazolamide** (Diamox), phenytoin (Dilantin), **primidone**, and propranolol (Inderal) may also adversely react with triagabine. Tiagabine should be used with other seizure prevention medications only if advised by a physician.

Many anticonvulsants may decrease the effectiveness of some forms of oral contraceptives (birth control pills).

Resources

BOOKS

Weaver, Donald F. *Epilepsy and Seizures: Everything You Need to Know.* Richmond Hill, ONT, Canada: Firefly Books, 2001.

OTHER

"Tiagabine." *Medline Plus.* National Library of Medicine. http://www.nlm.nih.gov/medlineplus/druginfo/uspdi/203392.html (March 20, 2004).

ORGANIZATIONS

American Epilepsy Society. 342 North Main Street, West Hartford, CT 06117-2507. http://www.aesnet.org.

Epilepsy Foundation. 4351 Garden City Drive, Landover, MD 20785-7223. Phone: (800) 332-1000. Tollfree phone: (800) 332-1000. http://www.epilepsyfoundation.org.

Adrienne Wilmoth Lerner

Tic douloureux *see* **Trigeminal neuralgia**

Tics

Definition

Tics are defined by the *Diagnostic and Statistical Manual of Mental Disorders*, fourth edition (DSM-IV), as "sudden, rapid, recurrent, nonrhythmic stereotyped motor movement[s] or vocalization[s]." The word "tic" itself is French, although its origin is unknown. These involuntary movements or noises, which occur mostly in children, can be found in a wide variety of disorders. *DSM-IV* goes on to define four tic disorders under the general heading of disorders usually first diagnosed in infancy, childhood, or adolescence: **Tourette syndrome** (TS; the most severe tic disorder), chronic motor or vocal tic disorder, transient tic disorder, and tic disorder not otherwise specified. Tic disorders are best understood as a spectrum or continuum ranging from transient simple tics at one end through chronic tic disorder to Tourette syndrome at the upper end.

New categories of tic disorder will be added to the forthcoming (2013) fifth edition of *DSM (DSM-5)*: substance-induced tic disorder and tic disorder due to a general medical condition. All tic disorders will be grouped under the subcategory of Motor Disorders, under the larger category of Neurodevelopmental Disorders.

Description

Tics are semi-voluntary repetitive (but nonrhythmic) patterns, and may be either motor tics (muscle movements) or vocal (phonic) tics. Most tics affect the neck and face primarily and may take such forms as coughing, snuffling, eye blinking, grimacing, shoulder shrugging or twitching, tongue clicking, and neck twisting. Although tics are not fully under control of the person's will, the individual with a tic disorder can often repress the tic for a period of time. Tics appear to be more likely to occur when the individual is under stress or concentrating on a task, such as reading or writing. Most tics diminish considerably or virtually disappear during sleep.

Both motor and vocal tics may be categorized as simple or complex, although the distinction between the two is not precise. Generally, a simple motor tic involves only one part of the body, such as eye blinking, finger flexing, or shoulder shrugging, while a complex tic is more involved and takes the form of some recognizable action, such as jumping up, hopping, making throwing motions with the arms, or twirling around. Complex motor tics also include imitating the actions of others and making involuntary obscene gestures. Simple vocal tics are usually just one sound or noise and may take the form of grunting, barking, or snuffling. Complex vocal tics involve recognizable words or animal sounds as opposed to simple noises. These may include the repetition of short phrases, such as "Oh, boy"; the repetition of a single word; repetition of the words of others, called echolalia; or involuntary swearing, known as coprolalia. Contrary to popular belief, only about 15% of patients diagnosed with TS have coprolalia.

Demographics

According to the American Academy of Pediatrics (AAP), tics and tic disorders affect about 20% of school-age children in North America. Tics are most common in children between the ages of seven and nine, although they have been diagnosed in children as young as two to three years. In terms of specific tic disorders, chronic motor tic disorder is thought to affect 1–2% of the population; transient tic disorder is much more common; and Tourette syndrome affects about 1% of the population. In other parts of the world doctors have reported rates for Tourette syndrome as high as 3%. It is not known as of 2011 whether different races and ethnic groups have different levels of risk for TS.

In most cases, tics disappear during adolescence, but they persist into adulthood in a few cases. There are also occasional cases of adult-onset tics, although these are usually associated with other neurological disorders.

Risk factors

As of 2011, there are three known risk factors for tics and tic disorders:

- family history of tic disorders, particularly Tourette syndrome—having a first-degree relative with TS increases a person's risk about tenfold
- sex—boys are two to five times more likely to develop Tourette syndrome than girls, and five times more likely to develop chronic motor tic disorder
- high levels of emotional stress in the family

Causes and symptoms

Causes

The causes of tics and tic disorders are not fully understood. At one time tics were thought to be symptoms of psychiatric illness, but most researchers now believe that tics result from a combination of genetic factors and differences in brain functioning. Some doctors also think that tics may simply be a byproduct of the immaturity of a child's **central nervous system** and that the ongoing maturation of the brain explains why many children simply outgrow their tics with no lasting complications.

Other researchers look for possible genetic causes for tic disorders. It is known that Tourette syndrome runs in families; however, no specific genes associated with the syndrome have been identified. Brain imaging studies suggest that children with TS have brains that are unusually sensitive to the neurotransmitter (brain chemical) dopamine and that the chemical activates parts of the brain that are responsible for the involuntary movements involved in tics. One finding that supports this theory is that medications that block the brain's uptake of dopamine are helpful in controlling tics.

Although parental criticism or nagging is not considered a direct cause of the tics, many pediatricians think that scolding to stop the tics can make them worse.

Symptoms

Tics may occur as isolated symptoms; they do not always indicate the presence of a tic disorder that meets *DSM-IV* criteria. They may also occur in patients with **autism**, developmental disorders, and stereotypic movement disorder. Persons who have had tics often report a strong premonitory (warning) urge resembling the urge to yawn or scratch an itch, and expressing the tic is experienced as a release of the tension caused by the urge. People with a tic disorder can sometimes control the premonitory urge until they can complete a task or go somewhere where expressing the tic will be less disruptive to others.

Tourette syndrome, the most severe tic disorder, often coexists with other neurological disorders such as attention-deficit/hyperactivity disorder (**ADHD**), various **sleep disorders**, and obsessive-compulsive disorder (OCD). About 40% of children diagnosed with TS have only TS; the remaining 60% have either TS plus ADHD or TS plus OCD. A few children with Tourette syndrome also suffer from disorders of impulse control, which may include aggressiveness, sexual acting-out, or rage attacks.

Diagnosis

Mild tics or tics that resolve quickly may not need any medical treatment. In other cases, the tics go away when the parents reduce pressures on the child or avoid over-scheduling the child's activities; however,

KEY TERMS

Coprolalia—The medical term for uncontrollable cursing or use of unacceptable words.

Echolalia—A vocal tic in which the person repeats the words or phrases of another person.

Gait—A person's habitual pattern of walking.

Involuntary—Not under the control of the will.

Neurotransmitters—Chemicals produced by the body that transmit nerve impulses across the gaps between nerve cells.

Premonitory urge—A feeling or sensation that warns a person with a tic disorder that tension is building up. Expressing the tic brings relief from the urge.

Tic—A sudden repetitive movement or utterance.

Transient—Brief and short-lived.

the AAP recommends that parents consult the child's doctor under the following circumstances:

- The tics are interfering with the child's schooling or friendships and are causing him or her anxiety or other emotional problems.

- The tics have lasted for more than a year.

- There are multiple tics that include tongue thrusting, chewing, sniffling, and snorting. These particular tics may indicate Tourette syndrome.

- There is a family history of tic disorders.

- The tics are becoming more intense or more frequent.

- The child is on medication for ADHD.

- Efforts to reduce emotional stress on the child have been unsuccessful.

Tics are not always visible during the child's first visit to the doctor's office. To improve diagnostic accuracy, the doctor may schedule a follow-up visit, obtain information about the tic from several sources (teachers as well as parents), or ask the parents to make a home video of the tics. The physical examination will include careful examination of the eyes (including eye movement), gait, postural stability, muscle tone, and any abnormal movements.

The diagnosis of a tic or tic disorder is clinical, meaning that it is based on the doctor's observation and judgment rather than test results. There are no laboratory or imaging tests as of 2011 that can be used to diagnose tic disorders, although the patient's doctor may order an electroencephalogram (EEG) or a blood test to rule out seizure disorders or thyroid problems. In some cases the doctor may also order a magnetic resonance image (MRI) or computed tomography (CT) scan to rule out **brain tumors** or head injuries. The health care professional will distinguish a tic disorder from other categories of involuntary movements, such as those that are related to other problems: medical conditions like epilepsy, alcohol or drug abuse; side effects of medication; or other behavioral, neurological, or psychological disorders. When a tic disorder has been diagnosed, further definition of the nature and scope of the tic will be made. Such factors as age at onset and duration of the tic will be taken into account according to the criteria listed in *DSM-IV*.

Transient tic disorder

As the name implies, transient tic disorder is characterized by motor or vocal tics that are not permanent and appear before age 18. The tic occurs many times a day for at least four weeks but dissipates after no more than 12 consecutive months. Persons with transient tic disorder experience impairment in social and school settings. When the tic lasts longer than 12 months, the diagnosis may be changed to Tourette syndrome or chronic motor or tic disorder.

Chronic motor or tic disorder

Chronic motor or vocal tic disorder features tics that persist for more than 12 consecutive months. The factor that distinguishes this disorder from Tourette is that only one type of tic—motor or vocal, but not both—is present. The other factors for diagnosis are the same. These include tics that first appear before age 18, occur many times a day, and persist for longer than one year. (Periods of up to three months with no tic occurrences do not rule out tic disorders). The person with chronic tic disorder is adversely affected in his or her ability to function in social or school settings because of the tic, although the impairment is usually less than for Tourette syndrome.

Tourette syndrome

Tourette syndrome, the most severe tic disorder, is named for Georges Gilles de la Tourette (1857–1904), a French neurologist who first described what he termed "une maladie des tics" in a study of nine patients published in 1884. The syndrome was later named for him. The diagnostic criteria used by the American Psychiatric Association for TS specify that the patient must:

- have several motor tics and at least one vocal tic for a period of a year, with no more than three consecutive months without a tic
- have been under 18 years of age when the tics started
- not be abusing alcohol or drugs or have any other disease or disorder that could be causing the tics

Treatment

Mild tics usually do not need any treatment. Although there are medications that can be prescribed to control severe tics, most doctors prefer to wait for a few months rather than prescribe medications right away. One reason is that the drugs given to control tics, including dopamine blockers such as fluphenazine (Prolixin), haloperidol (Haldol), pimozide (Orap), and risperidone (Risperdal), have side effects, particularly weight gain, drowsiness, and difficulty concentrating in school. Another reason for caution is that many children with tic disorders have periods when the tics are less severe.

A treatment that is sometimes recommended for children with simple vocal tics is botulinum Type A (Botox) injections. The Botox is injected into the vocal cords, temporarily paralyzing them and removing the urge to make the noise or sound.

In the case of Tourette syndrome, many doctors recommend psychotherapy for children with TS to help them cope with the social embarrassment and difficulties with schoolwork that they may be facing. Although TS does not cause **depression** or learning problems by itself, children may become depressed because of rejection by classmates due to the tics, or they may have trouble learning their lessons in school because their attention is focused on controlling the tics.

More recent forms of psychotherapy that show promise in treating tic disorders are awareness training and competing response training (sometimes called habit reversal training or HRT). In competing response training, children are asked to make some other kind of movement when they feel the urge to express the tic. Relaxation training is another behavioral strategy that has been shown to be helpful in treating patients with tic disorders.

A newer form of treatment for TS is **deep brain stimulation** (DBS). In DBS, a battery-operated device is implanted in the brain to deliver carefully targeted electrical stimulation to the parts of the brain that control movement. This procedure is recommended only for patients with extremely severe symptoms and should be done only in a specialized surgery center familiar with the procedure. In addition to clinical trials of DBS, other researchers are using functional magnetic resonance imaging (fMRI) and other advanced imaging techniques to study the parts of the brain involved in tics.

QUESTIONS TO ASK YOUR DOCTOR

- Is my child's tic serious enough to require further evaluation?
- What type of tic disorder does my child have?
- Will it go away by itself?
- If it does not, what treatment will you recommend?
- Will my child need imaging studies?
- What is your opinion of drug therapy for tic disorders?
- What is the prognosis?

Clinical trials

As of mid-2011 there were 98 clinical trials under way related to tics and tic disorders. Some are studies of medications for Tourette syndrome, including aripiprazole (Abilify), an atypical antipsychotic drug; **levetiracetam** (Keppra), a drug developed to treat epilepsy; and riluzole (Rilutek), a drug developed to prolong the survival of patients with Lou Gehrig's disease. Other studies are investigating the effectiveness of transcranial magnetic stimulation, habit reversal training, and other psychotherapies as treatments for tics. A few studies are looking into such dietary modifications as omega-3 fatty acids and the Atkins diet as treatments for tics. Information about current relevant clinical trials can be found at ClinicalTrials.gov.

Prognosis

As noted above, many mild tics in schoolchildren do not require detailed evaluation or formal medical treatment, and go away by themselves. Less than 1% of children develop long-lasting tics. Transient tic disorder, tic disorder not otherwise specified, and motor or vocal tic disorder usually resolve without complications, although if transient tic disorder lasts longer than a year, the diagnosis may be changed to Tourette syndrome.

Tourette syndrome is not usually a disabling condition although it can cause social embarrassment for affected children and teenagers. TS is often most severe in a patient's early teens, with symptoms improving in the later teens and improvement continuing into adult life. About one-third of adults find that their tics eventually go away; however, about 10% do not experience significant improvement in their 30s or even in their 40s.

People with Tourette syndrome have a normal life expectancy. The disorder does not affect individuals' basic intelligence or prevent them from completing their education once they are diagnosed; in fact, many people with Tourette syndrome have above-average intelligence. The chief problem confronting people with TS in adult life is an increased risk of depression, mood swings, and panic attacks compared to the general population.

Prevention

There is no way to prevent tics and tic disorders as of 2011 because their causes are not fully understood.

Resources

BOOKS

American Psychiatric Association. *Diagnostic and Statistical Manual of Mental Disorders.* 4th ed., text rev. Washington, DC: Author, 2000.

Buffolano, Sandra. *Coping with Tourette Syndrome: A Workbook for Kids with Tic Disorders.* Oakland, CA: Instant Help, 2008.

Shimberg, Elaine Fantle. *Tourette Syndrome: What Families Should Know.* Yarmouth, ME: Abernathy House, 2008.

Singer, Harvey S., et al. *Movement Disorders in Childhood.* Philadelphia: Saunders/Elsevier, 2010.

Woods, Douglas W., John C. Piacentini, and John T. Walkup, eds. *Treating Tourette Syndrome and Tic Disorders: A Guide for Practitioners.* New York: Guilford, 2007.

PERIODICALS

Bate, K.S., et al. "The Efficacy of Habit Reversal Therapy for Tics, Habit Disorders, and Stuttering: A Meta-analytic Review." *Clinical Psychology Review* 31 (July 2011): 865–71.

Bestha, D.P., et al. "Management of Tics and Tourette's Disorder: An Update." *Expert Opinion on Pharmacotherapy* 11 (August 2010): 1813–22.

Chadehumbe, M.A., et al. "Psychopharmacology of Tic Disorders in Children and Adolescents." *Pediatric Clinics of North America* 58 (February 2011): 259–72.

Debes, N.M., et al. "A Functional Magnetic Resonance Imaging Study of a Large Clinical Cohort of Children with Tourette Syndrome." *Journal of Child Neurology* 26 (May 2011): 560–69.

Franklin, S.A., et al. "Behavioral Interventions for Tic Disorders." *Psychiatric Clinics of North America* 33 (September 2010): 641–55.

Jankovic, J., and R. Kurlan. "Tourette Syndrome: Evolving Concepts." *Movement Disorders* 26 (May 2011): 1149–56.

Kurlan, R. "Clinical Practice: Tourette's Syndrome." *New England Journal of Medicine* 363 (December 9, 2010): 2332–38.

Lewis, K., et al. "Aripiprazole for the Treatment of Adolescent Tourette's Syndrome: A Case Report." *Journal of Pharmacy Practice* 23 (June 2010): 239–44.

Lim, E.C., and R.C. Seet. "Use of Botulinum Toxin in the Neurology Clinic." *Nature Reviews. Neurology* 6 (November 2010): 624–36.

Piacentini, J., et al. "Behavior Therapy for Children with Tourette Disorder: A Randomized Controlled Trial." *Journal of the American Medical Association* 303 (May 19, 2010): 1929–37.

Walkup, J.T., et al. "Tic Disorders: Some Key Issues for DSM-5." *Depression and Anxiety* 37 (June 2010): 600–10.

WEBSITES

"Facts for Families: Tic Disorders." American Academy of Child and Adolescent Psychiatry (AACAP). http://www. aacap.org/cs/root/facts_for_families/tic_disorders (accessed July 25, 2011).

"Health Issues: Tics, Tourette Syndrome, and OCD." Healthy Children. http://www.healthychildren.org/ English/health-issues/conditions/emotional-problems/ pages/Tics-Tourette-Syndrome-and-OCD.aspx (accessed July 25, 2011).

"Living with TS: Adult Issues." Tourette Syndrome Association (TSA). http://tsa-usa.org/People/LivingWithTS/ LivingTS.htm (accessed July 25, 2011).

"Neurodevelopmental Disorders." American Psychiatric Association. DSM-5 Development. http://www.dsm5. org/proposedrevision/pages/neurodevelopmentaldisor ders.aspx (accessed July 25, 2011).

"NINDS Tourette Syndrome Information Page." National Institute of Neurological Disorders and Stroke (NINDS). http://www.ninds.nih.gov/disorders/tourette/tourette.htm (accessed July 25, 2011).

Robertson Jr., William C. "Tourette Syndrome and Other Tic Disorders." Medscape Reference. http://emedicine. medscape.com/article/1182258-overview (accessed July 25, 2011).

"TIC Disorders in Children and Adolescents." Merck Manual Online. http://www.merckmanuals.com/professional/ sec20/ch318/ch318c.html (accessed July 25, 2011).

"Tourette Syndrome." Mayo Clinic. http://www.mayoclinic. com/health/tourette-syndrome/DS00541 (accessed July 25, 2011).

ORGANIZATIONS

American Academy of Child and Adolescent Psychiatry (AACAP), 3615 Wisconsin Avenue, NW, Washington, DC 20016-3007, (202) 966-7300, Fax: (202) 966-2891, http://www.aacap.org.

American Academy of Pediatrics (AAP), 141 Northwest Point Boulevard, Elk Grove Village, IL 60007-1098, (847) 434-4000, Fax: (847) 434-8000, http://www. aap.org.

National Institute of Neurological Disorders and Stroke (NINDS), P.O. Box 5801, Bethesda, MD 20824, (301) 496-5751, (800) 352-9424, http://www.ninds.nih.gov.

Tourette Syndrome Association (TSA), 42–40 Bell Boulevard, Suite 205, Bayside, NY 11361-2820, (718) 224-2999, Fax: (718) 279-9596, http://www. tsa-usa.org.

Rebecca J. Frey, PhD

Tinnitus

Definition

Tinnitus is noise—such as ringing, buzzing, whistling, roaring, clicking, chirping, or hissing—in one or both ears or the head.

Description

Tinnitus is a symptom of another condition, most often age-related **hearing loss**, called presbycusis; however, it can be a symptom of a problem in any part of the auditory system—the ear, the eighth or auditory cranial nerve that conducts signals from the inner ear to the brain, or the auditory cortex in the brain that processes and interprets sound.

The inner ear has thousands of hair cells that are moved by sound vibrations. These movements generate electrical signals within the cells that are carried to the brain. Bent or broken hairs or other cell damage may cause random auditory signals to be sent to the brain. Research suggests that tinnitus is most often caused by changes in the auditory cortex itself. Damage to hair cells may cause neural circuits in the auditory cortex to become increasingly sensitive to sound or changes to neural circuits may cause neurons to fire inappropriately, creating the illusion of sound. This may be similar to chronic pain syndrome, in which pain persists even after an injury has healed. Tinnitus can also affect the limbic system—the emotional center of the brain.

Most people experience occasional mild tinnitus. Transient tinnitus is often a brief tone heard in the quiet just before sleep or lasting an hour or so after attending a loud concert. If tinnitus is constant and intrusive, it can interfere with hearing, concentration, memory, or sleep. For some people, tinnitus is debilitating, causing **fatigue**, **depression**, or anxiety, and significantly interfering with the quality of life.

Tinnitus is usually subjective—meaning that no one else can hear the noise. Rarely, tinnitus is objective. A physician may be able to hear pulsatile tinnitus— sounds of blood pulsing or muscle spasms in the patient's ear.

Risks

Age-related hearing loss and exposure to loud noise are the most common causes of tinnitus in a world that is becoming an increasingly noisy. In addition to concerts and sports events, many people experience extreme noise on a daily basis at work. Firefighters and other emergency personnel, factory and construction workers, road crews, and musicians are among those at risk for tinnitus from noise-induced hearing loss. Firearm use, especially pistols and shotguns, can also cause tinnitus. Shock waves from explosions can damage the auditory cortex and tinnitus is one of the most common service-related disabilities in military personnel who served in Iraq and Afghanistan. People with post-traumatic stress disorder (PTSD) are susceptible to tinnitus, and it appears to be especially aggravated by loud noises in PTSD sufferers. In preteens and teenagers, tinnitus is usually associated with listening to personal music players and video games through ear buds. Some researchers believe that cell phone use may contribute to tinnitus.

Demographics

It is estimated that about one in five people have tinnitus, including up to 50 million Americans. As many as 12 million Americans have persistent tinnitus. An estimated 250 million people worldwide have a reduced quality of life because of tinnitus.

The incidence of tinnitus increases with age. It is particularly common in Caucasian men over age 65. Although it is relatively rare in children under 18, it may be underreported, especially in young children who are unable to communicate their symptoms. In children with certain types of congenital hearing loss, tinnitus may be so constant that they learn to ignore it.

Causes

The most common causes of tinnitus are:

- age-related hearing loss, which usually begins about age 60, worsens with increasing years, and is usually associated with damage to or loss of hair cells in the ears
- long-term exposure to loud noises, such as heavy equipment, chainsaws, firearms, and portable music players
- accumulation of hardened earwax that cannot be washed away, which irritates the eardrum and can cause hearing loss

More than 200 different medications can cause or worsen tinnitus in a dose-dependent manner. Some medications are ototoxic—directly toxic to the ear. Others have tinnitus as a side effect. Some medications cause tinnitus after they are discontinued. Medications that can cause tinnitus include:

- antibiotics
- diuretics (water pills)
- cancer drugs
- quinine and chloroquine for malaria
- aspirin at very high doses—12 or more daily

Less common causes of tinnitus include:

- middle ear or sinus infections
- foreign object in the ear
- ruptured eardrum
- loose hair in the ear canal that contacts the eardrum
- stiffening of the bones in the middle or inner ear, called otosclerosis
- Ménière's disease, an inner ear disorder that includes hearing loss and dizziness
- temporomandibular joint (TMJ) disorders, affecting the joint where the lower jawbone connects with the skull
- jaw misalignment
- head or neck injuries or conditions that affect the inner ear, auditory nerve, or auditory cortex
- acoustic neuroma or vestibular schwannoma—a noncancerous tumor on the auditory or nearby nerve
- meningiomas—noncancerous tumors in the tissue that protects the brain
- a brain tumor or aneurysm
- chronic brain syndromes
- thyroid problems
- allergies
- low blood pressure
- anemia
- hormonal changes in women
- various chronic health conditions

Objective or pulsatile tinnitus is caused by abnormalities in blood vessels or an inner ear bone condition. It also can be caused by muscle spasms in the tiny muscles attached to the middle ear bones, which can sound like intermittent clicks or crackling in the middle ear. Blood vessel disorders associated with tinnitus include:

- atherosclerosis, which can cause blood vessels near the middle and inner ear to lose elasticity
- high blood pressure or factors such as stress, alcohol, or caffeine that increase blood pressure and make tinnitus more noticeable
- turbulent blood flow due to a narrowing or kinking in the carotid artery or jugular vein of the neck
- head or neck tumors that press on blood vessels
- a vascular tumor near the middle or inner ear
- capillary malformations in the connections between arteries and veins, called arteriovenous malformations (AVMs)

Symptoms

The noise from tinnitus may be soft or loud, varying in pitch from a low roar to a high squeal. It is often loudest upon first awakening. Tinnitus is sometimes described as blowing, humming, or sizzling. It may sound like air escaping, water running, or musical notes. Although one study found that the sound is just barely above the hearing threshold, if it is high-pitched, it can seem much louder. Tinnitus may be constant or intermittent and may be unchanging or change in pitch over the course of the day.

Sometimes tinnitus is the first symptom of hearing loss from age or noise exposure. It is often associated with stress, fatigue, and depression, and these conditions appear to aggravate it.

Diagnosis

Tinnitus may be diagnosed by a primary-care physician, an audiologist, or an otolaryngologist—an ear, nose, throat (ENT) specialist. If possible, the underlying cause of the tinnitus is determined, sometimes by the type of noise:

- A temporary high-pitched ringing or buzzing can be caused by very loud noise or a blow to the ear.
- Continuous high-pitched ringing in both ears may indicate age-related hearing loss, long-term noise exposure, or medication effects.
- Continuous high-pitched ringing in one ear may suggest an acoustic neuroma.
- Low-pitched ringing in one ear may suggest Ménière's disease.
- Pulsatile tinnitus, or amplified heartbeat, may be due to high blood pressure, a tumor, or an aneurysm.
- Clicking that lasts a few seconds to minutes may be due to muscle contractions around the ear.

Diagnostic tests may include:

- a hearing exam—audiology or audiometry—to test for hearing loss in each ear
- effects on tinnitus of moving the eyes, jaw, neck, arms, and legs
- balance tests
- listening with a stethoscope against the neck or a tiny microphone in the ear canal for objective tinnitus
- imaging tests of the head, such as x rays, computed tomography (CT) scans, or magnetic resonance imaging (MRI)
- angiography—blood vessel studies

Treatment

Tinnitus treatment is sometimes a simple as removing accumulated earwax or discontinuing a medication. When tinnitus accompanies severe hearing loss, hearing aids or cochlear implants can enable outside sounds to drown out it out, especially if the tinnitus and hearing loss are in the same frequency range. Cochlear implants bypass the damaged portion of the inner ear, sending sound directly to the auditory nerve. Since they destroy remaining healthy hair cells, cochlear implants are only used in cases of deafness or near-deafness.

Counseling or support groups can help patients cope with tinnitus and associated problems. Cognitive-behavioral therapy, especially when coupled with other treatments, can help patients cope with emotional reactions to tinnitus.

Medications that are sometimes used for severe tinnitus include:

- tricyclic antidepressants, such as amitriptyline or nortriptyline
- antianxiety drugs, such as alprazolam
- vasodilators
- anticonvulsants
- antihistamines
- anesthetics, such as lidocaine
- drugs to treat irregular heart rhythms

Sound therapies

Masking or tinnitus retraining therapy (TRT) can reduce the contrast between the internal noise and the external world.

- Tinnitus masking devices or wearable sound generators are small electronics that are worn in the ear. They produce soft, continuous, pleasant sounds, random tones, or music, usually at a volume just above that of the tinnitus. Some hearing aids have build-in tinnitus maskers.
- TRT combines a masking device playing programmed tonal music at the tinnitus frequency with counseling to retrain the mind to ignore the tinnitus.
- White noise machines, bedside maskers, or tabletop sound generators, sometimes with pillow speakers, produce sounds such as falling rain or ocean waves to block tinnitus and promote relaxation and sleep.
- Acoustic neural stimulation delivers a broadband acoustic signal embedded in music and designed to change the neural circuits in the brain and desensitize the listener to tinnitus.

KEY TERMS

Atherosclerosis—Thickening and hardening of the inner layer of arteries, due to accumulation of plaque; a cause of pulsatile tinnitus.

Auditory nerve—The eighth cranial nerve that connects the inner ear to the brain.

Cochlea—The bony coiled labyrinth of the inner ear.

Otolaryngologist—An ear, nose, and throat (ENT) specialist.

Otosclerosis—A growth of spongy bone in the inner ear, causing progressive hearing loss.

Ototoxic—Damaging to the organs or nerves involved in hearing or balance.

Presbycusis—Hearing loss due to degenerative changes in the ear, usually associated with aging.

Pulsatile tinnitus—Objective tinnitus in which the pulse or heartbeat is heard in the ear.

Temporomandibular joint (TMJ) disorders—A disorder in the joint between the temporal bone above the ear and the lower jaw bone or mandible.

Tinnitus retraining therapy (TRT)—Tinnitus treatment that combines counseling with the use of a device that masks the tinnitus frequency.

Home remedies

Home remedies for tinnitus include:

- avoiding irritants, such as loud noise and nicotine
- managing stress
- reducing alcohol consumption
- stepwise elimination of other substances that can contribute to tinnitus, including sugar, salt, sweeteners, and caffeine
- sleeping with the head elevated, which can relieve congestion and make the noise less prominent
- meditation, biofeedback training, or other relaxation techniques
- using a fan, soft music, or low-level radio static to mask the noise

Alternative treatment

Alternative therapies that may help some patients include:

- acupuncture
- hypnosis
- craniosacral therapy

QUESTIONS TO ASK YOUR DOCTOR

- Is the noise in my head tinnitus?
- What could be causing my tinnitus?
- Do I have hearing loss?
- What treatments do you recommend?
- Can my tinnitus be cured?

- the herb ginkgo
- zinc or magnesium supplements
- melatonin
- B vitamins
- lipoflavonoid nutritional supplements
- homeopathic remedies
- magnets
- hyperbaric oxygen

Prognosis

Although treatment can often alleviate tinnitus, at least temporarily, there is no cure. Long-term exposure to loud noise can permanently damage hair cells, which cannot be repaired or replaced.

Prevention

The best prevention for tinnitus is to avoid ear damage from loud noise by using over-the-ear hearing protection. Various measures can prevent triggering or worsening tinnitus:

- listening to music at lower volume, especially when using headphones
- maintaining normal body weight and blood pressure with diet and exercise
- obtaining proper rest
- decreasing salt intake
- avoiding stimulants such as coffee, cola, tea, and tobacco
- learning to ignore head noise

Resources

BOOKS

Carmen, Richard. *The Consumer Handbook on Hearing Loss and Hearing Aids: A Bridge to Healing*. 3rd ed. Sedona, AZ: Auricle Ink, 2009.

Chasin, Marshall. *The Consumer Handbook on Hearing Loss and Noise*. Sedona, AZ: Auricle Ink, 2010.

Foy, George. *Zero Decibels: The Quest for Absolute Silence.* New York: Scribner, 2010.

Henry, James. *How to Manage Your Tinnitus: A Step-by-Step Workbook.* San Diego, CA: Plural, 2010.

Hogan, Kevin, and Jennifer Battaglino. *Tinnitus: Turning the Volume Down: A Decade of Specific Proven Strategies for Quieting the Noise in Your Head.* Rev. and expanded ed. Eagan, MN: Network 3000, 2010.

Jerger, James. *Audiology in the USA.* San Diego, CA: Plural, 2009.

Luxford, William M., M. Jennifer Derebery, and Karen I. Berliner. *The Complete Idiot's Guide to Hearing Loss.* New York: Alpha, 2010.

McKenna, Laurence, David Baguley, and Don J. McFerran. *Living with Tinnitus and Hyperacusis.* London: Sheldon, 2010.

PERIODICALS

Avery, Sarah. "Treatment Music to Some Sufferers' Ears." *Washington Post* (January 30, 2011): A3.

Beck, Melinda. "A Most Annoying Ringtone—Researchers Explore New Treatments to Silence the Persistent Din in the Ear." *Wall Street Journal* (December 14, 2010): D1.

De Ridder, Dirk, et al. "Phantom Percepts: Tinnitus and Pain as Persisting Aversive Memory Networks." *PNAS* 108, no. 20 (May 17, 2011): 8075–80.

Holmes, Susan, and Nigel D. Padgham. "More than Ringing in the Ears: A Review of Tinnitus and Its Psychosocial Impact." *Journal of Clinical Nursing* 18, no. 21 (November 2009): 2927–37.

"Ringing in the Brain." *Nature* 469, no. 7330 (January 20, 2011): 269.

Sweetow, Robert W., and Jennifer Henderson Sabes. "Effects of Acoustical Stimuli Delivered through Hearing Aids on Tinnitus." *Journal of the American Academy of Audiology* 21, no. 7 (July/August 2010): 461–73.

"Turn Down Tinnitus with Brain Alteration." *New Scientist* 209, no. 2795 (January 15–21, 2011): 16.

Zimmer, Carl. "The Brain." *Discover* 31, no. 8 (October 2010): 22.

WEBSITES

Shargorodsky, Josef, Gary C. Curhan, and Wildon R. Farwell. "Prevalence and Characteristics of Tinnitus among US Adults." *American Journal of Medicine* 123, no. 8 (August 2010): 711–18. http://www.amjmed.com/article/S0002-9343(10)00344-X/fulltext (accessed July 20, 2011).

"Tinnitus." American Academy of Otolaryngology—Head and Neck Surgery. http://www.entnet.org/HealthInformation/tinnitus.cfm (accessed July 20, 2011).

"Tinnitus." Mayo Clinic. July 31, 2010. http://www.mayoclinic.com/print/tinnitus/DS00365/ (accessed July 20, 2011).

"Tinnitus." MedlinePlus. http://www.nlm.nih.gov/medlineplus/tinnitus.html (accessed July 20, 2011).

"Tinnitus." National Institute on Deafness and Other Communication Disorders. http://www.nidcd.nih.gov/health/hearing/tinnitus (accessed July 20, 2011).

"Tinnitus Management." American Speech-Language-Hearing Association. http://www.asha.org/public/hearing/treatment/tinnitus_manage.htm (accessed July 20, 2011).

"Tinnitus—the Noise in Your Head That Won't Go Away." *Inside NIDCD Newsletter.* Winter 2010. http://www.nidcd.nih.gov/health/inside/wtr10/pg2.html (accessed July 20, 2011).

"Tips for Managing Tinnitus." American Tinnitus Association. http://www.ata.org/for-patients/tips (accessed July 20, 2011).

"Treatment Information." American Tinnitus Association. http://www.ata.org/for-patients/treatment (accessed July 20, 2011).

ORGANIZATIONS

American Academy of Otolaryngology—Head and Neck Surgery, 1650 Diagonal Road, Alexandria, VA 22314-2857, (703) 836-4444, http://www.entnet.org.

American Speech-Language-Hearing Association (ASHA), 2200 Research Boulevard, Rockville, MD 20850-3289, (301) 296-5700, Fax: (301) 296-8580, (800) 498-2071, actioncenter@asha.org, http://www.asha.org.

American Tinnitus Association, P.O. Box 5, Portland, OR 97207-0005, (503) 248-9985, (800) 634-8978, Fax: (503) 248-0024, tinnitus@ata.org, http://www.ata.org.

National Institute on Deafness and Other Communication Disorders (NIDCD), National Institutes of Health, 31 Center Drive, MSC 2320, Bethesda, MD 20892-2320, (301) 496-7243, (800) 241-1044, nidcdinfo@nidcd.nih. gov, http://www.nidcd.nih.gov/.

Margaret Alic, PhD

Todd's paralysis

Definition

Todd's paralysis is a brief period of paralysis that occurs in the aftermath of a seizure.

Description

The period of time directly following a seizure is called the "postictal state." During this time period, the individual's brain is still recovering from the major changes brought on by the seizure. Drowsiness and confusion are very common symptoms of the postictal state. In some cases, the symptoms are even more pronounced and dramatic and may even involve severe **weakness** or paralysis of a limb or one side of the body (hemiparesis), odd sensations such as numbness, or pronounced vision changes or blindness.

Demographics

Todd's paralysis usually strikes individuals who have epilepsy (recurrent seizures), although it may occur after any seizure.

Causes and symptoms

A seizure is an episode of abnormal electrical activity in a particular part of the brain. There are many kinds of seizures, and they may affect any specific part of the brain, or may spread to affect a wider distribution of the brain. The behavior of an individual suffering from a seizure may range from a simple, brief staring episode to complete loss of consciousness, with involuntary jerking of the muscles. The aftermath of a seizure is referred to as the postictal state. During the postictal period, although the seizure itself has ended, the brain is still recovering from the abnormal electrical discharges that precipitated the seizure activity. During this time period, the individual may be drowsy, less responsive than normal, or confused. Todd's paralysis is thought to occur due to depressed activity in the area of the brain that underwent the seizure.

The symptoms of Todd's paralysis depend on the area of the brain where the seizure took place. For example, if the seizure occurred in the motor cortex (that part of the brain responsible for purposeful movement of the muscles), Todd's paralysis may result in hemiparesis, an inability to move the muscles of one-half of the body. Because the occipital lobe (the lower back part of the brain) is responsible for vision, an occipital lobe seizure may result in visual change or outright blindness during the postictal phase. In fact, tracking the specific symptoms of Todd's paralysis may actually help the physician diagnose the specific area of the brain in which an individual's seizures are occurring.

The symptoms of Todd's paralysis are often gone within minutes or hours of their onset. In some, more rare cases, the symptoms may last as long as 48 hours. Ultimately, however, full function is restored.

Diagnosis

Diagnosis of Todd's paralysis is crucial, because the symptoms can closely resemble those of a stroke (injury to the brain due to oxygen deprivation after bleeding or a blockage of an artery). It is important to distinguish between Todd's paralysis and a stroke, because the treatments are quite different.

Generally, Todd's paralysis can be easily diagnosed when it occurs in the aftermath of a documented seizure. The quick resolution of symptoms is another clue pointing to Todd's paralysis. When the diagnosis is unclear,

KEY TERMS

Epilepsy—A condition in which an individual has recurrent seizures.

Hemiparesis—Severe weakness or paralysis affecting one side of the body.

Postictal—The time period immediately following a seizure.

Seizure—An episode of abnormal electrical activity in the brain.

however, tests may be run, including an electroencephalogram or EEG (a test that records information about the brain's electrical activity) or MRI. In the case of a seizure, the EEG may be abnormal, in the event of a stroke, the MRI may show an area of damage.

Treatment team

Todd's paralysis, like seizures and epilepsy, is usually treated by a neurologist.

Treatment

There is no specific treatment necessary for Todd's paralysis. The symptoms should fully resolve within minutes to hours or days.

Recovery and rehabilitation

Because of the quick and complete resolution of symptoms of Todd's paralysis, no rehabilitation is necessary.

Prognosis

The prognosis of Todd's paralysis is excellent, with full recovery to be anticipated.

Resources

BOOKS

Pedley, Timothy A. "The Epilepsies." In *Cecil Textbook of Internal Medicine,* edited by Lee Goldman, et al. Philadelphia: W.B. Saunders, 2000.

Pollack, Charles V., and Emily S. Pollack. "Seizures." In *Rosen's Emergency Medicine: Concepts and Clinical Practice,* 5th ed., edited by Lee Goldman, et al. St. Louis: Mosby, 2002.

PERIODICALS

Binder, D.K. "A history of Todd and his paralysis." *Neurosurgery* 54(2) (February 2004): 486–87.

Iriarte, J. "Ictal paralysis mimicking Todd's phenomenon" *Neurology* 59(3) August 2002): 464–65.

Kellinghaus, Christopher, and Prakash Kotagal. "Lateralizing value of Todd's palsy in patients with epilepsy." *Neurology* 62(2) (27 January 2004): 289–91.

Urrestarazu, E. "Postictal paralysis during video-EEG monitoring studies." *Review of Neurology* 35(5) (1 September 2002): 486–87.

WEBSITES

National Institute of Neurological Disorders and Stroke (NINDS). *Todd's Paralysis Fact Sheet*. Bethesda, MD: NINDS, 2003.

Rosalyn Carson-DeWitt, MD

Topiramate

Definition

Topiramate is an anticonvulsant indicated for the control seizures in the treatment of epilepsy (a neurological dysfunction in which excessive surges of electrical energy are emitted in the brain) and **Lennox-Gastaut syndrome** (a disorder which causes seizures and developmental delays).

Topiramate is also used for **migraine headache** prevention. In psychiatry, topiramate may be used in the treatment of bipolar **affective disorders**.

Purpose

Topiramate is thought to decrease and balance the abnormal electrical activity within the brain that may trigger seizures. While topiramate controls some types of seizures associated with epilepsy, there is no known cure for the disorder.

In patients with bipolar disorders, topiramate stabilizes mood without producing a euphoric feeling or inducing manic episodes.

Description

In the United States, topiramate is sold under the brand name Topamax.

Topiramate is most commonly prescribed to treat patients who do not respond to other anticonvulsant medications, or it is part of a combination of anticonvulsant medications used to treat intractable seizures. Although the precise mechanisms by which it exerts its therapeutic effects in epilepsy and other seizure disorders are unknown, topiramate has three specific seizure-reducing actions:

- decreases nerve cell excitation by blocking targeted neurotransmitters from binding to certain receptors in the brain
- blocks sodium channels in nerve cells, thus decreasing excessive nerve cell firing
- increases the availability of GABA, (gamma-aminobutyric acid), a neurotransmitter that inhibits nerve cell excitation in the brain

Recommended dosage

Topiramate is taken by mouth in tablet or sprinkle form. Topiramate is available in strengths of 25 mg, 100 mg, and 200 mg tablets, along with 15 mg and 25 mg sprinkle capsules. Patients usually take topiramate twice daily. Typical total daily doses are 200–400 mg for treatment of seizure disorders. For the treatment of bipolar disorders or migraine headache prevention, dosages vary.

Beginning a course of treatment which includes topiramate requires a gradual dose increasing regimen. The prescribing physician determines the proper beginning dosage and may raise a patient's daily dosage gradually over the course of several weeks. It may take several weeks to realize the full seizure-reducing benefits of topiramate.

A double dose of topiramate should not be taken to make up for a missed or forgotten dose. If a daily dose is missed, it should be taken as soon as possible, but if it is almost time for the next dose, the missed dose is skipped. When discontinuing treatment with topiramate, physicians typically direct patients to gradually taper their daily dosages. Stopping the medicine suddenly may cause seizures to return or occur more frequently.

In the treatment of bipolar disorders, persons should not stop taking topiramate without consulting the prescribing physician. Stopping the medicine suddenly may cause seizures, or severely and suddenly alter a patient's mood.

Precautions

Topiramate is not habit-forming. A physician should be consulted before combining topiramate with certain nonprescription medications. Patients should avoid alcohol and CNS depressants (medicines that can make one drowsy or less alert, such as antihistamines, sleep medications, and some pain medications) while taking topiramate. Because topiramate may cause drowsiness, persons should not drive or operate heavy machinery until they know how they will react to the drug.

Persons taking topiramate, particularly those with predisposing factors, should maintain an adequate fluid intake in order to minimize the risk of kidney stone formation. Approximately 1.5% of people taking topiramate develop kidney stones.

Topiramate may not be suitable for persons with a history of liver or kidney disease, mental illness, high blood pressure, angina (chest pain), irregular heartbeats, or other heart problems. Before beginning treatment with topiramate, patients should notify their physician if they consume a large amount of alcohol, have a history of drug use, are pregnant, or planning on becoming pregnant.

Topiramate may inhibit perspiration, causing body temperature to increase. Persons taking topiramate are at a greater risk for heat stroke and should use caution during strenuous exercise, prolonged exposure during hot weather, and while using saunas or hot tubs.

Topiramate may cause osteoporosis in adults and rickets in children. It may also slow the growth of children.

Topiramate may cause birth defects. Patients need to use effective birth control while taking topiramate. Patients who become pregnant while taking topiramate should contact their physician immediately.

Side effects

Patients and their physicians should weigh the risks and benefits of topiramate before beginning treatment. Topiramate is usually well tolerated but may cause a variety of usually mild side effects. **Dizziness** and drowsiness are the most frequently reported side effects of topiramate. Other possible side effects include:

- double vision
- tingling or prickly feeling of the extremities
- language problems, described as "trouble finding the right word"
- thinking and memory problems
- weight loss
- loss of appetite and nervousness (in children)

Many of these side effects disappear or occur less frequently during treatment as the body adjusts to the medication; however, if any symptoms persist or become too uncomfortable, the prescribing physician should be consulted.

Other, uncommon side effects of topiramate can lead to serious complications. A person taking topiramate who experiences any of the following symptoms should immediately contact their physician:

- blurred vision and eye pain
- glaucoma
- extreme mood or mental changes
- shakiness or unsteady walking
- kidney stones
- difficulty breathing
- chest pain
- irregular heartbeat
- faintness or loss of consciousness

Interactions

Topiramate may have negative interactions with some antihistimines, antidepressants, antibiotics, and monoamine oxidase inhibitors (MAOIs). Other medications such as **diazepam** (Valium), **phenobarbital** (Luminal, Solfoton), nefazodone, metronidazole, **acetazolamide** (Diamox), lanoxin (Digoxin, Digitek), phenytoin (Dilantin), **primidone**, and propranolol (Inderal) may also need to be adjusted and closely monitored if taken with topiramate. Topiramate, like many other anticonvulsant medications, may decrease the effectiveness of oral contraceptives (birth control pills).

Resources

BOOKS

Aminoff, Michael J., ed. *Neurology and General Medicine.* 4th ed. New York: Churchill Livingstone, 2007.

Devinsky, Orrin. *Epilepsy: Patient and Family Guide.* 3rd ed. New York: Demos Medical, 2007.

Diamond, Seymour, and Merle Lea Diamond. *A Patient's Guide to Headache and Migraine.* 2nd ed. Newtown, PA: Handbooks in Health Care, 2009.

George, Paulette. *Good Morning Beautiful: Winning the Battle Over Seizures.* Greenville, SC: Ambassador International, 2010.

Mauskop, Alex. *Migraine and Headache.* New York: Oxford University Press, 2009.

Panayiotopoulos, C.P. *Antiepileptic Drugs, Pharmacopoeia.* New York: Springer, 2010.

Patsalos, Philip N., and Blaise F.D. Bourgeois. *The Epilepsy Prescriber's Guide to Antiepileptic Drugs.* New York: Cambridge University Press, 2010.

Shorvon, Simon. *Handbook of Epilepsy Treatment.* 3rd ed. New York: Wiley-Blackwell, 2010.

Tatum, William O., Peter W. Kaplan, and Pierre Jallon. *Epilepsy A to Z: A Concise Encyclopedia.* 2nd ed. New York: Demos Medical, 2009.

Wootton, Tom, et al. *Bipolar In Order: Looking At Depression, Mania, Hallucination, and Delusion from the Other Side.* Tiburon, CA: Bipolar Advantage, 2010.

WEBSITES

"Seizure Medicines." Epilepsy.com. http://www.epilepsy.com/EPILEPSY/SEIZURE_MEDICINES (accessed July 20, 2011).

"Topiramate." MedlinePlus. http://www.nlm.nih.gov/medlineplus/druginfo/medmaster/a697012.html (accessed July 20, 2011).

ORGANIZATIONS

American Academy of Neurology (AAN), 1080 Montreal Avenue, Saint Paul, MN 55116, (651) 695-2717, (800) 879-1960, Fax: (651) 695-2791, memberservices@aan.com, http://www.aan.com.

American Epilepsy Society, 342 North Main Street, West Hartford, CT 06117-2507, (860) 586-7505, http://www.aesnet.org.

American Neurological Association, 5841 Cedar Lake Road, Suite 204, Minneapolis, MN 55416, (952) 545-6284, http://www.aneuroa.org.

American Psychiatric Association (APA), 1000 Wilson Boulevard, Suite 1825, Arlington, VA 22209-3901, (703) 907-7300, (888) 35-PSYCH, apa@psych.org, http://www.psych.org/.

Epilepsy Foundation, 8301 Professional Place, Landover, MD 20785-7223, (800) 332-1000, http://www.epilepsyfoundation.org.

Family Caregiver Alliance, 180 Montgomery Street, Suite 900, San Francisco, CA 94104, (415) 434-3388, (800) 445-8106, http://www.caregiver.org.

National Institute of Neurological Disorders and Stroke (NINDS), P.O. Box 5801, Bethesda, MD 20824, (301) 496-5751, (800) 352-9424, http://www.ninds.nih.gov.

National Institutes of Health (NIH), 9000 Rockville Pike, Bethesda, MD 20892, (301) 496-4000, NIHinfo@od.nih.gov, http://www.nih.gov/index.html.

U.S. Food and Drug Administration, 10903 New Hampshire Avenue, Silver Spring, MD 20993-0002, (888) 463-6332, http://www.fda.gov.

U.S. National Library of Medicine, 8600 Rockville Pike, Bethesda, MD 20894, (301) 594-5983, (888) 346-3656, Fax: (301) 402-1384, custserv@nlm.nih.gov, http://www.nlm.nih.gov.

Adrienne Wilmoth Lerner
Laura Jean Cataldo, RN, EdD

Tourette syndrome

Definition

Tourette syndrome (TS) is an inherited disorder of the nervous system that typically appears in childhood. The main features of TS are repeated movements and vocalizations called **tics**. TS can also be associated with behavioral and developmental problems.

Demographics

Tourette syndrome is a relatively common disorder found in all populations and all ethnic groups. TS is three to four times more common in males than females. The exact incidence of Tourette syndrome is unknown, but it is estimated to affect one to ten in 1,000 children. According to the National Institute for Neurological Disorders and Stroke (NINDS), an estimated 200,000 Americans have the most severe form

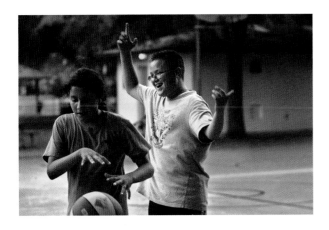

A pair of teenagers play basketball; the one on the right has Tourette syndrome. *(© s70/Zuma Press/newscom)*

of TS, and as many as one in 100 have milder symptoms such as chronic motor or vocal tics. Early TS symptoms are almost always noticed first in childhood, with the average onset between the ages of seven and ten years.

Description

Tourette syndrome is a variable disorder with onset in childhood. Though symptoms can appear anywhere between the ages of two and 18, typical onset is around age six or seven. Tics, which may be motor or vocal, tend to wax and wane (increase and decrease) in severity over time. The first references in the literature to what might today be classified as TS largely describe individuals who were wrongly believed to be possessed by the devil. In 1885, Gilles de la Tourette, a French neurologist, provided the first formal description of this syndrome, which he described as an inherited neurological condition characterized by motor and vocal tics.

Although vocal and motor tics are the hallmark of Tourette syndrome, other symptoms such as the expression of socially inappropriate comments or behaviors, obsessive compulsive disorder, attention-deficit disorder, self injuring behavior, **depression**, and anxiety also appear to be associated with Tourette syndrome. Symptoms usually intensify during teenage years and diminish in late adolescence or early adulthood. Patients may also develop co-occurring behavioral disorders, namely obsessive-compulsive disorder (OCD), attention-deficit/hyperactivity disorder (**ADHD**) or attention-deficit disorder (ADD), poor impulse control, and/or **sleep disorders**. Though some children have learning disabilities, intelligence is not impaired. TS is not degenerative and life span is normal.

Risk factors

As of 2011, TS risk factors are unknown, and researchers are studying risk factors before and after birth that may contribute to this complex disorder. Some of the suggested factors include severe psychological trauma, recurrent daily stresses, extreme emotional excitement, **PANDAS** (pediatric autoimmune neuropsychiatric disorder with streptococcal infection), and drug abuse.

Causes and symptoms

A variety of genetic and environmental factors likely play a role in causing TS. Studies suggest that the tics in Tourette syndrome are caused by an increased amount of a neurotransmitter called dopamine. A neurotransmitter is a chemical found in the brain that helps to transmit information from one brain cell to another. Other studies suggest that the defect in Tourette syndrome involves another neurotransmitter called serotonin or involves other chemicals required for normal functioning of the brain.

Genetic factors are believed to play a major role in the development of TS. Several chromosomal regions have been identified as possible locations of genes that confer susceptibility to TS. Some family studies have indicated that TS may be inherited in an autosomal dominant manner, but other studies have shown that this is not the case. Mutations involving the SLITRK1 gene have been identified in a small number of TS patients. This gene provides instructions for making a brain protein called SLITRK1. This protein probably plays a role in the development of nerve cells, including the growth of axons and dendrites that allow each nerve cell to communicate with nearby cells. It is unclear how mutations in the SLITRK1 gene can lead to this disorder. The inheritance pattern of Tourette syndrome remains unknown. Although the features of TS can cluster in families, many genetic and environmental factors are likely to be involved. Some researchers believe that Tourette syndrome has different causes in different individuals or is caused by changes in more than one gene. Further research is needed to establish the cause of Tourette syndrome.

Motor and vocal tics

The principal symptoms of Tourette syndrome include simple and complex motor and vocal tics. Simple motor tics are characterized by brief muscle contractions of one or more limited muscle groups. An eye twitch is an example of a simple motor tic. Complex motor tics tend to appear more complicated and purposeful than simple tics and involve coordinated contractions of several muscle groups. Some examples of complex motor tics include the act of hitting oneself and jumping. Copropraxia, the involuntary display of unacceptable/obscene gestures, and echopraxia, the imitation of the movement of another individual, are other examples of complex motor tics.

Vocal tics are actually manifestations of motor tics that involve the muscles required for vocalization. Simple vocal tics include **stuttering**, stammering, abnormal emphasis of part of a word or phrase, and inarticulate noises such as throat clearing, grunts, and high-pitched sounds. Complex vocal tics typically involve the involuntary expression of words. Perhaps the most striking example of this is coprolalia, the involuntary expression of obscene words or phrases, which occurs in fewer than one-third of people with Tourette syndrome. The involuntary echoing of the last word, phrase, sentence or sound vocalized by oneself (phalilalia) or of another person or sound in the environment (echolalia) are also classified as complex tics.

The type, frequency, and severity of tics exhibited varies tremendously between individuals with Tourette syndrome. Tourette syndrome has a variable age of onset and tics can start anytime between infancy and age 18. Initial symptoms usually occur before the early teens and the mean age of onset for both males and females is approximately seven years of age. Most individuals with symptoms initially experience simple muscle tics involving the eyes and the head. These symptoms can progress to tics involving the upper torso, neck, arms, hands, and occasionally the legs and feet. Complex motor tics are usually the latest onset muscle tics. Vocal tics usually have a later onset then motor tics. In some rare cases, people with Tourette syndrome suddenly present with multiple, severe, or bizarre symptoms.

Not only is there extreme variability in clinical symptoms between individuals with Tourette syndrome, but individuals commonly experience a variability in type, frequency, and severity of symptoms within the course of their lifetime. Adolescents with Tourette syndrome often experience unpredictable and variable symptoms, which may be related to fluctuating hormone levels and decreased compliance in taking medications. Adults often experience a decrease in symptoms or a complete end to symptoms.

A number of factors appear to affect the severity and frequency of tics. Stress appears to increase the frequency and severity of tics while concentration on another part of the body that is not taking part in a tic can result in the temporary alleviation of symptoms. Relaxation, following attempts to suppress the occurrence of tics, may result in an increased frequency of tics. An increased frequency and severity of tics can also result from exposure to drugs such as steroids, cocaine, amphetamines, and caffeine. Hormonal changes such as those that occur prior to the menstrual cycle can also increase the severity of symptoms.

Other associated symptoms

People with Tourette syndrome are more likely to exhibit non-obscene, socially inappropriate behaviors such as expressing insulting or socially unacceptable comments or socially unacceptable actions. It is not known whether these symptoms stem from a more general dysfunction of impulse control that might be part of Tourette syndrome.

Tourette syndrome appears to also be associated with ADD. ADD is a disorder characterized by a short attention span and impulsivity; in some cases, it also includes hyperactivity (ADHD). Researchers have found that 21–90% of individuals with Tourette syndrome also exhibit symptoms of ADD, whereas 2–15% of the general population exhibit symptoms of ADD.

People with Tourette syndrome are also at higher risk for having symptoms of OCD. OCD is a disorder characterized by persistent, intrusive, and senseless thoughts (obsessions) or compulsions to perform repetitive behaviors that interfere with normal functioning. A person with OCD, for example, may be obsessed with germs and may counteract this obsession with continual hand washing. Symptoms of OCD are present in 1.9–3% of the general population, whereas 28–50% of people with Tourette syndrome have symptoms of OCD.

Self-injurious behavior (SIB) is also seen more frequently in those with Tourette syndrome. Approximately 34–53% of individuals with Tourette syndrome exhibit some form of self-injuring behavior. The SIB is often related to OCD but can also occur in those with Tourette syndrome who do not have OCD.

Symptoms of anxiety and depression are also found more commonly in people with Tourette syndrome. It is not clear, however, whether these symptoms are symptoms of Tourette syndrome or occur as a result of having to deal with the symptoms of moderate to severe Tourette syndrome.

People with Tourette syndrome may also be at increased risk for having learning disabilities and personality disorders and may be more predisposed to behaviors such as aggression, antisocial behaviors, severe temper outbursts, and inappropriate sexual behavior. Further controlled studies need to be

KEY TERMS

Attention-deficit disorder (ADD)—Disorder characterized by a short attention span, impulsivity, and in some cases hyperactivity.

Autosomal dominant—A pattern of genetic inheritance where only one abnormal gene is needed to display the trait or disease.

Axon—The long extension of a nerve fiber that generally conducts impulses away from the body of the nerve cell.

Coprolalia—The involuntary expression of obscene words or phrases.

Copropraxia—The involuntary display of unacceptable/obscene gestures.

Decreased penetrance—Individuals who inherit a changed disease gene but do not develop symptoms.

Dendrites—Fibers of a brain cell that receive signals from other brain cells.

Dysphoria—Feelings of anxiety, restlessness, and dissatisfaction.

Echolalia—Involuntary echoing of the last word, phrase, or sentence spoken by someone else or sound in the environment.

Echopraxia—The imitation of the movement of another individual.

Neurotransmitter—Chemical in the brain that transmits information from one nerve cell to another.

Obsessive-compulsive disorder (OCD)—Disorder characterized by persistent, intrusive, and senseless thoughts (obsessions) or compulsions to perform repetitive behaviors that interfere with normal functioning.

Phalilalia—Involuntary echoing of the last word, phrase, sentence, or sound vocalized by oneself.

Tic—Brief and intermittent involuntary movement or sound.

performed to ascertain whether these behaviors are symptoms of Tourette syndrome.

Diagnosis

Examination

The TS diagnosis is made through observation and interview of the patient and discussions with other family members. The diagnosis of Tourette syndrome is complicated by a variety of factors. The extreme range of symptoms of this disorder makes it difficult to differentiate Tourette syndrome from other disorders with similar symptoms. Diagnosis is further complicated by the fact that some tics appear to be within the range of normal behavior. For example, an individual who only exhibits tics such as throat clearing and sniffing may be misdiagnosed with a medical problem such as allergies. In addition, bizarre and complex tics such as coprolalia may be mistaken for psychotic or "bad" behavior. Diagnosis is also confounded by individuals who attempt to control tics in public and in front of health care professionals and deny the existence of symptoms. Although there is disagreement over what criteria should be used to diagnosis Tourette syndrome, one aid in the diagnosis is the *Diagnostical and Statistical Manual of Mental Disorders*, fourth edition (*DSM-IV*). The *DSM-IV* outlines suggested diagnostic criteria for a variety of conditions including Tourette syndrome such as:

- Presence of both motor and vocal tics at some time during the course of the illness
- The occurrence of multiple tics nearly every day through a period of more than one year, without a remission of tics for a period of greater than three consecutive months
- Symptoms cause distress or impairment in functioning
- Age of onset of prior to 18 years of age
- Symptoms are not due to medications or drugs and are not related to another medical condition

Some physicians critique the *DSM-IV* criteria, citing that they do not include the full range of behaviors and symptoms seen in Tourette syndrome. Others criticize the criteria since they limit the diagnosis to those who experience a significant impairment, which may not be true for individuals with milder symptoms. For this reason many physicians use their clinical judgment as well as the *DSM-IV* criteria as a guide to diagnosing Tourette syndrome.

Tests

Patients may undergo blood tests, imaging studies such as magnetic resonance imaging (MRI), or an electroencephalogram (EEG) in order to rule out other possible explanations for the symptoms.

Treatment

There is no cure for Tourette syndrome, and treatment involves the control of symptoms through educational and psychological interventions and/or medications. The treatment and management of Tourette syndrome varies from patient to patient and is typically focused on the alleviation of the symptoms that are most bothersome to the patient or that cause the most interference with daily functioning.

Traditional

Psychological treatments such as counseling are not generally useful for the treatment of tics but can be beneficial in the treatment of associated symptoms such as OCD and ADD. Counseling may also help individuals to cope better with the symptoms of this disorder and to have more positive social interactions. Psychological interventions may also help people cope better with stressors that can normally be triggers for tics and negative behaviors; however, relaxation therapies may increase the occurrence of tics. Treatment is crucial in helping the affected child avoid depression, social isolation, and strained family relationships. The education of family members, teachers, and peers about Tourette syndrome can be helpful and may help to foster acceptance and prevent social isolation.

Drugs

Many people with mild symptoms of Tourette syndrome never require medication. Those with severe symptoms may require medication for all or part of their lifetime. No single or combination (more than one) drug therapy offers complete cessation of symptoms without adverse effects. The most effective treatment of tics associated with Tourette syndrome involves the use of drugs such as Haloperidol, Pimozide, Sulpiride, and Tiapride, which decrease the amount of dopamine in the body. Unfortunately, the incidence of side effects, even at low dosages, is quite high. The short-term side effects can include sedation, dysphoria, weight gain, movement abnormalities, depression, and poor school performance. Long-term side effects can include phobias, memory difficulties, and personality changes. These drugs are, therefore, better candidates for short-term rather than long-term therapy.

Tourette syndrome can also be treated with other drugs such as clonidine, clonazepam, and risperidone, but the efficacy of these treatments is unknown. In many cases, treatment of associated conditions such as ADD and OCD is often more of a concern than the tics themselves. Clonidine used in conjunction with stimulants such as Ritalin may be useful for treating people with Tourette syndrome who also have symptoms of ADD. Stimulants should be used with caution in individuals with Tourette syndrome since they can sometimes increase the frequency and severity of tics. OCD symptoms in those with Tourette syndrome are often treated with drugs such as Prozac, Luvox, Paxil, and Zoloft.

In many cases the treatment of Tourette syndrome with medications can be discontinued after adolescence. Trials should be performed through the gradual tapering off of medications and should always be done under a doctor's supervision. To date, no one medicine has been initially invented specifically for TS. One anomaly occurred in 2000 when Layton Biosciences received Food and Drug Administration (FDA) approval for a nicotine patch used to treat Tourette syndrome in combination with traditional drugs used to treat tics (e.g., Haldol).

A study conducted from 2005 to 2009 by Baylor College of Medicine, supported by the drug manufacturer, showed that the drug **Topiramate** effectively reduced tics in Tourette syndrome. Topiramate (Topamax) is a broad-spectrum antiepileptic, whose exact mechanism of action is unknown. According to the study, Topiramate had clear advantages over neuroleptic medications, the only approved medications for TS. Researchers plan to replicate the study on a larger population. Other effective medications that are used to treat some of the associated neurobehavioral disorders that can occur in patients with TS are methylphenidate and dextroamphetamine, which have been proven to lessen ADHD symptoms in people with TS without causing tics to become more severe.

Alternative

Clinical trials for the treatment of Tourette syndrome are currently sponsored by the National Institutes of Health (NIH) and other agencies. In 2009, NIH reported 22 ongoing or recently completed studies, including:

- A study to investigate how the sensitivity to touch and smell in patients with Tourette syndrome may differ from that of people without TS (NCT00368433)
- The evaluation of whether deep brain stimulation is effective at reducing tic frequency and severity in adults with Tourette syndrome (NCT00311909)
- A study using magnetic resonance imaging (MRI) and magnetic resonance spectroscopy (MRS) of the brain to try to gain a better understanding of the disease process in Tourette syndrome (NCT00030953)

In 2011, there were 14 different interventions being investigated in Tourette syndrome clinical trials. These clinical trials were conducted in 32 cities and were performed by 11 different clinical trial investigators, including studies conducted by Johns Hopkins Hospital and the National Institute of Neurological Disorders and Stroke (NINDS). These included studies of stimulant treatment of ADHD in TS and behavioral treatments for reducing tic severity in children

QUESTIONS TO ASK YOUR DOCTOR

- Is there any treatment for TS?
- What does it mean if a TS seems to run in my family?
- What medications will be prescribed?
- What are the side effects?

and adults. Information regarding current clinical trials can be found at ClinicalTrials.gov.

Prognosis

The prognosis for Tourette syndrome in individuals without associated psychological conditions is often quite good, and only approximately 10% of Tourette syndrome individuals experience severe tic symptoms. Approximately 30% of people with Tourette syndrome will experience a decrease in the frequency and severity of tics, and another 30–40% will experience a complete end of symptoms by late adolescence. The other 30–40% will continue to exhibit moderate to severe symptoms in adulthood. There does not appear to be a definite correlation between the type, frequency, and severity of symptoms and the eventual prognosis. Patients with severe tics may experience social difficulties and may isolate themselves from others in fear of shocking and embarrassing them. People with Tourette syndrome who have other symptoms such as OCD, ADD, and SIB usually have a poorer prognosis.

Prevention

There is no known way to prevent Tourette syndrome.

Resources

BOOKS

Buffolano, Sandra. *Coping with Tourette Syndrome: A Workbook to Help Kids with Tic Disorders*. Oakland, CA: Instant Help, 2008.

Buzbuzian, Denise. *Victory Over Tourette's Syndrome and Tic Disorders*. Truro, NS: Woodland, 2006.

Conners, Susan. *The Tourette Syndrome & OCD Checklist: A Practical Reference for Parents and Teachers*. Hoboken, NJ: Jossey-Bass, 2011.

Marsh, Tracy L., ed. *Children with Tourette Syndrome: A Parent's Guide*. 2nd ed. Bethesda, MD: Woodbine House, 2007.

Peters, Dylan. *Tic Talk: Living with Tourette Syndrome: A 9-Year-Old Boy's Story in His Own Words*. Chandler, AZ: Little Five Star, 2009.

Woods, Douglas W., et al. *Managing Tourette Syndrome: A Behaviorial Intervention Adult Workbook*. New York: Oxford University Press, 2008.

PERIODICALS

Altman, G., et al. "Children with Tourette Disorder: A Follow-Up Study in Adulthood." *Journal of Nervous and Mental Disease* 197, no. 5 (May 2009): 305–10.

Bernard, B.A., et al. "Determinants of Quality of Life in Children with Gilles de la Tourette Syndrome." *Movement Disorders* 24, no. 7 (May 2009): 1070–73.

Cavanna, A.E., et al. "The Behavioral Spectrum of Gilles de la Tourette Syndrome." *Journal of Neuropsychiatry and Clinical Neurosciences* 21, no. 1 (Winter 2009): 1–23.

Hedderick, E.F., et al. "Double-Blind, Crossover Study of Clonidine and Levetiracetam in Tourette Syndrome." *Pediatric Neurology* 40, no. 6 (June 2009): 420–25.

Jimenez-Shahed, J. "Tourette syndrome." *Neurologic Clinics* 27, no. 3 (August 2009): 737–55.

Verdellen, C.W., et al. "Habituation of Premonitory Sensations during Exposure and Response Prevention Treatment in Tourette's Syndrome." *Behavior Modification* 32, no. 2 (March 2008): 215–27.

WEBSITES

"Tourette Syndrome." Centers for Disease Control and Prevention. http://www.cdc.gov/ncbddd/tourette/index.html (accessed July 20, 2011)

"Tourette Syndrome." Genetics Home Reference. http://ghr.nlm.nih.gov/condition = tourettesyndrome (accessed July 20, 2011)

"Tourette Syndrome." Medline Plus. http://www.nlm.nih.gov/medlineplus/tourettesyndrome.html (accessed July 20, 2011)

"Tourette Syndrome: Frequently Asked Questions." Tourette Syndrome Association. http://www.tsa-usa.org/Medical/Faqs.html (accessed July 20, 2011)

ORGANIZATIONS

National Institute of Neurological Disorders and Stroke (NINDS), P.O. Box 5801, Bethesda, MD 20824, (301) 496-5751, (800) 352-9424, http://www.ninds.nih.gov.

Tourette Syndrome Association (TSA), 42–40 Bell Boulevard, Suite 205, Bayside, NY 11361-2820, (718) 224-2999, Fax: (718) 279-9596, http://www.tsa-usa.org.

Tourette Syndrome Foundation of Canada, 5945 Airport Road, Suite 195, MississaugaON, Canada, L4V 1R9, (905) 673-2255, (800) 361-3120, Fax: (905) 673-2638, tsfc@tourette.ca, http://www.tourette.ca.

Lisa Maria Andres, MS, CGC
Dawn J. Cardeiro, MS, CGC
Karl Finley
Monique Laberge, PhD

Transcranial doppler

Definition

Transcranial doppler (TCD) is a noninvasive form of ultrasound imaging that measures the velocity (speed) and direction of blood flow through the blood vessels in the brain. "Transcranial" comes from two Latin words meaning "across" or "through" and "skull." Doppler is the surname of Christian Doppler (1803–1853), an Austrian physicist and mathematician who first identified the effect that bears his name in 1842. The Doppler effect refers to the apparent change in frequency of sound waves or light waves, varying with the apparent velocity of the sound or light source and the observer. A common example of the Doppler effect is the way in which a car engine or ambulance siren sounds higher in pitch as the vehicle approaches an observer and decreases in pitch as the vehicle passes the observer and recedes in the distance.

Ultrasound medical imaging in general uses sound waves beyond the upper range of human hearing (whence the term "ultra") to create pressure waves in body tissues and fluids. The upper limit of human hearing is about 20,000 Hz (hertz; a measure of the number of sound wave cycles per second). Medical ultrasound generally uses frequencies in the range of 2 to 18 MHz (megahertz or 10^6 Hz), while TCD in particular usually uses 2 MHz. The sound waves penetrate a medium (a certain body region—in this case the skull and underlying blood vessels) and measure the reflection signature. The reflection signature reveals details about the inner structure of the medium, such as the condition of a fetus in the womb or, in the case of TCD, the speed and direction of blood flow in the arteries and veins of the brain.

Purpose

The purpose of TCD when it was first introduced in 1982 was to detect vasospasm (a condition in which blood vessels go into spasm and constrict, cutting down on the flow of blood to brain tissue) in cases of subarachnoid hemorrhage (SAH). SAH is a life-threatening condition in which there is bleeding into the space between the middle of the three **meninges** (layers of tissue covering the brain), which is called the arachnoid mater, and the innermost meninx, the pia mater. A subarachnoid hemorrhage may result from the spontaneous rupture of a blood vessel in the brain or from a **traumatic brain injury** (TBI).

TCD has also been used to evaluate and monitor patients with traumatic brain injuries (including mild traumatic brain injuries resulting from sports accidents), stroke, and other forms of cerebrovascular disease, and to screen children diagnosed with sickle cell disease for the risk of stroke. Other uses of TCD are:

- monitoring patients during brain surgery
- detection of emboli (free-floating masses of material or air/gas bubbles) in the blood vessels of the brain
- monitoring patients during radiation treatment of the central nervous system
- evaluating the effectiveness of thrombolytic (clot-dissolving) therapy
- assessing the effects of diseases or conditions that block or limit blood flow outside the brain on blood flow within the brain
- detection of subclavian steal syndrome (a condition in which blood is diverted or "stolen" from the brain to the upper arm when the artery that ordinarily supplies the upper arm is narrowed).
- detection of a patent foramen ovale (PFO); the foramen ovale ("oval opening" in Latin) is an opening between the two upper chambers of the heart that is present at birth but normally closes as the child grows older. If the foramen ovale does not close normally, it is said to remain open, or patent. Between 25–30% of adults have a PFO. Ordinarily it does not cause problems but may increase the risk of cryptogenic stroke (stroke of unknown cause) in patients younger than 55.

Description

A TCD instrument sends an ultrasound signal directly into an artery and analyzes the return signal to record blood flow velocity. The doctor, sonographer, or technologist places an ultrasound transducer (probe) at specific locations on the skull and back of the neck known as insonation windows. Because the bone in most areas of the skull is too thick to be penetrated by ultrasound waves, locations in which the bone is thinner must be used to obtain a reading. The four insonation windows are located on the temple above the cheekbone, through the eye, below the jaw, and on the back of the head. The probe emits a high-pitched sound above the range of human hearing, and the speed of the blood in the artery beneath the insonation window causes a change in the frequency of the wave displayed on a computer monitor. This change in frequency correlates directly with the speed of the blood flow and can be recorded for later analysis.

TCD has several advantages over other forms of diagnostic imaging and testing because the machine is portable, the procedure is noninvasive and does not require the use of dye or contrast agents, the cost is lower, and the risks to the patient are fewer than in

KEY TERMS

Arachnoid mater—The middle of the three meninges that cover and protect the central nervous system. It derives its name from its resemblance to a spider web.

Carotid arteries—Two large arteries, one on either side of the neck, that carry oxygenated blood from the heart to the brain.

Cerebrovascular—Referring to the blood vessels that supply the brain.

Cryptogenic stroke—Stroke of unknown cause; stroke that cannot be attributed to hardening of the arteries, clot formation, or emboli. Between 30–40% of all strokes are cryptogenic.

Embolus (plural, emboli)—A free-floating mass of material or an air/gas bubble floating in the bloodstream, capable of blocking a blood vessel.

Foramen ovale—A small opening between the two upper chambers of the heart that is present at birth but usually closes within the first three months after birth. An open (patent) foramen ovale has been linked to an increased risk of cryptogenic stroke in younger adults although the exact mechanism is not yet known.

Hematocrit—The percentage of blood volume occupied by red blood cells, normally about 45% for men and 40% for women; also known as the packed cell volume or PCV.

Hemodynamics—The study of blood flow in the body and the factors that influence it.

Insonation window—Any of four locations on the outside of the head and neck used for placement of the TCD probe.

Intracranial—Existing or occurring within the skull.

Lumen—The interior space of a tubular structure or organ, such as an artery or section of intestine.

Meninges (singular, meninx)—The three layers of membranous tissue that cover the brain and spinal cord. Transcranial doppler was originally developed to detect hemorrhages between the middle and the innermost meninges.

Plaque—A deposit of calcium, cholesterol, white blood cells, and other debris that can build up on the inner walls of arteries, leading to stenosis and eventual rupture of the artery or stroke.

Stenosis (plural, stenoses)—An abnormal narrowing in a blood vessel or other hollow tubular organ; also known as a stricture.

Transducer—Another word for the probe placed over the insonation windows in TCD.

Vasospasm—A condition in which a blood vessel goes into spasm and constricts, limiting the flow of blood to tissues. The lowered flow of blood can result in tissue death.

other diagnostic approaches. TCD can be done on an outpatient as well as inpatient basis.

Functional transcranial doppler

Functional transcranial doppler, or fTCD, is a form of TCD that can be used to track changes in blood flow velocity during the activation of nerve cells in the brain during various cognitive tasks. It is similar to functional magnetic resonance imaging (fMRI) in this regard. Since the early 1990s, fTCD has been used to map the organization of the left and right hemispheres of the brain in children as well as adults, yielding new information about language, color processing, facial recognition, and gender-related differences in brain organization.

Precautions

According to the American Academy of Neurology (AAN), TCD has a major limitation: It is most useful for evaluating the velocity of blood flow only in the larger intracranial blood vessels—although it is in these areas that disease is most likely to occur. In addition, TCD measures only changes in blood flow velocity; it does not provide the doctor with information about the internal anatomy of the blood vessels under examination. For example, an increase in blood velocity could result from an increase in the amount of blood flowing through the artery, a decrease in the diameter of the lumen (inner space) of the artery, or a combination of the two factors. TCD is often supplemented by another imaging procedure known as carotid ultrasonography or carotid duplex imaging, which provides information about any narrowing of the carotid arteries due to deposits of plaque.

Preparation

Prior to a TCD examination, the doctor takes a complete patient history, including the patient's age, sex, and race; current health status; any symptoms that may indicate cerebrovascular disease (numbness, tingling, difficulty speaking, **weakness, dizziness, fainting**, headaches); risk factors for cerebrovascular disease (diabetes, smoking, high blood pressure, other vascular disorders, family history of vascular disorders); medication history; and current laboratory values for blood pressure, intracranial pressure, heart rate, hematocrit, and hemoglobin content.

The actual TCD examination does not require any unusual preparation or removal of clothing on the patient's part. The patient lies on his or her back on an examining table while the operator places the probe on the insonation windows on the head and records the result. The patient will be asked to sit up or turn on one side when the insonation window at the back of the neck is examined. The full examination takes about half an hour.

Aftercare

No particular aftercare is needed for TCD.

Risks/side effects

There are several risks to TCD. One potential difficulty is that this imaging modality cannot be used with equal success on all patients because the thickness of the skull (and therefore the usefulness of the insonation windows) varies according to sex, race, and age; however, most examinations can be completed. Another difficulty is that TCD is heavily dependent on the skill and experience of the doctor using it. It can be performed by a physician or a sonographer but may require a neurologist (a doctor who specializes in diagnosing and treating disorders of the **central nervous system**) to interpret the results.

Mild side effects of TCD may include warming of the skin over the insonation windows (from the energy of the sound waves).

Clinical trials

There were 80 studies of TCD under way as of mid-2011, ranging from the effectiveness of TCD in monitoring stroke patients in intensive care and evaluating the outcome of patients with traumatic brain injuries to evaluating the effectiveness of clot-dissolving medications in stroke patients and monitoring children diagnosed with sickle cell disease. Other studies include research into the effects of vitamin C on blood flow in the brain and the effectiveness of aerobic exercise in improving blood flow to the brain in patients with diabetes. Information about current clinical trials can be found at ClinicalTrials.gov.

Resources

BOOKS

Allan, Paul, et al., ed. *Clinical Doppler Ultrasound*, 2nd ed. Oxford, UK: Churchill/Elsevier, 2006.

Baumgartner, R.W., ed. *Handbook on Neurovascular Ultrasound*. New York: Karger, 2006.

Reich, David L., et al., eds. *Monitoring in Anesthesia and Perioperative Care*. New York: Cambridge University Press, 2011.

PERIODICALS

Arkuszewski, M., et al. "Neuroimaging in Assessment of Risk of Stroke in Children with Sickle Cell Disease." *Advances in Medical Sciences* 55 (December 30, 2010): 115–29.

Drews, T., et al. "Transcranial Doppler Sound Detection of Cerebral Microembolism during Transapical Aortic Valve Implantation." *Thoracic and Cardiovascular Surgeon* 59 (June 2011): 237–42.

Forteza, A.M., et al. "Transcranial Doppler Detection of Cerebral Fat Emboli and Relation to Paradoxical Embolism: A Pilot Study." *Circulation* 123 (May 10, 2011): 1947–52.

Grocott, H.P., et al. "Monitoring of Brain Function in Anesthesia and Intensive Care." *Current Opinion in Anaesthesiology* 23 (December 2010): 759–64.

Len, T.K., and J.P. Neary. "Cerebrovascular Pathophysiology Following Mild Traumatic Brain Injury." *Clinical Physiology and Functional Imaging* 31 (March 2011): 85–93.

Misteli, M., et al. "Gender Characteristics of Cerebral Hemodynamics during Complex Cognitive Functioning." *Brain and Cognition* 76 (June 2011): 123–20.

Nicoletto, H.A., and L.S. Boland. "Transcranial Doppler Series Part V: Specialty Applications." *American Journal of Electroneurodiagnostic Technology* 51 (March 2011): 31–41.

Somers, M., et al. "The Measurement of Language Lateralization with Functional Transcranial Doppler and Functional MRI: A Critical Evaluation." *Frontiers in Human Neuroscience* 5 (March 28, 2011): 31.

Verlhac, S. "Transcranial Doppler in Children." *Pediatric Radiology* 41 (May 2011): Suppl. 1: S153–65.

WEBSITES

"Intracranial Cerebrovascular Evaluation: Transcranial Doppler." Society for Vascular Ultrasound. http://www.svunet.org/files/positions/0409-Intracranial.pdf (accessed July 26, 2011).

Pacific Vascular Institute for Continuing Medical Education (PVICME). "Transcranial Doppler and Imaging." YouTube. http://www.youtube.com/watch?v=wbV1p 66rXMo (accessed July 26, 2011).

"Transcranial Color Doppler." Online CME Course, GE Healthcare. http://www.gehealthcare.com/usen/ultra sound/products/cmetcd.html (accessed July 26, 2011).

Transcranial Doppler Educational Software Website. http://www.transcranial.com/index.html (accessed July 26, 2011).

"What Is Carotid Ultrasound?" National Heart, Lung, and Blood Institute (NHLBI). http://www.nhlbi.nih.gov/health/dci/Diseases/cu/cu_whatis.html (accessed July 26, 2011).

ORGANIZATIONS

American Academy of Neurology (AAN), 1080 Montreal Avenue, Saint Paul, MN 55116, (651) 695-2717, (800) 879-1960, Fax: (651) 695-2791, memberservices@aan.com, http://www.aan.com.

National Heart, Lung, and Blood Institute Health Information Center, P.O. Box 30105, Bethesda, MD 20824-0105, (301) 592-8573, Fax: (240) 629-3246, nhlbiinfo@nhlbi.nih.gov, http://www.nhlbi.nih.gov.

National Institute of Neurological Disorders and Stroke (NINDS), P.O. Box 5801, Bethesda, MD 20824, (301) 496-5751, (800) 352-9424, http://www.ninds.nih.gov.

Society for Vascular Ultrasound (SVU), 4601 Presidents Drive, Suite 260, Lanham, MD 20706-4831, (301) 459-7550, Fax: (301) 459-5651, svuinfo@ svunet.org, http://www.svunet.org.

Rebecca J. Frey, PhD

Transient global amnesia

Definition

Transient global amnesia (TGA) is a temporary short-term memory loss that may result from the deactivation of the brain's temporal lobes and/or thalamus (the part of the brain that serves as a center for the relay of sensory information). Usually occurring in otherwise healthy persons, TGA triggers memory loss from external stresses such as strenuous exertion, high levels of anxiety, sexual intercourse, immersion in water, and other similar conditions. The event may also be triggered by a condition called the Valsalva maneuver. During this maneuver, a person performs the "breathe-in-bear-down" movement that is automatically performed during strenuous exercise. It is thought that this maneuver temporarily siphons blood from the temporal lobes of the brain. The temporal lobes are where the memories are stored. This loss of blood may induce the loss of memory by persons experiencing TGA. While this hypothesis is still under review, it has been accepted as a logical explanation to a condition that currently has no generally accepted causal explanation.

Description

Transient global amnesia was first identified and described around 1960. Since that time, there have been extensive studies about the condition, but its etiology (causation) is still not clearly known or understood.

TGA affects memory function. People experiencing TGA can register information and there is no loss of social skills and sense of identity, but their ability to retain information is severely impaired. One of the puzzling associations with TGA is that many people who experience this disorder are also **migraine headache** sufferers. However, there is no report of a migraine prior to onset, nor is there any reported nausea, sensitivity to light or sound, or headache.

Demographics

There are no race or inherited conditions associated with TGA. Men experience the condition more often than women. In addition, the occurrence of this type of amnesia rarely happens before middle age, with about 12 out of 100,000 people ever experiencing the condition before age 50. The most likely ages in which to experience TGA are the 50s and 60s. About 3% of people who experience one episode of TGA will experience another episode sometime during their lifetime, but it is very rare for a person to experience more than three episodes of TGA.

The reason people in their 50s and 60s are more likely to experience TGA is not understood. No definitive links to any particular pathology or reaction to medication have been discovered. It is an elusive medical experience. For example, the connection of TGA with exposure to cold water, such as swimming in cold water or prolonged exposure to cold rain or snow, cannot be explained in any convincing way, but it is one of the condition's major triggers.

Causes and symptoms

The causes of this disorder are not yet fully understood. The hypotheses that the event is triggered by a temporary loss of blood to certain regions of the brain are most popular. In some cases, there is evidence of small strokes and local evidence of minor depressions on the surface of the brain. A well-accepted hypothesis suggests that blood is reduced to the temporal region of the brain during Valsalva, or weight-bearing movement.

People who have experienced TGA are also screened for current use of medications. Some drug interactions have been known to cause other types of amnesia, although not the type associated with TGA.

Another suggestion as a cause for TGA is that venous congestion (congested blood flow in the veins) inhibits blood flow to the thalamic or temporal regions of the brain. The support for this hypothesis is that increases in sympathetic nervous system activity and/or pressure within the thorax may exert pressure on the jugular veins. This, in turn, may disrupt arterial blood flow within the brain, resulting in ischemia (lack of oxygen) to memory centers or other areas of the brain. While the common precipitating factors have been discussed, why these events might trigger a TGA episode are not well understood.

Diagnosis

TGA is sometimes a difficult condition to diagnose. It is extremely helpful for an observer to contribute information to the physician. Some of the criteria for identifying the event are the impairment of memory, both newly learned and past. There is no loss of consciousness or personal identity. There must be no recent experience of head trauma. Patients must not be epileptics nor can they have experienced any form of a seizure in the last two years.

The episode usually lasts for only a few hours and is usually completely resolved by the end of 24 hours. However, rare cases have been documented in which the patient experiences the amnesia for up to a month.

Anterograde amnesia, which sometimes also follows head trauma, is a component of TGA. With the anterograde types of amnesia, the person experiences a memory loss of recent experiences, however, long-term memory persists. Persons with anterograde amnesia often ask questions and, after receiving a response, immediately ask the same question again. Physicians examining a person with amnesia will rule out retrograde amnesia, which is not a part of TGA. Retrograde amnesia is somewhat the opposite of anterograde amnesia, whereby the affected person can remember events that occur after the head trauma, but not before.

With TGA, a person experiences temporary confusion and lack of memory. The person is disoriented and confused, but no loss of personal identity occurs and long-term memories are intact. The person may be frightened and sometimes mildly delusional, but this passes soon and the incidence of recurrence is rare.

The initial kinds of tests a physician will request are those that rule out infection, stroke, brain injury, and other physiological conditions.

Blood tests such as a CBC with differential help to rule out infection. Another test often performed is running an electrolyte panel. Eletrolytes are common salt minerals such as potassium, calcium, magnesium, etc. Most professional and amateur athletes are aware of how important proper electrolyte balances are for proper body functioning. A lowering of electrolytes may cause some of the symptoms described by a person experiencing TGA. Other types of blood tests, including the search for clotting potentials, are often performed. To determine whether the patient may be prone to blood clotting, a physician may request a pothrombin time (PT) and activated partial thromboplastin time (aPTT). Quick clotting times could indicate a propensity towards thrombosis (blood clotting), which could lead to stroke.

Part of the diagnosis involves conducting several types of imaging tests. The uses of **positron emission tomography (PET)** and diffusion-weighted magnetic resonance imaging (MRI-DWI) have shown a small degree of ischemia (lack of blood flow) to certain areas of the brain with TGA. However, these same tests have shown conflicting results in other patients. At this writing, no definitive tests have been suggested to diagnose the condition.

Treatment team

Initially, most persons with TGA receive care from a physician in a hospital emergency department. A neurologist usually provides diagnosis and treatment. Both physicians usually order tests to differentiate TGA from other acute neurological events such as a stroke. As there is really no specific treatment for TGA, diagnosis and reassurance by a physician are important for a person experiencing TGA, as well as for family members.

Treatment

After ruling out trauma to the brain from accident, disease, or stroke, most people who have experienced TGA receive very little treatment because the

KEY TERMS

Amnesia—A general medical term for loss of memory that is not due to ordinary forgetfulness. Amnesia can be caused by head injuries, brain disease, or epilepsy, as well as by dissociation.

Anterograde amnesia—Amnesia for events that occurred after a physical injury or emotional trauma but before the present moment.

Retrograde amnesia—Amnesia for events that occurred before a traumatic injury.

Valsalva maneuver—A strain against a closed airway combined with muscle tightening, such as happens when a person holds his or her breath and tries to move a heavy object. Most people perform this maneuver several times a day without adverse consequences, but it can be dangerous for anyone with cardiovascular disease. Pilots perform this maneuver to prevent black-outs during high-performance flying.

condition is benign. A follow-up appointment with the neurologist is usually recommended.

Recovery and rehabilitation

Expected average times for recovery are within hours. A TGA patient rarely experiences the symptoms any longer than 24 hours. For most people, the condition lasts only 4–8 hours. Many people even report a shorter duration of one or two hours of disorientation and confusion. They may become frightened, but this is often alleviated with diagnosis and an explanation of the condition.

Prognosis

The prognosis for TGA patients is excellent. There are no debilitating side effects or any permanent loss of memory. TGA does not portend a serious stroke or similar condition involving the circulatory system. This is one of the reasons that TGA is such a perplexing syndrome for researchers; it is impossible to predict who will experience it. Because repeat occurrences are rare, numerous re-evaluations by a physician are usually not necessary.

Special concerns

It is important for people to be aware of the possibility of TGA. Seeking medical help, personal protection and reassurance are the beneficial to offer someone displaying TGA symptoms.

Resources

BOOKS

Adams, R. D., M. Victor, and A. H. Ropper. "Transient Global Amnesia." In *Principles of Neurology*. New York: McGraw-Hill, 1997.

PERIODICALS

Simons, Jon S., and John R. Hodges. "Previous Cases: Transient Global Amnesia." *Neurocases* (2000): 6, 211–30.

OTHER

Tuen, Charles. Neuroland. *Transient Global Amnesia*. January 4, 2004 (March 24, 2004). http://neuroland.com/sands/tga.htm.

ORGANIZATIONS

National Institute for Neurological Disorders and Stroke. P.O. Box 5801, Bethesda, MD 20824. Phone: (301) 496-5761. Tollfree phone: (800) 352-9424. http://www.ninds.nih.gov.

Brook Ellen Hall

Transient ischemic attack

Definition

A transient ischemic attack, or TIA, is often described as a mini-stroke. Unlike a stroke, the symptoms can disappear within a few minutes. TIAs and strokes are both caused by a disruption of the blood flow to the brain. In TIAs and most strokes, this disruption is caused by a blood clot blocking one of the blood vessels leading to the brain. The blockage produces symptoms such as sudden **weakness** or numbness on one side of the body, sudden dimming or loss of vision, and difficulty speaking or understanding speech. If the symptoms are caused by a TIA, they last less than 24 hours and do not cause brain damage. Stroke-associated symptoms, on the other hand, do not go away and may cause brain damage or death. TIAs can serve as an early warning sign of stroke and require immediate medical attention.

Demographics

About 240,000 people in the United States are diagnosed with a TIA each year; however, this number may be low because symptoms are transient and not everyone experiencing them will see a doctor. The risk of a TIA increases with age from about two per 10,000 people under age 35 to 1,500 people per 10,000 over age 85. Of people who have a TIA, roughly one-third will never have another, while the others will go on to have additional TIAs or a stroke. About 15% of people who have a stroke had a previous TIA.

Description

Strokes are the third leading cause of death in the United States and the leading cause of disability. Approximately 795,000 Americans have strokes annually; 20% die within one year. About 85% of these strokes are classified as ischemic. In ischemic stroke, a blood vessel leading to the brain becomes blocked and an area of the brain is deprived of oxygenated blood. (The other 15% of strokes are caused by bleeding from a blood vessel that has ruptured.) Without the blood supply, the cells in that area of the brain die. Since brain cells cannot grow back, the functions that are controlled by that brain area may be permanently lost.

Approximately 15% of strokes are preceded by one or more TIAs, and an estimated one-third of all TIAs are followed by a stroke within five years. They are considered a medical emergency and prompt medical attention is very important.

Risk factors for strokes and TIAs are very similar. The risk of a TIA or stroke is higher among men, African Americans, people over age 65, and people with heart disease or diabetes. Smokers, people with high blood pressure, and people who are overweight also have a greater risk for TIAs and strokes.

Causes and symptoms

A TIA is caused by a temporary blockage of one of the arteries that leads into the brain. Small blood clots, called microemboli, are the immediate cause of the blockage. The blockage forms because of damage or disease within the circulatory system. Blood clots can form in blood vessels because of artery damage, vascular disease, and other cardiovascular problems. For example, atherosclerosis is strongly associated with TIAs. Atherosclerosis is the build-up of fatty deposits or plaque at certain areas in the circulatory system. Clotting cells in blood, called platelets, tend to stick to atherosclerotic plaques or other damaged sites within blood vessels. Occasionally, a clot may grow large enough to block a blood vessel, or a piece of a clot may break off and circulate to other areas of the body. If a clot does not dissolve quickly enough, it can lodge in a blood vessel and block it. In TIAs, the microemboli dissolve within a short time.

Blood flows into the brain through two main pathways: the carotid arteries and the vertebrobasilar arteries. The carotid arteries are located on the front of the neck; the vertebrobasilar arteries are at the base of the skull at the back of the head. The symptoms produced by a TIA are determined by the arteries affected.

If a vertebrobasilar artery is blocked, common symptoms include double vision and **dizziness**, nausea and vomiting, difficulty speaking, and problems understanding and using spoken words. There may also be numbness around the mouth and a tingling sensation in the limbs. Blockage of a carotid artery produces complete loss of vision, dimmed or foggy vision, and paralysis or weakness on one side of the body. These symptoms also may be accompanied by language problems and speech difficulty. With either type of blockage, the microemboli dissolve within hours and full function returns.

Diagnosis

Examination

TIA is considered a medical emergency and individuals should get medical care right away, not wait to see if their symptoms resolve over time. Individuals having TIA symptoms should note the time the symptoms started, and are urged to remember that "time lost is brain lost."

The goal of diagnosis is to identify the precise cause of the TIA and to recommend treatment. Initial information that an individual can supply includes a medical history, what drugs are currently being taken and why, and a full description of the symptoms. Blood tests are ordered to screen blood counts—the numbers of specific blood cell types—and to measure glucose (sugar) and lipid (fats, including cholesterol) levels. Based on this information and a physical examination that includes blood pressure, pulse, and respiration measurements, one or more of the following imaging tests are ordered.

Tests

A computed tomography (CT) scan or a **magnetic resonance imaging** (MRI) scan usually is the first imaging test. CT or MRI can rule out other problems such as a tumor or **subdural hematoma** that can mimic the symptoms of a TIA. A **CT scan** also can uncover **aneurysms** and arteriovenous malformation, both of which are blood vessel abnormalities that can cause bleeding in the brain.

Another useful imaging test is carotid ultrasonography, a noninvasive procedure that allows examination of the interior of the carotid artery. This examination can detect **carotid stenosis**, a condition in which the artery is

KEY TERMS

Angioplasty—A medical procedure in which a catheter, or thin tube, is threaded through blood vessels. The catheter is used to place a balloon or stent (a small metal rod) at an area of stenosis and expand it mechanically.

Arteriography—A medical test in which an x-ray visible dye is injected into blood vessels. This dye allows the blood vessels to be imaged with x rays.

Atherosclerosis—A build-up of fatty tissue called plaque inside arteries that can impede or block blood flow.

Carotid artery—One of the major blood vessels leading to the brain; it runs up the front of the neck.

Echocardiography—A type of ultrasonography that is used to create an image of the heart and its functioning.

Endarterectomy—A surgical procedure in which diseased tissue and atherosclerotic plaque are removed from the inside of an artery.

Ischemia—A condition in which blood flow is cut off or restricted from a particular area. The surrounding tissue, starved of oxygen and nutrients, dies.

Microemboli—Small blot clots in the bloodstream.

Platelets—Tiny cells in the blood that help form blood clots.

Stenosis—The narrowing of an opening or passageway in the body. In arteries, stenosis is caused by a build-up of atherosclerotic plaque, disease, or other disorder.

Stroke—A condition in which blood flow to the brain has been blocked, thereby causing brain cells to die from lack of oxygen and nutrients; also called a "brain attack."

Ultrasonography—A medical test in which sound waves are directed against internal structures in the body. As sound waves bounce off the internal structure, they create an image on a video screen.

Vertebrobasilar arteries—Major blood vessels that lead to the brain. They are located at the base of the skull at the back of the head.

abnormally narrow because of atherosclerosis. Ultrasonography is very reliable in identifying stenosis, but it does not give enough information to accurately assess the degree of stenosis. Because treatment depends on the degree of stenosis, treatment decisions cannot be based

on ultrasonography. Another type of ultrasonography, called **transcranial Doppler** ultrasonography, is used to detect stenosis of the blood vessels within the brain and in the vertebrobasilar arteries.

Procedures

If stenosis is identified, a further test called cerebral arteriography may be done. This test is not done if the individual is in poor health, because it may be too risky. Arteriography involves injecting a special dye into the blood vessels that makes them visible on x rays. This procedure also is used to find suspected problems with blood vessels in the brain. Because it is an invasive procedure, complications can arise. Typically, these complications are minor and temporary. In a very small percentage of people with cardiovascular disease, the procedure may cause serious complications, such as stroke.

Although TIAs affect the brain, the ultimate cause of the problem may be found in the heart. Heart disease or damage to the heart's blood vessels is assessed by echocardiography. Echocardiography is a type of ultrasonography and is a noninvasive procedure.

Treatment

Treatment is aimed at preventing further TIAs and especially at preventing a stroke. The particular therapy depends on the root cause of the TIA and is not begun until this cause is identified. If possible, drug therapy is the preferred method of treating TIAs. Surgical intervention may be required if an individual's situation is not likely to respond to medication or if medication has failed.

Drugs

Anti-clotting drugs such as aspirin or cloplidgrel (Plavix) usually are given to reduce the chance of platelets forming clumps in the blood. These drugs are intended for long-term use. Anticoagulant (blood thinner) drugs such as warfarin (Coumadin) may be prescribed to keep blood from clotting. Other drugs may be prescribed to relax the smooth muscles of the arteries. Cholesterol-lowering drugs (statins) may be recommended, and conditions such as high blood pressure (hypertension) and diabetes mellitus that can worsen vascular disease will be treated.

Surgery

If carotid arteriography reveals at least a 70% blockage of the carotid artery, surgical treatment usually is recommended. The particular surgical method is called **carotid endarterectomy**. In endarterectomy, the artery is opened and the material clogging it is removed. Another procedure, called balloon angioplasty, has been suggested for treating carotid stenosis, but it is not as widely used. This procedure is performed by threading a thin tube through the blood vessel to the site that is clogged. A balloon or a stent (a slender rod) is then passed through the tube to mechanically widen the narrowed area. This procedure is successfully used in other blood vessels in the body, but there is some worry that using it close to the brain may be dangerous. Surgical treatment of blockage of the vertebrobasilar arteries is not usually recommended.

Home remedies and lifestyle changes

Treatment of TIAs also focuses on underlying problems. High blood pressure, heart disease, and high levels of blood lipids all require medical intervention. Condition-specific medications often are prescribed and lifestyle changes are strongly encouraged. These may include:

• losing weight if necessary and maintaining a healthy weight

• stopping smoking

• avoiding alcohol or consuming alcohol in moderation

• exercising moderately but regularly (5 days a week)

• eating a diet low in animal fats and sweets and high in fresh fruits, vegetables, and fiber

• controlling high blood pressure through salt (sodium) restriction, exercise, and medications as necessary

• controlling diabetes through exercise, diet, and medication as necessary by monitoring blood glucose levels regularly

Prognosis

One-third of TIAs are followed by stroke in the next five years; in the other two-thirds, the TIAs may either continue or disappear on their own; however, because of the risk of stroke-related disability and death, all TIAs should be treated as emergency medical situations.

Medical treatment significantly decreases the risk of stroke for people who experience one or more TIAs. Anti-platelet therapy reduces risk as much as 31%. Carotid endarterectomy also substantially reduces stroke risk. The procedure itself carries some risk, but the complication rate is less than 5%. The risk of complication can be lowered by choosing to have the procedure done in a facility experienced with carotid endarterectomy and by a surgeon with a low complication rate.

QUESTIONS TO ASK YOUR DOCTOR

• What are the indications that I may have had a TIA?

• What diagnostic tests are needed for a thorough assessment?

• What treatment options do you recommend for me?

• What other health conditions do I have that may affect the chance of another TIA or stroke?

• Are there any warning signs that a TIA is about to happen?

• Is it safe for me to drive now that I have had a TIA?

• What are the side effects associated with the medications you have prescribed for me?

• Will medications for a TIA interact with my current medications?

• Should I see a specialist? If so, what kind of specialist should I contact?

• If surgery is needed, what kind of surgical specialist should I contact?

• Since I am taking some of these drugs long term, will I need regular blood or other tests to check for their effectiveness?

• What tests or evaluation techniques will you perform to see if treatment has been beneficial for me?

• What lifestyle changes can I make to reduce the risk of another TIA or stroke?

• Does having a TIA put me at risk for other health conditions?

• What symptoms are important enough that I should seek immediate treatment?

• Can you recommend an organization that will provide me with additional information about TIAs?

Prevention

Treatment for TIAs is complemented by lifestyle changes. These practices also may prevent TIAs and strokes from ever occurring. Doctors and other health-care providers universally recommend that individuals stop smoking and consume alcohol in moderation. Regular health checkups can detect high blood pressure, heart disease, and other underlying problems. Adhering to treatment for these problems can help minimize TIA and stroke risks. Finally, maintaining a healthy weight and engaging in regular exercise as able are strongly recommended.

Resources

BOOKS

Ascheim, Deborah V., Robert Ascheim, and Penny Preston. *Heart Health Your Questions Answered*. New York: DK ADULT, 2009.

Blei, Francine, and Carlita Anglin. *100 Questions & Answers About Vascular Anomalies*. Sudbury, MA: Jones & Bartlett, 2010.

Caplan, Louis. *Stroke (What Do I Do Now?)*. New York: Oxford University Press, 2010.

Mant, Jonathan, and Marion F. Walker, eds. *ABC of Stroke*. Boston, MA: BMJ, 2011.

Pulsinelli, William A. "Ischemic Cerebrovascular Disease." In *Cecil Textbook of Medicine*, edited by Lee Goldman and Andrew I. Schafer. Philadelphia: W.B. Saunders, 2011.

WEBSITES

"Transient Ischemic Attack." MedlinePlus. http://www.nlm.nih.gov/medlineplus/transientischemicattack.html (accessed July 20, 2011).

Wedro, Benjamin C. "Transient Ischemic Attack (TIA, Mini-Stroke)." eMedicineHealth.com. http://www.emedicinehealth.com/transient_ischemic_attack_mini-stroke/article_em.htm (accessed July 20, 2011).

ORGANIZATIONS

American Academy of Neurology (AAN), 1080 Montreal Avenue, Saint Paul, MN 55116, (651) 695-2717, (800) 879-1960, Fax: (651) 695-2791, member services@aan.com, http://www.aan.com.

American Heart Association, 7272 Greenville Avenue, Dallas, TX 75231, (800) 242-8721, http://www.heart.org.

Centers for Disease Control and Prevention (CDC), 1600 Clifton Road, Atlanta, GA 30333, (800) CDC-INFO, cdcinfo@cdc.gov, http://www.cdc.gov.

National Heart, Lung, and Blood Institute Health Information Center, P.O. Box 30105, Bethesda, MD 20824-0105, (301) 592-8573, Fax: (240) 629-3246, nhlbiinfo@nhlbi.nih.gov, http://www.nhlbi.nih.gov.

National Institute of Neurological Disorders and Stroke (NINDS), P.O. Box 5801, Bethesda, MD 20824, (301) 496-5751, (800) 352-9424, http://www.ninds.nih.gov.

Society for Vascular Surgery, 633 North St. Clair, 22nd Floor, Chicago, IL 60611, (312) 334-2300, (800) 258-7188, Fax: (312) 334-2320, vascular@vascularsociety.org, http://www.vascularweb.org.

Julia Barrett, AM
Laura Jean Cataldo, RN, EdD

Transmissible spongiform encephalopathies *see* **Prion diseases**

Transverse myelitis

Definition

Transverse myelitis (TM) is an uncommon neurological syndrome caused by inflammation (a protective response which includes swelling, pain, heat, and redness) of the spinal cord, characterized by **weakness**, **back pain**, and bowel and bladder problems. It affects one to five persons per million.

Description

TM affects the entire thickness of the spinal cord, producing both sensory and movement problems. It is believed to be linked to the immune system, which may be prompted to attack the body's own spinal cord. Striking rapidly without warning, its effects can be devastating.

Causes and symptoms

Transverse myelitis has many different causes, often triggered by a variety of viral and bacterial infections (especially those associated with a rash such as measles or chickenpox). Once the infection subsides, the inflammation in the cord begins. About one-third of patients experience a flu-like illness with fever about the time they develop symptoms of TM. Sometimes, there appears to be a direct invasion of, and injury to, the spinal cord by an infectious agent (such as herpes zoster or the **AIDS** virus).

TM can also accompany a variety of diseases that break down tissue that surrounds and insulates the nerves (demyelinating diseases), such as **multiple sclerosis** (MS).

Some toxic substances, such as carbon monoxide, lead, or arsenic, can cause a type of myelitis characterized by inflammation followed by hemorrhage or bleeding that destroys the entire circumference of the spinal cord. Other types of myelitis can be caused by poliovirus; herpes zoster; rabies, smallpox or polio vaccination; or parasitic and fungal infections.

Many experts believe that TM can occur without any apparent cause, probably as the result of an autoimmune process. This means that a person's immune system attacks the spinal cord, causing inflammation and tissue damage.

Regardless of the cause of the myelitis, onset of symptoms is sudden and rapid. Problems with movement and sensation appear within one or two days after inflammation begins. Symptoms include soft (flaccid) paralysis of the legs, with pain in the lower legs or back, followed by loss of feeling and sphincter (muscles which close an opening, as in the anus) control. The earliest symptom may be a girdle-like sensation around the trunk.

The extent of damage occuring will depend on how much of the spinal cord is affected, but TM rarely involves the arms. Severe spinal cord damage also can lead to shock.

Diagnosis

A doctor will suspect transverse myelitis in any patient with a rapid onset of paralysis. Medical history, physical examination, brain and spinal cord scans, myelogram, spinal tap, and blood tests are used to rule out other neurological causes of symptoms, such as a tumor. If none of these tests suggests a cause for the symptoms, the patient is presumed to have transverse myelitis.

Treatment

There is no effective treatment for transverse myelitis, but any underlying infection must be treated. After this, the focus of care shifts from diagnosis and treatment to learning how to live with the effects of the syndrome. Patients are helped to cope psychologically with new limitations and are given physical rehabilitation.

Physical adaptations include learning to cope with bowel and bladder control, sexuality, inability to control muscles (**spasticity**), mobility, pain, and activities of daily living (such as dressing).

As nerve impulses from the spinal cord are often scrambled and misinterpreted by the brain as pain, painkillers are given to ease discomfort. Antidepressants or anticonvulsants may also help.

Prognosis

The prognosis depends on how much of the cord was damaged. Some people recover completely, while others have lasting problems and need help in learning how to cope with activities of daily living. People who develop spastic reflexes early in the course of the condition are more likely to recover than those who do not. If spinal cord tissue death (necrosis) occurs, the chance of a complete recovery is poor. Most recovery occurs within the first three months. A certain percentage of patients with TM go on to develop multiple sclerosis.

Resources

ORGANIZATIONS

Transverse Myelitis Association. 1787 Sutter Parkway, Powell, OH 43065-8806. (614) 766-1806. http://www.myelitis.org.

Carol A. Turkington

Traumatic brain injury

Definition

Traumatic brain injury (TBI) is the result of physical trauma to the head causing damage to the brain. This damage can be focal, or restricted to a single area of the brain, or diffuse, affecting more than one region of the brain. By definition, TBI requires that there be a head injury, or any physical assault to the head leading to injury of the scalp, skull, or brain, but not all head trauma is associated with TBI.

Description

TBI is sometimes known as acquired brain injury. The least severe and most common type of TBI is termed a concussion, which is technically defined as a brief loss of consciousness after a head injury without any physical evidence of damage on an imaging study such as a CT or MRI scan. In common parlance, concussion may refer to any minor injury to the head or brain.

Symptoms, complaints, and neurological or behavioral changes following TBI depend on the location(s) of the brain injury and on the total volume of injured brain. Usually, TBI causes focal brain injury involving a single area of the brain where the head is struck or where an object such as a bullet enters the brain. Although damage is typically worst at the point of direct impact or entry, TBI may also cause diffuse brain injury involving several other brain regions.

Closed head injury refers to TBI in which the head is hit by or strikes an object without breaking the skull. In a penetrating head injury, an object such as a bullet fractures the skull and enters brain tissue.

Diffuse brain damage associated with closed head injury may result from back and forth movement of the brain against the inside of the bony skull. This is sometimes called coup-contrecoup injury. "Coup," which is French for "blow," refers to the brain injury directly under the point of maximum impact to the skull. "Contrecoup," which is French for "against the blow," refers to the brain injury opposite the point of maximum impact.

For example, coup-contrecoup injury may occur in a rear-end collision, with high speed stops, or with violent shaking of a baby, because the brain and skull are of different densities and, therefore, travel at different speeds. The impact of the collision causes the soft, gelatinous brain tissue to jar against bony prominences on the inside of the skull.

Because of the location of these prominences and the position of the brain within the skull, the frontal lobes (behind the forehead) and temporal lobes (underlying the temples) are most susceptible to this type of diffuse damage. These lobes house major brain centers involved in speech and language, so problems with communication skills often follow closed head injuries of this type.

Depending on which areas of the brain are injured, other symptoms of closed head injury may include difficulty with concentration, memory, thinking, swallowing, walking, balance, and coordination; **weakness** or paralysis; changes in sensation; and alteration of the sense of smell.

Consequences of TBI can be relatively subtle or completely devastating, related to the severity and mechanism of injury. Diffuse axonal injury, or shear injury, may follow contrecoup injury even if there is no damage to the skull or obvious bleeding into the brain tissue. In this type of injury, damage to the part of the nerve that communicates with other nerves degenerates and releases harmful substances that can damage neighboring nerves.

When the skull cracks or breaks, the resulting skull fracture can cause a contusion, or an area of bruising of brain tissue associated with swelling and blood leaking from broken blood vessels. A depressed skull fracture occurs when fragments of the broken skull sink down from the skull surface and press against the surface of the brain. In a penetrating skull fracture, bone fragments enter brain tissue. Either of these types of skull fracture can cause bruising of the brain tissue, called a contusion. Contrecoup injury can also lead to brain contusion.

If the physical trauma to the head ruptures a major blood vessel, the resulting bleeding into or around the brain is called a hematoma. Bleeding between the skull and the dura, the thick, outermost layer covering the brain, is termed an **epidural hematoma**. When blood collects in the space between the dura and the arachnoid membrane, a more fragile covering underlying the dura, it is known as a **subdural hematoma**. An intracerebral hematoma involves bleeding directly into the brain tissue.

All three types of hematomas can damage the brain by putting pressure on vital brain structures. Intracerebral hematomas can cause additional damage as toxic breakdown products of the blood harm brain cells, cause swelling, or interrupt the flow of cerebrospinal fluid around the brain.

Demographics

Estimates for the number of Americans living today who have had a TBI range from between 2.5 and 6.5 million, making it a major public health problem costing the United States more than $48 billion annually. A recent review suggests that the incidence of TBI in the United States is between 180 and 250 per 100,000 population per year, with even higher incidence in Europe and South Africa.

Although TBI can affect anyone at any age, certain age groups are more vulnerable because of lifestyle and other risk factors. Males ages 15 to 24, especially those in lower socioeconomic levels, are most likely to become involved in high-speed or other risky driving, as well as physical fights and criminal activity. These behaviors increase the likelihood of TBI associated with automobile and motorcycle accidents or with violent crimes.

Infants, children under five years of age, and adults 75 years and older are also at higher risk for TBI than the general population because they are most susceptible to **falls** around the home. Other factors predisposing the very young and the very old to TBI include physical abuse, such as violent shaking of an infant or toddler known as the shaken-baby syndrome.

Causes and symptoms

Accidents, especially motor vehicle accidents, are the major culprit implicated in TBI. Because accidents are the leading cause of death or disability in men under age 35, and because over 70% of accidents involve injuries of the head and/or spinal cord, this is not surprising. In fact, transportation accidents involving automobiles, motorcycles, bicycles, and pedestrians account for half of all TBIs and for the majority of TBIs in individuals under the age of 75. At least half of all TBIs are associated with alcohol use. Sports injuries cause about 3% of TBIs; other accidents leading to TBI may occur at home, at work, or outdoors.

In those age 75 and older, falls are responsible for most TBIs. Other situations leading to TBI at all ages include violence, implicated in about 20% of TBIs. Firearm assaults are involved in most violent causes of TBI in young adults, whereas child abuse is the most common violent cause in infants and toddlers. In the **shaken baby syndrome**, a baby is shaken with enough force to cause severe contrecoup injury.

The symptoms of TBI may occur immediately or they may develop slowly over several hours, especially if there is slow bleeding into the brain or gradual swelling. Depending on the cause, mechanism, and extent of injury, the severity of immediate symptoms of TBI can be mild, moderate, or severe, ranging from mild concussion to deep **coma** or even death.

With concussion, the injured person may experience a brief or transient loss of consciousness, much like **fainting** or passing out, or merely an alteration in consciousness described as "seeing stars," feeling dazed, or "out of it." On the other hand, coma refers to a profound or deep state of unconsciousness in which the individual does not respond to the environment in any meaningful way.

When a person with TBI regains consciousness, some symptoms are immediately apparent, while others are not noticed until several days or weeks later. Symptoms which may be obvious right away after mild TBI include headache; changes in vision, such as blurred vision or tired eyes; nausea; **dizziness**; lightheadedness; ringing in the ears; bad taste in the mouth; or altered sense of smell, which is usually experienced as loss of the sense of taste.

Approximately 40% of patients with TBI develop postconcussion syndrome within days to weeks, with symptoms including headache, dizziness or a sensation of spinning (**vertigo**), memory problems, trouble concentrating, sleep disturbances, restlessness, irritability, **depression**, and anxiety. This syndrome may persist for a few weeks, especially in patients with depression, anxiety, or other psychiatric symptoms before the TBI.

With more severe injuries, there may also be immediate numbness or weakness of one or more limbs, blindness, deafness, inability to speak or understand speech, slurred speech, lethargy with difficulty staying awake, persistent vomiting, loss of coordination, disorientation, or agitation. In addition to some of these symptoms, young children with moderate to severe TBI may also experience prolonged crying and refusal to nurse or eat.

While the injured person is preoccupied with headache or pain related to other physical trauma, symptoms such as difficulty in thinking or concentrating may not be evident. Often these more subtle symptoms may appear only when the individual attempts to return to work or to other mentally challenging situations. Similarly, personality changes, depression, irritability, and other emotional and behavioral problems may initially be attributed to coping with the stress of the injury, and they may not be fully appreciated until the individual is recuperating at home.

Seizures may occur soon after a TBI or may first appear up to a year later, especially when the damage involves the temporal lobes. Other symptoms that may appear immediately or that may be noticed only while the individual is returning to usual activities are confusion, **fatigue** or lethargy, altered sleep patterns, and trouble with memory, concentration, attention, and finding the right words or understanding speech.

Diagnosis

Recognizing a serious head injury, starting basic first aid, and seeking emergency medical care can help the injured person avoid disability or even death. When encountering a potential TBI, it is helpful to find out what happened from the injured person, from clues at the scene, and from any eyewitnesses. Because spinal cord injury often accompanies serious head trauma, it is prudent to assume that there is also injury to the spinal cord and to avoid moving the person until the paramedics arrive. Spinal cord injury is a challenging diagnosis; nearly one-tenth of spinal cord injuries accompanying TBI are missed initially.

Signs apparent to the observer that suggest serious head injury and mandate emergency treatment include shallow or erratic breathing or pulse, drop in blood pressure, broken bones or other obvious trauma to the skull or face such as bruising, swelling or bleeding; one pupil larger than the other; or clear or bloody fluid drainage from the nose, mouth, or ears.

Symptoms reported by the injured person that should also raise red flags include severe headache, stiff neck, vomiting, paralysis or inability to move one or more limbs, blindness, deafness, or inability to taste or smell. Other ominous developments may include initial improvement followed by worsening symptoms; deepening lethargy or unresponsiveness; personality change, irritability, or unusual behavior; or incoordination.

When emergency personnel arrive, they will stabilize the patient, evaluate the above signs and symptoms, and assess the nature and extent of other

Cerebrospinal fluid (CSF)—A protective fluid surrounding and protecting the brain and spinal cord.

Closed head injury—TBI in which the head strikes or is struck by an object without breaking the skull.

Coma—A decreased level of consciousness with deep unresponsiveness.

Computed tomography (CT) scan—A neuroimaging test that generates a series of cross-sectional x rays of the head and brain.

Concussion—Injury to the brain causing a sudden, temporary impairment of brain function.

Contrecoup—An injury to the brain opposite the point of direct impact.

Contusion—A focal area of swollen and bleeding brain tissue.

Dementia pugilistica—"Punch-drunk" syndrome of brain damage caused by repeated head trauma.

Depressed skull fracture—A fracture in which fragments of broken skull press into brain tissue.

Diffuse axonal injury (shear injury)—Traumatic damage to individual nerve cells resulting in breakdown of overall communication between nerve cells in the brain.

Electroencephalogram (EEG)—A record of the tiny electrical impulses produced by the brain's activity. By measuring characteristic wave patterns, the EEG can help diagnose certain conditions of the brain.

Epidural hematoma—Bleeding into the area between the skull and the dura, the tough, outermost brain covering.

Glasgow coma scale—A measure of level of consciousness and neurological functioning after TBI.

Hematoma—Bleeding into or around the brain caused by trauma to a blood vessel in the head.

Intracerebral hematoma—Bleeding within the brain caused by trauma to a blood vessel.

Increased intracranial pressure—Increased pressure in the brain following TBI.

Magnetic resonance imaging (MRI)—A noninvasive neuroimaging test using magnetic fields to visualize water shifts in brain tissue.

Penetrating head injury—TBI in which an object pierces the skull and enters brain tissue.

Post-concussion syndrome—A complex of symptoms with headache following mild TBI.

Post-traumatic amnesia (PTA)—Difficulty forming new memories after TBI.

Post-traumatic dementia—Persistent mental deterioration following TBI.

Post-traumatic epilepsy—Seizures occurring more than one week after TBI.

Shaken baby syndrome—A severe form of TBI resulting from shaking an infant or small child forcibly enough to cause the brain to jar against the skull.

Subdural hematoma—Bleeding between the dura and the underlying brain covering.

Ventriculostomy—Surgery that drains cerebrospinal fluid from the brain to treat hydrocephalus or increased intracranial pressure.

---

injuries, such as broken bones, spinal cord injury, or damage to other organ systems. Medical advances in early detection and treatment of associated injuries have improved the overall outcome in TBI. The initial evaluation measures vital signs such as temperature, blood pressure, pulse, and breathing rate, while the neurological examination assesses reflexes, level of consciousness, ability to move the limbs, as well as pupil size, symmetry, and response to light.

These neurological features are standardized using the Glasgow Coma Scale, a test scored from 1 to 15 points. Each of three measures (eye opening, best verbal response, and best motor response) is scored separately, and the combined score helps determine the severity of

TBI. A total score of 3 to 8 reflects a severe TBI, 9 to 12 a moderate TBI, and 13 to 15 a mild TBI.

Imaging tests reveal the location and extent of brain injury and associated injuries and therefore help determine diagnosis and probable outcome. Sophisticated imaging tests can help differentiate the variety of unconscious states associated with TBI and can help determine their anatomical basis.

Until neck fractures or spinal instability have been ruled out with skull and neck x rays, and with head and neck computed tomography (CT) scans for more severe injuries, the patient should remain immobilized in a neck and back restraint.

By constructing a series of cross-sectional slices, or x ray images through the head and brain, the CT scan can diagnose bone fractures, bleeding, hematomas, contusions, swelling of brain tissue, and blockage of the **ventricular system** circulating cerebrospinal fluid around the brain. In later stages after the initial injury, it may also show shrinkage of brain volume in areas where neurons have died.

Using magnetic fields to detect subtle changes in brain tissue related to differences in water content, the magnetic resonance imaging (MRI) scan shows more detail than x ray or CT; however, it takes more time than the CT and is not as readily available, making it less suited for routine emergency imaging.

For patients with seizures or for those with more subtle episodic symptoms thought possibly to be seizures, the electroencephalogram (EEG) may reveal abnormalities in the electrical activity of the brain, or brain waves. Other diagnostic techniques that may be helpful include cerebral **angiography, transcranial Doppler** ultrasound, and single photon emission computed tomography (SPECT).

Treatment team

The first responder at the scene of TBI is usually a paramedic or emergency medical technician (EMT). In the emergency department, a trauma specialist may determine the extent of associated injuries. The neurologist is usually the primary treating physician assessing and managing the symptoms and consequences of TBI. Diagnostic technicians involved in TBI management include radiological and EEG technicians and audiologists who assess hearing.

If surgery is needed to remove blood clots or to insert a shunt to relieve increased pressure within the skull, a neurosurgeon is needed. After surgery, or for any patient with loss of consciousness, intensive care is managed by a specialized treatment team including neurologists, neurosurgeons, intensivists, respiratory therapists, and specialized nurses and technicians.

After the physical condition has stabilized, a speech therapist and/or neuropsychologist may evaluate swallowing, cognitive and behavioral abilities and carry out appropriate rehabilitation. Other specialized therapists include the occupational therapist, who addresses sensory deficits, hand movements, and the ability to perform activities of daily living such as dressing; and the physical therapist who directs exercise and other programs to rehabilitate weakness and loss of coordination. Vocational planners, psychologists, and psychiatrists may help the individual with TBI cope with returning to society and to gainful employment.

Treatment

Although no specific treatment may be needed for a mild head injury, it is crucial to watch the person closely for any developing symptoms over the next 24 hours. **Acetaminophen** or ibuprofen, available over-the-counter, may be used for mild headache, but aspirin should not be given because it can increase the risk of bleeding.

If the person is sleeping, he should be awakened every 2 to 3 hours to determine alertness and orientation to name, time, and place. Immediate medical help is needed if the person becomes unusually drowsy or disoriented, develops a severe headache or stiff neck, vomits, loses consciousness, or behaves abnormally.

Treatment for moderate or severe TBI should begin as soon as possible by calling 911 and beginning emergency care until the EMT team arrives. This includes stabilizing the head and neck by placing the hands on both sides of the person's head to keep the head in line with the spine and prevent movement which could worsen spinal cord injury. Bleeding should be controlled by firmly pressing a clean cloth over the wound unless a skull fracture is suspected, in which case it should be covered with sterile gauze dressing without applying pressure. If the person is vomiting, the head, neck, and body should be rolled to the side as one unit to prevent choking without further injuring the spine.

Although the initial brain damage caused by trauma is often irreversible, the goal is to stabilize the patient and prevent further injury. To achieve these goals, the treatment team must insure adequate oxygen supply to the brain and the rest of the body, maintain blood flow to the brain, control blood pressure, stabilize the airway, assist in breathing or perform CPR if necessary, and treat associated injuries.

About half of severely head-injured patients require **neurosurgery** for hematomas or contusions. Swelling of the injured brain may cause increased pressure within the closed skull cavity, known as increased intracranial pressure (ICP). ICP can be measured with a intraventricular probe or catheter inserted through the skull into the fluid-filled chambers (ventricles) within the brain. Placement of the ICP catheter is usually guided by CT scan. If ICP is elevated, ventriculostomy may be needed. This procedure drains cerebrospinal fluid from the brain and reduces ICP. Drugs that may decrease ICP include mannitol and barbiturates.

A recent review suggests that using intraventricular catheters coated with antibiotics reduces the risk for infection. Keeping the patient's body temperature low (hypothermia) also improves outcome after moderate to severe TBI. Increasing the level of oxygen in the blood beyond normal concentrations is also being explored as a treatment option for improving brain metabolism in TBI. Large, multicenter trials of these and other treatments, such as early surgery to relieve increased ICP, are still needed, and the quest continues for a therapy that could prevent nerve cell death in TBI.

Although some patients need medication for psychiatric and physical problems resulting from the TBI, prescribing drugs may be problematic because TBI patients are more sensitive to side effects.

Both in the immediate and later stages of TBI, rehabilitation is vital to optimal recovery of ability to function at home and in society.

Problems with orientation, thinking and communication problems should be addressed early, often during the hospital stay. The focus is typically on improving alertness, attention, orientation, speech understanding, and swallowing problems.

As the patient improves, rehabilitation should be modified accordingly. The panel suggested that physical therapy, occupational therapy, speech/language therapy, physiatry (physical medicine), psychology/ psychiatry, and social support should all play a role in TBI rehabilitation. Appropriate settings for rehabilitation may include the home, the hospital outpatient department, inpatient rehabilitation centers, comprehensive day programs, supportive living programs, independent living centers, and school-based programs. Families should become involved in rehabilitation, in modifying the home environment if needed, and in psychotherapy or counseling as indicated.

Clinical trials

The National Institute of Neurological Disorders and Stroke (NINDS) supports research on the biological mechanisms of brain injury, strategies to limit brain damage following head trauma, and treatments of TBI that may improve long-term recovery. Research areas include mechanisms of diffuse axonal injury; the role of calcium entry into damaged nerves causing cell death and brain swelling; the toxic effects of glutamate and other nerve chemicals causing excessive nerve excitability; natural processes of brain repair after TBI; the therapeutic use of cyclosporin A or hypothermia to decrease cell death and nerve swelling; and the use of stem cells to repair or replace damaged brain tissue.

NINDS-supported clinical research focuses on enhancing the ability of the brain to adapt to deficits after TBI; improving rehabilitation programs for TBI-related disabilities; and developing treatments for use in the first hours after TBI. Early treatments being investigated include hypothermia for severe TBI in children, magnesium sulfate to protect nerve cells after TBI, and lowering ICP and increasing blood flow to the brain.

To address the specific problems in thinking and communication following TBI, the NINDS is designing new evaluation tools for children, developing computer programs to help rehabilitate children with TBI, and determining the effects of various medications on recovery of speech, language, and cognitive abilities.

Information about current clinical trials can be found at ClinicalTrials.gov.

Prognosis

The Centers for Disease Control and Prevention (CDC) estimates that each year 1.7 million people sustain a traumatic brain injury. Of these, 52,000 die as a result of the TBI; 275,000 are hospitalized; and about 1.4 million visit and are released from an emergency room.

Outcomes vary with cause: 91% of TBIs caused by firearms, two-thirds of which may represent suicide attempts, are fatal, compared with only 11% of TBIs from falls. Low Glasgow Coma Scale scores predict a worse outcome from TBI than do high scores.

The Swedish Council on Technology Assessment in Health Care concluded that of 1,000 patients arriving at the hospital with mild head injury, one will die, nine will require surgery or other intervention, and about 80 will have abnormal findings on brain CT and will probably need to be hospitalized.

Immediate complications of TBI may include seizures, enlargement of the fluid-filled chambers within the brain (hydrocephalus or post-traumatic ventricular enlargement), leaks of cerebrospinal fluid, infection, injury to blood vessels or to the nerves supplying the head and neck, pain, bed sores, failure of multiple organ systems, and trauma to other areas of the body.

About one-fourth of patients with brain contusions or hematomas and about half of those with penetrating head injuries develop seizures within the first 24 hours of the injury. Those that do are at increased risk of seizures occurring within one week after TBI.

Hydrocephalus usually occurs within the first year of TBI, and it is associated with deteriorating neurological outcome, impaired consciousness, behavioral changes, poor coordination or balance, loss of bowel and bladder control, or signs of increased ICP.

Long-term survivors of TBI may suffer from persistent problems with behavior, thinking, and

QUESTIONS TO ASK YOUR DOCTOR

- What are the indications that my loved one may have traumatic brain injury?
- What diagnostic tests are needed for a thorough assessment?
- What treatment options do you recommend?
- What kind of changes can I expect to see with the medications you have prescribed?
- What are the side effects associated with the medications you have prescribed?
- Should I see a specialist? If so, what kind of specialist should I contact?
- If surgery is needed, what kind of surgical specialist should I contact?
- What tests or evaluation techniques will you perform to see if treatment has been beneficial?
- What physical limitations do you foresee?
- Will physical, occupational, or speech rehabilitation be beneficial?
- Does having traumatic brain injury put my loved one at risk for other health conditions?
- Can you recommend any support groups for me and my family?

communication disabilities, as well as epilepsy; loss of sensation, hearing, vision, taste, or smell; ringing in the ears (**tinnitus**), coordination problems, and/or paralysis. Recovery from cognitive deficits is most dramatic within the first six months after TBI, and less apparent subsequently.

Memory loss is especially common in severely head-injured patients, with loss of some specific memories and partial inability to form or store new memories. Anterograde post-traumatic amnesia refers to impaired memory of events that occurred after TBI, while retrograde post-traumatic amnesia refers to impaired memory of events that occurred before the TBI.

Personality changes and behavioral problems may include depression, anxiety, irritability, anger, apathy, paranoia, frustration, agitation, mood swings, aggression, impulsive behaviors or "acting out," social inappropriateness, temper tantrums, difficulty accepting responsibility, and alcohol or drug abuse.

Following TBI, patients may be at increased risk of other long-term problems such as **Parkinson's**

disease, **Alzheimer's disease**, "punch-drunk" syndrome (**dementia** pugilistica), and post-traumatic dementia.

Because of all the above problems, some patients may have difficulty returning to work following TBI, as well as problems with school, driving, sports, housework, and social relationships.

Special concerns

Unlike most other devastating neurological diseases, TBI can be prevented. Practical measures to decrease risk include wearing seatbelts; using child safety seats; wearing helmets for biking and other sports; safely storing firearms and bullets; using step-stools, grab bars, handrails, window guards, and other safety devices; making playground surfaces out of shock-absorbing material; and not driving under the influence of alcohol or other drugs that affect performance.

Because TBI follows trauma, it is often associated with injuries to other parts of the body, which require immediate and specialized care. Complications may include lung or heart dysfunction following blunt chest trauma, limb fractures, gastrointestinal dysfunction, fluid and hormonal imbalances, nerve injuries, deep vein thrombosis, excessive blood clotting, and infections.

Resources

BOOKS

Daisley, Audrey, Rachel Tams, and Udo Kischka. *Head Injury*. New York: Oxford University Press, 2009.

Huff, Eane. *Heads Up: Finding Possibility and Purpose with Head Injury*. Parker, CO: Outskirts, 2009.

Mason, Michael Paul. *Head Cases: Stories of Brain Injury and Its Aftermath*. New York: Farrar, Straus and Giroux, 2009.

PERIODICALS

Brady, Don, and Flo Brady. "Sport-related concussions: Myths and facts." *Communique* (June 2011): 32.

Gibbons, Susanne, Dina Kurzweil, and Dorraine D. Watts. "Mild traumatic brain injury: a survey of perceived knowledge and learning preferences of military and civilian nurses." *Journal of Neuroscience Nursing* (June 2011): 122.

Gould, Kate Rachel, et al. "Predictive and associated factors of psychiatric disorders after traumatic brain injury: a prospective study." *Journal of Neurotrauma* 28.7 (2011): 1155.

Jancin, Bruce. "Blast-Related brain injuries are turning up in civilian practices: expert analysis from the annual meeting of the American neuropsychiatric association." *Clinical Psychiatry News* (June 2011): 32.

McIlvoy, Laura, and Kimberly Meyer. "Nursing management of adults with severe traumatic brain injury." *Journal of Neuroscience Nursing* (August 2011): 233.

WEBSITES

Clinical Trials Website. http://www.clinicaltrials.gov (accessed July 21, 2011).

"Head Injury." MedlinePlus. http://www.nlm.nih.gov/medlineplus/ency/article/000028.htm (accessed July 21, 2011).

"NINDS Traumatic Brain Injury Information Page." National Institute of Neurological Disorders and Stroke. http://www.ninds.nih.gov/disorders/tbi/tbi.htm (accessed July 21, 2011).

ORGANIZATIONS

American Academy of Neurology (AAN), 1080 Montreal Avenue, Saint Paul, MN 55116, (651) 695-2717, (800) 879-1960, Fax: (651) 695-2791, memberservices@aan.com, http://www.aan.com.

American Academy of Physical Medicine and Rehabilitation, 9700 West Bryn Mawr Avenue, Suite 200, Rosemont, IL 60018-5701, (847) 737-6000, Fax: (847) 737-6001, info@aapmr.org, http://www.aapmr.org.

American Epilepsy Society, 342 North Main Street, West Hartford, CT 06117-2507, (860) 586-7505, http://www.aesnet.org.

American Neurological Association, 5841 Cedar Lake Road, Suite 204, Minneapolis, MN 55416, (952) 545-6284, http://www.aneuroa.org.

Brain Injury Association of America, 1608 Spring Hill Road, Suite 110, Vienna, VA 22182, (703) 761-0750, (800) 444-6443, Fax: (703) 761-0755, braininjuryinfo@biausa.org, http://www.biausa.org.

Brain Injury Resource Center, P.O. Box 84151, Seattle, WA 98124, (206) 621-8558, brain@headinjury.com, http://www.headinjury.com.

Family Caregiver Alliance, 180 Montgomery Street, Suite 900, San Francisco, CA 94104, (415) 434-3388, (800) 445-8106, http://www.caregiver.org.

Head Injury Association, 65 Austin Boulevard, Commack, NY 11725, (631) 543-2245, http://www.lihia.org.

Head Trauma Support Project, Inc., P.O. Box 215666, Sacramento, CA 95821, (916) 568-6660, info@headtraumasacramento.org, http://headtraumasacramento.org.

National Institute of Neurological Disorders and Stroke (NINDS), P.O. Box 5801, Bethesda, MD 20824, (301) 496-5751, (800) 352-9424, http://www.ninds.nih.gov.

National Institute on Deafness and Other Communication Disorders (NIDCD), National Institutes of Health, 31 Center Drive, MSC 2320, Bethesda, MD 20892-2320, (301) 496-7243, (800) 241-1044, nidcdinfo@nidcd.nih.gov, http://www.nidcd.nih.gov/.

National Institutes of Health (NIH), 9000 Rockville Pike, Bethesda, MD 20892, (301) 496-4000, NIHinfo@od.nih.gov, http://www.nih.gov/index.html.

U.S. National Library of Medicine, 8600 Rockville Pike, Bethesda, MD 20894, (301) 594-5983, (888) 346-3656, Fax: (301) 402-1384, custserv@nlm.nih.gov, http://www.nlm.nih.gov.

Laurie Barclay
Laura Jean Cataldo, RN, EdD

Tremor

Definition

Tremor is an unintentional (involuntary), rhythmic, alternating movement that may affect the muscles of any part of the body. It is the most common movement disorder in the general population worldwide. Tremor is caused by the rapid alternating contraction and relaxation of muscles and is a common symptom of diseases of the nervous system (neurologic disease).

Description

Occasional tremor is felt by almost everyone, usually as a result of fear or excitement; however, uncontrollable tremor or shaking is a common symptom of disorders that destroy nerve tissue, such as **Parkinson's disease** or **multiple sclerosis**. Tremor may also occur after stroke or head injury. Other types of tremor appear without any underlying illness.

Causes and symptoms

Tremor may be a symptom of an underlying disease, and it may be caused by drugs, including caffeine. It may also exist as the only symptom (essential tremor).

Underlying disease

Some types of tremor are signs of an underlying condition. As of 2011, about 500,000 Americans have Parkinson's disease (PD), a progressive disease that destroys nerve cells. About 50,000 new cases are reported each year in North America. Severe shaking is the most apparent symptom of Parkinson's disease. This coarse tremor features four to five muscle movements per second. The shaking is evident at rest—most often in a hand gesture called a pill-rolling tremor—but declines or disappears during movement. Unlike essential tremor, PD is more common in some racial and ethnic groups than others. The rates of PD in Europe and North America are about 56 to 234 per 100,000 people, compared to 14 to 148 per 100,000 in Asia.

Other disorders that cause tremor are multiple sclerosis, alcoholism, **peripheral neuropathy**, Wilson's disease, mercury poisoning, thyrotoxicosis, and liver **encephalopathy**.

A tremor that gets worse during body movement is called an intention tremor. This type of tremor is a sign that something is amiss in the **cerebellum**, a region of the brain concerned chiefly with movement, balance, and coordination.

Essential tremor

Many people have what is called essential tremor (ET), in which the tremor is the only symptom. ET is the most common single type of tremor. According to the International Essential Tremor Foundation (IETF), this type of shaking affects 10 million Americans, mostly older people. About 4–5% of people between the ages of 40 and 60 develop ET; the rate increases to 6–9% in adults over 60. ET is often misdiagnosed as Parkinson's disease. According to the National Institute of Neurological Disorders and Stroke (NINDS), about eight times as many people develop ET as have Parkinson's.

The cause of essential tremor is not known as of 2011, although it is an inherited problem in 60% of all cases. The genetic condition has an autosomal dominant inheritance pattern, which means that any child of an affected parent will have a 50% chance of developing the condition.

Essential tremor (ET) most often appears when the hands are being used, whereas a person with Parkinson's disease will most often have a tremor while walking or while the hands are resting. People with essential tremor will usually have shaking head and hands, but the tremor may also involve other parts of the body. The shaking often begins in the dominant hand and may spread to the other hand (usually within 3 years), interfering with eating, drinking, shaving, applying makeup, and writing. Some people also develop a quavering voice and partial **hearing loss**. ET may be triggered or increased in severity by strong emotion, stress, fever, physical exhaustion, or low blood sugar. Essential tremor may decrease in frequency as the person grows older, but may increase in severity when it does occur.

Essential tremor affects men and women equally and is found in all races and ethnic groups. The shaking often appears at about age 45, although the disorder may actually begin in adolescence or early adulthood. Essential tremor that begins very late in life is sometimes called senile tremor.

Drugs and tremor

Several different classes of drugs can cause tremor as a side effect. These drugs include amphetamines, antidepressant drugs, antipsychotic drugs, caffeine, and lithium. Tremor also may be a sign of withdrawal from alcohol or street drugs.

Psychogenic tremor

Psychogenic tremor—also called hysterical tremor—is a type of tremor caused by an underlying psychological rather than a physical disorder. Its location and intensity may vary, but in general it is characterized by sudden onset and remission; changes in the body part affected; tendency to worsen when the patient is stressed; and tendency to lessen in severity or disappear altogether when the patient's attention is distracted. Psychogenic tremor is sometimes seen in patients diagnosed with conversion disorder, a psychiatric disorder in which the patient's internal emotional conflicts are converted into physical symptoms.

Diagnosis

The diagnosis of tremor is clinical (based on the doctor's observations); there is no definitive laboratory or imaging test for tremor as of 2011. Close attention to where and how the tremor appears can help provide a correct diagnosis of the cause of the shaking. During the office examination, the doctor will look for such features as whether the tremor occurs during movement or at rest; whether it affects both sides of the body or only one; and whether it is worsened or lessened by changes in posture. The doctor will also check the patient for any sensory loss, **weakness** or muscle atrophy, or decreased reflexes.

The source of the tremor can be diagnosed when the underlying condition is found. Diagnostic techniques that make images of the brain, such as computed tomography scan (CT scan) or magnetic resonance imaging (MRI), may help form a diagnosis of multiple sclerosis or other tremor caused by disorders of the **central nervous system**. Blood and urine tests can rule out such metabolic causes as thyroid disease or drug side effects. A family history can help determine whether the tremor is inherited.

The patient may also be asked to complete some performance tests in order to evaluate the type and severity of the tremor as well as any limitations on the patient's functioning. These tests may include writing, drinking from a cup or glass, standing with the arms outstretched, touching the tip of the nose, or drawing a figure. A common test figure is the spiral of Archimedes, named for the Greek mathematician who devised it in the third century BC. Archimedes' spiral is a line generated over time by a point moving away from a fixed point with a constant speed along a line that rotates at a constant angular velocity. A person with tremor will typically produce a jagged-looking rather than a smooth curving line when they try to draw the spiral.

Other tests may include **electromyography**, a technique for measuring the electrical activity in skeletal muscles, both involuntary muscle activity and

Accelerometer—A specialized device attached to the index finger that records the frequency and amplitude (magnitude of change) of hand tremors.

Archimedes' spiral—A figure that is often used as a drawing test in the differential diagnosis of tremor.

Computed tomography (CT) scan—An imaging technique in which cross-sectional x rays of the body are compiled to create a three-dimensional image of the body's internal structures.

Electromyography—A technique for measuring involuntary muscle activity and muscle response to nerve stimulation.

Essential tremor—An uncontrollable (involuntary) shaking of the hands, head, and face. Also called familial tremor because it is sometimes inherited; it can begin in the teens or in middle age. The exact cause is not known.

Fetal tissue transplantation—A method of treating Parkinson's and other neurological diseases by grafting brain cells from human fetuses onto the affected area of the human brain. Human adults cannot grow new brain cells but developing fetuses can. Grafting fetal tissue stimulates the growth of new brain cells in affected adult brains.

Intention tremor—A rhythmic purposeless shaking of the muscles that begins with purposeful (voluntary) movement. This tremor does not affect muscles that are resting.

Liver encephalopathy—A condition in which the brain is affected by a buildup of toxic substances that would normally be removed by the liver. The condition occurs when the liver is too severely damaged to cleanse the blood effectively.

Magnetic resonance imaging (MRI)—An imaging technique that uses a large circular magnet and radio waves to generate signals from atoms in the body. These signals are used to construct images of internal structures.

Multiple sclerosis—A degenerative nervous system disorder in which the protective covering of the nerves in the brain are damaged, leading to tremor and paralysis.

Pallidotomy—A surgical procedure that destroys a small part of a tiny structure within the brain called the globus pallidus internus. This structure is part of the basal ganglia, a part of the brain involved in the control of willed (voluntary) movement of the muscles.

Parkinson's disease—A slowly progressive disease that destroys nerve cells. Parkinson's is characterized by shaking in resting muscles, a stooping posture, slurred speech, muscular stiffness, and weakness.

Psychogenic tremor—Tremor associated with a psychiatric disorder.

Thalamotomy—A surgical procedure that destroys part of a large oval area of gray matter within the brain that acts as a relay center for nerve impulses. The thalamus is an essential part of the nerve pathway that controls intentional movement. By destroying tissue at a particular spot on the thalamus, the surgeon can interrupt the nerve signals that cause tremor.

Thalamus—A large oval area of gray matter within the brain that relays nerve impulses from the basal ganglia to the cerebellum, both parts of the brain that control and regulate muscle movement.

Thyrotoxicosis—An excess of thyroid hormones in the blood, causing a variety of symptoms that include rapid heart beat, sweating, anxiety, and tremor.

Tremor control therapy—A method for controlling tremor by self-administered shocks to the part of the brain that controls intentional movement (thalamus). An electrode attached to an insulated lead wire is implanted in the brain; the battery power source is implanted under the skin of the chest, and an extension wire is tunneled under the skin to connect the battery to the lead. The patient turns on the power source to deliver the electrical impulse and interrupt the tremor.

Wilson's disease—An inborn defect of copper metabolism in which free copper may be deposited in a variety of areas of the body. Deposits in the brain can cause tremor and other symptoms of Parkinson's disease.

muscle response to nerve stimulation. The doctor may also use an accelerometer, which is a specialized device attached to the underside of the patient's index finger. The accelerometer produces a reading called a tremorgram, which records the frequency and amplitude (magnitude) of the tremor.

Treatment

Medications

Neither tremor nor most of its underlying causes can be cured. Most people with essential tremor respond to drug treatment, which may include propranolol, nadolol,

primidone, or a benzodiazepine tranquilizer. Other medications that benefit some patients with tremor include **topiramate**, **gabapentin**, and **zonisamide**. People with Parkinson's disease may respond to levodopa or other **antiparkinson drugs**. Newer medications for tremor that are considered investigational as of 2011 include 1-octanol, pregabalin, memantine, **levetiracetam** (drug used to treat epilepsy), and **sodium oxybate**. There are 153 clinical trials of therapies for tremor under way as of June 2011, most of them involving investigational medications or **deep brain stimulation**.

Research has shown that about 70% of patients treated with **botulinum toxin** A (Botox) have some improvement in tremor of the head, hand, and voice. Botulinum is derived from the bacterium *Clostridium botulinum*. This bacterium causes **botulism**, a form of food poisoning. It is poisonous because it weakens muscles. A very weak solution of the toxin is used in cases of tremor and paralysis to force the muscles to relax. Some patients experience unpleasant side effects with this drug and cannot tolerate effective doses. For other patients, the drug becomes less effective over time. About half of patients do not get any relief of tremor from medications.

Tremor control therapy

Tremor control therapy is a type of treatment using mild electrical pulses to stimulate the brain. These pulses block the brain signals that trigger tremor. In this technique, the surgeon implants an electrode into a large oval area of gray matter within the brain that acts as a relay center for nerve impulses and is involved in generating movement (thalamus). The electrode is attached to an insulated wire that runs through the brain and exits the skull where it is attached to an extension wire. The extension is connected to a generator similar to a heart pacemaker. The generator is implanted under the skin in the chest, and the extension is tunneled under the skin from the skull to the generator. The patient can control his or her tremor by turning on the generator with a handheld magnet to deliver an electronic pulse to the brain.

Some patients experience complete relief with this technique, but for others it is of no benefit at all. About 5% of patients experience complications from the surgical procedure, including bleeding in the brain. The procedure causes some discomfort, because patients must be awake while the implant is placed. Batteries must be replaced by surgical procedure every three to five years.

Other surgical treatments

A patient with extremely disabling tremor may find relief with a surgical technique called thalamotomy, in which the surgeon destroys part of the thalamus. The procedure is complicated by numbness, balance problems, or speech problems in a significant number of cases.

Pallidotomy is another type of surgical procedure sometimes used to decrease tremors from Parkinson's disease. In this technique, the surgeon destroys part of a small structure within the brain called the globus pallidus internus. The globus is part of the basal ganglia, another part of the brain that helps control movement. This surgical technique also carries the risk of disabling permanent side effects.

Fetal tissue transplantation (also called a nigral implant) is a controversial experimental method to treat Parkinson's disease symptoms. This method implants fetal brain tissue into the patient's brain to replace malfunctioning nerves. Unresolved issues include how to harvest the fetal tissue and the moral implications behind using such tissue, the danger of tissue rejection, and how much tissue may be required. Although initial studies using this technique looked promising, there has been difficulty in consistently reproducing positive results.

Small amounts of alcohol may temporarily (sometimes dramatically) ease the shaking. Some experts recommend a small amount of alcohol (especially before dinner). The possible benefits, of course, must be weighed against the risks of alcohol abuse.

Physical therapy

Patients with essential tremor may benefit from consulting a physical therapist for exercises to improve gait, coordination, and muscle control. For example, the therapist may teach the patient to brace the affected limb during the tremor or to hold an affected arm close to the body as a useful technique in improving motion control. The therapist may also recommend such devices as wrist weights or heavier glasses and food utensils to reduce the effects of tremor on daily activities.

Psychotherapy

Patients with psychogenic tremor may find that the tremor disappears completely when the underlying psychological problem is treated.

Alternative medicine

Some patients with essential tremor are helped by **acupuncture**, biofeedback, massage therapy, and hypnosis.

Relaxation guided imagery is reported to benefit some patients with Parkinson's disease.

Prognosis

Essential tremor and the tremor caused by neurologic disease (including Parkinson's disease) slowly get worse and can interfere with a person's daily life. While the condition is not life-threatening, it can severely disrupt a person's everyday experiences.

Prevention

Essential tremor and tremor caused by a disease of the central nervous system cannot be prevented as of 2011. Avoiding use of such stimulant drugs as caffeine and amphetamines can prevent tremor that occurs as a side effect of drug use.

Resources

BOOKS

Albanese, Alberto, and Joseph Jankovic. *Hyperkinetic Movement Disorders: Differential Diagnosis and Treatment.* Chichester, UK: John Wiley and Sons, 2012.

Chitnis, Shilpa, and Richard B. Dewey Jr., eds. *Movement Disorders.* New York: Oxford University Press, 2010.

Sirven, Joseph L., and Barbara L. Malamut, eds. *Clinical Neurology of the Older Adult.* 2nd ed. Philadelphia: Wolters Kluwer Health/Lippincott Williams and Wilkins, 2008.

PERIODICALS

Adler, C.H., et al. "Essential Tremor and Parkinson's Disease: Lack of a Link." *Movement Disorders* 26 (February 15, 2011): 372–77.

Bermejo-Pareja, F. "Essential Tremor—A Neurodegenerative Disorder Associated with Cognitive Defects?" *Nature Reviews Neurology* 7 (May 2011): 273–82.

Crawford, P., and E.E. Zimmerman. "Differentiation and Diagnosis of Tremor." *American Family Physician* 83 (March 15, 2011): 697–702.

Elbie, R., and G. Deuschl. "Milestones in Tremor Research." *Movement Disorders* 26 (May 2011): 1096–1105.

Fahn, S. "Classification of Movement Disorders." *Movement Disorders* 26 (May 2011): 947–57.

Peckham, E.L., and M. Hallett. "Psychogenic Movement Disorders." *Neurologic Clinics* 27 (August 2009): 801–19.

Puschmann, A., and Z.K. Wszolek. "Diagnosis and Treatment of Common Forms of Tremor." *Seminars in Neurology* 31 (February 2011): 65–77.

Sadeghi, R., and W.G. Ondo. "Pharmacological Management of Essential Tremor." *Drugs* 70 (December 3, 2010): 2215–28.

Schlesinger, I., et al. "Parkinson's Disease Tremor is Diminished with Relaxation Guided Imagery." *Movement Disorders* 24 (October 30, 2009): 2059–62.

Shah, R.S., et al. "Deep Brain Stimulation—Technology at the Cutting Edge." *Journal of Clinical Neurology* 6 (December 2010): 167–82.

WEBSITES

"Activa Tremor Control Therapy." Georgetown University Hospital. http://media.georgetownuniversityhospital.org/#/video/Tremor/Activa%20Tremor%20Control%20Therapy/ (accessed July 21, 2011).

"Essential Tremor." Mayo Clinic. http://www.mayoclinic.com/health/essential-tremor/DS00367 (accessed July 21, 2011).

"Essential Tremor Information." WE MOVE. http://www.wemove.org/et/ (accessed July 21, 2011).

"Essential Tremor Test." Mayo Clinic. http://www.mayoclinic.com/health/medical/IM00229 (accessed July 21, 2011).

"Facts about Essential Tremor." International Essential Tremor Foundation (IETF). http://www.essentialtremor.org/Facts-about-ET (accessed July 21, 2011).

"Tremor Fact Sheet." National Institute of Neurological Disorders and Stroke (NINDS). http://www.ninds.nih.gov/disorders/tremor/detail_tremor.htm (accessed July 21, 2011).

"Tremors." MedicineNet. http://www.medicinenet.com/tremor/article.htm (accessed July 21, 2011).

ORGANIZATIONS

American Academy of Neurology (AAN), 1080 Montreal Avenue, Saint Paul, MN 55116, (651) 695-2717, (800) 879-1960, Fax: (651) 695-2791, memberservices@aan.com, http://www.aan.com.

International Essential Tremor Foundation (IETF), P.O. Box 14005, Lenexa, KS 66285-4005, (913) 341-3880, (888) 387-3667, Fax: (913) 341-1296, info@essentialtremor.org, http://www.essentialtremor.org.

National Institute of Neurological Disorders and Stroke (NINDS), P.O. Box 5801, Bethesda, MD 20824, (301) 496-5751, (800) 352-9424, http://www.ninds.nih.gov.

Tremor Action Network (TAN), P.O. Box 5013, Pleasanton, CA 94566, (510) 681-6565, Fax: (925) 369-0485, http://www.tremoraction.org.

Worldwide Education and Awareness for Movement
  Disorders (WE MOVE), 5731 Mosholu Avenue, Bronx,
  NY, United States, 10471, (347) 843-6132, Fax: (718)
  601-5112, wemove@wemove.org, http://
  www.wemove.org.

Carol A. Turkington
Rebecca J. Frey, Ph.D.

Trigeminal neuralgia

Definition

Trigeminal neuralgia is a disorder of the trigemi-nal nerve that causes severe facial pain. It is also known as tic douloureux, Fothergill syndrome, or Fothergill's syndrome.

Description

Trigeminal neuralgia is a rare disorder of the sensory fibers of the trigeminal nerve (fifth cranial nerve), which innervate the face and jaw. The neu-ralgia is accompanied by severe, stabbing pains in the jaw or face, usually on one side of the jaw or cheek,

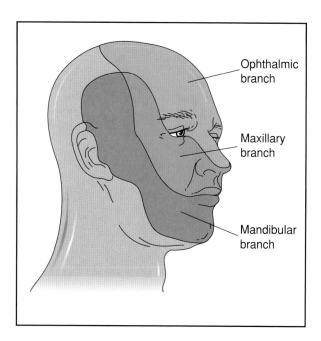

The pains of trigeminal neuralgia are usually extremely intense and are restricted to areas innervated by the trigeminal nerve. Areas where slight stimulation or irritation can trigger excruciating pain may be a few millimeters in size or large and diffuse. *(Illustration by Electronic Illustrators Group. Reproduced by permission of Gale, a part of Cengage Learning.)*

which usually last for some seconds. The pain before treatment is severe; however, trigeminal neuralgia as such is not a life-threatening condition. As there are actually two trigeminal nerves, one for each side of the face, trigeminal neuralgia often affects only one side of the face, depending on which of the two trigeminal nerves is affected.

Demographics

There have been no systematic studies of the prev-alence of trigeminal neuralgia, but the disorder is con-sidered rare. Onset is after the age of 40 in 90% of patients. Trigeminal neuralgia is slightly more com-mon among women than men.

Causes and symptoms

A number of theories have been advanced to explain trigeminal neuralgia, but none explains all the features of the disorder. The trigeminal nerve is made up of a set of branches radiating from a bulblike ganglion (nerve center) just above the joint of the jaw. These branches divide and subdivide to innervate the jaw, nose, cheek, eye, and forehead. Sensation is con-veyed from the surfaces of these parts to the upper spinal cord and then to the brain; motor commands are conveyed along parallel fibers from the brain to the muscles of the jaw. The sensory fibers of the trigeminal nerve are specialized for the conveyance of cutaneous (skin) sensation, including pain.

In trigeminal neuralgia, the pain-conducting fibers of the trigeminal nerve are somehow stimulated, perhaps self-stimulated, to send a flood of impulses to the brain. Many physicians assume that compression of the trigeminal nerve near the spinal cord by an enlarged loop of the carotid artery or of a nearby vein triggers this flood of impulses. Compression is thought to cause trigeminal neuralgia when it occurs at the root entry zone, a .19–.39 in. (0.5–1.0 cm) length of nerve where the type of myelination changes over from peripheral to central. Pressure on this area may cause demyelination, which in turn may cause abnor-mal, spontaneous electrical impulses (pain).

Compression is apparently the cause in some cases of trigeminal neuralgia, but not in others. Other theo-ries focus on complex feedback mechanisms involving the subnucleus caudalis in the brain. **Multiple sclero-sis**, which demyelinates nerve fibers, is associated with a higher rate of trigeminal neuralgia. **Brain tumors** can also be correlated with the occurrence of trigeminal neuralgia. Ultimately, however, the exactly mecha-nisms of trigeminal neuralgia remain a mystery.

Trigeminal neuralgia was first described by the Arab physician Jurjani in the eleventh century. Jurjani was also the first physician to advance the vascular compression theory of trigeminal neuralgia. French physician Nicolaus André gave a thorough description of trigeminal neuralgia in 1756 and coined the term tic douloureux. English physician John Fothergill also described the syndrome in the middle 1700s, and the disorder has sometimes been called after him. Knowledge of trigeminal neuralgia slowly grew during the twentieth century. In the 1960s, effective treatment with drugs and surgery began to be available.

The pains of trigeminal neuralgia have several distinct characteristics:

• They are paroxysmal, pains that start and end suddenly, with painless intervals between.
• They are usually extremely intense.
• They are restricted to areas innervated by the trigeminal nerve.
• As seen on autopsy, nothing is visibly wrong with the trigeminal nerve.
• About 50% of patients have trigger zones, areas where slight stimulation or irritation can bring on an episode of pain. Painful stimulation of the trigger zones is actually less effective than light stimulation in triggering an attack.
• The disorder comes and goes in an unpredictable way; some patients show a correlation of attack frequency or severity with stress or menstrual cycle.

Stimulation of the face, lips, or gums, such as talking, eating, shaving, tooth-brushing, touch, or even a current of air, may trigger the severe knifelike or shock-like pain of trigeminal neuralgia, often described as excruciating. Trigger zones may be a few square millimeters in size, or large and diffuse. The pain usually starts in the trigger zone, but may start elsewhere. Approximately 17% of patients experience dull, aching pain for days to years before the onset of paroxysmal pain; this has been termed pretrigeminal neuralgia.

The pain of trigeminal neuralgia is severe enough that patients often modify their behaviors to avoid it. They may suffer severe weight loss from inability to eat, become unwilling to talk or smile, and cease to practice oral hygiene. Trigeminal neuralgia tends to worsen with time, so that a patient whose pain is initially well-controlled with medication may eventually require surgery.

Diagnosis

Trigeminal neuralgia is a possible diagnosis for any patient presenting with severe, stabbing, paroxysmal pain in the jaw or face. However, the most common

causes of facial pain are dental problems and diseases of the mouth. Trigeminal neuralgia must also be differentiated from migraine headaches and from other cranial neuralgias (i.e., neuralgias affecting cranial nerves other than the trigeminal). Many persons with trigeminal neuralgia see multiple physicians before getting a correct diagnosis and may have multiple dental procedures performed in an effort to relieve the pain.

There is no definitive, single test for trigeminal neuralgia. Imaging studies such as computed tomography (CT) scans or magnetic resonance imaging (MRI) may help to rule out other possible causes of pain and to indicate trigeminal neuralgia. High-definition MRI **angiography** of the trigeminal nerve and brain stem is often able to spot compression of the trigeminal nerve by an artery or vein. Trial and error also has its place in the diagnostic process; the physician may initially give the patient **carbamazepine** (an anticonvulsant) to see if this diminishes the pain. If so, this is positive evidence for the diagnosis of trigeminal neuralgia.

Treatment team

Many different sorts of health care professionals may be consulted by patients with trigeminal neuralgia, including dentists, neurologists, neurosurgeons, oral surgeons, and ear, nose, and throat surgeons. A referral to a neurologist should always be sought, as trigeminal neuralgia is essentially a neurological problem.

Treatment

Treatment is primarily with drugs or surgery. Drugs are often preferred because of their lower risk, but may have intolerable side effects such as nausea or **ataxia** (loss of muscle coordination). The two most effective drugs are carbamazepine (an anticonvulsant often used in treating epilepsy), used for trigeminal neuralgia since 1962, and **gabapentin**. Drugs are prescribed initially in low doses and increased until an effective level is found. Other drugs in use for trigeminal neuralgia are phenytoin, baclofen, clonazepam, lamotrigine **topiramate**, and trileptal.

Carbamazepine, which inhibits the activity of sodium channels in the cell membranes of neurons (thereby reducing their excitability), is deemed the most effective medication for trigeminal neuralgia. Unfortunately, it has many side effects, including **vertigo** (**dizziness**), ataxia, and sedation (mental dullness). This may make it harder to treat elderly patients, who are more likely to have trigeminal neuralgia. Carbamazepine provides complete or partial relief for as many as 70% of patients. Phenytoin is also a sodium channel blocker, and also has adverse side effects, including hirsutism (increased facial hair), coarsening of facial features, and ataxia.

For patients whose pain does not respond adequately to medication, or who cannot tolerate the medication itself due to side effects, surgery is considered. Approximately 50% of trigeminal neuralgia patients eventually undergo surgery of some kind for their condition. The most common procedure is microvascular decompression, also known as the Jannetta procedure after its inventor. This involves surgery to separate the vein or artery compressing the trigeminal nerve. Teflon or polivinyl alcohol foam is inserted to cushion the trigeminal nerve against the vein or artery. This procedure is often effective, but some physicians argue that since other procedures that disturb or injure the trigeminal nerve are also effective, the benefit of microvascular decompression surgery is not relief of compression but disturbance of the trigeminal nerve, causing nonspecific nerve injury that leads to a change in neural activity.

Other surgical procedures are performed, some of which focus on destroying the pain-carrying fibers of the trigeminal nerve. The most high-tech and least invasive procedure is gamma-ray knife surgery, which uses approximately 200 convergent beams of gamma rays to deliver a high (and highly localized) radiation dose to the trigeminal nerve root. Almost 80% of patients undergoing this procedure experience significant relief with this procedure, although about 10% develop facial paresthesias (odd, non-painful sensations not triggered by any external stimulus).

Clinical trials

Information about current clinical trials can be found at ClinicalTrials.gov.

Prognosis

Trigeminal neuralgia is not life threatening. It tends, however, to worsen with time, and many patients who initially were successfully treated with medication must eventually resort to surgery. Some doctors advocate surgery such as microvascular decompression early in the course of the syndrome to forestall the demyelination damage. However, there is still much controversy and uncertainty about the causes of trigeminal neuralgia and the mechanism of benefit even in those treatments that provide relief for many patients.

Resources

BOOKS

Fromm, Gerhard H., and Barry J. Sessle, eds. *Trigeminal Neuralgia: Current Concepts Regarding Pathogenesis and Treatment.* Stoneham, MA: Butterworth-Heinemann, 1991.

Zakrzewska, Joanna M., and P. N. Patsalos. *Trigeminal Neuralgia.* London: Cambridge Press, 1995.

PERIODICALS

Brown, Cassi. "Surgical Treatment of Trigeminal Neuralgia." *AORN Journal* (November 1, 2003).

Mosiman, Wendy. "Taking the Sting out of Trigeminal Neuralgia." *Nursing* (March 1, 2001).

OTHER

Komi, Suzan, and Abraham Totah. "Understanding Trigeminal Neuralgia." *eMedicine.* April 30, 2004 (May 27, 2004). http://www.emedicine.com/med/topic2899.htm.

ORGANIZATIONS

Trigeminal Neuralgia Association. 2801 SW Archer Road, Gainesville, FL 32608. Phone: (352) 376-9955. Fax: (352) 376-8688. Email: tnanational@tna-support.org. http://www.tna-support.org.

Larry Gilman

Triptans

Definition

Triptans are a group of medications used to treat specific types of very painful headaches termed migraine and cluster headaches. The two main drugs are sumatriptan (Imitrex) and zolmitriptan (Zomig).

Purpose

Both migraine and cluster headaches are very painful medical conditions with distinct characteristics. Both sumatriptan and zolmitriptan are used as an abortive treatment for migraine headaches once the headache has already begun. Sumatriptan is also used to treat cluster headaches in a similar abortive manner. Triptan drugs do not prevent the occurrence of headaches, but rather shorten their duration. They are not used prophylactically, rather triptan treatment is simply a source of management to reduce the severity and length of the headache. While triptans are a major part of treatment for migraine and cluster headaches, these conditions are also treated with other drugs for both acute symptoms and to reduce the frequency of attacks. Lifestyle changes involving diet and sleep habits may also be a part of treatment.

Description

Migraine Characteristics

Migraine headaches are a chronic type of headache which have a genetic component. This means that they sometimes run in families. The pain of a **migraine headache** can range from mild to severe and can be debilitating. Migraines are caused by changes in the blood vessels located in the head. The arteries inside and around the skull first spasm and constrict, then rapidly dilate, causing the onset of pulsating pain. Inflammation of these blood vessels is also believed to play a role. Migraines may last anywhere from hours to days, are often unilateral near the eye or at the temples, throbbing, and made worse with exertion. Many migraines also involve painful light sensitivity, painful sound sensitivity, and non-pain symptoms such as nausea, vomiting, **fatigue**, and mood changes. Migraines may be precipitated by certain foods, stress, sleep deprivation, or extreme sensory stimuli such as a long day in bright sun, paint thinner fumes, or high levels of noise for long periods of time. Migraines are more common in women than men. Fluctuating estrogen levels, such as seen during the menstrual cycle, or menopause may trigger migraines. While many patients who suffer from migraines experience them a few times a month, migraines may happen as frequently as a few times a week or as infrequently as a couple times a year.

Migraines may occur with or without an aura (also known as a prodrome), which is a neurological phenomenon that comes on about ten to 30 minutes before the onset of migraine pain. The aura may be perceived by the patient as changes in vision such as flashing or shimmering light around objects or wavy lines in the visual field. Other types of aura include tingling and numbness in the face or the extremities, **dizziness**, irritability, or **weakness**. Traditionally migraine without aura was referred to as a "common migraine," migraine with aura was referred to as a "classic migraine," and migraine with more severe neurological symptoms such

as weakness or difficulty speaking was referred to as a "complex migraine"; however, these terms have fallen out of common use due to the fact that many patients do not experience migraines that fall consistently into one pattern type.

Cluster Headaches

Cluster headaches are excruciatingly sharp and painful headaches that come on quite suddenly. They are usually located in the region of the eye or temple on one side of the head, but pain may also radiate to other areas of the head or neck. Associated symptoms include a one-sided nasal stuffiness, and one-sided eye symptoms such as redness, tearing, swelling, pupillary constriction, or eyelid drooping. Sensitivity to light and nausea may occur with cluster headaches, similar to migraines but with light sensitivity being unilateral. They tend to appear in temporal clusters, meaning there are time periods where these headaches happen, often followed by periods with no **cluster headache**. Clusters may last from weeks to months, with periods of remission that last months or sometimes years. During a cluster the headaches usually occur every day (every 24 hours) at the same time and may last from 15 minutes to several hours. More than one attack may occur within a 24 hour time frame. Attacks tend to come on at night, are painful enough to wake a person with lancinating burning pain, and have earned the nickname "alarm clock headache." Generally cluster headaches are more common in men than women, unlike migraines.

The exact cause of cluster headaches is not well defined. Because cluster headaches occur at regular intervals of the season of the year as well as at the same time of day, it is believed that a part of the brain called the hypothalamus, which is involved in the cyclic biological clock of the body, may play a role. Seasonal effects include an increased frequency of cluster headaches around the periods of the year where daylight savings time changes occur. The hypothalamus is normally responsive to these day length and daily circadian rhythms. An abnormality in this system may be the reason the headaches follow such a pattern. Some clinical studies have demonstrated an increase in brain activity of the hypothalamus during a cluster headache.

Unlike migraines cluster headaches do not seem to be impacted by food or stress, but alcohol and the heart medication nitroglycerin taken in the same time period of a cluster seems to worsen attacks. Like migraines, cluster headaches also have a vascular component (involving blood vessels). Vasodilation (blood vessel dilation) that occurs as part of the abnormal syndrome may cause pressure and irritation to one of the major nerves responsible for sensation in the face.

This large nerve is called the trigeminal nerve, occurs on each side of the face, and has branches that reach around the temple and eye to convey touch and pain sensations to the brain. While pressure on this nerve from vasodilation may cause pain, the original cause of the abnormal physiological changes that led to vasodilation are less well understood.

Triptan Drugs

Triptan drugs such as sumatriptan (Imitrex) and zolmitriptan (Zomig) act directly on the blood vessels involved in an acute attack, to combat the vasodilation associated with the onset of migraine or cluster headache pain. These drugs both constrict blood vessels (vasoconstriction) and decrease inflammation of the vessels involved. Because these drugs act to constrict the blood vessels that dilated specifically in the acute setting of the headache onset, they are not used as a preventative. Triptans work because they activate a chemical receptor for the neurotransmitter serotonin on blood vessels. Neurotransmitters, like serotonin, are chemical messengers that mediate normal processes in the human body like blood vessel regulation. In this case, serotonin is the natural chemical the body would use to cause blood vessel constriction. Triptans mimic this natural chemical by binding to their receptor on the blood vessel surface. They are classified as serotonin receptor modulators. Triptans may also decrease activity of the trigeminal nerve itself, adding to its possible benefit in cluster headaches.

Recommended dosage

Triptan drugs are usually given as oral drugs but may also be given in a subcutaneous (under the skin) injection or nasal spray. For migraine headaches both drugs and all routes of administration are used. There is less information on the effectiveness of the nasal spray form of sumatriptan for cluster headache treatment, or for the use of zolmitriptan for cluster headaches. For cluster headaches injectable sumatriptan is preferred and approved by the Food and Drug Administration (FDA).

A usual oral dose of sumatriptan is between 25 to 100 mg taken at the onset of migraine pain. Zolmitriptan taken orally for migraines is used at a dose of 1.25 to 2.5 mg taken at the onset. Zolmitriptan also comes in orally disintegrating tablets taken in doses of 2.5 to 5 mg. Sumatriptan nasal spray is taken as 5 or 20 mg doses sprayed once in one nostril, or a 5 mg dose sprayed once in each nostril. Zolmitriptan is taken in a dose of 5 mg taken once in one nostril. If the migraine persists or recurs after two hours, a second oral or nasal spray dose may be taken. The maximum oral amount used within 24 hours is 200 mg for sumatriptan and 10 mg for zolmitriptan. The maximum dose for the sumatriptan nasal spray is 40 mg in 24 hours and for zolmitriptan is 10 mg per 24 hours. Subcutaneous injection doses of sumatriptan used for both migraine and cluster headaches are smaller than oral doses. Usually sumatriptan injection is 4 to 6 mg given once, that may be repeated after an hour for up to a maximum of 12 mg within a 24 hour time period. Patients with liver impairment may require lower doses of these drugs to prevent toxicity.

Precautions

Sensitivity to triptan drugs varies among patients, and some patients may find lower doses are more than their body system can tolerate. Triptan overdose may result in a condition known as serotonin syndrome, also called serotonin toxicity, serotonin poisoning, or serotonin storm. Serotonin overdose may be caused by taking multiple drugs that increase the amount of serotonin signaling in the body. While chemical signaling pathways are a part of normal brain function, over-activation can be dangerous. Drugs that increase serotonin signaling may do so by increasing the amount of natural serotonin available to bind to and activate receptors, or by directly activating serotonin receptors themselves. Antidepressants called monoamine oxidase inhibitors (MAOIs) increase the amount of serotonin present as a chemical messenger, and should not be used concurrently with triptans. Antidepressants called selective serotonin reuptake inhibitors (SSRIs) may also need to be avoided. These drugs can cause serotonin overdose if used at the same time or in time periods too close together. Symptoms of serotonin overdose may range from mild to life-threatening, depending on the individual situation. Symptoms may include high blood pressure, high fever, nausea, diarrhea, headache, sweating, increased heart rate, **tremor**, muscle twitching, **delirium**, shock, **coma**, and death.

Triptans may be contraindicated or may require caution in use in patients with uncontrolled hypertension, coronary artery disease, ischemic bowel disease, liver impairment, seizure disorder, vasospastic diseases, and in the elderly. The triptans are classified as category C during pregnancy, which means either there are no adequate human or animal studies or that adverse fetal effects were found in animal studies, but there is no available human data. The decision whether to use category C drugs in pregnancy is generally based on weighing the critical needs of the mother against the risk to the fetus. Other lower category agents are used whenever possible. Breastfeeding should be avoided for 12 hours after triptan use,

KEY TERMS

Aura—The prodrome set of sensory, neurological, and emotional indicators some patients experience about ten to 30 minutes before a migraine attack.

Cytochrome P450 (CYP450)—Enzymes present in the liver that metabolize drugs

Food and Drug Administration (FDA)—Government agency in the United States that regulates rules of use concerning medication.

Monoamine oxidase inhibitors (MAOIs)—Type of antidepressant medication that affects various kinds of neurotransmitters including serotonin.

Neurotransmitter—A chemical messenger that travels through the body and acts in the nervous system. Neurotransmitter signaling is responsible for a wide range of bodily processes and is often the target of medications involving the brain and cardiovascular system.

Neurotransmitter receptor—A physical recipient for chemicals called neurotransmitters. Receptors sit on the surface of cells that make up body tissues, and once bound to the neurotransmitter, they initiate the chemical signaling pathway associated with neurotransmitters.

Serotonin—A type of neurotransmitter involved in regulation of the blood vessels, brain processes, and disease states such as depression.

Serotonin syndrome—A potentially life threatening drug reaction involving an excess of the neurotransmitter serotonin, usually occurring when too many medications that increase serotonin are taken together such as antimigraine triptans and certain antidepressants.

Subcutaneous injection—Injection of a substance such as medication placed just under the surface of the skin.

Vasoconstriction—The narrowing or constriction of a blood vessel lumen.

Vasodilation—The widening or dilation of a blood vessel lumen.

and the drug's overall safety profile in breastfeeding is unknown.

Side effects

Triptan drugs are associated with many adverse reactions, the risk of which increase with dose. Common side effects include hot or cold sensations; jaw, neck, and chest pain, pressure, or tightness; dizziness; numbness and tingling in the extremities; and fatigue. Dry mouth, nausea, stomach discomfort, sweating, and **vertigo** may also occur. The injectable form of sumatriptan is specifically associated with injection site skin reactions, flushing, weakness, and drowsiness or sedation. Nasal sprays may cause throat pain, taste changes, and nasal irritation. Potential serious side effects of triptans that are less common include heart attack, life-threatening heart arrhythmias, severe hypertension crisis, cerebral blood vessel hemorrhaging, permanent blindness, seizures, and serotonin syndrome.

Interactions

Patients should make their doctor aware of any and all medications or supplements they are taking before using triptan medications. Using alcohol while taking these medications may create toxic reactions in the body. Alcohol should be avoided while taking triptan drugs. These medications are metabolized by a set of liver enzymes known as cytochrome P450 (CYP450). There are many subtypes of CYP450 enzymes and triptan drugs interact with multiple subtypes. Drugs that induce, or activate these enzymes may increase the metabolism of triptan drugs. This results in lower levels of therapeutic medication, thereby negatively affecting treatment. Drugs that act to inhibit the action of CYP450 may cause undesired increased levels of triptan drugs in the body. This could lead to increased side effects or even toxic doses. Likewise triptan medications may affect the metabolism of other drugs, leading to greater or lower doses than therapeutically desired. Although triptan drugs are taken for very short time frames, these concerns are still applicable and require guidance from a health care provider.

Triptan drugs activate serotonin receptors and should not be used at the same time as other medications that increase levels of the chemical messenger serotonin in the body. Too much serotonin release or chemical signaling may lead to serotonin syndrome, which can be severe and life threatening. The antidepressant MAOIs increase the amount of serotonin present as a chemical messenger, and should not be used concurrently with triptans. Antidepressant SSRIs may also need to be avoided. Multiple types of triptan drugs should not be used concurrently. The use of the herb St. John's wort while taking triptans may also cause toxicity due to too much serotonin release.

Another example of medications that have a type of additive effect with triptans are the anti-migraine

QUESTIONS TO ASK YOUR PHARMACIST

- Can I take the full dose the first time I use the medication or do I need to slowly increase the dose up to the full amount with use over time?

- What are the side effects I should watch for that tell me I have taken too much of this medication?

- Will this medication interact with any of my other prescription medications?

- Are there any over the counter medications I should not take with this medicine?

- Will this medicine interact with any of my herbal supplements?

- Can I drink alcoholic beverages in the same time frame as taking this medication?

medications called ergotamines and caffeine. Both of these drugs cause vasoconstriction and may have an additive effect with triptans causing adverse effects on the blood vessels. Other vasoconstrictors that should be avoided with triptan use include the commonly used herbs goldenseal, witch hazel, and ma huang. Feverfew, an herbal medication commonly used to treat migraines, may cause dangerous elevations in blood pressure and heart rate if combined with triptans.

Resources

BOOKS

Brunton, Laurence, Bruce A. Chabner, and Bjorn Knollman. *Goodman & Gilman's The Pharmacological Basis of Therapeutics.* 12th ed. New York: McGraw-Hill Professional, 2010.

Silberstein, Stephen D., and Michael J. Marmura. *Essential Neuropharmacology: The Prescriber's Guide.* New York: Cambridge University Press, 2010.

PERIODICALS

Eiland, Lea S., and Melissa O. Hunt. "The use of triptans for pediatric migraines." *Pediatric Drugs* 12.6 (2010): 379.

Johnston, Mollie M., and Alan M. Rapoport. "Triptans for the management of migraine." *Drugs* 70.12 (2010): 1505.

WEBSITES

Bajwa, Zahid H., and Ashraf Sabahat. "Acute Treatment of Migraine in Adults." UpToDate for Clinicians. http://www.uptodate.com/contents/acute-treatment-of-migraine-in-adults?source = search_result%selected Title = 1%7E45 (accessed July 21, 2011).

Cluster Headaches Worldwide Support Group. http://www.clusterheadaches.com (accessed July 21, 2011).

Dean, Laura. "Comparing Triptans." PubMed Health. http://www.ncbi.nlm.nih.gov/pubmedhealth/PMH0004934/ (accessed July 21, 2011).

Epocrates. https://online.epocrates.com (accessed July 21, 2011).

"Migraine: Treatment and Drugs." Mayo Clinic. http://www.mayoclinic.com/health/migraine-headache/DS00120/DSECTION = treatments-and-drugs (accessed July 21, 2011).

ORGANIZATIONS

American Headache Society, 19 Mantua Road, Mount Royal, NJ 08061, (856) 423-0043, Fax: (856) 423-0082, http://www.americanhead achesociety.org.

MAGNUM National Migraine Association, 100 North Union Street, Suite B, Alexandria, VA 22314, (703) 349-1929, http://www.migraines.org.

Maria Basile, PhD

Tropical spastic paraparesis

Definition

Tropical spastic paraparesis (TSP) is a slowly progressive spastic paraparesis caused by the human T-cell lymphotropic virus-1 (HTLV-1), with an insidious onset in adulthood. It has been found all around the world (except in the poles), mainly in tropical and subtropical regions.

Description

For several decades the term "tropical spastic paraparesis" (TSP) was used to describe a chronic and progressive clinical syndrome that affected adults living in equatorial areas of the world. Neurological and modern epidemiological studies found that in some individuals no one cause could explain the progressive **weakness**, sensory disturbance, and sphincter dysfunction that affected individuals with TSP. During the mid-1980s, an important association was established between the first human HTLV-1 virus and idiopathic TSP. Since then, this condition has been named HTLV-1 associated myelopathy/tropical spastic paraparesis or HAM/TSP and scientists now understand that it is a condition caused by a retrovirus that results in immune dysfunction. The main neurological features of HAM/TSP consist of **spasticity** and hyperreflexia (increased reflex action) of the lower extremities, urinary bladder disturbance, lower-extremity muscle weakness, sensory disturbances, and loss of coordination. Patients with HAM/TSP may also exhibit arthritis, lung changes, and inflammation of the skin.

Cofactors that may play a role in transmitting the disorder include being a recipient of transfusion blood products, breast milk feeding from an infected mother, intravenous drug use, or being the sexual partner of an infected individual for several years.

Demographics

Sporadic cases of TSP have been reported in the United States, mostly in immigrants from countries where this disease is endemic (naturally occurring). In the United States, the lifetime risk of an HTLV-1-infected person developing TSP/HAM has been calculated to be 1.7–7%, similar to that reported for United Kingdom, Africa, and the Caribbean.

The international incidence is difficult to estimate because of the insidious nature of this disease. HAM/TSP is common in regions of endemic HTLV-1, such as the Caribbean, equatorial Africa, Seychelles, southern Japan, and South America. However, it also has been reported from non-endemic areas, such as Europe and the United States. The prevalence in southern Japan is in the range of 8.6–128 per 100,000 inhabitants. An estimated 10–20 million individuals worldwide are carriers of HTLV-1.

HAM/TSP generally affects women more than men, with a female-to-male ratio of 3:1. This disease may occur at any age, with a peak in the third or fourth decade.

Causes and symptoms

Causes

The cause of HAM/TSP is still a matter of debate. Whereas only a small proportion of HTLV-1-infected individuals develop HAM/TSP, the mechanisms responsible for the progression of an HTLV-1 carrier state to clinical disease are not clear. However, three hypotheses are considered by scientists as the most likely cause of TSP: direct toxicity, autoimmunity, and bystander damage. The direct toxicity theory of HAM/TSP pathogenesis suggests that HTLV-I-infected cells are directly damaged by certain white blood cells. The autoimmunity theory postulates that the immune system attacks cells that react to HTLV-I infected cells. In the bystander damage hypothesis, circulating antivirus-specific cells migrating through the **central nervous system** produce damage to nearby cells that is directed against the infected cells.

Symptoms

Symptoms may begin years after infection. In response to the infection, the body's immune response may injure nerve tissue, causing various symptoms:

- Spasms and loss of feeling or unpleasant sensations in the lower extremities, accompanied by weakness
- Decreased sense of touch in mid-body areas
- A vibration sensation, especially in the lower extremities, resulting from spinal cord or peripheral nerve involvement
- Low lumbar pain with irradiation to the legs
- Increased reflexes of the upper extremities
- Increased urinary frequency and associated increased incidence of urinary tract infection

Less frequently observed symptoms include tremors in the upper extremities, optical nerve atrophy, deafness, abnormal eye movements, cranial nerve deficits, and absent or diminished ankle jerk reflex.

Diagnosis

During the clinical examination, it is important to exclude other disorders causing progressive spasticity and weakness in the legs. Diagnosis of HAM/TSP criteria typically involve documenting the following:

- Absence of a history of difficulty walking or running during school age
- Within 2 years of onset: increased urinary frequency, nocturia, or retention, with or without impotence; leg cramps or low back pain; symmetric weakness of the lower extremities
- Within 6 months of onset: complaints of numbness or dysesthesias of the legs or feet
- A clinical examination documenting increased reflexes; spasticity of both legs, abnormal gait (manner of walking), and absence of normal sensory level

Laboratory diagnosis using ELISA (enzyme-linked immunosorbent assay) detects the presence of antibodies against HTLV-I, confirmed by the western blot assay. Electrodiagnostic studies and magnetic resonance imaging may also be helpful to show evidence of active denervation, associated to HTLV-1.

Treatment team

Persons with TPS have multiple needs and the team should include a neurologist and a physical therapist. An occupational therapist can prescribe exercises designed to develop fine coordination or compensate for **tremor** or weakness, or suggest assistive devices. More advanced patients require continual nursing assistance.

Treatment

The U.S. Food and Drug Administration (FDA) has not officially approved any drug for the specific treatment of HAM/TSP in the United States. Many patients benefit from oral prednisolone or equivalent glucocorticoid therapy. A response rate of up to 91% has been reported in less advanced cases. Oral treatment with methylprednisolone may produced excellent to moderate responses in around 70% of patients. Plasmapheresis, interferon, oral azathiaprine, danazol, and vitamin C have been tried and also show transient effects. None of these treatments has been systematically studied in a controlled clinical trial. **Antiviral drugs** like AZT would be expected to help in reducing viral replication and associated direct cell injury.

Patients with HAM/TSP sometimes report neuropathic pain. Useful drugs include antiepileptics (e.g., **carbamazepine**, phenytoin, **gabapentin**, **topiramate**), baclofen, and tricyclic antidepressants. The dosages used usually are well bellow those used in the treatment of epilepsy. Physical therapy is commonly used in combination with medication for nerve pain.

Recovery and rehabilitation

The goal of a rehabilitation program for a person affected with HAM/TSP is to restore functions essential to daily living in individuals who have lost these capacities through injury or illness. Most rehabilitation programs are comprehensive in nature and have several different aspects.

Physical therapy is designed to help restore and maintain useful movements or functions and prevent complications such as frozen joints, contractures, or bedsores. Examples of physical therapy include:

• Stretching and range of motion exercises
• Exercises to develop trunk control and upper arm muscles
• Training in walking and appropriate use of assistive devices, such as ambulatory aids, braces, and wheelchairs
• Training in how to get from one spot to another, such as from the bed to a wheelchair or from a wheelchair to the car
• Training in how to fall safely in order to cause the least possible damage.

Occupational therapy focuses on specific activities of daily living that primarily involve the arms and hands. Examples include grooming, dressing, eating, handwriting, and driving.

KEY TERMS

Paraparesis—Weakness of the legs.

Retrovirus—An RNA virus containing an enzyme that allows the viruses' genetic information to become part of the genetic information of the host cell as the virus replicates.

Spastic—Involving uncontrollable, jerky contractions of the muscles.

Some rehabilitation centers have innovative programs designed to help people compensate for loss of memory or slowed learning ability. Rehabilitation may be carried out in a residential or an outpatient setting.

Clinical trials

Current information on clinical trials can be found at the National Institutes of Health website for clinical trials at www.clinicaltrials.gov.

Prognosis

HAM/TSP is usually a progressive neurological disorder, but it is rarely fatal. Most patients live for several decades after the diagnosis. Their prognosis improves if they take steps to prevent urinary tract infection and skin sore formation, and if they enroll in physical and occupational therapy programs.

Special concerns

An important component in the care of patients with TSP is the prevention of infections with the HTLV-1 virus. Several studies indicate that transmission of the HTLV-1 virus occurs through sexual or other intimate contact, intrauterine exposure, newborn exposure via breast milk, sharing of needles by drug abusers, and blood transfusion from infected persons. Transfusion of HTLV-1 antibody-positive blood causes infection in about 60% of recipients. Breastfeeding is contraindicated for mothers who are carriers of HTLV-1.

Resources

BOOKS

Parker, James N., and Philip M. Parker. *The Official Patient's Sourcebook on Tropical Spastic Paraparesis.* San Diego: Icon Group International, 2002.

PERIODICALS

Mora, Carlos A., et al. "Human T-lymphotropic Virus Type I-associated Myelopathy/Tropical Spastic Paraparesis: Therapeutic Approach." *Current Treatment Options in Infectious Diseases* 5 (2003): 443–55.

OTHER

"NINDS Tropical Spastic Paraparesis Information Page." *National Institute of Neurological Disorders and Stroke.* http://www.ninds.nih.gov/health_and_medical/disorders/tropical_spastic_paraparesis.htm (April 20, 2004).

"Tropical spastic paraparesis." *Dr. Joseph F. Smith Medical Library.* Thompson Corporation. http://www.chclibrary.org/micromed/00069230.html (April 20, 2004).

ORGANIZATIONS

National Organization for Rare Disorders (NORD). P.O. Box 1968 (55 Kenosia Avenue), Danbury, CT 06813-1968. Phone: (203) 744-0100. Fax: (203) 798-2291. Toll-free phone: (800) 999-NORD (6673). Email: orphan@rarediseases.org. http://www.rarediseases.org.

National Institute of Allergy and Infectious Diseases (NIAID). 31 Center Drive, Rm. 7A50 MSC 2520, Bethesda, MD 20892-2520. Phone: (301) 496-5717. Tollfree http://www.niaid.nih.gov.

Francisco de Paula Careta
Iuri Drumond Louro

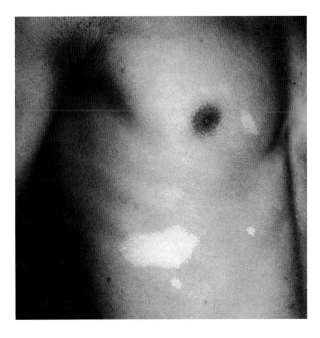

The irregular white blotches, called epiloia depigmentation areas, are typical of tuberous sclerosis. *(Wellcome Trust Library / Custom Medical Stock Photo).*

Tuberous sclerosis

Definition

Tuberous sclerosis (TS)—also known as tuberous sclerosis complex (TSC)—is a rare genetic neurological condition that affects persons of all ages. TS affects many organ systems, including the brain, skin, heart, kidneys, eyes, and lungs. Benign (noncancerous) growths or tumors called hamartomas form in various parts of the body, disrupting their normal functions. The name "tuberous" arises from the potato stem-shaped growths that occur in the brain, also known as tubers. These growths often involve overgrowth of nerves or the connective tissue within them, which is described by the term "sclerosis," which means "hardening." TS is also known as Bourneville's disease, after Désiré-Magloire Bourneville (1840–1909), the French neurologist who first identified it in 1880.

Demographics

Although tuberous sclerosis complex is considered to be a rare condition, estimates of the prevalence of the disorder have increased as clinical testing methods (particularly CT scans and ultrasound) have improved. In the United States, according to the Tuberous Sclerosis Alliance, as many as one child in 6,000 born is affected with TS and about 50,000 people are currently living with the disease. TS is seen in both sexes and all ethnic groups and populations; there are between one and two million cases of TS worldwide. The true incidence of TS may be higher than current statistics indicate because mildly affected individuals may not come to medical attention. TS is reported to affect all ethnic groups and races with equal frequency. Males and females are equally affected with the condition. About one-third of people with TS have an affected parent as well.

The most significant risk factor for TS is having a parent or other blood relative with the disorder. About two-thirds of people diagnosed with tuberous sclerosis have a new mutation in either of the two genes associated with the disorder rather than inheriting a defective gene.

Description

The term "tuberous sclerosis" by itself refers to the small tubers or knoblike growths in the brain of patients with TS that were found on autopsy and can be viewed using computed tomography (also called a CT scan). Persons with TS have a variety of symptoms ranging from very mild to severe; less than one-third of affected persons fit the classic constellation of TS symptoms. Some affected individuals may experience no serious health problems and, in the absence of a thorough clinical examination, may go through life without knowing that they are affected. Conversely, other patients with TS may have problems with behavioral, mental,

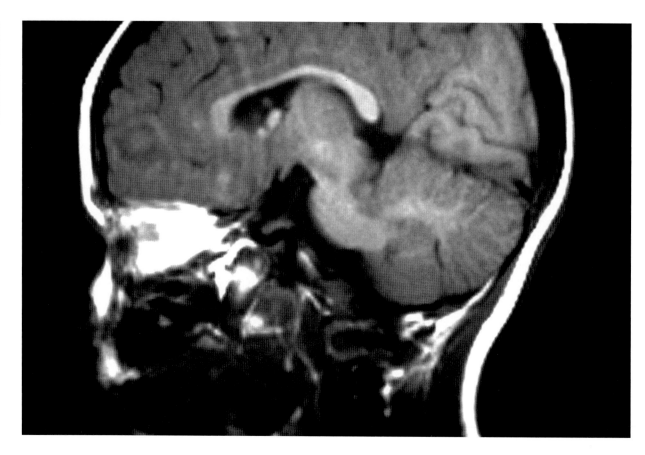

Sagital (side-view) MRI of a brain with tuberous sclerosis. The whitish areas toward the center represent the tubers (hamartomas). *(Living Art Enterprises, LLC / Photo Researchers, Inc.)*

and emotional functions as well as with their kidneys, heart, and eyes. Common symptoms of TS include kidney cysts, kidney growths, and heart tumors that may develop at a very young age or even before birth.

In addition, specific skin abnormalities, often medically insignificant, are among the most common symptoms of TS. Nearly everyone with TS has some symptoms affecting their skin. These include light-colored patches called ash-leaf spots; acne-type growths on the face, nail beds, and body; and areas of rough skin called shagreen patches.

Causes and symptoms

Causes

TS is an autosomal dominant genetic disorder caused by a single change or alteration in a gene called a mutation in either the TSC1 gene located on chromosome 9, or the TSC2 gene located on chromosome 16. These are the only genes known to be associated with TS as of 2011. Approximately two-thirds (66%) of patients with TS have it as the result of a new

mutation (change) in one of the TS genes; that is, it was not inherited from one of their parents. When a new mutation occurs, it most commonly occurs in the TSC2 gene. An individual must have a mutation in one of these two copies of a TS-causing gene in order to develop the condition. In addition, a person who has been diagnosed with TS and who therefore has a genetic mutation in one of the TS genes has a 50% chance of passing on the genetic mutation to his or her offspring. Laboratory testing for changes in the TS genes is available as of 2011; a list of laboratories offering mutation scanning for both genes is available on the Genetics Home Reference page listed under resources below. Prenatal testing of a pregnancy at risk for TS can be done by chorionic villus sampling (at 10 to 12 weeks) or amniocentesis (at 12 to 18 weeks).

The TSC1 gene is responsible for producing a protein called hamartin and TSC2, a protein called tuberin. Both genes are known as tumor suppressor genes, meaning that their normal function is to prevent the growth of tumors. Conversely, tumor growth results when gene function is altered. Research on how the disruption of either protein results in the clinical condition of TS is ongoing.

It is currently believed that every person who inherits or develops a mutation in either the TSC1 or TSC2 gene will develop some form of TS, but the severity of the disease, with its wide range of symptoms and complications, cannot accurately be predicted by identifying the specific gene mutation. Two people who have the same change in the same gene may have very different medical problems and symptoms.

Germline mosaicism can explain the sporadic occurrence of unaffected parents having more than one child with TS. Germline refers to the gonadal cells (sperm in males and eggs in females), while mosaicism refers to the presence of different cell lines in any given individual. A person with germline mosaicism for either the TSC1 or TSC2 gene is not affected with TS but may have an affected child. Unaffected parents of a child with TS have a 2% to 3% chance of having additional affected children. Typical genetic testing methods are performed on such somatic (non-germline) tissues as blood or skin and therefore will not detect germline mosaicism.

Symptoms

The basic underlying cause for illness and, less often, death due to tuberous sclerosis complex is the development of growths called hamartomas throughout the body. Hamartoma is a general term used to describe tumor-like growths that are not cancerous and are composed of cells usually found in that site but poorly developed. While these growths are typically benign (i.e., not cancerous), their presence often disrupts the normal functions of a particular organ system. The various hamartomas found in TS patients can be further distinguished and classified by their location and their histological properties—that is, their physical composition and characteristic appearance under a microscope. As each hamartoma comprises of different cellular elements, each one has a particular name. For example, although both are hamartomas, a fibroma is comprised of connective tissue whereas a lipoma is made up of fat cells.

While the organs affected vary from person to person, most people with TS have some type of skin irregularities called lesions. Some of the most commonly seen skin lesions are hypomelanotic macules—white or light patches sometimes in an ash-leaf shape and called ash-leaf spots. Many people in the general population have one or two light areas of skin, but the presence of three or more such macules in any one individual is considered a major diagnostic finding of

TS. A second major diagnostic feature of the condition is the appearance of small red bumps called fibromas, either on the face (facial angiofibromas) or around or under the finger- or toenails (ungual fibromas). In addition, patches of rough skin termed shagreen patches are highly specific to a diagnosis of TS. Finally, groups of small light circles called confetti spots are considered a minor feature of the disorder.

In contrast to skin lesions, brain lesions tend to be serious and are responsible for the neurological symptoms and cognitive impairment seen in severely affected individuals. There are four primary abnormalities that can be detected by **magnetic resonance imaging** (MRI) or computed tomography (CT) scanning, the first of which are cortical tubers—nodular growths found in the cortex of the brain—and give tuberous sclerosis (literally "hardened growths") its name. Subependymal nodules are growths found underneath the lining of the ventricles in the brain and may cause no problems for the patient unless they grow or begin to block the flow of the cerebral spinal fluid. In contrast, subependymal giant cell astrocytomas, noncancerous **brain tumors** comprised of star-shaped cells and found in about 5% of patients with TS, can, if untreated, result in blindness, hydrocephalus (fluid on the brain), and even death. Finally, cerebral white matter migration lines may be seen through radiographic (x ray) studies and are considered a minor diagnostic feature of TS.

About 85% of affected individuals develop epileptic seizures at some point in their lifetime, most beginning by the first year of life. Research suggests that early control of epilepsy by medication will decrease the chance of a child developing serious mental complications. Between one-half and two-thirds of people with TS have a range of mental abilities from normal to mild or moderate developmental delays and learning disabilities, to severe **mental retardation**. **Autism, attention deficit hyperactivity disorder (ADHD)**, and other behavioral problems are seen in affected individuals.

Fatty kidney tumors, known as renal angiomyolipomas, are one of the most common findings in TS patients, affecting 70–80% of older children and adults, and often cause serious renal malfunction. In addition, the presence of multiple renal cysts (fluid filled areas within the kidneys) is suggestive of the condition. In addition to these benign growths, malignant kidney tumors may also develop.

The most common cardiac symptom is one or more tumors (cardiac rhabdomyomas) in the heart. These tumors are almost exclusively seen in infants and young children and usually spontaneously disappear by late childhood, thereby avoiding the need for surgery. About 47–67% of infants and children with TS have heart tumors and some females develop the rhabdomyomas when they reach puberty.

Tuberous sclerosis affects the eyes in the form of retinal nodular hamartomas—multiple growths on the retina. A discoloration of the retina (retinal achromic patch) is also considered a minor feature of the condition.

In addition to the above, symptoms of TS may include dental pits in the teeth, growths in the rectum (hamartomatous rectal polyps), bone cysts, growths on the gums (gingival fibromas), and other non-specific growths (nonrenal hamartomas). Women with TS may develop lymphangiomyomatosis, a serious lung disease. Furthermore, all individuals with TS are at a higher risk over the general population for developing specific cancers, with 2% of patients developing a malignant tumor in one of the affected body tissues such as kidney or brain.

Diagnosis

Most tuberous sclerosis patients are diagnosed between ages 2 and 6 years, although there are a few cases of adults diagnosed as late as age 22. When a person exhibits signs of TS or has a family history of the condition, an evaluation by a medical geneticist, neurologist, or other qualified professional is recommended to confirm (or rule out) the diagnosis and to recommend screening and management options for the individual. In addition, speaking with a genetic counselor may help families understand the genetics behind the disorder, their recurrence risks (chances of having another affected family member), and the practical and psychosocial implications of the disease on their personal situation.

As a basic understanding of and testing methods for tuberous sclerosis have improved, the criteria used for confirming a diagnosis of tuberous sclerosis have been revised. The National Institutes of Health (NIH) has specified the following diagnostic criteria:

Major features:

• facial angiofibromas or forehead plaque
• nontraumatic ungual or periungual fibroma
• hypomelanotic macules (more than three)
• shagreen patch
• multiple retinal hamartomas
• cortical tuber
• subependymal nodule
• subependymal giant cell astrocytoma

• cardiac rhabdomyoma (one or more)
• lymphangiomyomatosis
• renal angiomyolipoma

Minor features:

• multiple randomly distributed dental pits
• hamartomatous rectal polyps
• bone cysts
• cerebral white matter migration lines
• gingival fibromas
• nonrenal hamartoma
• retinal achromic patch
• confetti skin lesions
• multiple renal cysts

A confirmed diagnosis of TS requires that a patient display two major features or one major and two minor features; a suspected diagnosis with one major and one minor feature; or a possible diagnosis with one major or two minor features in any one individual.

Examination

Detection of hypomelanotic macules (light patches on the skin) can be performed quickly and easily using a special ultraviolet lamp called a Wood's lamp. This light emphasizes the lightened areas on the skin that may otherwise be difficult to see using normal light. Other skin lesions called fibromas are easily visible and identifiable due to their characteristic smooth form, red color, and their even distribution on the face and/or their protrusions among the nails on the fingers and toes. Radiographic imaging using ultrasound, MRI, or CT technology can detect growths present in the brain, kidneys, heart, and eyes.

Tests

Optimal treatment for TS depends on proper disease management. The following tests should be performed on all patients with TS at the time of diagnosis to confirm a diagnosis of the disease as well as obtain baseline medical data for future evaluations:

• dermatologic (skin) examination
• fundoscopic (eye) examination
• renal (kidney) imaging study
• cardiac electrocardiogram (ECG) and echocardiogram (ECHO)
• brain magnetic resonance imaging (MRI)

Aneurysm—Increased size of a blood vessel like an artery, which may burst open.

Angiofibroma—Noncancerous growths on the skin, often reddish in color and filled with blood vessels.

Angiomyolipoma—Noncancerous growth in the kidney, most often found in tuberous sclerosis.

Bone cysts—Fluid- or air-filled space within the bones.

Computed tomography (CT) scan—Three-dimensional internal image of the body, created by combining x-ray images from different planes using a computer program.

Confetti skin lesions—Numerous light or white spots seen on the skin that resemble confetti.

Cortical tuber—Round (nodular) growth found in the cortex of the brain.

Dental pits—Small shallow holes or crevices in the tooth enamel.

Facial angiofibromas—Benign (non-cancerous) tumors of the face.

Forehead plaque—Flat, fibrous skin growth on the forehead.

Gingival fibromas—Fibrous growths found on the gums.

Hamartomatous rectal polyps—Benign (non-cancerous) growths found in the rectum.

Hypomelanotic macules—Patches of skin lighter than the surrounding skin.

Hypsarrhythmia—Typical brain wave activity found in infantile spasms.

Lymphangiomyomatosis—Serious lung disease characterized by the overgrowth of an unusual type of muscle cell resulting in the blockage of air, blood, and lymph vessels to and from the lungs.

Magnetic resonance imaging (MRI)—Three-dimensional internal image of the body, created using magnetic waves.

Mutation—A change in the order of deoxyribonucleic acid (DNA) bases that make up genes, akin to a misspelling.

Nonrenal hamartoma—Benign (non-cancerous) tumor-like growths not found in the kidneys that often disrupt the normal function of a particular organ system.

Nontraumatic ungual or periungual fibroma—Fibrous growth that appears around the fingernails and/or toenails

Plaque—Another term to describe angiofibromas on the forehead.

Renal cell carcinoma—A type of kidney cancer.

Retinal achromic patch—Small area on the retina of the eye that is lighter than the area around it.

Rhabdomyoma—Noncancerous growth in the heart muscle.

Sequencing—Genetic testing in which the entire sequence of deoxyribonucleic (DNA) bases that make up a gene is studied in order to detect a mutation.

Shagreen patches—Patches of skin with the consistency of an orange peel.

Skin tag—Abnormal outward pouching of skin, with a varying size.

Spasms—Sudden involuntary muscle movement or contraction.

Sporadic—Rare and scattered or random in occurrence.

Subependymal giant cell astrocytoma—Benign (non-cancerous) tumor of the brain comprised of star-shaped cells (astrocytes).

Subependymal nodule—Growth found underneath the lining of the ventricles in the brain.

Tubers—Firm growths in the brain, named for their resemblance in shape to potato stems.

Ultrasound—Two-dimensional internal image of the body, created using sound waves.

Vascular—Related to the blood vessels.

White matter radial migration line—White lines seen on a brain scan, signifying abnormal movement of neurons (brain cells) at that area.

Wood's lamp—A special lamp that uses ultraviolet light to detect certain types of skin lesions.

Treatment team

Treatment for people with TS is highly individualized, since symptoms vary greatly. The typical treatment team for someone with TS may include a neurologist, neurosurgeon, medical geneticist, genetic counselor, dermatologist, cardiologist, pulmonologist, nephrologist, ophthalmologist, social worker, and a primary care provider. Care providers in pediatric development are particularly important, including speech-language therapists and pediatric neuropsychologists.

Treatment

Since the characteristic feature of tuberous sclerosis is the growth of benign tumors, treatments are often focused on appropriate surgical interventions to arrest tumor growth or remove tumors whose growth has resulted in or may lead to medical complications, especially in the kidney or brain. Regular brain MRI studies should be performed in children and adults with previous findings as clinically indicated every one to three years in children and, less frequently, in adults without symptoms. In addition, periodic brain electroencephalogram (EEG) studies are recommended for both children and adult patients when clinically indicated.

Children without previous kidney findings should be offered renal imaging studies using ultrasound, MRI, or CT scanning every three years until they reach adolescence and then, every one to three years as adults. Likewise, asymptomatic adults should have imaging of their kidneys every one to three years. Both children and adults who have kidney symptoms should be monitored using imaging studies every six months to one year until the tumor growth stabilizes or decreases.

Any child with cardiac rhabdomyomas should be monitored every six months to one year until the tumor stabilizes or regresses completely. Adults with previous findings of cardiac tumors should be monitored as clinically recommended by their treating physician. While monitoring is important, cardiac rhabdomyomas, as well as retinal lesions and gingival fibromas, usually do not require treatment. In contrast to these benign tumors, cancerous tumors that develop in patients with TSC should be treated by an oncologist.

Facial angiofibromas and peri- and subungual fibromas on the nails are common symptoms in TSC patients. While they are generally not medically significant, they can cause skin irritations or be a cosmetic concern to the individual. Special techniques involving dermabrasion or laser therapy can be performed by a dermatologist or plastic surgeon to remove such growths.

Patients with seizure disorders are prescribed specific medications to control seizures. A newer anti-epileptic drug (vigabatrin) has been shown to be an effective medication in infants with seizures and has been shown to improve long-term outcomes in behavioral and intellectual areas. In addition to controlling seizures, early intervention programs that include special education, behavior modification, physical and occupational therapies, and speech therapy is

QUESTIONS TO ASK YOUR DOCTOR

- Does my child have TS? What diagnostic criteria have been used to make the diagnosis?
- What are the chances of having a second child with TS?
- What treatments do you recommend?
- How severe is my child's disease?
- What is the prognosis?

often recommended for individuals with learning disabilities, developmental delays, mental retardation, autism, and other mental and emotional disorders.

Neurodevelopmental testing is appropriate at the time of diagnosis for all children and should be performed every three years until adolescence and for any adult diagnosed with TS who displays signs of impairment. Subsequent evaluations should be done on both children and adults with previous findings of developmental delays or problems.

While present in only 1% of patients with TS, almost exclusively in females, lung complications can be serious and even fatal. Symptoms may include spontaneous pneumothorax (air in the chest cavity), dyspnea (difficult breathing), cough, hemoptysis (spitting of blood), and pulmonary failure. Therefore, a CT scan of the lungs is recommended for any TSC patient who has symptoms of lung disease or complications and for all female TSC patients at the age of 18. Clinical trials involving tamoxifen and progesterone treatments have shown positive results in some patients with lung disease.

The drug rapamycin (Rapamune) began to be used to treat TS on an experimental basis in 2011. Rapamycin is an immunosuppressant that appears to improve memory and learning in TS patients. As of mid-2011, there were 12 clinical trials under way of treating TS patients with rapamycin and 12 additional trials of a related drug called everolimus (Zortress). The Food and Drug Administration (FDA) approved the use of everolimus to treat subependymal giant cell astrocytomas in October 2010.

Prognosis

The life span of individuals with TS varies with the severity of the condition in any one person. Many affected people have normal life expectancies and a high quality of life, relatively free of symptoms or complications of the disease. Conversely, severely affected or disabled individuals may experience a shortened life span and a high rate of illness and medical complications; about 25% of severely affected infants die before age 10 and 75% die before age 25. Therefore, proper disease management, diagnostic monitoring, and follow-up are critical to achieving and maintaining optimal health in patients with TS.

Prevention

Apart from prenatal diagnosis, there is no effective way to prevent tuberous sclerosis as of 2011, particularly since so many cases involve new mutations of the TSC1 and TSC2 genes.

Resources

BOOKS

Ahmad, Shamim I. *Diseases of DNA Repair*. Austin, TX: Landes Bioscience, 2010.

Irivine, Alan, Peter Hoeger, and Albert Yan, eds. *Harper's Textbook of Pediatric Dermatology*. 3rd ed. Chichester, UK: Wiley-Blackwell, 2011.

Rowland, Lewis P., and Timothy A. Pedley, eds. *Merritt's Neurology*. 12th ed. Philadelphia: Lippincott Williams and Wilkins, 2010.

PERIODICALS

Berhouma, M. "Management of Subependymal Giant Cell Tumors in Tuberous Sclerosis Complex: The Neurosurgeon's Perspective." *World Journal of Pediatrics* 6 (May 2010): 103–10.

Borkowska, J., et al. "Tuberous Sclerosis Complex: Tumors and Tumorigenesis." *International Journal of Dermatology* 50 (January 2011): 13–20.

Chu-Shore, C.J., et al. "The Natural History of Epilepsy in Tuberous Sclerosis Complex." *Epilepsia* 51 (July 2010): 1236–41.

Lam, C., et al. "Rapamycin (Sirolimus) in Tuberous Sclerosis Associated Pediatric Central Nervous System Tumors." *Pediatric Blood and Cancer* 54 (March 2010): 476–79.

Numis, A.L., et al. "Identification of Risk Factors for Autism Spectrum Disorders in Tuberous Sclerosis Complex." *Neurology* 76 (March 15, 2011): 981–87.

Orlova, K.A., and P.B. Crino. "The Tuberous Sclerosis Complex." *Annals of the New York Academy of Sciences* 1184 (January 2010): 87–105.

Tiberio, D., et al. "Regression of a Cardiac Rhabdomyoma in a Patient Receiving Everolimus." *Pediatrics* 127 (May 2011): e1335–37.

Tsai, P., and M. Sahin. "Mechanisms of Neurocognitive Dysfunction and Therapeutic Considerations in Tuberous Sclerosis Complex." *Current Opinion in Neurology* 24 (April 2011): 106–13.

WEBSITES

Franz, David Neal. "Tuberous Sclerosis." Medscape Reference. http://emedicine.medscape.com/article/1177711-overview (accessed July 21, 2011).

"Information Sheets." Tuberous Sclerosis Alliance (TSA). http://www.tsalliance.org/pages.aspx?content = 522 (accessed July 21, 2011).

"NINDS Tuberous Sclerosis Information Page." National Institute of Neurological Disorders and Stroke (NINDS). http://www.ninds.nih.gov/disorders/tuberous_sclerosis/tuberous_sclerosis.htm (accessed July 21, 2011).

Northrup, Hope, and Au, Kit Sing. "Tuberous Sclerosis Complex." *GeneReviews*, edited by Roberta A. Pagon, et al. Seattle: University of Washington, 1993–2011. http://www.ncbi.nlm.nih.gov/books/NBK1220/ (accessed July 21, 2011).

"Tuberous Sclerosis Complex." Genetics Home Reference. http://ghr.nlm.nih.gov/condition/tuberous-sclerosis-complex (accessed July 21, 2011).

ORGANIZATIONS

National Institute of Neurological Disorders and Stroke (NINDS), P.O. Box 5801, Bethesda, MD 20824, (301) 496-5751, (800) 352-9424, http://www.ninds.nih.gov.

National Organization for Rare Disorders (NORD), 55 Kenosia Avenue, P.O. Box 1968, Danbury, CT 06813-1968, (203) 744-0100, (800) 999-6673, http://www.rarediseases.org.

Tuberous Sclerosis Alliance (TSA), 801 Roeder Road, Suite 750, Silver Spring, MD 20910-4467, (301) 562-9890, (800) 225-6872, Fax: (301) 562-9870, info@tsalliance.org, http://www.tsalliance.org/.

Tuberous Sclerosis Clinic, Children's Hospital Colorado, 13123 East 16th Avenue, Box B155, Aurora, CO 80045, (720) 777-6895, http://www.the childrenshospital.org/conditions/nervous/conditions/tuberous-sclerosis.aspx.

Deepti Babu, MS, CGC
Rebecca J. Frey, PhD

Ulnar neuropathy

Definition

Ulnar neuropathy is an inflammation or compression of the ulnar nerve, resulting in paresthesia (numbness, tingling, and pain) in the outer side of the arm and hand near the little finger.

Description

The ulnar nerve transmits impulses to muscles in the forearm and hand. The nerve is responsible for the proper sensing of touch, texture, and temperature throughout the fourth and fifth digits of the hand, the palm, and the underside of the forearm. Ulnar neuropathy arises most commonly because of damage to the nerve as it passes through the wrist. The elbow is also a frequent site of nerve damage. Ulnar neuropathy is variously known as bicycler's neuropathy, cubital tunnel syndrome, Guyon or Guyon's canal syndrome, and tardy ulnar palsy.

Demographics

Ulnar neuropathy that originates at the elbow is very common. Estimates are that 40 percent of Americans experience some form of this neuropathy at some point in their lives. While the ulnar nerve is structurally identical in men and women, men tend to develop ulnar neuropathy more than women. This is because men generally do not have as much fat overlaying the elbow, and so the underlying nerve can be more susceptible to irritation and damage.

The onset of ulnar neuropathy can occur slowly. As a result, many of those who are affected are middle-aged or older adults. Demographic risk factors include a family history of diabetes, alcoholism, and presence of human immunodeficiency virus. Because leaning on the elbows can trigger ulnar neuropathy, people such as telephone operators, receptionists, and those who operate computers for extended periods of time are at risk for developing the disorder.

Causes and symptoms

Ulnar neuropathy is caused by nerve damage. The nature of the nerve damage is varied and can result from inflammation or compression. Nerve damage at the elbow can result from compression of the nerve when sensation is obliterated during general anesthesia. A blow to the elbow or even too much leaning on the elbow can be damaging as well, as can diseases (rheumatoid arthritis) and metabolic disturbances (diabetes). Even malnutrition can be a factor, as protective fatty deposits and muscle mass waste away. Damage to the nerve at the wrist can be caused by a blow, tumors, and impinging of an artery.

The nerve damage that results in ulnar neuropathy can involve the main body of the nerve, the branching region at the end of the nerve known as the axon (which is involved in the movement of the nerve impulse to the adjacent nerve), and the protective myelin coating around the nerve. When the main body of the nerve is involved, the problem is usually a block in the passage of the impulse down the nerve. Axon damage typically decreases the movement of the nerve impulse away from the nerve or the wavelength of the impulse. As a result, the impulse may not reach the adjacent nerve or may not be recognized by the receptors of that adjacent nerve. Finally, damage to the myelin sheath (demyelination) also impedes the movement of signal down the body of the nerve.

Depending on the site of the neuropathy and whether the neuropathy arises suddenly (acute) or has been present for a long time (chronic), various symptoms can arise. Acute and chronic ulnar neuropathy of the elbow is always associated with numbness and **weakness**. Pain is present almost 40% of the time in the acute form of the disorder and almost 80% of the time in the chronic disorder. When the ulnar neuropathy involves the wrist, weakness is ever-present in a main muscle

KEY TERMS

Axon—The long, slender part of a nerve cell that carries electrochemical signals to another nerve cell.

Electromyogram—Often done after a nerve conduction velocity test, an electromyogram (EMG) is a diagnostic used test to evaluate nerve and muscle function.

Myelin sheath—Insulating layer around some nerves that speeds the conduction of nerve signals.

Nerve impulse—The electrochemical signal carried by an axon from one neuron to another neuron.

Neuron—A nerve cell.

Orthotic device—Devices made of plastic, leather, or metal which provide stability at the joints or passively stretch the muscles.

Paresthesia—Abnormal physical sensations such as numbness, burning, prickling, or tingling.

controlling wrist movement, generalized weakness in the absence of pain in 50% of those afflicted, and finger numbness occurs in about 25% of cases.

Other physical signs include the adoption of a clawed shape by the hand and the inability of the entire thumb to move to the forefinger in a single motion.

Diagnosis

Typically, the development of weakness in the elbow or wrist is the sign that alerts a clinician to the possibility of ulnar neuropathy. Follow-up tests can include ultrasound or magnetic resonance imaging to visualize cysts or structural abnormalities. The functioning of the nerve can be assessed in a nerve conduction test. Laboratory analyses of blood can be done to detect the presence of diabetes or infections that can damage nerves (such as **Lyme disease**, human immunodeficiency virus, hepatitis viruses).

Treatment team

Treatment can involve the family physician, family members, neurosurgeons, hand surgeon, pain specialist, and physical and occupational therapists. Therapists can often provide exercises that assist in maximizing muscular strength and orthotic devices to maintain proper positioning during repetitive or stressful movements, thereby reducing inflammation.

Treatment

Treatment can consist of the use of nonsteroidal anti-inflammatory drugs to control swelling around the nerve.

The use of splints or cushions can ease the discomfort and the stress on the ulnar nerve. For some, surgery is a useful option, when relief can be gained by removal of a cyst or correction of damage caused by a blow.

Recovery and rehabilitation

Sports and other normal activity can be resumed when the person is able to perform normal hand-gripping tasks such as opening a jar, forcefully grip a tennis racquet or bicycle handlebars, or work at a keyboard without pain or tingling in the elbow or hand. Braces and other orthotic devices, if worn consistently, often prevent reoccurrence of ulnar neuropathy.

Prognosis

If nerve damage has been caused by a blow or by trauma such as putting too much pressure on the elbow or wrist, recovery can be complete.

Resources

PERIODICALS

Hochman, M. G., and J. L. Zilberfarb. "Nerves in a pinch: imaging of nerve compression syndromes." *Radiology Clinics of North America* (January 2004): 221–45.

Kern, R. Z. "The electrodiagnosis of ulnar nerve entrapment at the elbow." *Canadian Journal of Neurological Science* (November 2003): 314–19.

OTHER

"Ulnar Neuropathy." *emedicine.com*. http://www.emedicine.com/neuro/topic387.htm (May 5, 2004).

ORGANIZATIONS

American Chronic Pain Association (ACPA). P.O. Box 850, Rocklin, CA 95677-0850. Phone: (916) 632-0922. Fax: (916) 632-3208. Tollfree phone: (800) 533-3231. Email: ACPA@pacbell.net. http://www.theacpa.org.

National Chronic Pain Outreach Organization (NCPOA). P.O. Box 274, Millboro, VA 24460. Phone: (540) 862-9437. Fax: (540) 862-9485. Tollfree Email: ncpoa@cfw.org. http://www.chronicpain.org.

National Institute for Neurological Diseases and Stroke. P.O. Box 5801, Bethesda, MD 20824. Phone: (301) 496-5751. Tollfree phone: (800) 352-9424. http://www.ninds/nih.gov.

National Institute of Arthritis and Musculoskeletal and Skin Diseases (NIAMS). 31 Centre Dr., Rm. 4Co2 MSC 2350, Bethesda, MD 20892-2350. Phone: (301) 496-8190. Tollfree phone: (877) 226-4267. Email: info@mail.nih.gov. http://www.niams.nih.gov.

Brian Douglas Hoyle, Ph.D.

Ultrasonography

Definition

Ultrasonography is the study of internal organs or blood vessels using high-frequency sound waves. The actual test is called an ultrasound scan or sonogram. Duplex ultrasonography uses Doppler technology to study blood cells moving through major veins and arteries. There are several types of ultrasound. Each is used in diagnosing specific parts of the body.

Purpose

An ultrasound is a noninvasive, safe method of examining a patient's eyes, pelvic or abdominal organs, breast, heart, or arteries and veins. It is often used to diagnosis disease, locate the source of pain, or look for stones in the kidney or gallbladder. Ultrasound produces images in real time. Images appear on the screen instantly. It may also be used to guide doctors who are performing a needle biopsy to locate a mass. (Needle biopsies are often used to obtain a sample of breast tissue to test for cancer cells.) Duplex/Doppler ultrasound aids in diagnosing a blockage in or a malformation of the vessel. Different color flows aid in identifying problem areas in smaller vessels. Endoscopic ultrasound combines a visual endoscopic exam, during which a flexible tube called an endoscope is threaded down the throat, with an ultrasound test. The ultrasound probe is attached to the end of the endoscope. An endoscopic ultrasound is helpful in determining how deeply a tumor has grown into normal tissues or the gastrointestinal tract. During a transvaginal ultrasound, the ultrasound probe is inserted into the vagina to obtain better images of the ovaries and uterus. Color flow Doppler imaging, using a transvaginal probe, is being performed to detect abnormal blood flow patterns associated with ovarian cancer.

Ultrasound applications in neurology are called neurosonography, which refers to ultrasound images of the brain and spinal column. These studies assess the blood flow within the brain and can be used to diagnose stroke, brain tumors, hydrocephalus, and other vascular problems in the brain and spinal column. Neurosonography can also delineate inflammatory processes, soft tissue masses, as well as ligamentous, muscular, and tendon injuries. Transcranial Doppler ultrasound provides images of the arteries and blood vessels in the neck, to assess blood flow and to quantify the risk of stroke.

Precautions

Ultrasound is considered safe with no known risks or precautions. The exam uses no radiation. Under

QUESTIONS TO ASK THE DOCTOR

- Did you see any abnormalities?
- What future care will I need?

normal circumstances the exam is normally painless; however, if the patient has a full bladder, pressure exerted during the exam may feel uncomfortable. An ultrasound conducted in conjunction with an invasive exam carries the same risks as the invasive exam.

Description

The patient will be asked to lie still on an exam table in a darkened room. The darkness helps the technician see images on a screen, which is similar to a computer monitor. Sometimes the patients are positioned so they can watch the screen. The technician will apply a lubricating gel to the skin over the area to be studied. Ultrasound uses high-frequency sound waves to produce an image. A small wand-like device called a transducer produces sound waves that are sent into the body when the device is pressed against the skin. The gel helps transmit the sound waves, which do not travel through the air. Neither the patient nor the technician can hear the sound waves. The technician moves the device across the skin in the area to be studied. The sound waves bounce off the fluids and tissues inside the body. The transducer picks up the return echo and records any changes in the pitch or direction of the sound. The image is immediately visible on the screen. The technician may print a still picture of any significant images for later review by the radiologist.

Preparation

Depending on the type of ultrasound ordered, patients may not need to do anything prior to the test. Other ultrasound studies may require that the patient not eat or drink anything for up to 12 hours prior to the exam, in order to decrease the amount of gas in the bowel. Intestinal gas may interfere in obtaining accurate results. The patient must have a full bladder for some exams and an empty bladder for others.

Aftercare

Remove any gel still left on the skin. No other aftercare is required following an ultrasound.

KEY TERMS

Biopsy—Removal of a tissue sample for examination under a microscope to check for cancer cells.

Endoscopy—Examination of the upper gastrointestinal tract using a thin, flexible instrument called an endoscope.

Radiologist—Doctor who has received special training and is experienced in performing and analyzing ultrasounds and other radiology exams.

Risks

Standard, diagnostic ultrasound is considered risk-free. Risks may be associated with invasive tests conducted at the same time, such as an endoscopic ultrasound or an ultrasound-guided needle biopsy.

Normal results

An ultrasound scan is considered normal when the image depicts normally shaped organs or normal blood flow.

Abnormal results

Abnormal echo patterns may represent a condition requiring treatment. Any masses, tumors, enlarged organs, or blockages in the blood vessel are considered abnormal. Additional testing may be ordered.

Resources

BOOKS

Bradley, W., et al. *Neurology in Clinical Practice*. 5th ed. Philadelphia: Butterworth-Heinemann, 2008.

Goetz, C.G. *Goetz's Textbook of Clinical Neurology*. 3rd ed. Philadelphia: Saunders, 2007.

PERIODICALS

Mehta, S. "Neuroimaging and transcranial ultrasonography in Parkinson's disease." *Current Neurology and Neuroscience Report* 8 (July 1, 2008): 297–303.

Tsivgoulis, G. "Advances in transcranial Doppler ultrasonography." *Current Neurology and Neuroscience Report* 9 (January 1, 2009): 46–54.

Debra Wood, RN
Rosalyn Carson-DeWitt, MD

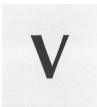

Valproic acid and divalproex sodium

Definition

Valproic acid is an anticonvulsant used to control seizures in the treatment of epilepsy, a neurological dysfunction in which excessive surges of electrical energy are emitted in the brain.

Valproic acid is closely related to divalproex sodium and valproate sodium. While these drugs are primarily used in the treatment of epilepsy, divalproex sodium is also indicated for the treatment of manic episodes (abnormally and persistently elevated mood) associated with bipolar disorder.

Purpose

Valproic acid is thought to depress activity in certain areas of the brain, suppressing the irregular firing of neurons to prevent seizures. Divalproex sodium is a stable coordination compound formed with valproic acid.

While valproic acid and divalproex sodium control the seizures associated with epilepsy, there is no known cure for the disease.

Description

In the United States, valproic acid and divalproex sodium are sold under the brand names Depekene and Depakote. Valproic acid is available in tablet and syrup form. Divalproex sodium is available in tablet, injection, or in sprinkle form.

Recommended dosage

Valproic acid usually requires two to four oral doses each day. The typical total daily dose is initiated at 15mg per kilogram (2.2 lb) of body weight and is increased in weekly intervals by 5–10 mg per kilogram of body weight until seizures are controlled. The frequency of adverse effects may increase with increasing doses; therefore, changes in dosage are made gradually. It may require several weeks of dosage titration (adjustment for maximum benefit and minimum risk) to realize the full benefits of valproic acid or divalproex sodium.

Persons should not take a double dose of anticonvulsant medications. If a daily dose is missed, it should be taken as soon as possible. However, if it is almost time for the next dose, the missed dose should be skipped.

When discontinuing treatment involving valproic acid or divalproex sodium, physicians typically direct patients to gradually reduce their daily dosages. Stopping the medicine suddenly may cause seizures to occur or become more frequent.

Precautions

Persons should avoid alcohol while taking valproic acid or divalproex sodium. It can exacerbate (heighten) the side effects of alcohol and other medications. A physician should also be consulted before individuals take valproic acid or divalproex sodium with certain non-prescription medications, such as medicines for asthma, appetite control, coughs, colds, sinus problems, allergies, and hay fever.

Valproic acid and divalproex sodium may not be suitable for persons with a history of liver or kidney disease, mental illness, high blood presure, angina (chest pain), irregular heartbeats, or other heart problems. Valproic acid and divalproex sodium may cause liver damage (hepatotoxicity), though the risk is low in adults. The prescribing physician may order routine blood tests to screen for liver damage.

Before beginning treatment with valproic acid or divalproex sodium, patients should notify their physician if they consume a large amount of alcohol, have a history of drug use, are pregnant, or plan to become pregnant.

Valproic acid and divalproex sodium may cause birth defects and has been linked to an increased risk of **spina bifida**. Physicians often counsel their patients to use effective birth control while taking either of these medications. Unlike many other anti-convulsant medications, valproic acid will not decrease the effectiveness of oral contraceptives (birth control pills). Patients who become pregnant while taking valproic acid or divalproex sodium should contact their physician immediately.

Side effects

Research indicates that valproic acid and divalproex sodium are generally well tolerated. In certain individuals and especially children under two years of age, however, valproic acid may cause severe damage to the liver or pancreas. It is important to keep all appointments with the physician and laboratory to monitor the body's response to valproic acid. Temporary nausea, vomiting, stomach cramps, weight gain, temporary hair loss, shaking, and an irregular menstural cycle are the most frequently reported side effects of valproic acid and divalproex sodium. Other possible side effects include:

• Nervousness
• Anxiety
• Dificulty with memory
• Double vision
• Loss of appetite
• Restlessness
• Sleepiness or sleeplessness
• Unusual drowsiness
• Diarrhea or constipation
• Heartburn or indigestion
• Aching joints and muscles or chills
• Unpleasant taste in mouth or dry mouth
• Tingling or prickly feeling on the skin

Many of these side effects disappear or occur less frequently during treatment as the body adjusts to the medication.

Other, uncommon side effects of valproic acid and divalproex sodium can be potentially serious. Patients taking valproic acid who experience any of the following symptoms should contact their physician:

• Jaundice (yellow tone to skin and eyes)
• Facial swelling
• Persistent fatigue
• Rash
• Mood or mental changes

• Depression
• Persistent trembling of the arms and hands
• Restlessness
• Excessive sleeplessness
• Hallucinations
• Difficulty breathing
• Chest pain
• Irregular heartbeat
• Faintness
• Persistant, severe headaches
• Persistant fever or pain

Interactions

Valproic acid and divalproex sodium may have negative interactions with some antacids, tricyclic antidepressants, antibiotics, monoamine oxidase inhibitors (MAOIs), and asprin and other non-steroidal anti-inflammatories NSAIDs. Other medications such as **diazepam** (Valium), **phenobarbital** (Luminal, Solfoton), nefazodone, metronidazole, **acetazolamide** (Diamox), phenytoin (Dilantin), **primidone**, propranolol (Inderal), and warfarin may also adversely react with volparic acid.

Volparic acid and divalproex sodium may react adversely with other anticonvulsants and anti-epilepsy drugs (AEDs). It should be used with other seizure prevention medications only if advised by a physician.

Resources

BOOKS

Weaver, Donald F. *Epilepsy and Seizures: Everything You Need to Know*. Richmond Hill, ONT, Canada: Firefly Books, 2001.

OTHER

American Society of Health-System Pharmacists, Inc. "Valproic acid." *Medline Plus*. http://www.nlm.nih.gov/medlineplus/druginfo/medmaster/a682412.html (March 20, 2004).

"Introduction to valproic acid." *Epilepsy.com*. The Epilepsy Project. http://www.epilepsy.com/medications/b_valproicacid_intro.html (March 20, 2004).

ORGANIZATIONS

Epilepsy Foundation. 4351 Garden City Drive, Landover, MD 20785-7223. Phone: (800) 332-1000. Tollfree phone: (800) 332-1000. http://www.epilepsyfoundation.org.

American Epilepsy Society. 342 North Main Street, West Hartford, CT 06117-2507. http://www.aesnet.org.

Adrienne Wilmoth Lerner

Vasculitic neuropathy

Definition

Vasculitic neuropathy refers to damage to the peripheral nerves (the nerves that are located outside the brain and spinal cord) as a consequence of **vasculitis** (a condition characterized by inflammation and destruction of blood vessels).

Description

Vasculitis refers to a number of conditions that cause inflammation in the blood vessels of the body. This inflammation can prevent sufficient blood flow from reaching various organs and tissues of the body. Because adequate blood flow is required to provide the organs and tissues with oxygen, vasculitis causes damage to oxygen-deprived organs and tissues. When peripheral nerves are oxygen-deprived due to vasculitis, vasculitic neuropathy ensues.

Peripheral neuropathy can occur as the only symptom of vasculitis, or it can be part of a symptom complex.

Demographics

About 60-70% of all patients with vasculitis will experience peripheral neuropathy. In fact, about 34% of all patients with vasculitis will manifest peripheral neuropathy as the sole manifestation of their vasculitis. The average age of an individual with vasculitic neuropathy is 62.

Causes and symptoms

Vasculitic neuropathy can accompany a number of types of vasculitis, including polyarteritis nodosa, Churg-Strauss syndrome, Wegener's granulomatosis, Sjogren's syndrome, rheumatoid vasculitis, and vasculitis due to infections (such as **Lyme disease**, hepatitis, HIV). Vasculitis occurs when the body's immune system accidentally misidentifies markers on the blood vessel walls as foreign. The immune system then begins to produce immune cells that attack and destroy the blood vessels. As the blood vessels become inflamed, blood flow through them is diminished, resulting in oxygen deprivation of the organs or tissues they normally serve. When the oxygen-deprived tissues are nerve cells, vasculitic neuropathy results.

Most people with vasculitic neuropathy notice pain and then **weakness** in a random, nonsymmetric distribution throughout their limbs; a smaller number (about one-third of all sufferers) notice pain and weakness that progress in a symmetric fashion, beginning with the feet or hands and progressing up the limbs. The pain of vasculitic neuropathy can include shooting, sharp pain, tingling, numbness, burning, and stinging. Some patients with vasculitic neuropathy will also experience fever, decreased appetite, weight loss, rash, **fatigue**, joint pain, and kidney problems.

Diagnosis

Examining a sample of an affected nerve cell (**biopsy**) will allow the diagnosis to be made. The biopsy will demonstrate the inflammation and destruction of blood vessel walls characteristic of vasculitis. Electrodiagnostic studies use needle electrodes to stimulate affected nerves or muscles, in order to demonstrate a slow or abnormal response.

Treatment team

Vasculitic neuropathy may be treated by a neurologist or a rheumatologist. Physical and occupational therapists can help optimize recovery of function.

Treatment

Treatment for vasculitic neuropathy involves medications that decrease inflammation and suppress the activity of the immune system. Such medications include cortciosteroids and cyclophosphamide. Physical and occupational therapy can help restore functioning and can provide strategies to help overcome any permanent disabilities caused by the vasculitic neuropathy.

Prognosis

Once treatment for vasculitic neuropathy has been initiated, symptom progression should halt, and the condition should stabilize. Some improvement in already established symptoms is possible; pain may decrease, and some degree of weakness may improve, although recovery of function is usually very slow and only partial.

Resources

BOOKS

Chalk, Colin. "Peripheral Neuropathies." In *Conn's Current Therapy 2004*, 56th edition, edited by Robert E. Rakel, et al. Philadelphia: Elsevier, 2004.

Griffin, John W. "Immune-Mediated Neuropathies." In *Cecil Textbook of Internal Medicine*, edited by Lee Goldman, et al. Philadelphia: W. B. Saunders, 2000.

PERIODICALS

Griffin, John W. "Vasculitic Neuropathies." *Rheumatic Diseases Clinics of North America* 27 (November 2001): 751–760

Nadeau, S. E. "Neurologic Manifestations of Systemic Vasculitis." *Neurologic Clinics* 20, no. 1 (February 2002): 123–50.

Pascuzzi, Robert M. "Peripheral Neuropathies in Clinical Practice." *Medical Clinics of North America* 87 (May 2003): 697–724.

Rosalyn Carson-DeWitt, MD

Vasculitis

Definition

Vasculitis refers to a varied group of disorders which all share a common underlying problem of inflammation of a blood vessel or blood vessels. The inflammation may affect any size blood vessel, anywhere

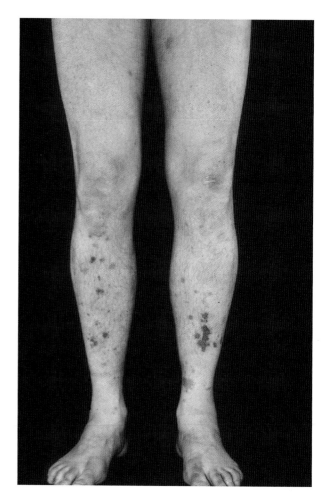

Some symptoms of vasculitis. (© *Custom Medical Stock Photo, Inc. Reproduced by permission.*)

in the body. It may affect either arteries and/or veins. The inflammation may be focal, meaning that it affects a single location within a vessel, or it may be widespread, with areas of inflammation scattered throughout a particular organ or tissue, or even affecting more than one organ system in the body.

Description

Inflammation is a process which occurs when the immune system of the body responds to either an injury or a foreign invader (virus, bacteria, or fungi). The immune system response involves sending a variety of cells and chemicals to the area in question. Inflammation causes blood vessels in the area to leak, causing swelling. The inflamed area becomes red, hot to the touch, and tender.

Antibodies are immune cells which recognize and bind to specific markers (called antigens) on other cells (including bacteria and viruses). These antibody-antigen complexes can then stimulate the immune system to send a variety of other cells and chemicals involved in inflammation to their specific location.

Some researchers believe that the damaging process of vasculitis is kicked off by such antibody-antigen complexes. These complexes are deposited along the walls of the blood vessels. The resulting inflow of immune cells and chemicals causes inflammation within the blood vessels.

The type of disease caused by vasculitis varies depending on a number of factors:

• the organ system or tissue in which the vasculitis occurs

• the specific type of inflammatory response provoked

• whether the affected vessels are veins (which bring blood to the heart) or arteries (which carry blood and oxygen from the heart to the organs and tissues)

• the degree to which blood flow within the affected vessel is reduced

Causes and symptoms

Some types of vasculitis appear to be due to a type of allergic response to a specific substance (for example, a drug). Other types of vasculitis have no identifiable initiating event. Researchers have not been able to consistently identify antibody-antigen complexes in all of the types of diseases caused by vasculitis. The types of antigens responsible for the initial immune response have often gone unidentified as well. Furthermore, not all people with such complexes deposited along the blood vessels go on to develop vasculitis. Some researchers believe that, in addition to the presence of immune complexes, an individual must have some other characteristics which make him or her susceptible to vasculitis. Many questions have yet to be answered to totally explain the development these diseases.

Symptoms

Symptoms of vasculitis depend on the severity of the inflammation and the organ system or systems affected. Some types of vasculitis are so mild that the only symptoms noted are small reddish-purple dots (called petechiae) on the skin due to tiny amounts of blood seeping out of leaky blood vessels. In more widespread types of vasculitis, the patient may have general symptoms of illness, including fever, achy muscles and joints, decreased appetite, weight loss, and loss of energy. The organ systems affected by vasculitis may include:

• Skin. Rashes, bumps under the skin, petechiae, larger reddish-purple circles (purpura), or bruising (ecchymoses) may appear. Areas of skin totally deprived of blood flow, and therefore of oxygen, may die, resulting in blackened areas of gangrene.

• Joints. In addition to joint pain, the joints themselves may become inflamed, resulting in arthritis.

• Brain and nervous system. Inflammation of the blood vessels in the brain can cause headaches, changes in personality, confusion, and seizures. If an area of the brain becomes totally deprived of oxygen, a stroke occurs. A **stroke** means that an area of brain tissue is either severely injured or completely dead from lack of oxygen. This may leave the individual with a permanent disability. If the vessels that lead to the eyes are affected, vision may become seriously disturbed. Nerves in the arms and legs may result in painful tingling sensations, loss of feeling, and weakness.

• Gastrointestinal system. Patients may have significant abdominal pain, vomiting, and diarrhea. If blood flow is completely cut off to an area of intestine, that part of the intestine will die off. The liver may be affected.

• Heart. This is an extremely serious type of vasculitis. The arteries of the heart (coronary arteries) may develop weakened areas, called aneurysms. The heart muscle itself may become inflamed and enlarged. With oxygen deprivation of the heart muscle, the individual may suffer a heart attack.

• Lungs. The patient may experience shortness of breath with chest pain, and may cough up blood. There may be wheezing.

• Kidney. Changes in the arteries of the kidney may result in high blood pressure. The kidneys may become increasingly unable to appropriately filter the blood, and kidney failure may occur.

Specific diseases

Multiple types of disease are associated with vasculitis. Many **autoimmune diseases** have vasculitis as one of their complications. These include systemic lupus erythematosus, rheumatoid arthritis, scleroderma, and **polymyositis**. Other types of diseases which have vasculitis as their major manifestations include:

• Polyarteritis nodosa is an extremely serious, systemic (affecting systems throughout the body) form of vasculitis. Small and medium arteries are involved, and the inflammation is so severe that the walls of the arteries may be destroyed. Any organ system, or multiple organ systems, may be affected. The most serious effects include kidney failure, complications involving the heart, gastrointestinal problems, and high blood pressure.

KEY TERMS

Aneurysm—A weakened area in the wall of a blood vessel which causes an outpouching or bulge. Aneurysms may be fatal if these weak areas burst, resulting in uncontrollable bleeding.

Antibody—Specialized cells of the immune system which can recognize organisms that invade the body (such as bacteria, viruses, and fungi). The antibodies are then able to set off a complex chain of events designed to kill these foreign invaders.

Antigen—A special, identifying marker on the outside of cells.

Autoimmune disorder—A disorder in which the body's antibodies mistake the body's own tissues for foreign invaders. The immune system therefore attacks and causes damage to these tissues.

Immune system—The system of specialized organs, lymph nodes, and blood cells throughout the body which work together to prevent foreign invaders (bacteria, viruses, fungi, etc.) from taking hold and growing.

Inflammation—The body's response to tissue damage. Includes hotness, swelling, redness, and pain in the affected part.

Petechia—A tiny, purplish-red spot on the skin. Caused by the leakage of a bit of blood out of a vessel and under the skin.

Purpura—A large, purplish-red circle on the skin. Caused by the leakage of blood out of a vessel and under the skin.

• Kawasaki's disease is an acute disease which primarily strikes young children. Fever and skin manifestations occur in all patients. While most patients recover completely, a few patients suffer from vasculitis in the heart. This is frequently fatal.

• Henoch-Schonlein purpura frequently occurs in children, but adults may also be affected. This disease tends to affect the skin, joints, gastrointestinal tract, and kidneys.

• Serum sickness occurs when an individual reacts to a component of a drug, for example penicillin. Symptoms of this are often confined to the skin, although fevers, joint pain, and swelling of lymph nodes may also occur.

• Temporal arteritis (also called giant cell arteritis) tends to involve arteries which branch off the major artery that leads to the head, called the carotid. An artery which feeds tissues in the area of the temple (the temporal artery) is often affected. Severe headaches are the most classic symptom. Other symptoms include fatigue, loss of appetite and then weight, fever, heavy sweating, joint pain, and pain in the muscles of the neck, shoulders, and back. If the vasculitis includes arteries which supply the eye, serious visual disturbance or even blindness may result.

• Takayasu's arteritis affects the aorta (the very large main artery that exits the heart and receives all of the blood to be delivered throughout the body), and arteries which branch off of the aorta. Initial symptoms include fatigue, fever, sweating at night, joint pain, and loss of appetite and weight. Every organ may be affected by this disease. A common sign of this disease is the inability to feel the pulse in any of the usual locations (the pulse is the regular, rhythmic sensation one can feel with a finger over an artery, for example in the wrist, which represents the beating of the heart and the regular flow of blood).

• Wegener's granulomatosis exerts its most serious effects on the respiratory tract. The vasculitis produced by this disease includes the formation of fibrous, scarring nodules called granulomas. Symptoms include nose bleeds, ear infections, cough, shortness of breath, and chest pain. There may be bleeding in the lungs, and a patient may cough up blood. The kidneys, eyes, and skin are also frequently involved.

Diagnosis

Diagnosis of any type of vasculitis involves demonstrating the presence of a strong inflammatory process. Tests which reveal inflammation throughout the body include erythrocyte sedimentation rate, blood tests which may reveal anemia and increased white blood cells, and tests to demonstrate the presence of immune complexes and/or antibodies circulating in the blood. An x-ray procedure, called **angiography**, involves injecting dye into a major artery, and then taking x-ray pictures to examine the blood vessels, in order to demonstrate the presence of inflammation of the vessel walls. Tissue samples (biopsies) may be taken from affected organs to demonstrate inflammation.

Treatment

Even though there are many different types of vasculitis, with many different symptoms based on the organ system affected, treatments are essentially the same. They all involve trying to decrease the activity of the immune system. Steroid medications (such as prednisone) are usually the first types of drugs used. Steroids work by interfering with the chemicals involved in the inflammatory process. More potent drugs for severe cases of vasculitis have more serious side effects. These include drugs like cyclophosphamide. Cyclophosphamide works by actually killing cells of the patient's immune system.

Prognosis

The prognosis for vasculitis is quite variable. Some mild forms of vasculitis, such as those brought on by reactions to medications, may resolve totally on their own and not even require treatment. **Temporal arteritis**, serum sickness, Henoch-Schonlein purpura, and Kawasaki's disease usually have excellent prognoses, although when Kawasaki's affects the heart, there is a high death rate. Other types of vasculitis were always fatal prior to the availability of prednisone and cyclophosphamide, and continue to have high rates of fatal complications. These include polyarteritis nodosa and Wegener's granulomatosis.

Prevention

Because so little is known about what causes a particular individual to develop vasculitis, there are no known ways to prevent it.

Resources

ORGANIZATIONS

Lupus Foundation of America. 1300 Piccard Dr., Suite 200, Rockville, MD 20850. (800) 558-0121. http://www.lupus.org.
Wegener's Foundation, Inc. 3705 South George Mason Drive, Suite 1813 South, Falls Church, VA 22041. (703) 931-5852.

Rosalyn Carson-DeWitt, MD

▌Vegetative state; minimally conscious state

Definition

A vegetative state is an unconscious condition in which patients are without awareness, thoughts, or behaviors, but have reflex responses and relatively normal sleep-wake cycles. A minimally conscious state (MCS) is one in which patient behavior indicates some small degree of awareness.

Description

Impaired states of consciousness are not well understood. Vegetative and minimally conscious states represent a range of conditions caused by damage to various regions of the brain. New technologies for detecting brain activity and responses are rapidly advancing the understanding of impaired consciousness.

During the 1970s, advances in intensive care significantly improved the survival rate of brain-injured **coma** patients. Within two to four weeks, patients usually emerged from totally unresponsive comas to either consciousness or an in-between state, which the neurologist Fred Plum named a persistent vegetative state (PVS). Although patients in a vegetative state are incapable of voluntary movements, are without cognitive function, and are unaware of themselves and their surroundings, they have reflex reactions, such as blinking, and appear to be awake. Their circulation, breathing, and sleep patterns are relatively intact.

During the 1990s, it was recognized that some patients did not meet the criteria for a vegetative state. They exhibited a slight degree of consciousness via voluntary or non-reflex movements and responses, although they could not consistently reproduce these behaviors. For example, they might follow objects with their eyes or answer "yes" to a question, although not necessarily appropriately. In 2002, Joseph Giacino and an international team of experts defined this as a minimally conscious state (MCS). MCS may be a direct consequence of brain damage or represent recovery from a vegetative state. Although popular media sometimes uses the terms "minimally conscious state" and "locked-in syndrome" interchangeably, the latter is a fully conscious condition in which patients are unable to move or communicate due to extensive paralysis.

Causes and symptoms

Although vegetative and minimally conscious states are rare, they can be caused by a wide variety of injuries or underlying illnesses, either directly or following a coma. **Traumatic brain injury** (TBI)—most often resulting from motor-vehicle accidents or violence, especially combat—is the most common cause of vegetative and minimally conscious states. Brain damage that leads to a vegetative state or MCS also can occur whenever the brain is deprived of blood flow or oxygen (hypoxia), as from a **stroke**, drowning, or heart attack. Other causes of vegetative and minimally conscious states include:

• prolonged high blood sugar (hyperglycemia) or low blood sugar (hypoglycemia) due to diabetes

- infections, such as encephalitis or meningitis, that cause inflammation of the central nervous system
- ongoing seizures
- poisoning with toxic drugs or carbon monoxide
- overdoses of medications, recreational drugs, or alcohol
- neurodegenerative disorders, such as Alzheimer's disease, in which loss of consciousness develops gradually

Vegetative and minimally conscious states result from injury to large areas of the cerebral hemispheres of the brain, which control thoughts and behaviors. The undamaged lower brain, thalamus, and brainstem—which control sleep cycles, breathing, blood pressure, heart rate, and body temperature—continue to function.

Unlike coma patients, those in vegetative or minimally conscious states open their eyes, have sleep/wake cycles, exhibit reflex responses, and may move or groan. They can breathe, suck, chew, swallow, gag, and cough. They may have a startle reaction to loud noises and sometimes even grimace, smile, laugh, or cry. In a vegetative state, these are reflex responses and the reflexes are usually abnormal, such as stiffening or jerking of the arms and legs. In contrast to a vegetative state, patients in an MCS often follow objects with their eyes and inconsistently recognize objects, follow simple instructions, communicate "yes" or "no" with words or gestures, and exhibit emotion. MCS patients sometimes speak words or phrases and may respond by smiling, crying, laughing, making sounds or gestures, or focusing with their eyes. They may reach for and try to hold an object. These actions are purposeful but are performed inconsistently.

Diagnosis

Diagnosis includes a physical exam to evaluate reflexes, pupil size, and response to painful stimuli, and a variety of laboratory tests and imaging studies to diagnose brain damage. If the cause of unconsciousness is unknown, information from family or friends is imperative, including:

- circumstances preceding the loss of consciousness
- the patient's medical history and conditions
- recent changes in the patient's health or behavior
- drug use, including prescription and over-the-counter medications and recreational drugs and alcohol

The FOUR (full outline of unresponsiveness) Score Coma Scale measures eye responses, motor responses, brainstem reflexes, and respiratory pattern. Eye responses include:

- pupillary reflex—contraction of the pupil in response to light
- corneal reflex—blinking when the cornea is touched with a piece of cotton or dripping water
- squirting ice-cold or warm water in the ear canals, which causes different types of reflexive eye movements depending on the type and cause of unconsciousness

The ability to respond to simple commands, such as squeezing a hand or looking up or down, is considered diagnostic of consciousness, although responses may be small or inconsistent. Following a person or object with one's eyes is often a first sign of regaining consciousness. Locating a painful stimulus, scratching one's nose, pulling at a feeding tube, smiling at a family member and not at someone else, or reacting to a joke are all considered signs of consciousness. Nevertheless, there are many possible causes for unresponsiveness other than a vegetative or minimally conscious state.

The Coma Recovery Scale-Revised (CRS-R) is designed to differentiate between vegetative and minimally conscious states. It uses standardized stimuli—such as a moving mirror held at a specified distance and angle for a specified number of trials to distinguish conscious eye tracking from spontaneous eye movement. The CRS-R includes auditory, visual, oromotor/verbal, communication, and arousal subscales, with a total score range of zero to 23. Functional object use or functional or accurate communication is indicative of emergence from an MCS. The following are diagnostic for an MCS rather than a vegetative state:

- reproducible or consistent movement in response to a command on the auditory function subscale
- fixation, visual pursuit (eye following), reaching for an object, or object recognition on the visual function subscale
- localization of noxious stimuli, object manipulation, or motor response on the motor function subscale
- intelligible vocalization on the oromotor/verbal subscale
- intentional nonfunctional communication

Electrophysiologic tests and imaging studies are particularly important for diagnosing unconscious states. Results that demonstrate activity in the brainstem, but little or no activity in the higher brain, are indicative of a vegetative state:

- Electroencephalography (EEG) measures electrical activity in the brain through electrodes on the scalp.
- Somatosensory evoked potential (SSEP) measures electrical signals in the brain in response to mild electrical stimulation in various parts of the body.

- Evoked potential (EP) studies measure brain activity in response to commands.
- Functional magnetic resonance imaging (fMRI) may be used to assess activity in specific brain regions in response to commands.

Treatment

Emergency treatment for vegetative and minimally conscious states may include immediate intravenous administration of glucose or antibiotics if diabetic shock or infection are suspected. Surgery may be required to relieve pressure from brain swelling. Other treatments may focus on the underlying cause or condition.

Ongoing treatment focuses on supportive care and maintaining general health with balanced nutrition and the prevention of infection and bedsores. Physical therapy is used to prevent permanent muscular contractions and bone, joint, and muscle deformities. Patients in an MCS receive more aggressive treatment and rehabilitation, since they may have better prospects for recovery. The Nociception Coma Scale has been developed for the purpose of assessing pain responses, so that MCS patients can be treated with pain medication if required.

New treatments for MCS are being actively investigated:

- Transcranial magnetic stimulation (TMS) involves exciting brain cells through an electromagnetic coil held over specific regions of the skull.
- Deep-brain stimulation (DBS) stimulates the central thalamus—which is crucial for arousal and wakefulness—through a surgically implanted electrode.
- Familiar vocal stimulation utilizes recordings of family members recounting events involving the patient.

Recovery and rehabilitation

Transition through stages of unconsciousness and recovery vary greatly depending on the type and severity of brain injury. Longer periods of unconsciousness usually mean more gradual emergence.

Clinical trials

Ongoing clinical trials of treatments for vegetative and minimally conscious states include:

- safety and effectiveness of the drug apomorphine following severe TBI
- effectiveness of bilateral electrical stimulation of the central thalamus for improving responsiveness in patients who have been in a vegetative or minimally conscious state for at least six months due to TBI, hypoxia, or ischemic stroke
- effectiveness of vagus nerve stimulation for increasing cerebral blood flow and brain metabolism following TBI
- effects of familiar voice stimulation during recovery from severe TBI

Prognosis

Prognosis for vegetative and minimally conscious states depends on the cause, site, and severity of brain damage and the patient's age. Younger brains are much better able to repair themselves and recover compared with brains of older patients. Patients in a vegetative state due to stroke, hypoxia, or certain types of severe illness are less likely to recover than patients with TBI.

Many people emerge from a vegetative state within a few weeks. About 60% of children and 50% of adults recover from vegetative states within the first six months, usually with varying degrees of permanent cognitive and physical impairments. The more prolonged a vegetative or minimally conscious state, the greater the disability, since the duration of the state corresponds to the extent and severity of brain damage. After 12 months in a PVS following a traumatic injury—and after three months following cardiac arrest—the likelihood of meaningful recovery is near zero. The diagnosis may be changed from PVS to permanent vegetative state and artificial hydration and nutrition may be withheld. Patients are extremely unlikely to awaken from a vegetative state that lasts more than three years. Some patients remain in vegetative states for years or decades, usually eventually dying of an infection, such as pneumonia, or respiratory failure.

Many MCS patients improve, although they almost always emerge in a state of confusion. They may regain their ability to comprehend and communicate, even many years later, but rarely regain normal functioning or the ability to live independently.

Special concerns

The identification and treatment of vegetative and minimally conscious states is evolving rapidly. New developments receive much media attention and can raise the hopes of family members, sometimes inappropriately. Despite some exceptional cases, very few patients in a prolonged vegetative state have the potential for even marginal recovery and difficult

KEY TERMS

Brainstem—The part of the brain that connects the forebrain and cerebrum to the spinal cord.

Coma—A severe state of unconsciousness from injury, disease, or poison.

Deep-brain stimulation (DBS)—Neurostimulation through an electrode surgically implanted in the brain; used to treat Parkinson's disease and other neurological conditions.

Electroencephalography (EEG)—The monitoring of electrical activity in the brain.

Evoked potential (EP)—Measurement of brain activity in response to stimuli.

Functional magnetic resonance imaging (fMRI)—Imaging of physical changes in the brain, such as blood flow, while performing mental tasks.

Hypoxia—Oxygen deficiency in a body tissue, such as cerebral hypoxia in the brain.

Ischemic stroke—A stroke caused by a blood clot in the brain.

Locked-in syndrome—A condition of full wakefulness and awareness but inability to communicate, except possibly with eye movements, due to paralysis.

Persistent vegetative state (PVS)—Severely impaired consciousness in which a patient is incapable of voluntary movement, but with sleep/wake cycles and eye opening; a coma lasting more than four weeks.

Stroke—Rupture or obstruction of a blood vessel in the brain.

Thalamus—The largest portion of the diencephalon of the brain, which relays impulses, especially sensory impulses, to and from the cerebral cortex, and which is critical for arousal and wakefulness.

Transcranial magnetic stimulation (TMS)—Stimulation of brain cells with an electromagnetic coil positioned over the skull.

Traumatic brain injury (TBI)—Damage to the brain from sudden trauma, most often from a motor-vehicle accident.

QUESTIONS TO ASK YOUR DOCTOR

- What tests will you perform to determine whether my family member is in a vegetative state or is minimally conscious?
- Is my family member in pain?
- What treatments can you suggest?
- What are signs that my family member may be recovering consciousness?
- What is my family member's prognosis?

suggesting at least some cognitive function and conscious awareness. Similar results have been reported with **positron emission tomography (PET)**. After extensive clinical testing, some of these patients have had their diagnoses upgraded from PVS to MCS. In response to low-level electrical shocks to the wrists of MCS patients, high activity has been detected in an area of the brain involved in processing pain, similar to activity seen in healthy volunteers; however, many experts are skeptical of these results.

An EEG study has found that healthy volunteers and MCS patients generate a much longer signal in response to irregular sounds, compared with patients in a vegetative state. Analysis indicated that both healthy subjects and the MCS patients sent signals in both directions between the higher-level frontal cortex of the brain and the temporal cortex responsible for auditory processing; however, patients in a vegetative state could pass signals only in one direction—from the auditory area to the frontal cortex. Such results may lead to clinical criteria for clearly distinguishing between vegetative and minimally conscious states.

These types of studies raise important medical and ethical issues:

- the frequency of diagnostic errors based on standard neurological tests

- the inadequacy of PVS and MCS classifications for conditions that presumably encompass a broad spectrum of brain injuries

- the suggestion that as many as 40% of patients diagnosed as in a vegetative state are actually conscious on some level

- difficulties with detecting small and fluctuating signs of consciousness in long-term-care patients

decisions concerning the maintenance of life support may be necessary.

A few TBI patients—mostly young people—in vegetative or minimally conscious states have been reported to show reactivity on fMRI to noxious stimuli, visual images, spoken words, or personal stories,

- the suggestion that at least some patients, especially those in an MCS, may be experiencing significant degrees of pain and suffering

Resources

BOOKS

Goodman, Kenneth W. *The Case of Terri Schiavo: Ethics, Politics, and Death in the 21st Century.* New York: Oxford University Press, 2010.

Jandial, Rahul, Charles B. Newman, and Samuel A. Hughes. *100 Questions & Answers About Head and Brain Injuries.* Sudbury, MA: Jones and Bartlett, 2009.

Laureys, Steven, and Guilio Tononi. *The Neurology of Consciousness: Cognitive Neuroscience and Neuropathology.* Boston: Elsevier Academic, 2009.

Schweiger, Avraham, Michael Frost, and Ofer Keren. "From Coma to Consciousness: Recovery and the Process of Differentiation." In *Process Approaches to Consciousness in Psychology, Neuroscience, and Philosophy of Mind,* edited by Michel Weber and Anderson Weekes. Albany, NY: SUNY Press, 2009.

Shepherd, Lois L. *If That Ever Happens to Me: Making Life and Death Decisions After Terri Schiavo.* Chapel Hill: University of North Carolina Press, 2009.

PERIODICALS

Billings, J. Andrew, Larry R. Churchill, and Richard Payne. "Severe Brain Injury and the Subjective Life." *Hastings Center Report* 40, no. 3 (May/June 2010): 17–21.

Boly, Melanie, et al. "Preserved Feedforward but Impaired Top-Down Processes in the Vegetative State." *Science* 332, no. 6031 (May 13, 2011): 858–62.

Fisher, Carl E., and Paul S. Appelbaum. "Diagnosing Consciousness: Neuroimaging, Law, and the Vegetative State." *Journal of Law, Medicine & Ethics* 38, no. 2 (Summer 2010): 374–85.

Iyer, V.N., et al. "Validity of the FOUR Score Coma Scale in the Medical Intensive Care Unit." *Mayo Clinic Proceedings* 84, no. 8 (August 2009): 32–47.

McGowan, Kat. "Back From the Brink." *Discover* 32, no. 2 (March 2011): 62.

McGowan, Kat. "Scans Unlock Hidden Life in Vegetative Brains." *Discover* 32, no. 1 (January/February 2011): 54.

Monti, Martin M., Steven Laureys, and Adrian M. Owen. "The Vegetative State." *British Medical Journal* 341, no. 7767 (August 7, 2010): 292.

Schiff, N.D., J.T. Giacino, and J.J. Fins. "Deep Brain Stimulation, Neuroethics, and the Minimally Conscious State: Moving Beyond Proof of Principle." *Archives of Neurology* 66, no. 6 (2009): 697–702.

Syd, L., and M. Johnson. "The Right to Die in the Minimally Conscious State." *Journal of Medical Ethics* 37 (March 2011): 175–78.

Zoroya, Gregg. "For Troops with Brain Trauma, a Long Journey Back." *USA Today* (July 29, 2010): A1.

WEBSITES

Boudry, Maarten, Roeland Termote, and Willem Betz. "Fabricating Communication: The Case of the Belgian Coma Patient." *Skeptical Inquirer* 34, no. 4 (July/August 2010): 12. http://www.csicop.org/si/show/fabricating_communication (accessed July 22, 2011).

Bruno, Marie-Aurélie, and Steven Laureys. "Uncovering Awareness: Medical and Ethical Challenges in Diagnosing and Treating the Minimally Conscious State." *Cerebrum.* Dana Foundation. http://www.dana.org/news/cerebrum/detail.aspx?id=28088 (accessed July 22, 2011).

de Lange, Catherine. "Sound Test Could Identify 'Locked-In' Patients." *New Scientist* May 12, 2011. http://www.newscientist.com/article/dn20471-sound-test-could-identify-lockedin-patients.html (accessed July 22, 2011).

Miller, Greg. "Is There Anybody There?" Science Now. http://news.sciencemag.org/sciencenow/2010/02/03-02.html?ref=hp (accessed July 22, 2011).

Monti, M.M., et al. "Willful Modulation of Brain Activity in Disorders of Consciousness." *New England Journal of Medicine* 362, no. 7 (February 18, 2010): 579–89. http://www.nejm.org/doi/pdf/10.1056/NEJMoa0905370 (accessed July 22, 2011).

"Research Highlights: Restoring Consciousness: Researcher Explores How to Aid Recovery from Coma." U.S. Department of Veteran Affairs. http://www.research.va.gov/news/research_highlights/consciousness-010609.cfm (accessed July 22, 2011).

Talan, Jamie. "Fanfare—and Caution—Greet Report that Patients with Consciousness Disorders Understand and Respond to Language." *Neurology Today* 10, no. 5 (March 4, 2010): 17, 21. http://www.aan.com/elibrary/neurologytoday/?event=home.showArticle&id=ovid.com:/bib/ovftdb/00132985-201003040-00006 (accessed July 22, 2011).

"Traumatic Brain Injury: Hope Through Research." National Institute of Neurological Disorders and Stroke. http://www.ninds.nih.gov/disorders/tbi/detail_tbi.htm (accessed July 22, 2011).

ORGANIZATIONS

American Academy of Neurology (AAN), 1080 Montreal Avenue, Saint Paul, MN 55116, (651) 695-2717, (800) 879-1960, Fax: (651) 695-2791, memberservices@aan.com, http://www.aan.com.

Brain Injury Association of America, 1608 Spring Hill Road, Suite 110, Vienna, VA 22182, (703) 761-0750, (800) 444-6443, Fax: (703) 761-0755, braininjuryinfo@biausa.org, http://www.biausa.org.

Coma/Traumatic Brain Injury Recovery Association, Inc., 8300 Republic Airport, Suite 106, Farmingdale, NY 11735, (631) 756-1826, http://www.comarecovery.org.

Dana Foundation and Dana Alliance for Brain Initiatives, 505 Fifth Avenue, 6th floor, New York, NY 10017, (212) 223-4040, Fax: (212) 317-8721, danainfo@dana.org, http://www.dana.org.

National Institute of Neurological Disorders and Stroke (NINDS), P.O. Box 5801, Bethesda, MD 20824, (301) 496-5751, (800) 352-9424, http://www.ninds.nih.gov.

Margaret Alic, PhD

Ventilatory assistance devices

Definition

Ventilatory assistance devices are mechanical devices that help a person breathe by replacing some or all of the muscular effort required to inflate the lungs.

Description

Ventilation is the process of inflating and deflating the lungs in order to breathe. Normally, a person uses several sets of muscles to accomplish this—the diaphragm at the base of the lungs, the muscles between the ribs (intercostals), and, to a small extent, the muscles of the lower neck and shoulder area. When these muscles are weakened through disease or injury, the ability to ventilate is impaired. As a result, a person cannot get sufficient oxygen into, and carbon dioxide out of, the lungs in order to maintain appropriate levels in the blood. In addition, weakened ventilation muscles also impair the ability to cough, which is an essential part of clearing lung secretions and preventing infection.

Ventilatory assistance devices may be needed for the following reasons:

- muscular dystrophies (progressive muscle weakening disorders)
- amyotrophic lateral sclerosis (ALS), a progressive disease causing muscle weakness)
- polio
- high spinal cord injury (injury to the spinal cord in the neck)
- Guillain-Barré syndrome (a rapidly progressive but reversible loss of muscle control)
- myasthenia gravis, acute crisis (muscle-weakening disease, in which patients may experience a "crisis" of rapid and dangerous loss of muscle strength)
- head trauma
- botulism (poisoning by botulinum toxin, usually from improperly preserved food)
- tetanus (poisoning by tetanus bacteria, usually by a deep puncture wound)

Nighttime ventilators are also used for people with obstructive sleep apnea. This is a condition in which breathing is impaired during sleep by obstructions in the airway, most often extra tissue at the rear of the throat.

Ventilatory assistance is not the same as supplying extra oxygen, as is done for people whose lungs are damaged. The person who needs ventilatory assistance generally has normal gas exchange capacity and simply needs help moving air in and out. Supplemental oxygen can worsen the situation in such cases, as it may depress the normal signals from the brain to stimulate breathing.

Ventilators

A ventilator is a machine that uses a tube to blow air into, and suck it out of, the body. The ventilator may be designed to deliver air at a set volume (volume ventilator), or at a set pressure (pressure ventilator).

Volume ventilator settings may be adjusted to deliver a variable volume of air depending on the patient's needs, and can either cycle automatically or be initiated by the patient's voluntary efforts.

Pressure ventilators come in two major styles. Continuous positive airway pressure (CPAP) delivers air at a steady pressure, which assists the patient while breathing in (inspiration) and resists breathing out (expiration). The purpose of CPAP is not to completely inflate the lungs but rather to maintain an open airway. This makes it most appropriate for use in sleep apnea, in which a patient's airway closes frequently during sleep. In contrast, bilevel positive airway pressure (BiPAP) delivers a higher pressure on inspiration in order to allow the patient to completely inflate the lungs, and then switches to a low pressure on expiration, to allow easy exhalation. BiPAP is a common choice for patients with neuromuscular disease, whose respiratory muscles are weakened.

There are other rarer devices in use, which surround a patient's chest cavity and abdomen with a rigid shell, and change the pressure within. By lowering the pressure, air rushes into the lungs. The iron lung is one such device; smaller and more portable cuirasses are occasionally used to similar effect.

Interfaces

The air from a ventilator is delivered to the patient either through a face mask or directly into the lungs through a tracheostomy (trach) tube. Each has its advantages and disadvantages.

A tracheostomy is an opening in the airway in the middle of the throat through which a tube is inserted to deliver air. The properly chosen trach tube will fit comfortably. A widespread misunderstanding about tracheostomy ventilation is that it prevents talking, but this does not have to be so. Trach tubes are available that do not interfere with speech, and patients contemplating tracheostomy should ensure that their respiratory specialist is familiar with them. Trach tubes may provide

Neuromuscular disease—Disease involving both the muscles and the nerves that control them.

the patient a greater sense of security and, unlike a face mask, it can easily be hidden from view with a well-placed scarf. Trach tubes do require daily lung hygiene, either by the patient or by a trained caregiver. This involves suctioning secretions from the lungs, which tend to be increased due to the presence of the tube.

Face masks fit snugly over the mouth and nose and are held on with a strap. Finding the right mask takes some time, but a well-fitting mask is comfortable and easy to tolerate for many hours per day. The mask usually must be removed to talk, but this does not present a problem for many patients who retain some use of their hands. The mask may also be used at night.

Other noninvasive interfaces are also available, including mouthpieces and nasal pillows that fit into one or the other orifice and are smaller than masks. These methods are usually chosen for patients who need fewer hours per day of ventilatory assistance.

Coughing

Patients with weakened respiratory muscles may be even more in need of cough assistance than they are of ventilatory assistance. Cough assistance may be delivered manually by a caregiver or by a machine (the in-exsufflator or cough assist) that is designed to inflate the lungs and then rapidly withdraw air, as occurs in a normal cough. This clears secretions that would otherwise accumulate and provide a locus for infection, as well as interfere with gas exchange.

Resources

BOOKS

Bach, J.R. *Noninvasive Mechanical Ventilation*. Philadelphia: Hanley & Belfus, 2002.

Kinnear, W.J.M. *Assisted Ventilation at Home: A Practical Guide*. Oxford: Oxford Medical, 1994.

WEBSITES

Muscular Dystrophy Association. "Assisted Ventilation." http://www.mdausa.org/publications/breathe/ventilation.html (accessed August 29, 2011).

National Heart, Lung, and Blood Institute. "What Is a Ventilator?" February 01, 2011. http://www.nhlbi.nih.gov/health/health-topics/topics/vent/ (accessed August 29, 2011).

Robinson, R. "Breathe Easy." *Quest Magazine* 5, no. 5 (October 1998). http://www.mdausa.org/publications/Quest/q55breathe.html (accessed August 28, 2011).

Robinson, R. "A Breath of Fresh Air." *Quest Magazine* 5, no. 6 (October 1998). http://www.mdausa.org/publications/Quest/q56freshair.html (accessed August 28, 2011).

ORGANIZATIONS

Muscular Dystrophy Association, 3300 East Sunrise Drive, Tucson, AZ 85718-3208, (520) 529-2000, (800) 572-1717, Fax: (520) 529-5300, mda@ mdausa.org, http://www.mda.org.

Richard Robinson
Rosalyn Carson-DeWitt, MD

Ventricular shunt

Definition

A ventricular shunt is a tube that is surgically placed in one of the fluid-filled chambers inside the brain (ventricles). The fluid around the brain and the spinal column is called cerebrospinal fluid (CSF). When infection or disease causes an excess of CSF in the ventricles, the shunt is placed to drain it and thereby relieve excess pressure.

Purpose

A ventricular shunt relieves hydrocephalus, a condition in which there is an increased volume of CSF within the ventricles. In hydrocephalus, pressure from the CSF usually increases. It may be caused by a tumor of the brain or of the membranes covering the brain (**meninges**), infection of or bleeding into the CSF, or inborn malformations of the brain. Symptoms of hydrocephalus may include headache, personality disturbances and loss of intellectual abilities (**dementia**), problems in walking, irritability, vomiting, abnormal eye movements, or a low level of consciousness.

Normal pressure hydrocephalus (a condition in which the volume of CSF increases without an increase in pressure) is associated with progressive dementia, problems walking, and loss of bladder control (urinary incontinence). Even though CSF is not thought to be under increased pressure in this condition, it may also be treated by ventricular shunting.

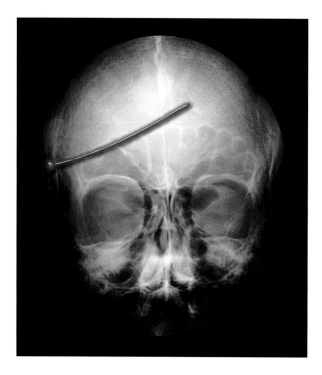

A digitally enhanced X ray of the skull of a nine-year-old boy showing the shunt that was placed into the ventricle of the brain. *(© Living Art Enterprises, LLC)*

Demographics

The congenital form of hydrocephalus is believed to occur at an incidence of approximately one to four out of every 1,000 births. The incidence of acquired hydrocephalus is not exactly known. The peak ages for the development of hydrocephalus are in infancy, between four and eight years, and in early adulthood. Normal pressure hydrocephalus generally occurs in patients over the age of 60.

Description

The ventricular shunt tube is placed to drain fluid from the **ventricular system** in the brain to the cavity of the abdomen or to the large vein in the neck (jugular vein). Therefore, surgical procedures must be done both in the brain and at the drainage site. The tubing contains valves to ensure that fluid can only flow out of the brain and not back into it. The valve can be set at a desired pressure to allow CSF to escape whenever the pressure level is exceeded.

A small reservoir may be attached to the tubing and placed under the scalp. This reservoir allows samples of CSF to be removed with a syringe to check the pressure. Fluid from the reservoir can also be examined for bacteria, cancer cells, blood, or protein, depending on the cause of hydrocephalus. The reservoir may also be used to inject antibiotics for CSF infection or chemotherapy medication for meningeal tumors.

Diagnosis/Preparation

The diagnosis of hydrocephalus should be confirmed by diagnostic imaging techniques, such as computed tomography scan (CT scan) or magnetic resonance imaging (MRI), before the shunting procedure is performed. These techniques will also show any associated brain abnormalities. CSF should be examined if infection or tumor of the meninges is suspected. Patients with dementia or **mental retardation** should undergo neuropsychological testing to establish a baseline psychological profile before the shunting procedure.

As with any surgical procedure, the surgeon must know about any medications or health problems that may increase the patient's risk. Because infections are both common and serious, antibiotics are often given before and after surgery.

Aftercare

To avoid infections at the shunt site, the area should be kept clean. CSF should be checked periodically by the doctor to be sure there is no infection or bleeding into the shunt. CSF pressure should be checked to be sure the shunt is operating properly. The eyes should be examined regularly because shunt failure may damage the nerve to the eyes (optic nerve). If not treated promptly, damage to the optic nerve causes irreversible loss of vision.

WHO PERFORMS THE PROCEDURE AND WHERE IS IT PERFORMED?

Ventricular shunting is performed in a hospital operating room by a neurosurgeon, a surgeon who specializes in the treatment of diseases of the brain, spinal cord, and nerves.

Risks

Serious and long-term complications of ventricular shunting are bleeding under the outermost covering of the brain (**subdural hematoma**), infection, **stroke**, and shunt failure. When a shunt drains to the abdomen (ventriculoperitoneal shunt), fluid may accumulate in the abdomen or abdominal organs may be injured. If CSF pressure is lowered too much, patients may have severe headaches, often with nausea and vomiting, whenever they sit up or stand.

Normal results

After shunting, the ventricles get smaller within three or four days. This shrinkage occurs even when hydrocephalus has been present for a year or more. Clinically detectable signs of improvement occur within a few weeks. The cause of hydrocephalus, duration of hydrocephalus before shunting, and associated brain abnormalities affect the outcome.

Of patients with normal pressure hydrocephalus who are treated with shunting, 25–80% experience long-term improvement. Normal pressure hydrocephalus is more likely to improve when it is caused by infection of or bleeding into the CSF than when it occurs without an underlying cause.

Morbidity and mortality rates

Complications of shunting occur in 30% of cases, but only 5% are serious. Infections occur in 5–10% of patients, and as many as 80% of shunts develop a mechanical problem at some point and need to be replaced.

Alternatives

In some cases of hydrocephalus, certain drugs may be administered to temporarily decrease the amount of CSF until surgery can be performed. In patients with hydrocephalus caused by a tumor, removal of the tumor often cures the buildup of

QUESTIONS TO ASK THE DOCTOR

- Why is a ventricular shunt recommended in my case?
- What is the cause of the hydrocephalus?
- What diagnostic tests will be performed prior to the shunt being placed?
- Where will the shunt be placed?
- Are there any alternatives to a ventricular shunt?

CSF. Approximately 25% of patients respond to therapies other than shunt placement.

Patients with normal pressure hydrocephalus may experience a temporary improvement in walking and mental abilities upon the temporary drainage of a moderate amount of CSF. This improvement may be an indication that shunting will improve their condition.

Resources

BOOKS

Aldrich, E. Francois, et al. "Hydrocephalus." In *Sabiston Textbook of Surgery,* edited by Courtney M. Townsend Jr. 16th ed. Philadelphia: W. B. Saunders, 2001.

Golden, Jeffery A., and Carsten G. Bonnemann. "Hydrocephalus." In *Textbook of Clinical Neurology,* edited by Christopher G. Goetz and Eric J. Pappert. Philadelphia: W. B. Saunders, 1999.

PERIODICALS

Hamid, Rukaiya K. A., and Philippa Newfield. "Pediatric Neuroanesthesia: Hydrocephalus." *Anesthesiology Clinics of North America* 19, no. 2 (June 1, 2001): 207–18.

OTHER

Dalvi, Arif. "Normal Pressure Hydrocephalus." *eMedicine,* January 14, 2002 [cited May 21, 2003]. http://www.emedicine.com/neuro/topic277.htm.

Hord, Eugenia-Daniela. "Hydrocephalus." *eMedicine,* January 14, 2002 [cited May 21, 2003]. http://www.emedicine.com/neuro/topic161.htm.

Sgouros, Spyros. "Management of Spina Bifida, Hydrocephalus, and Shunts." *eMedicine,* May 14, 2003. [cited May 21, 2003]. http://www.emedicine.com/ped/topic2976.htm.

ORGANIZATIONS

American Academy of Neurology. 1080 Montreal Ave., St. Paul, MN 55116. (800) 879-1960. http://www.aan.com.

Laurie Barclay, MD
Stephanie Dionne Sherk

Ventricular system

Definition

A ventricle is an internal cavity of the brain. Within the normal human brain, there is a connecting system of ventricles, commonly referred to as the ventricular system, which is filled with cerebrospinal fluid (CSF). The ventricular system within the brain develops from the cavity of the neural tube in the embryo.

Description

The ventricular system is composed of two lateral ventricles and two midline ventricles, referred to as the third and fourth ventricles. The chambers are connected to allow the flow of cerebrospinal fluid via two interventricular foramen (referred to as the foramen of Monro) and the cerebral aqueduct (referred to as the aqueduct of Sylvius).

The chambers of the ventricular system are lined or covered with ependymal cells and are continuous with the central canal enclosed within the spinal cord. Ependymal cells also line the central canal of the spinal cord.

Basic anatomy

The lateral ventricles

The lateral ventricles are separated by the septum pellucidum and do not communicate directly (i.e., do not allow the flow of cerebrospinal fluid) with each other. Cerebrospinal fluid within the individual lateral ventricles must flow to the third ventricle via the interventricular foramen associated with each lateral ventricle.

Lateral ventricles themselves are descriptively divided into a body with anterior, posterior, and inferior horns.

The third ventricle

The third ventricle is a narrow cavity or cleft located between the two thalami. The third ventricle also contains two saclike recesses called the anterior supraoptic recess and the infundibular recess. The massa intermedia, the neural tissue that connects both halves of the thalamus in some brains, runs through the third ventricle. Posteriorly, the third ventricle communicates with the fourth ventricle via the cerebral aqueduct, a narrow channel that allows the flow of cerebrospinal fluid from the third to the fourth ventricle. There is no choroids plexus within the cerebral aqueduct.

The fourth ventricle

The fourth ventricle is a wide and flattened space located just anterior to the **cerebellum** and posterior to the upper, or superior, half of the medulla oblongata and the pons. The fourth ventricle also has two lateral saclike pouches that are called the lateral recesses. The fourth ventricle is continuous with the upper (superior) terminal end of the central canal of the spinal cord. The fourth ventricle also connects with the subarachnoid space via three small foramina: the two foramina of Luschka (one in each of the lateral recesses) and the foramen of Magendie.

The subarachnoid space continues as the space between the arachnoid matter and the pia mater (meningal tissues that surround the brain and spinal cord) and is filled with CSF. The subarachnoid space also surrounds cranial and spinal nerves.

CSF flow and blockage of the ventricular system

The normal flow of cerebrospinal fluid—produced from brain surface tissue and the choroids plexuses within the ventricles—is from the two lateral ventricles through their respective interventricular foramina into the third ventricle. Then the CSF flows from the third ventricle through the cerebral aqueduct into the fourth ventricle and from there it can flow into the subarachnoid space where it is reabsorbed into the bloodstream.

Swellings or structures within the ventricular system may be due to congenital defect, trauma, or tumor.

If there is a blockage of the ventricular system, the flow of CSF is interrupted. If, for example, there is a blockage within the cerebral aqueduct, the normal flow of fluid formed in the lateral ventricles and the third ventricle is interrupted, and the lateral ventricles and third ventricle begin to swell with cerebrospinal fluid. The swelling or enlargement is termed hydrocephalus. Hydrocephalus can also result from the formation of CSF (as can occur with a tumor in one of the choroid plexuses) that exceeds the amount that can flow through the ventricular system, or from a downstream-diminished capacity to absorb cerebrospinal fluid.

A tumor in one of the interventricular foramen connecting a lateral ventricle to the third ventricle obstructs the flow of cerebrospinal fluid from the same side lateral ventricle and results in an asymmetrical swelling of the blocked lateral ventricle.

Blockage of the flow of CSF through the foramen connecting the fourth ventricle to the subarachnoid space usually produces asymmetrical swelling or dilation of the entire ventricular system. The entire ventricular system can also swell in cases of meningitis in which the flow of cerebrospinal fluid over the outer surface of the brain is obstructed.

Resources

BOOKS

Bear, M., et al. *Neuroscience: Exploring the Brain.* Baltimore: Williams & Wilkins, 1996.

Goetz, C. G., et al. *Textbook of Clinical Neurology.* Philadelphia: W.B. Saunders, 1999.

WEBSITES

"Development of the Ventricular System." *Temple University Department of Neuroanatomy.* May 10, 2004 (May 27, 2004). http://courses.temple.edu/neuroanatomy/lab/embryo/ventlate.htm.

Paul Arthur

Vertebrobasilar disease

Definition

Vertebrobasilar disease describes a broad spectrum of vascular abnormalities in the arterial supply to the brainstem.

Description

The vertebrobasilar circulation (VC; also called the posterior circulation) consists of the arterial supply to the brainstem, cerebellum, and occipital cortex. The vertebral arteries arise from the subclavian arteries in the neck. In the brain, the vertebral arteries lie deep in the base of the brain and unite in an area called the medullopontine junction to form the basilar artery. The basilar artery branches again to form the posterior cerebral arteries. Any interruption in blood flow in the VC may cause a broad spectrum of symptoms determined by the specific arterial branch or branches involved, and the degree of occlusion inside the blood vessels. The brainstem is a major area of neurologic activity since this area contains cranial nerves, neurosensory tracts, and the reticular activating system

(RAS). Problems in blood flow to the VC result in several overlapping clinical syndromes.

Demographics

In the United States, approximately 25% of strokes and TIAs (transient ischemic attacks or "mini" strokes) occur in the vertebrobasilar circulation. Research with magnetic resonance imaging (MRI) studies estimates that 40% of patients with vertebrobasilar TIAs (transient ischemic attacks) have brainstem infarction. The disease affects men twice as often as women. Vertebrobasilar ischemic disease occurs in late life, usually between 70–80 years of age. The incidence (number of new cases) is 20–30 cases per 1,000 for persons over age 75. In the United States, the death rate for **stroke** is higher among blacks than whites. A severe form of the disorder, called basilar artery syndrome, caused by complete obstruction of the vertebrobasilar circulation (inside the brain) is fatal in 75–85% of cases. Approximately 50% of persons who have infarctions in the vertebrobasilar area report TIA events within days or months prior to onset of permanent deficit.

Causes and symptoms

The cause of vertebrobasilar disease (VD) is atherosclerosis that affects the vertebrobasilar (posterior) circulation at intracranial (inside the cranium and includes the basilar artery) sites and extracranial (outside the cranium and includes the vertebral artery) sites. Partial or complete occlusion can occur in major arteries or smaller arterial branches. The cause of VD is atherosclerosis and vertebrobasilar insufficiency in the brain caused by blockage (occlusion), and is more common among patients with cardiovascular risk factors that typically include obesity, smoking, use of oral contraceptives, advanced age, diabetes mellitus, hypertension (high blood pressure). and dyslipidemias (abnormalities that cause an increase in lipids in the blood). Other causes of vertebrobasilar disease can include destruction to arteries such as fibrotic changes in the muscular layer of arteries (a condition called fibromuscular dysplasia) and arterial dissection or aneurysms.

The symptoms of TIA have a short duration and usually last approximately eight minutes. Vertigo is the hallmark symptom of vertebrobasilar insufficiency. Other symptoms include visual defects (diplopia), syncope (drop attacks), dysphagia (difficulty swallowing), dysarthria, hoarseness, and facial numbness, or paresthesias. Patients with early stage vertebrobasilar insufficiency have transient episodes of neurologic symptoms. Persons with more advanced disease to the vertebrobasilar circulation may have eye deficits, limb ataxia, loss of taste, limb/trunk dysesthesia, nystagmus, and deficit in temperature/pain perception.

Diagnosis

Neuroimaging studies are the primary diagnostic tool necessary to confirm vertebrobasilar disease. Other tests are also indicated and include analysis of blood, electrolytes, glucose, urinalysis, thyroid function tests, and erythrocyte sedimentation rate (a special blood test that rules out other possible disorders). Computed tomography (CT) scans help to detect mass defect, and MRIs can help visualize smaller areas of ischemia. Ultrasound studies can help assess and monitor vertebrobasilar patency (the degree of occlusion).

Treatment team

A neurologist is typically required as the specialist coordinator of treatment. A neurosurgeon is used for surgical evacuation of hemorrhages complicated by hydrocephalus. An interventional neuroradiologist may be required to provide thrombolytic agents (chemicals that dissolve clots) by intra-arterial infusion delivery (injecting a chemical directly in an artery located in the brain using TV monitor-guided imagery).

Treatment

Treatment can either be supportive or interventional if arterial patency is an option. Emergency treatment for a bleeding patient includes airway preservation, control of blood pressure, and assessment of neurologic and mental status, intravenous fluid management, prevention of vomiting, and antiplatelet agents to prevent arterial occlusion. Additionally, a stroke patient may require treatment for hypertension if present, and mouth feedings should be avoided since the patient may be unable to swallow or chew. Antiplatelet medications is the first line treatment for vertebrobasilar disease, but the usefulness is unclear. Anticoagulants (heparin) and antiplatelets (aspirin and ticlopidine, clopidogrel) are typically given to prevent recurrent or ongoing occlusion (caused by blood clots) of the posterior (vertebrobasilar) circulation.

KEY TERMS

Cranial nerves—The set of 12 nerves found on each side of the head and neck that control the sensory and muscle functions of the eyes, nose, tongue, face, and throat.

Dysarthria—Slurred speech.

Hydrocephalus—An abnormal accumulation of cerebrospinal fluid within the brain. This accumulation can be harmful by pressing on brain structures and damaging them.

Infarction—Death of tissue due to inadequate blood supply.

Nystagmus—An involuntary, rhythmic movement of the eyes.

Paresthesia—An abnormal sensation often described as burning, tickling, tingling, or "pins and needles."

Reticular activating system—A network of structures, including the brainstem, medulla, and thalamus, and nerve pathways, which function together to produce and maintain arousal.

Transient ischemic attack (TIA)—A brief interruption of the blood supply to part of the brain that causes a temporary impairment of vision, speech, or movement. Usually, the episode lasts for just a few moments, but it may be a warning sign for a full-scale stroke.

Surgical treatment options include endarterectomy, bypass grafting, angioplasty and stenting, and vertebral artery reconstruction.

Lifestyle modifications to treat vertebrobasilar disease include stopping smoking, regular **exercise**, a diet low in cholesterol (and cholesterol-lowering medications), and careful diabetic control.

Recovery and rehabilitation

Recovery is variable depending on the degree of occlusion in the vertebrobasilar circulation. Persons with the severe form, basilar artery occlusion, die in 75–85% of cases. Rehabilitation depends on the extent of damage and the deficits caused by permanent injury in the brain.

Clinical trials

Research in this area is diversified and abundant. The National Institute of Neurological Disorders and Stroke is investigating molecular mechanisms associated with neuronal injury. Research concerning the genetics of stroke and gene therapy is ongoing in experimental models. New research in high resolution neuroimaging techniques and rehabilitation have demonstrated compensatory mechanisms (recircuitry of neurons) as a result of stroke. Information about current relevant clinical trials can be found at ClinicalTrials.gov.

Prognosis

Vertebrobasilar TIAs have a favorable outcome since the chance for complete stroke is minimal. Collateral circulation from smaller blood vessels may help to improve the outcome.

Special concerns

Clinicians must be suspicious of vertebrobasilar insufficiency in elderly patients who suffer from vertigo. Hemorrhage has to be ruled out before blood thinner (anticoagulation) treatment is initiated. Additionally, it is important to take special precautions when feeding persons with brainstem infarction, because patients can develop problems with normal swallowing mechanisms that can cause aspiration pneumonia (caused by food lodged in the lungs).

Resources

BOOKS

Bradley, W., et al. *Neurology in Clinical Practice*. 5th ed. Philadelphia: Butterworth-Heinemann, 2008.
Goetz, C.G. *Goetz's Textbook of Clinical Neurology*. 3rd ed. Philadelphia: Saunders, 2007.

PERIODICALS

Costello, F. "Carotid artery dissection and vertebrobasilar insufficiency." *International Ophthalmology Clinics* 49 (July 1, 2009): 1– 14.
Kim, J. "Inner ear dysfunction due to vertebrobasilar ischemic stroke." *Seminars in Neurology* 29 (November 1, 2009):534–40.

WEBSITES

"Vertebrobasilar Circulatory Disorders." Medline Plus. http://www.nlm.nih.gov/medlineplus/ency/article/001423.htm (accessed August 28, 2011).

ORGANIZATIONS

National Stroke Association, 9707 East Easter Lane, Suite B, Centennial, CO 80112, (800) STROKES (787-6537), Fax: (303) 649-1328, info@stroke.org, http://www.stroke.org.

Laith Farid Gulli, MD
Alfredo Mori, MBBS
Nicole Mallory, MS, PA-C
Rosalyn Carson-DeWitt, MD

Vertigo, motion sickness

Definition

Vertigo is the medical term for a specific form of **dizziness** in which individuals feel as if the room (or environment) is spinning around them even though they are standing still. The name of the sensation comes from the Latin verb *verto*, which means "to turn around" or "to revolve." Vertigo is not a disorder by itself but rather a symptom of any of several disorders involving the vestibular system of the inner ear. The vestibular system is a group of organs in the inner ear that provide sensory input related to movement, orientation in space, and balance.

Motion sickness is a feeling of nausea or dizziness produced by conflicting information provided to the **central nervous system** by the various organs of sense perception. It is not a disorder or disease in the strict sense but a normal response to an abnormal situation, namely a disagreement between what the eyes see and what the organs of balance in the inner ear perceive.

Description

Motion sickness

Motion sickness is an ancient health issue for travelers, affecting seafarers for millennia and modern travelers by automobile, airplane, or spacecraft. It can also affect people on amusement park rides or playing computer simulation games. Motion sickness can even affect people riding on an animal. People vary in the intensity of the symptoms they experience during motion sickness. For most people it is only a minor problem, but some people become so sick that they are almost incapacitated. One difference between the nauseated feeling caused by motion sickness and that caused by other digestive disorders is that vomiting does not usually relieve the sick feeling in motion sickness; the person may continue to vomit without feeling better.

Vertigo

Vertigo is a sensation of one's surroundings whirling or spinning around; some people describe it as a sense of floating, "spaciness," or weightlessness. A few people experience vertigo as a feeling of being heavily weighted on one side of the body or pulled in one direction.

Demographics

Motion sickness

The demographics of people experiencing motion sickness vary somewhat depending on the mode of travel; almost 100% of people will get seasick on a boat in very rough waters but only about 30% will feel seasick sailing in relatively calm water. According to the Centers for Disease Control and Prevention (CDC), small boats and automobiles are the methods of travel most likely to produce motion sickness.

Some groups of people are more likely to develop motion sickness than others:

- children—about 50% of children between the ages of 2 and 12 get carsick
- people with migraine headaches
- women, particularly those who are pregnant or menstruating
- airline pilots—about 29% get airsick during flights; 70% experience motion sickness when training in flight simulators
- athletes—it is thought that athletes may be more susceptible to motion sickness because they have finely tuned senses and may be more aware of conflicting sensory input than most people
- astronauts—about 60% of American astronauts experience space sickness during their first shuttle flight. Motion sickness is thought to be more common in larger spacecraft because the astronauts can move around more freely.

Vertigo

Vertigo, like motion sickness, is a fairly common symptom in the general population even though it can have a number of different causes (described more fully below). About 5% of adults experience one or more episodes of vertigo in an average year; about 8% will experience vertigo at some point in their lives. Vertigo accounts for about 5–6% of all visits to doctors' offices and 2–3% of all visits to hospital emergency rooms in the United States and Canada each year. It is more common in adults than in children, twice as common in women as in men, and three times more common in the elderly than in younger adults. The most frequent single cause of vertigo is benign paroxysmal positional vertigo (BPPV), which accounts for at least 25% of cases. Vestibular neuronitis accounts for an additional 5%. Vertigo can be an unsettling experience for many people; fortunately, only about 5% of cases involve serious disorders.

Ménière's disease, a disorder of the inner ear that has vertigo as a prominent symptom, is known to run in families. The National Institute on Deafness and Other Communication Disorders (NIDCD) estimates that there are about 615,000 persons in the United States diagnosed with Ménière's disease as of 2011. Another

expert gives a figure of 1,000 cases per 100,000 population. About 55% of patients diagnosed with Ménière's have significant family histories of the disorder.

Causes and symptoms

Causes

MOTION SICKNESS. The basic cause of motion sickness is a disagreement between the eyes' perception of movement, the inner ear's perception of balance, and the body's orientation in space. The human sense of balance depends on the complex interaction of five different parts of the body:

- Inner ear's vestibular system. The vestibular system, as noted earlier, is a group of organs in the inner ear that provide sensory input related to movement, orientation in space, and balance. This system detects and monitors the motions of the head, such as rotation of the head on the neck or up-and-down, forward-and-backward, and side-to-side motions of the head.
- Eyes. The eyes help people locate themselves in space (whether they are upside down or right side up, for example) and identify the direction in which they are moving.
- Pressure receptors. These sensory receptors are located in the joints and spine; they tell the central nervous system what parts of the body are touching the ground.
- Sensory receptors in the muscles and joints. These receptors can tell what parts of the body are in motion.
- Central nervous system. The brain has to process inputs from the eyes, ears, pressure receptors, and muscle receptors, combine all this information, and interpret it.

If the combined sensory information is contradictory, the brain becomes confused. For example, someone riding in an airplane that has hit a patch of air turbulence may sense the up-and-down motion of the airplane through the pressure receptors in the body but not see any evidence of movement through the eyes. The brain receives messages that do not match or add up. One theory as to why this mismatch causes nausea and vomiting is that the part of the brain that resolves disagreements between what the eyes see and what the rest of the body feels is the same part that causes vomiting when a person eats something poisonous. This area is called the area postrema and is located in the lower part of the brain stem. This theory holds that when the eyes and the inner ear send the brain conflicting messages, the area postrema decides that one of the senses is mistaken, that the mistake is due to a poison, and that vomiting is necessary to get rid of the poison.

VERTIGO. Vertigo can be caused by a number of different disorders or conditions. The most common are:

• Benign paroxysmal positional vertigo (BPPV). BPPV is triggered by changes in the position of the head, such as lying down, tilting the head to one side, sitting up in bed, or bending over. It may also occur after a mild head injury. BPPV is caused by the migration of small crystals of calcium carbonate known as otoliths from the structures in which they are usually stored (the saccule and utricle) into one of the semicircular canals in the labyrinth of the inner ear. When the person changes head position, these otoliths (also called canaliths) displace some of the endolymph fluid in the inner ear and lead to the sensation of vertigo. Vertigo associated with BPPV usually lasts only 30 seconds to a minute and goes away once the person holds the head still. It is most common in adults over 60.

• Vestibular migraine. Vestibular migraine refers to vertigo associated with migraine headaches. The person typically experiences the vertigo along with the headache, but may also experience vertigo without a migraine episode.

• Head trauma (concussion). A skull fracture will often cause nausea and hearing loss as well as vertigo.

• Vestibular neuronitis. Vestibular neuronitis is a disorder of the vestibular system that may occur as a single brief episode or as a condition that lasts about 3 weeks and then resolves. It is associated with previous upper respiratory tract infections and is thought to represent a viral inflammation of the vestibular nerve that connects the ear to the brain. The virus most frequently associated with vestibular neuronitis is herpesvirus type 1, the type that causes cold sores in the mouth. Vestibular neuronitis is not associated with hearing loss.

• Ménière's disease. This is a disorder characterized by recurrent vertigo, sensory hearing loss, tinnitus (sensation of roaring or buzzing noises in the ear), and a feeling of fullness in the ear. It is named for the French physician Prosper Ménière, who first described the illness in 1861. People with Ménière's have periodic acute attacks that affect only one ear, in most cases. An attack is caused by fluctuating pressure in a fluid inside the inner ear known as endolymph. The endolymph is separated from another fluid called perilymph by thin membranes

containing nerves that govern hearing and balance. When the endolymph pressure increases, there is a sudden change in the rate of nerve cells firing, which leads to vertigo and a sense of fullness or discomfort inside the ear. An attack lasts from two or three to 24 hours.

• Heavy alcohol consumption.

• Medication side effects.

• Labyrinthitis resulting from allergies, bacterial infections, or viral infections that reach the inner ear, such as the common cold or influenza. Labyrinthitis differs from vestibular neuronitis in that it is accompanied by hearing loss. An acute episode of labyrinthitis lasts from one to six weeks.

• Repeated spinning of the body, as in certain childhood games or movements in classical ballet or figure skating. Vertigo due to this cause is usually brief and requires no treatment.

• Psychiatric disorders, most commonly panic attacks or depression.

Associated symptoms

As noted above, vertigo is itself a symptom rather than a disorder in its own right; however, vertigo is often accompanied by nausea, vomiting, and heavy perspiration. People with vertigo also frequently report feeling shaky or unsteady on their feet. Less common associated symptoms include blurred vision, **hearing loss**, and lowered level of consciousness. Patients with vestibular neuronitis may develop nystagmus, a form of involuntary eye movement.

Diagnosis

Patients with vertigo accompanied by any of the following symptoms should go to a hospital emergency room rather than their doctor, as these symptoms indicate a serious condition:

• dizziness or vertigo following a head injury

• stiff neck, fever over 101°F, or severe headache

• convulsions and vomiting that will not stop

• chest pain, heart palpitations, difficulty breathing, weakness, inability to move an arm or leg, or a change in vision or speech

• fainting or loss of consciousness

Diagnosis of motion sickness is usually based on the circumstances in which the person feels nauseated. Most people can tell when they are affected by motion sickness without consulting a doctor.

The most important part of the diagnostic process for vertigo is taking the patient history. While most people will first consult their primary care physician, he or she may refer the patient to an otolaryngologist, a specialist in ear, nose, and throat disorders. The doctor will ask about any recent infections, history of headaches, history of recent head injuries, medications taken, and a family history (if any) of vertigo. More specifically, the doctor will ask about the following:

• What was the severity of the first episode of vertigo?
• Onset: was it sudden or gradual?
• Length: how long did the episode last?
• Location: are both ears affected or only one?
• Recurrence: have there been several episodes of vertigo, how often do they occur, and how long do they last?
• Triggers: what triggers the vertigo, and what relieves it?
• Associated sensations in the ear: does the patient experience tinnitus, hearing loss, or a sense of fullness? Is the patient having a discharge from the ear?
• Other associated symptoms: has the patient experienced changes in vision or consciousness, nausea or vomiting, difficulty walking, or headache?
• Impact on the patient's life: Has the patient fallen, missed work, or stopped driving? Is the patient anxious or having panic attacks because of the vertigo?

The doctor will then examine the patient's eyes, ears, nose, and throat, perform some simple hearing tests, test the functions of the cranial nerves, take the patient's blood pressure, and ask the patient to stand up and walk a few steps to test gait and balance.

If the doctor suspects BPPV, he or she may perform the Dix-Hallpike positioning test. The patient is seated on the examining table with the legs extended in front. The doctor then turns the patient's head about 45° and then helps the patient lie down quickly with the head extended about 20° backward. The doctor then watches the patient's eyes to see whether nystagmus occurs. The patient may be asked to wear a special type of goggles called Frenzel goggles, which improve the sensitivity of the Dix-Hallpike test. A positive result indicates that BPPV is the most likely diagnosis.

A bedside test that can be done to test for loss of symmetry in the patient's vestibular system is called the caloric reflex test. The doctor first instills 1 mL of cold water at 86°F (30°C) into the patient's ear, followed by 1 mL of warm (111°F, 44°C) water. Instilling cold water into one ear will cause nystagmus toward the other ear, while instilling warm water will cause nystagmus toward the same ear. The caloric reflex test may be given as part of an electronystagmography (ENG) series of tests, which include measuring and recording the patient's eye movements in response to lights and similar stimuli as well as the caloric reflex test. ENG testing involves the attachment of electrodes around the patient's nose and measuring the movements of the eye in relation to the ground electrode.

Imaging tests are not usually useful in patients under 40 years of age. A computed tomography (CT) scan or magnetic resonance imaging (MRI) may be ordered if the doctor suspects a skull fracture, or a blood test to rule out syphilis or other infectious disorders that can affect the central nervous system. In severe cases of bacterial labyrinthitis, a culture of the infectious organism may be done.

Treatment

Treatment of vertigo and motion sickness depends on the cause(s) and the severity of the associated symptoms.

Medications

Treatment for motion sickness usually includes preventive measures, discussed below, and medications. The choice of medication depends on the length of the trip, any underlying medical conditions that the traveler may have, and concerns about drowsiness as a side effect. For example, airline pilots who have problems with airsickness are not allowed to take any medications that cause sleepiness or **visual disturbances** while they are in command of the plane.

Some medications for motion sickness, such as Benadryl, Bonine, and Dramamine, can be taken by mouth and are available without a prescription. They should be taken between 30 minutes to an hour before the trip in order to allow them to be absorbed through the digestive tract. Scopolamine, a prescription medication, is available in both an oral form and a transdermal patch. The patch is applied behind the ear four hours before the trip and can be replaced every three days if needed. The medication in the patch that prevents nausea is absorbed through the skin. All drugs taken to prevent motion sickness can cause drowsiness, dry mouth, blurred vision, and loss of coordination. People should use these medications with caution if they plan to drive, operate machinery, or go swimming or diving underwater. They should never combine these medications with alcohol.

Medications that are given to patients with Ménière's disease to treat the symptoms of an attack include drugs that help to control vertigo by numbing the brain's response to nerve impulses from the inner ear. These include such benzodiazepine tranquilizers as **diazepam** (Valium) or alprazolam (Xanax), and such antinausea drugs as prochlorperazine (Compazine). The doctor may also prescribe steroid medications to reduce inflammation in the inner ear.

Vestibular migraine is treated with the same medications used to prevent or treat migraine headaches.

Vestibular neuronitis is most commonly treated with a three-week course of methylprednisolone (Medrol, an anti-inflammatory steroid drug) to bring down the inflammation. The vertigo associated with the disorder may be treated with Dramamine, Benadryl, Antivert (meclozine, a medication that blocks the conduction of nerve impulses from the vestibular system to the brain), or Phenergan.

Labyrinthitis is treated in its early stages with **antiviral drugs**, often acyclovir, or with a corticosteroid drug like prednisone. Bacterial labyrinthitis is treated with a broad-spectrum antibiotic. Prochlorperazine (Compazine) may be given to relieve the patient's vertigo and nausea. Because labyrinthitis causes acute anxiety in many patients, a selective serotonin reuptake inhibitor (SSRI) like Prozac may also be prescribed.

Surgery

Ménière's disease can be treated with surgery if the patient does not respond to medications or psychotherapy. About 40% of patients with Ménière's disease are helped only by surgery. The surgeon may remove excess endolymphatic fluid; remove the entire labyrinth of the inner ear (the most radical procedure); inject an antibiotic into the middle ear through an incision in the ear drum; or operate on the internal canal of the ear, separating the nerve bundles governing hearing from the nerve bundles that govern the sense of balance, in order to control the patient's vertigo without sacrificing hearing. This procedure is called vestibular nerve sectioning.

Patients with BPPV who do not respond to canalith repositioning (described below) may be treated surgically by canal plugging. In canal plugging, the surgeon inserts a bone plug to block a portion of the inner ear. The plug prevents the fluid in the semicircular canal from responding to the shifting of calcium carbonate particles during head movement.

Psychotherapy

Patients with Ménière's disease whose attacks are triggered by emotional stress may be helped by therapists who teach biofeedback, meditation, or other techniques of stress reduction. Cognitive behavioral therapy is also reported to benefit patients with Ménière's.

Psychotherapy is also the treatment of choice for patients whose vertigo is associated with panic attacks, **depression**, anxiety disorders, or other psychiatric disorders.

Physical therapy

Canalith repositioning, also known as the Epley maneuver, is a procedure that is done in the doctor's office to relieve the symptoms of BPPV by moving the loose particles of calcium carbonate back into the utricle. There they are usually reabsorbed by the fluid in the inner ear. The doctor or physical therapist has the patient recline and turn the head to a 45° angle. Next, the doctor or therapist turns the patient's head in the opposite direction to a 90° angle. In the third step, the patient is asked to turn on the side of the nonsymptomatic ear and hold the head slightly downward. In the final step, the patient sits upright with the head tilted slightly forward. The patient is asked to avoid lying flat or placing the treated ear below shoulder level for the rest of the day. That night, the patient should sleep with the head elevated on two pillows.

The Epley maneuver can be repeated if necessary, and the patient can also be taught to perform it at home.

Patients with long-term vertigo following a severe episode of labyrinthitis may be helped by vestibular rehabilitation therapy (VRT). VRT is an individualized program of exercises designed by a physical therapist or occupational therapist for each patient. The therapist evaluates the patient's posture, balance, and gait, and measures the patient's eye/head coordination (how well the patient's eyes can track a moving object without moving the head). The therapist then devises a set of eye, head, and body exercises to be done at home as well as in the clinic. In essence, VRT retrains the brain to recognize and process signals from the vestibular system and coordinate them with information from the eyes and the body's sense of its orientation in space. VRT is often recommended as postsurgical treatment when a patient has had an operation for a vestibular disorder.

KEY TERMS

Area postrema—The part of the brain stem that controls vomiting.

Audiologist—A healthcare professional who specializes in diagnostic testing of hearing impairments and rehabilitation of patients with hearing problems.

Brain stem—The lower part of the brain that joins the spinal cord. It controls breathing, pain perception, and other vital functions.

Canalith—The name for a calcium carbonate crystal that has migrated into one of the semicircular canals of the ear.

Electronystagmography (ENG)—A series of diagnostic tests for vestibular disorders that involves recording the patient's eye movements while the examiner moves the head into various positions or instills warm or cold water into the patient's ear canal.

Endolymph—The fluid contained inside the membranous labyrinth of the inner ear.

Idiopathic—Of unknown cause or spontaneous origin.

Labyrinth—The inner ear. It consists of the membranous labyrinth (a system of sacs and ducts made of soft tissue) and the osseous or bony labyrinth (which surrounds and contains the membranous labyrinth).

Labyrinthitis—Acute inflammation of the inner ear, which may be caused by bacteria, viruses, or allergies.

Nystagmus—A periodic rhythmic involuntary movement of the eyes.

Otolaryngology—The branch of medicine that treats disorders of the ear, nose, and throat.

Otolith organs—Two small structures (saccule and utricle) that contain calcium carbonate crystals which can cause vertigo if they enter one of the semicircular canals and displace endolymph fluid when the person changes head position.

Otology—The branch of medicine that specializes in medical or surgical treatment of ear disorders.

Perilymph—The fluid that lies between the membranous labyrinth of the inner ear and the bony labyrinth.

Prophylaxis—A measure taken to prevent disease or an acute attack of a chronic disorder.

Tinnitus—A sensation of ringing, buzzing, roaring, or clicking noises in the ear.

Transdermal—Referring to a type of drug that enters the body by being absorbed through the skin.

Vertigo—An illusory feeling that either one's self or the environment is revolving. It is usually caused either by diseases of the inner ear or disturbances of the central nervous system.

Vestibular system—The group of organs in the inner ear that provide sensory input related to movement, orientation in space, and balance.

Alternative

There are a few types of alternative treatments that work for some people with motion sickness; they include drinking ginger tea or chewing on candied ginger. Ginger has long been used in traditional Chinese medicine to prevent nausea and is commonly recommended for morning sickness in pregnant women. Ginger also has the advantage of not causing drowsiness as a side effect. Another alternative treatment that benefits some travelers is the use of wrist bands or electric devices that stimulate a point on the wrist called the P6 point in **acupuncture**. The point is located about an inch and a half below the crease where the wrist meets the hand.

According to the NIDCD, acupuncture, tai chi, niacin, and gingko biloba have been tried as treatments for Ménière's disease, but there is no evidence as of 2011 that these treatments are effective.

Clinical trials

There were 39 clinical trials under way for vertigo as of mid-2011. One is a trial of functional magnetic resonance imaging (fMRI) as a way to diagnose vertigo. Others are trials of the Epley maneuver in treating BPPV, vestibular rehabilitation therapy in treating the long-term effects of severe labyrinthitis, and various medications in treating vestibular neuronitis and vestibular migraine. Information about current relevant clinical trials can be found at ClinicalTrials.gov.

Prognosis

Motion sickness

The prognosis for motion sickness is very good. Most people who experience motion sickness feel better fairly quickly after their trip is over, although some people who suffer from severe seasickness may feel sick for two or three days after reaching land.

Many people who travel frequently often develop a tolerance for the particular types of motion associated with a specific method of transportation; sailors sometimes speak of "getting one's sea legs" as a way of describing getting used to the motions of a ship without getting seasick.

Vertigo

The prognosis for vertigo depends on the cause. BPPV has no cure as of 2011 but can usually be managed well with canalith repositioning, which is effective in about 80% of cases. Canal plugging surgery is successful in about 90% of cases.

Ménière's disease is not fatal; however, there is no cure for it as of 2011. Medical treatment between attacks and/or surgery are intended to lower the patient's risk of further hearing loss. Although patients with milder forms of the disorder may be able to control their symptoms through dietary changes alone, the long-term results of Ménière's disease typically include progressive loss of hearing, increasing vertigo, or permanent **tinnitus**.

Vestibular neuronitis has a very good prognosis; most cases clear up completely in about three weeks. A small minority of patients experience recurrent episodes of vertigo following rapid head movement for several years afterward.

Labyrinthitis can lead to long-term episodes of vertigo or dizziness, particularly if it is not treated promptly. Bacterial labyrinthitis is the cause of one-third of all cases of hearing loss in later life. In a few cases, labyrinthitis can lead to Ménière's disease.

Prevention

Motion sickness

In addition to taking medications to prevent or minimize motion sickness, the CDC recommends the following preventive measures:

- Choose a seat that will provide a smoother ride—a seat where the eyes will see the same motion that the body and inner ears feel. These are the front seats of cars, the forward cars of trains, the center of a boat, and the seats over the wings of an airplane.
- Focus on the scenery outside the vehicle or the distant horizon rather than trying to read or looking at objects inside the vehicle.
- Minimize motions of the head and close the eyes. If possible, lie flat on the back or take a nap.
- Eat a light meal without fatty or spicy foods before traveling; do not eat a heavy meal before a trip or travel on a completely empty stomach.
- Do not drink alcoholic beverages or smoke.
- Try to minimize emotional stress and anxiety.
- If possible, open a nearby window or vent and breathe in some fresh air.

Vertigo

Prevention of vertigo caused by Ménière's disease involves prophylaxis (prevention of acute attacks) as well as direct treatment of symptoms. Prophylactic treatment begins with diet and nutrition. A low-salt diet is recommended for almost all patients with Ménière's, as reducing salt intake helps to lower the body's overall fluid volume. Lowered fluid volume in turn reduces the amount of fluid in the inner ear. Patients should avoid foods with high sodium content, including pizza, smoked or pickled fish, and other preserved foods. Other foods that commonly trigger acute attacks include chocolate; beverages containing caffeine or alcohol, particularly beer and red wine; and foods with high carbohydrate or high cholesterol content. Since nicotine also triggers Ménière's attacks, patients are advised to stop smoking. The doctor may also prescribe a diuretic, usually Dyazide or Diamox, to lower the fluid pressure in the inner ear. Diuretic medications help to prevent acute attacks but will not stop an attack once it has begun.

Vestibular migraine is preventable by taking medications intended to ward off migraine headaches. Verapamil (Isoptin) is the medication most often prescribed, although some patients benefit from methysergide (Sansert). A low-sodium diet such as the one recommended for Ménière's disease is reported to help about 30% of patients with vestibular migraine.

Vestibular neuronitis and labyrinthitis can be prevented by prompt treatment of ear infections, colds, flu, sinus congestion, and other respiratory tract infections.

Resources

BOOKS

Andreoli, Thomas E., et al., eds. *Andreoli and Carpenter's Cecil Essentials of Medicine.* 8th ed. Philadelphia: Saunders/Elsevier, 2010.

Blitzer, Andrew, et al. *Oxford American Handbook of Otolaryngology.* New York: Oxford University Press, 2008.

Hickey, Sue. *Finding Balance: Healing from a Decade of Vestibular Disorders.* New York: Demos Health, 2011.

Lindqvist, Agnes, and Gjord Nyman, eds. *Dizziness: Vertigo, Disequilibrium and Lightheadedness.* New York: Nova Biomedical, 2009.

PERIODICALS

Benun, J. "Balance and Vertigo in Children." *Pediatrics in Review* 32 (February 2011): 84–85.

Bisdorff, A.R. "Management of Vestibular Migraine." *Therapeutic Advances in Neurological Disorders* 4 (May 2011): 183–91.

Bronstein, A.M., and T. Lempert. "Management of the Patient with Chronic Dizziness." *Restorative Neurology and Neuroscience* 28 (January 2010): 83–90.

Clarke, A.H. "Laboratory Testing of the Vestibular System." *Current Opinion in Otolaryngology and Head and Neck Surgery* 18 (October 2010): 425–30.

Gottschall, K.R., et al. "Early Vestibular Physical Therapy Rehabilitation for Meniere's Disease." *Otolaryngologic Clinics of North America* 43 (October 2010): 1113–19.

Huppert, D., et al. "Which Medication Do I Need to Manage Dizzy Patients?" *Acta Oto-laryngologica* 131 (March 2011): 228–41.

Kaski, D., and B.M. Seemungal. "The Bedside Assessment of Vertigo." *Clinical Medicine* 10 (August 2010): 402–05.

Kutz Jr., J.W. "The Dizzy Patient." *Medical Clinics of North America* 94 (September 2010): 989–1002.

Post, R.E., and L.M. Dickerson. "Dizziness: A Diagnostic Approach." *American Family Physician* 82 (August 15, 2010): 361–69.

Sismanis, A. "Surgical Management of Common Peripheral Vestibular Diseases." *Current Opinion in Otolaryngology and Head and Neck Surgery* 18 (October 2010): 431–35.

WEBSITES

American Academy of Otolaryngology—Head and Neck Surgery. "Chapter 7: Dizziness." In *Primary Care Otolaryngology.* ENTnet.org. http://www.entnet.org/EducationAndResearch/loader.cfm?csModule = security%2fgetfile&pageid = 9667 (accessed July 26, 2011).

"Asking Your Audiologist about Vertigo." American Speech-Language-Hearing Association (ASHA). http://www.asha.org/uploadedFiles/aud/InfoSeries Vertigo.pdf (accessed July 26, 2011).

"Benign Paroxysmal Positional Vertigo (BPPV)." Mayo Clinic. http://www.mayoclinic.com/health/vertigo/DS00534 (accessed July 26, 2011).

Carroll, I. Dale. "Motion Sickness." Centers for Disease Control and Prevention (CDC). http://wwwnc.cdc.gov/travel/yellowbook/2012/chapter-2-the-pre-travel-consultation/motion-sickness.htm (accessed July 26, 2011).

"Dix-Hallpike Test and Epley Maneuver." YouTube. http://www.youtube.com/watch?v = 59EIKztATiw&feature = related (accessed July 26, 2011).

"Dizziness and Motion Sickness." American Academy of Otolaryngology—Head and Neck Surgery. http://www.entnet.org/HealthInformation/dizzinessMotionSickness.cfm (accessed July 26, 2011).

"Dizziness and Vertigo." Merck Manual Online. http://www.merckmanuals.com/professional/sec08/ch091/ch091e.html (accessed July 26, 2011).

Marill, Keith A. "Vestibular Neuronitis." Medscape Reference. http://emedicine.medscape.com/article/794489-overview (accessed July 26, 2011).

"Ménière's Disease." National Institute on Deafness and Other Communication Disorders (NIDCD). http://www.nidcd.nih.gov/health/balance/meniere.html (accessed July 26, 2011).

"Possible Symptoms of Vestibular Disorders." Vestibular Disorders Association (VEDA). http://www.vestibular.org/vestibular-disorders/symptoms.php (accessed July 26, 2011).

Samy, Hesham M. "Dizziness, Vertigo, and Imbalance." Medscape Reference. http://emedicine.medscape.com/article/1159385-overview (accessed July 26, 2011).

Shoup, Angela G. "Electronystagmography." Medscape Reference. http://emedicine.medscape.com/article/836028-overview (accessed July 26, 2011).

"Slide Show: Canalith Repositioning Procedure." Mayo Clinic. http://www.mayoclinic.com/health/canalith repositioning-procedure/MY01322 (accessed July 26, 2011).

ORGANIZATIONS

American Academy of Otolaryngology—Head and Neck Surgery, 1650 Diagonal Road, Alexandria, VA 22314-2857, (703) 836-4444, http://www.entnet.org.

American Speech-Language-Hearing Association (ASHA), 2200 Research Boulevard, Rockville, MD 20850-3289, (301) 296-5700, (800) 498-2071, Fax: (301) 296-8580, actioncenter@asha.org, http://www.asha.org.

Centers for Disease Control and Prevention (CDC), 1600 Clifton Road, Atlanta, GA 30333, (800) CDC-INFO, cdcinfo@cdc.gov, http://www.cdc.gov.

National Institute on Deafness and Other Communication Disorders (NIDCD), National Institutes of Health, 31 Center Drive, MSC 2320, Bethesda, MD 20892-2320, (301) 496-7243, (800) 241-1044, nidcdinfo@nidcd.nih.gov, http://www.nidcd.nih.gov.

Vestibular Disorders Association (VEDA), P.O. Box 13305, Portland, OR 97213, (800) 837-8428, Fax: (503) 229-8064, https://vestibular.org.

Rebecca J. Frey, Ph.D.

Vestibular schwannoma

Definition

A vestibular schwannoma is a type of benign (non-cancerous) tumor that affects the eighth cranial nerve.

Description

The eighth cranial nerve is involved in both hearing (the auditory or acoustic component of the nerve) and balance (the vestibular component of the nerve). Like all cranial nerves, the eighth cranial nerve (also called the acoustic or auditory nerve) is paired, meaning that there is one on each side of the body. Each eighth cranial nerve runs from the inner ear to the brain, passing through a bony canal called the internal auditory canal. This canal is shared with the seventh cranial nerve, the facial nerve.

Like many nerve fibers, the eighth cranial nerve is wrapped in a sheath composed of specialized Schwann cells that serve to speed the transmission of information along the nerve. When the Schwann cells grow in an uncontrolled fashion, they can develop into a tumor, called schwannoma or neuroma. Although a vestibular schwannoma is not malignant (cancerous), it can still result in serious symptoms caused by pressure on the eighth cranial nerve or on surrounding tissues or the adjacent facial nerve. Most cases of vestibular schwannoma are unilateral; that is, only one of the two eighth cranial nerves is affected.

Demographics

About 100,000 people in the United States develop vestibular schwannoma. Most people who develop a vestibular schwannoma are between the ages of 30 and 50; children rarely develop vestibular schwannoma. Women are slightly more likely than men to develop a vestibular schwannoma.

There is an increased risk of developing a vestibular schwannoma in individuals who have a disease called **neurofibromatosis**. In these cases, the tumors tend to develop on both sides (bilaterally). In fact, about 10% of all cases of vestibular schwannoma occur in individuals who have neurofibromatosis. People with neurofibromatosis who develop vestibular schwannoma may do so at a younger age, sometimes in their teens or early adulthood.

Causes and symptoms

No one knows exactly why some people develop a vestibular schwannoma. Most seem to occur sporadically, with no identifiable cause. There is an increased risk of developing a vestibular schwannoma in individuals with neurofibromatosis, and some research has suggested that individuals who are chronically exposed to loud noise may have an increased risk of developing a vestibular schwannoma.

The initial symptoms of vestibular schwannoma are caused by pressure on the eighth cranial nerve, and include gradually progressive one-sided **hearing loss**, buzzing in the ears (**tinnitus**), **dizziness**, and difficulty with balance. In particular, the hearing impairment greatly affects the ability to understand speech (speech discrimination). When the vestibular schwannoma puts pressure on the seventh cranial nerve, pain and numbness in the face may develop. Eventually, the facial muscles may become paralyzed. The individual may also experience difficulty chewing and/or swallowing, ear pain, and headache. When left untreated, hearing impairment may eventually lead to complete deafness in the affected ear. If the tumor begins to encroach on other brain tissues, the person may experience nausea, vomiting, fever, vision changes, and difficulty walking.

Diagnosis

A careful neurologic examination will reveal the deficits that are characteristic of vestibular schwannoma. Computed tomography (CT) or magnetic resonance imagaing (MRI) scan may help pinpoint the tumor. Audiometry and brainstem auditory evoked potential tests are performed to establish the degree of hearing deficit prior to treatment. Audiometry assesses hearing acuity by evaluating the ability to hear various volumes and tones. A brainstem auditory evoked potential test evaluates brain wave responses to clicking sounds, in order to assess the functioning of the auditory (hearing) pathways in the brain.

Treatment team

When an individual is suspected of having a vestibular schwannoma, an otorhinolaryngologist and/or neurologist may be consulted to arrive at a diagnosis. An otorhinolaryngologist will be called upon if surgery is required.

Treatment

Surgery is nearly always necessary to treat vestibular schwannoma. There are several different types of surgery that are used to remove a vestibular schwannoma, classified by the anatomical pathway used to reach the tumor (called the "approach"). The surgeon will choose the approach based on tumor size, preoperative hearing acuity, and the patient's ability to tolerate surgical risk. In some cases, it is not possible to remove the entire vestibular schwannoma without considerable risk of damage to adjacent structures. In these cases, only part of the vestibular schwannoma may be removed, and the rest may be left in place (called "partial resection").

When a patient is medically frail, the surgeon may choose to simply monitor the growth of the vestibular schwannoma, delaying surgery until it becomes absolutely necessary. Occasionally, very small vestibular schwannoma may be treated with radiation therapy; when partial resection is necessary, surgery may be followed by radiation treatment.

Newer treatment techniques are called stereotactic radiosurgery or gamma knife surgery. Three-dimensional imaging allows the exact location of the tumor to be defined. The patient's head is held in a frame that allows high-dose radiation to be delivered from multiple angles directly at the tumor site.

Recovery and rehabilitation

In patients for whom the hearing impairment is not total, a hearing aid may be helpful. In patients who have completely lost hearing in one ear, a system called contralateral routing of sound (CROS) sends sound from the deaf ear through a microphone to the hearing ear, improving overall hearing acuity.

Prognosis

Without treatment, vestibular schwannoma will nearly always result in permanent deafness. Although surgery carries a high risk of hearing loss and facial nerve impairment, about 66% of patients who have small- to medium-sized vestibular schwannoma have improved hearing acuity following surgery.

Resources

BOOKS

Janus, Todd J., and W. K. Alfred Yung. "Primary Neurological Tumors." In *Textbook of Clinical Neurology*, edited by Christopher G. Goetz. Philadelphia: W. B. Saunders, 2003.

Ng, James J. "Acoustic Neuroma." In *Ferri's Clinical Advisor: Instant Diagnosis and Treatment*, edited by Fred F. Ferri. St. Louis: Mosby, 2004.

Sagar, Stephen M., and Mark A. Israel. "Primary and Metastatic Tumors of the Nervous System." In *Harrison's Principles of Internal Medicine*, edited by Eugene Braunwald, et al. New York: McGraw-Hill Professional, 2001.

Seidman, Michael D., George T. Simpson, and Mumtaz J. Khan. "Common Problems of the Ear." In *Noble: Textbook of Primary Care Medicine*, edited by John Noble, et al. St. Louis: W. B. Saunders, 2001.

PERIODICALS

Ho, S. Y. "Acoustic Neuroma: Assessment and Management." *Otolaryngology Clinics of North America* 35, no. 2 (1 April 2002): 393–404.

ORGANIZATIONS

Acoustic Neuroma Association. 600 Peachtree Pkwy, Suite 108, Cumming, GA 30041-6899. Phone: (770) 205-8211. Fax: (770) 205-0239. Email: ANAUSA@aol.com. http://anausa.org/.

National Institute on Deafness and Other Communication Disorders, National Institutes of Health. 31 Center Drive, MSC 2320, Bethesda, MD 20892-2320. Phone: (301) 496-7243 . Fax: (301) 402-0018. Email: nidcdinfo@nidcd.nih.gov. http://www.nidcd.nih.gov/health/hearing/acoustic_neuroma.asp.

Rosalyn Carson-DeWitt, MD

Visual disturbances

Definition

Visual disturbances are abnormalities of sight. Visual disturbances associated with neurological disorders often include double vision (diplopia), moving or blurred vision due to nystagmus (involuntary rapid movements of the eyes), reduced visual acuity, reduced visual field, and partial or total loss of vision as in papilledema, a swelling of the optic disc, or in blindness. Visual disturbances are often symptoms of other disorders, in particular neurological disorders, but can also occur due to muscular disorders, vascular diseases, cancer, or trauma. Additionally, diseases such as diabetes and hyperthyroidism can contribute to the visual abnormalities. Some visual disturbances arise from congenital conditions that are often hereditary.

Description

Diplopia

Diplopia, or double vision, causes a person to see two objects instead of one. There are two main reasons for diplopia: one is a physical change in the lens, conjuctiva, or retinal surface; the second reason involves an inability of the brain to overlay the images seen with both eyes, which happens in a person with normal vision. The first type usually involves only one eye and is not corrected by covering of the eye. Scars or other physical defects in the eye cause the split of a single image, thus resulting in double vision. In contrast, the second type usually involves both eyes (binocular) and is corrected when one eye is covered. Binocular diplopia arises when the eye movement in one direction is prevented, and is often a congenital (present at birth) condition. Binocular diplopia is usually caused by misalignment of the eyes, which can be nerve or muscle related.

Abnormalities in eye movement can result from conditions such as cranial nerve paralysis (paresis), neuromuscular disease (e.g., **myasthenia gravis**), **multiple sclerosis**, infection, **stroke**, overactive thyroid (Graves' disease), or direct trauma to the eye. Diplopia can also be a result of a growing tumor, which presses on the nerves involved in eye movements.

The nerves involved in diplopia include three cranial nerves: the oculomotor nerve (third cranial nerve), the abducens nerve (sixth cranial nerve), and the trochlear nerve (fourth cranial nerve). These three nerves direct the movements of six extraocular muscles. Four muscles are innervated by the third cranial nerve, and the other two are innervated exclusively by either the fourth or the sixth cranial nerve. This arrangement allows the physician to determine the cause of visual disturbances observed in a patient. Misalignment of the eyes can be in any direction: inward, outward, upward, downward, or a combination. Damage to the third cranial nerve can cause outward and downward turning of the affected eye and the inability to pass midline in either of the two directions. Fourth cranial nerve damage will result in vertical diplopia, which is compensated by head tilting. Head turning is used to compensate for sixth cranial nerve damage that prevents outward movement of the eye.

Nystagmus

A different type of visual disturbance, nystagmus, is caused by abnormal eye movements and often results in blurred vision. Normal control of the eye movements depends on the neuronal connections between the eyes, brainstem, and the **cerebellum**. Changes in the **central nervous system** or peripheral labyrinthine apparatus can cause the uncontrolled, repetitive eye movements known as nystagmus. There are many types and subtypes of nystagmus depending on the underlying cause and movement involved. The most common form involves a jerking motion from side to side (horizontal nystagmus). The rapid eye movements can also appear in a vertical direction, usually indicating a problem with the central nervous system. Rotary movements are also sometimes observed in nystagmus.

Although nystagmus by itself does not cause loss of vision, it is often associated with poor vision. Nystagmus can develop in early childhood or in adulthood. Childhood nystagmus can be associated with eye defects (cataract or retinal disorders) or result from unknown causes (congenital idiopathic nystagmus). Most cases of congenital nystagmus are not caused by a disease process and are familial.

If nystagmus develops later in life, it can be a sign of a serious underlying problem such as stroke, multiple sclerosis, or complication from head trauma. The direction of the eye movement can help the physician to diagnose the underlying neurological problem. For example, in an unconscious person, vertical nystagmus can indicate brainstem damage. This illustrates that eye movements not only cause visual disturbances but are also an important diagnostic tool to determine if the brain is still alive.

The presence of the occulocephalic reflex (doll's eye movements) in people with **coma** shows that the brainstem is intact. The physician turns the patient's head from side to side or left to right to elicit the reflex. When the reflex is present, the eyes appear to move freely in the opposite direction from the direction the head was turned, thus moving in relation to the head. When the eyes remain fixated, a lack of cerebral activity is indicated. Another important diagnostic test is the cold caloric test. The cold caloric test traces the direction of nystagmus to assess the oculovestibular reflex. An unconscious person's ear is injected with cold water, causing slow horizontal movement of the eyes towards the stimulation, which is followed by a fast return of the eyes to the midline.

Blindness

Blindness is the partial or complete loss of vision. The leading causes of blindness are glaucoma, cataracts, and diabetic retinopathy. Blindness can also result from eye diseases, optic nerve disorders, or brain diseases involving visual pathways or the occipital lobe of the brain. The patterns of visual field reduction depend on the area that is being affected by disease. Damage to visual pathways as a result of macular degeneration, retinal detachment, or optic nerve atrophy can affect one or both eyes. In contrast, damage to the optic nerve chiasm or the pathway beyond it affects both eyes. There are many eye diseases that can cause visual abnormalities or/and blindness, including retinal detachment, cataracts, retinal disorders (often inherited), and macular degeneration.

Macular degeneration is the leading cause of blindness for those over age 55 in the United States. The macula is the central portion of the retina that records images and sends them from the eye to the brain via the optic nerve. If the macula deteriorates, the eye loses the ability to see in fine detail. The cause of macular degeneration is not fully understood, but risks for the disorder increase with age. Other abnormalities in the central retina can lead to blurry vision or can affect color perception. Color blindness can also originate from the lack of one or more type of cones, a type of light receptor on the eye. Total color blindness (monochromatic vision) is very rare; most commonly, varying levels of single color deficits are found among people with color blindness. Central vision can also be destroyed by small hemorrhages in the retina as a result of the aging process or diabetic retinopathy.

The neuronal diseases affecting the optic nerve and causing blindness can result from developmental abnormalities (hereditary or sporadic), abnormalities in the blood vessels causing an insufficient blood supply to the eyes or optic nerve, glaucoma, and demyelinating and inflammatory diseases such as multiple sclerosis, tumors, toxic agents, and trauma.

Optic nerve damage

Papilledema, the swelling of the optic nerve, can result from increased intracranial pressure or optic nerve deterioration (optic neuropathy). Inflammation,

lack of adequate blood supply to the optic nerve, and certain diseases such as multiple sclerosis can cause the optic nerve to deteriorate. A brain tumor, bleeding or blood clots in the brain, brain swelling due to **encephalitis** or trauma, or a blockage in cerebrospinal fluid circulation can cause an increase in pressure inside the skull (intracranial pressure). The condition is often life threatening, and correct diagnosis of papilledema is important.

Papilledema arising from increased intracranial pressure is often accompanied by other symptoms, including diplopia, nausea, headache, and reduction of the visual field. When diagnosing papilledema, the physician looks for swelling of the optic disc (the area where the optic nerve enters the eye). The early signs include slight changes in appearance of the edge of neural tissue. Later, the disc rises from the retinal surface and can appear pale or can show signs of hemorrhages in severe cases. Persistent, chronic papilledema can cause atrophy of the optic nerve head and result in blindness.

The optic nerve can also be damaged by increased intraocular pressure (IOP) as in glaucoma. The pressure develops in aqueous area of the eye and is transmitted to the back of the eye, causing an initial reduction in peripheral vision and leading eventually to blindness. Glaucoma is often a complication arising from diabetes.

Additionally, optic neuritis, or inflammation of the optic nerve, can cause permanent loss of vision. Demyelinating diseases such as multiple sclerosis, systemic infections, diabetes, and hereditary factors can cause optic neuritis. Optic neuritis can also be a secondary complication of diseases such as **meningitis**, sinusitis, or tuberculosis, or reactions to toxins or trauma.

Other important causes of blindness are tumors affecting the optic chiasm (the area in the brain where the optic nerves cross) such as gliomas, cerebral tumors, and pituitary adenomas. In these cases, the transfer of visual stimuli through the optic nerve and visual pathways is directly affected and results in blindness.

Resources

BOOKS

Acheson, James, and Paul Riordan-Eva. *Fundamentals of Clinical Ophthalmology: Neuro-Ophthalmology*. London: BMJ Books, 1999.

Glaser, J. D., ed. *Neuro-ophthalmology*, 3rd ed. Philadelphia: Lippincott Williams and Wilkins, 1999.

OTHER

"Double Vision (Diplopia)." *InteliHealth Inc*. February 28, 2004 (June 3, 2004). http://www.intelihealth.com/IH/ihtIH/WSIHW000/9339/23796.html.

"Understanding Nystagmus." *Royal National Institute of the Blind*. February 28, 2004 (June 3, 2004). http://www.rnib.org.uk/xpedio/groups/public/documents/public website/public_rnib003659.hcsp.

ORGANIZATIONS

National Eye Institute. 2020 Vision Place, Bethesda, MD 20892-3655. Phone: (301) 496-5248. http://www.nei.nih.gov/.

Agnieszka Maria Lichanska, PhD

Vitamin/nutritional deficiency

Definition

Vitamins are substances that the human body requires but is unable to synthesize and, therefore, must obtain externally. Deficiencies in three B vitamins, B1 or thiamine, B3 or niacin and B12 or cobalamin are known to cause neurological disorders. Thiamine deficiencies result in **beriberi**, which causes peripheral neurological dysfunction and cerebral neuropathy. Niacin deficiencies cause a wasting disease known as pellagra, which affects the skin, mucous membranes, gastrointestinal tract as well as the brain, spinal cord and peripheral nerves. Cobalamin deficiencies most often result in pernicious anemia. Neurological symptoms of pernicious anemia include numbness in the extremities, impaired coordination, and a ringing in the ears.

Description

Thiamine deficiency

Thiamine was the first water-soluble vitamin to be discovered and is, therefore, also known as vitamin B1. Thiamine deficiency, or beriberi, manifests itself as both wet beriberi, which affects the cardiovascular system, and dry beriberi, which causes neurological dysfunction. People suffering from beriberi exhibit muscle atrophy or wasting (especially in the legs), edema (swelling), mental confusion, intestinal discomfort, and an enlarged heart. Severe cases of dry beriberi may result in Wernicke-Korsakoff syndrome, and acute cases of wet beriberi may cause shoshin beriberi. Both of these extreme forms of the disease are sometimes fatal. In most cases, administering thiamine successfully reverses symptoms associated with thiamine deficiencies.

Niacin deficiency

Niacin deficiency results in pellagra. The major symptoms of pellagra are dermatitis, **dementia** (loss of intellectual functions), and diarrhea. Pellagra means "rough skin" in Italian, and it was named because of the characteristic roughened skin of people who have the disease. Skin lesions generally appear on both sides of the body (bilaterally) and are found in regions exposed to sunlight. The disease also affects mucous membranes of the mouth, vagina, and urethra. Gastrointestinal discomfort is an early symptom, followed by nausea, vomiting, and diarrhea, often bloody. Neurological dysfunctions associated with niacin deficiencies include memory loss, confusion, and confabulation (imagined memory). Although treatment with niacin usually reverses all of the symptoms, untreated niacin deficiencies can result in multiple organ failure.

Vitamin B12 deficiency

Vitamin B12, also called cobalamin or cyanocobalamin, has the most complex chemical structure of all vitamins. It is unique in that it contains a cobalt atom embedded in a ring, similar to the iron atom in hemoglobin. The cobalt gives the molecule a dark red color. Vitamin B12 is found bound to animal protein and is very rare in vegetables. A deficiency of vitamin B12 results in a blood disorder, also called an anemia, which enlarges red blood cells so that the immune system destroys them at an increased rate. Because the blood cells are enlarged, the disease is characterized as a macrocytic anemia. Vitamin B12 functions in many important cellular processes, including synthesis of red blood cells, DNA synthesis and the formation of the myelin sheath that acts as insulation around nerve cells. One of the most common causes of vitamin B12 deficiency is pernicious anemia, which is itself caused by a lack of a glycoprotein called intrinsic factor that is required for absorption of vitamin B12. Intrinsic factor is secreted by the stomach, where it binds to the vitamin and transports it to the small intestine for absorption. Symptoms of vitamin B12 deficiency progress from **weakness** and **fatigue** to neurological disorders including numbness in the extremities, poor coordination, and eventually, to hallucinations and psychosis. Vitamin B12 deficiencies are usually treated with intramuscular injections of vitamin B12 initially and oral vitamin B12 supplements on an ongoing basis.

Demographics

Thiamine deficiency

Thiamine deficiencies have no sex or racial predilection. Thiamine deficiency is more common in developing countries where poor nutrition occurs frequently, although no accurate statistics on its occurrence are available. In many of these countries, cassava or milled rice acts as a major staple of the diet. While cassava does contain some thiamine, it contains so much carbohydrate relative to the thiamine, that eating cassava actually consumes thiamine. Most of the thiamine in rice is found in the husk. When the husk is removed from the rice during milling, the result is a diet staple that is an extremely poor source of thiamine.

Beriberi is often associated with alcoholism, likely because of low thiamine intake, impaired ability to absorb and store thiamine and acceleration in the reduction of thiamine diphosphate. People who strictly follow fad diets, people undergoing starvation, and people receiving large amounts of intravenous fluids are all susceptible to beriberi. Some physical conditions such as hyperthyroidism, pregnancy, or severe illness may cause a person to require more thiamine than normal and may put a person at risk for deficiency.

A form of beriberi specific to infants known as infantile beriberi can occur in babies between two and four months old that are fed only breast milk from mothers who are thiamine deficient.

Niacin deficiency

Pellagra is most common when maize is a major part of the diet. Although maize does contain niacin, it is not biologically available unless it is treated with basic compounds, such as lime. This process occurs in the making of tortillas, so populations in Mexico and Central America do not usually suffer from pellagra. Maize is also deficient in tryptophan, a precursor to niacin.

In the early 1900s, pellagra was epidemic in the southern United States because of the large amount of corn in the diet. After niacin was discovered to prevent pellagra in 1937, flour was fortified with niacin and reports of pellagra decreased dramatically. Currently, incidence rates of pellagra in the United States are unknown. People at risk for pellagra include alcoholics, people on fad diets, and people with gastrointestinal absorption dysfunction.

The group of people who most commonly suffer from pellagra live in the Deccan Plateau of India. Their diet is rich in millet or sorghum, which contains tryptophan, but also large concentrations of another amino acid, leucine. It is thought that leucine inhibits the conversion of tryptophan to niacin.

Vitamin B12 deficiency

Pernicious anemia is most common in patients of northern European descent and African Americans and less frequent in people of southern European descent and Asians. There is no sex predilection. Vitamin B12 deficiency occurs in 3%–43% of people over the age of 65. A form of pernicious anemia is also found in children under the age of ten. It is more frequent in patients with other immune disorders such as Grave's disease or Crohn's disease. There is some evidence that relatives of people who have pernicious anemia are more likely to get the disorder, indicating some genetic component to the disease. Because vitamin B12 only occurs in animal proteins, vegetarians are susceptible to the disease and should take vitamin B12 supplements.

Causes and symptoms

Thiamine deficiency

Thiamine deficiencies are caused by an inadequate intake of thiamine. In most developed countries getting enough thiamine is not a problem since it is found in all vegetables, especially the outer layer of grains. It is not present in refined sugars or fats and is not found in animal tissue. Diets rich in foods that contain thiaminases, enzymes that break down thiamine, such as milled rice, shrimp, mussels, clams, fresh fish and raw meat may be associated with thiamine deficiencies.

Thiamine is absorbed through the digestive tract by a combination of active and passive absorption. It is stored in the body as thiamine diphosphate, also called thiamine pyrophosphate, and thiamine triphosphate.

Thiamine diphosphate is the active form and it is used as a coenzyme in several steps in cellular respiration. Thiamine may also have an important role in the function of nerve cells independent of cellular respiration. It is found in the cell membranes of nerve axons, and electrical stimulation of nerve cells causes a release of thiamine.

Early thiamine deficiency produces fatigue, abdominal pain, constipation, irritation, loss of memory, chest pain, anorexia and sleep disturbance. As the deficiency progresses, it can be classified as dry beriberi or wet beriberi depending on the activity of the patient. Many persons experience a mixture of the two types of beriberi, although pure forms do occur.

When caloric intake and physical activity are low, thiamine deficiency produces neurological dysfunction termed dry beriberi. Symptoms occur with equal intensity on both sides of the body and usually start in the legs. Impaired motor and reflex function coupled with pain, numbness and cramps are symptomatic of the disease. As the disease advances, ankle and knee jerk reactions will be lost, muscle tone in the calf and thigh will atrophy and eventually the patient will suffer from **foot drop** and toe drop. The arms may begin to show symptoms of neurological dysfunction after the legs are already symptomatic. Histological (tissue) tests may indicate patchy degradation of myelin in muscle tissues.

Wernicke-Korsadoff syndrome, also called cerebral beriberi, occurs in extreme cases of dry beriberi. The early stage is called Korsakoff's syndrome and is characterized by confusion, the inability to learn, amnesia, and telling stories that bear no relation to reality. Wernicke's **encephalopathy** follows with symptoms of vomiting, nystagmus (rapid horizontal or vertical eye movement), opthalmoplegia (inability to move the eye outwards) and ptosis (eyelid droop). If untreated, Wernicke's encephalopathy may progress to **coma** and eventually death.

If a person has a high caloric intake and reasonable levels of activity, but has a diet with insufficient thiamine, myocardial dysfunction, termed wet beriberi, may result. This disease consists of vasodilatation and high cardiac output, retention of salt and water, and eventual damage to the heart muscle. A person suffering from wet beriberi will exhibit rapid heartbeat (tachycardia), swelling (edema), high blood pressure, and chest pain.

Shoshin beriberi is a more acute form of wet beriberi and is characterized by damage to the heart muscle accompanied by anxiety and restlessness. If no treatment is received, the damage to the heart may be fatal.

Niacin deficiency

Niacin, also called vitamin B3, is a general term for two molecules: nicotinic acid and nicotinamine. Nicotinic acid is very easily converted into biologically important molecules including nicotinamide adenine dinucleotide (NAD or coenzyme I) and nicotinaminamide adenine dinucleotide phosphate (NADP or coenzyme II), both of which are crucial to oxidation-reduction reactions in cellular metabolism. These reactions play key roles in glycololysis, the generation of high-energy phosphate bonds, and metabolism of fatty acids, proteins, glycerol and pyruvate. Because niacin plays such an important role in so many different cellular functions, the effect of niacin deficiencies on the body is extremely broad.

The amino acid, tryptophan is a precursor to niacin, and therefore, niacin deficiency can be averted if tryptophan is included in the diet. Some of the psychological symptoms of pellagra are thought to be related to decreased conversion rates of tryptophan to serotonin (a neurotransmitter) in the brain.

Causes of pellagra include diets that are deficient in niacin or its precursor, tryptophan. These diets often rely heavily on unprocessed maize. Other diets that may cause pellagra contain amino acid imbalances. For example, diets that rely on sorghum as a staple contain excessive amounts of the amino acid leucine, which interferes with tryptophan metabolism. Other causes of pellagra include alcoholism, fad diets, diabetes, cirrhosis of the liver, and digestive disorders that prevent proper absorption of niacin or tryptophan. One such disorder is called Hartnup disease, which is a congenital defect that interferes with tryptophan metabolism.

Symptoms of pellagra occur in the skin, in mucous membranes, the gastrointestinal tract and the **central nervous system**. Skin symptoms are usually bilaterally symmetric. They include lesions characterized by redness and crusting, thickening of the skin and skin inelasticity. Secondary infections are common, especially after exposure to the sun. Mucus membranes are also affected by pellagra. Typically, the tongue becomes bright red first and then the mouth becomes sore, coupled with increased salivation and edema of the tongue. Eventually, ulcers may appear throughout the mouth. Gastrointestinal symptoms include burning of the mouth and esophagus and abdominal pain. Later symptoms include vomiting and diarrhea, often bloody.

The central nervous system is also affected by niacin deficiencies. Early symptoms include memory loss, disorientation, confusion, **hallucination**. More severe symptoms are characterized by loss of consciousness, rigidity in the extremities and uncontrolled sucking and grasping.

Vitamin B12 deficiency

Vitamin B12 is required for the biochemical reaction that converts homocysteine to methionine, one of the essential amino acids required to synthesize proteins. Because vitamin B12 impairs DNA translation, cell division is slow, but the cytoplasm of the cell develops normally. This leads to enlarged cells, especially in cells that usually divide quickly, like red blood cells. In addition, there is usually a high ration of RNA to DNA in these cells. Enlarged red blood cells are more likely to be destroyed by the immune system in the bone marrow, causing a deficit of red blood cells in the blood. Methionine is also required to produce choline and choline-containing phospholipids. Choline and choline-containing phospholipids are a major component of cell membranes and acetocholine, which is crucial to nerve function.

Vitamin B12 requires several binding proteins in order to be absorbed properly. After ingestion into the stomach, it forms a complex with R binding protein, which moves into the small intestine. The stomach secretes another protein, intrinsic factor, which binds with vitamin B12 after R binding factor is digested in the small intestine. Intrinsic factor bound with vitamin B12 adheres to specialized receptors in the ileum, where it is brought inside of cells that line the intestinal wall. Vitamin B12 is then transferred to another protein, transcobalamin II, which circulates through the blood plasma to all parts of the body. Another protein, transcobalamin I, is found bound to vitamin B12; however, its function is not well understood.

Because of the complexity of the steps required for vitamin B12 absorption, there are many different ways that deficiencies could arise. First, a person could have inadequate intake of vitamin B12. This is extremely rare, since it is found in most animal proteins, but it does occur in some strict vegetarians. If any of the proteins that usher vitamin B12 through the body are unavailable or damaged, vitamin B12 deficiencies could arise. The most common such problem is associated with inadequate production of intrinsic factor, which results in pernicious anemia. Inadequate production of intrinsic factor can occur because of atrophy (wasting) of the stomach lining, the removal of the part of the stomach that produces intrinsic factor, or in rare cases because of a congenital defect. Rare cases of intestinal parasites such as a fish tapeworm and bacterial infections may also result in vitamin B12 deficiencies. Finally, acid is often required to hydrolyze vitamin B12 from animal proteins in the stomach. If the stomach is not sufficiently acidic, for example, in the presence of antacid medicines, quantities of vitamin B12 available for absorption may be deficient.

The liver stores large amounts of vitamin B12. It is estimated that if vitamin B12 uptake is suddenly stopped, it would take three to five years to completely deplete the stores in a typical adult. As a result, vitamin B12 deficiencies develop over many years. Initial symptoms include weakness, fatigue, lightheadedness, weight loss, diarrhea, abdominal pain, shortness of breath, sore mouth and loss of taste, and tingling in the fingers and toes.

As the disease progresses, neurological symptoms begin to appear. These include forgetfulness, **depression**, confusion, difficulty thinking and impaired judgment. Eventually, a person with vitamin B12 deficiency will have numbness in the fingers and toes, impaired balance and poor coordination, ringing in the ears, changes in reflexes, hallucinations and psychosis.

Diagnosis

Thiamine deficiency

A patient with bilateral symmetric neurological symptoms, especially in the lower extremities may be suffering from thiamine deficiency, especially if there is an indication that the diet may be poor. Diseases with symptoms that are similar to beriberi include diabetes and alcoholism. Other neuropathies, such as sciatica, are often not symmetric and are not usually associated with beriberi.

Laboratory tests may show high concentrations of pyruvate and lactate in the blood and low concentrations of thiamine in the urine. Because the disease responds so well to thiamine, it is often used as a diagnostic tool. After administration of thiamine diphosphate, an increase in certain enzyme activity in red blood cells is an excellent indicator of thiamine deficiency.

Niacin deficiency

There are no diagnostic tests currently available to detect niacin deficiencies. Concentrations of niacin and tryptophan in the urine of patients suffering from pellagra are low but not lower than other patients with malnutrition. Diagnosis must be made given a patient's symptoms and dietary history. Because replacement of niacin is so effective, it may be used as a diagnostic tool.

Vitamin B12 deficiency

A person suspected of suffering from vitamin B12 deficiency will be subjected to a physical examination along with blood tests. These blood tests will include a complete blood count (CBC). If blood analyses indicate that the red blood cells are enlarged, vitamin B12 deficiency may be diagnosed. Other disorders that exhibit enlarged red blood cells (macrocytes) include alcoholism, hypthyroidism, and other forms of anemia. White

KEY TERMS

Amino acid—An organic compound composed of both an amino group and an acidic carboxyl group. Amino acids are the basic building blocks of proteins. There are 20 types of amino acids (eight are "essential amino acids" which the body cannot make and must, therefore, be obtained from food).

Anemia—A condition in which there is an abnormally low number of red blood cells in the bloodstream. It may be due to loss of blood, an increase in red blood cell destruction, or a decrease in red blood cell production. Major symptoms are paleness, shortness of breath, unusually fast or strong heart beats, and tiredness.

Vitamins—Small compounds required for metabolism that must be supplied by diet, microorganisms in the gut (vitamin K), or sunlight (UV light converts pre-vitamin D to vitamin D).

blood cells with segmented nuclei also indicate vitamin B12 deficiency. Other blood tests include a vitamin B12 test and folic acid tests. Low concentrations of both may indicate vitamin B12 deficiencies. Elevated levels of homocysteine, methylmalonic acid (MMA) or lactate dehydrogenase (LDH) indicate vitamin B12 deficiencies. Finally, tests that indicate the presence of antibodies against intrinsic factor may indicate pernicious anemia.

Once a vitamin B12 deficiency has been established in a patient, the severity of the disease can be evaluated using a Schilling test. The patient is orally administered radioactive cobalamin and then an injection of unlabeled cobalamin is given intramuscularly. The ratio of radioactive to unlabeled cobalamin in the urine during the next 24 hours gives information on the absorption rate of cobalamin by the patient. If the rates are abnormal, pernicious anemia is diagnosed. As a final check, the patient is given cobalamin bound to intrinsic factor. With this, the patient's absorption rates should become normal if pernicious anemia is the cause of the symptoms.

Treatment

Thiamine deficiency

In most cases, rapid administration of intravenous thiamine will reduce symptoms of thiamine deficiency. Continued dosages of the vitamin should be continued for several weeks accompanied by a nutritious diet. Following recovery, a diet containing one to two times the recommended daily allowance of thiamine (1–1.5 mg per day) should be maintained. Shoshin beriberi requires cardiac support as well. Thiamine has not been found to be toxic for people with normal kidney function, even at high doses.

Niacin deficiency

Niacin deficiency can be treated effectively with replacement of niacin in the diet. In the case of Hartnup disease, large quantities of niacin may be required for effective reversal of symptoms.

Vitamin B12 deficiency

Vitamin B12 deficiency responds well to administration of cobalamin. Because absorption in the small intestine is often part of the problem, the best way to administer cobalamin is by intramuscular injection on a daily basis. After 6 weeks, the injections can be decreased to monthly for the rest of the patient's life. Usually, response to this treatment alleviates all symptoms of the disease. In severe cases, a blood transfusion may be needed and neurological conditions may not be completely reversed.

Resources

BOOKS

Garrison, Robert H., Jr. and Elizabeth Somer. *The Nutrition Desk Reference*. New Canaan, CT: Keats, 1985.

Peckenpaugh, Nancy J. and Charlotte M. Poleman. *Nutrition: Essentials and Diet Therapy*. Philadelphia: W. B. Saunders 1999.

OTHER

Lovinger, Sarah Pressman. "Beriberi" *MEDLINE plus*. National Library of Medicine. http://www.nlm.nih.gov/medlineplus/ency/article/000339.htm#Symptoms (February, 8 2004).

"Niacin deficiency." *The Merck Manual*.http://www.merck.com/mrkshared/mmanual/section1/chapter3/3l.jsp (January 16, 2004).

"Thiamine deficiency and dependency." *The Merk Manual*. http://www.merck.com/mrkshared/mmanual/section1/chapter3/3j.jsp (January 16, 2004).

ORGANIZATIONS

NIH/National Digestive Diseases Information Clearinghouse. 2 Information Way, Bethesda, MD 20892-3570. Phone: (301) 654-3810. Fax: (301) 907-8906. Tollfree phone: (800) 891-5389. Email: nddic@info.niddk.nih.gov. http://www.niddk.nih.gov.

National Heart, Lung, and Blood Institute (NHLBI). P.O. Box 30105, Bethesda, MD 20824-0105. Phone: (301) 592-8573. Fax: (301) 592-8563. Email: NHLBIinfo@rover.nhlbi.nih.gov. http://www.nhlbi.nih.gov.

Juli M. Berwald, Ph.D.

Vitamin B$_{12}$ deficiency *see* **Vitamin/ nutritional deficiency**

von Economo disease *see* **Encephalitis lethargica**

Von Hippel-Lindau disease

Definition

Von Hippel-Lindau disease (VHL) is a hereditary condition that involves cancer and can affect people of all ages. It was named in 1964 after the physicians to first describe aspects of the condition in the early 1900s, German ophthalmologist Eugen von Hippel and Swedish pathologist Arvid Lindau.

Description

VHL often involves symptoms in the **central nervous system** (CNS) and includes hemangioblastomas of the **cerebellum**, spinal cord, brainstem, and nerve root. Retinal hemangioblastomas and endolymphatic sac tumors are CNS tumors that can also be seen. The kidneys, adrenal gland, pancreas, epididymis, and female broad ligaments may also be affected.

Behavioral and learning problems are not usually associated with VHL, but may be if the CNS tumors are quite significant. Symptoms of VHL do not usually cause concerns in very early childhood. However, VHL is a hereditary cancer syndrome for which screening is appropriate in late childhood and adolescence for those at risk.

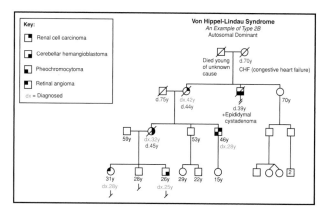

See Symbol Guide for Pedigree Charts. *(Illustration by Argosy, Inc. Reproduced by permission of Gale, a part of Cengage Learning.)*

Demographics

Studies from 1991 indicated an incidence of VHL of about 1 in 36,000 live births in eastern England. The condition affects people of all ethnic groups worldwide, with an equal proportion of males and females.

In 1993, the gene for VHL was identified. The majority of people with VHL also have an affected parent, but in about 20% of cases there is no known family history of VHL.

Causes and symptoms

Causes

Mutations in the VHL gene on chromosome 3 are now known to cause the condition. VHL is inherited in an autosomal dominant manner, meaning that an affected individual has a 50% chance to pass a disease-causing mutation to offspring, regardless of their gender.

VHL is a tumor-suppressor gene, or one whose normal function is to prevent cancer by controlling cell growth. Mutations in the VHL gene potentially cause uncontrolled cell growth in the gene, which is why a person with a VHL mutation is prone to developing cancer and other growths.

Symptoms

Hemangioblastomas of the CNS are the most common tumor in VHL; about 60–80% of people with VHL develop these tumors. The average age for CNS hemangioblastomas to develop is 33 years. The tubors are a frequent cause of death in people with VHL because they can disturb normal brain functioning. They can occur anywhere along the brain/spine areas, and swelling or cysts are often associated. The most common locations for CNS hemangioblastomas are in the spinal cord and cerebellum.

Symptoms from CNS hemangioblastomas depend on their size and exact location. Common symptoms include headaches, vomiting, gait disturbances, and **ataxia**, especially when the cerebellum is involved. Spinal hemangioblastomas often bring pain, but sensory and motor loss may develop only if the tumor is so large that it is pressing into the spinal cord. Some hemangioblastomas never cause symptoms, and are only seen with special imaging techniques.

Retinal hemangioblastomas are seen in as many as 60% of people, and many times may be the first sign of VHL. There may be multiple hemangioblastomas in one eye or even in both eyes. The average age for these to develop is about 25 years, but some

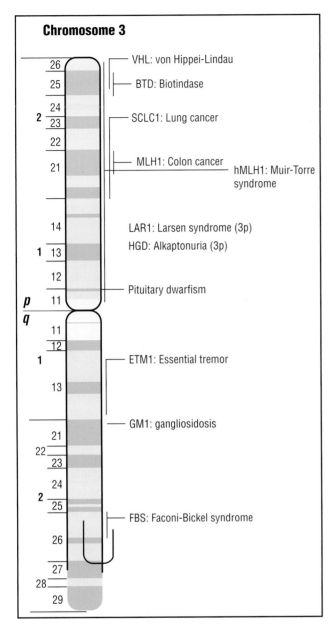

Chromosome 3

26 — VHL: von Hippel-Lindau

25 —— BTD: Biotindase

24

2 23 — SCLC1: Lung cancer

22

21 — MLH1: Colon cancer — hMLH1: Muir-Torre syndrome

14 — LAR1: Larsen syndrome (3p)

1 13 — HGD: Alkaptonuria (3p)

12

p 11 — Pituitary dwarfism

q

11

12

1 — ETM1: Essential tremor

13

— GM1: gangliosidosis

21

22

23

24

2 25

— FBS: Faconi-Bickel syndrome

26

27

28

29

von Hippel-Landau disease, on chromome 3. *(Illustration by Argosy, Inc. Reproduced by permission of Gale, a part of Cengage Learning.)*

develop in people younger than 10 years of age. When in the early stages and quite small, retinal hemangioblastomas may not cause symptoms. As they progress, they can cause retinal detachment, with partial or total vision loss.

Endolymphatic sac tumors are seen in about 11% of people with VHL, but are very rare in the general population. The first sign of this form of tumor may be partial **hearing loss**, which may progress to total hearing loss. Other symptoms can be **tinnitus** (buzzing in

the ear), **dizziness**, and facial paresis. These tumors often erode or expand the inner bones of the ear, a major reason for the hearing loss.

Kidney involvement occurs in about 60% of people with VHL, which usually includes renal cell carcinoma and kidney cysts. The typical age that these symptoms develop is 39 years. One or both kidneys may be diseased, with multiple cysts or growths that may be seen in each kidney. Renal cell carcinoma is a major cause of death in VHL. Kidney disease may not cause symptoms, or may not cause a reduction in kidney function. In severe cases blood in the urine, a mass or pain may be felt in an affected person's side.

Adrenal gland pheochromocytomas occur in 10–20% of people with VHL; the average age of diagnosis is 30 years, though they have been seen in children under the age of 10. There may be a single tumor present or multiple tumors. For people with a subset of VHL called type 2C, a pheochromocytoma is the only symptom they have. Five percent of all pheochromocytomas are cancerous, requiring treatment. Symptoms of pheochromocytomas may include intermittent or continuous high blood pressure, heart palpitations, a quickened heart rate, headaches, sweating episodes, nausea, and paleness of the skin. Pheochromocytomas may also cause the level of catecholamines to be elevated in urine.

Of all people with VHL, 35–70% have a pancreatic tumor, cyst, or cystadenoma. The masses often develop in the mid-30s and are usually without symptoms. Pancreatic involvement is important to diagnose VHL, but is difficult to identify on its own because it may cause no medical problems.

Men with VHL have epididymal cystadenomas 25–60% of the time. There may be multiple masses, occurring in both sides. If occurring in both sides, in rare cases they may lead to infertility. Epididymal cystadenomas are non-cancerous and may show up in the teenage years. In women, a similar tumor to the epididymal cystadenoma in men is that of the broad ligaments. These are not very common, so the true frequency and age of development is unknown in VHL. They are noncancerous and usually cause no specific symptoms.

Diagnosis

Until the discovery of the VHL gene, the diagnosis of the condition was made on a clinical basis. People with a family history of VHL need only have a CNS hemangioblastoma (including retinal), pheochromocytoma, or renal cell carcinoma to be given a diagnosis. Those without a family history must have two or more CNS hemangioblastomas, or one CNS and a visceral finding (with the exception of epididymal and renal cysts) to have a diagnosis.

There has been the creation of subtypes within VHL. Type 1 families are at a very low risk for pheochromocytomas, but have the typical risk for all other tumors that are seen. All type 2 families have a risk for pheochromocytomas; type 2A families have a low risk for renal cell carcinoma, while type 2B families have a high risk for it; type 2C families only have pheochromocytomas and no other signs of VHL.

Hemangioblastomas of the brain and spine are typically found through magnetic resonance imaging (MRI) scans. Those found in the retina can be seen by examination of the dilated eye by an ophthalmologist. Endolymphatic tumors may be visualized using computed tomography (CT) and MRI scans of the internal ear canals. Audiograms can also be done to identify and track hearing loss.

Renal and pancreatic involvement is often found through abdominal CT scans, MRI scans, or ultrasounds of the kidneys and pancreas. Pheochromocytomas can be seen on CT or MRI scans, and occasionally meta-iodobenzylguanidine (MIBG) scintigraphy is required to detect them. Epididymal cystadenomas are usually felt by a physical examination and confirmation through an ultrasound. Broad ligament cystadenomas can be diagnosed by CT scans or an ultrasound.

Genetic testing is available for VHL through gene sequencing and other methods. Testing is useful for confirming a clinical diagnosis or for family testing when there is an identified VHL mutation in the family. Analysis of the VHL gene is not perfect, but it detects about 90% of mutations that cause VHL. An informative test result is one that identifies a known mutation in the gene, and this confirms that the person has VHL. A negative test result means a mutation was not found in the gene. This either means that the tested individual does not have VHL or instead has a mutation that cannot be found through testing but actually has the diagnosis.

Genetic testing for children at risk for VHL is recommended because some symptoms can show up in childhood. Earlier screening may reduce the chance of serious future complications. As with all genetic testing in people who have no symptoms, the risks, benefits, and limitations of testing should be discussed through proper genetic counseling.

Treatment team

Treatment for people with VHL is often specific to the person. A multi-disciplinary team and approach are essential. A treatment team for someone with VHL may include a neurologist, neurosurgeon, medical geneticist, genetic counselor, endocrinologist, pulmonologist, nephrologist, ophthalmologist, social worker, urologist, and a primary care provider. Often there are pediatric specialists in these fields who aid in the care for children. The key is good communication between the various specialists to coordinate medical care.

Treatment

There is no cure for von Hippel-Lindau disease. Treatment and management are often based on symptoms. Genetic testing has helped to identify individuals without symptoms, so medical screening may begin earlier than usual.

Most brain and spine hemangioblastomas can be treated by removal through surgery. Radiation therapy is sometimes used, if surgery is not possible. Growth patterns of these tumors can be unpredictable, so monitoring through regular imaging is important. Screening by MRI is recommended yearly, beginning at age 11.

Treatment for retinal tumors varies. Many tumors respond to laser therapy or cryotherapy. In rare cases, removal of the eye is needed to reduce severe pain or the risk for irreversible glaucoma. The key is early diagnosis and monitoring to prevent vision loss or blindness. For this reason, an ophthalmology exam is recommended first in infancy, and yearly thereafter.

Surgery may be quite successful for endolymphatic sac tumors, often preserving the hearing of a person with VHL. Radiation therapy is sometimes used for treatment, but its effectiveness is still unknown. CT and MRI scans of the internal ear canals and audiology exams are recommended if any typical symptoms develop.

Treatment for renal cell carcinoma often includes surgery, depending on the size of the affected area. Percutaneous ablation or cryoablation are experimental treatments that may work well because they are less invasive than other therapies. An abdominal ultrasound is first recommended at age eight, and then an MRI if necessary, and yearly thereafter. An abdominal CT scan is first recommended at age 18 or earlier if needed, and yearly thereafter.

Treatment for pheochromocytomas is most often by surgical removal, with an attempt to keep as much of the adrenal gland as possible. Medications such as corticosteroids are used as a treatment. Since pheochromocytomas can cause significant symptoms, it is important for the person with VHL to be screened prior to any surgery or delivery of a child. Blood or

Ataxia—Uncoordinated muscular movement; often causes difficulty with walking and other voluntary movements.

Brainstem—The entire unpaired subdivision of the brain (rhombencephalon, mesencephalon, and diencephalon).

Catecholamines—Chemicals such as epinephrine, dopa, and norepinephrine; often at high levels in the urine if a pheochromocytoma is present.

Cerebellum—Large area in the posterior of the brain (above the pons and below the cerebrum) responsible for functions like coordination.

Chemotherapy—Chemical treatment often used for cancer.

Computed tomography (CT) scan—Three-dimensional internal image of the body, created by combining x-ray images from different planes using a computer program.

Corticosteroids—Steroid normally produced by the adrenal gland.

Cryoablation—Using very cold temperatures to remove a foreign substance or body.

Cryotherapy—Using very cold temperatures to treat a disease.

Cyst—Sac of tissue filled with fluid, gas, or semi-solid material.

Cystadenoma—Noncancerous growth, in which fluid-filled, gas, or semi-solid areas may be present.

Endolymphatic sac tumor—Growths that develop within inner ear structures called endolymph sacs.

Epididymis—Male genital structure usually connected to the testis; an area where sperm collects.

Gait—The way in which one walks.

Glaucoma—Condition of the eye with increased internal pressure, often causing vision problems.

Hemangioblastoma—Tumor often found in the brain, as in von Hippel-Lindau disease.

Magnetic resonance imaging (MRI) scan—Three-dimensional internal image of the body, created using magnetic waves.

Meta-iodobenzylguanidine (MIBG) scintigraphy—A procedure for looking at the amount of a radioactive chemical, meta-iodobenzylguanidine, injected into the body to find growths such as pheochromocytomas.

Metanephrine—A byproduct of epinephrine, found elevated in urine if a pheochromocytoma is present.

Mutation—A change in the order of deoxyribonucleic acid (DNA) bases that make up genes.

Nerve root—Two groups of nerves that run from the spinal cord to join and form the spinal nerves.

Palpitation—A heartbeat that is more pronounced, often felt physically.

Paresis—Partial or total loss of movement or sensation.

Percutaneous ablation—A method for removing a foreign body by a method just above the skin, as in using an ointment.

Pheochromocytoma—Noncancerous growth in the adrenal gland.

Renal cell carcinoma—A type of kidney cancer.

Retina—Structure in the eye that receives and processes light.

Sequencing—Genetic testing in which the entire sequence of deoxyribonucleic (DNA) bases that make up a gene is studied, in an effort to find a mutation.

Tinnitus—Abnormal noises in the ear, like ringing.

Ultrasound—Two-dimensional internal image of the body, created using sound waves.

Visceral—Generally related to the digestive, respiratory, urogenital, or endocrine organs.

24-hour checks of urine catecholamine and metanephrine levels are recommended beginning at age two, and yearly thereafter. They are also recommended if a person's blood pressure is raised.

Surgery is the typical treatment for pancreatic growths and cysts, depending on their specific location and size. A goal is to keep as much of the pancreas as possible. If the tumors spread, chemotherapy is

sometimes necessary. As with screening of the kidneys, abdominal ultrasounds are recommended beginning at age eight, and yearly thereafter; abdominal CT scans are recommended beginning at age 18, and yearly thereafter.

Both epididymal and broad ligament cystadenomas are non-cancerous and usually cause no symptoms. Therefore, treatment for both is only recommended if symptoms arise. There are no routine screening recommendations for either type. Ultrasounds can be used to find epididymal cystadenomas, and to monitor their growth over time. Ultrasounds or CT scans can be used to identify and monitor broad ligament cystadenomas.

Recovery and rehabilitation

Though VHL typically does not affect a person's thinking, learning, or behavior, the disease can have a significant impact on a person's life. Medical appointments can be frequent, and the pain from tumors may be considerable. Feelings of guilt associated with passing a disease-causing mutation to children have been reported in families. Professional therapy or family counseling may be helpful for some people.

Clinical trials

Trials are conducted at several institutions, including the National Cancer Institute and National Institute of Neurological Disorders and Stroke. Information on current clinical trials can be found at ClinicalTrials.gov.

Prognosis

Prognosis for someone with von Hippel-Lindau disease is highly dependent on symptoms. Those people who die may do so as a result of significant complications with tumors. Renal cell carcinomas and CNS hemangioblastomas have been the greatest causes for death in people with VHL.

The outlook for people with VHL has improved significantly. Before the advent of comprehensive medical screening, the median survival of patients with the condition was less than 50 years of age. Genetic testing now helps identify people at risk before they even develop symptoms, so screening can begin as early as possible. This has helped to reduce the risk of complications and increase the quality of life for many. Medical screening may be further tailored to the individual as scientific studies identify medical complications associated with specific VHL mutations in families.

Resources

BOOKS

Parker, James N., and Philip M. Parker. *The Official Patient's Sourcebook on von Hippel-Lindau Disease: A Revised and Updated Directory for the Internet Age.* San Diego: Icon Health Publishers, 2002.

PERIODICALS

Couch, Vicki, et al. "Von Hippel-Lindau Disease." *Mayo Clinic Proceedings* (2000) 75: 265–72.

Hes, F. J., et al. "Molecular Genetic Aspects of von Hippel-Lindau (VHL) Disease and Criteria for DNA Analysis in Subjects at Risk." *Netherlands Journal of Medicine* (2001) 59: 235–43.

Lonser, Russell R., et al. "Von Hippel-Lindau Disease." *Lancet* 361 (June 14, 2003): 2059–67.

WEBSITES

National Institute of Neurological Disorders and Stroke. http://www.ninds.nih.gov/index.htm (April 27, 2004).

*Online Mendelian Inheritance in Man.*http://www.ncbi.nlm.nih.gov/omim/ (April 27, 2004).

ORGANIZATIONS

Kidney Cancer Association. 1234 Sherman Avenue, Suite 203, Evanston, IL 60202-1375. Phone: (847) 332-1051. Fax: (847) 332-2978. Tollfree phone: (800) 850-9132. Email: office@kidneycancerassociation.org. http://www.kidneycancerassociation.org.

VHL Family Alliance. 171 Clinton Avenue, Brookline, MA 02455-5815. Phone: (617) 277-5667. Fax: (617) 734-8233. Tollfree phone: (800) 767-4VHL. Email: info@vhl.org. http://www.vhl.org.

Deepti Babu, MS, CGC

von Recklinghausen disease *see*
Neurofibromatosis

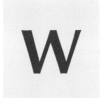

Walker *see* **Assistive mobile devices**

Wallenberg syndrome

Definition

Wallenberg syndrome is a type of brainstem stroke manifested by imbalance, **vertigo**, difficulty swallowing, hoarseness of voice, and sensory disturbance. It is caused by blockage in one of the arteries supplying the medulla and **cerebellum**.

Description

The first clinical description of Wallenberg syndrome was given by Gaspard Viesseux in 1808 and published by Alexander John Gaspard Marcet in 1811. But it was in 1895 that Adolf Wallenberg eloquently described the different symptoms and signs and confirmed the findings during autopsy. The syndrome is also known as lateral medullary infarct (LMI) or posterior inferior cerebellar artery syndrome (PICA).

It usually affects people over 40 years of age. They tend to have vascular risk factors such as hypertension, high cholesterol, and diabetes. Wallenberg syndrome can also occur in younger people, but the underlying causes are different.

Demographics

Wallenberg syndrome is rare, and accurate estimates about incidence are unavailable. In a large stroke registry in Sweden gathered by Norving and Cronquist in 1991, only about 2% of all strokes over a six-year period were caused by LMI.

Causes and symptoms

Causes

The stroke occurs in the medulla and cerebellum. The medulla controls such important functions as swallowing, speech articulation, taste, breathing, strength, and sensation. The cerebellum is important for coordination. The blood supply to these areas is via a pair of vertebral arteries and its branch, called the PICA.

Initially, the PICA was thought to be the blocked major artery, but this has been disproved from autopsy studies. In eight out of 10 cases, it is the vertebral artery that is occluded due to plaque buildup or because of a clot traveling from the heart. In younger patients, the vertebral artery dissection causes the infarct. The area of the stroke is only about 0.39 in. (1 cm) vertically in the lateral part of the medulla and does not cross the midline.

Symptoms

Fully 50% of patients report transient neurological symptoms for several weeks preceding the stroke. During the first 48 hours after the stroke, the neurological deficit progresses and fluctuates. **Dizziness**, vertigo, facial pain, double vision, and difficulty walking are the most common initial symptoms. The facial pain can be quite bizarre with sharp jabs or jolts around the eye, ear, and forehead. Patients feel "seasick" or "off-balance" with nausea and vomiting. Objects appear double, tilted, or swaying. Along with gait imbalance, it becomes nearly impossible for the patient to walk despite good muscle strength. Other symptoms include hoarse voice, slurred speech, loss of taste, difficulty swallowing, hiccups, and altered sensation in the limbs of the opposite side.

The eye on the affected side has a droopy eyelid and a small pupil. The eyes jiggle when the person moves around, a condition called nystagmus. There is decreased pain and temperature perception on the same side of the face. The limbs on the opposite side show decreased sensory perception. Voluntary movements of the arm on the affected side are clumsy. Gait is "drunken," and patients lurch and veer to one side.

Diagnosis

Accurate diagnosis usually requires the expertise of a neurologist or a stroke specialist. It is common for an inexperienced physician to dismiss the symptoms of nausea, vomiting, and vertigo as being caused by an ear infection or viral illness. Diagnosis requires a thorough physical exam and neuroimaging. CAT scans are insensitive and can detect only a large stroke or bleed in the cerebellum. Magnetic resonance imaging (MRI) scans are far superior, with the stroke showing up as a tiny bright spot in the medulla.

Treatment team

The team includes a neurologist or stroke specialist for initial diagnosis, workup, and medical management. Rehabilitation requires a physical therapist, occupational therapist, and speech therapist. Depending on whether complications arise, a neurosurgeon and a critical care physician may be involved.

Treatment

Treatment for Wallenberg syndrome is mostly symptomatic. The size of the underlying blocked artery is too small to allow any mechanical or chemical re-opening. Aim of treatment is to alleviate symptoms, modify underlying risk factors, and prevent complications and future strokes.

Medical therapy

Blood thinners such as heparin are given intravenously in some patients for the first few days to stop further formation and propagation of the clot. Following that, the patient usually has to take other blood thinners such as aspirin for life. Medications are also used to control high blood pressure and cholesterol. Pain in Wallenberg syndrome can sometimes be quite severe and disabling. A variety of analgesics or narcotics are used. Some patients need anti-seizure medications like **gabapentin** for pain management. Medications are also used for symptomatic treatment of vomiting and hiccups.

Surgical therapy

If the stroke is sufficiently large, the dead tissue swells up and can push the medulla downwards, impairing its vital functions and causing death. In this case, a

KEY TERMS

Brain stem—The stalk-like portion of the brain that connects the cerebral hemispheres and the spinal cord. The brain stem receives sensory information and controls such vital functions as blood pressure and respiration.

Cerebellum—Part of the brain that consists of two hemispheres, one on each side of the brainstem. It acts as a fine tuner for muscle tone, co-ordination of movement, posture, gait and skilled voluntary movement.

Dissection—Tear in the wall of an artery that causes blood from inside the artery to leak into the wall and thereby narrows the lumen of the blood vessel.

Infarct—Dead tissue resulting from lack of blood supply to brain; also called a stroke.

Medulla—The lowermost portion of the brainstem that controls vital functions such as respiration, blood pressure, swallowing, and heart rate.

Nystagmus—Involuntary, uncontrollable, rapid, and repetitive movements of the eyeballs.

Stroke—Also called as cerebrovascular accident (CVA) or cerebral infarction, it occurs when there is interruption of blood supply to a portion of the brain or spinal cord, resulting in damage or death of the tissue.

Vertigo—Dizziness with a sense of spinning of self and/or surroundings with resultant loss of balance, nausea, and vomiting. Occurs due to a problem in the inner ears or the cerebellum and brainstem.

neurosurgeon can remove a part of the skull to allow for the brain to swell.

Recovery and rehabilitation

Physical therapy focuses on improving balance and coordination. Assistive devices such as a cane, walker, or wheelchair may be used. Occupational therapy is used to help with daily activities like eating, which may be difficult due to clumsiness and incoordination. Speech training helps with articulation that has been impaired due to vocal cord paralysis. Special attention should be paid to food consistency to prevent aspiration. Initially, patients require pureed or semi-solid food. After initial treatment in the hospital, patients will need short-term placement in a nursing home or rehabilitation facility before going home. Modifications in living environment may include for example, hand rails and non-slip rugs.

Prognosis

Prognosis is usually quite encouraging both in the short and the long term. Symptoms such as nausea and vomiting disappear within a week. Clumsiness, difficulty swallowing, and gait imbalance improve over six months to a year. However, there is a 10% death rate due to complications such as aspiration pneumonia, breathing difficulty, and cardiac arrhythmias.

Special concerns

Social and emotional needs

Depression is very common among stroke survivors who face quite a challenge resulting from the abrupt change in lifestyle. They benefit from counseling, social support, and using antidepressant medications. Stroke support groups help patients and their families cope with the stroke and its aftermath.

Resources

BOOKS

"Vertebrobasilar Occlusive Disease." Chapter 22 in *Stroke—Pathophysiology, Diagnosis, and Management*, edited by Henry J. M. Barnett, et al. New York: Churchill Livingstone, 1998.

"Medullary Infarcts and Hemorrhages." Chapter 41 in *Stroke Syndromes*, edited by Julien Bogousslavsky, et al. New York: Cambridge University Press, 2001.

Parker, James N., and Philip M. Parker, eds. *The Official Patient's Sourcebook on Wallenberg's Syndrome: A Revised and Updated Directory for the Internet Age.* San Diego, CA: ICON Health Publications, 2002.

PERIODICALS

Kim, J. S. "Pure Lateral Medullary Infarction: Clinical-radiological Correlation of 130 Acute, Consecutive Patients." *Brain* 126 (May 2003): 1864–72.

ORGANIZATIONS

American Stroke Association. 7272 Greenville Avenue, Dallas, TX 75231. Phone: (800) 242-8721. Tollfree phone: (888) 4STROKE. http://www.strokeassociation.org.

National Rehabilitation Information Center. 4200 Forbes Blvd, Suite 202, Lanham, MD 20706-4829. Phone: (301) 562-2400. Fax: (301) 562-2401. Tollfree phone: (800) 346-2742. Email: naricinfo@heitechservices.com. http://www.naric.com.

National Stroke Association. 9707 East Easter Lane, Englewood, CO 80112. Phone: (303) 649-9299. Fax: (303) 649-1328. Email: info@stroke.org. http://www.stroke.org.

Chitra Venkatasubramanian, MBBS, MD

Weakness

Definition

Weakness is a symptom of a disease or a disorder rather than a disease in its own right. It refers to reduced strength in one or more muscles. Weakness may be general (global), affecting the entire body, or localized (focal). Weakness can also be categorized as either subjective (perceived by the person who feels weak) or objective (true weakness as measured by laboratory tests of muscular strength). Subjective weakness is commonly associated with infectious diseases that cause fever, like influenza or mononucleosis; the patient lacks energy and may feel weak all over. In some cases subjective weakness may be associated with **depression** or another psychiatric disturbance known as conversion disorder. Objective weakness can result from a variety of physical conditions, described more fully below.

Description

To understand muscle weakness, it is helpful to review the workings of the neuromuscular system in the human body. There are four basic components in the system, and weakness can result from dysfunction in any one of them:

- Upper motor neurons are the nerve cells located in a part of the brain known as the cerebral motor cortex. These upper motor neurons transmit nerve impulses to lower motor neurons.
- Lower motor neurons are located in the spinal cord. This set of motor neurons in turn pass nerve impulses to the muscles at the neuromuscular junction.
- Neuromuscular junction (NMJ) is a synapse (junction) that allows a motor neuron to transmit the nervous impulse to voluntary muscles.
- Voluntary muscles can fail to function normally causing weakness.

Muscular weakness has different characteristics according to the part of the neuromuscular pathway that is affected. Dysfunction of upper motor neurons leads to loss of control over lower motor neurons, resulting in increased muscle tone (**spasticity**) and overactive or over-responsive reflexes. Disorders affecting the lower motor neurons lead to decreased muscle tone (flaccidity), abnormally slow reflexes, and muscle twitches under the skin known as fasciculations. **Myasthenia gravis**, the most common disorder of the neuromuscular junction, is characterized by weakness that gets worse with exercise or activity and improves with rest. Dysfunction of the voluntary muscle itself, known as **myopathy**, tends to be most noticeable in the largest muscle groups, those in the arms and legs.

The doctor will need to distinguish muscle weakness from two other conditions that may coexist with it but are not identical with it. One is asthenia, a sense of weariness in the absence of a physical muscular disorder. Asthenia is common in patients with **sleep disorders**; chronic **fatigue** syndrome; depression; or chronic heart, lung, and kidney disorders. The other condition is fatigue, which refers to the inability to continue performing a muscular movement after a number of repetitions. By contrast, a person with muscle weakness cannot perform the first repetition of the movement.

Demographics

Weakness is one of the most common symptoms that leads patients to consult their primary care doctor; however, asthenia and fatigue are far more common in the general population than primary muscle weakness, and the doctor will need to ask the patient what he or she means by "feeling weak." Patients who are suffering from fatigue rather than muscle weakness will typically say that they "feel tired all the time" without any clear onset or timing pattern or that they feel weak "all over" without identifying any specific parts of the body that are affected or tasks that are difficult to perform (such as lifting heavy objects or climbing stairs). The cause of primary muscle weakness may be apparent in some cases, but in many other cases the doctor will need to conduct a variety of tests as well as ask the patient detailed questions about the location and other characteristics of the weakness in order to uncover the cause(s).

Causes and symptoms

There are various causes of true muscle weakness, as distinct from subjective feelings of weakness.

Causes

There are many possible causes of muscle weakness; one source lists 464 separate disorders that may affect muscle strength. They can be grouped together as follows:

• Infectious diseases. Contagious diseases that can cause muscle weakness include Epstein-Barr virus (EBV), HIV infection, Lyme disease, influenza, trichinosis, polio, bacterial or viral meningitis, syphilis, rabies, and toxoplasmosis. Severe diarrhea associated with cholera or food poisoning due to bacterial contamination can also cause muscle weakness.

• Neurological disorders. These include stroke, brain tumors, amyotrophic lateral sclerosis (Lou Gehrig's disease), Guillain-Barré syndrome, Bell's palsy, multiple sclerosis, spinal cord injury, and degenerative disk disease (pinched spinal nerve).

• Neuromuscular disorders. These include myasthenia gravis, botulism, and Lambert-Eaton syndrome.

• Exposure to toxins. Insecticides, nerve gas, heavy metals (lead, arsenic, bismuth, thallium, cadmium), and paralytic shellfish poisoning can all cause muscle weakness.

• Metabolic disorders. These include thyrotoxicosis, hyperparathyroidism, hypocortisolism (Addison's disease), hypercortisolism (Cushing's syndrome), and disorders of potassium balance.

• Rheumatologic disorders. The two most common rheumatologic disorders that cause muscle weakness are systemic lupus erythematosus (SLE) and rheumatoid arthritis.

• Genetic disorders. These include Becker muscular dystrophy, myotonic dystrophy type 1, and limb/girdle muscular dystrophies.

• Drugs and medications. Drugs of abuse and medications are one of the most common causes of muscle weakness in adults. They include alcohol; cocaine; some heart medications; some drugs given to treat thyroid conditions; some antiretroviral drugs (used to treat AIDS); cancer chemotherapy drugs; penicillin; nonsteroidal anti-inflammatory drugs (NSAIDs such as ibuprofen, naproxen, and aspirin, available as over-the-counter pain relievers); sulfonamide antibiotics; statins (used to lower blood cholesterol levels); and corticosteroids.

• Deconditioning caused by prolonged bed rest.

• Starvation.

Symptoms

Muscle weakness is itself a symptom with different characteristics depending on its cause:

• General weakness. Also called global weakness, general weakness affects the entire body. The most common causes of generalized weakness are muscle wasting due to long stays in an ICU (sometimes called ICU myopathy); myopathies due to alcoholism, potassium imbalance, or corticosteroid medications; and the use of paralytic drugs in an ICU patient.

• Localized or focal weakness. The most common cause of weakness on one side of the body is stroke. Bell's palsy, multiple sclerosis, and nerve disorders caused by entrapment (such as carpal tunnel syndrome), or spinal cord compression due to metastatic cancer or trauma are other common causes of localized muscle weakness.

- Acute onset. Infectious diseases and stroke are common causes of sudden muscle weakness.
- Gradual onset. Drugs, electrolyte imbalances, and rheumatologic disease are common causes of gradual muscle weakness.
- Progressive (worsening over time) weakness. This pattern of weakness is characteristic of genetic and metabolic disorders.

Diagnosis

Individuals should consult a doctor if they develop muscle weakness with any of the following characteristics:

- The weakness has been present for some time and does not have an obvious cause.
- The weakness has come on suddenly, is localized in one part or side of the body, and is not accompanied by fever.
- The patient has difficulty breathing, talking, or swallowing.
- The patient is too weak to lift the head against gravity.
- The weakness has come on suddenly following a viral illness.
- The weakness is limited to one part of the body.

A diagnosis of weakness begins in the doctor's office with a careful family history as well as the patient's medical, occupational, sexual, and psychological history. A family history may suggest a genetic disorder or other disorders known to run in families, such as lupus or rheumatoid arthritis; it may also help in evaluating the possibility of stroke. Occupational history may suggest such work-related causes as exposure to insecticides, heavy metals, or other toxins; a back injury; or such repetitive stress disorders as **carpal tunnel syndrome**. A sexual history may point to HIV infection or syphilis. A complete list of all medications that the patient takes on a regular basis, including NSAIDs and other over-the-counter preparations, is essential; likewise a history of the patient's use of alcohol and/or other drugs of abuse. Given that undiagnosed depression is present in many patients complaining of weakness, many primary care doctors screen patients for this mood disorder with a short depression inventory that the patient can complete in the office. A patient with conversion disorder, however, may require referral to a neurologist as well as a psychiatrist to clarify the diagnosis.

The doctor will ask the patient (or caregiver) some questions about the weakness intended to narrow down the possible cause:

- Timing: when the weakness appeared; whether it came on suddenly or gradually; whether it is worse at certain times of the day; whether it is constant or comes and goes; whether it followed an infection, trip abroad, or vaccination
- Quality: Whether the weakness moves from one part of the body to another; whether there is numbness, pain, or tingling associated with the weakness; whether specific activities (breathing, writing, walking, talking, chewing, swallowing, climbing stairs, lifting objects, etc.) are affected by the weakness
- Location of the weakness in the body: whether it is general or focal
- Factors that make the weakness worse, if any: physical activity, rest, weather, hunger, pain, and emotional stress
- Factors that relieve the weakness, if any: rest, eating, and taking a pain reliever
- Other symptoms present with the weakness, if any: fever, diarrhea, nausea and vomiting, headache, visual disturbances, weight loss, pain, dizziness, changes in mental status, and changes in the temperature or skin color of the affected area of the body

Neurological examination

The next step in evaluating weakness is a thorough examination of the patient's nervous system. The doctor may test the patient's sight, hearing, and other senses; test the reflexes; look closely at the face for signs of asymmetry or drooping of the eyelids; and ask the patient to sit, stand, squat, walk a short distance, write a few sentences, raise the arms above shoulder level, turn the head against resistance, shrug the shoulders, blink repeatedly, and perform other actions intended to determine whether the weakness affects the **central nervous system**, the **peripheral nervous system** (the portion of the nervous system that lies outside the brain and spinal cord), or both. The doctor may use the following rating scale to measure the strength of the patient's large muscles:

- 0: no visible contraction of the muscle
- 1: muscle visibly contracts but limb does not move
- 2: patient can move the limb but not against the force of gravity
- 3: patient can move the limb against gravity but not against resistance
- 4: muscle moves against resistance but only weakly
- 5: muscle has full strength

If the neurological examination does not point to a definite cause, the doctor will examine such other organ systems as the skin, respiratory tract, endocrine system, or cardiovascular system for possible causes.

Laboratory tests

Laboratory tests (blood and urine samples) may be ordered if the doctor suspects a metabolic disorder, electrolyte imbalance, sexually transmitted and other infectious diseases, an autoimmune disorder, food poisoning or exposure to toxins, alcoholism, chronic liver disease, or kidney disorders. A **lumbar puncture** may be done to test the cerebrospinal fluid for evidence of **meningitis**. The doctor may also order a thyroid function test if a thyroid disorder is suspected, or if the patient has been taking thyroid-suppressing medication.

Imaging studies

Imaging studies are performed when the doctor suspects stroke or other cerebrovascular disorders, head injuries, **multiple sclerosis**, or **brain tumors**. Computed tomography (CT) scans and magnetic resonance imaging (MRI) are the imaging studies most often used. MRI can also be used to diagnose inflammation of the muscles and damage to the spinal cord.

Muscle testing and nerve conduction studies

Direct testing of the muscles may be done if the doctor suspects a motor neuron or neuromuscular junction disorder. One technique is **electromyography** (EMG), which involves the stimulation of skeletal muscles by an electrode in order to measure and record the level and frequency of electrical activity in the muscle. There are two types of EMG: intramuscular EMG, in which a fine wire electrode is inserted through the skin directly into the muscle; and surface EMG, in which the electrode is placed on the surface of the skin. The patient may feel slight soreness afterward in the area of the muscles that are tested. The test usually takes 30–45 minutes.

Nerve conduction studies (NCSs) are often performed at the same time as EMGs. An NCS is usually done when the patient has pain, tingling, or numbness associated with weakness, or when the doctor has other reasons to suspect such disorders as carpal tunnel syndrome, myasthenia gravis, Lambert-Eaton syndrome, **Guillain-Barré syndrome**, **peripheral neuropathy**, or a damaged spinal disk. To perform an NCS, the doctor will place patches containing electrodes resembling those used for an electrocardiogram (EKG) over the skin at the locations supplied by the nerves to be tested. The electrodes in the skin patches convey mild electric impulses that stimulate the nerve. The electrical

KEY TERMS

Asthenia—A general term for a lack or loss of energy; an overall sense of weariness.

Axon—The long slender projection of a neuron that carries the nerve impulse away from the cell body to another neuron, muscle, or gland tissue.

Congenital—Present at birth.

Conversion disorder—A psychiatric disorder in which the patient's emotional distress takes the form of (is converted into) various neurological and motor symptoms that mimic a neuromuscular disorder but have no neurological explanation.

Deconditioning—The loss of normal body functioning (including muscle strength) in a normally demanding environment due to adaptation to a less demanding environment. Deconditioning can result from prolonged bed rest, aging, paralysis, being placed in a body cast, or other reasons for a decrease in physical activity.

Electromyography—A technique for measuring and recording the electrical activity of skeletal muscle.

Fasciculation—A small localized involuntary contraction and relaxation of muscles visible under the skin.

Flaccidity—Abnormally low muscle tone without an obvious cause (such as trauma).

Motor neuron—Any neuron in the central nervous system with an axon that projects outside the CNS and controls muscles either directly or indirectly.

Myasthenia—Muscle weakness.

Myasthenia gravis—An autoimmune disorder of the muscles in which muscles become progressively weaker during periods of activity and improve during periods of rest.

Myopathy—Any disorder of muscle tissue that results in weakness.

Neuromuscular junction—The synapse between the axon of a motor neuron and muscle fiber.

Peripheral neuropathy—Damage to nerves that lie outside the brain and spinal cord.

Spasticity—Abnormally high muscle tone in skeletal muscle, often caused by damage to upper motor neurons in the central nervous system.

Synapse—The junction between a neuron and its target cell.

impulses then given off by the nerve are recorded by another electrode. The time it takes for the impulse to travel between the two electrodes is used to measure the speed of the nerve impulse. The patient may feel some discomfort from the electric shock but should not feel pain after the NCS is completed.

Muscle biopsy

A muscle **biopsy** may be performed if the doctor suspects that muscle tissue has been damaged by an infectious disease (toxoplasmosis, trichinosis), a traumatic accident, muscular dystrophy, congenital myopathy, wasting of muscle tissue, or a metabolic disorder affecting the muscle. The biopsy, which is usually done on an outpatient basis, may be performed either by inserting a hollow needle into the muscle to withdraw a sample of tissue; or by open biopsy, in which the doctor makes a small incision into the skin over the muscle and removes a small piece of muscle. The patient will be given a local anesthetic prior to either type of biopsy. There may be some bruising and a small amount of bleeding afterward as well as soreness in the area of the biopsy that lasts about a week.

Treatment

The treatment of muscle weakness depends on the diagnosis of the cause. Patients with depression or conversion disorder require psychiatric evaluation and treatment. Patients with acute life-threatening illnesses related to their muscular symptoms may need to be put on a ventilator. Patients with weakness caused by medication side effects may need to have their dosage adjusted or another drug substituted. Patients with weakness caused by occupational injuries, stress, or toxic chemicals may need to consider a change in employment. Physical therapy and rehabilitation are beneficial to all patients with muscle disorders no matter what the cause.

Clinical trials

There were 571 clinical trials of muscle weakness under way as of mid-2011. They range from investigations of muscle weakness related to prolonged stays in the ICU and studies of weakness associated with medications to research into the effectiveness of exercise programs and physical therapy in relieving weakness. A few clinical studies are concerned with gaining improved understanding of rare neuromuscular disorders.

Prognosis

The prognosis of muscle weakness depends on the cause.

Resources

BOOKS

Burkman, Kip. *The Stroke Recovery Book: A Guide for Patients and Families.* 2nd ed. Omaha, NB: Addicus, 2011.

Hilton-Jones, David, Jane Freebody, and Jane Stein. *Neuromuscular Disorders in the Adult: A Practice Manual.* New York: Oxford University Press, 2011.

Mahadevan, S.V., and Gus M. Garmel, eds. *Introduction to Clinical Emergency Medicine.* 2nd ed. New York: Cambridge University Press, 2011.

PERIODICALS

Chawla, J., and G. Gruener. "Management of Critical Illness Polyneuropathy and Myopathy." *Neurologic Clinics* 28 (November 2010): 961–77.

Dupuis, L., et al. "Skeletal Muscle in Motor Neuron Diseases: Therapeutic Target and Delivery Route for Potential Treatments." *Current Drug Targets* 11 (October 2010): 1250–61.

Kumar, V., and H.J. Kaminski. "Treatment of Myasthenia Gravis." *Current Neurology and Neuroscience Reports* 11 (February 2011): 89–96.

Logan, L.R. "Rehabilitation Techniques to Maximize Spasticity Management." *Topics in Stroke Rehabilitation* 18 (May/June 2011): 203–11.

Peterson, M.D., and P.M. Gordon. "Resistance Exercise for the Aging Adult: Clinical Implications and Prescription Guidelines." *American Journal of Medicine* 124 (March 2011): 194–98.

Puthucheary, Z., et al. "Skeletal Muscle Dysfunction in Critical Care: Wasting, Weakness, and Rehabilitation Strategies." *Critical Care Medicine* 38 (October 2010): Suppl. 10: S676–82.

Selcen, D. "Myofibrillar Myopathies." *Neuromuscular Disorders* 21 (March 2011): 161–71.

Stone, J., and A. Carson. "Functional Neurologic Symptoms: Assessment and Management." *Neurologic Clinics* 29 (February 2011): 1–18.

Tobin, M.J., et al. "Narrative Review: Ventilator-induced Respiratory Muscle Weakness." *Annals of Internal Medicine* 153 (August 17, 2010): 240–45.

Wee, C.D., et al. "The Genetics of Spinal Muscular Atrophies." *Current Opinion in Neurology* 23 (October 2010): 450–58.

WEBSITES

"EMG Test." YouTube. http://www.youtube.com/watch?v=k0uSpYd_Ics (accessed July 26, 2011).

Huff, J. Stephen, and Chris Ghaemaghami. "Chapter 10: Weakness and Numbness." In *Approach to Common Neurological Symptoms in Internal Medicine.* American Academy of Neurology (AAN). http://www.aan.com/go/education/curricula/internal/chapter10 (accessed July 26, 2011).

Marshall, Scott A. "Conversion Disorders." Medscape Reference. http://emedicine.medscape.com/article/287464-overview (accessed July 26, 2011).

"Neuromuscular Diseases in the MDA Program." Muscular Dystrophy Association (MDA). http://www.mda.org/disease/ (accessed July 26, 2011).

"NINDS Congenital Myopathy Information Page." National Institute of Neurological Disorders and Stroke (NINDS). http://www.ninds.nih.gov/disorders/myopathy_congenital/myopathy_congenital.htm (accessed July 26, 2011).

"Weakness." MedlinePlus. http://www.nlm.nih.gov/medlineplus/ency/article/003174.htm (accessed June 18, 2011).

"Weakness." Merck Manual Online. http://www.merckmanuals.com/professional/sec17/ch216/ch216c.html (accessed July 26, 2011).

ORGANIZATIONS

American Academy of Neurology (AAN), 1080 Montreal Avenue, Saint Paul, MN 55116, (651) 695-2717, (800) 879-1960, Fax: (651) 695-2791, memberservices@aan.com, http://www.aan.com.

Muscular Dystrophy Association, 3300 East Sunrise Drive, Tucson, AZ 85718-3208, (520) 529-2000, (800) 572-1717, Fax: (520) 529-5300, mda@mdausa.org, http://www.mda.org.

National Institute of Arthritis and Musculoskeletal and Skin Diseases (NIAMS), 1 AMS Circle, Bethesda, MD 20892-3675, (301) 495-4484, (877) 226-4267, NIAMSinfo@mail.nih.gov, http://www.niams.nih.gov.

National Institute of Neurological Disorders and Stroke (NINDS), P.O. Box 5801, Bethesda, MD 20824, (301) 496-5751, (800) 352-9424, http://www.ninds.nih.gov.

Rebecca J. Frey, Ph

Werdnig-Hoffman disease *see* **Spinal muscular atrophy**

Wernicke-Korsakoff syndrome *see* **Beriberi**

West Nile virus

Definition

West Nile virus is a mosquito-borne virus that causes viral illnesses of varying seriousness, ranging from no symptoms or mild influenza-like symptoms to **encephalitis** or **meningitis**.

Description

The primary hosts of West Nile virus (WNV) are birds, in which the virus numbers multiply before being transmitted by mosquitoes to the next victim. Over 140 species of birds can be infected with WNV. Besides birds, the virus can infect other vertebrates, including humans and horses. West Nile virus belongs to the genus *Flavivirus*. It belongs to the Japanese encephalitis serocomplex, which includes St. Louis encephalitis, Murray Valley encephalitis, and Kunjin virus. Infections occur generally between late summer and early fall in temperate areas and throughout the year in southern climates. Although typical manifestation of WNV is asymptomatic, the virus can cross the blood-brain barrier and cause severe illness and paralysis.

WNV was originally isolated in a feverish woman living in the West Nile District of Uganda during 1937. The virus was ecologically characterized in Egypt during the 1950s and later linked to severe human meningoencephalitis in elderly patients during a 1957 outbreak in Israel. Since 1937, subsequent outbreaks of WNV have

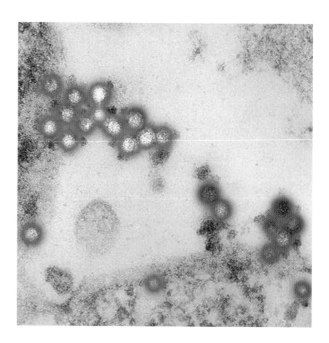

The **West Nile virus.** (© *Scott Camazine/Photo Researchers, Inc.*)

been reported in Africa, Asia, Australia, Oceania, Western Europe, and the Middle East.

In the summer of 1999, WNV was first reported in the New York City area and then spread rapidly across the entire continent. It is still unknown how the WNV reached the United States, but it is suspected that the transport of infected birds or the international travel of infected humans may have been to blame. After its arrival in the New York area, the virus spread across the United States, northward into Canada, and southward into Mexico. In 2002, a severe outbreak of WNV in the United States killed 284 people and caused 2,944 cases of severe brain damage. By 2005, the Center for Disease Control and Prevention (CDC) had recorded avian or animal WNV infections in every state except Alaska, Hawaii, and Washington. Since 2005, the number of cases has eased somewhat. In 2010, the CDC documented a total of 1,021 cases and reported no human infections in seven states.

Life Cycle and Transmission

Like most flaviviruses, WNV is maintained in a natural host-vector-host cycle, where the primary vector is the mosquito. The zoonotic cycle begins with a reservoir host, which is most commonly avian. When a mosquito feeds on the infected bird, the virus is passed to the insect along with the blood meal. The virus then multiplies rapidly within the mosquito's body and salivary glands over the next few days. When the insect feeds on another animal or human, the virus can be transmitted through the bite and cause serious illness.

Most mosquitoes can become infected with the WNV, but female mosquitoes of the *Culex pipiens* species are of particular concern, as they live in suburban and urban areas, can survive through the winter, prefer to feed on birds, and frequently bite humans. The *Culex pipiens*, also known as the house mosquito, is also the most common vector for WNV transmission. *Culex restuan*, *Culex quinquefasciatus*, *Aedes Albopictus*, and *Aedes Vexans* are also common carriers of the WNV.

Common food sources for mosquitoes, birds represent the primary WNV reservoir species. A continent-wide study published in 2007 suggests that WNV has severely affected bird populations associated with human habitats in North America, showing that WNV is indeed the main factor behind the observed large-scale declines in bird populations. For instance, in 2005, crow populations declined regionally by up to 45% from 1998 levels, although they had increased steadily for two decades. American crow declines have been positively correlated with the intensity of human

WNV epidemics within each region studied. Similar correlations between human infections and impacts on bird species were strongest for house wrens and eastern bluebirds. The virus has also been identified in more than 250 bird species in the United States, including blue jays, ravens, magpies, sparrows, and starlings. Many in the scientific community believe that the rapid spread of WNV in North America may be due in part to the migratory nature of birds. Infected birds carry the virus with them as they travel in summer and winter, thus acting as reservoirs in their new nesting sites.

Most vertebrates, such as alligators, bats, chipmunks, skunks, squirrels, and rabbits, can also be infected with WNV. Horses, in particular, are commonly infected with WNV, although a vaccine against equine WNV exists. Like humans, the majority of horses suffer either no or mild symptoms, but severe illness and death can and does occur. There are relatively few cases of dogs and cats becoming infected with WNV. Animals of all species exhibiting fever, **weakness**, poor coordination, spasms, seizures, and/or personality changes may be infected with WNV.

There is no evidence of WNV transmission from person-to-person through touch, kissing, or other contact. However, there is evidence of WNV transplacental (mother-to-child) transmission, and possible viral transmission through breastfeeding. As such, pregnant mothers should be aware of the presence of WNV in their area and take appropriate precautions. The transmission of WNV has also been evidenced in blood transfusions and organ transplants; although the current blood supply is now tested for the presence of the WNV and the risk of infection via blood is very low. People that are immunocompromised (from disease or chemotherapy, for example) and people aged 50 and older represent the highest risk group for serious WNV infection.

Demographics

In the United States, the CDC monitors and records human WNV infections. In 2010, 1,021 cases were reported, including 57 deaths, 15 of which were in Arizona. Washington, Montana, Maine, Vermont, Delaware, West Virginia, and North Carolina reported no human cases. WNV is common in Africa, Asia, and the Middle East. Outbreaks have occurred in France, Russia, Romania, and the Czech Republic.

Only about 1% of people infected with West Nile virus become seriously ill. Among those with severe illness, fatality rates range from 3–15% and are highest among people age 75 and older.

Causes and symptoms

The exact mechanism of WNV-caused illnesses remains unclear. However, it is suspected that the virus enters the host's blood stream and multiples. It can then develop to the point where it crosses the blood brain-barrier, which separates the blood from the **central nervous system**. When this occurs, the virus can infect the brain, spinal cord, and other vital systems, creating a potentially deadly inflammatory response.

The incubation period for WNV after infection typical ranges between 3 to 14 days. Eighty percent of infected persons will exhibit no clinically apparent symptoms whatsoever. Roughly 20% of infected persons will exhibit a series of mild flu-like symptoms, also known as West Nile Fever. These mild symptoms can persist for 3 to 6 days, possibly weeks, and include:

• eye pain

• fever

• headache

• loss of appetite

• lymphadenopathy (abnormal enlargement of the lymph nodes)

• malaise (nonspecific bodily discomfort)

• myalgia (nonspecific muscular pain/tenderness)

• nausea

• rash (on the neck, torso, and limbs)

• vomiting

In approximately one in 100 cases (about 1%), WNV can cross the blood-brain barrier and develop into a severe neuroinvasive disease. Immunocompromised and elderly (older than 50) patients are at an increased risk for developing more severe syndromes; a 20-fold increase in incidence among older patients. Symptoms indicating the possible presence of severe West Nile-related syndromes include:

• severe headache

• high fever

• acute muscle weakness

• neck stiffness

• convulsions and tremors

• disorientation and stupor

• paralysis

• coma

People exposed to WNV infection, especially the immunocompromised and elderly, should contact their health provider immediately if they develop a severe headache accompanied by high fever.

Typically, severe WNV syndromes manifest as one of three syndromes: West Nile encephalitis (inflammation of the brain); West Nile meningitis (inflammation of the **meninges** of the brain and spinal cord); or West Nile meningoencephalitis (inflammation of both the brain and the meninges). These three syndromes can cause severe brain damage and even death. Severe WNV disease carries a mortality rate ranging between 3% and 15%, with elderly patients suffering the highest mortality rate. The majority of these deaths result from complications attributable to West Nile meningoencephalitis. Additionally, severe WNV disease can cause acute vision loss due to inflammatory disorders of the eye, such as chorioretinitis, optic neuritis, retinal **vasculitis**, uveitis, and vitritis. Less frequently, the patient can exhibit acute flaccid paralysis, similar to **poliomyelitis** (polio) or **Guillain-Barré syndrome**, caused by inflammation of the spinal cord and/or damage to the peripheral nerves. In some severe cases, this acute flaccid paralysis can disrupt muscles that control breathing and result in respiratory failure.

Diagnosis

A proper diagnosis of WNV infection depends heavily upon clinical presentation, laboratory testing, and patient history. Patients with a known susceptibility to WNV (the elderly and immunocompromised) that exhibit symptoms during the late spring to early fall, or at any time in warmer climates, should be tested for WNV and other arboviral infections. Additionally, health providers should remain constantly aware of the local presence of WNV activity, such as reports of recent animal and/or human cases. Similarities of symptoms and serological cross-reactivity of WNV and other flaviviruses may lead to confusion and an incorrect diagnosis. Health providers must use thorough laboratory testing to differentiate WNV antibodies from those of other arboviruses.

Symptomatic WNV infection can be classified as either non-neuroinvasive or neuroinvasive, with each being identified according to certain criteria.

Non-neuroinvasive

The majority of WNV infections are asymptomatic. In approximately 20% of WNV cases, clinically recognizable symptoms can manifest. To be clinically classified as non-neuroinvasive West Nile disease, the following must be true:

• no neuroinvasive symptomology

• presence of fever without other recognizable cause

• four-fold or greater increase in serum antibody titer

- virus isolated from and or demonstrated in blood, tissue, cerebrospinal fluid (CSF), or other bodily fluid
- virus-specific immunoglobulin M (IgM) antibodies demonstrated in CSF through antibody-capture methods

Neuroinvasive

In the rare cases (about 1%) of West Nile disease, the virus crosses the blood-brain barrier and manifests in severe and life-threatening symptomology. Clinical confirmation of neuroinvasive disease requires the presence of a fever and at least one of the following:

- acutely altered mental status, such as disorientation, stupor, or coma
- acute central or peripheral neurological difficulties, such as paralysis, nerve palsy, sensory deficits, and abnormal muscle function
- an increased white blood cell concentration in the CSF coupled with symptoms of meningitis, such as severe headache and neck pain

Treatment

Currently, there is no specific treatment for WNV infection. Instead, supportive care is used to treat the varying symptoms and syndromes associated with the various West Nile diseases. Although milder symptoms can be treated at home, severe symptoms can require hospitalization. Treatment of severe symptoms may require the use of intravenous infusions, airway and respiratory management and support, and use of preventative measures against secondary infection.

Clinical trials

As of 2011, several clinical trials for the study and treatment of WNV were underway. Information on clinical trials currently recruiting patients can be found at http://www.clinicaltrials.gov. There is no cost to the patient to participate in a clinical trial.

Prognosis

The majority of WNV infections are asymptomatic. West Nile fever offers an excellent prognosis associated with quick recovery and no adverse side effects. The majority of symptoms resolve within a few days or weeks of manifestation.

However, the prognosis is not as positive for patients experiencing the more severe syndromes attributable to WNV infection. Symptoms of West Nile encephalitis, West Nile meningitis, and West Nile meningoencephalitis can last for several weeks and cause severe and permanent neurological damage. Inflammation

can interfere with the brain and central nervous system and result in death, especially amongst the elderly population. Patients may experience prolonged muscle weakness and loss of motor control. Long-term rehabilitation is typically required and a full recovery is not assured. If the muscles used for breathing are affected, death from respiratory failure may result.

Prevention

Although there is a WNV vaccine for horses and exotic birds in zoos, there is no WNV vaccine for humans as of 2011.

Prevention techniques of WNV typically coincide with avoidance measures against mosquito bites; the primary source of the virus. These include the use of insect repellant (with 5–20% DEET) on exposed body parts, wearing loose-fitting clothes over the limbs and torso while outdoors, using mosquito coils and/or citronella candles outdoors, and limiting outdoor activities during peak biting periods and/or in areas with high mosquito density. While camping outdoors, knockdown spray or bed netting with pyrethrum is suggested. Mosquito eradication programs have been instituted in some cities. Public health authorities can use United States Environmental Protection Agency-approved "adulticidies" in areas suspected of the presence of WNV.

The *Culex pipiens* mosquito is the primary vector of WNV transmission and also commonly live and feed in urban areas. Special precautions should be taken to reduce exposure to these potentially infected insects. Screen doors and enclosed porches can help keep mosquitoes from coming into the house. It should be noted that studies have shown that mosquito control devices such as "bug zappers" and CO_2-baited traps do not significantly reduce the risk of being bitten.

Removing potential mosquito breeding areas from near the home and from the neighborhood can further reduce the risk of bites. Any container that can collect half an inch of standing water can become a potential breeding site in as little as five days. Old tires, empty plant pots, and empty trashcans should be removed, while water sources like ponds or birdbaths should be cleaned regularly. Standing water on any property should be drained, such as from clogged eves. Swimming pools and hot tubs should be properly covered and chlorinated to prevent mosquitoes breeding in them.

The CDC recommends that individuals who find a dead bird not handle the bird with their bare hands. Instead, they should call their local public health department to report the bird and then follow any instructions given by the health department.

Resources

BOOKS

Beltz, Lisa A. *Emerging Infectious Disease: A Guide to Diseases, Causative Agents, and Surveillance*. San Francisco: Jossey-Bass, 2011.

Oldstone, Michael B. *Viruses, Plagues, and History: Past, Present, and Future*. New York: Oxford University Press, 2010.

Sfakianos, Jeffrey, and Alan Hecht. *West Nile Virus*. 2nd ed. New York: Chelsea House, 2009.

WEBSITES

Salinas Jr., Jess D. "West Nile Virus." Medscape Reference. http://emedicine.medscape.com/article/312210-overview (accessed July 22, 2011).

"Understanding West Nile Virus," National Institute of Allergy and Infectious Diseases. ttp://www.niaid.nih.gov/topics/westNile/understanding/Pages/default.aspx (accessed July 22, 2011).

"West Nile Virus." MedlinePlus. http://www.nlm.nih.gov/medlineplus/westnilevirus.html (accessed July 22, 2011).

"West Nile Virus: Questions and Answers." United States Centers for Disease Control and Prevention. http://www.cdc.gov/ncidod/dvbid/westnile/q&a.htm (accessed July 22, 2011).

ORGANIZATIONS

Centers for Disease Control and Prevention (CDC), 1600 Clifton Road, Atlanta, GA 30333, (800) CDC-INFO, cdcinfo@cdc.gov, http://www.cdc.gov.

National Institute of Allergy and Infectious Diseases (NIAID), 6610 Rockledge Drive, MSC 6612, Bethesda, MD 20892-6612, (301) 496-5717, (866) 284-4107, Fax: (301) 402-3573, ocpostofficer@niaid. nih.gov, http://www.niaid.nih.gov.

Jason Fryer,
Monique Laberge, PhD
Tish Davidson, AM

West syndrome *see* **Infantile spasms**

Wheelchair *see* **Assistive mobile devices**

Whiplash

Definition

Whiplash is the mechanism that causes the neck injury often suffered in a rear-end automobile collision. People also use the same term, whiplash, to mean the resultant neck injury itself. Whiplash produces a wide range of symptoms, but almost all victims experience pain. About 1,000,000 whiplash injuries occur in the United States every year.

Description

An occupant of a car struck suddenly from the rear undergoes rapid acceleration and deceleration. The head and neck swing freely while the body remains supported by the seat and seatbelts. The rapid movement of the head causes variable amounts of hyperextension, hyperflexion, stretching, and twisting of neck structures, in a fashion similar to the snapping of a whip.

The structures often affected include muscles, ligaments, nerves, intervertebral disks, and spinal joints. Specific damage may range from minimal strains to complicated tears, hemorrhage, and joint injury, as shown by animal studies and autopsies of accident victims.

Causes and symptoms

Besides motor vehicle accidents, causes of whiplash include sports and other recreational activities, **falls**, and fights. Women tend to have more persistent symptoms than men do, perhaps because women's smaller neck muscles are more vulnerable.

Symptoms following a whiplash injury may begin immediately or any time up to a few days later. Symptoms include variable combinations of:

- pain or stiffness in the neck, jaw, shoulders, arms, or back
- dizziness
- headache
- loss of feeling in the upper extremities
- problems with vision or hearing
- problems with concentration
- depression, anxiety, or other changes in mood

Symptoms may last for no more than a day or two or may persist for months or years.

Diagnosis

Many patients with whiplash receive evaluation by emergency medical technicians (EMTs) at the scene of an accident, always starting with the ABCs of resuscitation: airway, breathing, and circulation. At the same time, in head or neck trauma, initial care providers always worry about the possibility of dangerous injury to the spine bones or spinal cord. Often, the EMTs will immobilize the neck in a stiff brace and strap the patient flat on a board, until a physician determines that it is safe for the neck to move. This minimizes the risk that any serious injury could progress and cause irreversible nerve damage. Unfortunately, this immobilization is usually very uncomfortable for the patient.

When such a patient arrives at the emergency department (ED), the nurse will further assess the patient for stable vital signs, proper alertness, and good ability to move and feel the extremities. A patient strapped to a spine immobilization board often demands to remove the neck brace and get up, but the nurse must ensure that the patient remains still until cleared by the physician. The nurse quickly asks the doctor to examine the patient.

Another danger is that a patient may vomit while immobilized. This presents a risk for aspiration of stomach contents, which can threaten breathing. The nurse must be alert to quickly turn the patient on the side, while still immobilized and with the neck brace still in place, to prevent this complication.

The physician obtains the patient's description of the event, then looks for injury to other organs, especially in the head, chest, abdomen, and back. The doctor will check for bony tenderness or limitation of movement, and examine the functions of deep tendon reflexes plus motor and sensory nerves. When the physician is confident that no injury threatens the spinal cord the patient is "cleared." The physician will remove the brace and free the patient from the rigid board.

The physician may order x-ray studies to exclude fracture or displacement of bone, but in typical whiplash these tests rarely show any abnormality. When there is severe or persistent pain or numbness, magnetic resonance imaging (MRI) may detect more subtle damage.

Treatment

Patients should apply ice in the first 24-48 hours. Physicians prescribe medicines such as ibuprofen (Motrin, Advil) or aspirin, **acetaminophen**, muscle relaxants, or narcotics (codeine, hydrocodone, Vicodin).

Use of soft cervical collars is controversial. Many doctors prescribe them, but some studies have shown that these devices prolong the return to normal activities. Physical therapy or exercises may reduce pain or limitation of movement.

Many patients use balms or salves, and seek alternative treatments such as chiropractic manipulation, biofeedback, **acupuncture**, or acupressure. In cases of protracted symptoms, patients may benefit from traction, ultrasound treatments, local injections of cortisone, or use of a nerve stimulator.

Prognosis

The course of an individual whiplash injury is unpredictable. Most people improve within a month, but 20% or more have symptoms that last longer than a year. The risk of greater symptoms increases for an unrestrained victim of a rear-end collision, or for one whose head is turned or tilted at the time of injury.

Controversy surrounds the role that accident-related litigation plays in delaying recovery from whiplash. An April 2000, article in the *New England Journal of Medicine* examined this issue. The authors showed a decreased incidence and improved prognosis of whiplash injury when the province of Saskatchewan changed to a new insurance claim system that eliminated payments for pain and suffering. However, other authors downplay the effect of psychosocial factors on recovery from whiplash.

Health care team roles

The EMT performs rescue, assessment, and initial treatment at the scene of an accident. A nurse in the ED or medical office also assesses the patient with whiplash. The nurse carries out physician orders for medication and treatments, monitors the patient throughout the stay, and instructs the patient and caregivers before discharge. The aide assists the nurse.

A radiology technician performs the x-ray or MRI studies. A physical therapist helps with exercise, massage, ultrasound, and other treatments. A social worker may coordinate later care.

Prevention

Proper adjustment of the automobile headrest is important to reduce the severity of a whiplash injury, because a headrest that does not come up behind the head offers no protection. Driving habits that reduce the frequency of abrupt stops make it less likely that a driver will suffer a rear-end collision.

Resources

BOOKS

Clark, Charles R., et al, ed. *The Cervical Spine*. Philadelphia: Lippincott-Raven, 1998.

Goetz, Christopher G., and Eric J. Pappert. *Textbook of Clinical Neurology*. Philadelphia: W. B. Saunders, 1999.

PERIODICALS

Cassidy, J. David, et al. "Effect of Eliminating Compensation for Pain and Suffering on the Outcome of Insurance Claims for Whiplash Injury." *New England Journal of Medicine* 342, no. 16 (April 20, 2000): 1179-86.

ORGANIZATIONS

American Academy of Orthopaedic Surgeons. 6300 North River Road, Rosemont, IL 60018-4262. (800) 346-AAOS. http://www.aaos.org.

Kenneth J. Berniker, M.D.

Whipple's disease

Definition

Whipple's disease is a rare infectious disorder that can affect many areas of the body, including the gastrointestinal and central nervous systems. Caused by the bacteria *Tropheryma whipplei*, it is typically diagnosed from malabsorption symptoms such as diarrhea and weight loss. If the **central nervous system** is infected, Whipple's disease can cause impairment of mental

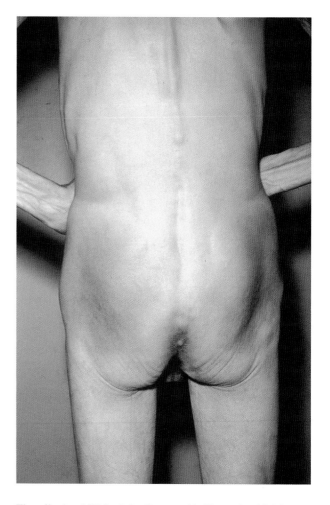

The effects of Whipple's disease. *(© Phototake. All rights reserved.)*

faculties and lead to **dementia**. It can be treated successfully with antibiotic therapy, but up to one-third of patients suffer relapse.

Description

Whipple's disease, also known as intestinal lipodystrophy, was first reported in 1907 by George Hoyt Whipple (1878–1976). An autopsy on a thirty-seven year old male missionary revealed a granular accumulation of fatty acids in the walls of the small intestine and lymph nodes.

Historically, Whipple's disease has been considered an gastrointestinal disorder; however, in the 1960s, it was realized that other organs could be involved, with or without intestinal infection. It is now considered a systemic infection with a wide range of possible symptoms.

Demographics

The disorder typically affects middle-aged men of European descent. Most cases have been reported in North America and Europe. Many texts suggest the disorder affects eight times as many males as females, although there is some evidence to suggest the rate in females is rising.

The disease is extremely rare and no reliable estimate of incidence is known. Farmers and other rural people are most often diagnosed with Whipple's disease, but as yet, no specific environmental factors have been linked to the disorder.

Causes and symptoms

The bacterium that causes Whipple's disease was only successfully cultured in 1997. *Tropheryma whipplei* belongs to the high G+C phylum of gram-positive bacteria, and its genome was sequenced in 2003.

Whipple's disease has traditionally been regarded as a malabsorption disease of the small intestine, but in most cases the first symptoms are arthritic joints, which can precede the malabsorption symptoms of Whipple's disease by many years. Commonly, the disease progresses to the small intestine. Symptoms then include diarrhea, anemia, weight loss, and there is often fat present in the stool, all due to the bacteria disrupting absorption of fat and nutrients. If untreated, other malabsorption problems, such as reductions in the levels of calcium and magnesium, may result. Fever and night sweats are common, as well as general **weakness**. There are many further possible symptoms depending on the organs affected.

In cases where the central nervous system is affected, there may be a decrease in intellectual abilities, insomnia, **hearing loss** or **tinnitus** (ringing in the ears), and uncontrolled muscle movements (**ataxia**) or eye movements. If untreated, the disorder can lead to dementia and progressive brain cell death, leading to **coma** and death over a period of months to years.

Diagnosis

Diagnosis of Whipple's disease is difficult and is commonly suspected only if the patient presents with malabsorption symptoms. Then, a small-bowel **biopsy** can be made to locate the presence of the bacteria and confirm the diagnosis. However, symptoms can vary greatly depending on the areas of the body that are affected, and up to one-third of sufferers do not present with malabsorption ailments.

Treatment team

Once diagnosed, the treatment of Whipple's disease is often straightforward and can be monitored with minor hospital procedures. However, due to the rarity of the disease and the recent developments in studying the disorder, it is recommended that contact be made with specialized centers of research or a neurologist.

Treatment

Whipple's disease generally responds well to antibiotic therapy. The recommended treatment is two weeks of intravenous antibiotics followed by a year or more of oral antibiotics. If the malabsorption symptoms are pronounced, the patient may require intravenous fluids and electrolytes, and other dietary supplements. A diet high in calories and protein is often recommended and should be monitored by a physician.

Recovery and rehabilitation

When treated, symptoms such as diarrhea and fever can resolve within days, and most symptoms typically improve within a few weeks. In most cases, symptoms of the disorder are lessened or ameliorated by treatment. The progress of therapy can be checked by biopsy of the small intestine. In about one third of cases, the disease relapses and is more likely to affect the central nervous system than the initial infection. Periodic monitoring over several years, therefore, is essential to prevent neurological damage.

Clinical trials

There are no ongoing clinical trials in the United States specific for Whipple's disease, the National Institute of Diabetes and Digestive and Kidney Diseases supports research for similar disorders. Information regarding current clinical trials can be found at ClinicalTrials.gov.

Prognosis

If untreated Whipple's disease can be fatal, but when treated with antibiotic therapy most patients experience rapid recovery and lasting remission. However, up to a third of patients may suffer a relapse.

Special concerns

Knowledge of Whipple's disease is rapidly evolving, and there have been many recent developments that may lead to new diagnostic options and new treatments in the near future.

Resources

PERIODICALS

Marth, Thomas, and Dider Raoult. "Whipple's disease," *Lancet* 361, no. 9353 (January 18, 2003): 239–47.

OTHER

"NINDS Whipple's Disease Information Page." National Institute of Neurological Disorders and Stroke. http://www.ninds.nih.gov/health_and_medical/disorders/whipples.htm (March 10, 2004).
"Whipple's Disease." *National Digestive Diseases Information Clearinghouse*.http://digestive.niddk.nih.gov/ddiseases/pubs/whipple/index.htm (March 10, 2004).

ORGANIZATIONS

National Organization for Rare Disorders (NORD). P.O. Box 1968 (55 Kenosia Avenue), Danbury, CT 06813-1968. Phone: (203) 744–0100. Fax: (203) 798–2291. Tollfree phone: (800) 999–NORD (6673). Email: orphan@rarediseases.org. http://www.rarediseases.org.

David Tulloch

Chromosome 7

GCK: Diabetes

ELN: Williams syndrome

Autistic disorder (7q)

Pendrin: Pendred syndrome

CFTR: Cystic fibrosis

OB: Obesity

Pancreatic cancer

Williams syndrome, on chromosome 7. *(Illustration by Argosy, Inc. Reproduced by permission of Gale, a part of Cengage Learning.)*

Williams syndrome

Definition

Williams syndrome is a genetic disorder caused by a deletion of a series of genes on chromosome 7q11. Individuals with Williams syndrome have distinctive facial features, mild **mental retardation**, heart and blood vessel problems, short stature, unique personality traits, and distinct learning abilities and deficits.

Description

Williams syndrome, also known as Williams Beuren syndrome, was first described in 1961 by Dr. J. C. P. Williams of New Zealand. At that time it was noted that individuals with Williams syndrome had an unusual constellation of physical and mental findings. The physical features include a characteristic facial appearance, heart and cardiovascular problems, high blood calcium levels, low birth weight, short stature, and other connective tissue abnormalities. The intellectual problems associated with Williams include a mild mental retardation and a specific cognitive profile. That is, individuals with Williams syndrome often have the same pattern of learning abilities and disabilities, as well as many similar personality traits.

The findings in Williams syndrome are variable—that is, not all individuals with Williams syndrome will have all of the described findings. In addition to being variable, the physical and mental findings associated with Williams syndrome are progressive—they change over time.

Genetic profile

Williams syndrome is a genetic disorder due to a deletion of chromosome material on the long arm of chromosome 7. A series of genes are located in this region. Individuals with Williams syndrome may have some or all of these genes deleted. Because of this, Williams syndrome is referred to as a contiguous gene deletion syndrome. Contiguous refers to the fact that these genes are arranged next to each other. The size of the deletion can be large or small, which may explain why some individuals with Williams syndrome are more severely affected than others. If one thinks of these genes as the letters of the alphabet, some individuals with Williams syndrome are missing A to M, some are missing G to Q and others are missing A to R. While there are differences in the amount of genetic material that can be deleted, there is a region of overlap. Everyone in the above example was missing G to M. It is thought that the missing genes in this region are important causes of the physical and mental findings of Williams syndrome.

Two genes in particular, ELN and LIMK1, have been shown to be important in causing some of the characteristic symptoms of Williams syndrome. The ELN gene codes for a protein called elastin. The job of elastin in the human body is to provide elasticity to the connective tissues such as those in the arteries, joints and tendons. The exact role of the LIMK1 gene is not known. The gene codes for a substance known as lim kinase 1 that is active in the brain. It is thought that the deletion of the LIMK1 gene may be responsible for the visuospatial learning difficulties of individuals with Williams syndrome. Many other genes are known to be in the deleted region of chromosome 7q11 responsible for Williams syndrome and much work is being done to determine the role of these genes in Williams syndrome.

Williams syndrome is an autosomal dominant disorder. Genes always come in pairs and in an autosomal dominant disorder, only one gene need be missing or altered for an individual to have the disorder. Although Williams syndrome is an autosomal disorder, most individuals with Williams syndrome are the only people in their family with this disorder. When this is the case, the chromosome deletion that causes Williams syndrome is called *de novo*. A *de novo* deletion is one that occurs for the first time in the affected individual. The cause of *de novo* chromosome deletions is unknown. Parents of an individual with Williams syndrome due to a *de novo* deletion are very unlikely to have a second child with Williams syndrome. However, once an individual has a chromosome deletion, there is a 50% chance that that person will pass it on to their offspring. Thus individuals with Williams syndrome have a 50% chance of passing this deletion (and Williams syndrome) to their children.

Demographics

Williams syndrome occurs in one in 20,000 births. Because Williams syndrome is an autosomal dominant disorder, it affects an equal number of males and females. It is thought that Williams syndrome occurs in people of all ethnic backgrounds equally.

Signs and symptoms

Williams syndrome is a multi-system disorder. In addition to distinct facial features, individuals with Williams syndrome can have cardiovascular, growth, joint and other physical problems. They also share unique personality traits and have intellectual differences.

Infants with Williams syndrome are often born small for their family and 70% are diagnosed with failure to thrive during infancy. These growth problems continue throughout the life of a person with Williams syndrome and most individuals with Williams syndrome have short stature (height below the third percentile). Infants with William syndrome can also be extremely irritable and have "colic-like" behavior. This behavior is thought to be due to excess calcium in the blood (hypercalcemia). Other problems that can occur in the first years include strabismus (crossed eyes), ear infections, chronic constipation, and eating problems.

Individuals with Williams syndrome can have distinct facial features sometimes described as "elfin" or "pixie-like." While none of these individual facial features is abnormal, the combination of the different features is common for Williams syndrome. Individuals with Williams syndrome have a small upturned nose, a small chin, long upper lip with a wide mouth, small widely spaced teeth and puffiness around the eyes. As an individual gets older, these facial features become more pronounced.

People with Williams syndrome often have problems with narrowing of their heart and blood vessels. This is thought to be due to the deletion of the elastin gene and is called elastin arteriopathy. Any artery in the body can be affected but the most common narrowing is seen in the aorta of the heart. This condition is called supravalvar aortic stenosis (SVAS) and occurs in approximately 75% of individuals with Williams syndrome. The degree of narrowing is variable. If left untreated, it can lead to high blood pressure, heart disease and heart failure. The blood vessels that lead to the kidney and other organs can also be affected.

Deletions of the elastin gene are also thought to be responsible for the loose joints of some children with Williams syndrome. As individuals with Williams syndrome age, their heel cords and hamstrings tend to tighten, which can lead to a stiff awkward gait and curving of the spine.

Approximately 75% of individuals with Williams syndrome have mild mental retardation. They also have a unique cognitive profile (unique learning abilities and disabilities). This cognitive profile is independent of their IQ. Individuals with Williams syndrome generally have excellent language and memorization skills. They can have extensive vocabularies and may develop a thorough knowledge of a topic that they are interested in. Many individuals are also gifted musicians. Individuals with Williams syndrome have trouble with concepts that rely on visuospatial ability. Because of this, many people with Williams syndrome have trouble with math, writing, and drawing.

People with Williams syndrome also often share personality characteristics. They are noted to be very talkative and friendly—sometimes inappropriately—and they can be hyperactive. Another shared personality trait is a generalized anxiety.

Diagnosis

The diagnosis of Williams syndrome is usually made by a physician familiar with Williams syndrome and based upon a physical examination of the individual and a review of his or her medical history. It is often made in infants after a heart problem (usually SVAS) is diagnosed. In children without significant heart problems, the diagnosis may be made after enrollment in school when they are noted to be "slow learners."

While a diagnosis can be made based upon physical examination and medical history, the diagnosis can now be confirmed by a DNA test.

Williams syndrome is caused by a deletion of genetic material from the long arm of chromosome 7. A specific technique called fluorescent in situ hybridization testing, or FISH testing, can determine whether there is genetic material missing. A FISH test will be positive (detect a deletion) in over 99% of individuals with Williams syndrome. A negative FISH test for Williams syndrome means that no genetic material is missing from the critical region on chromosome 7q11.

Prenatal testing (testing during pregnancy) for Williams syndrome is possible using the FISH test on DNA sample obtained by chorionic villus sampling (CVS) or by amniocentesis. Chorionic villus sampling is a prenatal test that is usually done between 10 to 12 weeks of pregnancy and involves removing a small amount of tissue from the placenta. Amniocentesis is a prenatal test that is usually performed at 16–18 weeks of pregnancy and involves removing a small amount of the amniotic fluid that surrounds the fetus. DNA is obtained from these samples and tested to see if the deletion responsible for Williams syndrome is present. While prenatal testing is possible, it is not routinely performed. Typically, the test is only done if there is a family history of Williams syndrome.

Treatment and management

Because Williams syndrome is a multi-system disorder, the expertise of a number of specialists is required for management of this disorder.

The height and growth of individuals with Williams syndrome should be monitored using special growth curves developed specifically for individuals with Williams syndrome. Individuals who fall off these growth curves should be worked up for possible eating or thyroid disorders.

A cardiologist should evaluate individuals with Williams syndrome yearly. This examination should include measurement of blood pressure in all four limbs and an echocardiogram of the heart. An echocardiogram is a special form of ultrasound that looks at the structure of the heart. Doppler flow studies, which look at how the blood flows into and out of the heart, should also be done. Individuals with supravalvar stenosis may require surgery to fix this condition. The high blood pressure caused by this condition may be treated with medication. Examinations should take place yearly as some of these conditions are progressive and may worsen over time.

Individuals with Williams syndrome should also have a complete neurological examination. In addition, the blood calcium levels of individuals with Williams syndrome should be monitored every two years. High levels of calcium can cause irritability, vomiting, constipation, and muscle cramps. An individual found to have a high level of calcium should consult a nutritionist to make sure that their intake of calcium is not higher than 100% of the recommended daily allowance (RDA). Because vitamin D can increase calcium levels, individuals with Williams syndrome and high calcium should not take multivitamins containing vitamin D. If calcium levels remain high after limiting vitamin D and decreasing dietary intake of calcium, an individual with hypercalcemia should see a nephrologist for further management and to monitor kidney function.

Strabismus (crossed eyes) can be treated by patching or by surgery. Ear infections can be treated with antibiotics and surgical placement of ear tubes.

KEY TERMS

de novo deletion—A deletion that occurs for the first time in the affected individual. The cause of de novo deletions is not known.

Hypercalcemia—High levels of calcium in the blood.

Stellate—A star-like, lacy white pattern in the iris. Most often seen in light-eyed individuals.

The developmental differences of individuals with Williams syndrome should be treated with early intervention and special education classes. Specific learning strategies that capitalize on the strengths of individuals with Williams syndrome should be used. Physical, occupational, and speech therapy should be provided. Behavioral counseling and medication may help with behavioral problems such as hyperactivity and anxiety.

Prognosis

The prognosis for individuals with Williams syndrome is highly dependent on the medical complications of a particular individual. Individuals with Williams syndrome who have no heart complications, or very minor ones, have a good prognosis. Good medical care and treatment of potential problems allows most individuals with Williams syndrome to lead a long life. The prognosis for individuals with more serious medical complications such as severe heart disease or hypertension is more guarded. Since the medical conditions associated with Williams syndrome are progressive rather than static, it is very important that individuals with Williams syndrome have yearly medical examinations with a health care provider familiar with Williams syndrome.

The range of abilities among individuals with Williams syndrome is very wide and the ultimate functioning of an individual is dependent on his or her abilities. While individuals with Williams syndrome do well in structured environments such as school, their unique abilities and disabilities do not permit them to do as well in unstructured surroundings. Some individuals with Williams syndrome live independently but most live with their parents or in a supervised setting. Many individuals with Williams syndrome can gain employment in supervised settings and do well at tasks that do not require mathematics or visuo-spatial abilities. It is important to encourage individuals with Williams syndrome toward independence but to recognize that their

friendly and outgoing personalities may lead them into abusive situations.

Resources

BOOKS

Bellugi, Ursula, and Marie St. George. *Journey from Cognition to Brain to Gene: Perspectives from Williams Syndrome.* Cambridge, MA: MIT Press, 2001.

PERIODICALS

Van Herwegen, J., et al. "Variability and Standardized Test Profiles in Typically Developing Children and Children with Williams Syndrome." *The British Journal of Developmental Psychology* 29 (November 2011): 883–94.

ORGANIZATIONS

Williams Syndrome Association. PO Box 297, Clawson, MI 48017-0297. (248) 541-3630. Fax: (248) 541-3631. TMonkaba@aol.com. http://www.williams-syndrome.org/.

Williams Syndrome Foundation. University of California, Irvine, CA 92679-2310. (949)824-7259. http://www.wsf.org/.

Kathleen Fergus, MS, CGC

Wilson disease

Definition

Wilson disease, or WD, is a rare inherited disorder that causes excess copper to accumulate in the body. It is also known as hepatolenticular degeneration. Steadily increasing amounts of copper circulating in the blood are deposited primarily in the brain, liver, kidneys, and the cornea of the eyes. WD is fatal if it is not recognized and treated. It is named for an American neurologist, Samuel A. K. Wilson, who first described it in 1912.

Description

Under normal conditions, copper that finds its way into the body through the diet is processed within the liver. This processed form of copper is then passed into the gallbladder, along with the other components of bile (a fluid produced by the liver, which enters the small intestine in order to help in digestive processes). When the gallbladder empties its contents into the first part of the small intestine (duodenum), the copper in the bile enters and passes through the intestine with the waste products of digestion. In healthy individuals, copper is then passed out of the body in stool.

In Wilson disease, copper does not pass from the liver into the bile, but rather begins to accumulate within the liver. As copper levels rise in the liver, the damaged organ begins to allow copper to flow into the

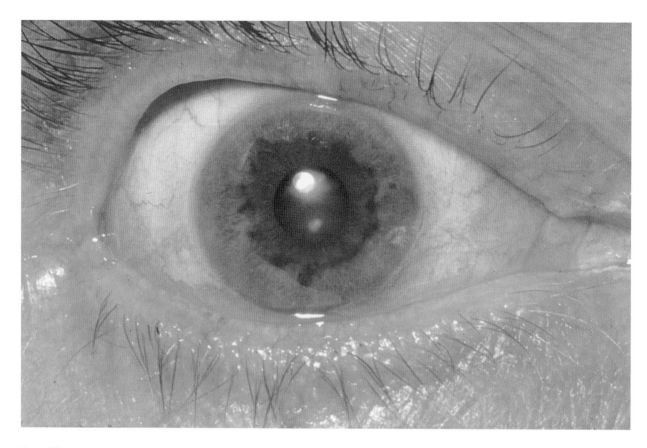

Eye afflicted with a Kayser-Fleischer ring, a brownish ring overlying the outer rim of the iris of the eye, which is caused by Wilson's disease. *(© SPL/Photo Researchers, Inc.)*

bloodstream, where it circulates. Copper is then deposited throughout the body, building up primarily in the kidneys, the brain and nervous system, and the eyes. Wilson disease, then, is a disorder of copper poisoning occurring from birth.

Wilson disease affects approximately one in 30,000 to one in 100,000 individuals and can affect people from many different populations. Approximately one in 90 individuals are carriers of the gene for Wilson disease.

Causes and symptoms

Wilson disease is inherited in an autosomal recessive manner. Autosomal recessive refers to the pattern of inheritance where each parent carries a gene for the disease on one of his or her chromosome pairs. When each parent passes on the chromosome with the gene for Wilson disease, the child will be affected with the disease. Both males and females can be affected with Wilson disease. If individuals are carriers of the Wilson disease gene they do not have any symptoms of this disease. In order to be affected, an individual must inherit two copies of the gene, one from each parent. Many cases

of Wilson disease may not be inherited but occur as a spontaneous mutation in the gene.

The gene for Wilson disease is located on chromosome number 13. The name of the gene is called ATP7B and is thought to be involved in transporting copper. Over 200 different mutations of this gene have been identified, making diagnosis by genetic testing difficult.

Symptoms typically present between the ages of three and 60, with age 17 considered to be the average age a diagnosis is made. About half of all patients experience their first symptoms in the liver. The illness causes swelling and tenderness of the liver, sometimes with fever, mimicking more common disorders, such as viral hepatitis and infectious mononucleosis. Abnormal levels of circulating liver enzymes reveal that the liver is being seriously damaged. This form of damage is referred to as fatty degeneration. Without medical intervention, the liver damage will progress to actual cirrhosis. An often-fatal manifestation of liver disease is called fulminant hepatitis. This extremely severe inflammation of the liver (hepatitis) results in jaundice, fluid leaking into the abdomen, low protein circulating

Wilson Disease
Autosomal Recessive

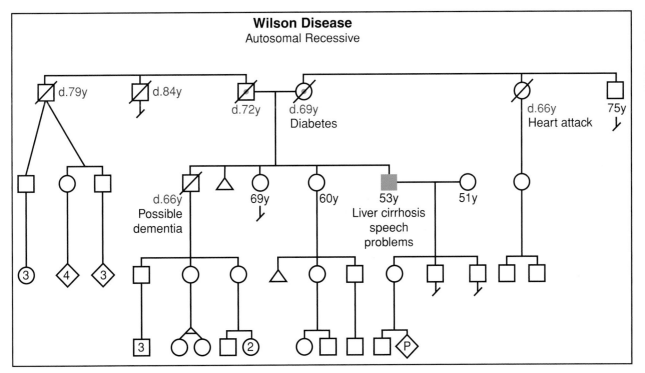

See Symbol Guide for Pedigree Charts. *(Illustration by Argosy, Inc. Reproduced by permission of Gale, a part of Cengage Learning.)*

in the blood, abnormalities of the blood clotting system, swelling of the brain, and anemia due to the abnormal destruction of red blood cells.

Neurological symptoms are the first to occur in half of all patients due to copper accumulation in the brain and nervous system. The average age of onset for neurological symptoms is 21. These symptoms include tremors of the hands, uncontrollable movements of the limbs, stiffness, drooling, difficulty swallowing, difficulty talking, and headache. There is no change in patient's intelligence.

About one-third of all patients with Wilson disease have a variety of psychiatric symptoms as the first signs of the disease. These symptoms include inability to cope, **depression**, irritability, increased anger, and inappropriate behavior. Often times patients have trouble completing tasks at work or in school.

Other symptoms that can affect patients with Wilson disease and may occur before or after a diagnosis has been made include joint disorders, symptoms of arthritis and skeletal problems such as osteoporosis. Patients have occasionally been affected with kidney stones, abnormal handling of glucose in their body and women have menstrual cycle irregularities, including stopping their regular cycle temporarily.

Diagnosis

The diagnosis of Wilson disease can be performed relatively easily through several different tests; however, because Wilson disease is so rare, diagnosis is often unfortunately delayed. The tests used to diagnose Wilson disease can be performed on patients who have and who have not already shown symptoms of the disease. It is extremely important to make a diagnosis as soon as possible since liver damage can occur before there are any signs of the disease.

An easy way to diagnose Wilson disease is to measure the amount of a glycoprotein found in the blood called ceruloplasmin. Low levels of ceruloplasmin can diagnose the disease in about 80% of affected patients. This procedure is not as effective for women taking birth control pills, pregnant women, or infants younger than six months of age.

A second test involving an eye examination to detect a characteristic ring of copper deposited in a membrane of the cornea (referred to as Kayser-Fleischer rings) is very easy to perform and is very useful in diagnosing patients who have already exhibited symptoms. This test is not as effective in persons without symptoms. This diagnostic test cannot be used by itself to make a diagnosis because some patients with liver disease but not Wilson disease will test positive.

KEY TERMS

Anemia—A blood condition in which the level of hemoglobin or the number of red blood cells falls below normal values. Common symptoms include paleness, fatigue, and shortness of breath.

Bile—A substance produced by the liver and concentrated and stored in the gallbladder. Bile contains a number of different substances, including bile salts, cholesterol, and bilirubin.

Biopsy—The surgical removal and microscopic examination of living tissue for diagnostic purposes.

Cell—The smallest living units of the body, which group together to form tissues and help the body perform specific functions.

Ceruloplasmin—A protein circulating in the bloodstream that binds with copper and transports it.

Chelation therapy—A method of removing copper or other heavy metals from the body by giving medications that bind to the metal and allow it to be excreted.

Chromosome—A microscopic thread-like structure found within each cell of the body and consists of a complex of proteins and DNA. Humans have 46 chromosomes arranged into 23 pairs. Changes in either the total number of chromosomes or their shape and size (structure) may lead to physical or mental abnormalities.

Cirrhosis—A chronic degenerative disease of the liver, in which normal cells are replaced by fibrous tissue. Cirrhosis is a major risk factor for the later development of liver cancer.

Deoxyribonucleic acid (DNA)—The genetic material in cells that holds the inherited instructions for growth, development, and cellular functioning.

Gallbladder—A small, pear-shaped organ in the upper right hand corner of the abdomen. It is connected by a series of ducts (tube-like channels) to the liver, pancreas, and duodenum (first part of the small intestine). The gallbladder receives bile from the liver and concentrates and stores it. After a meal, bile is squeezed out of the gallbladder into the intestine, where it aids in digestion of food.

Gene—A building block of inheritance, which contains the instructions for the production of a particular protein and is made up of a molecular sequence found on a section of DNA. Each gene is found on a precise location on a chromosome.

Glucose—One of the two simple sugars, together with galactose, that makes up the protein, lactose, found in milk. Glucose is the form of sugar that is usable by the body to generate energy.

Hepatitis—A viral disease characterized by inflammation of the liver cells (hepatocytes). People infected with hepatitis B or hepatitis C virus are at an increased risk for developing liver cancer.

Jaundice—Yellowing of the skin or eyes due to excess of bilirubin in the blood.

Toxic—Poisonous.

A third test for diagnosing Wilson disease involves measuring the amount of copper in the liver. This can be accomplished by sampling a portion of the liver, called a **biopsy**. This is one of the most effective ways in which to diagnose Wilson disease; however, the procedure itself is more difficult to perform than the others.

Other tests are also useful, for example, measuring the amount of copper passed into the urine daily (high in Wilson disease). Another lab test measures the ability of a patient's ceruloplasmin to bind with a form of copper (decreased in Wilson disease). And finally, as discussed under genetic profile, some patients can be diagnosed through a DNA test to determine whether they carry two genes for Wilson disease. This test does not always prove to be useful in certain patients and is of most use when used to test the brothers and sisters of affected patients.

Molecular genetic testing is not particularly valuable in diagnosing WD because of the large number of possible gene mutations.

Treatment

Treatment involves life-long administration of either D-penicillamine (Cuprimine, Depen) or trientine hydrochloride (Syprine). Both of these drugs remove copper deposits throughout the body by binding to the copper which then leaves the body in the urine. This type of treatment is called chelation therapy. Zinc acetate (Galzin) and a low copper diet are other ways in which to treat Wilson disease.

Penicillamine has a number of serious side effects:

- joint pain
- neurological problems
- systemic lupus erythematosus

- decreased production of all blood elements
- interference with clotting
- allergic reactions

Careful monitoring is necessary. When patients have side effects from penicillamine, the dose can sometimes be lowered to an effective level that causes fewer difficulties. Alternatively, steroid medications may be required to reduce certain sensitivity reactions. Trientine has fewer potential side effects, but must still be carefully monitored.

Treatment with zinc acetate is also an effective way to remove excess copper from the body. Zinc is a metal that works to block copper absorption and bind copper in the intestinal cells until it is all released into the stool approximately one week later. The benefit of treatment with zinc is there are no toxic side effects however the zinc is a slower acting agent than the other drugs. It takes four to eight months for the zinc to be effective in reducing the overall amount of copper in the body.

Finally, patients with Wilson disease are encouraged to follow a diet low in copper, with an average copper intake of 1.0 mg/day. Foods to be avoided for the high levels of copper include liver and shellfish. Patients are also instructed to monitor their drinking water for excess levels of copper and drink distilled water instead.

Patients may be given a liver transplant in the event of liver failure as a complication of WD. Liver transplantation has been reported to have a relatively favorable outcome, in some cases decreasing the patient's neurologic symptoms.

Prognosis

Without treatment, Wilson disease is always fatal. With treatment, symptoms may continue to worsen for the first six to eight weeks. After this time, definite improvement should begin to be seen. However, it may take several years (two to five) of treatment to reach maximal benefit to the brain and liver. Even then, many patients are not returned to their original level of functioning. Patients with Wilson disease need to maintain some sort of anticopper treatment for the rest of their lives in order to prevent copper levels from rising in the body. Interruptions in treatment can result in a relapse of the disease, which is not reversible and can ultimately lead to death.

Resources

BOOKS

Beers, Mark H., and Robert Berkow, eds. "Mineral Deficiency and Toxicity." In *The Merck Manual of Diagnosis and Therapy*. Whitehouse Station, NJ: Merck Research Laboratories, 2004.

PERIODICALS

Daniel, K. G., R. H. Harbach, W. C. Guida, and Q. P. Dou. "Copper Storage Diseases: Menkes, Wilsons, and Cancer." *Frontiers in Bioscience* 9 (September 1, 2004): 2652–62.

Georghe, L., I. Popescu, S. Iacob, et al. "Wilson's Disease: A Challenge of Diagnosis. The 5-Year Experience of a Tertiary Centre." *Romanian Journal of Gastroenterology* 13 (September 2004): 179–85.

Gow, P.J., et al. "Diagnosis of Wilson's Disease: An Experience Over Three Decades." *Gut* 46 (March 2000): 415–19.

Robertson, W.M. "Wilson's Disease." *Archives of Neurology* 57, no. 2 (February 2000): 276–77.

Velez-Pardo, C., M. J. Rio, S. Moreno, et al. "New Mutation (T1232P) of the ATP-7B Gene Associated with Neurologic and Neuropsychiatric Dominance Onset of Wilson's Disease in Three Unrelated Colombian Kindred." *Neuroscience Letters* 367 (September 9, 2004): 360–64.

ORGANIZATIONS

American Liver Foundation. 1425 Pompton Ave., Cedar Grove, NJ 07009. (800) 223-0179. http://www.liverfoundation.org.

National Organization for Rare Disorders (NORD). 55 Kenosia Avenue, P. O. Box 1968, Danbury, CT 06813-1968. (203) 744-0100. Fax: (203) 798-2291. http://www.rarediseases.org.

Wilson's Disease Association. 4 Navaho Dr., Brookfield, CT 06804. (800) 399-0266.

OTHER

Carter, Beth A., MD. "Wilson Disease." eMedicine June 17, 2004. http://www.emedicine.com/ped/topic2441.htm.

Wilson's Disease Association. http://www.medhelp.org/wda/wil.htm.

Katherine S. Hunt, MS
Rebecca J. Frey, PhD

X

X-linked spinal and bulbar muscular atrophy
see **Kennedy disease**

Z

Zellweger syndrome

Definition

Zellweger syndrome is a severe and fatal genetic disorder affecting the brain, liver, and kidneys. It can be inherited by children of individuals that carry mutations for a specific gene.

Description

Zellweger syndrome is a fatal disorder that damages the brain, liver, and kidneys. There are related syndromes that have Zellweger-like symptoms and involve defects in the distinct cytoplasm organelles of cells called the peroxisomes; these include neonatal **adrenoleukodystrophy**, infantile **Refsum disease**, and hyperpipecolic acidemia. Zellweger syndrome is the most severe of these related syndromes.

Demographics

The incidence of Zellweger syndrome worldwide is roughly 1 in 100,000 births.

Causes and symptoms

Mutations in one of the many genes that cause Zellweger syndrome lead to a dysfunctional protein that is important for the cells' ability to import newly synthesized proteins into small cytoplasmic organelles called peroxisomes. Zellweger syndrome is characterized by the reduction or absence of these peroxisomes. Key enzymes that are critical for various chemical reactions, in particular oxidation, are contained within the peroxisomes.

Functional and structural abnormalities of the peroxisomes can lead to the disease development observed in Zellweger syndrome. Because peroxisomes are abundant in the liver and the kidney, these organs are affected in Zellweger syndrome. Toxic molecules that enter the bloodstream are detoxified by the peroxisomes, although there are additional mechanisms for detoxification. For example, when large amounts of ethanol from alcoholic beverages are consumed, roughly 5–25% of the ethanol can be oxidized by the peroxisomes. Peroxisomes can also function in the organic creation of key compounds and play important roles in the various chemical reactions.

Zellweger syndrome is caused by mutations in any one of several different genes involved in the function of the peroxisome. These include peroxin-1 (PEX1), peroxin-2 (PEX2), peroxin-3 (PEX3), peroxin-5 (PEX5), peroxin-6 (PEX6), and peroxin-12 (PEX12). Each of these gene locations are biochemically and genetically distinct and are found on different chromosomes.

The observable clinical features of Zellweger syndrome can include facial, developmental, and ocular (eye) defects. Characteristic features commonly include a high forehead, upslanting eyes, and skin folds, called epicanthal folds, along the medial (nasal) borders of the palpebral fissures (space between upper and lower eyelids) of the eyes. Typically, babies with Zellweger syndrome have severe **weakness**, hyptonia (loss of muscle tone), and often have neonatal seizures. There are also several ocular abnormalities that can affect eyesight.

Diagnosis

Absent peroxisomes in the liver and kidney was initially demonstrated by American pathologist S. L. Goldfischer in 1985. The absence of these organelles in the liver is currently thought to be the hallmark of this disorder. Patients with Zellweger syndrome have been found to have remarkably fewer peroxisomes in both the brain and cultured skin fibroblasts. Fibroblasts are a type of skin cell, and, in Zellweger syndrome, these cells appear to have ghost-like peroxisomes, which are caused by an absence of specific proteins inside the organelles that are recruited into the membranes.

Peroxisomes play an important role in organ development. Brain abnormalities can be explained by the

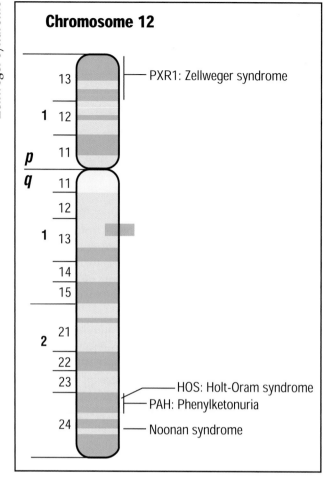

Chromosome 12

13 — PXR1: Zellweger syndrome

1 12

p 11

q 11

12

1 13

14

15

21

2 22

23 — HOS: Holt-Oram syndrome
   — PAH: Phenylketonuria

24 — Noonan syndrome

Zellweger syndrome, on chromosome 12. *(Illustration by Argosy, Inc. Reproduced by permission of Gale, a part of Cengage Learning.)*

fluid of the amnion, a process called amniocentesis. Thus, pregnant mothers who have previously had an affected baby can opt to have prenatal diagnosis to determine if the fetus is affected.

Treatment team

Physicians, nurses, and therapists provide the basis of the treatment team for a person with Zellweger's syndrome. Geneticists also provide diagnostic and genetic counseling services. Support services are available for families.

Treatment

There is no cure for Zellweger syndrome and treatment is based solely on lessening the symptoms and supporting the involved organs.

Recovery and rehabilitation

Physical, occupational, respiratory, and speech therapists can provide supportive strategies and devices to maintain posture, independent breathing, speech, eating, and other daily activities according to the infant or child's developmental stage for as long as practically possible.

Clinical trials

A clinical trial was sponsored in 2004 by the FDA Office of Orphan Products Development for the treatment of Zellweger syndrome (which is under review by the National Institutes of Health). It involved determining the effectiveness of giving oral bile acids (cholic acid, chenodeoxycholic acid, and ursodeoxycholic acid) as therapy for affected individuals.

Prognosis

Persons with Zellweger syndrome rarely live more than one year after diagnosis, with death due mostly to severe feeding difficulties, liver complications, respiratory distress, and cardiac defects.

disrupted migration of nerve cells called neurons (or neuroblasts at this stage of development) around the third month of gestation. This defect occurs in a specific area of the brain called the cerebrum and leads to small or thick convolutions in brain tissue. This brain abnormality allows Zellweger syndrome to be distinguished from other diseases that involve brain abnormalities. Other tissues involved in the disease development include the liver, kidney, cartilage, heart, and muscle. Most patients have cysts on their kidneys.

Zellweger syndrome is diagnosed by measuring metabolic compounds in blood samples from patients. Various fatty acids, plasmalogens, pipecolic acid, and bile acid intermediates are usually studied. Aside from plasmalogen levels, which are diminished, these compounds are typically increased in affected individuals. It is also possible to detect fatty acid levels and plasmalogen synthesis before birth by obtaining cells in the

Special concerns

Because Zellweger syndrome is usually fatal within the first year of life, genetic counseling and prenatal diagnosis are usually assigned a high priority for parents identified or concerned that they may be at risk for having a baby with the syndrome.

Resources

PERIODICALS

Depreter, M., M. Espeel, and F. Roels. "Human Peroxisomal Disorders." *Microsc Res Tech* (2003) 61: 203–23.

Gootjes, J., et al. "Biochemical Markers Predicting Survival in Peroxisome Diogenesis Disorders." *Neurology* (2002) 59: 1746–9.

OTHER

Johns Hopkins University School of Medicine. *The Peroxisome.* January 3, 2004 (March 2, 2004). http://www.peroxisome.org/Layperson/layperson.html.

National Institute of Neurological Disorders and Stroke. *NINDS Zellweger Syndrome Information Page* January 3, 2004 (March 2, 2004). http://www.ninds.nih.gov/health_and_medical/disorders/zellwege_doc.htm.

ORGANIZATIONS

National Organization for Rare Disorders. P.O. Box 1968, Danbury, CT 06813-1968. Phone: (203) 744-0100. Email: orphan@rarediseases.org. http://www.rarediseases.org.

United Leukodystrophy Foundation, Inc. 2304 Highland Drive, Sycamore, IL 60178. Phone: (800) 728-5483. Fax: (815) 895-2432. Email: ulf@tbcnet.com. http://www.ulf.org.

Bryan Richard Cobb

Zonisamide

Definition

Zonisamide is an anticonvulsant used to control seizures in the treatment of epilepsy, a neurological dysfunction in which excessive surges of electrical energy are emitted in the brain.

Purpose

Zonisamide decreases abnormal activity and excitement within the brain that may trigger seizures. While zonisamide controls the partial seizures (focal seizures) associated with epilepsy, there is no known cure for the disease.

Some physicians have also used zonisamide in the treatment of mood disorders. Zonisamide is additionally under study for the treatment of migraine headaches and neuropathic (nerve) pain.

Description

In the United States, zonisamide is sold under the brand name Zonegran. Zonisamide is classified as a sulfonamide anticonvulsant. The precise mechanisms by which it works are unknown.

Recommended dosage

Zonisamide is taken by mouth in tablet form. It is prescribed by physicians in varying dosages, usually from 100mg to 400mg daily.

Beginning a course of treatment that includes zonisamide requires a gradual dose-increasing regimen. Adults and teenagers 16 years or older typically take 100 mg per day for the first two weeks. Daily dosages of zonisamide may then be increased 100mg once every two weeks until reaching the full daily dose (usually not more than 400mg.) It may take several weeks to realize the full benefits of zonisamide.

Persons should not take a double dose of anticonvulsant medications. If a daily dose is missed, it should be taken as soon as possible. However, if it is almost time for the next dose, the missed dose should be skipped.

When discontinuing treatment with zonisamide, physicians typically direct patients to gradually reduce their daily dosages. Stopping the medicine suddenly may cause seizures to occur or become more frequent.

Precautions

Persons taking zonisamide should avoid alcohol and **central nervous system** depressants (medications including antihistimines, sleep medications, and some pain medications). Combining these substances with zonisamide can exacerbate (heighten) the side effects of alcohol and other medications.

A physician should be consulted before taking zonisamide with certain non-perscription medications, such as medicines for asthma, appetite control, coughs, colds, sinus problems, allergies, and hay fever.

Zonisamide may inhibit perspiration, causing body temperature to increase during physical activity. Persons taking zonisamide are at a greater risk for heat stroke. Caution should be used during strenuous exercise, prolongued exposure during hot weather, and while using saunas or hot tubs.

Zonisamide may not be suitable for persons with a history of liver or kidney disease, mental illness, high blood presure, angina (chest pain), irregular heartbeats, or other heart problems.

Before beginning treatment with zonisamide, patients should notify their physician if they consume a large amount of alcohol, have a history of drug use, are pregnant, or plan to become pregnant. Most physicians recommend using effective birth control while taking zonisamide, as it may cause defects to a developing fetus. Patients who become pregnant while taking zonisamide should contact their physician immediately.

Side effects

Research indicates that zonisamide is generally well tolerated. However, it may cause a variety of usually mild side effects. Headache, nausea and **fatigue**, and **weakness** are the most frequently reported side effects of zonisamide. Other possible side effects include:

• Difficulty sleeping
• Nervousness
• Anxiety
• Abdominal pain
• Dificulty with memory
• Double vision
• Loss of appetite
• Restlessness
• Drowsiness
• Diarrhea or constipation
• Indigestion
• Aching joints and muscles
• Unpleasant taste in mouth or dry mouth
• Tingling or prickly feeling on the skin

Many of these side effects disappear or occur less frequently during treatment as the body adjusts to the medication. However, if any symptoms persist or become too uncomfortable, the prescribing physician should be consulted.

Other, uncommon side effects of zonisamide can be serious. A patient taking zonisamide who experiencs any of the following symptoms should contact their physician:

• Rash or bluish patches on the skin
• Discouragement, feeling sad or empty
• Mood or mental changes
• Shakiness or unsteady walking
• Lack of appetite

KEY TERMS

Epilepsy—A disorder associated with disturbed electrical discharges in the central nervous system that cause seizures.

Seizure—A convulsion, or uncontrolled discharge of nerve cells that may spread to other cells throughout the brain.

Sulfonamides—A group of antibiotics used to treat a wide range of bacterial infections.

• Kidney stones
• Difficulty breathing
• Chest pain
• Slow or irregular heartbeat
• Faintness
• Confusion or loss of consciousness
• Persistant, severe headaches
• Persistant fever or pain

Interactions

Zonisamide may have negative interactions with some antifungal medications, antihistimines, antidepressants, antibiotics, and monoamine oxidase inhibitors (MAOIs). Other medications such as **diazepam** (Valium), fluoxetine (Prozac, Sarafem), fluvoxamine (Luvox), HIV protease inhibitors (indinavir), ritonavir (Norvir), ipratropium (Atrovent), isoniazid, **phenobarbital** (Luminal, Solfoton), nefazodone, metronidazole, **acetazolamide** (Diamox), phenytoin (Dilantin), **primidone**, propranolol (Inderal), and rifampin (Rifadin, Rimactane) may also adversely react with Zonisamide.

Zonisamide is sometimes prescribed as part of a combination of drugs to prevent seizures. The physician will carefully monitor the combination drug therapy, as sometimes zonisamide will potentiate (enhance) the effects of other anticonvulsant medications.

Zonisamide may decrease the effectiveness of some forms of oral contraceptives (birth control pills).

Zonisamide should not be taken by those allergic to sulfa drugs.

Resources

BOOKS

Weaver, Donald F. *Epilepsy and Seizures: Everything You Need to Know*. Richmond Hill, ONT, Canada: Firefly Books, 2001.

OTHER

"Zonisamide." *Medline Plus*. National Library of Medicine. http://www.nlm.nih.gov/medlineplus/druginfo/uspdi/500137.html (March 20, 2004).

ORGANIZATIONS

American Epilepsy Society. 342 North Main Street, West Hartford, CT 06117-2507. Phone: (860) 586-7505. Tollfree http://www.aesnet.org.

Epilepsy Foundation. 4351 Garden City Drive, Landover, MD 20785-7223. Phone: (800) 332-1000. Tollfree phone: (800) 332-1000. http://www.epilepsyfoundation.org.

Adrienne Wilmoth Lerner

Zonisamide

GLOSSARY

A

AADC INHIBITORS. Drugs that block the amino acid decarboxylase; one type of enzyme that breaks down dopamine. Also called DC inhibitors, they include carbidopa and benserazide.

ABRASION. A wound caused by superficial damage to the skin caused by contact with a rough surface. A skinned knee from a fall is an example of an abrasion.

ABSCESS. A localized collection of pus or infection that is walled off from the rest of the body.

ABSENCE SEIZURE. A type of generalized seizure in which a person may temporarily appear to be staring into space or have jerking or twitching muscles. Previously called a petit mal seizure.

ABSTINENCE. The voluntary refraining from satisfying an appetite, craving, or indulgence (e.g., avoiding drugs, alcohol, or sexual activity).

ACALCULIA. The inability to perform basic calculation (addition, subtraction, multiplication, division).

ACCELEROMETER. A specialized device attached to the index finger that records the frequency and amplitude (magnitude of change) of hand tremors.

ACETYLCHOLINE. The neurotransmitter, or chemical, that works in the brain to transmit nerve signals involved in regulating muscles, memory, mood, and sleep.

ACETYLSALICYLIC ACID. Aspirin; an analgesic, antipyretic, and antirheumatic drug prescribed to reduce fever and for relief of pain and inflammation.

ACHALASIA. An esophageal disease of unknown cause, in which the lower sphincter or muscle is unable to relax normally, resulting in obstruction, either partial or complete.

ACID MALTASE. The enzyme that regulates the amount of glycogen stored in muscle cells. When too much glycogen is present, acid maltase is released to break it down into waste products.

ACIDOSIS. A condition of decreased alkalinity resulting from abnormally high acid levels (low pH) in the blood and tissues. Usually indicated by sickly sweet breath, headaches, nausea, vomiting, and visual impairments.

ACOUSTIC. A term that refers to hearing.

ACOUSTIC NEUROMA. A benign tumor that grows on the nerve leading from the inner ear to the brain. As the tumor grows, it exerts pressure on the inner ear and causes severe vertigo.

ACOUSTIC TRAUMA. Permanent damage to the hair cells in the cochlea caused by a one-time exposure to an extremely loud noise, such as an explosion or military shellfire.

ACQUIRED IMMUNE DEFICIENCY SYNDROME (AIDS). HIV infection that has led to certain opportunistic infections, cancers, or a CD4+ T-lymphocyte (helper cell) blood cell count lower than 200/mL.

ACROCEPHALOPOLYSYNDACTYLY SYNDROMES. A collection of genetic disorders characterized by cone shaped abnormality of the skull and partial fusing of adjacent fingers or toes.

ACROCEPHALY. An abnormal cone shape of the head.

ACROPARESTHESIAS. Painful burning sensation in hands and feet.

ACTION POTENTIAL. The wave-like change in the electrical properties of a cell membrane, resulting from the difference in electrical charge between the inside and outside of the membrane.

ACUITY. Sharpness.

ACUPRESSURE. A form of massage using acupuncture points.

ACUTE DISSEMINATED ENCEPHALOMYELITS (ADEM). An autoimmune disease that causes inflammation of the brain and spinal cord.

ACUTE MOUNTAIN SICKNESS (AMS). Illness, including cerebral edema, that can affect people at high altitudes, usually above 14,000 ft (4,267 m).

ACUTE PAIN. Pain in response to injury or another stimulus that resolves when the injury heals or the stimulus is removed.

ACUTE RETROVIRAL SYNDROME (ARS). A syndrome that develops in about 30% of HIV patients within a few weeks of infection. ARS is characterized by nausea, vomiting, fever, headache, general tiredness, and muscle cramps.

ACYCLOVIR. An antiviral drug that is available in oral, intravenous, and topical forms and that blocks replication of the varicella zoster virus.

ADENOMA. A type of noncancerous (benign) tumor that often involves the overgrowth of certain cells of the type normally found within glands.

ADRENAL. A pair of glands located on top of the kidneys that secrete substances or hormones, like steroids and adrenaline, which regulate various functions, such as water balance and stress response.

ADRENAL INSUFFICIENCY. Problems with the adrenal glands that can be life threatening if not treated. Symptoms include sluggishness, weakness, weight loss, vomiting, darkening of the skin, and mental changes.

ADRENOCORTICOTROPIC HORMONE (ACTH). A pituitary hormone that stimulates the cortex of the adrenal glands to produce adrenal cortical hormones.

ADVANCED BONE AGE. The bones, on x ray, appear to be those of an older individual.

AEROBIC EXERCISE. Any exercise that increases the body's oxygen consumption and improves the functioning of the cardiovascular and respiratory systems.

AFFECT. In psychology, a feeling or emotion that occurs prior to cognition or thinking. Affective disorders are those involving the emotions (particularly anxiety or sadness) as contrasted to thought disorders. Affective disorders are also known as mood disorders.

AFFECTIVE FLATTENING. A loss or lack of emotional expressiveness. It is sometimes called blunted or restricted affect.

AFFERENT. Refers to peripheral nerves that transmit signals to the spinal cord and the brain. These nerves carry out sensory function.

AGITATION. Excessive restlessness or emotional disturbance that is often associated with anxiety or psychosis; common in middle-stage AD.

AGNOSIA. Inability to recognize familiar people, places, objects, or body parts.

AGRANULOCYTOSIS. An acute febrile condition marked by severe depression of the granulocyte-producing bone marrow, and by prostration, chills, swollen neck, and sore throat, sometimes with local ulceration.

AGRAPHIA. The inability to write.

AIDED COMMUNICATION SYSTEMS. Any of a number of communication systems that involve tools or equipment of some kind in addition to the human body.

AIDS. Acquired Immune Deficiency Syndrome is a sexually transmitted disease caused by the Human Immunodeficiency Virus (HIV). It weakens the immune system and makes a person susceptible to many infections and malignancies.

AIDS DEMENTIA COMPLEX (ADC). A type of brain dysfunction caused by HIV infection resulting in difficulty thinking, confusion, and loss of muscular coordination.

AKATHISIA. Agitated or restless movement, usually affecting the legs and accompanied by a sense of discomfort. It is a common side effect of neuroleptic medications.

AKINESIA. A loss of the ability to move; freezing in place.

ALEXANDER TECHNIQUE. A form of movement therapy that emphasizes correct posture and the proper positioning of the head with regard to the spine.

ALEXIA. Aphasia characterized by the loss of reading ability.

ALEXITHYMIA. An inability to identify and express feelings or emotions.

ALLERGEN. Any substance that irritates only those who are sensitive (allergic) to it.

ALLOGENEIC. Donor cells or tissues that are genetically distinct from those of the recipient.

ALPHA-FETOPROTEIN (AFP). A chemical substance produced by the fetus and found in the fetal circulation. AFP is also found in abnormally high concentrations in most patients with primary liver cancer.

ALTERNATING HEMIPLEGIA (AH); ALTERNATING HEMIPLEGIA OF CHILDHOOD (AHC). A rare and often progressive neurological disorder characterized by repeated, transient paralysis on alternating sides of the body.

ALZHEIMER'S DISEASE. A progressive, neurodegenerative disease characterized by loss of function and death of nerve cells in several areas of the brain, leading to loss of mental functions such as memory and learning. Formerly called presenile dementia.

AMENORRHEA. The absence or abnormal stoppage of menstrual periods.

AMINO ACID. An organic compound composed of both an amino group and an acidic carboxyl group. Amino acids are the basic building blocks of proteins. There are 20 types of amino acids (eight are "essential amino acids" which the body cannot make and must therefore be obtained from food).

AMNESIA. A general medical term for loss of memory that is not due to ordinary forgetfulness. Amnesia can be caused by head injuries, brain disease, or epilepsy, as well as by dissociation. Includes: 1) Anterograde amnesia: inability to retain the memory of events occurring after the time of the injury or disease which brought about the amnesic state. 2) Retrograde amnesia: inability to recall the memory of events which occurred prior to the time of the injury or disease which brought about the amnesic state.

AMNIOCENTESIS. A procedure performed at 16–18 weeks of pregnancy in which a needle is inserted through a woman's abdomen into her uterus to draw out a small sample of the amniotic fluid from around the baby. Either the fluid itself or cells from the fluid can be used for a variety of tests to obtain information about genetic disorders and other medical conditions in the fetus.

AMNIOTIC FLUID. The fluid which surrounds a developing baby during pregnancy.

AMYGDALA. An almond-shaped brain structure of the limbic system that is activated in stressful situations and triggers fear.

AMYLOID. A waxy, translucent, starch-like protein that is deposited in tissues during the course of certain chronic diseases such as rheumatoid arthritis and Alzheimer's disease.

AMYLOIDOSIS. The accumulation of amyloid deposits in various organs and tissues in the body so that normal functioning is compromised. Primary amyloidosis usually occurs as a complication of multiple myeloma. Secondary amyloidosis occurs in patients suffering from chronic infections or inflammatory diseases such as tuberculosis, rheumatoid arthritis, and Crohn's disease.

AMYOTROPHIC LATERAL SCLEROSIS (ALS). A neurodegenerative disease that is caused by degeneration of the motor fibers and neurons in the brain and spinal cord, leading to stiffness, weak muscles, respiratory failure, and death. Also known as Lou Gehrig's disease.

AMYOTROPHY. A type of neuropathy resulting in pain, weakness, and/or wasting in the muscles.

ANALGESIA. A decrease in the perception of pain. Analgesic medications are used for pain relief.

ANALGESIC. A medication that relieves pain without causing loss of consciousness; over-the-counter analgesics include aspirin and NSAIDs.

ANEMIA. A condition in which there is an abnormally low number of red blood cells in the bloodstream. It may be due to loss of blood, an increase in red blood cell destruction, or a decrease in red blood cell production. Major symptoms are paleness, shortness of breath, unusually fast or strong heart beats, and tiredness.

ANEURYSM. A weakened area in the wall of a blood vessel that causes an outpouching or bulge. Aneurysms may be fatal if the weak areas burst.

ANGINA (ANGINA PECTORIS). Chest pain caused by an insufficient supply of oxygen and decreased blood flow to the heart muscle. Angina is frequently the first sign of coronary artery disease.

ANGIOFIBROMA. Noncancerous growths on the skin, often reddish in color and filled with blood vessels.

ANGIOGRAPHY. A technique for visualizing blood vessels by threading a catheter through a large vein in the patient's arm or leg, injecting a contrast material when the catheter reaches the desired location, and taking images by standard radiography or a CT scan. Angiography of the blood vessels in the brain is called cerebral angiography.

ANGIOKERATOMA. A skin rash comprised of red bumps. The rash most commonly occurs between the navel and the knees.

ANGIOMA. A tumor (such as a hemangioma or lymphangioma) that mainly consists of blood vessels or lymphatic vessels.

ANGIOMYOLIPOMA. Noncancerous growth in the kidney, most often found in tuberous sclerosis.

ANGIOPLASTY. A technique for mechanically widening a narrowed or blocked blood vessel by inserting a balloon catheter, inflating the balloon to crush the fatty deposits obstructing the blood vessel, and deflating the balloon and withdrawing the catheter.

ANGULAR GYRUS. A particular ridge (outfolding) in the parietal lobe of the brain.

ANOMIC APHASIA. A condition characterized by either partial or total loss of the ability to recall the names of persons or things as a result of a stroke, head injury, brain tumor, or infection.

ANOREXIA. Lack or loss of appetite. The psychophysiological disorder called *anorexia nervosa* is characterized by food aversion, fear of obesity, and distorted self-image.

ANOREXIANT. A drug that suppresses appetite.

ANOXIA. Lack of oxygen.

ANTERIOR FONTANELLE. The soft-spot on the skull of an infant that is located in the center of the head just behind the hairline.

ANTERIOR HORN CELLS. Subset of motor neurons within the spinal cord.

ANTERIOR VITREITIS. Inflammation of the corpus vitreum, which surrounds and fills the inner portion of the eyeball between the lens and the retina.

ANTEROGRADE AMNESIA. Amnesia for events that occurred after a physical injury or emotional trauma but before the present moment.

ANTIBODY. Specialized cells of the immune system which can recognize organisms that invade the body (such as bacteria, viruses, and fungi). The antibodies are then able to set off a complex chain of events designed to kill these foreign invaders.

ANTICHOLINERGIC. Related to the ability of a drug to block the nervous system chemical acetylcholine. When acetylcholine is blocked, patients often experience dry mouth and skin, increased heart rate, blurred vision, and difficulty in urinating. In severe cases, blocking acetylcholine may cloud thinking and cause delirium.

ANTICIPATION. The apparent tendency of certain inherited diseases to appear at increasingly earlier ages in successive generations and with increasing severity.

ANTICONVULSANT DRUGS. Drugs used to prevent convulsions or seizures. They often are prescribed in the treatment of epilepsy.

ANTIDEPRESSANTS. A type of medication that is used to treat depression; it is also sometimes used to treat autism.

ANTIEMETIC. A drug that helps stop nausea and vomiting.

ANTIEPILEPTIC DRUG (AED). Anticonvulsant drug; a medication to prevent epileptic seizures.

ANTIGEN. A substance that stimulates the immune system to produce antibodies.

ANTIOXIDANT. A molecule that prevents oxidation. In the body antioxidants attach to other molecules called free radicals and prevent the free radicals from causing damage to cell walls, DNA, and other parts of the cell.

ANTIPSYCHOTICS. A group of drugs used to treat schizophrenia. The older antipsychotic drugs are also called neuroleptics.

ANTITOXIN. A substance that inactivates a poison (e.g., toxin) and protects the body from being injured by it.

ANTIVIRAL. A drug that prevents viruses from replicating and therefore spreading infection.

ANXIETY. Worry or tension in response to real or imagined stress, danger, or dreaded situations. Physical reactions, such as fast pulse, sweating, trembling, fatigue, and weakness may accompany anxiety.

ANXIETY DISORDER. A psychiatric disorder involving the presence of anxiety that is so intense or so frequently present that it causes difficulty or distress for the individual.

AORTA. The major artery that carries oxygenated blood from the heart to be delivered by arteries throughout the body.

APHASIA. Loss of the ability to use or understand language, usually as a result of brain injury or disease.

APHERESIS. The process of withdrawing blood, removing one or more blood components, and transfusing the remaining blood back into the donor.

APNEA. An irregular breathing pattern characterized by abnormally long periods of the complete cessation of breathing.

APOLIPOPROTEIN E (APOE). A protein that transports cholesterol throughout the body. One form of this protein, APOE e4, is associated with a 60% risk of late-onset AD.

APRAXIA. Difficulty performing a voluntary movement, although the muscles necessary are all functional.

AQUAPORIN-4 (AQP4). Channels through which water enters cells in the brain and which appear to be involved in brain edema.

ARACHNOID MEMBRANE. One of the three membranes that sheath the spinal cord and brain; the arachnoid is the middle membrane. Also called the arachnoid mater. It derives its name from its resemblance to a spider web (spiders are arachnids).

ARBOVIRUSES. Viruses harbored by arthropods (mosquitoes and ticks) and transferred to humans by their bite. Arboviruses are one cause of encephalitis.

ARCHIMEDES' SPIRAL. A figure that is often used as a drawing test in the differential diagnosis of tremor.

AREA POSTREMA. The part of the brain stem that controls vomiting.

AREFLEXIA. Absence of a reflex; a sign of possible nerve damage.

ARNOLD-CHIARI MALFORMATION. A condition in which the cerebellum, a structure in the brain, protrudes into the spinal canal.

ARTERIOGRAM. An x-ray study of an artery that has been injected with a contrast dye.

ARTERIOGRAPHY. A medical test in which an x-ray visible dye is injected into blood vessels. This dye allows the blood vessels to be imaged with x rays.

ARTERIOSCLEROSIS. Hardening of the arteries caused by high blood cholesterol and high blood pressure.

ARTERIOVENOUS MALFORMATION (AVM). An abnormal connection between veins and arteries, usually congenital. A cerebral AVM may result in epilepsy; severe headache; bleeding into the brain; difficulties with speech, movement or coordination; or hallucinations, memory problems, and confusion.

ARTERY. Blood vessel with muscular walls that carries blood from the heart and lungs to oxygenate the body tissues.

ARTHRALGIA. Joint pain.

ASPERGER SYNDROME. A developmental disorder of childhood characterized by autistic behavior but without the same difficulties acquiring language that children with autism have.

ASPHYXIA. Lack of oxygen. In the case of cerebral palsy, lack of oxygen to the brain.

ASPIRATION. Inhalation of food or saliva.

ASSISTIVE DEVICE. A general term for canes, walkers, crutches, reachers, and other helps for people with mobility difficulties and other disabilities.

ASTHENIA. A general term for a lack or loss of energy; an overall sense of weariness and muscle weakness.

ASTHMA. A condition characterized by spasms of the lung's airways that causes breathing difficulties.

ASTROCYTES. Large, star-shaped glial cells in the brain that support nerve cells and appear to be involved in cerebral edema.

ASYMMETRIC. Not occurring equally on both sides of the body.

ATAXIA. A deficiency of muscular coordination, especially when voluntary movements are attempted, such as grasping or walking.

ATHEROSCLEROSIS. A disease characterized by the buildup of fatty deposits on the insides of artery walls, which results in thickening and hardening of the arteries and the narrowing of space for the passage of blood; also known as arteriosclerosis and hardening of the arteries, it can lead to high blood pressure, stroke, and heart attack.

ATHETOSIS. A symptom of movement disorders that consists of slow, writhing, wavelike movements, usually in the hands or feet. It is also known as mobile spasm. It may occur together with chorea; the combined symptom is called choreoathetosis.

ATONIC SEIZURE. A seizure characterized by a sudden loss of muscle tone, causing the individual to fall to the floor.

ATRIAL FIBRILLATION. A disorder of the heart beat associated with a higher risk of stroke. In this disorder, the heart beats rapidly and irregularly, and the upper chambers (atria) do not completely empty, which can allow blood clots to form.

ATROPHY. The progressive wasting and loss of function of any part of the body.

ATTENTION-DEFICIT HYPERACTIVITY DISORDER (ADHD). A condition in which a person (usually a child) has an unusually high activity level and a short attention span. People with the disorder may act impulsively and may have learning and behavioral problems.

AUDIOLOGIST. A healthcare professional who specializes in diagnostic testing of hearing impairments and rehabilitation of patients with hearing problems.

AUDITORY. Pertaining to the sense of hearing.

AUDITORY NERVE. The eighth cranial nerve that connects the inner ear to the brain.

AURA. The set of sensory, neurological, and emotional indicators some patients experience about ten to 30 minutes before a migraine attack.

AURICULAR ACUPUNCTURE. Acupuncture using only points found on the ears.

AUTISM. A syndrome characterized by a lack of responsiveness to other people or outside stimulus. Often occurs in conjunction with a severe impairment of verbal and non-verbal communication skills.

AUTISTIC PSYCHOPATHY. Hans Asperger's original name for Asperger syndrome. It is still used occasionally as a synonym for the disorder.

AUTOANTIBODIES. Antibodies that attack the body's own cells or tissues.

AUTOIMMUNE DISORDER. A disorder characterized by abnormal functioning of the immune system that causes the body to produce antibodies against its own tissues.

AUTOLOGOUS. A transplant in which the patient is both the donor and recipient.

AUTOMATISMS. Movements during a seizure that are semi-purposeful but involuntary.

AUTONOMIC. Refers to peripheral nerves that carry signals from the brain and that control involuntary actions in the body, such as the beating of the heart.

AUTONOMIC FAILURE. Refers to failure in the autonomic nervous system, which comprises two divisions called the parasympathetic nervous system, which slows heart rate, increases intestinal and gland activity, and relaxes sphincter muscles, and the sympathetic nervous system, which accelerates heart rate, raises blood pressure, and constricts blood vessels.

AUTONOMIC NERVOUS SYSTEM. The part of the nervous system that controls involuntary functions such as breathing and heart beat.

AUTOSOMAL. Relating to any chromosome besides the X and Y sex chromosomes. Human cells contain 22 pairs of autosomes and one pair of sex chromosomes.

AUTOSOMAL DOMINANT. A pattern of inheritance in which only one of the two copies of an autosomal gene must be abnormal for a genetic condition or disease to occur. A person with an autosomal dominant disorder has a 50% chance of passing it to his or her offspring.

AUTOSOMAL RECESSIVE. A pattern of inheritance in which both copies of an autosomal gene must be abnormal for a genetic condition or disease to occur. When both parents have one abnormal copy of the same gene, they have a 25% chance with each pregnancy that their offspring will have the disorder.

AXON. The long, slender part of a nerve cell that carries electrochemical signals to another nerve cell.

AXONOTMESIS. Damage to the axon of a nerve cell (often from compression or crushing) that does not completely destroy its protective sheath (endoneurial sheath) so that regeneration can occur.

B

B VITAMINS. This family of vitamins consists of thiamine (B_1), riboflavin (B_2), niacin (B_3), pantothenic acid (B_5), pyridoxine (B_6), biotin, folic acid (B_9), and cobalamin (B_{12}). They are interdependent and involved in converting glucose to energy.

BABESIOSIS. A disease caused by protozoa of the genus *Babesia* characterized by a malaria-like fever, anemia, vomiting, muscle pain, and enlargement of the spleen. Babesiosis, like Lyme disease, is carried by a tick.

BALANCED CHROMOSOME TRANSLOCATION. A rearrangement of the chromosomes in which two chromosomes have broken and exchanged pieces without the loss of genetic material.

BALLISMUS. Involuntary violent flinging movements that may take the form of uncontrollable flailing. It is also called ballism. Ballismus that occurs with chorea is known as choreoballismus or choreoballism.

BAR. A unit of pressure roughly equal to the pressure of the earth's atmosphere at sea level, about 14.5 pounds per square inch (psi).

BARBITURATE. A class of drugs including phenobarbital that have sedative properties and depress respiratory rate, blood pressure, and nervous system activity.

BARORECEPTORS. Sensors located in the blood vessels that detect the pressure of blood flowing through them. These sensors send messages to the nervous system as part of the physiological blood pressure regulation mechanism.

BAROTRAUMA. The medical term for physical injury to the ear or other body tissues caused by a difference in pressure between an air space inside or beside the body and the surrounding fluid (water or air).

BASAL GANGLIA. The four deeply imbedded masses of gray matter in each cerebral hemisphere, including the caudate nucleus and the amygdala, that govern movement as well as emotion and certain aspects of cognition (thinking).

BECKER MUSCULAR DYSTROPHY (BMD). A type of muscular dystrophy that affects older boys and men, and usually follows a milder course than Duchenne muscular dystrophy.

BELL'S PALSY. Facial paralysis or weakness with a sudden onset, caused by swelling or inflammation of the seventh cranial nerve, which controls the facial muscles. Disseminated Lyme disease sometimes causes Bell's palsy.

BENIGN. Nonmalignant; not cancerous.

BENZODIAZEPINES. A class of tranquilizers or anti-anxiety drugs, used to treat a variety of conditions including epileptic seizures.

BETA-AMYLOID PLAQUES. Also known as senile plaques, these structures in the brain, composed of dead or dying nerve cells and cell debris surrounding deposits of beta-amyloid protein, are diagnostic of AD. Beta-amyloid forms when amyloid precursor protein (APP) is not broken down properly.

BICEPS MUSCLE. Muscle in the arm which helps to flex the arm.

BILATERAL. Occurring on both sides of the body.

BILE. A substance produced by the liver, and concentrated and stored in the gallbladder. Bile contains a number of different substances, including bile salts, cholesterol, and bilirubin.

BIOPSY. The surgical removal and microscopic examination of living tissue for diagnostic purposes or to follow the course of a disease. Most commonly the term refers to the collection and analysis of tissue from a suspected tumor to establish malignancy.

BIOPSYCHOSOCIAL MODEL. An approach to human health that holds that a combination of biological, psychological, and social factors should be taken into account when evaluating a patient rather than physical factors alone.

BIOTRANSFORMATION. The conversion of a compound from one form to another by the action of enzymes in the body of an organism.

BIPOLAR DISORDER. A psychiatric disorder marked by alternating episodes of mania and depression. Also called bipolar illness or manic-depressive illness.

BLASTOCYST. A very early embryo, consisting of a ball of 150–200 cells with an inner cell mass from which embryonic stem cells are derived.

BLOOD VESSELS. General term for arteries, veins, and capillaries that transport blood throughout the body.

BLOOD-BRAIN BARRIER. A blockade of cells separating the circulating blood from elements of the central nervous system (CNS); it acts as a filter, preventing many substances from entering the central nervous system.

BLOOD-BRAIN BARRIER. The protective membrane that separates circulating blood from brain cells, allowing some substances to enter while others (including certain toxic substances, infectious agents, and some drugs) are prevented from entering brain tissue.

BONE CYSTS. Fluid- or air-filled space within the bones.

BONE MARROW TRANSPLANT (BMT). The infusion of blood-forming stem cells for incorporation into the recipient's bone marrow or bone cavities.

BOTULINUM TOXIN (BOTOX). Any of a group of potent bacterial toxins or poisons produced by different strains of the bacterium *Clostridium botulinum*. The toxins cause muscle paralysis and the relaxation of muscles in spasm.

BRACHIAL PLEXUS. A group of nerves that exit the cervical (neck) and upper thoracic (chest) spinal column to provide muscle control to the shoulder, arms, and hands.

BRACHYCEPHALY. An abnormal thickening and widening of the skull.

BRADYCARDIA. Slower than normal heart rate, usually defined as a resting heart rate of 60 beats per minute or less.

BRADYKINESIA. Extremely slow movement.

BRAINSTEM. The stalk of the brain that connects the two cerebral hemispheres with the spinal cord. It is involved in controlling vital functions, movement, sensation, and nerves supplying the head and neck.

BREECH PRESENTATION. Buttocks presentation during delivery.

BROCA'S APHASIA. A condition characterized by either partial or total loss of the ability to express oneself, either through speech or writing. Hearing comprehension is not affected. This condition may result from a stroke, head injury, brain tumor, or infection.

BRUXISM. Habitual clenching and grinding of the teeth, especially during sleep.

BULBAR MUSCLES. Muscles that control chewing, swallowing, and speaking.

BUNION. A bulge on the first joint of the big toe, caused by the swelling of a fluid sac under the skin.

BUSPIRONE. An anxiolytic drug that does not affect GABA, but instead modifies serotonin neuro-transmission. Unlike benzodiazepines, it may take 3–6 weeks for buspirone to reach maximal effectiveness. As a result, the drug is only used to treat generalized anxiety disorder.

C

CACHEXIA. Severe malnutrition, emaciation, muscle wasting and debility associated with the inability to absorb the nutritional value of food eaten.

CALCIFICATION. A process in which tissue becomes hardened due to calcium deposits.

CANALITH. The name for a calcium carbonate crystal that has migrated into one of the semicircular canals of the ear.

CAPILLARY BED. A dense network of tiny blood vessels that enables blood to fill a tissue or organ.

CAPSAICIN. An active ingredient from hot chili peppers that is used in topical ointments to relieve pain. It appears to work by reducing the levels of a chemical substance involved in transmitting pain signals from nerve endings to the brain.

CARBIDOPA. A drug combined with levodopa to slow the breakdown of the levodopa, used to treat the symptoms of Parkinson's disease.

CARBON MONOXIDE. A colorless, odorless, highly poisonous gas.

CARBONIC ANHYDRASE. An enzyme that shifts the rate of reaction to favor the conversion of carbon dioxide and water into carbonic acid, bicarbonate ions, and free protons.

CARCINOGEN. A substance known to cause cancer.

CARDIOMYOPATHY. A disease of the heart muscle that leads to generalized deterioration of the muscle and its pumping ability.

CARDIOPULMONARY RESUSCITATION (CPR). A procedure for restoring normal breathing that includes clearing air passages, mouth-to-mouth artificial respiration, and heart massage by exerting pressure on the chest.

CAROTID ARTERIES. Two large arteries, one on either side of the neck, that carry oxygenated blood from the heart to the brain.

CAROTID ENDARTERECTOMY. Surgical procedure designed to reduce the accumulation of plaque in the carotid artery and thus, prevent stroke.

CARPAL TUNNEL. A passageway in the wrist, created by the bones and ligaments of the wrist, through which the median nerve passes.

CARRIER. A person who possesses a gene for an abnormal trait without showing signs of the disorder. The person may pass the abnormal gene on to offspring.

CATALYZE. Facilitate. A catalyst lowers the amount of energy required for a specific chemical reaction to occur. Catalysts are not used up in the chemical reactions they facilitate.

CATAPLEXY. A sudden and dramatic loss of muscle strength without loss of consciousness; one symptom of narcolepsy.

CATATONIA. A condition in which a person sits motionless for long periods of time and does not respond to others.

CATECHOLAMINES. Chemicals such as epinephrine, dopa, and norepinephrine; often at high levels in the urine if a pheochromocytoma is present.

CATHETER. Tube inserted into a body cavity or blood vessel to allow drainage of fluids (as in a urinary catheter), injection of drugs, or insertion of a surgical instrument.

CAUDA EQUINA. The collection of spinal nerve roots that lie inside the spinal column below the end of the spinal cord. The name comes from the Latin for "horse's tail."

CAUDA EQUINA SYNDROME (CES). A group of symptoms characterized by numbness or pain in the legs and/or loss of bladder and bowel control, caused by compression and paralysis of the nerve roots in the cauda equina. CES is a medical emergency.

CD4. A type of protein molecule in human blood. HIV infects cells with CD4 surface proteins and, as a result, depletes the number of T cells, B cells, natural killer cells, and monocytes in the patient's blood.

CELL. The smallest living units of the body which group together to form tissues and help the body perform specific functions.

CENTRAL NERVOUS SYSTEM (CNS). The part of the nervous system comprised of the brain and spinal cord.

CEPHALALGIA. The medical term for headache.

CEREBELLAR. Involving the part of the brain (cerebellum) that controls walking, balance, and coordination.

CEREBELLAR ATAXIA. Unsteadiness and lack of coordination caused by a progressive degeneration of the part of the brain known as the cerebellum.

CEREBELLUM. The lower back part of the brain that consists of two hemispheres, one on each side of the brainstem. It acts as a fine tuner for muscle tone, coordination of movement, posture, gait, and skilled voluntary movement.

CEREBRAL ANEURYSM. An abnormal, localized bulge in a blood vessel that is usually caused by a congenital weakness in the wall of the vessel.

CEREBRAL COLLATERAL BLOOD FLOW. Anatomical and physiological mechanisms that allow blood destined for one hemisphere of the brain to crossover and nourish tissue on the other side of the brain when the supply to the other side of the brain is impaired.

CEREBRAL CORTEX. The layer of gray matter that makes up the surface of cerebral hemispheres of the brain. It is responsible for controlling sensation, movement, and higher cognitive functions.

CEREBRAL DOMINANCE. The preeminence of one cerebral hemisphere over the other in the control of cerebral functions.

CEREBRAL EMBOLISM. A blockage of blood flow through a vessel in the brain by a blood clot that formed elsewhere in the body and traveled to the brain.

CEREBRAL HERNIATION. Herniation or shifting of the brain from its normal position within the skull or down through the opening at the bottom of the skull.

CEREBRAL ISCHEMIA. Lack of oxygen to the brain, which may result in tissue death.

CEREBRAL PALSY (CP). A movement disorder caused by a permanent brain defect or an injury present at birth, or shortly after. It is frequently associated with premature birth. Cerebral palsy is not progressive.

CEREBRAL THROMBOSIS. A blockage of blood flow through a vessel in the brain by a blood clot that formed in the brain itself.

CEREBRAL VASCULAR ACCIDENT. Damage to brain cells caused by lack of blood flow in the brain from emboli (clots) plaque, or hemorrhage.

CEREBROSIDES. Fatty carbohydrates that occur in the brain and nervous system.

CEREBROSPINAL FLUID (CSF). The fluid that circulates through the central nervous system protecting and maintaining uniform pressure on the brain and spinal cord.

CEREBROVASCULAR. Referring to the blood vessels that supply the brain.

CEREBRUM. The upper and largest part of the brain, consisting of the two cerebral hemispheres and connecting structures; it is responsible for conscious mental processes.

CERULOPLASMIN. A protein circulating in the bloodstream that binds with copper and transports it.

CERVICAL. Pertaining to a neck.

CERVICAL VERTEBRAE. The seven vertebrae of the neck.

CERVICO–MEDULLARY JUNCTION. The area where the brain and spine connect.

CHARLES BONNET SYNDROME (CBS). A disorder characterized by visual hallucinations following a sudden age-related deterioration in a person's vision, most commonly glaucoma or macular degeneration. CBS is named for a Swiss doctor who first described it in his visually impaired grandfather in 1780.

CHELATION THERAPY. A method of removing copper or other heavy metals from the body by giving medications that bind to the metal and allow it to be excreted.

CHEMOTHERAPY. Chemical medical treatment often used for cancer.

CHI. Basic life energy.

CHIARI II ANOMALY. A structural abnormality of the lower portion of the brain (cerebellum and brain stem) associated with spina bifida. The lower structures of the brain are crowded and may be forced into the foramen magnum, the opening through which the brain and spinal cord are connected.

CHIROPRACTIC. A system of therapy based on the notion that health and disease are related to the interactions between the brain and the nervous system. Treatment involves manipulation and adjustment of the segments of the spinal column. Chiropractic is considered a form of alternative medicine.

CHOLESTEROL. A fat-soluble steroid alcohol (sterol) found in animal fats and oils and produced in the body from saturated fats. High cholesterol levels contribute to the development of cardiovascular disease.

CHOLINESTERASE INHIBITORS. Drugs that may slow the progression of AD by inhibiting the enzymes that break down acetylcholine.

CHOREA. A term that is used to refer to rapid, jerky, involuntary movements of the limbs or face that characterize several different disorders of the nervous system, including chorea of pregnancy and Huntington's chorea as well as Sydenham's chorea.

CHOREA GRAVIDARUM. Chorea occurring in the early months of pregnancy.

CHOREIFORM. Movements resembling chorea; spasmodic movements of the limb or facial muscles.

CHORIONIC VILLUS SAMPLING (CVS). A procedure used for prenatal diagnosis at 1–12 weeks gestation. Under ultrasound guidance a needle is inserted either through the mother's vagina or abdominal wall and a sample of cells is collected from around the early embryo. These cells are then tested for chromosome abnormalities or other genetic diseases.

CHOROID. A vascular membrane that covers the back of the eye between the retina and the sclera and serves to nourish the retina and absorb scattered light.

CHOROID PLEXUS. Specialized cells located in the ventricles of the brain that produce cerebrospinal fluid.

CHROMOSOME. A microscopic thread-like structure found within each cell of the human body that consists of a complex of proteins and DNA. Humans have 46 chromosomes arranged into 23 pairs. Chromosomes contain the genetic information necessary to direct the development and functioning of all cells and systems in the body. They pass on hereditary traits from parents to child and determine whether the child will be male or female.

CHRONIC. A word used to describe a long-lasting condition. Chronic conditions often develop gradually and involve slow changes.

CHRONIC PAIN. Pain that lasts beyond the term of an injury or painful stimulus. Can also refer to cancer pain, pain from a chronic or degenerative disease, and pain from an unidentified cause.

CHRONOTHERAPY. A sleep disorder treatment that involves adjusting sleep and wake times to reset one's biological clock.

CIRCADIAN RHYTHM. An approximately 24-hour cycle of physiological and behavioral activity.

CIRCADIAN RHYTHM SLEEP DISORDER (CRSD). A disruption of the circadian rhythm sleep-wake cycle.

CIRCLE OF WILLIS. Also known as the circulus arteriosus; formed by branches of the internal carotid arteries and the vertebral arteries.

CIRRHOSIS. A chronic degenerative disease of the liver, in which normal cells are replaced by fibrous tissue. Cirrhosis is a major risk factor for the later development of liver cancer.

CLAUDICATION. Cramping or pain in a leg caused by poor blood circulation. This condition is frequently caused by hardening of the arteries (atherosclerosis). Intermittent claudication occurs only at certain times, usually after exercise, and is relieved by rest.

CLEFT PALATE. An opening or hole in the roof of the mouth that occurs at birth when the roof fails to fully develop in the infant.

CLINICAL TRIAL. All new drugs undergo clinical trials before approval. Clinical trials are carefully conducted tests in which effectiveness and side effects are studied, with the placebo effect eliminated.

CLONIC. A type of seizure characterized by rhythmic jerking of the arms and legs.

CLONUS. A sustained series of involuntary rhythmic jerks following quick stretch of a muscle.

CLOSED HEAD INJURY. TBI in which the head strikes or is struck by an object without breaking the skull.

CLOT. The end product of the clotting cascade, clots are a semisolid mass of blood cells and products that seal wounds in blood vessel walls to prevent the loss of blood.

CLOTTING CASCADE. Set of chemical reactions involving multiple chemical mediators that result in the formation of a blood clot.

CLUSTER HEADACHE. A painful recurring headache associated with the release of histamine from cells.

COAGULATION. Process by which a blood clot is formed.

COAGULOPATHY. A disorder in which blood is either too slow or too quick to coagulate (clot).

COCHLEA. The bony, labyrinthine, fluid-filled, coiled chamber in the inner ear.

COENZYME. A substance needed by enzymes to produce many of the reactions in energy and protein metabolism in the body.

COGNITION. The mental activities associated with thinking, learning, and memory.

COGNITIVE-BEHAVIORAL THERAPY (CBT). A type of psychotherapy that involves recognizing and changing negative and self-defeating patterns of thinking and behavior.

COLLAGEN. The fibrous protein of cartilage, connective tissue, tendon, skin, and bone.

COMA. A state of deep unconsciousness lasting longer than six hours caused by disease, injury, drug overdose, or poison.

COMMAND HALLUCINATION. A type of auditory hallucination in which the person hears voices ordering him or her to perform a specific act.

COMORBID. Referring to the presence of one or more diseases or disorders in addition to the patient's primary disorder.

COMPUTED TOMOGRAPHY (CT) SCAN. An imaging technique in which cross-sectional x rays of the body are compiled to create a three-dimensional image of the body's internal structures.

COMT INHIBITORS. Drugs that block catechol-o-methyl transferase, an enzyme that breaks down dopamine. COMT inhibitors include entacapone and tolcapone.

CONCUSSION. Injury to the brain causing a sudden, temporary impairment of brain function.

CONDITIONING. Bone marrow preparation; also known as myeloablation or immunosuppressive therapy; the destruction of bone marrow by chemotherapy and/or radiation in preparation for a stem cell transplant.

CONDUCT DISORDER. A behavioral and emotional disorder of childhood and adolescence. Children with a conduct disorder act inappropriately, infringe on the rights of others, and violate societal norms.

CONDUCTION APHASIA. A condition characterized by the inability to repeat words, sentences, or phrases as a result of a stroke, head injury, brain tumor, or infection.

CONFABULATION. In psychiatry, the filling-in of gaps in memory with false information that the patient believes to be true. It is not deliberate telling of lies.

CONFETTI SKIN LESIONS. Numerous light or white spots seen on the skin that resemble confetti.

CONFUSION. In medicine, a condition in which a person is disoriented with respect to time, place, and personal identity, and generally does not function mentally at their normal level.

CONGENITAL. Present at birth.

CONSTRUCTIONAL APRAXIA. Difficulty or inability to copy a drawing.

CONTINUOUS POSITIVE AIRWAY PRESSURE (CPAP). A ventilation system that blows a gentle stream of air into the nose to keep the airway open.

CONTRACTURE. An abnormal and usually permanent shortening and contraction of a muscle or tendon that causes a deformity or subnormal range of movement.

CONTRAST (AGENT, MEDIUM). A substance injected into the body that delineates certain structures that would otherwise be hard or impossible to see on the radiograph (film).

CONTRAST MATERIAL. Any material introduced into the body that has a different opacity from soft tissue and can be used in radiography, magnetic resonance imaging, or CT scans to help the radiologist visualize internal body structures. Contrast materials are also known as contrast media or contrast agents.

CONTRECOUP. An injury to the brain opposite the point of direct impact.

CONTUSION. The medical term for a bruise.

CONVERSION DISORDER. A psychiatric disorder in which the patient's emotional distress takes the form of (is converted into) various neurological and motor symptoms that mimic a neuromuscular disorder but have no neurological (physical) explanation.

CONVULSION. Involuntary contractions of body muscles that accompany a seizure episode.

COPROLALIA. The involuntary expression of obscene words or phrases.

COPROPRAXIA. The involuntary display of unacceptable/obscene gestures.

CORDOTOMY. Surgery to relieve pain by destroying bundles of nerve fibers on one or both sides of the spinal cord.

CORNEA. The transparent structure of the eye over the lens that is continuous with the sclera in forming the outermost protective layer of the eye.

COROLLARY DISCHARGE. A mechanism in the brain that allows one to distinguish between self-generated and external stimuli or perceptions.

CORPUS CALLOSUM. A thick bundle of nerve fibers deep in the center of the forebrain that provides communications between the right and left cerebral hemispheres.

CORTICAL TUBER. Round (nodular) growth found in the cortex of the brain.

CORTICOSPINAL NEURONS. Nerve cells with axons that extend from the cerebral cortex to, and down, the spinal cord.

CORTICOSPINAL TRACT. A tract of nerve cells that carries motor commands from the brain to the spinal cord.

CORTICOSTEROIDS. A group of drugs similar to natural corticosteroid hormones produced by the adrenal glands. The drugs have a wide variety of applications, including use for inflammatory disorders and swelling. Examples include cortisone and prednisone.

CORTISOL. A hormone secreted by the cortex of the adrenal gland. Cortisol regulates the function of nearly every organ and tissue in the body.

CRANIAL NERVES. The set of 12 nerves found on each side of the head and neck that control the sensory and muscle functions of the eyes, nose, tongue, face, and throat.

CRANIAL SUTURE. Any one of the seven fibrous joints between the bones of the skull.

CRANIOFACIAL. Relating to or involving both the head and the face.

CRANIOSYNOSTOSIS. A birth defect of the brain characterized by the premature closure of one or more of the cranial sutures, the fibrous joints between the bones of the skull.

CRANIOTOMY. Any surgical procedure in which a piece of bone is temporarily removed from the skull in order to gain access to the brain.

CRANIUM. Skull; the bony framework that holds the brain.

CREATANINE PHOSPHOKINASE. A chemical normally found in the muscle fibers, and released into the bloodstream when the muscles undergo damage and breakdown.

CREATINE PHOSPHOKINASE. A muscle enzyme present in various skeletal muscles and the heart which is released due to any type of muscle injury and this can be measured in the blood.

CREUTZFELDT-JAKOB DISEASE (CJD). A degenerative disease of the central nervous system caused by a prion, an abnormally folded protein.

CRYOABLATION. Using very cold temperatures to remove a foreign substance or body.

CRYOTHERAPY. Using very cold temperatures to treat a disease.

CRYPTOGENIC STROKE. Stroke of unknown cause; stroke that cannot be attributed to hardening of the arteries, clot formation, or emboli. Between 30–40% of all strokes are cryptogenic.

CT SCAN. The abbreviated term for computed or computerized axial tomography. The test may involve injecting a radioactive contrast into the body. Computers are used to scan for radiation and create cross-sectional images of internal organs.

CUTANEOUS. Relating to the skin.

CUTANEOUS DISORDERS. Disorders affecting the skin.

CYCLOOXYGENASE. An enzyme in the body that contributes to the formation of prostaglandins.

CYCLOPIA. A rare form of holoprosencephaly in which the orbits of the eye fail to form two normal eye cavities. There is one central eye with a malformed and nonfunctional nose; in some cases, the face is completely missing.

CYST. Sac of tissue filled with fluid, gas, or semi-solid material.

CYSTADENOMA. Non-cancerous growth, in which fluid-filled, gas, or semi-solid areas may be present.

CYSTICERCOSIS. Medical condition in which a patient has cystic lesions formed by pork tapeworm larvae in the tissues of the body, after the ingestion of eggs that hatch inside the host.

CYSTICERCUS (PLURAL CYSTICERCI). A cystic lesion formed by pork tapeworm larvae in tissue of the body.

CYTOCHROME P450 (CYP450). Enzymes present in the liver that metabolize drugs.

CYTOKINE. A protein associated with inflammation that, at high levels, may be toxic to nerve cells in the developing brain.

CYTOMEGALOVIRUS. A member of the herpes virus group found throughout all geographic locations and socioeconomic groups; virus usually remains dormant throughout life, reactivating when the body's immune system is severely debilitated. The virus attacks and enlarges certain cells in the body.

CYTOPLASM. The substance within a cell including the organelles and the fluid surrounding the nucleus.

CYTOSKELETON. A network of filaments that give structure and shape to the cell.

D

DANDY-WALKER MALFORMATION (OR SYNDROME). A complex structural abnormality of the brain frequently associated with hydrocephalus, or accumulation of excess fluid in the brain. Abnormalities in other areas of the body may also be present. Individuals with Dandy-Walker malformation have varying degrees of mental handicap or none at all.

DE NOVO DELETION. A deletion that occurs for the first time in the affected individual. The cause of de novo deletions is not known.

DE NOVO MUTATION. Genetic mutations that are seen for the first time in the affected person, not inherited from the parents.

DE QUERVAIN'S SYNDROME. Inflammation of the tendons contained within the wrist, associated with aching pain in the wrist and thumb. Named for the Swiss surgeon who first described it in 1895, the syndrome is sometimes called washerwoman's sprain because it is commonly caused by overuse of the wrist.

DECIBEL (DB). A unit of measurement for expressing the relative intensity of sounds.

DECOMPRESSION. Any surgical procedure done to relieve pressure on a nerve or other part of the body. A laminectomy is sometimes called an open decompression.

DECOMPRESSION SICKNESS. A group of symptoms that occur when a person is exposed to a rapid drop in pressure (as in coming up from a dive or climbing to high altitude in a spacecraft), and gases previously dissolved in the blood form bubbles in body tissues and organs. Symptoms include muscle and joint pain ("the bends"), headaches, itchy or swollen skin, loss of balance, difficulty breathing, seizures, and leg paralysis.

DECONDITIONING. The loss of normal body functioning (including muscle strength) in a normally demanding environment due to adaptation to a less demanding environment. Deconditioning can result from prolonged bed rest, aging, paralysis, being placed in a body cast, or other reasons for a decrease in physical activity.

DECREASED PENETRANCE. Individuals who inherit a changed disease gene but do not develop symptoms.

DEEP BRAIN STIMULATION (DBS). Neurostimulation through an electrode surgically implanted in the brain; used to treat Parkinson's disease and other neurological conditions.

DEFICIT. In medicine, the loss or impairment of a function or ability.

DEGENERATION. Gradual, progressive loss of nerve cells.

DEGENERATIVE DISC DISEASE. Narrowing of the disc space between the spinal bones (vertebrae).

DEGRADATION. Loss or diminishing.

DELIRIUM. A disturbance of consciousness marked by confusion, inattention, delusions, hallucinations, and agitation. It is distinguished from dementia by its relatively sudden onset and variation in the severity of symptoms.

DELIRIUM TREMENS. A complication that may accompany alcohol withdrawal. The symptoms include body shaking (tremulousness), insomnia, agitation, confusion, hearing voices or seeing images that are not really there (hallucinations), seizures, rapid heart beat, profuse sweating, high blood pressure, and fever.

DELTOID MUSCLE. A muscle near the clavicle bone which is responsible for arm movement.

DELUSION. A persistent false belief held in the face of strong contradictory evidence.

DEMENTIA. A progressive loss of intellectual functions without impairment of consciousness or perception. The condition is often associated with brain disease and persons exhibit symptoms such as disorientation and impaired memory, judgment, and intellect.

DEMENTIA PUGILISTICA. "Punch-drunk" syndrome of brain damage caused by repeated head trauma.

DEMYELINATING DISEASES. A group of diseases characterized by the breakdown of myelin, the fatty sheath surrounding and insulating nerve fibers. This breakdown interferes with nerve function, and can result in paralysis. Multiple sclerosis is a demyelinating disorder.

DEMYELINATION. Loss of the myelin sheath that surrounds and insulates the axons of nerve cells and is necessary for the proper conduction of neural impulses.

DENDRITES. Fibers of a brain cell that receive signals from other brain cells.

DENTAL PITS. Small shallow holes or crevices in the tooth enamel.

DEOXYRIBONUCLEIC ACID (DNA). The genetic material in cells that holds the inherited instructions for growth, development, and cellular functioning.

DEPOLARIZATION. Occurs when a neuron exchanges ions, causing an influx of sodium and calcium inside the cell and an efflux of potassium out of the cell.

DEPOT. A type of drug preparation and administration that involves the slow, gradual release from an area of the body where the drug has been injected.

DEPOT DOSAGE. A form of medication that can be stored in the patient's body tissues for several days or weeks, thus minimizing the risk of the patient forgetting daily doses. Haloperidol and fluphenazine can be given in depot form.

DEPRESSED SKULL FRACTURE. A fracture in which fragments pieces of broken skull press into brain tissue.

DEPRESSION. A psychiatric disorder in which the mood is low for a prolonged period of time, and feelings of hopelessness and inadequacy interfere with normal functioning..

DERMATOME. An area of skin that receive sensations through a single nerve root.

DESMIN. A protein that provides part of the structure to heart, skeletal, and smooth muscle cells.

DETRUSOR. Muscle in the wall of the bladder that contracts to push urine out into the urethra.

DEVELOPMENTAL DELAY. The failure to meet certain developmental milestones, such as sitting, walking, and talking, at the average age. Developmental delay may indicate a problem in development of the central nervous system.

DIABETES MELLITUS. Disease characterized by the inability of the body to produce or respond properly to insulin, required by the body to convert glucose to energy.

DIALYSIS. Process by which special equipment purifies the blood of a patient whose kidneys have failed.

DIETITIAN. A health care professional who specializes in individual or group nutritional planning, public education in nutrition, or research in food science. To be licensed as a registered dietitian (RD) in the United States, a person must complete a bachelor's degree in a nutrition-related field and pass a state licensing examination. Dietitians are also called nutritionists.

DIFFERENTIATION. The process by which a cell increases in complexity and specialization of function.

DIFFUSE AXONAL INJURY (SHEAR INJURY). Traumatic damage to individual nerve cells resulting in breakdown of overall communication between nerve cells in the brain.

DIFFUSION TENSOR IMAGING (DTI). A refinement of magnetic resonance imaging that allows the doctor to measure the flow of water and track the pathways of white matter in the brain. DTI is able to detect abnormalities in the brain that do not show up on standard MRI scans.

DIPLEGIA. Paralysis affecting like parts on both sides of the body, such as both arms or both legs.

DIPLOPIA. Also known as double vision, a visual disorder due to unequal action of the eye muscles causing two images of a single object to be seen.

DIRECT SELECTION. Any method of using an AAC device that involves the use of a body part or object attached to a body part to select an item from a speech-generating device or communication board.

DISCECTOMY. Surgery to relieve pressure on a nerve root caused by a bulging disc or bone spur.

DISCOGRAPHY. A test in which dye is injected into a disc space thought to be causing back pain, allowing the surgeon to confirm that an operation on that disc will be likely to relieve pain.

DISEASE ERADICATION. A status whereby no further cases of a diseases occur anywhere, and continued control measures are unnecessary.

DISFLUENCY. An inability to speak fluently.

DISSECTION. Tear in the wall of an artery that causes blood from inside the artery to leak into the wall and thereby narrows the lumen of the blood vessel.

DISSEMINATED. Scattered or distributed throughout the body. Lyme disease that has progressed beyond the stage of localized EM is said to be disseminated.

DISSOCIATION. A reaction to trauma in which the mind splits off certain aspects of the traumatic event from conscious awareness. Dissociation can affect the patient's memory, sense of reality, and sense of identity.

DISSOCIATIVE DISORDER. A reaction in which the mind splits off aspects of a traumatic event from conscious awareness and which can affect memory, sense of reality, and sense of identity.

DISTAL MUSCULAR DYSTROPHY (DD). A form of muscular dystrophy that usually begins in middle age or later, causing weakness in the muscles of the feet and hands.

DIURETIC DRUGS. A group of medications that increase the amount of urine produced and relieve excess fluid buildup in body tissues. Diuretics may be used in treating high blood pressure, lung disease, premenstrual syndrome, and other conditions.

DNA. Deoxyribonucleic acid; the genetic material in cells that holds the inherited instructions for growth, development, and cellular functioning.

DNA TESTING. Analysis of DNA (the genetic component of cells) in order to determine changes in genes that may indicate a specific disorder.

DONEPEZIL HYDROCHLORIDE (ARICEPT). A drug that increases the levels of acetylcholine in the brain.

DOPAMINE. A brain chemical (neurotransmitter) responsible for carrying messages throughout the nervous system, particularly messages regarding movement.

DOPAMINE RECEPTOR AGONISTS (DAS). The older class of antipsychotic medications, also called neuroleptics. These primarily block the site on nerve cells that normally receive the brain chemical dopamine.

DORSAL. Pertaining in direction to the back or upper surface of an organ or structure.

DORSAL COLUMNS. This refers to nerve fiber tracts that run in the portion of the spinal cord that is closest to the back. It carries sensory information like position sense and deep pain from the legs and arms to the brain.

DORSAL RHIZOTOMY. A surgical procedure that cuts nerve roots to reduce spasticity in affected muscles.

DORSAL ROOT ENTRY ZONE OPERATION (DREZ). Surgery to relieve pain by severing spinal neurons.

DORSAL ROOT GANGLIA. The subset of neuronal cells controlling impulses in and out of the brain.

DOWN SYNDROME. A genetic disorder characterized by an extra (third) chromosome 21 (the syndrome is also called trisomy 21). Symptoms include mental retardation and susceptibility to early-onset Alzheimer's disease.

DUCHENNE MUSCULAR DYSTROPHY (DMD). The most severe form of muscular dystrophy, DMD usually affects young boys and causes progressive muscle weakness, usually beginning in the legs.

DURA MATER. The outermost and toughest of the three membranes or meninges that cover the brain and spinal cord. The arteries that supply the dura mater and the portion of the dura mater at the base of the skull are sensitive to pain.

DYNATOME. An area in which pain is felt when a given spinal nerve is irritated.

DYSARTHRIA. Imperfect articulation of speech due to muscular weakness resulting from damage to the central or peripheral nervous system.

DYSAUTONOMIA. A disorder or dysfunction of the autonomic nervous system.

DYSCALCULIA. Difficulty with basic arithmetic and calculations.

DYSESTHESIA. Painful feeling of numbness, tingling, or burning.

DYSGRAPHIA. Impaired writing ability due to brain damage.

DYSKINESIA. Impaired ability to make voluntary movements.

DYSKINESIAS. A group of disorders characterized by involuntary movements of muscles.

DYSLEXIA. A learning disability characterized by lack of proficiency in reading, spelling, and writing.

DYSPHAGIA. The medical term for difficulty in swallowing.

DYSPHONIA. Disordered phonation or voice production.

DYSPHORIA. Feelings of anxiety, restlessness, and dissatisfaction.

DYSTHYMIA. A psychological condition of chronic depression that is not disabling, but prevents the sufferer from functioning at his or her full capacity.

DYSTONIA. A neuromuscular disorder characterized by sustained muscle contractions that cause twisting and repetitive movements or abnormal body postures.

DYSTROPHIN. A protein that helps muscle tissue repair itself. Both Duchenne muscular dystrophy and Becker muscular dystrophy are caused by flaws in the gene that instructs the body how to make this protein.

E

ECHOCARDIOGRAPHY. A type of ultrasonography that is used to create an image of the heart and its functioning.

ECHOLALIA. A vocal tic in which the person repeats the words or phrases of another person.

ECHOPRAXIA. The imitation of the movement of another individual.

ECTOPIC. In an abnormal position.

EDEMA. An excess accumulation of fluid in cells and tissues.

EFFERENT. Refers to peripheral nerves that carry signals away from the brain and spinal cord. These nerves carry out motor and autonomic functions.

ELBOW EXTENSION. Movement away from the body at a jointed point.

ELECTROCARDIOGRAM (ECG, EKG). A test that uses electrodes attached to the chest with an adhesive gel to transmit the electrical impulses of the heart muscle to a recording device.

ELECTROCONVULSIVE THERAPY (ECT). A psychological treatment in which a series of controlled electrical impulses are delivered to the brain in order to induce a seizure within the brain.

ELECTROENCEPHALOGRAM (EEG). A procedure that uses electrodes on the scalp to record electrical activity of the brain. Used for detection of epilepsy, coma, and brain death.

ELECTROMYOGRAM, ELECTROMYOGRAPHY (EMG). A diagnostic used test to evaluate nerve and muscle function. In the test, small electrodes are placed on or in the skin; the patterns of electrical activity are projected on a screen or over a loudspeaker. This procedure is used to test for muscle disorders, including muscular dystrophy.

ELECTRON. One of the small particles that make up an atom. An electron has the same mass and amount of charge as a positron, but the electron has a negative charge.

ELECTRONYSTAGMOGRAM, ELECTRONYSTAGMOGRAPHY (ENG). A series of diagnostic tests for vestibular disorders that involves recording the patient's eye movements while the examiner moves the head into various positions or instills warm or cold water into the patient's ear canal.

EMBOLISM. A blood clot, air bubble, or clot of foreign material that travels and blocks the flow of blood in an artery. When blood supply to a tissue or organ is blocked by an embolism, infarction (death of the tissue the artery feeds) occurs. Without immediate and appropriate treatment, an embolism can be fatal.

EMBOLIZATION. The deliberate introduction of a metal coil or gelatin sponge into a blood vessel to stop bleeding or to seal off a tumor or aneurysm.

EMBOLUS (PLURAL EMBOLI). A blood clot that broke free from the inner surface of the blood vessel and has traveled to other parts of the body, where it may lodge and occlude blood flow.

EMBRYO. The stage of development between a fertilized egg and a fetus.

EMBRYONIC STEM CELL (ESC); HUMAN EMBRYONIC STEM CELL (HESC). Cells from the inner cell mass of a blastocyst that can reproduce themselves indefinitely and differentiate into any cell type in the body.

ENCEPHALITIS. Inflammation of the brain, usually caused by a virus. The inflammation may interfere with normal brain function and cause seizures, sleepiness, confusion, personality changes, weakness in one or more parts of the body, and even coma.

ENCEPHALOGRAM. Machine that detects brain activity by measuring electrical activity in the brain.

ENCEPHALOPATHIC. Widespread brain disease or dysfunction.

ENCEPHALOPATHY. A disease of the brain, particularly involving an alteration in brain structure.

ENDARTERECTOMY. A surgical procedure in which diseased tissue and atherosclerotic plaque are removed from the inside of an artery.

ENDOCRINE. Pertaining to a gland that secretes directly into the bloodstream.

ENDODONTIST. A dentist who specializes in the treatment of diseases and injuries that affect the tooth root, dental pulp, and the tissues surrounding the tooth root.

ENDOLYMPH. The fluid contained inside the membranous labyrinth of the inner ear.

ENDOLYMPHATIC SAC TUMOR. Growths that develop within inner ear structures called endolymph sacs.

ENDORPHINS. A class of peptides in the brain that are produced during exercise and bind to opiate receptors, resulting in pleasant feelings and pain relief.

ENDOSCOPE. A device made of a tube and an optical system for observing the inside of the body.

ENDOSCOPY. A clinical technique using an instrument called an endoscope, used for visualization of structures within the body.

ENDOTHELIUM. A layer of cells called endothelial cells that lines the inside surfaces of body cavities, blood vessels, and lymph vessels.

ENDOVASCULAR. Referring to any procedure or treatment performed within a blood vessel.

ENTRAPMENT NEUROPATHY. A disorder of the peripheral nervous system in which a nerve is damaged by compression as it passes through a bony or fibrous passage or canal. Many repetitive motion disorders are associated with entrapment neuropathies.

ENZYMATIC REPLACEMENT THERAPY. A treatment method used to replace missing enzymes. It is possible to synthesize enzymes and then inject them intravenously into patients.

ENZYME. A protein that catalyzes a biochemical reaction or change without changing its own structure or function.

ENZYME REPLACEMENT THERAPY. Giving an enzyme to a person who needs it for normal body function. It is given through a needle that is inserted into the body.

EPIDIDYMIS. Male genital structure usually connected to the testis; an area where sperm collect.

EPIDURAL HEMATOMA. Bleeding into the area between the skull and the dura, the tough, outermost brain covering.

EPIDURAL SPACE. The space immediately surrounding the outermost membrane (dura mater) of the spinal cord.

EPIGLOTTIS. A thin layer of cartilage behind the tongue that helps block food from entering the windpipe.

EPILEPSY. A disorder associated with disturbed electrical discharges in the central nervous system that cause seizures.

EQUINUS. Excess contraction of the calf, causing toe walking.

ERB POINT. A point 2–3 centimeters above the clavicle.

ERECTILE DYSFUNCTION (ED). The consistent inability to achieve or maintain a penile erection; psychogenic ED may be acquired (PAED) or lifelong (PLED).

ERGONOMICS. The branch of science that deals with human work and the efficient use of energy, including anatomical, physiological, biomechanical, and psychosocial factors.

ERGOT; ERGOTAMINE. Drugs derived from ergot fungi that are used to treat migraine.

ERYTHEMA. Redness of the skin due to congestion of the capillaries, usually due to injury, infection, or inflammation.

ERYTHEMA MIGRANS (EM). A red skin rash that is one of the first signs of Lyme disease in about 75% of patients.

ERYTHROCYTE SEDIMENTATION RATE. The speed at which red blood cells sink in a tube of freshly drawn blood, which is a rough measure of clotting disorders or inflammation.

ESSENTIAL TREMOR. An uncontrollable (involuntary) shaking of the hands, head, and face. Also called familial tremor because it is sometimes inherited; it can begin in the teens or in middle age. The exact cause is not known.

EUTHYROID. State of normal function of the thyroid gland.

EVOKED POTENTIAL (EP). Measurement of brain activity in response to stimuli.

EVOKED POTENTIALS. Measurements of brain activity in response to stimuli.

EVOKED POTENTIALS. Tests that measure the brain's electrical response to stimulation of sensory organs (eyes or ears) or peripheral nerves (skin). These tests may help confirm the diagnosis of MS.

EXACERBATION. The appearance of new symptoms or the aggravation of old symptoms.

EXCESSIVE DAYTIME SLEEPINESS (EDS). A persistent sense of mental cloudiness, a lack of energy, a depressed mood, or extreme state of exhaustion.

EXCISION. Surgical removal.

EXECUTIVE FUNCTIONS. A term used to describe a set of brain functions that control or manage other cognitive processes, such as planning for the future, choosing among different possible courses of behavior, and abstract thinking or reasoning.

EXON. The expressed portion of a gene. The exons of genes are those portions that actually chemically code for the protein or polypeptide that the gene is responsible for producing.

EXPANSION. Growing cells in laboratory culture to increase their numbers.

EXTENSIVE SUPPORT. Ongoing daily support required to assist an individual in a specific adaptive area, such as daily help with preparing meals.

EXTRA-LARYNGEAL. Actions of muscles outside the larynx, but usually in its vicinity, which influence its functioning.

EXTRAPYRAMIDAL. Refers to brain structures located outside the pyramidal tracts of the central nervous system.

EXTRAPYRAMIDAL SYMPTOMS (EPS). A group of side effects associated with antipsychotic medications. EPS include parkinsonism, akathisia, dystonia, and tardive dyskinesia.

EXTRAPYRAMIDAL SYSTEM. Functional, rather than anatomical unit, comprised of nuclei and nerve fibers that are chiefly involved with subconscious, automatic aspects of motor coordination, but which also assist in regulation of postural and locomotor movements.

EXTRINSIC PATHWAY. One of two initial pathways of the clotting cascade.

F

FACIAL ANGIOFIBROMAS. Benign (non-cancerous) tumors of the face.

FACIAL NERVE. A cranial nerve that controls the muscles in the face.

FACIOSCAPULOHUMERAL MUSCULAR DYSTROPHY (FSH). This form of muscular dystrophy, also known as Landouzy-Dejerine condition, begins in late childhood to early adulthood and affects both men and women, causing weakness in the muscles of the face, shoulders, and upper arms.

FACTITIOUS DISORDER. A type of mental disturbance in which patients intentionally act physically or mentally ill without obvious benefits. It is distinguished from malingering by the absence of an obvious motive, and from conversion disorder by intentional production of symptoms.

FAILURE TO THRIVE. Significantly reduced or delayed physical growth.

FAMCICLOVIR. An oral antiviral drug that blocks the replication of the varicella zoster virus.

FAMILIAL. Tending to occur in more members of a family than expected by chance alone.

FAMILIAL HEMIPLEGIC MIGRAINE (FHM). An inherited type of migraine headache characterized by temporary hemiparesis.

FASCICULATION. A small localized involuntary contraction and relaxation of muscles (twitching) visible under the skin.

FAST FOURIER TRANSFER. A digital processing of the recorded signal resulting in a decomposition of its frequency components.

FATAL FAMILIAL INSOMNIA. A rare, progressive neurological disease that is believed to be transmitted via an abnormal protein called a prion.

FEBRILE CONVULSION. Seizures occurring mainly in children between three months and five years of age that are triggered by fever.

FEMORAL ARTERY. An artery located in the groin area that is the most frequently accessed site for arterial puncture in angiography.

FETAL. Refers to the fetus. In humans, the fetal period extends from the end of the eighth week of pregnancy to birth.

FETAL ALCOHOL SYNDROME. Syndrome characterized by distinct facial features and varying mental retardation in an infant due to impaired brain development resulting from the mother's consumption of alcohol during pregnancy.

FETAL TISSUE TRANSPLANTATION (FTT). A method of treating Parkinson's and other neurological diseases by grafting brain cells from human fetuses onto the affected area of the human brain. Human adults cannot grow new brain cells but developing fetuses can. Grafting fetal tissue stimulates the growth of new brain cells in affected adult brains.

FETUS. The term used to describe a developing human infant from approximately the third month of pregnancy until delivery. The term embryo is used prior to the third month.

FIBRIN. Elastic protein that acts when blood coagulates to form a net structure to trap platelets and other blood cells and form a clot.

FIBRINOGEN. Precursor of fibrin.

FIBROBLAST. Cells that form connective tissue fibers like skin.

FIBROMYALGIA. A fairly common chronic condition associated with musculoskeletal pain, fatigue, morning stiffness, and other nonspecific symptoms.

FILUM TERMINALE. The strand of elastic, fibrous tissue that secures the lower end of the spinal cord.

FINGER AGNOSIA. Inability to identify a particular finger.

FLACCID. Weak, soft, floppy.

FLACCID PARALYSIS. Paralysis characterized by limp, unresponsive muscles.

FLACCIDITY. Abnormally low muscle tone without an obvious cause (such as trauma).

FLAIL. To swing freely.

FLASHBACK. A vivid sensory or emotional experience that happens independently of the initial event or experience. Flashbacks resulting from the use of LSD are sometimes referred to as hallucinogen persisting perception disorder, or HPPD.

FLAVIVIRUS. An arbovirus that can cause potentially serious diseases, such as dengue, yellow fever, Japanese encephalitis, and West Nile fever.

FLUENT. Speaking, reading, and/or writing smoothly and rapidly with ease.

FLUORESCEIN DYE. An orange dye used to illuminate the blood vessels of the retina in fluorescein angiography.

FLUOROSCOPE. An imaging device that displays "moving x rays" of the body. Fluoroscopy allows the radiologist to visualize the guide wire and catheter he or she is moving through the patient's artery.

FOLIC ACID. One of the B vitamins important for healthy growth of the fetus. It is essential to the normal development of a baby's spine, brain and skull, especially during the first four weeks of pregnancy.

FONTANELLE. One of the two soft areas on a baby's scalp; a membrane-covered gap between the bones of the skull.

FOOD AND DRUG ADMINISTRATION (FDA). Government agency in the United States that regulates rules of use concerning medication.

FOOT DROP. A condition in which the person has difficulty moving the toes and forefoot upward due to weakness, damage to the muscles of the lower leg, or damage to the peroneal nerve. The person's toes typically point downward when he or she tries to walk.

FORAMEN (PLURAL, FORAMINA). The medical term for a natural opening or passage. The foramina of the spinal column are openings between the vertebrae for the spinal nerves to branch off from the spinal cord.

FORAMEN OVALE. A small opening between the two upper chambers of the heart that is present at birth but usually closes within the first three months after birth. An open (patent) foramen ovale has been linked to an increased risk of cryptogenic stroke in younger adults although the exact mechanism is not yet known.

FORAMINOTOMY. Surgery to enlarge the bony hole, or foramen, where a nerve root enters or exits the spinal canal.

FOREHEAD PLAQUE. Flat, fibrous skin growth on the forehead.

FRACTURE. Any break in the continuity of a human bone. Fractures may be classified as open or closed, partial or complete, and according to the part of the body affected.

FRAGILE X SYNDROME. A genetic condition related to the X chromosome that affects mental, physical, and sensory development.

FREE RADICAL. A molecule with an unpaired electron that has a strong tendency to react with other molecules in DNA (genetic material), proteins, and lipids (fats), resulting in damage to cells. Free radicals are neutralized by antioxidants.

FRONTAL LOBE. The largest, most forward-facing part of each side or hemisphere of the brain.

FRONTAL PLAGIOCEPHALY. An abnormal condition of the skull in which the front is more developed on one side than it is on the other side.

FUNCTIONAL DISORDER. A condition that affects psychological or physical function without affecting organic structure.

FUNCTIONAL MAGNETIC RESONANCE IMAGING (FMRI). Imaging of physical changes in the brain, such as blood flow, while performing mental tasks.

G

GADOLINIUM. A very rare metallic element useful for its sensitivity to electromagnetic resonance, among other things. Traces of it can be injected into the body to enhance the MRI pictures.

GAIT. Manner in which a person walks.

GALLBLADDER. A small, pear-shaped organ in the upper right hand corner of the abdomen. It is connected by a series of ducts (tube-like channels) to the liver, pancreas, and duodenum (first part of the small intestine). The gallbladder receives bile from the liver, and concentrates and stores it. After a meal, bile is squeezed out of the gallbladder into the intestine, where it aids in digestion of food.

GAMMA RAY. A high-energy photon emitted by radioactive substances.

GAMMA-GLOBULIN. An extract of human blood that contains antibodies.

GANGLION. A mass of nerve tissue outside of the central nervous system.

GANGLIOSIDE. A fatty (lipid) substance found within the brain and nerve cells.

GANTRY. A name for the portion of a CT scanner which houses the x-ray tube and detector array used to capture image information and send it to the computer.

GAS GANGRENE. A potentially fatal infection in which bacteria form bubbles of gas in skin or muscle tissue that is already dead.

GELASTIC SEIZURES. Seizures manifesting with brief involuntary laughter.

GENE. A building block of inheritance, which contains the instructions for the production of a particular protein, and is made up of a molecular sequence found on a section of DNA. Each gene is found in a precise location on a chromosome.

GENERALIZED ANXIETY DISORDER. An anxiety disorder characterized by excessive worry or fear about a number of activities or events.

GENETIC DISEASE. A disease caused by genes inherited from one or both parents.

GENETIC HETEROGENEITY. A condition where the clinical features of a specific disease can be caused by mutations in several different genes.

GENIOPLASTY. An operation performed to reshape the chin. Genioplasties are often done to treat OSA because the procedure changes the structure of the patient's upper airway.

GENOME. The entire collection of genes of an individual.

GENOTYPE. The structure of DNA that determines the expression of a trait. Genotype is the genetic constitution of an organism, as distinguished from its physical appearance or phenotype.

GERSTMANN'S SYNDROME. A rare disorder that includes agraphia, as well as loss of simple arithmetic skills, the ability to distinguish left and right, recognition of one's fingers, and often other communicative skills.

GERSTMANN-STRÄUSSLER-SCHEINKER SYNDROME. A rare, progressive neurological disease that is believed to be transmitted via an abnormal protein called a prion.

GILLBERG'S CRITERIA. A six–item checklist for Asperger syndrome developed by Christopher Gillberg, a Swedish researcher. It is widely used as a diagnostic tool.

GINGIVAL FIBROMAS. Fibrous growths found on the gums.

GINKGO. An herb from *Ginkgo biloba*, a shade tree native to China with fan-shaped leaves and fleshy seeds with edible kernels. Some alternative practitioners recommend ginkgo extract for preventing and treating AD.

GLAND. A collection of cells whose function is to release certain chemicals (hormones) that are important to the functioning of other, sometimes distantly located, organs or body systems.

GLASGOW COMA SCALE. A measure of level of consciousness and neurological functioning after TBI.

GLAUCOMA. Condition of the eye with increased internal pressure, often causing vision problems.

GLIAL CELL. Nerve tissue of the central nervous system other than the signal-transmitting neurons. Glial cells are interspersed between neurons and providing support and insulation. There are three main types of neuroglia: astrocytes, oligodendrocytes, and microglia.

GLIOMA. A tumor that originates in the cells supporting and nourishing brain neural tissue (glial cells).

GLOBAL APHASIA. A condition characterized by either partial or total loss of the ability to communicate verbally or using written words as a result of widespread injury to the language areas of the brain. This condition may be caused by a stroke, head injury, brain tumor, or infection. The exact language abilities affected vary depending on the location and extent of injury.

GLOBOID CELLS. Large cells containing excess toxic metabolic "waste" of galactosylceramide and psychosine.

GLOBOID-CELL LEUKODYSTROPHY (GLD). Krabbe disease; a rare, inherited, and usually fatal disorder that causes demyelination of nerves in the central nervous system.

GLUCOCEREBROSIDE. A cerebroside that contains glucose in the molecule.

GLUCOCORTICOIDS. General class of adrenal cortical hormones that are mainly active in protecting against stress and in protein and carbohydrate metabolism.

GLUCOSE. One of the two simple sugars, together with galactose, that makes up the protein lactose, found in milk. Glucose is the form of sugar that is usable by the body to generate energy.

GLYCOGEN. The chemical substance used by muscles to store sugars and starches for later use. It is composed of repeating units of glucose.

GOITER. A swelling or enlargement of the thyroid gland.

GRAFT-VERSUS-HOST DISEASE (GVHD). A condition in which immune system cells from a stem cell transplant react against recipient cells and tissues.

GRAPHEME. A minimal unit of a writing system, such as a letter or group of letters that represents a single sound.

GRAY MATTER. Areas of the brain and spinal cord that are comprised mostly of unmyelinated nerves; it is the myelin that gives the rest of the brain its whitish appearance.

GRIEF REACTION. The normal depression felt after a traumatic major life occurrence such as the loss of a loved one.

GROUP A BETA-HEMOLYTIC *STREPTOCOCCUS* (GAS, GABHS). Bacteria commonly found in the throat and on the skin, which most often cause no symptoms or a mild illness such as strep throat.

GROWTH FACTOR. Any substance occurring naturally in the body that stimulates cell growth. Most growth factors are either proteins or steroid hormones.

GUIDE WIRE. A wire that is inserted into an artery to guide a catheter to a certain location in the body.

GUILLAIN-BARRÉ SYNDROME. A disorder in which the body's immune system attacks part of the peripheral nervous system. Weakness, tingling, and abnormal sensations in the arms and upper body can progress until the muscles become totally disabled and the patient is effectively paralyzed.

GUSTATORY. Pertaining to the sense of taste.

H

HAIR CELLS. Special cells in the cochlea that convert the movement of the fluid inside the cochlea into electrical signals that travel to the brain via the auditory nerve.

HALF-LIFE. The time required for half of the atoms in a radioactive substance to decay.

HALLUCINATION. False sensory perceptions, including hearing sounds or seeing people or objects that are not present. Hallucinations can also affect the senses of smell, touch, and taste.

HALLUCINOGEN. A drug or other substance that induces hallucinations.

HAMARTOMATOUS RECTAL POLYPS. Benign (noncancerous) growths found in the rectum.

HANDEDNESS. The preference of either the right or left hand as the dominant hand for the performance of tasks such as writing.

HAPTIC. Pertaining to the sense of touch; sometimes called tactile hallucinations.

HEIMLICH MANEUVER. An action designed to expel an obstructing piece of food from the throat. It is performed by placing the fist on the abdomen, underneath the breastbone, grasping the fist with the other hand (from behind), and thrusting it inward and upward.

HEMANGIOBLASTOMA. Tumor often found in the brain, as in von Hippel-Lindau disease.

HEMATOCRIT. The percentage of blood volume occupied by red blood cells, normally about 45% for men and 40% for women. It is also known as the packed cell volume or PCV.

HEMATOMA. A localized collection of blood, often clotted, in body tissue or an organ, usually due to a break or tear in the wall of blood vessel.

HEMATOPOIETIC STEM CELL TRANSPLANT (HSCT). Infusion of blood-forming stem cells from donor bone marrow, circulating blood, or umbilical cord blood.

HEMATOPOIETIC STEM CELLS. Cells in the blood and bone marrow that can differentiate into various types of blood cells.

HEMICHOREA. Chorea that affects only one side of the body.

HEMICRANIA CONTINUA. A continuous or chronic one-sided headache that responds to treatment with indomethacin.

HEMIPARESIS. Muscle weakness or partial paralysis on one side of the body.

HEMIPLEGIA. Paralysis of one side of the body.

HEMISPHERE. One of the two halves or sides—the left and the right—of the brain.

HEMODYNAMICS. The study of blood flow in the body and the factors that influence it.

HEMORRHAGE. Severe, massive bleeding that is difficult to control. The bleeding may be internal or external.

HEMOSTASIS. Process by which the flow of blood is slowed or stopped.

HEMOSTATIC PLUG. A clot that arrests or slows bleeding.

HEPATITIS. A viral disease characterized by inflammation of the liver cells (hepatocytes). People infected with hepatitis B or hepatitis C virus are at an increased risk for developing liver cancer.

HEPATOSPLENOMEGALY. Enlargement of the liver and spleen.

HEPATOTOXICITY. Damaging or destructive to the liver.

HEREDITARY SPASTIC PARAPLEGIA (HSP). Familial spastic paraparesis; a spectrum of inherited neurological disorders that can cause paraplegia.

HERNIATED DISK. A blisterlike bulging or protrusion of the contents of the disk out through the fibers that normally hold them in place. It is also called a ruptured disk, slipped disk, or displaced disk.

HERNIATION. Movement or rupture of tissue or fluid from its normal position.

HERPES SIMPLEX. A virus that causes sores on the lips (cold sores) or on the genitals (genital herpes).

HERPES VARICELLA ZOSTER VIRUS. The virus that typically causes chicken pox in children; then may reactivate later in life to cause shingles.

HIB DISEASE. An infection caused by *Haemophilus influenza* type b (Hib). This disease mainly affects children under the age of five. In that age group, it is the leading cause of bacterial meningitis, pneumonia, joint and bone infections, and throat inflammations.

HIGH-ALTITUDE CEREBRAL EDEMA (HACE). Brain swelling caused by spending periods of time at high altitudes; severe or end-stage acute mountain sickness.

HIGH-FUNCTIONING AUTISM (HFA). A subcategory of autistic disorder consisting of children diagnosed with IQs of 70 or higher.

HIGHLY ACTIVE ANTIRETROVIRAL THERAPY (HAART). An individualized combination of three or more antiretroviral drugs used to treat patients with HIV infection. It is sometimes called a drug cocktail.

HIPPOCAMPUS. A part of the brain that is involved in memory formation and learning. The hippocampus is shaped like a curved ridge and is part of the limbic system.

HISTAMINE. A substance released by immune system cells in response to the presence of an allergen. It stimulates widening of blood vessels and increased porousness of blood vessel walls so that fluid and protein leak out from the blood into the surrounding tissue, causing localised inflammation of the tissue.

HISTOLOGIC. Pertaining to histology, the study of cells and tissues at the microscopic level.

HISTOLOGY. The study of tissue structure.

HIV. Acronym for human immunodeficiency virus, the virus that causes AIDS.

HLA. Human leukocyte antigen; the major tissue compatibility complex, which determines whether transplanted donor cells will be compatible with those of the recipient.

HOLOPROSENCEPHALY. Brain, cranial, and facial malformations present at birth that are caused by incomplete cleavage of the brain during embryologic development.

HORMONE. Chemical substance produced by certain endocrine glands that are released into the bloodstream where they control and regulate functioning of several other tissues.

HUNTINGTON DISEASE. A midlife-onset inherited disorder characterized by progressive dementia and loss of control over voluntary movements. It is sometimes called Huntington's chorea.

HYDROCEPHALUS. A condition marked by an abnormal accumulation of cerebrospinal fluid within the ventricles of the brain. Untreated hydrocephalus can lead to enlargement of the head, vision disorders, convulsions, mental disabilities, and even death.

HYDROGEN. The simplest, most common element known in the universe. It is composed of a single electron (negatively charged particle) circling a nucleus consisting of a single proton (positively charged particle). It is the nuclear proton of hydrogen that makes MRI possible by reacting resonantly to radio waves while aligned in a magnetic field.

HYPERBARIC. Pertaining to an environment in which the pressure of the air (or other gases) is greater than one bar.

HYPERCALCEMIA. High levels of calcium in the blood.

HYPEREXTENSION. Overstretching toward the back.

HYPERFLEXION. Overstretching toward the front.

HYPERFUNCTION. Term used to describe excess effort or strain involved in producing an action.

HYPERHIDROSIS. Excessive sweating. Hyperhidrosis can be caused by heat, overactive thyroid glands, strong emotion, menopause, or infection.

HYPERPIGMENTATION. An abnormal condition characterized by an excess of melanin in localized areas of the skin, which produces areas that are much darker than the surrounding unaffected skin.

HYPERREFLEXIA. An increased reaction to reflexes.

HYPERSOMNIA. Episodes of sleeping excessively, followed by periods of normal sleep.

HYPERTENSION. The medical term for high blood pressure.

HYPERTHERMIA. Elevated body temperature.

HYPERTHYROID. State of excess thyroid hormone in the body.

HYPERTHYROIDISM. Abnormally high levels of thyroid hormone. About 2% of patients with this condition develop chorea.

HYPERTONIA. Excessive muscle tone or tension, causing resistance of muscle to being stretched.

HYPNAGOGIC. Pertaining to drowsiness; refers to hallucinations that occur as a person falls asleep.

HYPNAGOGIC HALLUCINATIONS. Dream–like auditory or visual hallucinations that occur while falling asleep.

HYPNOPOMPIC. Persisting after sleep; refers to hallucinations that occur as a person awakens.

HYPNOTICS. A class of drugs that are used as a sedatives and sleep aids.

HYPOCALCEMIA. Abnormally low levels of calcium in the blood.

HYPOCRETIN. A brain chemical that promotes wakefulness; low levels are associated with narcolepsy.

HYPOGLYCEMIA. An abnormally low glucose (blood sugar) concentration in the blood.

HYPOKALEMIA. Decreased levels of the electrolyte potassium in the blood.

HYPOMELANOTIC MACULES. Patches of skin lighter than the surrounding skin.

HYPONATREMIA. A deficiency of sodium in the blood.

HYPOPITUITARISM. A condition characterized by underactivity of the pituitary gland.

HYPOPLASIA. Incomplete or underdevelopment of a tissue or organ.

HYPOTELORISM. A birth defect in which the eyes are set abnormally close together.

HYPOTHALAMUS. The lowermost part of the diencephalon, containing several nuclei, nerve tracts, and the pituitary gland; it is the regulatory seat of the autonomic nervous system, controling heartbeat, body temperature, thirst, hunger, blood pressure, blood sugar levels, and other functions.

HYPOTHERMIA. The medical term for loss of body heat to the point that the core body temperature drops below the temperature for normal metabolic processes (about 95°F).

HYPOTONIA. Decreased muscle tone.

HYPOXEMIA. Abnormally low blood oxygen.

HYPOXIA. Oxygen deficiency in a body tissue, such as cerebral hypoxia in the brain.

HYPSARRHYTHMIA. Typical brain wave activity found in infantile spasms.

IATROGENIC. Referring to disease transmission or injury caused by a medical procedure.

ICHTHYOSIS. Rough, dry, scaly skin that forms as a result of a defect in skin formation.

ICTAL EEG. An EEG done to determine the type of seizure characteristic of a person's disorder. During this EEG, seizure medicine may be discontinued in an attempt to induce as seizure during the testing period.

ICTHYOSIS. A disease condition where the skin becomes rough, thick, and scaly like that of a fish.

IDOPATHIC. A disease or condition of unknown cause or origin.

ILLUSION. A false interpretation of a real sensory image or impression.

IMMUNE RESPONSE. A response from the body to an antigen that occurs when the antigen is identified as foreign and that induces the production of antibodies and lymphocytes capable of destroying the antigen or making it harmless.

IMMUNE SYSTEM. The system of specialized organs, lymph nodes, and blood cells throughout the body which work together to prevent foreign invaders (bacteria, viruses, fungi, etc.) from taking hold and growing.

IMMUNOADSORPTION. A procedure that can remove harmful antibodies from the blood.

IMMUNOCOMPROMISED. An abnormal condition in which the body's ability to fight infection is decreased due to a disease process, certain medications, or a condition present at birth.

IMMUNOGLOBULIN. A protein in the blood that is the component part of an antibody.

IMMUNOSUPPRESSANT. A drug that reduces the body's natural immunity by suppressing the natural functioning of the immune system.

IMMUNOSUPPRESSED. Suppression of the immune system by medications during the treatment of diseases such as cancer or following an organ transplantation.

IMMUNOSUPPRESSIVE THERAPY. Destruction of the immune system with chemotherapy and/or radiation treatment to prevent rejection of transplanted cells; drug treatment to suppress the donor immune system following a stem cell transplant, to prevent graft-versus-host disease.

IN VITRO FERTILIZATION (IVF). A procedure in which an egg cell is fertilized with sperm in a laboratory and allowed to form an embryo, which can be implanted in a woman to initiate pregnancy.

INBORN ERROR OF METABOLISM. One of a group of rare conditions characterized by an inherited defect in an enzyme or other protein. Inborn errors of metabolism can cause brain damage and mental retardation if left untreated. Phenylketonuria, Tay-Sachs disease, and galactosemia are inborn errors of metabolism.

INCISION. A surgical cut or gash.

INCLUSION BODY. A small intracellular body found within the cytoplasm or nucleus of another cell, characteristic of disease.

INCONTINENCE. Inability to control excretory functions such as defecation and urination.

INCREASED INTRACRANIAL PRESSURE. Pressure inside the cranium (skull) that is higher than normal.

INDICATION. The basis for beginning treatment for a disease or giving a diagnostic test.

INDUCED PLURIPOTENT STEM CELL (IPS CELL). A specialized cell, such as a skin cell, that has been induced or reprogrammed to return to a pluripotent or non-specialized state similar to an embryonic stem cell.

INDUCTION. Process in which one tissue (the prechordal plate, for example) changes another tissue (for example, changes tissue into neural tissue).

INFANTILE SPASMS. Clusters of rapid jerks followed by stiffening or jackknife movements. Usually starts in the first year of life and stops by age 4.

INFARCT. Tissue death due to lack of oxygen resulting from a blood clot, plaque, or inflammation that blocks an artery.

INFLAMMATION. The body's response to tissue damage. Includes warmth, swelling, redness, and pain in the affected part.

INHERITANCE PATTERN. Refers to dominant or recessive inheritance.

INNERVATION. Distribution or supply of nerves to a structure.

INSIDIOUS. Progressing gradually and inconspicuously, but with serious effects. Sydenham's chorea may have an insidious onset.

INSOMNIA. Prolonged or abnormal inability to obtain adequate sleep.

INSONATION WINDOW. Any of four locations on the outside of the head and neck used for placement of the TCD probe.

INTENTION TREMOR. A rhythmic purposeless shaking of the muscles that begins with purposeful (voluntary) movement. This tremor does not affect muscles that are resting.

INTERFERON. A naturally occuring immune system protein.

INTERFERON ALFA. A potent immune-defense protein that is used as an anti-cancer drug.

INTERNATIONAL NORMALIZED RATIO (INR). Laboratory measurement that is indicative of the clotting ability of the blood.

INTERPERSONAL THERAPIES. Also called talk therapy, this type of psychological counseling is focused on determining how dysfunctional interpersonal relationships of the affected individual may be causing or influencing symptoms of depression.

INTERVENTION. In medicine, any action that produces an effect or is intended to change the course of a disease process.

INTERVENTIONAL NEURORADIOLOGY. The subspecialty of neuroradiology that involves treatment of patients utilizing minimally invasive interventional techniques as well as performing diagnostic imaging. It is also known as neurointerventional surgery.

INTERVERTEBRAL DISCS. Gelatinous structures separating the spinal vertebrae and acting as shock absorbers.

INTRACEREBRAL HEMATOMA. Bleeding within the brain caused by trauma to a blood vessel.

INTRACEREBRAL HEMORRHAGE. A cause of some strokes in which vessels within the brain begin bleeding.

INTRACRANIAL. Existing or occurring within the skull.

INTRACRANIAL HYPERTENSION. Condition in which there is elevated pressure within the cranium, or skull, leading to increased brain pressure; can be dangerous.

INTRACRANIAL PRESSURE (ICP). The overall pressure within the skull.

INTRAGENIC. Occuring within a single gene.

INTRAOCULAR. Inside the eye.

INTRAVENOUS IMMUNOGLOBULINS (IVIG). Treatment with pooled antibodies from donor sera to treat autoimmune disorders or immune system deficiencies.

INTRAVENTRICULAR HEMORRHAGE. Bleeding into the brain, specifically into the ventricles.

INTRINSIC PATHWAY. One of two initial pathways of the clotting cascade.

INTRON. That portion of the DNA sequence of a gene that is not directly involved in the formation of the chemical that the gene codes for.

INTUBATION. The placement of a flexible tube into a patient's trachea (windpipe) to maintain an open airway or to administer certain drugs.

INVOLUNTARY. Not under the control of the will.

ION CHANNELS. Gateways present on the surface of neurons that allow the flow of ions such as sodium through the neuronal surface membrane, propagating an electrical signal that allows parts of the brain to communicate and function.

IONIZING RADIATION. Electromagnetic radiation that can damage living tissue by disrupting and destroying individual cells. All types of nuclear decay radiation (including x rays) are potentially ionizing. Radio waves do not damage organic tissues they pass through.

IRIS. The colored part of the eye, containing pigment and muscle cells that contract and dilate the pupil.

IRITIS. Inflammation of the iris, the membrane in the pupil, the colored portion of the eye. It is characterized by photophobia, pain, and inflammatory congestion.

IRRITATIVE HALLUCINATIONS. Hallucinations caused by abnormal electrical activity in the brain.

ISCHEMIA. A condition in which blood flow is cut off or restricted from a particular area. The surrounding tissue, starved of oxygen and nutrients, dies.

ISCHEMIC EVENT. Condition in which a vital organ such as the brain is deprived of oxygen for a period of time.

ISCHEMIC STROKE. A stroke caused by a blood clot in the brain.

J

JAUNDICE. Yellowing of the skin or eyes due to excess of bilirubin in the blood.

JOINT CONTRACTURES. Stiffness of the joints that prevents full extension.

K

KAPOSI'S SARCOMA. A cancer of the connective tissue that produces painless purplish-red (in people with light skin) or brown (in people with dark skin) blotches on the skin. It is a major diagnostic marker of AIDS.

KARYOTYPE. A standard arrangement of photographic or computer-generated images of chromosome pairs from a cell in ascending numerical order, from largest to smallest.

KORSAKOFF'S SYNDROME. A disorder of the central nervous system resulting from long-term thiamin deficiency. It is characterized by amnesia, confusion, confabulation, and unsteady gait; it is most commonly seen in alcoholics.

KURU. A prion disease associated with the cannibalism formerly practiced by the Fore people of Papua New Guinea. Its name comes from a word in the Fore language that means "to shake" or "to tremble."

KYPHOSIS (DOWAGER'S HUMP). A pronounced rounding of the normal forward curve of the upper back.

L

LABYRINTH. The inner ear. It consists of the membranous labyrinth (a system of sacs and ducts made of soft tissue) and the osseous or bony labyrinth (which surrounds and contains the membranous labyrinth).

LABYRINTHITIS. Acute inflammation of the inner ear, which may be caused by bacteria, viruses, or allergies.

LACINATING PAIN. Piercing, stabbing, or darting pain.

LAMBERT-EATON MYASTHENIC SYNDROME (LEMS). An autoimmune disease that affects neuromuscular junctions and is often associated with cancer elsewhere in the body.

LAMINAE (SINGULAR, LAMINA). The broad plates of bone on the upper surface of the vertebrae that fuse together at the midline to form a bony covering over the spinal canal.

LAMINOTOMY. A less invasive alternative to a laminectomy in which a hole is drilled through the lamina.

LARYNGEAL STRIDOR. Constriction of the voice box, causing vocal hoarseness.

LATERAL FLEXION. To flex toward a side.

LEARNING DISABILITY. Any of various disorders that interfere with a child's ability to learn, resulting in problems with language, reasoning, and academic skills; believed to be caused by deficits in processing and integrating information.

LEFT VENTRICULAR ENLARGEMENT. Abnormal enlargement of the left lower chamber of the heart.

LENNOX-GASTAUT SYNDROME. A severe form of epilepsy in children, resulting in intractable (difficult to control) seizures and developmental delays.

LEPTOMENINGEAL ANGIOMA. A swelling of the tissue or membrane surrounding the brain and spinal cord, which can enlarge with time.

LESION. A defective or injured section or region of an organ.

LEUCOPENIA. A condition in which the number of leukocytes circulating in the blood is abnormally low, most commonly due to a decrease in new cell production in conjunction with development of an infectious disease as a reaction to a drug or other chemical.

LEUKEMIA. A cancer of blood cells characterized by the abnormal increase in the number of white blood cells in the tissues. There are many types of leukemias and they are classified according to the type of white blood cell involved.

LEUKOCYTOSIS. An elevated white blood cell count.

LEUKODYSTROPHY. Any of several inherited diseases characterized by the degeneration of myelin in the brain, spinal cord, and peripheral nerves.

LEUKOMALACIA. Softening of the brain's white matter.

LEVODOPA (L-DOPA). A substance used in the treatment of Parkinson's disease. Levodopa can cross the blood-brain barrier that protects the brain. Once in the brain, it is converted to dopamine and thus can replace the dopamine lost in Parkinson's disease.

LEWY BODIES. Areas of injury found on damaged nerve cells in certain parts of the brain associated with dementia.

LIGAMENTA FLAVA (SINGULAR, LIGAMENTUM FLAVUM). A series of bands of tissue that are attached to the vertebrae in the spinal column. They help to hold the spine straight and to close the spaces between the laminar arches. The Latin name means "yellow band(s)."

LIMB-GIRDLE MUSCULAR DYSTROPHY (LGMD). Form of muscular dystrophy that begins in late childhood to early adulthood and affects both men and women, causing weakness in the muscles around the hips and shoulders.

LIMB-GIRDLE MYOPATHY. A muscular dystrophy-type disorder characterized by weakness in the muscles of the shoulders trunk, and pelvic girdle, often progressing to respiratory or cardiac failure.

LIMBIC SYSTEM. A complex of nerve tracts and nuclei that function as the seat of memory and emotions, containing the fornix, hippocampus, amygdala, and the cingulate gyrus.

LIMITED SUPPORT. A predetermined period of assistance required to deal with a specific event, such as training for a new job.

LIPIDS. Organic compounds not soluble in water, but soluble in fat solvents such as alcohol. Lipids are stored in the body as energy reserves and are also important components of cell membranes. Commonly known as fats.

LIPODYSTROPHY. The medical term for redistribution of body fat in response to HAART, insulin injections in diabetics, or rare hereditary disorders.

LIPOPIGMENTS. Substances made up of fats and proteins found in the body's tissues.

LIPOPROTEINS. Compounds of protein that carry fats and fat-like substances such as cholesterol in the blood.

LIVER ENCEPHALOPATHY. A condition in which the brain is affected by a buildup of toxic substances that would normally be removed by the liver. The condition occurs when the liver is too severely damaged to cleanse the blood effectively.

LOADING DOSE. Initial dose of medication intended to raise levels of drug in the blood stream to a therapeutic level.

LOCKED-IN SYNDROME. A condition of full wakefulness and awareness but inability to communicate, except possibly with eye movements, due to paralysis.

LOCOMOTOR. Means of or pertaining to movement or locomotion.

LORDOSIS. Anterior curvature of the spine, creating a swayback appearance.

LORDOSIS (SWAYBACK). An exaggeration of the normal backward arch in the lower back.

LUMBAR. Pertaining to the part of the back between the chest and the pelvis.

LUMBAR PUNCTURE. A procedure in which a small amount of cerebrospinal fluid is removed from the lower spine. Examination of this fluid helps diagnose certain illnesses.

LUMBAR VERTEBRAE. The five vertebrae below the thoracic vertebrae and above the sacrum.

LUMEN. The interior space of a tubular structure or organ, such as an artery or section of intestine.

LYME BORRELIOSIS. Another name for Lyme disease.

LYMPHANGIOMYOMATOSIS. Serious lung disease characterized by the overgrowth of an unusual type of muscle cell resulting in the blockage of air, blood, and lymph vessels to and from the lungs.

LYMPHOCYTIC MENINGITIS. Benign infection of the protective coverings of the brain (the meninges).

LYMPHOMA. A blood cancer in which lymphocytes, a variety of white blood cells, grow at an unusually rapid rate.

LYSERGIC ACID DIETHYLAMIDE (LSD). The first synthetic hallucinogen, discovered in 1938.

LYSOSOME. Membrane-enclosed compartment in cells, containing many hydrolytic enzymes; where large molecules and cellular components are broken down.

M

MAGNETIC FIELD. The three-dimensional area surrounding a magnet, in which its force is active. During MRI, the patient's body is permeated by the force field of a superconducting magnet.

MAGNETIC RESONANCE IMAGING (MRI). An imaging technique that utilizes the properties of magnetism to create nondestructive, three-dimensional, internal images of the soft tissues of the body, including the brain, spinal cord, and muscle.

MAJOR DEPRESSION. A psychological condition in which the patient experiences one or more disabling attacks of depression that lasts two or more weeks.

MAJOR TRANQUILIZERS. The family of drugs that includes the psychotropic or neuroleptic drugs, sometimes used to help autistic people. They carry significant risk of side effects, including parkinsonism and movement disorders, and should be prescribed with caution.

MALABSORPTION. The inability to adequately or efficiently absorb nutrients from the intestinal tract.

MALABSORPTION SYNDROME. A condition characterized by indigestion, bloating, diarrhea, loss of appetite, and weakness caused by poor absorption of nutrients from food as a result of HIV infection itself, giardiasis, or other opportunistic infections of the digestive tract, or certain surgical procedures involving the stomach or intestines.

MALINGERING. Knowingly pretending to be physically or mentally ill to avoid some unpleasant duty or responsibility, or for economic benefit.

MANDIBLE. The medical term for the lower jaw. One type of oral appliance used to treat OSA pushes the mandible forward in order to ease breathing during sleep.

MANIA. A period of excess mental activity, often accompanied by elevated mood and disorganized behavior.

MAO-B INHIBITORS. Inhibitors of the enzyme monoamine oxidase B. MAO-B helps break down dopamine; inhibiting it prolongs the action of dopamine in the brain. Selegiline is an MAO-B inhibitor.

MARFAN SYNDROME. An inherited condition that affects connective tissue throughout the body including weakening the connective tissue found in arteries.

MEASLES ENCEPHALITIS. A serious complication of measles occurring in about one out of every 1,000 cases, causing headache, drowsiness, and vomiting seven to ten days after the rash appears. Seizures and coma can follow, which may lead to retardation and death.

MEDIAN NERVE. A nerve which runs through the wrist and into the hand. It provides sensation and some movement to the hand, the thumb, the index finger, the middle finger, and half of the ring finger.

MEDICAL TOURISM. Traveling to a foreign country for a medical treatment that is not available in one's home country.

MEDICATION-OVERUSE HEADACHE (MOH). A chronic daily headache caused by frequent use of pain-relievers or headache medications.

MEDULLA OBLONGATA. The lower part of the brainstem that borders the spinal cord and regulates breathing, heartbeat, and blood flow.

MELATONIN. A hormone involved in regulation of the sleep-wake cycle and other circadian rhythms.

MENINGES. A series of membranous, pain-sensitive layers of connective tissue that protect the central nervous system (brain and spinal cord). Damage or infection to the meninges, such as in meningitis, can cause serious neurological damage and even death. In order from outermost to innermost, the meninges are the dura mater, arachnoid mater, and pia mater.

MENINGITIS. An infection or inflammation of the membranes that cover the brain and spinal cord. It is usually caused by bacteria or a virus.

MENTAL STATUS EXAMINATION (MSE). A clinical evaluation in which the doctor assesses the patient's external appearance, attitude, behavior, mood and affect, speech, thought processes, thought content, perception, cognition, insight (or lack thereof), and judgment.

MERIDIAN. A channel through which chi travels in the body.

META-IODOBENZYLGUANIDINE (MIBG) SCINTIGRAPHY. A procedure to look at the amount of a radioactive chemical, meta-iodobenzylguanidine, injected into the body to find growths like pheochromocytomas.

METABOLIC ACIDOSIS. Overly acidic condition of the blood.

METABOLIC EQUIVALENT OF TASK (MET). The energy cost of a physical activity, measured as a multiple of the resting metabolic rate, which is defined as 3.5 milliliters of oxygen consumed per kilogram (kg) of body weight per minute, equivalent to 1 kilocalorie per kg per hour.

METABOLISM. All the physical and chemical changes that take place within an organism.

METANEPHRINE. A byproduct of epinephrine, found elevated in urine if a pheochromocytoma is present.

METASTASIS. The spread of cancer from one part of the body to another. Cells in the metastatic (secondary) tumor are like those in the original (primary) tumor.

MICROCEPHALY. A condition in which a person's head is abnormally small for his or her age and sex.

MICROEMBOLI. Small blot clots in the bloodstream.

MICROFORM HPE. A term that refers to persons with a very mild form of HPE (as evidenced in minor facial deformities) who do not have any noticeable brain damage when tested by conventional brain imaging.

MICROTIA. Small or underdeveloped ears.

MIGRAINE. A type of headache caused by a cascade of events in the brain, including initial dilatation or widening of blood vessels, followed by chemical release and then painful spasms of blood vessels in the brain. Often associated with nausea, vomiting, and sensitivity to light and noise; can be episodic or chronic.

MILD COGNITIVE IMPAIRMENT (MCI). A transitional phase of memory loss in older people that precedes dementia or AD.

MINERALOCORTICOID. A steroid hormone, like aldosterone, that regulates the excretion of salt, potassium, and water.

MITOCHONDRIA. Spherical or rod-shaped structures within the cytoplasm of a cell. Mitochondria contain genetic material (DNA and RNA) and are responsible for converting food to energy.

MITOCHONDRIAL DNA (MTDNA). The genetic material found in mitochondria, the organelles that generate energy for the cell. Because reproduction is by cloning, mtDNA is usually passed along female lines, as part of the egg's cytoplasm.

MITRAL VALVE PROLAPSE. A heart defect in which one of the valves of the heart (which normally controls blood flow) becomes floppy. Mitral valve prolapse may be detected as a heart murmur, but there are usually no symptoms.

MONOAMINE OXIDASE (MAO) INHIBITORS. A class of antidepressants used to treat certain types of mental depression. Monoamine oxidase inhibitors are especially useful in treating people whose depression is combined with other problems such as anxiety, panic attacks, phobias, or the desire to sleep too much.

MONONEUROPATHY. Disorder involving a single nerve.

MOTOR. Refers to peripheral nerves that control voluntary movements, such as moving the arms and legs.

MOTOR FUNCTION. The ability to produce body movement by complex interaction of the brain, nerves, and muscles.

MOTOR NERVES. Motor or efferent nerve cells carry impulses from the brain to muscle or organ tissue.

MOTOR NEURON DISEASE. A neuromuscular disease, usually progressive, that causes degeneration of motor neuron cells and loss or diminishment of voluntary muscle control.

MOTOR UNIT ACTION POTENTIALS. Spikes of electrical activity recorded during an EMG that reflect the number of motor units (motor neurons and the muscle fibers they transmit signals to) activated when the patient voluntarily contracts a muscle.

MOTOR UNITS. Functional connection with a single motor neuron and muscle.

MOXIBUSTION. Acupuncture technique which involves burning the herb moxa or mugwort.

MUCOPOLYSACCHARIDE. A complex molecule made of smaller sugar molecules strung together to form a chain. Found in mucous secretions and intercellular spaces.

MULTI-INFARCT DEMENTIA (MID). Dementia caused by damage to brain tissue resulting from a series of blood clots or clogs in the blood vessels. It is also called vascular dementia.

MULTIPLE SCLEROSIS (MS). A progressive, autoimmune disease of the central nervous system characterized by damage to the myelin sheath that covers nerves. The disease, which causes progressive paralysis, is marked by periods of exacerbation and remission.

MULTIPLE SLEEP LATENCY TEST (MSLT). A measurement of brain activity during daytime naps.

MULTIPOTENT STEM CELL. A stem cell that has the potential to differentiate into several types of cells found in a specific organ or tissue, but not into all cell types. For example, blood stem cells can differentiate into various types of blood cells, but not into cells of other tissues or organs.

MUSCLE TONE. Also termed tonus; the normal state of balanced tension in the tissues of the body, especially the muscles.

MUSCULAR DYSTROPHY. A group of inherited diseases characterized by progressive wasting of the muscles.

MUTATION. A permanent change in the genetic material that may alter a trait or characteristic of an individual, or manifest as disease. This change can be transmitted to offspring.

MYASTHENIA. The medical term for muscle weakness.

MYASTHENIA GRAVIS. A chronic autoimmune disease characterized by fatigue and muscular weakness, especially in the face and neck, that results from a breakdown in the normal communication between nerves and muscles caused by the deficiency of acetylcholine at the neuromuscular junction.

MYELIN. The substance that is wrapped around nerves. Myelin is responsible for speed and efficiency of impulses traveling through those nerves. When the myelin sheath is damaged, nerve communication is disrupted.

MYELITIS. Inflammation of the spinal cord.

MYELOGRAPHY, MYELOGRAM. A technique for imaging abnormalities of the spinal cord and spinal nerves by injecting a contrast material into the cerebrospinal fluid inside the spinal cord and then making a radiographic image. A myelogram is usually followed by a CT scan.

MYELOMENINGOCELE. A sac that protrudes through an abnormal opening in the spinal column.

MYELOPATHY. A disorder in which the tissue of the spinal cord is diseased or damaged.

MYOCLONUS. Involuntary contractions of a muscle or an interrelated group of muscles. Also known as myoclonic seizures.

MYOFILAMENT. Ultrastructural microscopic unit of a muscle that is made up of proteins that contract.

MYOGLOBINURIA. Reddish urine caused by excretion of myoglobin, a breakdown product of muscle.

MYOPATHY. Any abnormal condition or disease of muscle tissue, characterized by muscle weakness and wasting.

MYOSITIS. Inflammation of a muscle.

MYOTONIC DYSTROPHY. A form of muscular dystrophy, also known as Steinert's condition, characterized by delay in the ability to relax muscles after forceful contraction, wasting of muscles, as well as other abnormalities.

N

NARCOLEPSY. A life-long sleep disorder marked by four symptoms: sudden brief sleep attacks, cataplexy (a sudden loss of muscle tone usually lasting up to 30 minutes), temporary paralysis, and hallucinations. The hallucinations are associated with falling asleep or the transition from sleeping to waking.

NASAL POLYPS. Drop-shaped overgrowths of the nasal membranes.

NECROSIS. Cellular or tissue death; skin necrosis may be caused by multiple, consecutive doses of radiation from fluoroscopic or x-ray procedures.

NEGATIVE SYMPTOMS. Symptoms of schizophrenia characterized by the absence or elimination of certain behaviors. DSM-IV specifies three negative symptoms: affective flattening, poverty of speech, and loss of will or initiative.

NEOPLASM. An abnormal growth of tissue or cells (a tumor) that may be either malignant (cancerous) or benign.

NERVE BIOPSY. A medical test in which a small portion of a damaged nerve is surgically removed and examined under a microscope.

NERVE CONDUCTION. The speed and strength of a signal being transmitted by nerve cells. Testing these factors can reveal the nature of nerve injury, such as damage to nerve cells or to the protective myelin sheath.

NERVE CONDUCTION VELOCITY TESTING (NCV). A type of test that uses an electromyography unit to evaluate electrical potentials from peripheral nerves by measuring how long it takes for a nerve impulse to reach a muscle after stimulation with an electrical current.

NERVE IMPULSE. The electrochemical signal carried by an axon from one neuron to another neuron.

NERVE ROOT. Two groups of nerves that run from the spinal cord to join and form the spinal nerves.

NERVE SIGNALING. The pathway by which neurons communicate; can be electrical or chemical.

NERVOUS TIC. A repetitive, involuntary action, such as the twitching of a muscle or repeated blinking.

NEURAL. Referring to any tissue with nerves, including the brain, the spinal cord, and other nerves.

NEURAL PROSTHESES. A general term for devices implanted in neurosurgery to help restore the structure or function of the central nervous system. They include stents, artificial spinal disks, platinum coils to treat aneurysms, vagus nerve stimulators, deep brain stimulators, and similar devices.

NEURAL TUBE. A hollow column of ectodermal tissue that forms in early embryonic development and goes on to become the spinal cord and spinal column.

NEURAL TUBE DEFECT (NTD). A birth defect caused by abnormal closure or development of the neural tube, the embryonic structure that gives rise to the central nervous system.

NEURALGIA. Pain along the pathway of a nerve.

NEUROBLASTOMA. A malignant tumor of nerve cells that strikes children.

NEUROCYSTICERCOSIS (NCC). Medical condition in which a patient has cystic lesions formed by pork tapeworm larvae specifically in the brain or spinal cord.

NEURODEGENERATION. The deterioration of nerve tissues.

NEUROFIBRILLARY TANGLES. Accumulations of twisted protein fragments inside nerve cells in the brain that are diagnostic of AD.

NEUROFIBROMA. A soft tumor usually located on a nerve.

NEUROFIBROMATOSIS. Also called Von Recklinghausen's disease; a disease in which tumors grow on nerve cells throughout the body.

NEUROGENIC. Caused by nerves; originating in the nerves.

NEUROGENIC PAIN. Pain originating in the nerves or nervous tissue.

NEUROLEPTIC. Another name for the older type of antipsychotic medications given to schizophrenic patients.

NEUROLOGIC DISORDERS. Disorders affecting the nervous system.

NEUROLOGICAL. Relating to the brain and central nervous system.

NEUROMUSCULAR. Involving both the muscles and the nerves that control them.

NEUROMUSCULAR DISEASE. Disease involving both the muscles and the nerves that control them.

NEUROMUSCULAR JUNCTION. The site at which nerve impulses are transmitted to muscles.

NEUROMYELITIS OPTICA (NMO). An autoimmune disease that destroys myelin and damages fibers of the optic nerve and spinal cord.

NEURON. A cell specialized to conduct and generate electrical impulses and to carry information from one part of the brain to another.

NEURONAL CEROID LIPOFUSCINOSES. A family of four progressive neurological disorders.

NEURONAL MIGRATION. A step of early brain development in which nerve cells travel over large distances to different parts of the brain.

NEURONAL SIGNALING. The communication between neurons, nerve cells that act to accomplish many bodily processes and recognize stimuli from the outside environment such as pain.

NEUROPATHY. A condition affecting the nerves supplying the arms and legs. Typically, the feet and hands are involved first. If sensory nerves are involved, numbness, tingling, and pain are prominent, and if motor nerves are involved, the patient experiences weakness.

NEUROPSYCHIATRIC DISORDER. A disorder with both neurological and psychiatric components.

NEUROSURGEON. A surgeon who specializes in surgery of the nervous system, including the brain and nerves.

NEUROSYPHILIS. The slowly progressive destruction of the brain and spinal cord caused by untreated tertiary syphilis. It can be asymptomatic or cause different disorders such as tabes dorsalis, general paresis and meningovascular syphilis.

NEUROTRANSMITTER. One of a group of chemicals secreted by a nerve cell (neuron) to carry a chemical message to another nerve cell, often as a way of transmitting a nerve impulse. Examples of neurotransmitters include acetylcholine, dopamine, serotonin, and norepinephrine.

NEW DAILY PERSISTENT HEADACHE (NDPH). A treatment-resistant chronic headache that begins abruptly and may last for years.

NEW VARIANT CREUTZFELDT-JAKOB DISEASE. A more newly identified type of Creutzfeldt-Jakob disease that has been traced to the ingestion of beef from cows infected with bovine spongiform encephalopathy. Known in the popular press as Mad Cow Disease.

NOCICEPTOR. A neuron that is capable of sensing pain.

NOCTURIA. Excessive need to urinate at night. Nocturia is a symptom of OSA and often increases the patient's daytime sleepiness.

NON-NUCLEOSIDE REVERSE TRANSCRIPTASE INHIBITORS. The newest class of antiretroviral drugs that work by inhibiting the reverse transcriptase enzyme necessary for HIV replication.

NONRENAL HAMARTOMA. Benign (non-cancerous) tumor-like growths not found in the kidneys that often disrupt the normal function of a particular organ system.

NONSTEROIDAL ANTI-INFLAMMATORY DRUGS (NSAIDS). A class of pain relief medications that also decreases inflammation, including ibuprofen (Advil), naproxen (Aleve), and acetylsalicylic acid (Aspirin).

NONTRAUMATIC UNGUAL OR PERIUNGUAL FIBROMA. Fibrous growth that appears around the fingernails and/or toenails.

NONVERBAL LEARNING DISABILITY (NLD). A learning disability syndrome identified in 1989 that may overlap with some of the symptoms of Asperger syndrome.

NOREPINEPHRINE. A hormone released by nerve cells and the adrenal medulla that causes constriction of blood vessels. Norepinephrine also functions as a neurotransmitter.

NOTOCHORD. A flexible rod-shaped body found in the embryos of all vertebrates that eventually forms the spinal column.

NUCLEIC ACIDS. The cellular molecules DNA and RNA that act as coded instructions for the production of proteins and are copied for transmission of inherited traits.

NUCLEIC DNA (NDNA). The genetic material found in the nucleus of the cell.

NUCLEOSIDE ANALOGUES. The first group of effective anti-retroviral medications. They work by interfering with the AIDS virus' synthesis of DNA.

NUCLEOTIDE. Any of a group of organic molecules that link together to form the building blocks of DNA or RNA.

NYSTAGMUS. An involuntary, rhythmic movement of the eyes.

O

OBESITY. Excessive weight due to accumulation of fat, usually defined as a body mass index (BMI) of 30 or above or body weight greater than 30% above normal on standard height-weight tables.

OBSESSIVE-COMPULSIVE DISORDER (OCD). A psychoneurotic disorder characterized by obsessions and/or compulsions and anxiety or depression.

OCCIPITAL NERVES. Two pairs of nerves that originate in the area of the second and third vertebrae of the neck, and are part of a network that innervate the neck, upper back, and head.

OCCLUSION. Blockage.

OCULOPHARYNGEAL MUSCULAR DYSTROPHY (OPMD). Form of muscular dystrophy affecting adults of both sexes, and causing weakness in the eye muscles and throat.

OFF-LABEL USE. Drugs in the United States are approved by the Food and Drug Administration (FDA) for specific uses, periods of time, or dosages based on the results of clinical trials. It is legal for physicians to administer these drugs for other "off-label" or non-approved uses. It is not legal for pharmaceutical companies to advertise drugs for off-label uses.

OFFAL. The entrails and internal organs of a butchered animal. Its use as human or animal food makes it one means of transmitting some types of spongiform encephalopathies.

OLFACTORY. Pertaining to the sense of smell.

OPEN-LABEL STUDY. A type of study in which both the researchers and the subjects are aware of the drug or therapy that is being tested.

OPHTHALMOPARESIS. Paralysis of one or more of the muscles of the eye.

OPHTHALMOPLEGIA. Paralysis of the motor nerves of the eye.

OPIATE. A drug derived from opium, such as morphine, codeine, or heroin. Opiates are very effective at alleviating pain.

OPIATE BLOCKERS. A type of drug that blocks the effects of natural opiates in the system. This makes some people, including some people with autism, appear more responsive to their environment.

OPIOID. A synthetic drug, such as methadone, that has narcotic properties similar to opiates but is not derived from opium.

OPPORTUNISTIC INFECTION. An infection caused by an organism that does not cause disease in a person with a healthy immune system.

OPPOSITIONAL DEFIANT DISORDER. A disorder characterized by hostile, deliberately argumentative, and defiant behavior toward authority figures.

OPSOCLONUS. Often called "dancing eyes," this symptom involves involuntary, quick darting movements of the eyes in all directions.

OPTHALMOPLEGIA. Paralysis of the muscles that control eye movements.

OPTIC NERVE. The bundle of nerve fibers that carry visual messages from the retina to the brain.

OPTIC NEURITIS. Inflammation of the optic nerve, often accompanied by vision loss.

OREXIN. Another name for hypocretin, a chemical secreted in the hypothalmus that regulates the sleep/wake cycle. Narcolepsy is sometimes described as an orexin deficiency syndrome.

ORGANELLE. A specialized structure within a cell that is separated from the rest of the cell by a membrane composed of lipids and proteins. Organelles carry out metabolic functions.

ORGANIC BRAIN SYNDROME. A brain disorder that is caused by defective structure or abnormal functioning of the brain.

ORIENTATION. In psychiatry, the ability to locate oneself in one's environment with respect to time, place, and people.

ORTHOSTATIC HYPOTENSION. A sudden decrease in blood pressure upon sitting up or standing. May be a side effect of several types of drugs.

ORTHOTIC DEVICE. A device made of plastic, leather, or metal which provides stability at the joints or passively stretches the muscles.

OSSICLES. A group of three small bones in the middle ear that transmit sound waves to the cochlea. The three bones are called the malleus (hammer), incus (anvil), and stapes (stirrup).

OSTEOARTHRITIS. A chronic disease characterized by damage to the cartilage in the joints. The joints become inflamed, deformed, and enlarged, and movement becomes painful.

OSTEOPATHY. A system of therapy that uses standard medical and surgical methods of diagnosis and treatment while emphasizing the importance of proper body alignment and manipulative treatment of musculoskeletal disorders. Osteopathy is considered mainstream primary care medicine rather than an alternative system.

OSTEOPOROSIS. A disorder involving loss of calcium and density in the bones, resulting in brittle bones and changes in posture.

OTOLARYNGOLOGIST. A physician who specializes in medical and surgical treatment of disorders of the ear, nose, throat, and larynx. An ENT.

OTOLARYNGOLOGY. The branch of medicine that treats disorders of the ear, nose, and throat.

OTOLITH ORGANS. Two small structures (saccule and utricle) that contain calcium carbonate crystals which can cause vertigo if they enter one of the semicircular canals and displace endolymph fluid when the person changes head position.

OTOLOGY. The branch of medicine that specializes in medical or surgical treatment of ear disorders.

OTOSCLEROSIS. A growth of spongy bone in the inner ear, causing progressive hearing loss.

OTOTOXIC. Damaging to the organs or nerves involved in hearing or balance.

OVER-THE-COUNTER (OTC). A drug that can be purchased without a doctor's prescription.

OXYGEN TOXICITY. A condition marked by disorientation, breathing problems, and vision changes, caused by overexposure to molecular oxygen at elevated partial pressures. It is also known as oxygen poisoning or oxygen intoxication.

P

PAIN DISORDER. A psychiatric disorder in which pain in one or more parts of the body is caused or made worse by psychological factors. The lower back is one of the most common sites for pain related to this disorder.

PALLIDOTOMY. A surgical procedure that destroys a small part of a tiny structure within the brain called the globus pallidus internus. This structure is part of the basal ganglia, a part of the brain involved in the control of willed (voluntary) movement of the muscles.

PALPITATION. A heartbeat that is more pronounced, often felt physically.

PALSY. Paralysis or uncontrolled movement of muscles.

PANDAS DISORDERS. A group of childhood disorders associated with such streptococcal infections as scarlet fever and "strep throat." The acronym stands for Pediatric Autoimmune Neuropsychiatric Disorders Associated with Streptococcal Infections. Sydenham's chorea is considered a PANDAS disorder.

PANDEMIC. An infectious disease that spreads across a large region or even worldwide.

PANIC DISORDER. A series of unexpected attacks, involving an intense, terrifying fear similar to that caused by a life-threatening danger.

PAPILLOEDEMA. Edema or swelling in the optic disk (a portion of the optic nerve that collects nerves from the light sensitive layer of the eye, also called the retina).

PARALYSIS. The inability to use a muscle because of injury to or disease of the nerves leading to the muscle.

PARANEOPLASTIC NEUROLOGICAL DISORDER (PND). An autoimmune response to cancer cells that are producing proteins normally produced only in the brain or nervous system.

PARANEOPLASTIC SYNDROME. A syndrome in which substances produced by cancer cells prompt abnormalities in the body at a distance from the actual site of the malignancy.

PARAPARESIS. Muscle weakness or partial paralysis of the lower limbs.

PARAPHASIA. Aphasia characterized by the use of wrong words or senseless combinations of sounds or words.

PARAPLEGIA. Paralysis of the lower half of the body involving both legs and usually due to disease or injury to the spinal cord.

PARASITE. An organism that lives and feeds in or on another organism (the host) and does nothing to benefit the host.

PARASYMPATHETIC NERVOUS SYSTEM. A branch of the autonomic nervous system that tends to induce secretion, increase the tone and contraction of smooth muscle, and cause dilation of blood vessels.

PARATHYROID GLANDS. A pair of glands adjacent to the thyroid gland that primarily regulate blood calcium levels.

PARESIS. Partial or total loss of movement or sensation.

PARESTHESIA. Abnormal subjective sensations like numbness, tingling, pain, burning, or prickling that occur due to neuropathy.

PARIETAL LOBE. The middle portion of each cerebral hemisphere of the brain; associated with bodily sensations.

PARKINSON'S DISEASE. A neurological disorder caused by a deficiency of dopamine, a neurotransmitter, which is a chemical that assists in transmitting messages between the nerves within the brain. It is characterized by slowness of voluntary movements, mask-like facial expression, and a rhythmic tremor of the limbs and stooped posture.

PARKINSONIAN. Related to symptoms associated with Parkinson's disease.

PARKINSONISM. A set of symptoms originally associated with Parkinson's disease that can occur as side effects of neuroleptic medications. The symptoms include trembling of the fingers or hands, a shuffling gait, and tight or rigid muscles.

PARTIAL SEIZURE. A seizure that starts in one particular part of the brain. The abnormal electrical activity may remain confined to that area, or may spread to the entire brain. Also called a focal seizure.

PARTIAL THROMBOPLASTIN TIME (APTT). Laboratory value that measures the effectiveness of the intrinsic pathway of coagulation as well as the final common pathway.

PATHOGEN. A disease-causing organism.

PATHOPHYSIOLOGY. The changes in body functions associated with a disorder or disease.

PENETRANCE. The degree to which individuals possessing a particular genetic mutation express the trait that this mutation causes. One hundred percent penetrance is expected to be observed in truly dominant traits.

PENETRATING HEAD INJURY. A traumatic brain injury (TBI) in which an object pierces the skull and enters brain tissue.

PERCUTANEOUS ABLATION. Attempting to remove a foreign body by a method just above the skin, like using an ointment.

PERILYMPH. The fluid that lies between the membranous labyrinth of the inner ear and the bony labyrinth.

PERIODIC LIMB MOVEMENT DISORDER (PLMD). A neurological disorder that often accompanies restless legs syndrome.

PERIODIC LIMB MOVEMENTS IN SLEEP (PLMS). Random movements of the arms or legs that occur at regular intervals of time during sleep.

PERIPHERAL BLOOD STEM CELLS (PBSC). Blood-cell-forming stem cells in circulating blood.

PERIPHERAL NERVES. Nerves outside the brain and spinal cord (throughout the body) that carry information to and from the spinal cord.

PERIPHERAL NERVOUS SYSTEM (PNS). One of the two major divisions of the nervous system. PNS nerves link the central nervous system with sensory organs, muscles, blood vessels, and glands.

PERIPHERAL NEUROPATHY. Any disease of the nerves outside of the spinal cord, usually resulting in weakness and/or numbness.

PERIVENTRICULAR. Located around the brain's ventricles.

PEROXISOME. A cellular organelle containing different enzymes responsible for the breakdown of waste or other products.

PERSEVERATION. Continuous involuntary repetition of speech or behavior.

PERSISTENT VEGETATIVE STATE (PVS). Severely impaired consciousness in which a patient is incapable of voluntary movement, but with sleep/wake cycles and eye opening; a coma lasting more than four weeks.

PERVASIVE DEVELOPMENTAL DISORDER (PDD). The term used by the American Psychiatric Association for individuals who meet some but not all of the criteria for autism.

PETECHIA. A tiny, purplish-red spot on the skin. Caused by the leakage of a bit of blood out of a vessel and under the skin.

PEYER'S PATCHES. Clumps of lymphoid tissue found in the lower section of the small intestine that function to protect the intestines from dangerous microorganisms. There are about 30 Peyer's patches in the human small intestine. The patches are named for their discoverer, Johann Conrad Peyer (1653–1712), a Swiss anatomist.

PHALILALIA. Involuntary echoing of the last word, phrase, sentence, or sound vocalized by oneself.

PHARYNGITIS. Inflammation of the throat, accompanied by dryness and pain. Pharyngitis caused by a streptococcal infection is the usual trigger of Sydenham's chorea.

PHARYNX. The muscular cavity that leads from the mouth and nasal passages to the larynx and esophagus.

PHENOTYPE. The externally observable characters of an organism due to genetic and environmental effects on development. The physical expression of an individual's genes.

PHENYLKETONURIA (PKU). An inborn error in metabolism that prevents the body from using phenylalanine, an amino acid necessary for normal growth and development.

PHEOCHROMOCYTOMA. Non-cancerous growth in the adrenal gland.

PHOBIA. A persistent abnormal fear of an object, experience, or place.

PHOBIC DISORDER. Persistent fear of social situations, objects, or specific situations.

PHONEME. A basic unit of sound in a language.

PHONOLOGICAL. Language sounds.

PHOTON. A light particle.

PHYSICAL ACTIVITY. Any activity that involves moving the body and burning calories.

PHYSICAL FITNESS. A combination of muscle strength, cardiovascular health, and flexibility that is usually attributed to regular exercise and good nutrition.

PHYTANIC ACID. A substance found in various foods that, if allowed to accumulate, is toxic to various tissues. It is metabolized in the peroxisome by phytanic acid hydroxylase.

PHYTANIC ACID HYDROXYLASE. A peroxisomal enzyme responsible for processing phytanic acid. It is defective in Refsum disease.

PIA MATER. The innermost of the three meninges covering the brain.

PICK'S DISEASE. A rare type of primary dementia that affects the frontal lobes of the brain. It is characterized by a progressive loss of social skills, language, and memory, leading to personality changes and sometimes loss of moral judgment.

PINNA. The visible part of the outer ear.

PITCH. The property of sound that is determined by the frequency of sound wave vibrations reaching the ear.

PITUITARY GLAND. The most important of the endocrine glands (glands that release hormones directly into the bloodstream), the pituitary is located at the base of the brain. Sometimes referred to as the "master gland," it regulates and controls the activities of other endocrine glands and many body processes including growth and reproductive function. Also called the hypophysis.

PLAQUE. A deposit of calcium, cholesterol, white blood cells, and other debris that can build up on the inner walls of arteries, leading to stenosis and eventual rupture of the artery or stroke.

PLASMA. The clear yellowish liquid portion of blood.

PLASMAPHERESIS. The removal, treatment, and return of blood plasma; used to remove autoantibodies or immune complexes from the blood.

PLATELETS. Blood cells that are a critical part of hemostasis and clot formation.

PLURIPOTENT STEM CELL. A stem cell that can differentiate into any of the cell types found in an organism.

POINT OF VIEW. In a person with dyslexia, this term is used to describe the angle from which their mind's eye views an object. This point of view may be unanchored and moving about, as if several different people were telling what they see all at the same time.

POLYDACTYLY. The presence of extra fingers or toes.

POLYDIPSIA. Excessive thirst.

POLYGENIC. A trait or disorder that is determined by several different genes. Most human characteristics, including height, weight, and general body build, are polygenic. Schizophrenia and late-onset Alzheimer's disease are considered polygenic disorders.

POLYMORPHISM. A difference in DNA sequence among individuals; genetic variation.

POLYSOMNOGRAPHY, POLYSOMNOGRAM (PSG). A group of tests administered to analyze heart, blood, and breathing patterns during sleep.

POLYURIA. Excessive production and excretion of urine.

POOR MUSCLE TONE. Muscles that are weak and floppy.

PORT-WINE STAIN. Dark-red birthmarks seen on the skin, named after the color of the dessert wine.

PORTAL HYPERTENSION. A condition caused by cirrhosis of the liver. It is characterized by impaired or reversed blood flow from the portal vein to the liver, an enlarged spleen, and dilated veins in the esophagus and stomach.

PORTAL VEIN THROMBOSIS. The development of a blood clot in the vein that brings blood into the liver. Untreated portal vein thrombosis causes portal hypertension.

POSITIVE SYMPTOMS. Symptoms of schizophrenia that are characterized by the production or presence of behaviors that are grossly abnormal or excessive, including hallucinations and thought-process disorder.

POSITRON. One of the small particles that make up an atom. A positron has the same mass and amount of charge as an electron, but the positron has a positive charge.

POSITRON EMISSION TOMOGRAPHY (PET). A diagnostic technique in which computer-assisted x rays are used to track a radioactive substance inside a patient's body. Biochemical activity of the brain can be studied using PET.

POST-CONCUSSION SYNDROME. A complex of symptoms including headache following mild TBI.

POST-EXPOSURE PROPHYLAXIS (PEP). A four-week course of antiretroviral drugs given to people immediately following exposure to HIV infection from rape, unprotected sex, needlestick injuries, or sharing needles.

POST-HERPETIC NEURALGIA (PHN). Long-lasting nerve pain caused by herpes zoster.

POST-TRAUMATIC AMNESIA (PTA). Difficulty forming new memories after traumatic brain injury (TBI).

POST-TRAUMATIC DEMENTIA. Persistent mental deterioration following traumatic brain injury (TBI).

POST-TRAUMATIC EPILEPSY. Seizures occurring more than one week after traumatic brain injury (TBI).

POSTERIOR COLUMN. Long fiber tracts that run in the spinal cord, carrying vibratory and position sense from the limbs to the brain.

POSTERIOR FOSSA. Area at the base of the skull attached to the spinal cord.

POSTICTAL. The time period immediately following a seizure.

POSTMORTEM. After death.

POSTURAL DRAINAGE. The use of positioning to drain secretions from the bronchial tubes and lungs into the trachea or windpipe.

POSTURAL HYPOTENSION. A condition in which a person's blood pressure drops sharply when they stand or rise suddenly. It is characterized by dizziness, difficulty keeping one's balance, lightheadedness, and occasional headache. It is sometimes called orthostatic hypotension.

POSTUROGRAPHY. A technique for assessing balance disorders by having the patient stand on a platform that can be moved or tilted in various directions while a computer records the patient's body movements as he or she attempts to maintain balance.

POVERTY OF SPEECH. A negative symptom of schizophrenia, characterized by brief and empty replies to questions. It should not be confused with shyness or reluctance to talk.

PRECHORDAL PLATE. A thickened region of endodermal tissue located toward the head end of the developing embryo.

PREDNISONE. A corticosteroid often used to treat inflammation.

PREGNANCY CATEGORY. A system of classifying drugs according to their established risks for use during pregnancy. Category A: Controlled human studies have demonstrated no fetal risk. Category B: Animal studies indicate no fetal risk, but no human studies; or adverse effects in animals, but not in well-controlled human studies. Category C: No adequate human or animal studies; or adverse fetal effects in animal studies, but no available human data. Category D: Evidence of fetal risk, but benefits outweigh risks. Category X: Evidence of fetal risk. Risks outweigh any benefits.

PREMONITORY URGE. A feeling or sensation that warns a person with a tic disorder that tension is building up. Expressing the tic brings relief from the urge.

PRENATAL TESTING. Testing for a disease, such as a genetic condition, in an unborn baby.

PRESBYCUSIS. Hearing loss due to degenerative changes in the ear, usually associated with aging.

PRESENILE DEMENTIA. The original name for Alzheimer's disease.

PRESENILIN (PSEN). Presenilin 1 and presenilin 2 are proteins that are involved in processing amyloid precursor protein (APP). Mutations in the genes encoding these proteins can cause early-onset AD.

PRESYNAPTIC. Before the synapse.

PREVALENCE. The number of cases of a specific disease in a population at a specific point in time, divided by the total number of individuals in the population.

PRIMARY CRANIOSYNOSTOSIS. Abnormal closure of the cranial sutures caused by an abnormality in the sutures themselves.

PRIMARY HEADACHE. A headache that has no identifiable underlying cause.

PRIMARY HEMOSTASIS. The initial activities that occur in response to blood vessel damage that initiate clot formation.

PRIMARY PROGRESSIVE. A pattern of symptoms of MS in which the disorder progresses without remission, or with occasional plateaus or slight improvements.

PRIMARY TUMOR. Abnormal growths that originated in the location where they have are diagnosed.

PRION. An infectious agent consisting of protein in a misfolded form. Its name is a combination of "protein" and "infection."

PROBIOTICS. Treatment with beneficial microbes, either by ingestion or through a rectal or vaginal suppository, to restore a healthy balance of bacteria to the body.

PRODROME. A symptom or group of symptoms that appears shortly before an acute attack of illness. The term comes from a Greek word that means "running ahead of."

PROGENITOR. A cell that has differentiated from a stem cell and is committed to developing into a specific cell type.

PROGLOTTID. Section of growth of an adult pork tapeworm that contains both male and female reproductive capacity, is released from the adult with the ability to independently function, and then exits the body and produces eggs.

PROGRESSIVE SUPRANUCLEAR PALSY. A rare disease that shows some of the same features of PD, but differs in several ways. People with progressive supranuclear palsy usually do not develop tremors, but they have rigidity, bradykinesia (slow movements), and falls. The disorder gradually destroys nerve cells in the parts of the brain that control eye movements, breathing, and muscle coordination. The loss of nerve cells causes palsy (paralysis) that slowly gets worse as the disease progresses. The palsy affects the ability to move the eyes vertically (up and down) at first. Their eye movements then become even more restrictive (ophthalmoplegia). The ability to relax the muscles is lost, as is control over balance.

PROJECTILE VOMITING. Forceful vomiting that is not preceded by nausea. It is usually associated with increased pressure inside the head.

PRONATION. The motion of the forearm to turn the palm downwards.

PROPHYLACTIC. Guarding from or preventing the spread or occurrence of disease or infection.

PROPHYLAXIS. A measure taken to prevent disease or an acute attack of a chronic disorder. Migraine prophylaxis refers to medications taken to reduce the frequency of migraine attacks.

PROPRIOCEPTION. A person's normal sense of posture, balance, direction of movement, and location in space.

PROPRIOCEPTION. The ability to sense the location and postion and orientation and movement of the body and its parts.

PROPTOSIS. Bulging eyeballs.

PROSENCEPHALON. The medical term for the forebrain.

PROSTAGLANDIN. Chemical substance that participates in a wide range of body functions including the production of pain and fever associated with inflammation, the protection of stomach lining, and blood clot formation.

PROSTAGLANDINS. A group of hormonelike molecules that exert local effects on a variety of processes including fluid balance, blood flow, and gastrointestinal function. They may be responsible for the production of some types of pain and inflammation.

PROTEASE INHIBITORS. The second major category of drug used to treat AIDS that works by suppressing the replication of HIV.

PROTEIN. Important building blocks of the body, composed of amino acids, involved in the formation of body structures and controlling the basic functions of the human body.

PROTEINURIA. Excess protein in the urine.

PROTHROMBIN TIME. Measurement of the clotting tendency of blood, specifically the extrinsic aspect of the clotting cascade.

PROTHROMBOTIC STATE. Physiological state in which the blood will tend to clot more.

PSEUDODEMENTIA. Depression with symptoms resembling those of dementia. The term "dementia of depression" is now preferred.

PSYCHODYNAMIC THERAPIES. A form of psychological counseling that seeks to determine and resolve the internal conflicts that may be causing an individual to be suffering from the symptoms of depression.

PSYCHOGENIC NON-EPILEPTIC SEIZURES (PNES). Pseudoseizures, non-epileptic events, non-epileptic paroxysmal events, psychogenic non-epileptic status epilepticus (PNESE), or psychogenic non-epileptic attacks (PNEA); seizures, episodes, or events that resemble epilepsy but which are caused by psychological factors rather than by brain abnormalities.

PSYCHOGENIC TREMOR. Tremor associated with a psychiatric disorder.

PSYCHOMOTOR RETARDATION. Slowing of movement and speech.

PSYCHOSIS. A severe mental disorder characterized by loss of contact with reality. Hallucinations are associated with such psychotic disorders as schizophrenia and brief psychotic disorder.

PSYCHOTHERAPY. Psychological counseling that seeks to determine the underlying causes of a patient's depression. The form of this counseling may be cognitive/behavioral, interpersonal, or psychodynamic.

PTOSIS. Eyelid droop.

PULMONARY EMBOLISM. Condition in which the main artery of a lung is blocked by an embolus that has traveled from elsewhere in the body.

PULSATILE TINNITUS. Objective tinnitus in which the pulse or heartbeat is heard in the ear.

PURKINJE'S CELLS. Large branching cells of the nervous system.

PURPURA. A large, purplish-red circle on the skin. Caused by the leakage of blood out of a vessel and under the skin.

PUSTULE. A pus-filled lesion of the skin that resembles the "pimples" of adolescent acne.

PYRIDOSTIGMINE BROMIDE (MESTINON). An anticholinesterase drug used in treating myasthenia gravis.

Q

QUADRIPARESIS. Partial or incomplete paralysis of all four limbs.

QUADRIPLEGIA. Permanent paralysis of the trunk, lower and upper limbs. It is caused by injury or disease affecting the spinal cord at the neck level.

QUINACRINE. An antimalarial drug that is being tested as a possible treatment for prion diseases.

R

RADICULONEURITIS. Inflammation of a spinal nerve.

RADICULOPATHY. A bulging of disc material often irritating nearby nerve structures resulting in pain and neurologic symptoms. A clinical situation in which the radicular nerves (nerve roots) are inflamed or compressed. This compression by the bulging disc is referred to as a radiculopathy. This problem tends to occur most commonly in the neck (cervical spine) and low back (lumbar spine).

RADIO WAVES. Electromagnetic energy of the frequency range corresponding to that used in radio communications, usually 10,000 cycles per second to 300 billion cycles per second. Radio waves are the same as visible light, x rays, and all other types of electromagnetic radiation, but are of a higher frequency.

RADIOGRAPHY. The use of x rays to create photographic records on specially sensitized plates or films.

RADIOISOTOPE. One of two or more atoms with the same number of protons but a different number of neutrons. In nuclear scanning, radioactive isotopes are used as diagnostic agents.

RADIOLOGIST. A medical doctor specially trained in radiology (x-ray) interpretation and its use in the diagnosis of disease and injury.

RADIOTHERAPY. The use of x rays or other radioactive substances to treat disease.

RANGE OF MOTION (ROM). The range of motion of a joint from full extension to full flexion (bending) measured in degrees like a circle.

RAYNAUD'S PHENOMENON. A disorder characterized by episodic attacks of loss of circulation in the fingers or toes. Most cases of Raynaud's are not work-related; however, the disorder occasionally develops in workers who operate vibrating tools as part of their job, and is sometimes called vibration-induced white finger.

REBOUND HEADACHE. A type of primary headache caused by overuse of migraine medications or pain relievers. It is also known as analgesic abuse headache.

RECEPTOR. A structure located on the outside of a cell's membrane that causes the cell to attach to specific molecules; the molecules are then internalized, taken inside the cell.

RECESSIVE. Producing little or no phenotypic effect when occurring in heterozygous condition with a contrasting allele.

RECESSIVE GENE. A type of gene that is not expressed as a trait unless inherited by both parents.

RECOMBINANT HUMAN GROWTH HORMONE. A synthetic form of growth hormone that can be given to a patient to help skeletal growth.

RED BLOOD CELL (RBC). Part of the blood responsible for its red color and oxygen transport to body tissues.

REFERRED PAIN. Pain felt at a site different from the location of the injured or diseased part of the body. Referred pain is due to the fact that nerve signals from several areas of the body may "feed" the same nerve pathway leading to the spinal cord and brain.

REFLEX SEIZURE. Seizure brought on by specific sensory stimuli.

RELAPSE. Recurrence of an illness after a period of improvement.

RELAPSING-REMITTING. A pattern of symptoms of MS in which symptomatic attacks occur that last 24 hours or more, followed by complete or almost complete improvement.

RELEASE HALLUCINATIONS. Hallucinations that develop after partial loss of sight or hearing, and represent images or sounds formed from memory traces rather than present sensory input. They are called "release" hallucinations because they would ordinarily be blocked by incoming sensory data.

REM. Rapid eye movement; a stage of the normal sleep cycle characterized by rapid eye movements, increased forebrain and midbrain activity, and dreaming.

REM SLEEP BEHAVIOR DISORDER (RBD). The acting out of wild or violent dreams and hallucinations during REM sleep; an early symptom of Parkinson's disease.

REMISSION. When active symptoms of a chronic disease are absent.

RENAL CELL CARCINOMA. A type of kidney cancer.

RESONATOR. As used in regard to the human speech mechanism, it is the cavity extending from the vocal folds to the lips, which selectively amplifies and modifies the energies produced during speech and voice production. It is synonymous with the term vocal tract.

RESTENOSIS. The repeated narrowing of blood vessels.

RESTLESS LEGS SYNDROME (RLS). A neurological disorder characterized by aching, burning, or creeping sensations in the legs and an urge to move the legs, often resulting in insomnia.

RETICULAR ACTIVATING SYSTEM. A network of structures, including the brainstem, medulla, and thalamus, and nerve pathways, which function together to produce and maintain arousal.

RETICULAR ACTIVATING SYSTEM. Ascending arousal system; a nerve network extending from the brainstem through the cerebral cortex that controls the degree of activity in the central nervous system, maintaining sleep and wakefulness and controlling transitions between states of consciousness.

RETINA. Light-sensitive tissue on the back of the eye that receives images and converts them into nerve impulses to be sent to the brain by way of the optic nerve.

RETINAL ACHROMIC PATCH. Small area on the retina of the eye that is lighter than the area around it.

RETINITIS PIGMENTOSA. A family of genetically linked retinal diseases that cause progressive deterioration of peripheral vision and eventually blindness.

RETINOPATHY. Noninflammatory or degenerative condition involving the retina of the eye.

RETRACTOR. An instrument used during surgery to hold an incision open and pull back underlying layers of tissue.

RETROGRADE AMNESIA. Amnesia for events that occurred before a traumatic injury.

RETROVIRUS. A group of viruses that contain RNA and the enzyme reverse transcriptase. These viruses produce DNA that they add to the genetic material of infected cells. Many viruses in this family cause tumors. The virus that causes AIDS is a retrovirus.

REVIEW OF SYSTEMS (ROS). A systematic checklist of the various organ systems in the human body, used to ensure that all relevant physical signs and symptoms have been taken into account during a medical or psychiatric evaluation.

REYE'S SYNDROME. A life-threatening illness in children that usually follows the flu or chickenpox and is often associated with the use of aspirin and an underlying disorder of fatty acid metabolism.

RHABDOMYOLYSIS. Breakdown of muscle fibers resulting in release of muscle contents into the blood.

RHABDOMYOMA. Noncancerous growth in the heart muscle.

RHEUMATIC DISEASE. A type of disease involving inflammation of muscles, joints, and other tissues.

RHEUMATIC FEVER. Chiefly childhood disease marked by fever, inflammation, joint pain, and Sydenham's chorea. It is often recurrent and can lead to heart valve damage.

RHINITIS. Inflammation and swelling of the nasal membranes.

RHIZOTOMY. Surgery to relieve pain by cutting the nerve root near its point of entry to the spinal cord.

RODENTICIDES. Chemical that kills rodents.

ROMBERG TEST. A balance test that evaluates a person's proprioception and the condition of their vestibular system. The person is asked to stand upright on both feet with the eyes closed for a timed period of one minute. The test is positive if the person sways or falls within the timed period.

RUBELLA. Also known as German measles. When a woman contracts rubella during pregnancy, her developing infant may be damaged. One of the problems that may result is autism.

S

SACCULAR ANEURYSM. A type of aneurysm that resembles a small sack of blood attached to the outer surface of a blood vessel by a thin neck.

SACROILIAC JOINT. The joint between the triangular bone below the spine (sacrum) and the hip bone (ilium).

SACRUM. An area in the lower back, below the lumbar region.

SCANNING. A method of item selection on an AAC device in which a light beam, another type of visual indicator, or communication partner moves over (scans) the items on a communication board. When the indicator reaches the desired item, the user operates a switch or nods the head to select the item.

SCAPHOCEPHALY. An abnormally long and narrow skull.

SCAPULA. The bone also known as the shoulder blade.

SCHIZOPHRENIA. A severe mental disorder in which a person loses touch with reality and may have illogical thoughts, delusions, hallucinations, behavioral problems, and other disturbances.

SCHWANN CELL. A type of supportive cell in the nervous system that compose the myelin sheath around nerve fibers.

SCIATICA. A common form of nerve pain related to compression of fibers from one or more of the lower spinal nerve roots, characterized by burning low back pain radiating to the buttock and back of the leg to below the knee or even to the foot.

SCLERA. The tough white membrane that forms the outer layer of the eyeball.

SCOLEX. Head portion of the pork tapeworm with hooks and suckers to attach to body tissues.

SCOLIOSIS. A medical condition in which the spine is curved abnormally from side to side as well as from front to back. Scoliosis may be congenital, idiopathic (of unknown cause), or the result of a neuromuscular disorder.

SEASONAL AFFECTIVE DISORDER (SAD). A mood disorder related to major depressive disorder in which the patient's symptoms are correlated with changes in the length and intensity of daylight over the course of the changing seasons.

SECONDARY CRANIOSYNOSTOSIS. Abnormal closure of the cranial sutures caused by a failure of the brain to grow and expand.

SECONDARY HEADACHE. A headache caused by an underlying condition or disease.

SECONDARY HEMOSTASIS. A later stage of hemostasis where a formed clot is stabilized and blood vessels constrict to conserve blood loss.

SECONDARY PROGRESSIVE. A pattern of symptoms of MS in which there are relapses and remissions, followed by more steady progression of symptoms.

SEDATIVE. A medication that has a calming effect and may be used to treat nervousness or restlessness. Sometimes used as a synonym for hypnotic.

SEDENTARY. Inactivity and lack of exercise; a lifestyle that is a major risk factor for becoming overweight or obese and developing chronic diseases.

SEIZURE. A convulsion, or uncontrolled discharge of nerve cells that may spread to other cells throughout the brain, resulting in abnormal body movements or behaviors.

SELECTIVE RELAXANT BINDING AGENTS (SRBAS). A new class of drugs that can be used to reverse the effects of neuromuscular blockers. Sugammadex is the first drug in this category. It was discovered in Scotland in 2007.

SELECTIVE SEROTONIN REUPTAKE INHIBITOR (SSRI). A type of antidepressant, such as fluoxetine, that inhibits the inactivation of the neurotransmitter serotonin by blocking its reuptake by neurons.

SELF-RENEWAL. The process by which stem cells divide and replace themselves indefinitely.

SEMANTIC COMPACTION. A way to represent language in an AAC system that involves the use of short sequences of icons or pictorial symbols to form words. It is sometimes referred to as Minspeak.

SENSORIUM. The place in the brain where external expressions are localized and processed before being perceived.

SENSORY. Refers to peripheral nerves that transmit information from the senses to the brain.

SENSORY ATAXIA. A form of ataxia in which the person has not lost cerebellar control of movement but has lost sensory input into control of movement.

SENSORY NERVES. Sensory or afferent nerves carry impulses of sensation from the periphery or outward parts of the body to the brain. Sensations include feelings, impressions, and awareness of the state of the body.

SEPSIS. The presence of infection-causing organisms or associated toxins in the blood or within body tissues.

SEPTUM PELLUCIDUM. Two-layered thin wall separating the right and the left anterior horn of lateral ventricle.

SEQUENCING. Genetic testing in which the entire sequence of deoxyribonucleic (DNA) bases that make up a gene is studied in order to detect a mutation.

SERIAL CASTING. A series of casts designed to gradually move a limb into a more functional position.

SEROCONVERSION. The development of detectable specific antibodies in a patient's blood serum as a result of infection or immunization.

SEROTONIN. 5-Hydroxytryptamine; a neurotransmitter that occurs throughout the body, including in blood platelets, the lining of the digestive tract, and the brain. It causes very powerful contractions of smooth muscle and is associated with mood, attention, emotions, and sleep. Low serotonin levels are associated with mood disorders, particularly depression and obsessive-compulsive disorder.

SEROTONIN DOPAMINE ANTAGONISTS (SDA). The newer second-generation antipsychotic drugs, also called atypical antipsychotics. SDAs include clozapine (Clozaril), risperidone (Risperdal), aripiprazole (Abilify), and olanzapine (Zyprexa).

SEROTONIN SYNDROME. A potentially life-threatening drug reaction involving an excess of the neurotransmitter serotonin, usually occurring when too many medications that increase serotonin are taken together such as antimigraine triptans and certain antidepressants.

SERUM. The fluid part of the blood that remains after blood cells, platelets, and fibrogen have been removed. Also called blood serum.

SERUM CK TEST. A blood test that determines the amount of the enzyme creatine kinase (CK) in the blood serum. An elevated level of CK in the blood indicates that muscular degeneration has occurred and/or is occurring.

SHAGREEN PATCHES. Patches of skin with the consistency of an orange peel.

SHAKEN BABY SYNDROME. A severe form of TBI resulting from shaking an infant or small child forcibly enough to cause the brain to jar against the skull.

SHINGLES. An disease caused by an infection with the herpes zoster virus, the same virus that causes chickenpox. Symptoms of shingles include pain and blisters along one nerve, usually on the face, chest, stomach, or back.

SHOULDER DYSTOCIA. Difficult shoulder delivery.

SHUNT. A channel through which blood or another body fluid is diverted from its normal path by surgical reconstruction or the insertion of a synthetic tube.

SICKLE CELL DISEASE. An inherited disorder characterized by a genetic flaw in hemoglobin production. (Hemoglobin is the substance within red blood cells that enables them to transport oxygen.) The hemoglobin that is produced has a kink in its structure that forces the red blood cells to take on a sickle shape, inhibiting their circulation and causing pain. This disorder primarily affects people of African descent.

SKIN TAG. Abnormal outward pouching of skin, with a varying size.

SLEEP APNEA. Temporary cessation of breathing while sleeping.

SLEEP PARALYSIS. An abnormal episode of sleep in which the patient cannot move for a few minutes, usually occurring on falling asleep or waking up. Often found in patients with narcolepsy.

SLOW-WAVE SLEEP. Deep, usually dreamless sleep, that occurs regularly between intervals of REM sleep.

SOMATIZATION DISORDER. A chronic condition in which psychological stresses are converted into physical symptoms that interfere with work and relationships. Lower back pain is a frequent complaint of patients with somatization disorder.

SOMATOFORM DISORDERS. A group of psychological disorders characterized by physical complaints for which no physiological explanation can be found and which probably involve psychological factors.

SOMNAMBULISM. Motor actions, such as walking, during sleep.

SOMNILOQUY. Sleep talking.

SONIC HEDGEHOG (SHH). The shorthand term for a protein involved in the mammalian signaling pathway that plays a critical role in organ development and the organization of the brain. It was named for a character in a 1991 video game.

SPASMS. Sudden involuntary muscle movement or contraction.

SPASTIC. Involving uncontrollable, jerky contractions of the muscles.

SPASTIC HEMIPLEGIA. A form of cerebral palsy that effects the arm and leg on one side of the body; also known as spastic hemiparesis.

SPASTIC PARAPLEGIA GENE (SPG). One of a number of different genes in which mutations can cause hereditary spastic paraplegia.

SPASTIC QUADRIPLEGIA. Inability to use and control movements of the arms and legs.

SPASTICITY. Abnormally high muscle tone, stiffness, in skeletal muscle, often caused by damage to upper motor neurons in the central nervous system.

SPEECH SYNTHESIS. The artificial production of human speech through combining stored units of speech in the user's native language to produce individualized messages.

SPEECH SYNTHESIZER. A computerized device that accepts input, interprets data, and produces audible language.

SPEECH-GENERATING DEVICE (SGD). A dedicated electronic device that allows an AAC user to produce audible speech, either by selecting from a digitized collection of messages or by producing new messages through speech synthesis.

SPEECH-LANGUAGE PATHOLOGIST. A non-physician health care provider who evaluates and treats disorders of communication and swallowing.

SPHENOIDAL ELECTRODES. Fine wire electrodes that are implanted under the cheek bones, used to measure temporal seizures.

SPIKE WAVE DISCHARGE. Characteristic abnormal wave pattern in the electroencephalogram that is a hallmark of an area that has the potential of generating a seizure.

SPINA BIFIDA. A birth defect in which the neural tube fails to close during fetal development and a portion of the spinal cord and nerves fail to develop properly.

SPINA BIFIDA OCCULTA. A relatively mild form of spina bifida in which the defect is not visible from the surface.

SPINAL CORD. The part of the central nervous system that extends from the base of the skull and runs through the vertebral column in the back. It acts as a relay to convey information between the brain and the periphery.

SPINAL DEGENERATION. Wear and tear on the intervertebral discs, which can narrow the spinal canal and cause back stiffness and pain.

SPINAL FUSION. A surgical procedure that stabilizes the spine and prevents painful movements, but with resulting loss of flexibility.

SPINAL LAMINECTOMY (SPINAL DECOMPRESSION). Surgical removal of a piece of the bony roof of the spinal canal known as the lamina to increase the size of the spinal canal and reduce pressure on the spinal cord and nerve roots.

SPINAL STENOSIS. Narrowing of the canals in the vertebrae or around the nerve roots, causing pressure on the spinal cord and nerves.

SPINAL TAP. A procedure by which a needle is inserted into the space between two lumbar vertebrae to obtain fluid that circulates around the spinal cord. Also called a lumbar puncture.

SPIRAL CT. Also referred to as helical CT, this method allows for continuous 360-degree x-ray image capture.

SPIROCHETE. A spiral-shaped bacterium. The bacteria that cause Lyme disease and syphilis, for example, are spirochetes.

SPONDYLITIS. Inflammation of the spinal joints, characterized by chronic back pain and stiffness.

SPONDYLOLISTHESIS. A more extreme form of spondylosis, with slippage of one vertebra relative to its neighbor.

SPONDYLOSIS. A degenerative condition of the cervical spine, causing narrowing of the bony canal through which the spinal cord passes.

SPORADIC. Occurring at random.

SPORES. A state of "suspended animation" that some bacteria can adopt when conditions are not ideal for growth. Spores are analogous to plant seeds and can germinate into growing bacteria when conditions are right.

ST. VITUS' DANCE. Another name for Sydenham's chorea. St. Vitus was a fourth-century martyr who became the patron saint of dancers and actors during the Middle Ages. He was also invoked for protection against nervous disorders, epilepsy, and the disease that bears his name.

STATIC ENCEPHALOPATHY. A disease of the brain that does not get better or worse.

STATINS. A group of medications given to lower blood cholesterol levels that work by inhibiting an enzyme involved in cholesterol formation. Statins are also known as HMG-CoA reductase inhibitors.

STATUS EPILEPTICUS. An acute prolonged brain seizure lasting 30 minutes or more.

STATUS MIGRAINOSUS. The medical term for an acute migraine headache that lasts 72 hours or longer.

STELLATE. A star-like, lacy white pattern in the iris. Most often seen in light-eyed individuals.

STENOSIS (PLURAL, STENOSES). An abnormal narrowing in a blood vessel or other hollow tubular organ. It is also known as a stricture.

STENT. A wire tube or tube-like device placed in a blood vessel to keep it permanently open.

STEROID. A naturally occurring hormone, and a large class of drugs that chemically resemble cholesterol. Among the more common types of steroids, anabolic steroids are sometimes used illegally in athletics, and glucocorticoid steroids are used to reduce inflammation.

STIMULANT. Any chemical or drug that has excitatory actions in the central nervous system.

STIMULUS. A factor capable of eliciting a response in a nerve.

STOKES-ADAMS SYNDROME. Recurrent episodes of temporary loss of consciousness (fainting) caused by an insufficient flow of blood from the heart to the brain. This syndrome is caused by a very rapid or a very slow heartbeat.

STRABISMUS. Deviation of one eye from parallelism with the other.

STREP INFECTION. An infection, such as strep throat, caused by the bacteria known as group A *Streptococcus*.

STREPTOCOCCUS (PLURAL, STREPTOCOCCI). A genus of spherical-shaped anaerobic bacteria occurring in pairs or chains. Sydenham's chorea is considered a complication of a streptococcal throat infection.

STRESS TEST. An electrocardiogram recorded before, during, and after a period of increasingly strenuous cardiovascular exercise, usually on a treadmill or stationary bicycle.

STRIATUM. Structure inside the forebrain comprised of the caudate nucleus and the lentricular nucleus. The term is sometimes used to include the putamen and the globus pallidus.

STRIDOR. A high-pitched sound made when breathing caused by the narrowing of the airway.

STROKE. Also called as cerebrovascular accident (CVA) or cerebral infarction, it occurs when there is interruption of blood supply to a portion of the brain or spinal cord, resulting in damage or death of the tissue.

STRUCTURED INTERVIEW. A type of interview often used by researchers or clinicians to gather data, in which subjects (or patients) are asked a series of standardized questions in the same order with the same wording. The questions are usually closed-ended (meaning the choice of answers is fixed in advance), although some structured interviews include a few open-ended questions.

STUPOR. A decreased level of consciousness in which a person responds only to painful stimuli.

STUTTERING. Speech disorder characterized by speech that has more dysfluencies than is considered average.

SUBARACHNOID. The space underneath the layer of meningeal membrane called the arachnoid.

SUBARACHNOID HEMORRHAGE. A cause of some strokes, bleeding that occurs underneath the arachnoid membrane, a layer of the meninges.

SUBARACHNOID SPACE. The space between two membranes surrounding the spinal cord and brain, the arachnoid and pia mater.

SUBCLAVIAN. Located beneath the collarbone (clavicle).

SUBCORTICAL. The neural centers located below (inferior to) the cerebral cortex.

SUBCORTICAL APHASIA. A condition characterized by either partial or total loss of the ability to communicate verbally or use written words as a result of damage to non language-dominated areas of the brain. This condition may be caused by a stroke, head injury, brain tumor, or infection.

SUBCUTANEOUS INJECTION. Injection of a substance such as medication placed just under the surface of the skin.

SUBDURAL ELECTRODES. Strip electrodes that are placed under dura mater (the outermost, toughest, and most fibrous of the three membranes [meninges] covering the brain and spinal cord). They are used to locate foci of epileptic seizures prior to epilepsy surgery.

SUBDURAL HEMATOMA. A collection of blood or a clot trapped under the dura matter, the outermost membrane surrounding the brain and spinal cord, often causing neurological damage due to pressure on the brain.

SUBEPENDYMAL GIANT CELL ASTROCYTOMA. Benign (non-cancerous) tumor of the brain comprised of star-shaped cells (astrocytes).

SUBEPENDYMAL NODULE. Growth found underneath the lining of the ventricles in the brain.

SUBSTANTIA NIGRA. A structure in the midbrain that plays a role in eye movement, learning, reward seeking, and addiction. The death of dopaminergic nerve cells in the substantia nigra is the primary cause of Parkinson's disease. The name of the structure means "black substance" in Latin.

SULFONAMIDES. A group of antibiotics used to treat a wide range of bacterial infections.

SUNSETTING. Confusion or agitation in the evening.

SUPERIOR OBLIQUE MUSCLE. One of six extraocular muscles concerned with eye movement. The superior oblique muscle pushes the eye down, turns it inward and rotates it outward.

SYDENHAM CHOREA (SD). Saint Vitus dance; an autoimmune neurological disorder of childhood resulting from a group A *Streptococcus* infection and characterized by abnormal involuntary movements.

SYLVIAN FISSURE. The lateral fold separating the brain hemisphere into the frontal and temporal lobes.

SYMPATHETIC NERVOUS SYSTEM. A branch of the autonomic nervous system that regulates involuntary reactions to stress such as increased heart and breathing rates, blood vessel contraction, and reduction in digestive secretions.

SYMPATHETIC SKIN RESPONSE. Minute change of palmar and plantar electrical potential.

SYNAPSE. A junction between two neurons. At a synapse the neurons are separated by a tiny gap called the synaptic cleft.

SYNCOPE. A loss of consciousness over a short period of time, caused by a temporary lack of oxygen in the brain.

SYNEGENEIC. A transplant in which the donor and recipient are identical twins or triplets.

SYPHILIS. Sexually transmitted disease caused by a corkscrew shaped bacterium called Treponema pallidum. It is characterized by three clinical stages namely primary, secondary and tertiary or late syphilis.

SYRINGOMYELIA. A chronic disease involving abnormal accumulations of fluid within the spinal column.

SYRINX. Abnormal fluid-filled cavities within the spinal cord.

SYSTEMIC LUPUS ERYTHEMATOSUS (SLE). A chronic, inflammatory, autoimmune disorder in which the individual's immune system attacks, injures, and destroys the body's own organs and tissues. It may affect many organ systems including the skin, joints, lungs, heart, and kidneys.

SYSTOLIC. Referring to the rhythmic contraction of the heart (systole) as the blood in the chambers is forced out. Systolic blood pressure is blood pressure measured during the systolic phase.

T

T CELL. A type of white blood cell produced in the thymus gland that regulates the immune system's response to diseased or malignant cells. It is possible that a subcategory of T cells known as CD4 cells plays a role in Ménière's disease.

T-LYMPHOCYTE. A type of white blood cell, also known as a T-helper cell, a T_h cell, an effector T cell, or a CD4+ T cell, whose numbers in a blood sample can be used to monitor the progression of HIV infection.

TACHYCARDIA. Elevated heart rate.

TACHYPNEA. Elevated breathing rate.

TARDIVE DYSKINESIA. A movement disorder that may result from long-term treatment with the older antipsychotic drugs. Its symptoms include uncontrollable tongue thrusting, lip smacking, and facial grimacing.

TARGET HEART RATE. The heart rate, in beats per minute (bpm), that should be maintained during cardiovascular exercise by an individual of a given age.

TAU PROTEIN. A protein involved in maintaining the internal structure of nerve cells. Tau protein is damaged in AD and forms neurofibrillary tangles.

TELANGIECTASES. Spidery red skin lesions caused by dilated blood vessels.

TELANGIECTASIA. Abnormal dilation of capillary blood vessels leading to the formation of telangiectases or angiomas.

TEMPORAL LOBE. The part of each side or hemisphere of the brain that is on the side of the head, nearest the ears.

TEMPOROMANDIBULAR JOINT (TMJ). The small joint in front of the ear in humans where the mandible (lower jaw) is attached to the skull.

TEMPOROMANDIBULAR JOINT (TMJ) DISORDERS. A disorder in the joint between the temporal bone above the ear and the lower jaw bone or mandible.

TEMPOROMANDIBULAR JOINT (TMJ) SYNDROME. Symptoms, such as headache, that are related to a disorder in the joints between the temporal bone above the ear and the lower jaw bone or mandible.

TENDINITIS. Inflammation of a tendon.

TENDON REFLEX. This is a simple circuit that consists of a stimulus like a sharp tap delivered to a tendon and the response is one of the appropriate muscle contraction. It is used to test the integrity of the nervous system.

TENOTOMY. A surgical procedure that cuts the tendon of a contracted muscle to allow lengthening.

TENSILON TEST. A test for diagnosing myasthenia gravis. Tensilon is injected into a vein and, if the person has MG, their muscle strength will improve for about five minutes.

TENSION-TYPE HEADACHE (TTH). A band-like or squeezing primary headache that can be episodic or chronic.

TERATOGEN. Any drug, chemical, maternal infection, or environmental factor known to cause birth defects.

TETRAPLEGIA. Paralysis of all four limbs. Also called quadriplegia.

THALAMOTOMY. A surgical procedure that destroys part of a large oval area of gray matter within the brain that acts as a relay center for nerve impulses. The thalamus is an essential part of the nerve pathway that controls intentional movement. By destroying tissue at a particular spot on the thalamus, the surgeon can interrupt the nerve signals that cause tremor.

THALAMUS. A large oval area of gray matter within the brain that relays nerve impulses from the basal ganglia to the cerebellum, both parts of the brain that control and regulate muscle movement.

THERMOGRAPHY. A test using infrared sensing devices to measure differences in temperature in body regions thought to be the source of pain.

THIAMINE. A B vitamin essential for the body to process carbohydrates and fats. Alcoholics may suffer complications (including Wernike-Korsakoff syndrome) from a deficiency of this vitamin.

THIAMINE PYROPHOSPHATE (TPP). The coenzyme containing thiamine that is essential in converting glucose to energy.

THORACIC. Refers to the chest area. The thorax runs between the abdomen and neck and is encased in the ribs.

THROMBIN. Important factor in blood clot and fibrin formation, also known as coagulation factor II.

THROMBOXANE. Chemical mediator of platelet aggregation.

THROMBUS (PLURAL THROMBI). A stationary blood clot formed on the inner surface of damaged blood vessels or inside the heart, which may occlude blood flow.

THYMUS. A gland located in the front of the neck that coordinates the development of the immune system.

THYROTOXICOSIS. An excess of thyroid hormones in the blood, causing a variety of symptoms that include rapid heart beat, sweating, anxiety, and tremor.

THYROXINE. Hormone produced by the thyroid gland.

TIC. A brief and intermittent involuntary movement or sound.

TINNITUS. A sensation of ringing, buzzing, roaring, or clicking noises in the ear.

TINNITUS RETRAINING THERAPY (TRT). Tinnitus treatment that combines counseling with the use of a device that masks the tinnitus frequency.

TISSUE PLASMINOGEN ACTIVATOR (TPA). A clot-dissolving enzyme that is used to prevent or reduce neurological damage from ischemic stroke and heart muscle damage from a heart attack.

TISSUE-SPECIFIC STEM CELL. Adult or somatic stem cell; a multipotent stem cell that can differentiate into the specialized cell types of the tissue from which it was derived.

TITER. The concentration of a specific antibody in blood serum.

TOMOGRAPHY. A technique for producing a focused three-dimensional image of body structures at a precise depth, while blurring details at other depths. The process involves gathering a series of two-dimensional cross-section images and combining them using tomographic reconstruction software processed by a computer.

TONIC-CLONIC SEIZURE. A seizure involving the entire body characterized by unconsciousness, muscle contraction, and rigidity. Also called grand mal or generalized seizures.

TONIFICATION. Acupuncture technique for strengthening the body.

TONSILLITIS. Inflammation of the tonsils, which are in the back of the throat.

TOPICAL. For application to the surface of the skin.

TORTICOLLIS. Twisting of the neck to one side that results in abnormal carriage of the head and is usually caused by muscle spasms. Also called wryneck.

TOTAL BODY IRRADIATION; TBI. Whole-body irradiation therapy; used for conditioning to destroy bone marrow prior to a stem cell transplant.

TOURETTE SYNDROME (TS). An abnormal condition that causes uncontrollable facial grimaces and tics, and arm and shoulder movements. Tourette syndrome is best known, perhaps, for uncontrollable vocal tics that include grunts, shouts, and use of obscene language (coprolalia). Also known as Gilles de la Tourette syndrome.

TOXIC. Poisoinous.

TOXIN. A poisonous substance produced by a microorganism, plant, or animal.

TOXOPLASMOSIS. Infection by the parasite *Toxoplasma gondii*, which can damage the central nervous system.

TRACHEOSTOMY. The procedure used to open a hole in the neck to the trachea, or windpipe. It is sometimes used in conjunction with a respirator.

TRACHEOTOMY. A surgical procedure in which a small hole is cut into the trachea, or windpipe, below the level of the vocal cords.

TRACTION. Spinal stretching using weights applied to the spine, once thought to decrease pressure on the nerve roots but now seldom used.

TRANSCORTICAL APHASIA. A condition characterized by either partial or total loss of the ability to communicate verbally or use written words that does not affect an individual's ability to repeat words, phrases, and sentences.

TRANSCRANIAL MAGNETIC STIMULATION (TMS). Stimulation of brain cells with an electromagnetic coil positioned over the skull.

TRANSCRIPTION. The process by which genetic information on a strand of DNA is used to synthesize a strand of complementary RNA.

TRANSCRIPTION FACTOR. A protein that acts to regulate the expression of genes.

TRANSCUTANEOUS ELECTRICAL NERVE STIMULATION (TENS). A form of pain therapy administered via a TENS unit. This therapy utilizes electrodes that adhere to the skin and deliver varying frequencies of electric current. Some patients find minimal to moderate pain relief when this therapy is done on a frequent and ongoing basis.

TRANSDERMAL. Referring to a type of drug that enters the body by being absorbed through the skin.

TRANSDUCER. Another word for the probe placed over the insonation windows in TCD.

TRANSIENT. Brief and short-lived.

TRANSIENT ISCHEMIC ATTACK (TIA). A brief interruption of the blood supply to part of the brain that causes a temporary impairment of vision, speech, or movement. Usually, the episode lasts for just a few moments, but it may be a warning sign for a full-scale stroke.

TRANSMISSIBLE SPONGIFORM ENCEPHALOPATHY. A term that refers to a group of diseases, including kuru, Creutzfeldt-Jakob disease, Gerstmann-Sträussler-Scheinker syndrome, fatal familial insomnia, and new variant Creutzfeldt-Jakob disease. These diseases share a common origin as prion diseases, caused by abnormal proteins that accumulate within the brain and destroy brain tissue, leaving spongy holes.

TRANSVERSE MYELITIS. Inflammation and scarring across the entire width of one segment of the spinal cord, disrupting nerve transmission to parts of the body served by nerves from that segment and below.

TRAPEZIUS MUSCLE. Muscle of the upper back that rotates the shoulder blade, raises the shoulder, and flexes the arm.

TRAUMATIC BRAIN INJURY (TBI). Damage to the brain from sudden trauma, most often from a motor-vehicle accident.

TREMOR. Involuntary rhythmic movements, which may be intermittent or constant, involving an entire muscle or only a circumscribed group of muscle bundles.

TREMOR CONTROL THERAPY. A method for controlling tremor by self-administered shocks to the part of the brain that controls intentional movement (thalamus). An electrode attached to an insulated lead wire is implanted in the brain; the battery power source is implanted under the skin of the chest, and an extension wire is tunneled under the skin to connect the battery to the lead. The patient turns on the power source to deliver the electrical impulse and interrupt the tremor.

TREPANATION. A surgical procedure in which a circular piece of bone is removed from the skull by a special saw-like instrument called a trephine or trepan. The operation is also known as trephination or trephining.

TRICEPS. Muscle of the back of the upper arm, primarily responsible for extending the elbow.

TRIGEMINAL NERVE. The main sensory nerve of the face and motor nerve for chewing muscles.

TRIGEMINAL NEURALGIA. A disorder affecting the trigeminal nerve (the 5th cranial nerve), causing episodes of sudden, severe pain on one side of the face.

TRIGGER FINGER. An overuse disorder of the hand in which one or more fingers tend to lock or "trigger" when the patient tries to extend the finger.

TRIGLYCERIDES. Neutral fats; lipids formed from glycerol and fatty acids that circulate in the blood as lipoprotein. Elevated triglyceride levels contribute to the development of cardiovascular disease.

TRIGONOCEPHALY. An abnormal development of the skull characterized by a triangular shaped forehead.

TRINUCLEOTIDE. A sequence of three nucleotides.

TRINUCLEOTIDE REPEAT EXPANSION. A sequence of three nucleotides that is repeated too many times in a section of a gene.

TRIPTANS. A class of drugs that bind to and activate serotonin receptors in the brain; used to treat migraines.

TRISOMY. An abnormality in chromosomal development. Chromosomes are the structures within a cell that carry its genetic information. They are organized in pairs. Humans have 23 pairs of chromosomes. In a trisomy syndrome, an extra chromosome is present so that the individual has three of a particular chromosome instead of the normal pair. An extra chromosome 18 (trisomy 18) causes mental retardation.

TUBEROUS SCLEROSIS. A genetic disease that causes skin problems, seizures, and mental retardation. Autism occurs more often in individuals with tuberous sclerosis.

TUBERS. Firm growths in the brain, named for their resemblance in shape to potato stems.

TUMOR. An abnormal growth of cells. Tumors may be benign (noncancerous) or malignant (cancerous).

TUMOR GRADING. Tumor grade refers to the degree of abnormality of cancer cells compared with normal cells. Establishing a grade allows the physician to determine further courses of treatment.

TUMORIGENESIS. Formation of tumors.

TYPE I INCONTINENTIA PIGMENTI. Sporadic IP. This disorder is caused by mutations in the gene at Xp11. These mutations are not inherited from the parents, they are *de novo* mutations. This type of IP probably represents a different disease than type II IP.

TYPE II INCONTINENTIA PIGMENTI. Familial, male-lethal type IP. This type of IP is the "classic" case of IP. It is caused by mutations in the NEMO gene located at Xq28. Inheritance is sex-linked recessive.

TZANCK PREPARATION. A procedure in which skin cells from a blister are stained and examined under the microscope.

U

ULNAR NERVE. The nerve that supplies some of the forearm muscles, the elbow joint, and many of the short muscles of the hand.

ULTRASONOGRAPHY (ULTRASOUND). A process that uses the reflection of high-frequency sound waves to make an image of structures deep within the body. Ultrasonography is routinely used to detect fetal abnormalities.

UNAIDED COMMUNICATION SYSTEMS. Ways of communicating other than speech that involve only the human body. Gestures, sign language, and body language are all forms of unaided communication systems.

UNILATERAL. Occurring on only one side of the body.

URINARY INCONTINENCE. unable to control urinary excretion.

URINARY SPHINCTER. The muscles used to control the flow of urine out of the urinary bladder. When contracted urine remains in the bladder, and when relaxed urine is allowed to flow into the urethra and out of the body.

URINARY URGENCY. A strong desire to urinate that can be difficult to control.

UVEITIS. Inflammation of all or part the uvea. The uvea is a continuous layer of tissue in the eye that consists of the iris, the ciliary body, and the choroid. The uvea lies between the retina and sclera.

UVULOPALATOPHARYNGOPLASTY (UPPP). An operation to remove excess tissue at the back of the throat to prevent it from closing off the airway during sleep.

V

VAGINISMUS. An involuntary spasm of the muscles surrounding the vagina, making penetration painful or impossible.

VAGUS NERVE. the thenth cranial nerve, that is, a nerve connected to the brain. The vagus nerve has branches to most of the major organs in the body, including the larynx, throat, windpipe, lungs, heart, and most of the digestive system.

VALACYCLOVIR. An oral antiviral drug that blocks the replication of the varicella zoster virus.

VALSALVA MANEUVER. A strain against a closed airway combined with muscle tightening, such as happens when a person holds his or her breath and tries to move a heavy object. Most people perform this maneuver several times a day without adverse consequences, but it can be dangerous for anyone with cardiovascular disease. Pilots perform this maneuver to prevent black-outs during high-performance flying.

VASCULAR. Pertaining to the veins, arteries, and organs in the body's circulatory system.

VASCULITIS. A condition in which inflammation of the blood vessels deprives organs and tissues of oxygen, resulting in damage.

VASOCONSTRICTION. The narrowing or constriction of a blood vessel lumen.

VASODILATION. The widening or dilation of a blood vessel lumen.

VASODILATOR. Any drug that relaxes blood vessel walls.

VASOSPASM. A condition in which a major blood vessel goes into spasm and suddenly constricts, cutting off or restricting blood supply to an organ or body part. Vasospasm in a cerebral artery can lead to stroke.

VECTOR. An animal carrier that transfers an infectious organism from one host to another. The vector that transmits Lyme disease from wildlife to humans is the deer tick or black-legged tick.

VECTOR-BORNE DISEASE. A disease that is delivered from one host to another by a vector or carrier organism.

VEIN. Blood vessel in which blood flows from the tissues toward the heart and lungs for oxygenation.

VENTILATOR. Respirator; breathing machine; a life-support device for maintaining artificial respiration.

VENTRAL. Pertaining in direction to the front or lower surface of an organ.

VENTRICLES. The four fluid-filled chambers, or cavities, found in the two cerebral hemispheres of the brain, at the center of the brain, and between the brain stem and cerebellum. They are linked by channels, or ducts, allowing cerebral fluid to circulate through them.

VENTRICULOPERITONEAL SHUNT. A tube equipped with a low-pressure valve, one end of which is inserted into a cerebral ventricle, the other end of which is routed into the peritoneum, or abdominal cavity.

VENTRICULOSTOMY. A surgical opening into a ventricle of the brain to drain cerebrospinal fluid; used to treat hydrocephalus and brain edema.

VERMIS. The central portion of the cerebellum, which divides the two hemispheres. It functions to monitor and control movement of the limbs, trunk, head, and eyes.

VERTEBRA (PLURAL, VERTEBRAE). One of the bones of the spinal column. There are 33 vertebrae in the human spine.

VERTEBROBASILAR ARTERIES. Major blood vessels that lead to the brain. They are located at the base of the skull at the back of the head.

VERTEX PRESENTATION. Head presentation during delivery.

VERTIGO. Dizziness with a sense of spinning of self and/or surroundings with resultant loss of balance, nausea, and vomiting. Occurs due to a problem in the inner ears or the cerebellum and brainstem.

VERY LONG CHAIN FATTY ACIDS (VLCFA). A type of fat that is normally broken down by the peroxisomes into other fats that can be used by the body.

VESICLE. A small, raised lesion filled with clear fluid.

VESTIBULAR SYSTEM. The group of organs in the inner ear that provide sensory input related to movement, orientation in space, and balance.

VIRAL LOAD. A measure of the severity of HIV infection, calculated by estimating the number of copies of the virus in a milliliter of blood.

VIRUS. A tiny, disease-causing structure that can reproduce only in living cells and causes a variety of infectious diseases.

VISCERAL. Generally related to the digestive, respiratory, urogenital, or endocrine organs.

VITAMINS. Small compounds required for metabolism that must be supplied by diet, microorganisms in the gut (vitamin K), or sunlight (UV light converts pre-vitamin D to vitamin D).

VOIDING. The act of urinating.

VOLUNTARY. An action or thought undertaken or controlled by a person's free will or choice.

VOLUNTARY MUSCLE. A muscle under conscious control, such as arm and leg muscles.

W

WASTING SYNDROME. A combination of weight loss and change in composition of body tissues that occurs in patients with HIV infection. Typically, the patient's body loses lean muscle tissue and replaces it with fat as well as losing weight overall.

WERNICKE'S APHASIA. A condition characterized by either partial or total loss of the ability to understand what is being said or read. The individual maintains the ability to speak, but speech may contain unnecessary or made-up words.

WERNICKE-KORSAKOFF SYNDROME. A combination of symptoms, including eye-movement problems, tremors, and confusion, that is caused by a lack of the B vitamin thiamine and may be seen in alcoholics.

WESTERN BLOT. A procedure that uses electrical current passed through a gel containing a sample of tissue extract in order to break down the proteins in the sample and detect the presence of antibodies for a specific disease. The Western blot method is used in HIV testing to confirm the results of an initial screening test.

WHITE MATTER. A substance, composed primarily of myelin fibers, found in the brain and nervous system that protects nerves and allows messages to be sent to and from the brain and various parts of the body. Also called white substance.

WHITE MATTER RADIAL MIGRATION LINE. White lines seen on a brain scan, signifying abnormal movement of neurons (brain cells) at that area.

WILD-TYPE VIRUS. A virus occurring naturally in the environment or a population in its original form.

WILSON'S DISEASE. An inborn defect of copper metabolism in which free copper may be deposited in a variety of areas of the body. Deposits in the brain can cause tremor and other symptoms of Parkinson's disease.

WINDOW PERIOD. The period of time between a person's getting infected with HIV and the point at which antibodies against the virus can be detected in a blood sample.

WITHDRAWAL SYMPTOMS. A group of physical or mental symptoms that may occur when a person suddenly stops using a drug on which he or she has become dependent.

WOOD'S LAMP. A special lamp that uses ultraviolet light to detect certain types of skin lesions.

WORD SALAD. Speech that is so disorganized that it makes no linguistic or grammatical sense.

X

X-LINKED GENE. A gene carried on the X chromosome, one of the two sex chromosomes.

XANTHOCHROMIA. Presence of red blood cell breakdown products.

Y

YIN/YANG. In Chinese philosophy, the universal characteristics of the natural world. Yin and yang comprise the substance of nature and the mind, and they represent the process of harmonization that maintains a constant and dynamic balance among all things. Yoga is deeply influenced by these concepts.

Z

ZOONOSIS (PLURAL, ZOONOSES), OR ZOONOTIC DISEASE. Any disease of animals that can be transmitted to humans under natural conditions. Lyme disease and babesiosis are examples of zoonoses, as are some prion diseases.

ZYGOMATIC ARCH. Cheekbone; a quadrilateral bone forming the prominence of the cheek. It articulates (touches or moves) with the frontal, sphenoid, and maxillary, and temporal bones.

INDEX

Numbers before a colon indicate volume. Numbers after a colon indicate page references. **Boldface** page numbers indicate the main essay for a topic. *Italicized* page numbers indicate photographs or illustrations.

A

A-P diameter, 1:315
A-T. *See* Ataxia-telangiectasia
A-T Project Foundation, 1:143
AAB-001. *See* Bapineuzumab
AAC. *See* Assistive communicative technologies
AADC (Amino acid decarboxylase) inhibitors, 1:108, 2:827
AAMA (American Academy of Medical Acupuncture), 1:8
AAMI (Age-associated memory impairment), 1:345–346, 348
AAMR (American Association on Mental Retardation), 2:674
AAN (American Academy of Neurology), 1:228, 2:768, 1077
AANS (American Association of Neurological Surgeons), 2:786
AAOS (American Academy of Orthopaedic Surgeons), 1:459, 613–614
AAP (American Academy of Pediatrics), 1:10, 159, 396, 2:1058, 1059
AAP (American Academy of Pediatrics), 1:10, 159, 396, 2:1058, 1059
ABA (Applied behavior analysis), 1:159
Abacavir, 1:35
ABCR drugs, 2:717
ABCs (Airway, breathing and circulation) of Resuscitation, 2:1171
Abdominal region, definition of, 1:75
Abducens nerve palsy. *See* Sixth nerve palsy
Abduction, 1:75
Abetalipoproteinemia. *See* Bassen-Kornzweig syndrome
Abilify. *See* Aripiprazole
Abitrate. *See* Clofibrate
ABNS (American Board of Neurological Surgery), 2:789
Abscess, subarachnoid, 2:673

Absence seizures, 2:942
  Lennox-Gastaut syndrome, 1:622, 623
  prognosis, 1:438
  status epilepticus with, 2:996
  symptoms, 1:432, 2:942, 943
  treatment, 2:809–810, 944, 1025–1027
Abstract thinking, 1:347
Abulia, 1:**1–2**
Abuse
  child, 2:946–948, 1087, 1088
  physical, 2:1087
  See also Alcohol abuse; Substance abuse
Abusive head trauma. *See* Shaken baby syndrome
Academic achievement, 1:618
Acadians, 1:475
Acanthocytosis.
  See Bassen-Kornzweig syndrome
Accelerometer, 2:1095
Accidental falls. *See* Falls
Accreditation Council for Graduate Medical Education (ACGME), 2:781, 789
ACE inhibitors, 1:98, 449–450, 2:802
Acephaly. *See* Anencephaly
Acephate, 1:292
Acetaminophen
  for back pain, 1:176
  for carpal tunnel syndrome, 1:252
  for febrile seizures, 1:467
  headaches from, 1:513
  for idiopathic neuropathy, 1:577
  for migraine headaches, 1:105–107, 509, 523
  for pain, 2:813
  phenobarbital interactions, 2:855
  platelet inhibitor interactions, 1:98
  for tabes dorsalis, 2:1039
  for traumatic brain injuries, 2:1090
  for whiplash, 2:1171
Acetaminophen, aspirin, plus caffeine, 1:523
Acetaminophen with codeine, 1:176, 311

Acetaminophen with hydrocodone, 1:176, 215, 2:1171
Acetate, 1:42
Acetazolamide, 1:**2–3**
  for hydrocephalus, 1:558
  lamotrigine interactions, 1:616
  for Ménière's disease, 2:1143
  for olivopontocerebellar atrophy, 2:797
  for periodic paralysis, 2:836–837
  primidone interactions, 1:103
  for pseudotumor cerebri, 2:891
  topiramate interactions, 2:1070
  valproic acid interactions, 2:1120
  zonisamide interactions, 2:1188
Acetyl-CoA-alpha-glucosaminide acetyltransferase, 2:708
Acetyl-L-carnitine, 1:59, 351
Acetylcholine (ACh)
  Alzheimer's disease, 1:51
  amantadine, 1:63–65
  anticholinergics, 1:91
  autonomic nervous system, 2:839
  botulism, 1:211
  cholinergic stimulants, 1:290
  cholinesterase inhibitors, 1:291–292
  congenital myasthenia, 1:304–305
  Lambert-Eaton myasthenic syndrome, 2:823
  Lewy body dementia, 1:637
  motor neuron diseases, 2:692
  myasthenia gravis, 1:164, 2:731
  neuromuscular blockers, 2:769
  Parkinson's disease, 1:91, 2:953
  role of, 1:507, 2:790, 791, 839
Acetylcholine (ACh) receptors, 1:162, 163, 286
Acetylcholinesterase, 2:731
Acetylcholinesterase inhibitors.
  See Cholinesterase inhibitors
Acetylsalicylic acid. *See* Aspirin
ACGME (Accreditation Council for Graduate Medical Education), 2:781, 789
ACh. *See* Acetylcholine
ACh (Acetylcholine) receptors, 1:162, 163, 286

Index

Index

Disorganized schizophrenia, 2:932–933

Disorientation, 1:341–342

Disputed thoracic outlet syndrome, 2:1050

Dissociative disorders, 2:892

Dissociative identity disorder (DID), 2:931

Distal end, 1:75

Distal muscular dystrophy (DD), 2:722–731

Distance therapy, 1:357

Disulfiram, 1:342

Ditropan. *See* Oxybutynin

Diuretics
   for beriberi, 1:198
   interactions, 1:3, 2:771
   for Ménière's disease, 2:1143
   for periodic paralysis, 2:837
   side effects
      falls, 1:458
      hearing loss, 1:527
      myopathy, 2:740
      orthostatic hypotension, 2:802
      tinnitus, 2:1063
   for subdural hematoma, 2:1025
   thiazide, 2:837

Divalproex sodium, 1:104, **2:1119–1121**
   for chronic daily headaches, 1:515
   for epilepsy, 1:437, 2:1119–1121
   interactions, 2:1119, 1120–1121
   for migraine headaches, 1:523
   neural tube defects from, 2:979

Dix-Hallpike test, 1:194, 2:1140

Dizziness, *1:378*, **378–381**
   causes, 1:273, 378–379, 2:669, 718
   chronic subjective, 2:893
   diagnosis, 1:379–380
   psychogenic, 2:893–896
   treatment, 1:380

DLL1 (Delta-like 1) gene, 1:544

DM1 (Myotonic dystrophy type 1), 2:742–743

DM2 (Myotonic dystrophy type 2), 2:742, 743, 744

DMD (Duchenne muscular dystrophy), 2:722–731, 740, 741

DMG (Dimethylglycine), 1:160

DNA (Deoxyribonucleic acid)
   gene therapy, 1:487
   mitochondrial, 1:46, 2:683–685, 686
   nuclear, 2:684, 685, 686
   recombinant, 1:484
   role of, 1:483
   synthetic, 1:487

DNA methylation studies, 1:82–83

DNA testing
   Canavan disease, 1:240–241
   encephalitis, 1:418
   Gaucher disease, 1:482

Gerstmann-Straussler-Scheinker disease, 1:489, 490
   Krabbe disease, 1:601
   meningitis, 1:418
   myopathy, 2:741
   Niemann-Pick disease, 2:794
   Rett syndrome, 2:922
   Williams syndrome, 2:1176
   Wilson disease, 2:1180
   See also Genetic testing

Docosahexanoic acid (DHA), 1:12, 147

Docusate sodium, 2:718

Dogs, *1:433,* 2:1167

Dolasetron, 1:606

Dominant inheritance. *See* Autosomal dominant inheritance

Dominant Spinocerebellar Ataxias (DSCAs), 1:146

Donepezil, 1:292–293
   for Alzheimer's disease, 1:58, 59, 350
   for Binswanger disease, 1:202
   for Lewy body dementia, 1:637

Dong quai, 1:98

Dopamine
   abulia, 1:1
   ADHD, 1:152
   amantadine, 1:63–65
   anticholinergics, 2:828
   atomoxetine, 1:150
   chorea, 1:294
   COMT inhibitors, 1:255
   Huntington disease, 1:550
   migraine headache, 1:507, 523
   neuroleptic malignant syndrome, 2:761, 762
   Parkinson's disease, 1:91, 108, 2:827
   progressive supranuclear palsy, 2:888
   restless legs syndrome, 2:918
   role of, 1:16, 2:791, 825
   secretion of, 2:814
   tics, 2:1059

Dopamine agonists. *See* Dopamine receptor agonists

Dopamine antagonists, 1:382

Dopamine receptor agonists, 1:109–111, **381–383**
   for chorea, 1:294
   for corticobasal degeneration, 1:313
   for dystonia, 1:402
   for parkinsonism, 2:722
   for Parkinson's disease, 1:109–111, 381–383, 2:827–828
   for progressive supranuclear palsy, 2:888
   for restless legs syndrome, 2:919
   for schizophrenia, 2:936
   side effects, 1:382, 2:827–828, 936
   for tics, 2:1060

Dopaminergics. *See* Dopamine receptor agonists

Dopergine. *See* Lisuride

Doppler, Christian, 2:1076

Doppler ultrasonography, 2:1117
   aneurysm, 1:79
   brain death determination, 1:229
   carotid stenosis, 1:246
   transcranial, 2:1076–1079, 1083, 1117

Dorsal nerve roots, 1:221

Dorsal rhizotomy, 1:283

Dorsal root entry zone (DREZ) operation, 1:177

Dorsal root ganglia, 1:595, 2:949, 950

Dorsal simultanagnosia, 1:24

Dorsiflecos muscles, 1:471

Dorsomedial thalamic nuclei, 1:372

Dostinex. *See* Cabergoline

Double-blind study, 1:299

Double cortex syndrome, 1:641, 2:773

Double vision, 2:1146–1149
   emergency care for, 2:764
   fourth nerve palsy, 1:472–474
   myasthenia gravis, 2:732
   prisms for, 1:473–474, 2:955, 1050
   sixth nerve palsy, 2:954, 955
   third nerve palsy, 2:1049

Double voiding, 2:807

Dowager's hump. *See* Kyphosis

Down syndrome, 1:52, 55, 635, 2:675, 676–677

Doxacurium, 1:91, 2:769–771

Doxepin, 1:104, 357, 2:813

Doxycyline, 1:243, 654

DQB1 gene, 2:748

Drainage, 2:835

DRB1 gene, 2:748

DREZ (Dorsal root entry zone) operation, 1:177

Driving, 1:101, 531

DRM (Desmin-related myopathy), 2:737

Drop attacks, 1:622, 623, 624
   See also Atonic seizures

Drop foot. *See* Foot drop

Droperidol, 1:105–107

DRPLA, 1:148

Drug Enforcement Administration (DEA), 1:114

Drug-induced myopathy (DIM), 2:740–741

Drug-induced paralysis, 2:769–772

Drug overdose. *See* Overdose

Drug receptors, 2:852

Drug therapy. *See* Pharmacotherapy

Drug tolerance, 1:196, 2:854

Dry beriberi, 1:197, 2:1149

Dry eye, 1:192, 207

Dry mouth, 1:393

H

Hallucinations, 1:**499–504**
    auditory, 1:500, 502–503, 2:748,
        932, 933
    causes, 1:500–501
        Alzheimer's disease, 1:52, 53
        delirium, 1:342
        schizophrenia, 2:933
    demographics, 1:490–500
    haptic (tactile), 1:500
    hypnagogic, 1:500
    irritative, 1:501
    release, 1:501
    during sleep, 2:964
    treatment, 1:503
    visual, 1:500, 636, 2:748
Hallucinosis, alcoholic, 1:499,
    501–502
Haloperidol
    for Alzheimer's disease, 1:59
    carbamazepine interactions, 1:243
    for delirium, 1:344
    for dementia, 1:350
    for schizophrenia, 2:936
    side effects, 1:108, 2:825, 1074
    for tics, 2:1060
    for Tourette syndrome, 2:1074
Halstead-Reitan Battery, 2:777
HAM/TSP (HTLV-1 associated
    myelopathy/tropical spastic
    paraparesis). *See* Tropical spastic
    paraparesis
Hamartomas, 2:1107, 1109–1110
Hamilton Depression Rating Scale
    (HDRS), 1:17, 355
Hand-eye coordination, 1:133
Happy Puppet syndrome, 1:81
Haptic (tactile) hallucinations, 1:500
Harada-Ito procedure, 1:474
Hard HBOT chambers, 1:563
Hartnup disease, 2:1153
HBOT (Hyperbaric oxygen therapy),
    1:283, **561–565**, *562*, 2:1065
HDRS (Hamilton Depression Rating
    Scale), 1:17, 355
Head and neck cancers, 2:780, 960
Head circumference
    megalencephaly, 2:665
    microcephaly, 2:680–682
    Sotos syndrome, 2:971, 972, 973
    Sturge-Weber syndrome, 2:1019
Head injuries
    anatomy of, 2:672
    closed, 1:409, 2:1086
    complications
        benign positional vertigo, 1:194
        brain death, 1:228
        coma, 1:300
        dementia, 1:346
        demographics, 1:120
        dysarthria, 1:384
        epidural hematoma, 1:430
        epilepsy, 1:433
        headaches, 1:506

    tinnitus, 2:1063
    traumatic brain injuries,
        2:1086–1093
    vertigo, 2:1139
    emergency care for, 2:764–765
    penetrating, 2:1086, 1087
    prevention, 1:121, 438
    ventilatory assistance devices for,
        2:1130
    See also Brain injuries; Traumatic
        brain injuries
Head pointers, 1:387
Head-tilting exercises, 1:194–195
Headaches, 1:*504*, **504–512**
    causes, 1:505–506, 507, 513, 517
        aneurysm, 1:78, 79
        Arnold-Chiari malformation,
            1:127
        arteriovenous malformations,
            1:130
        Lyme disease, 1:653
        neurocysticercosis, 2:756
        paroxysmal hemicrania,
            2:829–831
        syringomyelia, 2:1032
    chronic daily, 1:505, 507, 509–510,
        512–516
    cluster, 1:505–511, 516–520, *517,*
        517t, 2:1100–1104
    demographics, 1:506–507, 513,
        516–517
    diagnosis, 1:508, 514
    hypnic, 1:513
    inflammatory, 1:505
    medication-overuse, 1:512, 513,
        515
    new daily persistent, 1:512, 513,
        514, 515
    prevention, 1:515–516, 519
    primary, 1:504–505, 512, 513
    prognosis, 1:519
    rebound, 1:505, 509, 512
    secondary, 1:504, 505–506, 512,
        513, 515
    sinus, 1:505
    symptoms, 1:507
    tension, 1:368–370, *504,* 505–511,
        513–514, 2:795
    traction, 1:505
    treatment, 1:508–511, 515, 519
        acupuncture, 1:5, 515
        alternative medicine,
            1:510–511, 515
        dichloralphenazone, iso-
            metheptene, acetaminophen
            combination, 1:368–370
    See also Migraine headache
Healing. *See* Wound healing
Health care costs. *See* Costs
Health history. *See* Medical history
Hearing aids, 1:527–528, 2:1146
Hearing comprehension, 1:118
Hearing disorders, 1:**524–530**

Hearing loss, 1:**524–530,** *525*
    age-related, 1:527, 2:1062, 1064
    causes, 1:527
        ataxia, 1:147
        Ménière's disease, 2:668, 669
        Ramsay-Hunt syndrome
            type II, 2:902
        Refsum disease, 2:908
        vestibular schwannoma,
            2:1145, 1146
    classification, 1:524–525
    conductive, 1:524, 527–528
    demographics, 1:525–526
    diagnosis, 1:528
    hereditary, 1:525, 527
    noise-induced, 1:525, 527, 528–529
    prevention, 1:528–529
    prognosis, 1:528
    sensorineural, 1:524, 527, 528
    sudden sensorineural, 1:524, 525
    symptoms, 1:527–528
    treatment, 1:528–529
Hearing tests, 1:528
    benign positional vertigo, 1:194
    dizziness, 1:380
    Ménière's disease, 2:669
    neurofibromatosis, 2:760
    tinnitus, 2:1064
Hearing therapy, 1:316
Heart attacks
    anticoagulant/antiplatelet drugs
        for, 1:92
    coma after, 1:302
    encephalopathy from, 1:426
    prevention, 1:248
    risk factors, 1:442, 444, 462, 2:1123
    stem cell therapy for, 2:999
Heart disease, 1:476, 2:661, 1029
Heart muscle, 2:837
Heart muscle weakness. *See*
    Cardiomyopathy
Heart rate, 1:441, 492, 2:837
Heart transplantation, 2:729
Heart valve disease, 1:92, 2:1029, 1030
Heartburn, 1:83
    See also Gastroesophageal reflux
        disease
Heat stroke, 2:1069
Heat therapy, 2:813, 874, 913
Heavy metals, 1:16, 347, 2:843
Heerfordt syndrome, 2:784
Heinrich, Wilhelm, 1:213
Helical CT scans. *See* Spiral CT scans
Helmets, 2:672
Hemangioblastomas, 1:224,
    2:1154–1158
Hemangiopericytomas, 1:224
Hematocrit, 1:95
Hematomas
    causes, 2:673
        angiography, 1:88
        lumbar puncture, 1:646

I

IgG (Immunoglobulin G), 2:700
IHS (International Headache Society), 1:504, 505, 521
ILAE (International League Against Epilepsy), 1:433–434, 2:941
Illiteracy, functional, 1:396
Illusions, *vs.* hallucinations, 1:499
Imagery. *See* Guided imagery
Imaging studies
    aphasia, 1:118
    autoimmune diseases, 1:163
    back pain, 1:612
    brain and spinal tumors, 1:224–225
    Brown-Séquard syndrome, 1:246
    central cord syndrome, 1:257
    chorea, 1:294
    chronic daily headaches, 1:514
    headaches, 1:508
    hemiplegia, 1:535
    hydrocephalus, 1:558
    hydromyelia, 1:560
    hypotonia, 1:571
    lupus, 1:649
    paraplegia, 1:535
    paroxysmal hemicrania, 2:830
    piriformis syndrome, 2:858
    porencephaly, 2:870
    repetitive motion disorders, 2:912–913
    seizures, 2:943
    spina bifida, 2:980
    susceptibility weighted, 1:201
    tinnitus, 2:1064
    Tourette syndrome, 2:1073
    weakness, 2:1164
    See also Brain imaging; CT scans; Magnetic resonance imaging; Positron emission tomography; Single photon emission computed tomography; Ultrasonography; X rays
Imipramine, 1:154, 357, 365, 2:717, 845
Imitrex. *See* Sumatriptan
Immersive virtual reality, 2:850
Immobilization
    Brown-Séquard syndrome, 1:246
    Parsonage-Turner syndrome, 2:833
    spinal cord injuries, 2:986
    traumatic brain injuries, 2:1089, 1090
    whiplash, 2:1171
Immune globulin. *See* Immunoglobulins
Immune-mediated encephalomyelitis. *See* Acute disseminated encephalomyelitis
Immune response, 1:589, 2:1122
Immunization. *See* Vaccinations
Immunoadsorption, 2:798–799

Immunocompromised patients
    cytomegalic inclusion body disease, 1:333, 334
    foscarnet for, 1:112
    progressive multifocal leukoencephalopathy, 2:886
    shingles, 2:949, 951, 952
    West Nile virus, 2:1167, 1168
Immunoglobulin G (IgG), 2:700
Immunoglobulins, 1:164, 297
    See also Intravenous immunoglobulin
Immunosuppressant drugs
    for acute disseminated encephalomyelitis, 1:9
    for autoimmune diseases, 1:164
    for Behcet's syndrome, 1:190
    for chronic inflammatory demyelinating polyneuropathy, 1:297
    for dermatomyositis, 1:360, 2:865
    for Lambert-Eaton myasthenic syndrome, 1:508
    for myasthenia gravis, 2:734
    for neurosarcoidosis, 2:784
    for polymyositis, 2:865
    for Schilder's disease, 2:927
    for stem cell transplants, 2:1003
Immunosuppression. *See* Immunocompromised patients
Implantable electrodes, 1:408, 2:1096
Implanted pulse generator (IPG), 1:338, 339
Impotence. *See* Erectile dysfunction
Imprinting, 1:81, 82
Impulsive behavior
    ADHD, 1:153, 154, 155
    atomoxetine for, 1:149–151
    cognitive behavioral therapy for, 1:154
    tic disorders, 2:1059
In-home respite, 2:916
In vitro fertilization (IVF), 1:601, 2:999
Inactivated polio virus (IPV), 2:863
Inactivity, 1:439, 462
Inapsine, 1:105–107
Inattention, 1:149–151, 152–153, 155
Incisional biopsy, 1:203–205
Inclusion bodies, 1:577, 2:1008
Inclusion body myositis (IBM), 1:**577–580,** 586–589, 2:740
Incontinence. *See* Fecal incontinence; Urinary incontinence
Incontinentia pigmenti (IP), 1:**580–583,** 584
Indacin. *See* Indomethacin
Indameth. *See* Indomethacin
Independence 3000 IBOT Transporter, 1:406
Independent living skills, 2:676, 984, 1177

Inderal. *See* Propranolol
India, 1:156
Indians. *See* Native Americans
Indinavir, 1:35, 616, 2:1188
Indirect bypass, 2:704
Individualized education plans (IEP)
    ADHD, 1:155
    agenesis of the corpus callosum, 1:22–23
    congenital myopathies, 1:309
    dyslexia, 1:395, 396–397
    Friedreich ataxia, 1:477
    megalencephaly, 2:666
    mental retardation, 2:676
    Moyamoya disease, 2:704–705
    See also Special education
Individuals with Disabilities Education Act (IDEA), 1:395
Indocin. *See* Indomethacin
Indomethacin, 1:509, 515, 2:830
Industrialization, 2:910
Infant botulism, 1:210–212
Infantile Alexander disease, 1:43–46
Infantile beriberi, 1:197, 198, 2:1150
Infantile hemiplegia, 1:534
Infantile hypotonia. *See* Hypotonia
Infantile Krabbe disease, 1:600, 601, 629
Infantile metachromatic leukodystrophy, 2:678, 679
Infantile Refsum disease, 2:907, 1185
Infantile spasms, 1:**583–586,** 623
Infantile spongy degeneration. *See* Canavan disease
Infants
    Alexander disease, 1:43–46
    arachnoid cysts, 1:122–124
    ataxia-telangiectasia, 1:143–144
    Bassen-Kornzweig syndrome, 1:184–187
    Canavan disease, 1:240
    cardiac rhabdomyomas, 2:1109–1110
    cerebral palsy, 1:278, 281–282
    febrile seizures, 1:465–468
    Gaucher disease, 1:482
    hearing tests, 1:528
    hemiplegia, 1:533, 534
    hydrocephalus, 1:556–558, 557
    hypotonia, 1:570–572
    incontinentia pigmenti, 1:581, 582
    Krabbe disease, 1:600
    Leigh disease, 1:620–622
    lissencephaly, 1:640–642
    metachromatic leukodystrophy, 2:678, 679
    Niemann-Pick disease, 2:792–794
    pain scales, 2:812
    periodic paralysis, 2:836
    pseudotumor cerebri, 2:891
    Rett syndrome, 2:921, 922
    Sandhoff disease, 2:925–927

Index

Index

Index

O

Pandemics, AIDS, 1:30

Panencephalitis, subacute sclerosing, 2:1023–1024

Panic attacks, 2:893–896, 1139

PANK2 (Pantothenate kinase 2), 2:820

Pantothenate kinase 2 (PANK2), 2:820

Pantothenate kinase-associated neurodegeneration (PKAN), 2:**820–821**

PAPAW (Pushrimactivated power-assisted wheelchair), 1:406

Papilledema, 2:890, 1148

Parageusia, 1:391

Paralysis
acute motor, 2:841
causes
alternating hemiplegia, 1:48–49
Brown-Séquard syndrome, 1:246
cerebral palsy, 1:278
locked-in syndrome, 1:642–643
Parsonage-Turner syndrome, 2:832
poliomyelitis, 2:861, 862, 863, 874
schizencephaly, 2:929, 930
spina bifida, 2:979
spinal cord injuries, 2:985, 987
transverse myelitis, 2:1086
West Nile virus, 2:1168
chronic sensorimotor, 2:841
demographics, 1:534
drug-induced, 2:769–772
facial, 1:*191*, 191–193
flaccid, 2:699, 862
ipsilateral, 1:246
Klumke's, 2:751, 752
obstetrical brachial plexus, 1:213–216, *214*
periodic, 1:285, 2:835–837
sleep, 2:748, 964
subacute sensorimotor, 2:841
thyrotoxic periodic, 2:1054
Todd's, 2:1066–1068
treatment, 2:987
See also Hemiplegia; Paraplegia

Paralytic chorea, 2:1031

Paramyotonia congenita, 2:**821–822**

Paraneoplastic syndromes, 1:162, 266–267, 507, 2:798, **822–823**

Paranoia, 1:53

Paranoid schizophrenia, 2:932

Paraparesis, tropical spastic, 1:547, 2:1104–1107

Paraphenylenediamine, 1:647

Paraplegia, 1:**533–537**
causes, 1:534–535
diagnosis, 1:535, 2:697
hereditary spastic, 1:534, 535, 538–541
spastic, 1:630
treatment, 1:535, 2:770

Parasagittal planes, 1:74

Parasitic disorders, 1:38, 233

Parasomnias, 2:**963–969**

Parasympathetic nervous system, 1:91, 166, 221, 222, 290, 2:837

Parcopa. *See* Levodopa plus carbidopa

Parental age, 2:933

Parental therapy, 1:17

Paresthesias, 1:388–389, 390, 2:912

Parietal lobe, 1:25, 219, 490

Parkinson, James, 2:824

Parkinsonism
causes, 2:699, 825
antiviral drugs, 1:113
chlorpromazine, 1:108, 2:825
dopamine receptor agonists, 2:936
Fahr disease, 1:453, 454
multiple system atrophy, 1:167, 2:720–722
prevention, 2:701–702
symptoms, 2:699
treatment, 1:63–65, 108–111, 2:702, 722

Parkinson's disease, 1:346–352, 2:*824*, **824–829**
acetylcholine in, 2:953
causes, 1:108, 2:696, 824, 825
vs. corticobasal degeneration, 1:313
demographics, 1:337–338, 2:699, 824
diagnosis, 1:55, 2:826
drug therapy, 1:108–111, 2:827–828, 1096
anticholinergics, 1:91, 109–111, 2:828
antioxidants, 2:825, 827, 828
botulinum toxin, 2:699
cholinesterase inhibitors, 1:109–111, 2:827
COMT inhibitors, 1:109–111, 255–256, 2:828
dopamine receptor agonists, 1:109–111, 381–383, 2:827–828
levodopa, 1:91, 108–111, 381–383, 2:699, 827
MOA-B inhibitors, 1:109–111, 2:827
vs. Lewy body dementia, 1:635
vs. multiple system atrophy, 1:167, 2:721
vs. progressive supranuclear palsy, 2:888
symptoms, 2:699, 825–826
dysarthria, 1:385
festinating gait, 1:180
hallucinations, 1:502
tremor, 2:825, 1093, 1094, 1096

treatment, 2:700–701, 826–827
deep brain stimulation, 1:337–341, 2:700, 816
guided imagery, 2:1097
Lee Silverman voice treatment, 1:619–620
pallidotomy, 1:340, 2:*814*, 814–816, 828, 1096
stem cell transplant, 2:1002
thalamotomy, 1:340

Parlodel. *See* Bromocriptine

Parnate. *See* Tranylcypromine

Parosmia, 1:89

Paroxetine
for Alzheimer's disease, 1:59
antimigraine drug interactions, 1:107
for dementia, 1:350
for depression, 1:357
hallucinations from, 1:501
for migraine headaches, 1:104
for multiple sclerosis, 2:718
for Tourette syndrome, 2:1074

Paroxysmal and Myokymia syndrome. *See* Episodic Ataxia Type 1

Paroxysmal hemicrania (PH), 2:**829–831**

Parsonage-Turner syndrome, 2:**831–834**

Partial seizures, 1:432, 434, 435, 2:941
causes, 1:623, 2:942, 1044
complex, 1:605, 623, 2:941, 942, 944, 996, 1044
febrile, 1:466
simple, 1:605, 2:941, 942, 1044
status epilepticus with, 2:995, 996
symptoms, 2:942
treatment, 2:944
gabapentin, 1:479–480
lacosamide, 1:605–607
levetiracetam, 1:632–635
succinamides, 2:1026
tiagabine, 2:1056–1057

Partial spinal sensory syndrome. *See* Brown-Séquard syndrome

Partial thromboplastin time (PTT), 1:94

Passiflora incarnata. See Passionflower

Passionflower, 2:951, 968

Passive range of motion (PROM), 2:833, 904

Patches, eye, 1:192, 2:955, 956

Patent foramen ovale (PFO), 2:1076

Paternal age, 1:157

Patient-controlled anesthesia (PCA), 1:613

Patient education, 1:252–254

Patient history. *See* Medical history

Pavulon. *See* Pancuronium

Paxil. *See* Paroxetine

PCA (Patient-controlled anesthesia), 1:613

PCP (Phencyclidine), 1:181, 342, 501, 2:740, 934

PCR (Polymerase chain reaction), 1:34, 2:886, 950

PD. *See* Parkinson's disease

Pearson syndrome, 2:683

Pediatric autoimmune neuropsychiatric disorders associated with streptococcus (PANDAS), 1:162, 2:**816–819**, 1030

Pediatric neuroradiology, 2:778, 780

Pediatric neurosurgery, 2:786, 787

Pediatric traumatic brain injury. *See* Shaken baby syndrome

Peer pressure, 1:133, 155

Pegasys. *See* Interferon alpha

Pelizaeus-Merzbacher disease (PMD), 1:630–631

Pellagra, 2:1149–1153

Pelvic floor muscles, 2:806

Pelvic muscle rehabilitation, 2:807

Pelvic region, 1:75

PEM (Protein-energy malnutrition), 1:462–463

PEMA (Phenylmethylmalonamide), 2:877

Pemoline, 1:134, 153, 396, 2:717

Penetrance (genetics), 1:543

Penetrating head injuries, 2:1086, 1087

Penicillamine, 2:1180–1181

Penicillin G, 1:654, 2:1038

Penicillins, 1:290, 419, 2:1030, 1031, 1162

Pentam-300. *See* Pentamidine

Pentamidine, 1:35, 422

Pentanucleotide repeat, 2:992

Pentobarbital, 2:670

PEO (Progressive external ophthalmoplegia), 2:683

PEP (Post-exposure prophylaxis), 1:34

Peppermint, 2:951

Percocet. *See* Oxycodone

Percutaneous aspiration, 1:560

Percutaneous discectomy, 1:375–376

Perencephaly. *See* Porencephaly

Performance-Oriented Assessment of Mobility (POAM), 1:181

Pergolide, 1:109–111, 2:828, 919

Perinatal hypoxia, 1:571

Perineural cysts, 2:**834–835**

Perineural lymphatics, 2:673

Periodic limb movements in sleep (PLMS), 2:918, 919, 920, 968

Periodic paralysis (PP), 1:285, 2:**835–837**

Peripheral blood stem cell transplants, 2:1003

Peripheral myelin protein 22 (PMP22), 1:287, 288, 289

Peripheral nerve roots, 2:984

Peripheral nervous system, 2:**837–840** anatomy and function, 1:220–222, *259*, 2:837–841 balance and gait disorders, 1:179 Charcot Marie Tooth disease, 1:287 spinal cord injuries, 2:984–985

Peripheral nervous system disorders. *See* Peripheral neuropathy

Peripheral neuropathy, 2:839–840, **840–846** alcoholic, 1:42, 43 causes, 2:840, 842–843 autoimmune diseases, 1:161 neurosarcoidosis, 2:782–783 Refsum disease, 2:907–908 repetitive motion disorders, 2:910 vasculitic neuropathy, 2:1121 classification, 2:841–842 demographics, 2:840 diagnosis, 2:843–844 diffuse, 1:363 idiopathic, 1:575–577 lupus with, 1:648 prevention, 2:845–846 restless legs syndrome with, 2:918 *vs.* sciatic neuropathy, 2:939 symptoms, 1:388, 389, 2:842 treatment, 2:844–845

Periventricular heterotopia, 2:772, 773

Periventricular leukomalacia, 2:**847–848**

Permanent vegetative state, 2:1127

Permax. *See* Pergolide

Pernicious anemia, 2:1150–1153

Peroneal muscular atrophy. *See* Charcot Marie Tooth disease

Peroxin (PX) genes, 2:1185

Peroxisomes, 1:10, 2:1185–1186

Persantine. *See* Dipyridamole

Persistent Lyme disease (PLD), 1:653

Persistent Lyme encephalopathy, 1:427

Persistent vegetative state (PVS) causes, 1:276 *vs.* coma, 1:300 definition of, 1:230, 2:1125 ethical issues, 2:1128–1129 *vs.* minimally conscious state, 2:1128 *vs.* permanent vegetative state, 2:1127 prognosis, 1:302

Personal hygiene, 1:52, 60, 2:934

Personality disorders, 1:653, 2:856, 1072, 1092, 1176

Perspiration, 2:1187

Pertofane. *See* Desipramine

Pervasive developmental disorder not otherwise specified (PPD-NOS), 1:156–157

Pervasive support mental retardation, 2:674

Pesticides, organophosphate, 1:292

PET. *See* Positron emission tomography

Petadolex, 1:510

Petasites hybridus. See Butterbur root

Petit mal seizures. *See* Absence seizures

Petroleum jelly, 2:952, 958

Petrosal sinus sampling, 1:331

PEX7 gene, 1:630

Peyer's patches, 1:322

Peyote, 1:499

Pfeiffer syndrome, 1:315

PFO (Patent foramen ovale), 2:1076

PH (Paroxysmal hemicrania), 2:**829–831**

pH level, 1:2

Phalen's sign, 1:252

Phalilalia, 2:1072

Phantom limb, 2:812, **848–851**

Phantosmia, 1:89

Pharmacodynamics, 2:852

Pharmacoepideconomics, 2:853

Pharmacoepidemiology, 2:853

Pharmacogenetics, 2:852

Pharmacogenomics, 2:852

Pharmacokinetics, 2:852

Pharmacotherapy, 2:**851–854**

Phase I clinical trials, 1:299

Phase II clinical trials, 1:299

Phase III clinical trials, 1:299

Phase IV clinical trials, 1:299

Phenazopyridine, 2:718

Phencyclidine (PCP), 1:181, 342, 501, 2:740, 934

Phendimetrazine, 1:262–264

Phenelzine, 1:107, 357, 382

Phenergan, 2:1141

Phenobarbital, 1:99–103, 2:**854–855** for epilepsy, 1:437, 2:854–855 interactions, 1:102, 103, 2:855 carbamazepine, 1:243 dexamethasone suppression test, 1:331 modafinil, 2:688 sodium oxybate, 2:971 succinamides, 2:1027 tiagabine, 2:1057 topiramate, 2:1070 valproic acid, 2:1120 zonisamide, 2:1188

Index

Q

R

neuroleptic malignant syndrome
from, 2:761–763
for schizophrenia, 2:936
for tics, 2:1060
for Tourette syndrome, 2:1074
Ritalin. *See* Methylphenidate
Ritonavir, 1:35, 616, 2:1188
Rivastigmine, 1:58, 109–111,
292–293, 350, 2:827
Rizatriptan, 1:105–107, 509
RLS (Restless legs syndrome), 1:463,
2:**917–921,** 964–968
Robaxin. *See* Methocarbamol
Robitussin. *See* Dextromethorphan
Rocephin. *See* Ceftriaxone
Rocuronium, 1:91, 2:769–771
Roentgen, Wilhelm, 2:778
Rofecoxib, 1:176
Role playing, 1:158
Romberg test, 1:182, 458
Ropinirole, 1:109–111, 381–383,
2:827, 919
ROS (Reactive oxygen species), 2:684
ROS (Review of systems), 1:181
Rosemary, 1:59
Rosenthal fibers, 1:44, 629
RRMS (Relapsing-remitting multiple
sclerosis), 1:260, 261, 2:715, 717, 719
RSNA (Radiological Society of
North America), 1:7
RSV (Respiratory syncytial virus),
1:112
Rubella, 1:279
Rufen. *See* Ibuprofen
Ryanodine receptor, 1:286, 307, 308
RYR1 gene, 1:307, 308

S

Sabin, Alvert, 2:863
Sabin vaccine, 2:693, 863
Saccular aneurysms, 1:130
Sacks, Oliver, 2:768
Sacral nerve cysts. *See* Perineural
cysts
Sacral radiculopathy.
See Radiculopathy
Sacral vertebrae, 2:939, 984–985
SAD (Seasonal affective disorder),
1:14–19, 353–359
SAD (Sporadic Alzheimer's disease),
1:51, 54
Saffron, 1:357
Sagittal craniosynostosis, 1:314, 315
Sagittal planes, 1:74
Sagittal sinuses, 1:219
Sagittal sutures, 1:74
SAH. *See* Subarachnoid hemorrhage

Saiko-keishi-to-shakuyaku, 1:59
Saint Vitus Dance. *See* Sydenham's
chorea
Salicylates, 1:342, 523, 2:924
Salicylic acid. *See* Aspirin
Salicylic acid gel, 2:958
Saliva, 1:393, 2:1027
Salivary gland disease.
See Cytomegalic inclusion body
disease
Salivation disorders, 2:694
Salk vaccine, 2:863
Salon sink radiculopathy, 2:900
Salt. *See* Sodium
Sanctura. *See* Trospium chloride
Sandhoff disease, 2:**925–927,** 1002
Sandimmune. *See* Cyclosporine
Sanfilippo syndrome.
See Mucopolysaccharidoses III
Sanfilippo syndrome type A.
See Mucopolysaccharidoses IIIA
Sanfilippo syndrome type B.
See Mucopolysaccharidoses IIIB
Sanfilippo syndrome type C. *See*
Mucopolysaccharidoses IIIC
Sanfilippo syndrome type D.
See Mucopolysaccharidoses IIID
Sansert. *See* Methysergide
Saquinavir, 1:35, 606
Sarafem. *See* Fluoxetine
Sarcoglycans, 2:725
Sarcoidosis, 2:782–785
Sarcomas, Kaposi's, 1:33
SBMA (Spinobulbar muscular
atrophy), 2:988
SCA-1 gene, 2:797
SCA-2 gene, 2:797
SCA1 (Spinocerebellar ataxia type 1),
1:146
SCA2 (Spinocerebellar ataxia type 2),
1:146
SCA3 (Spinocerebellar ataxia type 3).
See Machado-Joseph disease
SCA4 (Spinocerebellar ataxia type 4),
1:146
SCA5 (Spinocerebellar ataxia type 5),
1:147
SCA6 (Spinocerebellar ataxia type 6),
1:147
SCA7 (Spinocerebellar ataxia type 7),
1:147
SCA10 (Spinocerebellar ataxia
type 10), 1:147
SCA11 (Spinocerebellar ataxia
type 11), 1:147
Scanning, 1:137, 530, 531
Scarlet fever, 2:818
SCAs (Spinocerebellar ataxias),
1:146–148, 2:797 **991–995**

Scheie syndrome.
See Mucopolysaccharidoses I S
Schilder-Addison disease. *See*
Adrenoleukodystrophy
Schilder's disease, 1:239, 2:**927–928**
Schilling test, 2:1153
Schistosomiasis, 1:29
Schizencephaly, 2:772, 773, **928–931,**
929
Schizophrenia, 2:**931–938,** *932*
adult-onset, 1:500
causes, 1:16, 2:933
vs. delirium, 1:343–344
demographics, 1:15, 2:931
diagnosis, 2:931, 934–936
prognosis, 2:937
symptoms, 1:500, 501, 502–503,
2:932, 933–934
treatment, 2:936–937
types, 2:932–933
Schwann cells, 1:286, 2:841, 1145
Schwannomas, 1:222–223, 2:1063,
1145–1146
Sciatic nerve, 2:857–859, 938–939
Sciatic neuropathy, 1:173, 374, 375,
609, 2:**938–941**
Sciatica. *See* Sciatic neuropathy
SCID (Structured Clinical Interview
for DSM-IV), 1:17, 355
Scintigraphy, meta-
iodobenzylguanidine, 2:1156
Scissors gait, 1:180, 280
Sclerosis
primary lateral, 2:693–694,
875–876
tuberous, 1:436, 2:*1107,*
1107–1113, *1108*
See also Amyotrophic lateral
sclerosis; Multiple sclerosis
Scoliosis
back pain from, 1:173
cerebral palsy, 1:282
clinical trials, 1:283
Friedreich ataxia, 1:476
Klippel-Feil syndrome, 1:598
muscular dystrophy, 2:726, 729
myofibrillar myopathy, 2:738
Rett syndrome, 2:921
spinal fusion for, 1:476
syringomyelia, 2:1033
Scooters, 1:405–407, *406*
Scopolamine, 1:91, 92, 109–111,
2:670, 1140–1141
Scrapie, 1:321–322, 2:878–884
Screening Test for Autism in
Two-Year-Olds, 1:158
Screening tests, 1:158, 299
SDAs (Serotonin dopamine
antagonists), 2:936–937
SDR (Selective dorsal rhizotomy),
2:975
Seafood poisoning, 1:145, 390

Strabismus
  botulinum toxin for, 1:208
  incontinentia pigmenti, 1:582
  Moebius syndrome, 2:689
  septo-optic dysplasia, 2:945
  vs. sixth nerve palsy, 2:954
  Williams syndrome, 2:1176
Straight leg-raising test, 1:174, 375
Strattera. *See* Atomoxetine
Strength training, 1:440
Strep culture, 2:818
Strep throat, 2:816–819, 1029, 1030, 1031
Streptococcus pneumoniae, 1:416, 418, 419, 420
Streptococcus sp., 1:416
Streptomycin, 1:291, 2:670, 735
Stress, 1:16–17, 173, 463, 2:912, 937
Stress urinary incontinence, 2:806, 806*t*
Stretching, 1:440
  back pain, 1:178, 614–615
  cerebral palsy, 1:282
  disc herniation, 1:376
  muscular dystrophy, 2:729
  myofibrillar myopathy, 2:738
  piriformis syndrome, 2:858
  postpolio syndrome, 2:874
  primary lateral sclerosis, 2:876
  repetitive motion disorders, 2:913
Stria medullaris, 1:371
Striatonigral degeneration, 2:721, **1008–1011**
Striatum, 2:1008, 1009
Striopallidodentate calcinosis. *See* Fahr disease
Stroke, 1:260, 2:*1011,* **1011–1018**
  causes, 2:1011, 1012–1013
  complications
    agraphia, 1:25, 26, 28
    Alzheimer's disease, 1:51
    aphasia, 1:115–116
    apraxia, 1:120
    central pain syndrome, 1:264
    cerebral edema, 1:233, 573
    coma, 1:300, 302
    dysarthria, 1:384
    dysesthesias, 1:389
    dyslexia, 1:394
    epilepsy, 1:433
    fourth nerve palsy, 1:473
    Gerstmann syndrome, 1:490
    hemiplegia, 1:533, 534
    locked-in syndrome, 1:642
    movement disorders, 2:697–698
  demographics, 1:245, 249, 275, 2:1011, 1082
    children, 1:275, 2:1011, 1013, 1016
    mortality, 1:247–248, 249, 260, 2:1011, 1016, 1082
  diagnosis, 2:1013–1014
  fetal, 1:279

  hemorrhagic, 1:245, 275, 2:698, 1011, 1012–1013, 1014–1015, 1016
  prevention, 1:248, 2:701, 702, 1016–1017
  prognosis, 2:1016
  recurrence, 2:1015
  risk factors, 1:120, 260, 2:1012
    Binswanger disease, 1:201
    carotid endarterectomy, 1:247
    carotid stenosis, 1:249, 250
    cerebral hematomas, 1:275
    headaches, 1:506
    lupus, 1:648
    Moyamoya disease, 2:703
    neurocysticercosis, 2:756
    shingles, 2:950
    temporal arteritis, 2:1042
    transient ischemic attacks, 2:1012, 1017, 1082, 1084
    vasculitis, 2:1123
    vertebrobasilar disease, 2:1135, 1137
    Wallenberg syndrome, 2:1159–1161
  symptoms, 1:260, 2:765, 1013
  vs. Todd's paralysis, 2:1067
  vs. transient ischemic attacks, 2:1081
  treatment, 1:260, 2:779, 1014–1016
    anticoagulant/antiplatelet drugs, 1:92, 2:702, 1014, 1017
    carotid endarterectomy, 1:245–248
    emergency care, 2:763–764, 1012, 1015, 1016
    stem cell therapy, 2:999
  See also Ischemic stroke; Transient ischemic attacks
Structured Clinical Interview for DSM-IV (SCID), 1:17, 355
Strumpell-Lorrain syndrome. *See* Hereditary spastic paraplegia
Stump pain, 2:849
Stupor, 1:230
Sturge-Weber syndrome (SRS), 2:*1018,* **1018–1020**
Stuttering, 2:893, **1020–1024**
Subacute sclerosing panencephalitis, 2:**1023–1024**
Subacute sensorimotor paralysis, 2:841
Subarachnoid abscess, 2:673
Subarachnoid hemorrhage (SAH)
  causes, 1:78, 2:673
    diagnosis, 1:645, 2:1076
    emergency care, 2:763–764, 765
Subarachnoid space, 1:124, 2:672, 673, 1134–1135
Subclavian steal syndrome, 2:1076
Subcortical aphasia, 1:117
Subcortical arterioslcerotic encephalitis. *See* Binswanger disease
Subcortical dementia, 1:199–203

Subdural, definition of, 2:672
Subdural electrodes, 1:408
Subdural hematoma, 2:*1024,* **1024–1025**
  causes, 2:673, 1024
    head injuries, 1:430, 2:673, 1087
    shaken baby syndrome, 2:947, 1024
    ventricular shunts, 2:1133
  vs. epidural hematoma, 1:429
  treatment, 2:1025
Subependymal giant cell astrocytomas (SEGA), 1:222, 2:1109, 1112
Subependymal nodules, 2:1109
Subjective weakness, 2:1161
Submucous plexus, 1:221–222
Subspecialties, 2:768, 778, 786
Substance abuse
  acupuncture for, 1:5
  ADHD with, 1:155
  adverse effects
    affective disorders, 1:16
    AIDS transmission, 1:31
    delirium, 1:342
    dementia, 1:347
    hallucinations, 1:500, 501
    septo-optic dysplasia, 2:945
    tremor, 2:1094
    weakness, 2:1162
  schizophrenia with, 2:933, 934, 937
  spinal cord injuries with, 2:984
  See also Alcohol abuse
Substance P, 2:811
Substantia nigra
  deep brain stimulation, 1:337
  hypokinetic dysarthria, 1:385
  movement disorders, 2:696
  nigra cell implants, 2:1096
  Parkinson's disease, 1:108, 2:814, 825
  striatonigral degeneration, 2:1008, 1009
Subthalamic nucleus (STN), 1:337, 339, 402
Subthalamus, 1:372
Succinamides, 2:**1025–1027**
Succinylcholine. *See* Suxamethonium
Sucralfate, 1:554
Sudafed. *See* Pseudoephedrine
Sudden cardiac death, 1:462
Sudden infant death syndrome, 1:212
Sudden sensorineural hearing loss (SSHL), 1:524, 525
Sugammadex, 2:770
Sugar diabetes. *See* Diabetes mellitus
Sugar intake, 1:152
Sugar tests. *See* Blood sugar tests
Suicide
  ADHD, 1:155
  affective disorders, 1:15, 19
  anxiolytic overdose, 1:114

Index

U

VLOFA (Very late onset Friedreich ataxia), 1:475

VNS (Vagus nerve stimulation), 1:438, 624, 2:944, 1045, 1127

Vocal fold spasticity, 2:800, 801

Vocal tics, 2:1058, 1060, 1061, 1071–1072

VOCAs (Voice output communication aids), 1:138

Vocational counseling, 1:13, 165, 2:922

Voice-activated software, 1:289, 491

Voice disorders, 2:799–801

Voice output communication aids (VOCAs), 1:138

Voice production test, 2:800

Voice therapy, 2:895

Voice volume, 1:619–620

Volkmann contractures, 1:389

Voluntary muscle disorders. *See* Myopathy

Voluntary muscles, 2:731, 988–989, 1006–1008, 1161–1162

Vomiting, 1:37–38, 466, 467, 621, 2:1137

Von Basedow myopathy. *See* Thyrotoxic myopathy

von Economo's disease. *See* Encephalitis lethargica

Von Hipple-Lindau (VHL) disease, 1:224, 2:*1154*, **1154–1158**, *1155*

von Strumpell, Adolf, 1:538

VRT (Vestibular rehabilitation therapy), 2:1141, 1142

Vyvanse. *See* Lisdexamfetamine dimesylate

VZV vaccine, 2:952

W

Wada test, 1:311

Waddling gait, 1:180

Walker, Arthur E., 1:335, 2:786

Walker-Warburg syndrome, 1:640

Walkers, 1:141–143, 148, 2:888, 995

Walking, 1:440

Wallenberg syndrome, 2:**1159–1161**

Warfarin, 1:93–98

dosage, 1:94, 2:852

interactions, 1:96, 98

antiepileptic drugs, 1:98, 2:943

carbamazepine, 1:98, 102, 243

hydantoins, 1:554

lamotrigine, 1:616

phenobarbital, 1:103, 2:855

phenytoin, 1:103

valproic acid, 2:1120

side effects, 1:96

for stroke, 2:702, 1014, 1017

for transient ischemic attacks, 2:1083

Warm-up period, 1:443–444

Warrington Memory Test, 1:24

Wasting. *See* Atrophy

Wasting syndrome, AIDS-related, 1:38

Water (Chinese traditional medicine), 1:6

Water pills. *See* Diuretics

Watson, JAmes D., 1:486

WBRT (Whole-brain radiation therapy), 1:233

Weakness, 2:**1161–1166**

causes, 2:1162

Bell's palsy, 1:*191*, 191–193

cerebral palsy, 1:282

congenital myasthenia, 1:304–305

dermatomyositis, 1:359–361

Friedreich ataxia, 1:474

hereditary spastic paraplegia, 1:541

HTLV-1 associated myelopathy, 1:547–549

Huntington disease, 1:550

hypotonia, 1:572

inclusion body myositis, 1:577–580

inflammatory myopathy, 1:586–589

Joubert syndrome, 1:592

Kennedy disease, 1:595–597

Lambert-Eaton myasthenic syndrome, 1:607–609

mitochondrial myopathies, 2:685

Moebius syndrome, 2:688–690

monomelic amyotrophy, 2:690–692

motor neuron diseases, 2:693

multiple sclerosis, 2:716

muscular dystrophy, 2:726, 727

myasthenia gravis, 2:731–736

myofibrillar myopathy, 2:737–739

myopathy, 2:740–741

Parsonage-Turner syndrome, 2:832

periodic paralysis, 2:836

polymyositis, 2:864

Pompe disease, 2:867

postpolio syndrome, 2:874

primary lateral sclerosis, 2:875–876

spinal muscular atrophy, 2:989

thyrotoxic myopathy, 2:1053

diagnosis, 1:411–413, 2:1163–1165

foot drop from, 1:471–472

objective *vs.* subjective, 2:1161

symptoms, 2:1162–1163

treatment, 2:764, 1165

Webbed neck, 1:598

Wechsler Intelligence Scales, 2:675

Wechsler Preschool and Primary Scale of Intelligence, 2:675

Weekend warriors, 1:172

Wegener's granulomatosis, 2:1124, 1125

Weight-bearing exercise, 1:457

Weight gain, 2:892

Weight loss, 2:891, 959, 962

Wellbutrin. *See* Buproprion

Wender Utah Rating Scale, 1:153

Werdnig-Hoffman disease. *See* Type II SMA

Wernicke encephalopathy, 1:41, 2:996, 1151

Wernicke, Karl, 2:776

Wernicke-Korsakoff syndrome, 1:41, 197, 198, 2:1149, 1151

Wernicke's aphasia, 1:26, 27, 117

Wernicke's area, 1:25, 219, 274

Wernicke's syndrome, 1:43

West Indies, 2:783

West Nile virus (WNV), 1:417, 419, 2:*1166*, **1166–1170**

West syndrome, 1:624

West, W. J., 1:583–586

Western Aphasia Battery, 1:117

Western blot test, 1:34, 2:1006

Western equine encephalitis, 1:417

Wet beriberi, 1:197, 2:1149, 1151

Wheelchair athletes, 1:143

Wheelchairs, 1:141–143, 148

dysarthria modifications, 1:387

electric powered, 1:143, 405–406, *406*

Friedreich ataxia, 1:477

myotonic dystrophy, 2:745

spinocerebellar ataxias, 2:995

striatonigral degeneration, 2:1010

stroke, 2:1016

See also Assistive mobile devices

Whiplash, 2:**1170–1172**

Whiplash shaken infant syndrome. *See* Shaken baby syndrome

Whipple, George Hoyt, 2:1172

Whipple's disease, 2:*1172*, **1172–1174**

White blood cell count, 1:297, 418, 2:1005

White blood cells, 1:490, 2:1041

White matter, 1:216, 2:847, 886, 1019, 1109

White noise machines, 2:1064

White vinegar, 2:951

Whites. *See* Caucasians

WHO. *See* World Health Organization

Whole-body vibration, 2:912

Whole-brain radiation therapy (WBRT), 1:233

Will, loss of, 1:1–2

Williams Beuren syndrome. *See* Williams syndrome

Williams, J. C. P., 2:1174

X

Y

Index

Z

Zanamivir, 1:111–113

Zarontin. *See* Ethosuximide

Zea mays. See Maize

Zellweger syndrome, 1:630–631, 2:772, 773, **1185–1187,** *1186*

Zemeron. *See* Rocuronium

Ziagen. *See* Abacavir

ZIC2 gene, 1:543

Zidovudine, 1:35, 350, 2:887, 1106

Zinc
    for Alzheimer's disease, 1:59
    for anosmia, 1:90

    for dementia, 1:351
    for Lyme disease, 1:654
    for polymyositis, 2:865
    for tinnitus, 2:1065

Zinc acetate, 2:1180, 1181

Zinc deficiency, 1:466

Zocor. *See* Simvastatin

Zolmitriptan, 1:105–107, 509, 519, 522, 2:1100–1104

Zoloft. *See* Sertraline

Zolpidem, 1:501

Zomig. *See* Zolmitriptan

Zomig-ZMT. *See* Zolmitriptan

Zone therapy. *See* Reflexology

Zonegran. *See* Zonisamide

Zonisamide, 1:99–103, 2:**1187–1189**
    for epilepsy, 1:99–103, 437, 2:1187–1189
    interactions, 1:103, 2:1187, 1188
    for migraine headache, 1:509, 2:1187
    side effects, 1:102, 2:1188
    for tremor, 2:1096

Zoonosis, 1:651, 2:1167

Zortress. *See* Everolimus

Zostavax. *See* VZV vaccine

Zostrix, 2:951

Zovirax. *See* Acyclovir

Zyloprim. *See* Allopurinol

Zyprexa. *See* Olanzapine